D0147039

Exercise Testing and Prescription

A HEALTH-RELATED APPROACH

Exercise Testing and Prescription

A HEALTH-RELATED APPROACH

SIXTH EDITION

David C. Nieman
Appalachian State University

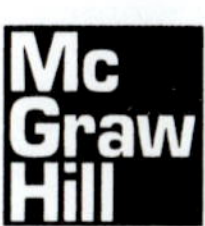

Boston Burr Ridge, IL Dubuque, IA Madison, WI New York San Francisco St. Louis
Bangkok Bogotá Caracas Kuala Lumpur Lisbon London Madrid Mexico City
Milan Montreal New Delhi Santiago Seoul Singapore Sydney Taipei Toronto

McGraw-Hill Higher Education

A Division of The ***McGraw-Hill*** *Companies*

EXERCISE TESTING AND PRESCRIPTION: A HEALTH-RELATED APPROACH
Published by McGraw-Hill, a business unit of The McGraw-Hill Companies, Inc., 1221 Avenue of the Americas, New York, NY, 10020.

This book is printed on acid-free paper.

3 4 5 6 7 8 9 0 QPD/QPD 0 9 8

ISBN 978-0-07-304474-3
MHID 0-07-304474-1

Vice president and editor-in-chief: *Emily Barrosse*
Publisher: *William R. Glass*
Sponsoring editor: *Christopher Johnson*
Executive marketing manager: *Pamela S. Cooper*
Director of development: *Kathleen Engelberg*
Developmental editor: *Beth Baugh, Carlisle Publishing Services*
Developmental editor for technology: *Julia D. Ersery*
Senior media project manager: *Ron Nelms, Jr.*
Media producer: *Michele Borrelli*
Project manager: *Valerie Heffernan, Carlisle Publishing Services*
Lead production supervisor: *Randy Hurst*
Design manager: *Preston Thomas*
Media supplement manager: *Kathleen Boylan*
Cover image: *Glenn Migsui*

This text was set in 9/12 Palatino by Carlisle Publishing Services, and printed on 45# New Era Matte Plus by Quebecor World Printing, Dubuque, Iowa.

Library of Congress Cataloging-in-Publication Data

Nieman, David C., 1950-
Exercise testing and prescription : a health-related approach / David C. Nieman.—6th ed.
p. cm.
Includes bibliographical references and index.
ISBN 0-07-304474-1
1. Exercise—Physiological aspects. 2. Physical fitness. 3. Sports medicine. 4. Exercise tests. 5. Exercise therapy. I. Title.
QP301.N53 2007
613.7—dc22

2005054338

Photographs are reprinted with permission of Robert O. Parriott.

The Internet addresses listed in the text were accurate at the time of publication. The inclusion of a website does not indicate an endorsement by the authors or McGraw-Hill, and McGraw-Hill does not guarantee the accuracy of the information presented at these sites.

www.mhhe.com

To my wife Cathy—
dietitian, editor, loving companion,
and award-winning quilter

Brief Contents

Contents

Preface

This textbook describes knowledge, skills, and abilities for exercise testing and prescription and reviews the health-related benefits of regular physical activity. Detailed information and norms are given for various tests of body composition and for aerobic and musculoskeletal fitness. Exercise prescription guidelines and physical activity benefits are provided for a wide variety of conditions—including obesity; coronary heart disease; stroke; colon, breast, and prostate cancer; hypertension; dyslipidemia; metabolic syndrome; type 1 and type 2 diabetes; arthritis; osteoporosis; and anxiety and depression—and for different types of individuals, such as children and youth, the elderly, pregnant women, and athletes.

The first edition of this book was published in 1986 to assist readers in preparing for certification from the American College of Sports Medicine (ACSM). Because this is still a major purpose of this book, the basic structure has been retained to ensure successful preparation for certification and the ACSM's new registry for the clinical exercise physiologist (RCEP).

Since the 1980s, much progress has been made in advancing our understanding of exercise testing and prescription, the health-related benefits of regular physical activity, clinical exercise physiology, and public policy issues. This new edition presents the most current information available on each of these topics. The content is supported by more than 500 new references for a total of over 2,400 references. Figures, tables, and boxes have been updated and have been added to complement and support the book's new content.

ORGANIZATION

As in previous editions, the chapters are organized to present a natural progression of information. The reader will find it most satisfactory to start with Chapter 1 and continue chapter by chapter to the end of the book. The book is divided into four parts. Part I deals with public policy issues in physical activity, trends in physical activity patterns and wellness, and basic definitions. Part II describes the various tests for each of the major elements of physical fitness: cardiorespiratory endurance, body composition, and musculoskeletal fitness. Part III reviews the basics of exercise physiology, the process of writing exercise prescriptions, and the relationship between nutrition and performance. Part IV summarizes current understanding regarding the association of physical activity and heart disease, obesity, aging, osteoporosis, arthritis, psychological health, diabetes, cancer, and other concerns. In addition, a complete review of exercise risks is presented in Chapter 16. The appendix material includes numerous tables of physical fitness testing norms (which complement those found within the chapters), photos of basic calisthenics, anatomical diagrams, and a detailed listing of the energy cost of human physical activities.

NEW TO THIS EDITION

Updated content. This text is fully updated and integrated with new information from *ACSM's Guidelines for Exercise Testing and Prescription* (7th edition) (2006), *USDA Dietary Guidelines for Americans* (2005), and MyPyramid (2005). It covers new facts and trends, and it includes updated classification tables for fitness testing (see Appendix A), obesity, diabetes, cancer, hypertension, heart disease, osteoporosis, and arthritis. Specific updates include the ACSM physical activity recommendations for school-aged youth; the National High Blood Pressure Education Program (NIH) guidelines for the detection, classification, prevention, and treatment of hypertension; American Cancer Society guidelines for the prevention of cancer; American Diabetes Association guidelines for the screening of diabetes in adults and children; guidelines on the prevention and delay of type 2 diabetes; Institute of Medicine guidelines for confronting the epidemic of childhood obesity and Institute of Medicine equations for estimating resting metabolic rate and total energy expenditure; a summary of research on high-protein, low-carbohydrate diets for weight loss; nutrition and physical activity guidelines from the USDA for weight loss and sustaining weight loss; surgeon general recommendations for the prevention and treatment of osteoporosis; ACSM guidelines for physical activity and bone health; and American College of Obstetricians and Gynecologists guidelines for exercise during pregnancy.

Focus on prevention. This edition emphasizes the prevention guidelines for all major diseases, including diabetes, cancer, heart disease, osteoporosis, and arthritis.

Boxed material. Throughout the text, boxes have been added to highlight exercise testing and prescription for a wide variety of individuals and patients.

New practical information. This new edition features several new Physical Fitness Activities that offer students the opportunity to build skills and apply what they are learning.

SUCCESSFUL FEATURES

Preparation for ACSM exams. The content and focus of this text continually prepare the student for the key topics that need to be mastered to achieve ACSM certification. The book also serves as a valuable reference throughout a career in an applied fitness setting.

Health-related context. Exercise testing and prescription are presented in a health-related context that features the latest research findings on exercise and nutrition, obesity, heart disease, diabetes, cancer, and aging.

Illustrations, photographs, tables, and graphs. One of the key strengths of this book is the visually engaging presentation of material, which makes it clear and appealing to students.

Sports Medicine Insight boxes. These boxes highlight issues of current interest, such as methods of determining body composition, physical fitness in children and youth, and ACSM certification tracks.

Physical Fitness Activity feature. This tool promotes hands-on learning by encouraging the student to take part in activities such as readiness for exercise, precertification screening questionnaires, cardiorespiratory endurance testing, and assessment of muscular fitness.

Review Questions. Each chapter ends with Review Questions and Answers that encourage students to review the key points of the chapter. The answers are listed following the questions so that students can gain immediate feedback.

Website resources. This book includes the website addresses of many professional organizations and resources for information on health and fitness, nutrition, and many other topics.

NEW OR EXPANDED TOPICS

This new edition has been significantly revised and updated. The following list is a sampling of the topics that are either new to this edition or covered in greater depth than in the previous edition.

Chapter 1: Health and Fitness

- Updated statistics on physical education trends for children and adolescents
- Trends in overweight for children and adolescents
- Trends in numbers of health/fitness clubs

Chapter 2: Physical Fitness Defined

- American College of Sports Medicine physical activity recommendations for school-aged youth

Chapter 3: Testing Concepts

- American College of Sports Medicine updated guidelines for risk stratification, risk factors, recommendations for medical examination and exercise testing, and contraindications to exercise testing.
- Updated preparticipation physical evaluation form from the American College of Sports Medicine
- Information on organizations that provide certification in the health/fitness industry
- American College of Sports Medicine certification and registry programs, including the new "Certified Physical Trainer" program

Chapters 4–6: Cardiorespiratory Fitness; Body Composition; Musculoskeletal Fitness

- Classification of blood pressure for adults, including the new "prehypertension" category
- Recommendations for follow-up based on initial blood pressure measurements
- Five new Physical Fitness Activities, including measurement of resting heart rate and blood pressure, estimation of $\dot{V}O_{2max}$ using an equation, the 1-mile walk test, and a step test for college students
- Mean body mass index values for men and women across five age groups

Chapter 8: Exercise Prescription

- Review of new physical activity recommendations from the Institute of Medicine and the U.S. Department of Agriculture

- Integration of the 2006 *ACSM's Guidelines for Exercise Testing and Prescription*
- Use of pedometers and walking 10,000 steps a day

Chapter 9: Nutrition and Performance

- Detailed review of the 2005 *Dietary Guidelines for Americans*
- Description of the new MyPyramid food intake pattern, with detailed figures and tables
- Updated information on the Dietary Reference Intakes (DRIs)
- Review of chemical performance-enhancement products for athletes
- Description of a new method of blood doping using blood substitutes
- New Physical Fitness Activities using *MyPyramid.gov* and *MyPyramidTracker.gov*
- Review of water balance information from the Institute of Medicine

Chapter 10: Heart Disease

- Updated statistics on cardiovascular disease in the United States and prevalence of risk factors
- Table on current smoking prevalence in the United States by race/ethnicity, education level, age group, and poverty level
- Detailed review of the 2003 National High Blood Pressure Education Program of the National Heart, Lung, and Blood Institute
- New table of antihypertensive medications
- Classification and management of blood pressure for adults from the Joint National Committee on Detection, Evaluation, and Treatment of High Blood Pressure
- Update on lifestyle modifications to manage hypertension
- New summary of lifestyle modifications to lower LDL-cholesterol levels and raise HDL-cholesterol levels

Chapter 11: Cancer

- Update on basic cancer facts and figures from the American Cancer Society (ACS)
- Revised ACS recommendations for the early detection of cancer in asymptomatic people
- Current ACS cancer prevention guidelines
- Sunlight and skin cancer
- Update on physical activity and cancer relationships

Chapter 12: Diabetes

- Type 2 diabetes in children
- New standards for diagnosing pre-diabetes and diabetes
- Updated guidelines on screening and risk factors for diabetes, including criteria for testing in children
- Current guidelines for gestational diabetes mellitus
- Steps to control diabetes for life
- Prevention, delay, and treatment of type 2 diabetes
- Updated Physical Fitness Activity on adding up risk factors for diabetes

Chapter 13: Obesity

- New prevalence data on overweight/obesity in children, youth, and adults
- Institute of Medicine recommendations to confront the epidemic of childhood obesity
- Institute of Medicine equations to estimate basal energy expenditure and total energy expenditure
- Update on high-protein, low-carbohydrate diet plans for weight loss

Chapter 14: Psychological Health

- Current data on suicide
- New data on prevalence of frequent mental distress and serious psychological distress among adults in the United States
- National Sleep Foundation guidelines for improved sleep, and sleep requirements over the life cycle
- New Physical Fitness Activities on measurement of serious psychological distress and determination of sleep problems

Chapter 15: Aging, Osteoporosis, and Arthritis

- Summary of 15 indicators related to older adult health status, behaviors, preventive care and screening, and injuries, and *Healthy People 2010* targets
- Guidelines for bone mineral density testing

- Five steps for prevention of osteoporosis
- Risk factors for osteoporosis from the National Osteoporosis Foundation and the Office of the Surgeon General
- Update on therapeutic medications for osteoporosis prevention and treatment from the National Institutes of Health
- Current diet recommendations for optimal bone health
- Physical activity and osteoporosis recommendations from the Office of the Surgeon General
- ACSM guidelines on physical activity and bone health
- Update on prevalence of arthritis in the United States
- Current risk factors for arthritis from the Centers for Disease Control and Prevention
- Update on medications for arthritis from the U.S. Food and Drug Administration
- New Physical Fitness Activity on determining risk for developing osteoporosis
- New Physical Fitness Activity on calculating calcium intake

Chapter 16: Exercise Risks

- Current guidelines for exercise during pregnancy from the American College of Obstetricians and Gynecologists (ACOG)
- Updated prevalence data for asthma from the Asthma and Allergy Foundation of America (AAFA)

Appendix A

- Updated physical fitness test norms from the Cooper Institute and the Canadian Society of Exercise Physiology
- Updated anthropometric tables from the National Center for Health Statistics

Online Ancillaries

Online ancillaries that accompany this text include test bank questions and detailed, comprehensive PowerPoint slides. These resources can be accessed by visiting the book's website at www.mhhe.com/nieman6e.

NutritionCalc Plus

Also available is NutritionCalc Plus (ISBN 0-07-292126-9), a dietary analysis program with an easy-to-use interface that allows users to track their nutrient and food group intake, energy expenditures, and weight control goals. The program analyzes food intakes and activity levels based on the user's personal profile information and generates reports, graphs, and summaries for comparison and analysis. The database includes thousands of ethnic foods, supplements, fast foods, and convenience foods, and users can add their own foods to the food list. NutritionCalc Plus is available on CD-ROM (Windows only) or online.

ACKNOWLEDGMENTS

I appreciate the help provided by the following reviewers, who offered many good suggestions that were useful in developing both this revision and the previous edition.

LaGary Carter
Valdosta State University

Inza L. Fort
University of Arkansas

Ellen L. Glickman
Kent State University

Alexander Joseph Koch
Truman State University

Lisa Lloyd
Texas State University–San Marcos

Frank Bosso
Youngstown State University

Susan Fox
Oregon State University

Steve Glass
Wayne State College

Mark Kasper
Valdosta State University

David Pavlat
Central College

Tonya Skalon
Ball State University

David C. Nieman

part I

Trends and Definitions

chapter 1

Health and Fitness Trends

The 1990s brought a historic new perspective to exercise, fitness, and physical activity by shifting the focus from intensive vigorous exercise to a broader range of health-enhancing physical activities. Research has demonstrated that virtually all individuals will benefit from regular physical activity.

—U.S. Department of Health and Human Services, *Healthy People 2010*

TRENDS IN HEALTH

The most notable, and undoubtedly still the most influential, definition of health is that of the World Health Organization (WHO).[1] The definition appeared in the preamble of its constitution in 1948: "*Health* is a state of complete physical, mental, and social well-being, and not merely the absence of disease."

This definition stemmed from a conviction of WHO organizers that the security of future world peace would lie in the improvement of physical, mental, and social health. The definition suggests that health goes beyond the mere avoidance of disease and extends to how one feels and functions physically, mentally, and socially.

This definition was criticized by some as difficult to measure. In response, WHO in 1984 added that any measure of health must take into account "the extent to which an individual or a group is able to realize aspirations and satisfy needs, and to change or cope with the environment." Health in this sense is seen as a "resource for everyday life." Health also involves an ability to perform within society, and to accommodate stresses, whether physical or mental.

Wellness is an approach to personal health that emphasizes individual responsibility for well-being through the practice of health-promoting lifestyle behaviors. In other words, wellness is an all-inclusive concept that encourages good health behaviors to improve quality of life and reduce the risk of premature disease. *Health behavior* is defined as the combination of knowledge, practices, and attitudes that together contribute to motivate the actions people take regarding health and wellness. *Health promotion*, a term that gained favor during the 1970s, is defined as the science and art of helping people change their lifestyle to move toward a state of optimal health.[1,2]

The Dimensions of Health

Health has three dimensions: mental, physical, and social. Each individual is a complex mixture of mental, physical, and social factors, all of which interact and are dependent on each other.[1] When one of the dimensions is neglected or overemphasized, the other areas are negatively influenced.

The three dimensions of health are tightly interdependent, and quality of life demands that each receives balanced attention (see Figure 1.1).

- Mental health refers to both the absence of mental disorders (e.g., depression, anxiety, and dependence on drugs) and the individual's ability to negotiate the daily challenges and social interactions of life without experiencing mental, emotional, or behavioral problems. Mental health is enhanced as people learn and grow intellectually and cope with daily circumstances and emotions in a positive, optimistic, and constructive manner.
- Physical health is defined as the absence of physical disease (e.g., premature heart disease or cancer), while having energy and vigor to perform moderate to vigorous levels of physical activity without undue fatigue and the capability of maintaining such ability throughout life. This energy and vigor is

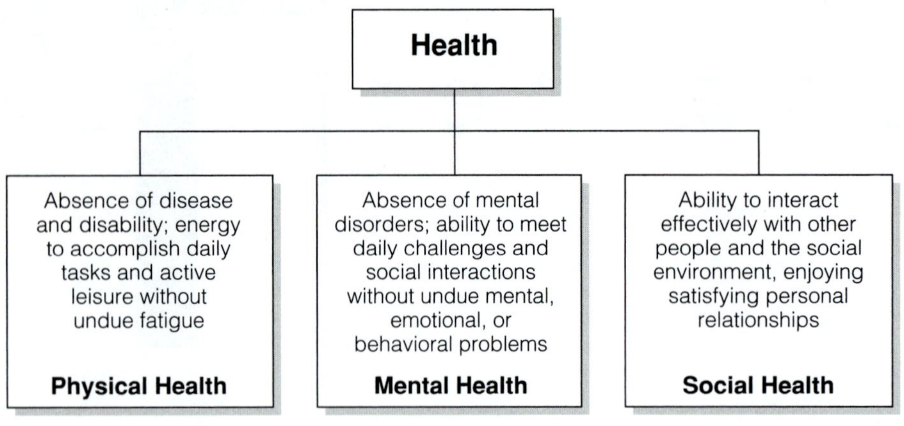

Figure 1.1 According to the World Health Organization, "Health is physical, mental, and social well-being, not merely the absence of disease and infirmity."

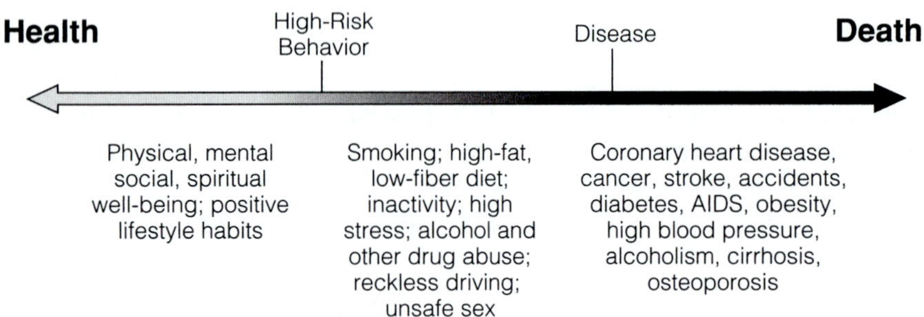

Figure 1.2 The health continuum. The health continuum shows that between optimal health and death lies disease, which is preceded by a prolonged period of negative lifestyle habits.

gained by following several good health habits such as getting regular sleep and physical activity, keeping body fat down and the muscles in good tone, and eating a balanced diet.

- Social health refers to the ability to interact effectively with other people and the social environment (e.g., social groups and networks), engaging in satisfying personal relationships. To gain social health, people should avoid social isolation and instead become involved with family, friends, neighbors, clubs, a church, and other social groups and organizations.

The Health Continuum

Health and wellness imply that individuals are engaged in behaviors that enhance quality of life. This process is illustrated in the health continuum (see Figure 1.2). On the left side of the continuum is health, a state earned through the adoption and practice of good health habits. The reward for such behavior is a high-quality life. The absence of health is death, as depicted on the right side. For most people, before death comes disease, which itself is preceded by a long period of high-risk behaviors. The bulk of Americans dwell in the high-risk behavior zone of the wellness continuum, reluctant to move to the left because bad habits have them strapped in and full of denial about the fact that soon they will be drifting right toward premature disease and death. According to government health officials, individual behaviors and environmental factors are responsible for about 70% of all premature deaths in the United States.

The *Healthy People* Initiative

Healthy People is the prevention agenda for the nation, a road map to better health for all. Since 1980, the U.S. Department of Health and Human Services has used health-promotion and disease-prevention objectives to improve our health.

This agenda started in 1979 with the release of *Healthy People: The Surgeon General's Report on Health Promotion and Disease Prevention.*[3] Noting that the nation's first public health revolution against infectious diseases had been very successful, the surgeon general issued a challenge to begin a second public health revolution—this time against chronic disease, or the lifestyle-related diseases such as heart disease, cancer, stroke, chronic obstructive pulmonary disease, and diabetes. Today, chronic disease accounts for about two thirds of all deaths, whereas in 1900, only about 1 in 10 people died from these causes (see Figure 1.3).

The surgeon general's call for action was followed up with the first set of national health objectives, *Promoting Health/Preventing Disease: Objectives for the Nation*, which

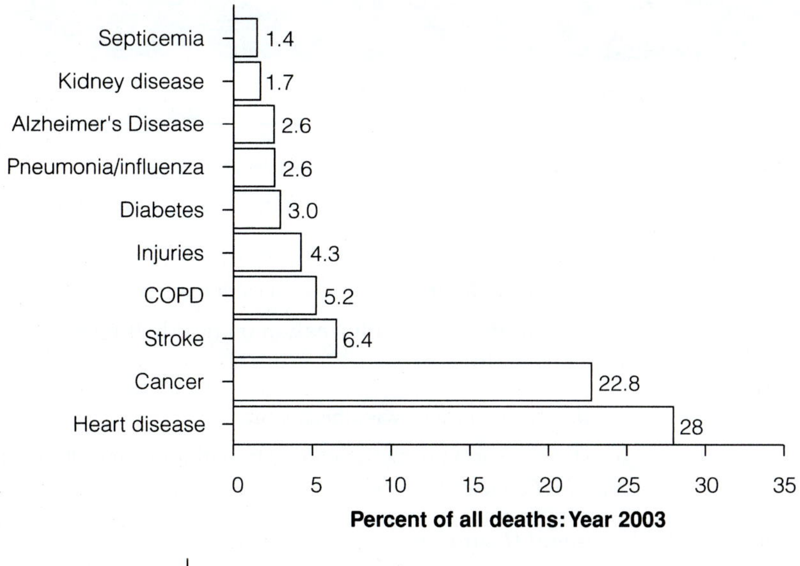

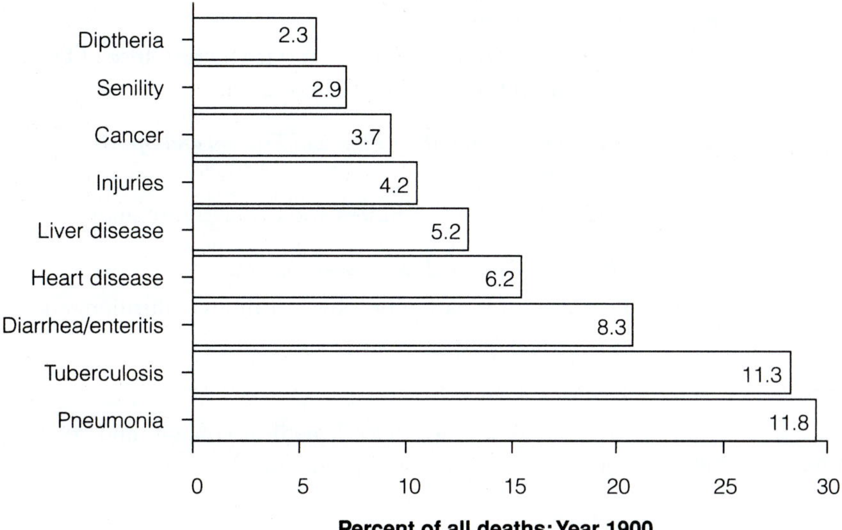

Figure 1.3 Major causes of death in the United States in 1900 and 2003. Source: U.S. Department of Health and Human Services. *Healthy People 2010.* Washington, DC: National Center for Health Statistics, January 2000.

was published in 1980.[4] It set out 226 health objectives for 1990, emphasizing 15 focus areas for health improvement. This was the first time that health promotion received attention by the nation's highest health official.

In 1990, another set of objectives was published to improve the health of the nation, *Healthy People 2000*.[5] The 310 health objectives were divided into 22 focus areas, with three overarching goals: to increase years of healthy life, reduce disparities in health among different population groups, and achieve access to preventive health services for all. This framework provided good direction for individuals to change personal health behaviors and for health organizations to support good health through health-promotion policies. Of the 13 physical activity and fitness objectives, 1 was met (increasing worksite fitness programs), and 4 showed solid gains, indicating that the message about increased physical activity was reaching some segments of the U.S. population.

The current national health objectives for the year 2010 were published in 2000. *Healthy People 2010* is the United States' contribution to WHO's Health for All strategy.[6] *Healthy People 2010* has two major goals:

- *Goal 1: Increase quality and years of healthy life.* A healthy life means that individuals have a full range of function from infancy through old age, allowing them to enter into satisfying relationships with other people and to work and play. Currently, the average baby born can expect to live 77 years, but only 64 of these years will be healthy. By the year 2010, it is hoped by government health officials that this healthy life expectancy will rise to 66 years.
- *Goal 2: Eliminate health disparities.* There are many barriers to good health, but it is unfortunate that in America gender, race, income, education, age, disability, and sexual orientation often interfere with

Box 1.1

Important Internet Sites on Health and Fitness

There are thousands of Internet sites devoted to health and fitness. Here is a sampling of Internet sites that provide high-quality information. See the chapters on nutrition and specific diseases to get Internet lists for those areas. MEDLINE*plus* is an excellent free resource of consumer health and fitness information and is managed by the National Library of Medicine (NLM). MEDLINE*plus* is available on the Internet from the NLM home page (http://www.nlm.nih.gov/) or directly at MEDLINE*plus* (http://www.nlm.nih.gov/medlineplus).

American College of Sports Medicine (www.acsm.org)

Information on health and fitness, and links to other sites

American Council on Exercise (www.acefitness.org)

Consumer information on fitness equipment and programs; certification of professionals

American Heart Association, Fitness Center (www.justmove.org)

A comprehensive resource for fitness information and news

Centers for Disease Control and Prevention (www.cdc.gov)

Provides a wealth of health information for consumers and professionals

Consumer Information Center (www.pueblo.gsa.gov)

Scores of downloadable documents on health, fitness, and diet

Government HealthFinder (www.healthfinder.gov)

Links to authoritative information on health, fitness, nutrition, and disease

Health Government (www.health.gov)

The primary government health site with information on *Healthy People 2010*

National Health Information Center (www.health.gov/nhic/)

A health information referral service of the Office of Disease Prevention and Health Promotion

President's Council on Physical Fitness and Sports (www.fitness.gov)

Authoritative site on fitness and health information

Shape Up America! (www.shapeup.org)

Provides information on physical fitness, nutrition, and safe weight management

WebMD (www.webmd.com)

Provides news, health and medical content, and references for consumers and professionals

access to quality health care and opportunities to practice good health habits. By the year 2010, government health officials plan to eliminate these disparities.

The nation's progress in achieving the two goals of *Healthy People 2010* will be monitored through 467 objectives in 28 focus areas. As depicted in Figure 1.4, the objectives are based on the determinants of health, primarily individual behaviors and environmental factors. Individual biology and behaviors influence health through their interaction with each other and with the individual's social and physical environments. Policies and interventions can improve health by targeting factors related to individuals and their environments, including access to quality health care. In *Healthy People 2010*, 10 leading health indicators receive special attention: physical activity, overweight and obesity, tobacco, substance abuse, responsible sexual behavior, mental health, injury and violence, environmental quality, immunization, and access to health care. The complete report can be found on the Internet. See Box 1.1 for this and other Internet sites dealing with health and fitness.

Healthy People 2010 focus area 22, "physical activity and fitness," has one primary goal: improve health, fitness, and quality of life through daily physical activity. According to *Healthy People 2010*, research has shown that virtually all individuals will benefit from regular physical activity, and 15 objectives have been formulated to encourage Americans to adopt and maintain an active lifestyle. Some key *Healthy People 2010* physical activity and fitness objectives are listed in Table 1.1.

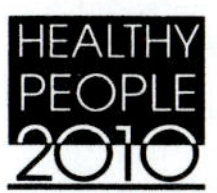

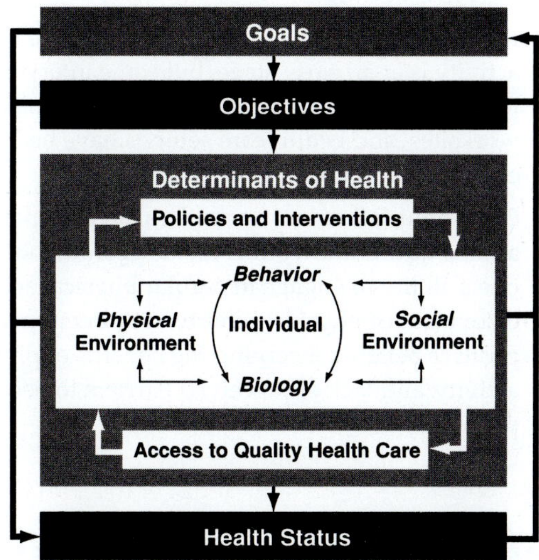

Figure 1.4 The goals and objectives of *Healthy People 2010*. Source: U.S. Department of Health and Human Services. *Healthy People 2010*. Washington, DC: January 2000. http://www.health.gov/healthypeople/.

TABLE 1.1 Physical Activity and Fitness, *Healthy People 2010* Objectives

Objective 22-1: Reduce to 20% the proportion of adults who engage in no leisure-time physical activity. (In 1997, this proportion was 40%.)

Objective 22-2: Increase to at least 30% the proportion of adults who engage regularly, preferably daily, in moderate physical activity for at least 30 minutes per day. (In 1997, 15% met this goal.)

Objective 22-3: Increase to at least 30% the proportion of adults who engage in vigorous physical activity that promotes the development and maintenance of cardiorespiratory fitness three or more days per week for 20 or more minutes per occasion. (In 1997, 23% met this goal.)

Objective 22-4: Increase to at least 30% the proportion of adults who perform physical activities that enhance and maintain muscular strength and endurance. (In 1998, 18% met this goal.)

Objective 22-5: Increase to at least 43% the proportion of adults who perform physical activities that enhance and maintain flexibility. (In 1998, 30% met this goal.)

Objective 22-6: Increase to at least 35% the proportion of adolescents who engage in moderate physical activity for at least 30 minutes on five or more of the previous seven days. (In 1999, 27% met this goal.)

Objective 22-7: Increase to at least 85% the proportion of adolescents who engage in vigorous physical activity that promotes cardiorespiratory fitness three or more days per week for 20 or more minutes per occasion. (In 1999, 65% met this goal.)

Objective 22-8: Increase the proportion of the nation's public and private schools that require daily physical education for all students. (Target: 25%, middle and junior high schools, compared to 17% in 1994; 5% for senior high schools compared to 2% in 1994.)

Objective 22-9: Increase to at least 50% the proportion of adolescents who participate in daily school physical education. (In 1999, 29% met this goal.)

Objective 22-10: Increase to at least 50% the proportion of adolescents who spend at least 50% of school physical education class time being physically active. (In 1999, 38% met this goal.)

Objective 22-11: Increase to at least 75% the proportion of adolescents who view television two or fewer hours on a school day. (In 1999, 57% met this goal.)

Objective 22-12: Increase the proportion of the nation's public and private schools that provide access to their physical activity spaces and facilities for all persons outside of normal school hours.

Objective 22-13: Increase to at least 75% the proportion of worksites offering employer-sponsored physical activity and fitness programs. (In 1998–1999, 46% of worksites met this goal.)

Objective 22-14: Increase to at least 25% the proportion of trips made by walking (adults). (In 1995, 17% of trips of 1 mile or less were made by walking.)

Objective 22-15: Increase to at least 2% the proportion of trips made by bicycling (adults). (In 1995, 0.6% of trips of 5 miles or less were made by bicycling.)

Objective 19-1: Increase to at least 60% the proportion of adults who are at a healthy weight. (In 1988–1994, 42% met this goal.)

Objective 19-2: Reduce to less than 15% the proportion of adults who are obese. (In 1988–1994, 23% were obese.)

Source: U.S. Department of Health and Human Services. *Healthy People 2010*. Washington, DC: January 2000. http://www.health.gov/healthypeople/.

THE SURGEON GENERAL'S REPORT ON PHYSICAL ACTIVITY AND HEALTH*

In 1994, the Office of the Surgeon General authorized the Centers for Disease Control and Prevention (CDC) to serve as the lead agency for preparing the first report on physical activity and health by the surgeon general.[7] This landmark review of the research on physical activity and health was published in 1996 and has helped initiate a new awareness of the importance of regular exercise. The main message of the surgeon general's first report on physical activity and health was that "Americans can substantially improve their health and quality of life by including moderate amounts of physical activity in their daily lives."

The report's major conclusions included the following:

- People of all ages, both males and females, benefit from regular physical activity.
- People can obtain significant health benefits by including a moderate amount of physical activity (e.g., 30 minutes of walking briskly or raking leaves, 15 minutes of running, or 45 minutes of playing volleyball) on most, if not all, days of the week. Through a modest increase in daily activity most Americans can improve their health and quality of life.
- People can gain additional health benefits through greater amounts of physical activity. People who can maintain a regular regimen of activity that is of longer duration or of more vigorous intensity are likely to derive greater benefit.
- Physical activity reduces the risk of premature mortality in general, and of coronary heart disease, hypertension, colon cancer, and diabetes mellitus in particular. Physical activity also improves mental health and is important for the health of muscles, bones, and joints.
- More than 60% of American adults are not regularly physically active. In fact, 25% of all adults are not active at all. Physical inactivity is more prevalent among women than men, among blacks and Hispanics than whites, among older than younger adults, and among the less affluent than the more affluent.
- The most popular leisure-time physical activities among adults are walking and gardening or yard work.
- Nearly half of American youths 12–21 years of age are not vigorously active on a regular basis. Moreover, physical activity declines dramatically during adolescence.
- Daily attendance in physical education classes has declined among high school students from 42% in 1991 to 25% in 1995.
- Research on understanding and promoting physical activity is at an early stage, but some interventions to promote physical activity through schools, worksites, and health-care settings have been evaluated and found to be successful.
- Consistent influences on physical activity patterns among adults and youths include confidence in one's ability to engage in regular physical activity, enjoyment of physical activity, support from others, positive beliefs concerning the benefits of physical activity, and lack of perceived barriers to being physically active.

*Additional information on the surgeon general's report can be obtained at this site on the Internet: www.cdc.gov.

EXERCISE AND PHYSICAL FITNESS IN AMERICA

Although the modern-day fitness movement falls short in attracting the majority of Americans, it has been a major force in shaping societal norms and standards. In addition, the contemporary movement has roots in various events dating from the previous century.

A Brief Historical Review

During the mid- to late 1800s, as America experienced increasing urbanization and industrialization, the health of Americans became a growing concern of many leaders.[8,9] The new nation grew from 17 million people in 1840 to more than 50 million in 1880, becoming more urban in the process. Many farmers became factory workers, travel changed from horses to trains, and the invention of the telegraph vastly accelerated communication. Greatly expanded numbers of industrial laborers worked 12 to 16 hours a day, six days a week.

In response to these changing conditions, America's first health and fitness reform movement took shape, led by social reformers such as Oliver Wendell Holmes, Sr., Catharine Beecher, and Dioclesian Lewis, and by health reformers such as Sylvester Graham and William Alcott. The reform movement was directed at the increasingly poor health of the general population, particularly in the cities. Gymnasiums opened, and various organizations such as the YMCA, YWCA, and settlement houses organized exercise programs. The health reformers also urged people to pay attention to improving their diets and avoid the abuse of drugs such as alcohol—themes still embraced today.

In the schools, several progressive colleges hired medical doctors—including Edward Hitchcock (Amherst), Dudley Allen Sargent (Harvard), Edward Hartwell (Johns Hopkins), and William Anderson (Yale)—to teach students about health, gymnastic exercises with light dumbbells and other apparatus, weight lifting, European gymnastics, and anthropometric measurements. Most of the programs were based on German and Swedish gymnastic programs, which consisted of marching, free exercises with rings and clubs, and work with apparatus such as the balance board, rings, and vaulting box.[10] These programs emphasized the health-related values of proper physical exercise, with muscular strength and size seen as most important.

Dioclesian Lewis, a medical doctor, gave up his medical practice to become a leading figure in the health and fitness movement from 1850 to 1880. An animated and inspirational speaker (it was said people could "inhale hygiene in his presence"), he developed a system of "New Gymnastics" that swept the country in the early 1860s.[8] His exercise program was structured around several sets of light exercises, including beanbag games; calisthenic movements with 6-inch wooden rings, wooden dumbbells, and wands; and dancing and marching to musical accompaniment (the original aerobic-dance system).

Catharine Beecher warned against the poor health of women and against the societal conventions that limited women's participation in physical activity; her stand was supported strongly by Lewis and other reformers.[9] Her famous brother, the Reverend Henry Ward Beecher of Brooklyn, was an advocate of the "muscular Christianity movement," which aimed at "breadth of shoulders as well as of doctrines." He favored vigorous outdoor recreation and urged that churches and other Christian associations provide opportunities for young adults of the city to exercise in wholesome environments.

In 1845, when Alexander Cartwright and his friends took what was essentially a child's game and turned it into an adult male sport called "baseball," they initiated America's love affair with sports.[9] Other games were organized into sports during the latter half of the 1800s, and a growing public interest in sports spread onto the college campus.

At the same time that Amherst, Harvard, Johns Hopkins, and Yale were hiring medical doctors to maintain and improve students' health, the growing popularity of intercollegiate sport introduced thousands of students to the fun and stimulation of vigorous games and athletics. The students began to organize a series of intercollegiate sporting contests. The relatively dull routine of gymnastic drills paled in comparison to sport participation, and soon after the turn of the century, sports surpassed gymnastics as the students' exercise of choice; the trend was supported by such educational leaders as John Dewey, William Kilpatrick, and Thomas Wood.

Schools gradually shifted from medical doctors to "physical educators" who promoted sports and games as the best way to develop intellectual awareness, character, and improved moral and social behavior, along with physical fitness.[10] John Dewey, for example, believed that to be effective centers of learning, schools must be interesting and must emphasize the role of play in the education of the student. Luther Gulick stressed the role of sports in the "toughening of the individual for the achievements of life." Many educators melded these viewpoints, believing that the objectives of physical education could best be met through a "sports for all" program, therefore shifting the curriculum from the goal of health through gymnastics to the goals of character, sportsmanship, and fitness through sport.

According to some critics, however, the promotion of physical fitness became secondary to the development of game and sport skills (motor fitness), and the attainment of psychosocial goals. This was the beginning of a furious debate that has continued to this day—should physical education emphasize health-related physical activities (exercises that develop the heart, lungs, and musculoskeletal systems), or should it emphasize motor-fitness–related activities (exercises that develop coordination, balance, agility, speed, and power)?[11]

Between World War I and World War II, the United States became a nation in which sport was a part of its very being, as entertainment, as an integral part of education, and as an accepted and worthwhile way for all Americans to spend leisure time.

The Contemporary Fitness Movement

In the 1940s and 1950s, several major events prompted Americans to take a closer look at both school physical education programs and adult fitness.

For one thing, statistics on draftees during World War II spurred the media to report that school sports programs were not adequately enhancing students' physical fitness. Out of 9 million registrants examined for the armed services in early 1943, almost 3 million (one third) were rejected for physical and mental reasons.[10] The chief of Athletics and Recreation of the Services Division of the U.S. Army responded by recommending at the 1943 War Fitness Conference that "physical education through play must be discarded and a more rugged program substituted."

Later, in 1953, the shocking results of the Kraus–Weber tests of minimum muscular fitness of schoolchildren were released, arousing massive public and official concern.[12] The tests consisted of six simple movements of key muscle groups. Among U.S. children, 57.9% failed while only 8.7% of European children failed. When President Eisenhower's attention was called to the report of this study, he immediately called for a special White House Conference on the subject, which was finally held in June 1956. As a result, the President's Council on Youth Fitness and a President's Citizens Advisory Committee on the Fitness of American Youth were formed.

Among adults in the general population, the stage was being set for the second popular fitness movement. After World War II, heart disease had reached epidemic proportions, obesity had become a major public health problem, and health-care costs had begun to skyrocket. A growing sentiment among some health researchers and administrators was that technological advances in transportation, communication, and industry had created a society in which physical activity was no longer necessary or even likely, so if people were to get adequate exercise, they would have to make an effort to interject it into their normal sedentary routine.

Finally, the late 1960s brought a sudden change in adult fitness awareness. In 1967, Oregon track coach Bill Bowerman toured New Zealand and discovered "jogging." He returned to America and wrote *Jogging,*[13] igniting the first running boom in the United States, with his book selling more than 300,000 copies.

In 1968, Kenneth H. Cooper, a medical doctor for the U.S. Air Force, published his book *Aerobics,*[14] followed 2 years later by *The New Aerobics.*[15] In these books, Cooper challenged Americans to take personal charge of their lifestyles and to counter the epidemics of heart disease, obesity, and rising health-care costs by engaging in regular exercise.

To Cooper, the best form of exercise is "aerobic," a word he coined to represent activities that stimulated the heart, lungs, and blood vessels. Stated Cooper: "The best exercises are running, swimming, cycling, walking, stationary running, handball, basketball, and squash, and in just about that order. . . . Isometrics, weight lifting, and calisthenics, though good as far as they go, don't even make the list, despite the fact that most exercise books are based on one of these three, especially calisthenics."[14]

These two books provided the necessary theoretical fuel for an adult fitness revolution that soon zoomed across the country. Millions took up the aerobic challenge and began jogging, cycling, walking, and swimming programs.[16] Ken Cooper's wife, Mildred Cooper, joined her husband in 1972 in writing *Aerobics for Women.*[17] Within 9 years, these three books on aerobics sold more than 6 million copies and were translated into 15 foreign languages and into braille.

In 1972, Frank Shorter won the Olympic marathon gold medal in Munich. The extensive television coverage of this marathon and Shorter's silver-medal effort in 1976 (Montreal) helped to spawn the road-racing movement that has since become so popular.[18]

Running, which quickly became a symbol of the American exercise movement, was promoted by a spate of successful books by Henderson,[19] Ullyot,[20] Sheehan,[21] and others, climaxing in *The Complete Book of Running* by Jim Fixx,[22] which topped the best-seller lists for nearly 2 years. In the space of one year, 1977 to 1978, the magazine *Runner's World* more than tripled its circulation from 85,000 to 270,000.[18]

Just as the running movement was starting, another popular form of adult exercise, aerobic dance, emerged. By making exercise fun and socially oriented, aerobic dance attracted millions who otherwise might not have joined the fitness movement.[23] Aerobic dance, now one of the most popular, organized fitness activities for women in the United States, traces its origins to Jacki Sorenson, the wife of a naval pilot, who began conducting exercise classes at a U.S. Navy base in Puerto Rico in 1969. The growth of aerobic dance has been stimulated more recently by the production of recorded dance exercise programs (see Figure 1.5).

The original aerobic-dance programs consisted of an eclectic combination of various dance forms, including ballet, modern jazz, disco, and folk, as well as calisthenic-type exercises. More recent innovations include water aerobics (done in a swimming pool), non-impact or low-impact aerobics (one foot on the ground at all times), specific types of dance aerobics, step aerobics (using a low stool), and assisted aerobics (with weights worn on the wrists and/or ankles).

The fitness movement experienced strong growth during the 1970s and 1980s but appears to have plateaued dur-

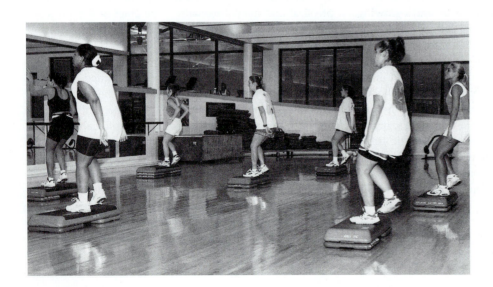

Figure 1.5 Aerobic dance is one of the most popular forms of exercise for women.

ing the 1990s. The most popular fitness activity continues to be fitness walking, followed by gardening or yard work, stretching exercises, bicycling, strengthening exercises, stair climbing, jogging or running, aerobic dancing, and swimming.

Health clubs (as we know them today) evolved in the mid- to late 1970s when racquetball, tennis, and aerobic dance grew in popularity.[24] Many of the early clubs were not run professionally, and some unscrupulous operators crowded their clubs with too many members while delivering little service (or in some instances, closing shop and leaving town after receiving "lifetime" membership dues).

To combat this problem and ensure quality control over the fitness movement, universities have developed sophisticated graduate-degree programs, and various professional groups provide certification and continuing education programs. In 1988, the International Health, Racquet and Sportsclub Association (IHRSA) and a health-club-industry trade group adopted a code of conduct and, in 1993, established a list of minimum standards.[24] In 1992, the American College of Sports Medicine (ACSM) published an exhaustive standards manual, which listed 353 mandatory policies and procedures and 397 guidelines that were strongly recommended for health clubs.[25] In 1997, the ACSM published a revised list of standards and guidelines for health and fitness facilities[26] The ACSM standards emphasized that every program offered in a facility be held in a safe environment by a trained, professional staff. Memberships at commercial clubs grew strongly during the past 20 years, with huge gains being recorded among members age 65 and older. According to Figure 1.6, in 1982, IHRSA reported that there were 6,211 health and fitness clubs, a number that more than quadrupled to 26,830 in 2005. IHRSA estimates that by the year 2010, club memberships will reach 40 million.

Also joining the fitness movement have been many hospitals and corporations that provide programs for their employees, employees' families, and, in most instances, the community.[24] Government surveys indicate that about half of worksites with 50 or more employees offer employer-sponsored physical activity and fitness programs.[6]

Current Activity Levels of American Adults

Since the early 1990s, many surveys of the activity levels of American adults have attempted to evaluate the magnitude of the present adult fitness revolution in the United States.[6,7] Measurement of physical activity is difficult, and no single technique is suitable for all purposes. More than 30 methods for assessment of physical activity have been described, and these can be divided into three broad categories: self-report surveys, mechanical and electronic monitors, and physiological measurement.

Time and cost restraints have led to the predominant use of self-report surveys in national studies investigating the physical activity patterns of American adults.[7] All of the other techniques are simply too burdensome and costly for a general population survey. Self-report survey methods include telephone or mail questionnaires using short- or long-term recall of typical habits, and personal diaries, which are used for varying lengths of time (e.g., activities recorded every 15 minutes for 3 days in a row).

Three government-sponsored national surveys have provided the most useful data on the physical activity habits of American adults: (1) the National Health Interview Survey of Health Promotion and Disease Prevention (NHIS) from the National Center for Health Statistics (NCHS); (2) the Behavioral Risk Factor Surveillance System (BRFSS), administered in cooperation with the CDC; and (3) the National Health and Nutrition Examination Survey (NHANES) of U.S. adults.[7]

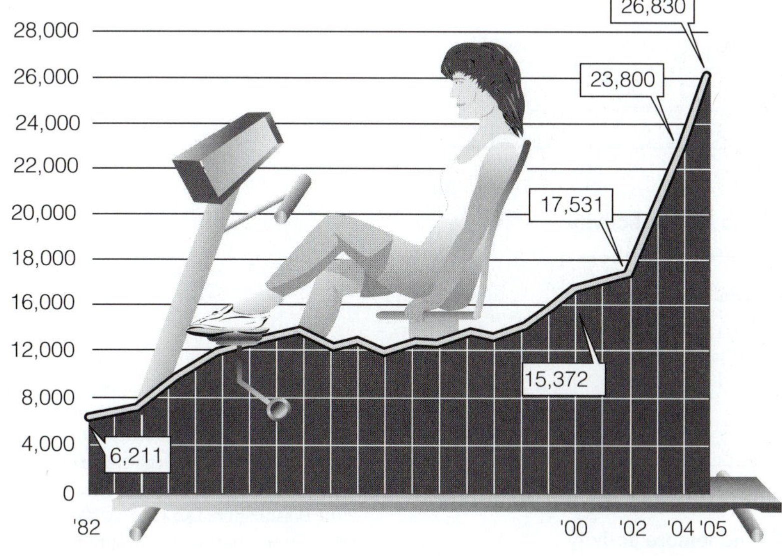

Figure 1.6 The number of health and fitness clubs has more than quadrupled between 1982 and 2005. Source: International Health, Racquet, and Sports Club Association.

The NHIS assessed the frequency, duration, and intensity of physical activity. Data were collected on a national representative sample of a large number of American adults, representing one of the best current sources of descriptive information on American physical activity habits.[6,7,27,28]

The BRFSS consists of annual random-digit-dialed telephone surveys conducted by state health departments in cooperation with the CDC. These surveys routinely collect risk-factor data, including the prevalence of sedentary lifestyles.[29]

In the NHANES, adults were asked questions about the type and frequency of their physically active hobbies, sports, and exercises.[6,7,30]

Based on these surveys, several important conclusions can be drawn.[6,7,27,28]

1. Few Americans engage in appropriate levels of physical activity. Only 23% of American adults report exercising vigorously (at an intensity of at least 50% VO_{2max}, for 20 or more minutes a session, three or more times per week), the level generally recommended for cardiovascular benefit. As stated earlier, the year 2010 goal has been set at 30% (see Figure 1.7).[6]

   Approximately 17% of Americans report they exercise moderately for 30 minutes or more five or more times per week, while 38% report essentially sedentary lifestyles. The rest of Americans (22%) report exercising irregularly (see Figure 1.7).

2. Physical inactivity rises with increase in age.[28] As summarized in Figure 1.8, the proportion of adults who engage in no leisure-time physical activity

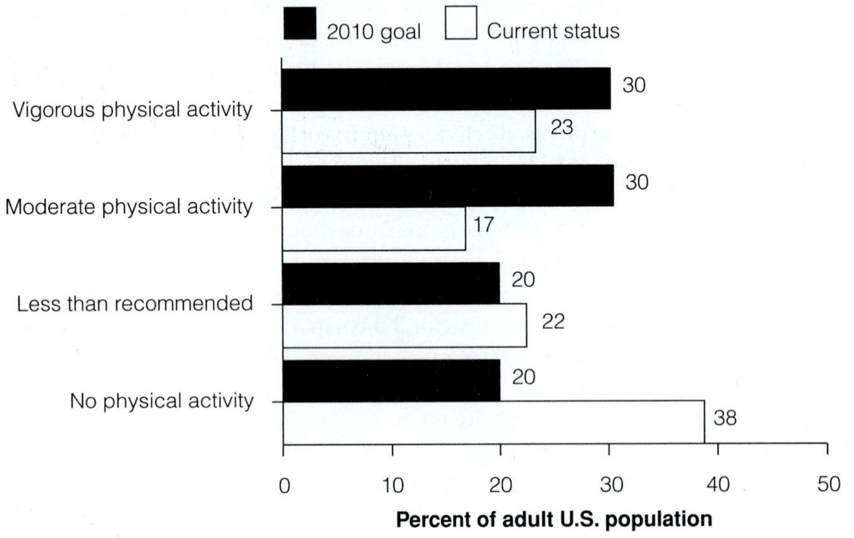

Figure 1.7 Comparison of *Healthy People 2010* goals and current accomplishments. Source: U.S. Department of Health and Human Services. *Healthy People 2010.* Washington, DC: January 2000. http://www.health.gov/healthypeople/.

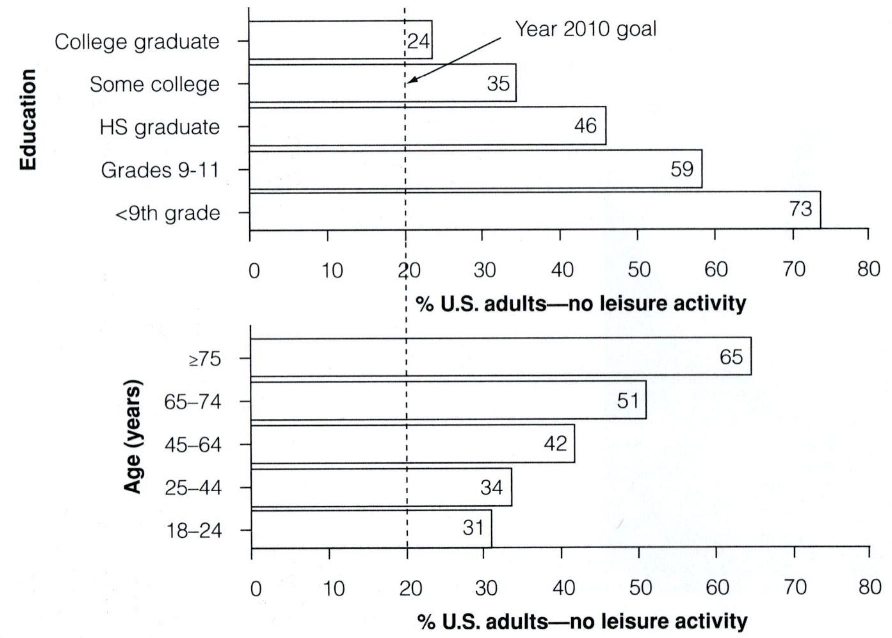

Figure 1.8 Changes in physical activity patterns with education and aging. Source: U.S. Department of Health and Human Services. *Healthy People 2010.* Washington, DC: January 2000. http://www.health.gov/healthypeople/.

TABLE 1.2 Percentage of Adults Who Exercise on a Regular Basis (Five or More Times a Week for 30 or More Minutes per Session), by Education Level and Income

Characteristic	Percentage of All Adults
Education level	
<12 years	15.6
12 years	17.8
13–15 years	22.7
>15 years	23.5
Income	
<$10,000	17.6
$10,000–$19,999	18.7
$20,000–$34,999	20.3
$35,000–$49,999	20.9
≥ $50,000	23.5

Source: Physical Activity and Health: A Report of the Surgeon General, 1996.

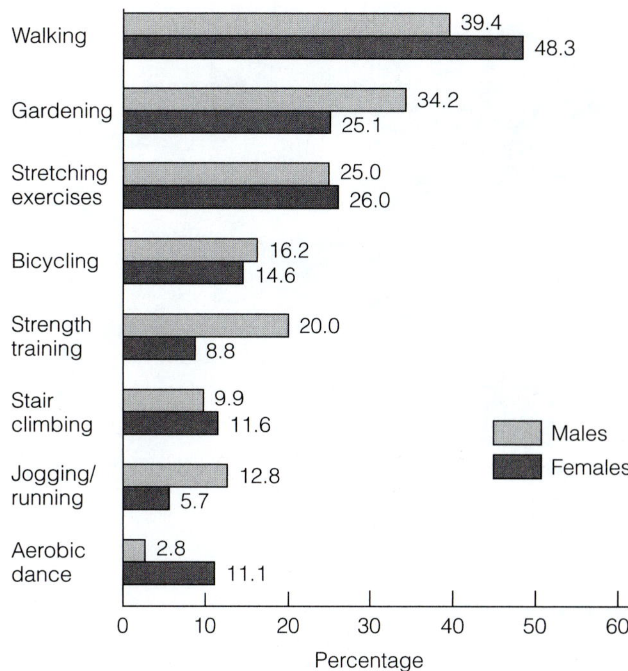

Figure 1.9 Percentage of adults reporting participation in selected activities. Americans tend to engage in physical activities that are low cost, convenient, and easy to schedule.[7]

doubles between the ages of 18–24 and ≥ 75 years.[6,7] At all ages, inactivity is higher among women than men.[28]

3. People with higher incomes and more education tend to exercise more often (see Table 1.2 and Figure 1.8).[6,7,30] People of higher socioeconomic status (SES) (as indicated by income, education, and occupation) are more likely to be physically active (especially when considering total time devoted to physical exercise) than are those of lower SES (see Table 1.2). In general, managers and professionals are more active in their leisure time than are other white-collar workers, who in turn exercise more frequently than do blue-collar workers. Other disparities in levels of physical activity exist among population groups. Inactivity is higher among African Americans and Hispanics than whites, and higher among people with disabilities and certain health conditions.[6]
4. Walking and other convenient activities are most popular. The most popular physical activity reported by both Americans and Canadians is walking (see Figure 1.9). Other activities that consistently account for large numbers of participants include gardening, calisthenics, bicycling, exercising with indoor equipment (such as stationary bicycles, stair climbers, treadmills, weights), aerobic dancing, and jogging/running.[6,7] These activities have several important features in common, including low cost, casual scheduling, and convenience.
5. A greater proportion of people in the western states exercise (see Figure 1.10).[7,27,28] Regionally, the northeast and the south have the lowest proportion of physically active residents; the midwest and west have the highest proportion who have "regular, sustained activity."[7]
6. The exercise boom appears to have plateaued. Unfortunately, there is no adequate series of statistics available to gauge trends in activity since the mid-1950s or so in America. One problem is that no satisfactory definition of physical activity has been consistently used in comparable national surveys. Nonetheless, using various national probability samples by Gallup (1961 to 1984), Louis Harris and Associates (1979 to present), the CDC (1982 to present, BRFSS), and the NCHS, the data suggest that at any given age, the proportion of people who exercise regularly tended to increase strongly throughout the 1970s and early 1980s, before plateauing during the late 1980s and 1990s.[6,7,31]
7. Few American adults are building muscular fitness. Only about one in five adults perform physical activities that enhance muscular strength and endurance two or more days per week.[6,7] (The *Healthy People 2010* target is 30%). About 30% of adults perform flexibility exercises, below the 2010 target of 40%.
8. Americans use their cars instead of their legs for short trips. The U.S. Department of Transportation reports that over 75% of all trips less than 1 mile are made by automobile.[6] In addition, the number of walking trips as a percentage of all trips taken has declined over the years.

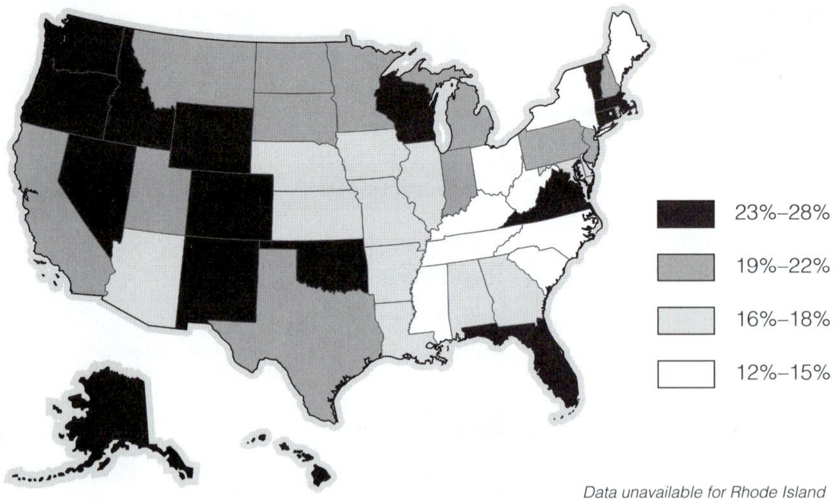

Figure 1.10 Regular, sustained activity by American adults. Adults from the western half of the nation tend to be more active than their eastern counterparts. Source: Behavioral Risk Factor Surveillance System.

Future Challenges

Results from these surveys point out some very basic problems with the modern-day fitness movement. In particular, despite all of the media hype, the majority of Americans are *not* exercising. Less than 40% of Americans are exercising appropriately. Physical inactivity is more common among those with less education and income, the elderly, and females.[6,7,28,29]

Perhaps two principles from the national surveys discussed in this chapter stand out: (1) Americans appear more inclined to exercise if it can be done at moderate- versus high-intensity levels, suggesting that we more strongly emphasize activities such as walking in our public health endeavors rather than activities such as running; (2) we should direct more attention to helping people exercise during their regular daily routine instead of seeking time and energy to add exercise to an already crowded schedule.

YOUTH FITNESS STUDIES

There is a perceived fitness crisis among American children and youths. In general, most experts feel that American children and youths are less healthy, active, and physically fit than is recommended.[6,7] Baseline data on the health-related fitness level of school-age children were made available in 1984 with the release of the First National Children and Youth Fitness Study (NCYFS I);[32] in 1985 with the President's Council on Physical Fitness and Sports School Population Fitness Survey;[33] in 1987 with the Second National Children and Youth Fitness Study (NCYFS II);[34–36] from the national school-based Youth Risk Behavior Survey of youths in grades 9–12;[37] from the NHIS, Youth Risk Behavior Survey of all young people ages 12–21; and from CDC's Youth Media Campaign Longitudinal Survey.[7,38] Results from these six surveys have caused much public concern about the fitness of American youths (see Figure 1.11).

In general, although some experts differ on their interpretation of the test results, the general perception is that American children and youths are less active and physically fit than is recommended for optimal protection against future chronic disease.[39] The habits of youth typically track into college and adulthood. See Box 1.2 for a summary of the fitness habits of American college students.

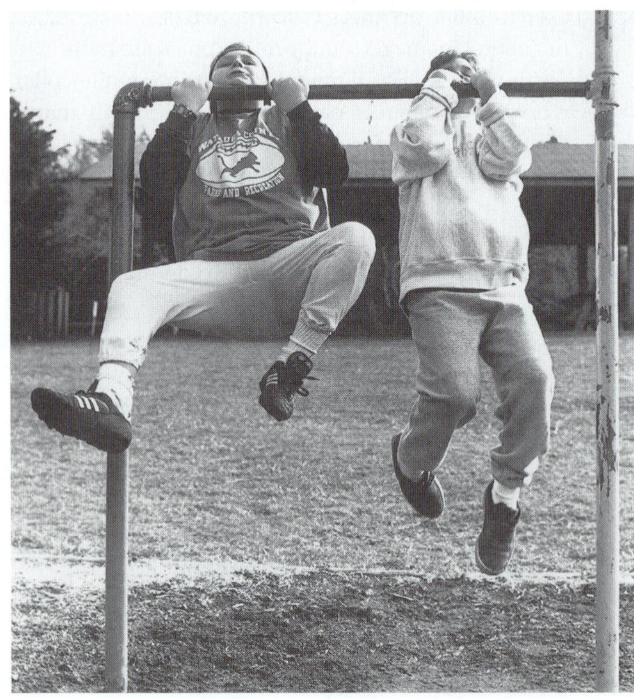

Figure 1.11 National surveys on the fitness status of American children and youths have aroused much public concern.

Box 1.2

National College Health Risk Behavior Survey

Fitness Habits

A CDC survey of college students nationwide revealed that the majority do not exercise on a regular basis, with a significant proportion worried about their body weight.

- Nationwide, 20.5% of college students are classified as being overweight.
- Six in ten female college students, and 3 in 10 males report they are attempting to lose weight at any given time.
- Less than 4 in 10 college students participate in aerobic activities that make them sweat and breathe hard for at least 20 minutes on three or more days each week. Male students (44%) are more likely than female students (33%) to report vigorous physical activity.
- One in three college students stretch on a regular basis.
- Nationwide, 30% of college students (34% of males, 27% of females) engage in strengthening exercises on three or more days weekly.
- One in five students enroll in physical education classes during the collegiate school year.
- Nationwide, 18% of students (27% of males, 10% of females) participate in one or more college or university sports teams (intramural or extramural).

Source: Centers for Disease Control and Prevention. Youth Risk Behavior Surveillance: National College Health Risk Behavior Survey—United States, 1995. *CDC Surveillance Summaries. MMWR* 46(No. SS-6), 1997.

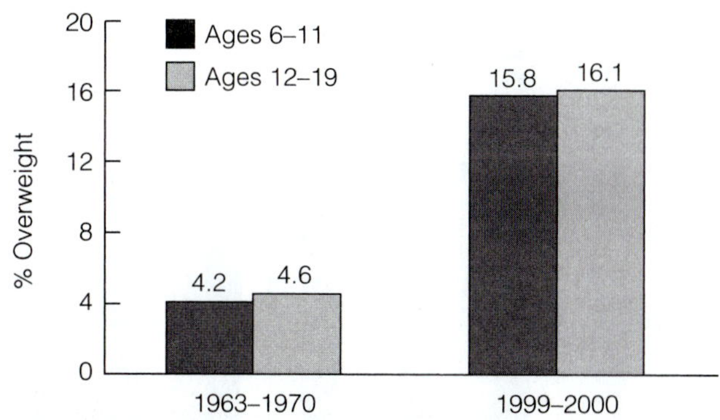

Figure 1.12 The percentage of overweight children and adolescents has more than tripled since the 1960s.

Important findings from these six surveys include the following:

- Youths are increasingly overweight. As depicted in Figure 1.12, the percentage of young people who are overweight has more than tripled since 1963–1970.[6,7] This finding is disturbing because a high proportion of overweight youths end up obese as adults (about half of obese school-age children become obese adults, and more than 80% of obese adolescents remain obese into adulthood) (see Chapter 13).
- Only 65% of adolescents exercise vigorously.[6] *Healthy People 2010* proposed to increase to at least 85% the proportion of adolescents who engage regularly in vigorous aerobic physical activity. As Figure 1.13 shows, this proportion falls sharply with increasing age.
- Only 28% of teenagers attend physical education classes daily. Children and youths need daily physical education (PE) to keep fit and healthy, and to help them gain the knowledge, attitudes, and skills they need to engage in lifelong physical activity. Schools are failing to meet this need. According to the CDC, only 56% of high school students are enrolled in a PE class, 28% attend PE classes daily, and 39% are physically active for more than 20 minutes during PE classes.[37] These proportions have declined since 1991, and are lower among female students and students in higher grades (Figure 1.14). Children and teenagers spend about 4 hours a day on average doing sedentary activities such as watching television, playing video games, or using a computer.
- Girls exercise less than boys. Activity levels of girls are below those of boys and tend to drop sharply as age or grade in school increases (see Figure 1.13).
- Upper body strength is poor for many children and youths. For example, among girls ages 9–17, about half cannot perform more than one pull-up. For boys ages 6–12, 40% cannot do more than one pull-up, while 25% cannot do any. About one half of males and two thirds of females, ages 12–21 years do not participate regularly in strengthening or toning activities (e.g., push-ups, sit-ups, or weight lifting).
- Aerobic (heart and lung) fitness is lower than recommended for many young people. About half of girls ages 6–17 and 60% of boys ages 6–12

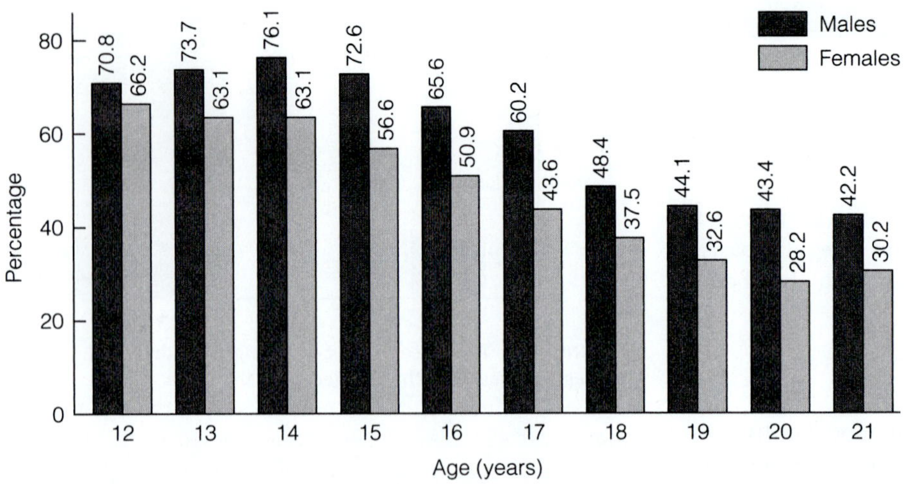

Figure 1.13 Vigorous exercise among young people during three or more of the seven days preceding the survey. Female young people exercise vigorously less often than males, and the percentage for both males and females falls sharply with increasing age.[7]

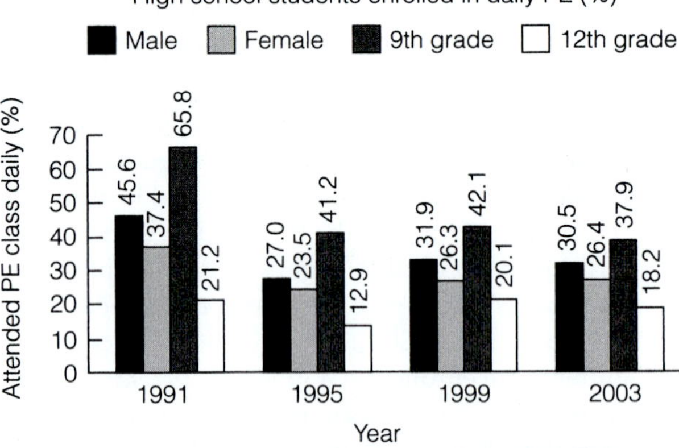

Figure 1.14 The proportion of high school students enrolled in PE has decreased since 1991 and is lower among female students and those in higher grades. Source: Centers for Disease Control and Prevention. Physical activity among children aged 9–13 years—United States, 2002.

cannot run a mile in less than 10 minutes, for example.

- Many young people have disease risk factors.[39] About 13% of children and youths ages 12–17 smoke, with the proportion rising to 35% among high school seniors. Close to one in three children and adolescents have serum cholesterol levels that exceed 170 milligrams per deciliter (mg/dl), the level deemed "acceptable" by the National Cholesterol Education Program. A national survey by the CDC revealed that 63% of adolescents have two or more of five major risk factors for chronic disease. Risk factors tend to cluster and show tracking from childhood and adolescence to adulthood meaning that every attempt should be made to bring risk factors under control while people are young.

GUIDELINES FOR PROMOTING LIFELONG PHYSICAL ACTIVITY AMONG YOUNG PEOPLE

Children and youths need daily physical activity to keep fit and healthy.[6,7,32,40,41] Chapter 8 outlines some specific recommended exercise prescriptions for young people. In general, parents and teachers are urged to provide many opportunities for play and simple sports for children and youths.[40,41] Enjoyment and excitement have been identified as major reasons why children and youths engage in physical activity such as sports. Physically active parents and role models provide support for children to be active. The American Academy of Pediatrics has emphasized that children need active play, good physical education programs, parental involvement, and generally active lifestyles, rather than specific vigorous exercise training.

In 1997, the CDC released guidelines urging schools and communities to encourage physical activity among young people so that they will continue to engage in physical activity in adulthood and will obtain the health benefits of physical activity throughout life.[42] The CDC guidelines included recommendations about nine aspects of school and community programs.

In 2000, the Secretary of Health and Human Services and the Secretary of Education released their report, "Promoting Better Health for Your People Through Physical Activity and Sports."[39] Ten strategies were described to promote lifelong participation in enjoyable and safe physical activity and sports. These focused on the roles of families, school and after-school programs, youth sports and recreation programs, community environments, and the media.

1. Include education for parents and guardians as part of youth physical activity promotion initiatives.
2. Help all children, from pre-kindergarten through grade 12, to receive quality, daily physical

education. Help all schools to have certified physical education specialists; appropriate class sizes; and the facilities, equipment, and supplies needed to deliver quality, daily physical education.

3. Publicize and disseminate tools to help schools improve their physical education and other physical activity programs.
4. Enable state education and health departments to work together to help schools implement quality, daily physical education and other physical activity programs.
   a. With a full-time state coordinator for school physical activity programs
   b. As part of a coordinated school health program
   c. With support from relevant governmental and nongovernmental organizations
5. Enable more after-school care programs to provide regular opportunities for active, physical play.
6. Help provide access to community sports and recreation programs for all young people.
7. Enable youth sports and recreation programs to provide coaches and recreation program staff with the training they need to offer developmentally appropriate, safe, and enjoyable physical activity experiences for young people.
8. Enable communities to develop and promote the use of safe, well-maintained, and close-to-home sidewalks, crosswalks, bicycle paths, trails, parks, recreation facilities, and community designs featuring mixed-use development and a connected grid of streets.
9. Implement an ongoing media campaign to promote physical education as an important component of a quality education and long-term health.
10. Monitor youth physical activity, physical fitness, and school and community physical activity programs in the nation and each state.

WORKSITE HEALTH-PROMOTION AND FITNESS ACTIVITIES

Since the mid-1970s, there have been major changes in employer attitudes toward workplace health-promotion programs. Interest in worksite health programs has increased, fueled in part by a supportive science base and a desire to help contain spiraling health-care costs while improving productivity and morale and reducing employee absenteeism and turnover.[43]

There are several advantages in using the workplace as a setting for health and fitness programs, including convenience, easy accessibility, supportive company policies and incentives, and the opportunity to affect the lives of family members. Also, the worksite is an effective location for offering health screening and educational programs otherwise inaccessible to at-risk persons.

In 1985 and 1992, the Office of Disease Prevention and Health Promotion, Public Health Service, conducted national surveys to determine the extent of health-promotion activities in the private sector.[43] Overall, the 1992 survey of more than 1,500 worksites revealed an increase in worksite health-promotion activities since 1985 and substantial progress toward achieving many of the worksite-related health objectives for the year 2000. The 1992 survey found that 81% of worksites offered at least one health-promotion activity, compared with 66% in 1985.

Worksite size is a strong indicator of health-promotion activity, with the larger companies more involved than the smaller ones.[43] Seventy-two percent of worksites allow employees to use official company time to participate in health-promotion activities, and 45% allow the use of flextime. Employers use several types of incentives to encourage healthy practices, including flexible spending accounts and risk-rated health insurance premiums. Some also offer subsidized discounts or reduced fees for participation in community-based health programs.

The eight benefits cited most frequently by worksites offering health-promotion programs in the 1992 survey were[43]

1. Improved employee health—28%
2. Improved employee morale—26%
3. Reduced health insurance cost—19%
4. Reduced absenteeism—19%
5. Increased output/productivity—16%
6. Reduced accidents on the job—9%
7. Improved education on health issues—7%
8. Reduced workers' compensation claims—4%

The three most common barriers to implementing worksite health promotion were cost, lack of management support, and lack of interest by employees.[43]

In response to financial pressures, employer-based health-promotion programs are emphasizing activities most likely to save money *and* improve health. Employers are paying increased attention to (1) identifying those employees at greatest risk of health-care utilization and (2) using social marketing strategies to engage them in health-promotion programs. Box 1.3 describes a recommended strategy for improving the health status of employees at worksite settings.[44] Studies show that a comprehensive health-promotion program focused on high-risk individuals can achieve long-term positive health effects.[44–49]

Benefits of Worksite Exercise Programs

A growing number of companies, especially large ones, have worksite physical fitness programs. Since 1985,

Box 1.3

Wellness Outreach at Work

Wellness Outreach at Work was developed by the Worker Health Program, a research unit of the Institute of Labor and Industrial Relations at the University of Michigan. The program offers comprehensive risk-reduction services to all employees at a workplace. It encompasses screening for cardiovascular risks, referral for medical treatment, follow-up counseling, and health-improvement programs. The program has been implemented in more than 100 worksites and has reached more than 75,000 employees in organizations ranging in size from 5 employees to 6,000 employees, both blue collar and white collar, at an average cost of about $100 per employee each year.

The Wellness Outreach at Work Program consists of three main components: planning, implementation, and evaluation.

1. *Planning.* This component involves appointing a wellness committee and hiring wellness professionals, setting goals, promoting the program, and establishing procedures to ensure confidentiality. Based on information from 100 worksites and 75,000 employees, employee risk factors typically are as follows:

   a. Exercise fewer than three times a week (65–72%)

   b. Have high or borderline-high cholesterol (≥ 200 mg/dl) (45–60%)

   c. Smoke cigarettes (18–45%)

   d. Are overweight by 20% or more (26–40%)

   e. Have high blood pressure (≥ 140/90 mm Hg) (22–38%)

   f. Report high levels of stress (21–35%)

2. *Implementation.* This component consists of five major tasks:

   a. *Screening and referral.* Five waves of screening are recommended to identify high-risk employees.

   b. *Follow-up and counseling of employees.* The keys to a successful wellness program are persistent and long-term one-to-one outreach and follow-up counseling to encourage adherence, promote changes in lifestyle, and prevent relapse. Experts urge contacting employees at least every 6 months throughout their careers at the worksite. People with several health risks, people in key positions, and those in need of medical evaluation should receive the highest priority.

   c. *Follow-up with physicians.* Inform the physician or clinic of each employee who has gone through screening, and supply basic results.

   d. *Health-improvement programs.* Offer three types of programs—classes, minigroups, and guided self-help.

   e. *Organizing worksite activities.* Organize and support activities and worksite policies that promote a healthy work environment.

3. *Evaluation.* The final component involves monitoring the programs to find out what is working and how to refine the various programs. Achievable objectives for most worksites for the first year include the following:

   a. At least 70% of the employees participate in initial screening.

   b. At least 80% of the employees with targeted health risks receive follow-up counseling by a wellness counselor.

   c. At least 50% of the employees interviewed by a counselor begin a risk-reduction program.

Following the implementation of the Wellness Outreach at Work Program, typical results include these changes:

- About 50% of workers with high blood pressure bring it under control.
- About 55% of those with high cholesterol reduce it by 20 mg/dl or more.
- About 28% of overweight employees lose at least 10 pounds and keep it off.
- About 25% of smokers quit and do not relapse.
- About 50% of all workers exercise at least three times a week.
- About 30% of all workers make changes in their lives to reduce stress.

Source: Erfurt JC, Foote A, Heirich MA, Brock BM. *The Wellness Outreach at Work Program: A Step-by-Step Guide.* NIH Publication No. 95-3043, August 1995.

physical fitness programs have showed the most impressive gains of all worksite health-promotion programs.[43] In fact, the year 2000 goals were exceeded for each worksite size category.

Table 1.3 outlines the *Healthy People 2010* objective for worksite fitness programs.[6] About half of all worksites with 50 or more employees offer fitness programs, with this proportion rising to 68% among the largest worksites. The *Healthy People 2010* target is 75%.

What benefits can be expected from worksite exercise programs? In general, the research results support the notion that worksite exercise programs improve fitness and help reduce health risks.[6,49] The findings consistently show improvements in aerobic capacity and exercise habits, as well as in other fitness-related measures. In most cases, health risk factors such as smoking and elevated blood lipids also respond to the worksite programs. The impact of these programs on job performance, including productivity and job-related attitudes, and the effect on health-care costs, are less well established.

A major challenge for worksite fitness directors is employee adherence to on-site programs, with most studies showing that less than 20% of employees became long-term participants.[48] Often these participants were generally active to begin with, and thus were at lower risk for chronic disease than nonparticipants.

Predicted Future Growth for Worksite Health Programs

Projections for the next decade indicate that worksite health programs will continue to grow in importance.[44,50] Most experts are predicting, however, that construction of on-site fitness facilities will decline as companies attempt to make better use of existing facilities and community resources and encourage self-help programs in the employees' homes, and as other alternative health-promotion programs are offered.[50] Physical activities that can be built into the normal day of the employee (e.g., walking or cycling to and from work) may prove more acceptable and more cost-effective than formal classes at the worksite.

TABLE 1.3 ***Healthy People 2010:*** **Worksite Physical Activity and Fitness Programs**

Objective 22-13. Increase the proportion of worksites offering employer-sponsored physical activity and fitness programs.
Target. 75%
Baseline. 46% of worksites with 50 or more employees offered physical activity and/or fitness programs at the worksites or through their health plans in 1998–1999.

Worksite Size (no. of employees)	Worksite or Health Plan, %	Health Plan, %	Worksite, %
50–99	38	21	24
100–249	42	20	31
250–749	56	25	44
≥ 750	68	27	61
Total (≥ 50)	46	22	36

Data source: National Worksite Health Promotion Survey, Association for Worksite Health Promotion (AWHP).
Source: U.S. Department of Health and Human Services. *Healthy People 2010.* Washington, DC: January 2000.

STRATEGIES FOR INCREASING PHYSICAL ACTIVITY IN AMERICA

The challenges set forth in *Healthy People 2010* are directed to people throughout the nation—health professionals, community groups, employers, the media, professional organizations, government agencies, and individuals. Meeting these challenges and objectives will require both individual and collective effort. No single person, family, business, organization, or government has the resources to bring about the changes needed to implement the broad and far-reaching physical activity objectives for the year 2010.

Regular physical activity is associated with a wide array of health benefits. This association legitimizes the development of national directives to promote physical activity across all segments of this society, as an aid to preventing chronic disease and improving the quality of life. As an example, sedentary living is estimated to cause one third of deaths due to coronary heart disease, colon cancer, and diabetes.[51] Therefore, encouraging people to become physically active would do much to reduce mortality and enhance quality of life.

Tremendous challenges lie ahead if the physical activity and fitness objectives for the year 2010 are to be met. To meet these objectives, Americans need population-based strategies that seek to reach all Americans, using tools such as mass media and community organization (e.g., environmental change).

Population-Based Strategies

The goal of population- or community-based interventions is to achieve risk reduction across a broad segment of the population.[52–54] A variety of strategies are utilized to focus on four targets of change: (1) the person, (2) organizations (e.g., worksites), (3) the environment (e.g., development of fitness trails), and (4) public policies (e.g., federal or state reimbursement for preventive services). The key concept here is that multifaceted intervention strategies are needed to reach a wide variety of people.

Specific strategies include the following:

- Enhancement of physical activity throughout the day by encouraging stair climbing and exercise breaks, providing trails and paths for transportation-related activity, and increasing the number of parks and recreation areas for leisure-time activity
- Support of legislative and regulatory policies that promote physical activity at school, at the worksite, and in the community
- Increases in funding for school, worksite, and community health/fitness programs; for research that supports physical activity for all Americans; and for insurance reimbursement of health/fitness activities.
- Use of electronic and print media to repeatedly transmit relevant information
- Cooperation among community leaders and power structures involving the private sector, organizations of health professionals, the mass media, schools, and other community groups, to promote behavioral change
- Development of community programs tailored to the needs and preferences of specific target groups (especially those at high risk and various minority groups)

Of particular usefulness are community and worksite risk-factor screening programs, with an emphasis on measurement, immediate counseling, and referral of high-risk individuals. Such programs have proven to be an effective way of reaching large numbers of people.[45,46]

To enhance people's long-term participation in regular physical activity, several factors should be considered, especially those that pertain to the person, the exercise regimen itself, and the environment.[52–54]

Personal Factors

Factors such as gender, age, occupational status, health status, education, and prior exercise experience should be considered when helping establish community-based exercise programs.[52–54] In general, women tend to participate in less strenuous activities than men. Older people are less active and appear to enjoy such activities as walking and gardening more than young people. Blue-collar workers are less formally active than white-collar workers, overweight people and smokers are less active, and less-educated people tend to exercise less than those with more education. Common reasons adults cite for not adopting more physically active lifestyles include lack of time, lack of self-motivation, find the exercise boring and inconvenient, fear of injury, low self-efficacy, insufficient trails, parks, sidewalks, and paths, and lack of support from family and friends.[52]

The Exercise Regimen

The 1996 surgeon general's report on physical activity and health places emphasis on reducing inactivity and increasing light-to-moderate physical activity.[7] Moderate-intensity, longer-duration activities, such as walking, are being promoted more and more by fitness leaders because these types of activities are more acceptable to the average person, increasing the likelihood of a permanent change in lifestyle.

Also, the musculoskeletal risks are less, and studies show that health benefits are still realized, especially when the total caloric expenditure averages at least 1,000 calories per week. It has been demonstrated that people tend to adhere better to moderate-intensity than to vigorous-intensity physical activity programs, and that injuries from high-intensity workouts are a major cause of relapse from exercise.[52]

SPORTS MEDICINE INSIGHT

Wellness Success Stories

Since 1979 when the *Healthy People* process began, many positive changes in the health of Americans have been measured. A major goal of this book is to help you follow the *Healthy People* road map to wellness. Wellness highlights of the past quarter-century include the following successes:

- Life expectancy or the number of years one is expected to live at birth has increased from about 47 years in 1900 to a current 77 years, the highest ever in U.S. history. Most of this increase is attributable to widespread vaccination, control of infectious diseases from cleaner water and improved sanitation, safer and healthier foods, safer workplaces and motor vehicles, a decline in deaths from coronary heart disease and stroke from improvements in personal behavior and lifestyles, and a recognition of tobacco use as a health hazard.
- Stroke and coronary heart disease death rates reached epidemic levels about 50 years ago but have been falling ever since. Since 1950, the

(continued)

SPORTS MEDICINE INSIGHT *(continued)*

Wellness Success Stories

American death rate for stroke decreased 70%, and for heart disease, 55%. This is one of the greatest health success stories of the past half-century and is due to improvements in American health habits and medical care.

- Cancer death rates decreased during the 1990s after decades of concern over increases. As with heart disease, much of the decrease is because of improvements in lifestyles (especially better diets and less smoking), and an emphasis on early screening for cancer.
- Cigarette consumption has decreased. In 1965, 52% of men and 34% of women smoked. Now only 23% of all Americans smoke.
- Diets have improved. Fat intake has decreased from over 40% of total calories in the 1960s to a current 33% of calories. Americans are consuming more poultry, fish, and low-fat dairy products, and less beef, pork, eggs, and whole milk.
- Alcohol consumption has fallen. Since the 1980s, alcohol intake has decreased due in part to the public's increasing awareness of alcohol's associated dangers.
- Prevalence of high blood pressure, a major risk factor for stroke and coronary heart disease, has fallen from 39% in the 1960s to a current 26% of Americans.
- Prevalence of high blood cholesterol, another risk factor for heart disease, has fallen from 32% in the 1960s to a current 17%.

KEY WELLNESS CHALLENGES FOR THE FUTURE

Despite the successes, some important health-related areas still need improvement:

- Too many Americans, about 65%, are overweight and obese. Despite a nationwide obsession with ideal body weight, government studies over the past 40 years have shown that Americans are losing the war. The prevalence of being overweight has tripled among children and adolescents since the 1960s.
- Too few American young people and adults exercise regularly. As emphasized in this chapter, about 6 in 10 adults do not engage in sufficient exercise despite the common knowledge that inactivity is related to heart disease, certain types of cancer, obesity, osteoporosis, and frailty in old age. One third of American teenagers do not exercise vigorously on a regular basis, with this proportion rising dramatically as they enter adulthood.
- Disease risk factors are still too widely prevalent among both adults and adolescents. One in four Americans smoke, one in four have high blood pressure, and one in five have high blood cholesterol. About two in three adolescents have two or more of five major risk factors for chronic disease, and these often remain into adulthood.
- Mental stress levels are high. About 6 in 10 American adults report that they experience moderate to high levels of stress, posing one of the greatest health challenges for the next century.

The Environment

In general, more people tend to participate in physical activity when community facilities and conducive environments are nearby and available.[7,52] Time is a major obstacle to regular physical activity, and greater availability of community exercise facilities, trails, and parks that are close to homes is a major factor in helping people become more involved. Thus, community efforts are more effectively applied when promoting low-cost, home- or near-home-based physical activity patterns than when trying to encourage people to join programs that involve substantial travel time.

Programs that emphasize the availability of appropriate exercise facilities can have a substantial impact on the health of the community.[7] This is the essence of effective public health intervention, and officials should consider the potential positive effects of altering policies related to the distribution of exercise facilities and trails in the community.

The family is a powerful influence on several health-promoting behaviors, including physical activity.[7,52] Support from a variety of sources—including family members and spouse, exercise partners and staff, and co-workers and employers—can have a positive impact on long-term adherence to exercise.

Environmental support also includes the use of federal, state, and county public health departments to provide economic support and to establish public policies to facilitate local community efforts.

SUMMARY

1. The year 2010 health objectives for the nation were reviewed, with emphasis on the physical activity and fitness objectives. The objectives were evaluated in relation to adult exercise habits, youth fitness, and worksite exercise programs.
2. The problem of inactivity in this country can be viewed in a historical context, showing how concepts of healthful exercise have changed. A turning point in adult fitness awareness took place in 1968, with the publication of Ken Cooper's first book, *Aerobics*.
3. National surveys have tried to evaluate the magnitude of the present fitness revolution. Only one in four Americans is exercising at levels generally recommended for basic aerobic fitness.
4. Those exercising effectively tend to be of upper socioeconomic status, young, male, and from the western region of the nation.
5. Several major surveys of child and youth fitness have been conducted during the 1980s and 1990s. They show that large numbers of American children and youths exercise at less than desirable levels. Of particular concern are test results showing poor upper-body strength and cardiorespiratory fitness.
6. Studies show that through worksite exercise programs, fitness status can be improved, and absenteeism and health risks and costs can be lowered.
7. Population strategies to increase physical activity in America should be multifaceted, with an emphasis on four targets of change—the person, organizations, the environment, and public policies.

Review Questions

1. *According to the World Health Organization, ____ is physical, mental, and social well-being, and not merely the absence of disease and infirmity.*

   A. Exercise **B.** Physical fitness
   C. Cardiovascular endurance **D.** Health
   E. Energy

2. *____ is the leading cause of death in the United States today, followed by ____.*

   A. Cancer/heart disease
   B. Influenza/heart disease
   C. Heart disease/accidents
   D. Cancer/liver disease
   E. Heart disease/cancer

3. *In 1968, Dr. ____, a medical doctor for the U.S. Air Force, published his book,* **Aerobics**, *which helped spawn the modern-day health and fitness movement.*

   A. Bill Bowerman **B.** Ken Cooper
   C. Luther Gulick **D.** Catharine Beecher
   E. Alexander Cartwright **F.** None of these

4. *Which one of the following statements regarding the fitness of American youths is true?*

   A. American youths have become fatter since the 1960s.
   B. A majority of American youths take daily physical education classes.
   C. American youths obtain enough exercise in physical education classes.
   D. The upper body strength of American youths is unusually high.

5. *Which personal factor predicts improved adherence to exercise?*

   A. Cigarette smoking (versus nonsmoking)
   B. Little education (versus high education)
   C. Blue-collar worker (versus white-collar worker)
   D. Old age (versus young)
   E. Normal weight (versus overweight)

6. *Which one of the following statements regarding the wellness revolution is not true?*

   A. Life expectancy is now about 84 years, the highest ever.
   B. Heart disease and stroke death rates are falling.
   C. Cigarette consumption is down to a prevalence of 23% of the population.
   D. Diets are improving, with animal fat consumption down.
   E. The majority of Americans are not exercising at appropriate levels.

7. *Seventeen percent of Americans have high blood cholesterol, which is defined as above a threshold of ____ mg/dl.*

   A. 160 **B.** 200 **C.** 240 **D.** 300

8. *____ health is the absence of disease and disability, while having sufficient energy and vitality to accomplish daily tasks and active recreational pursuits without undue fatigue.*

   A. Mental **B.** Physical
   C. Social **D.** Emotional
   E. Spiritual

9. *____ health is one's ability to interact effectively with other people, engaging in satisfying personal relationships.*

   A. Mental **B.** Physical
   C. Social **D.** Emotional
   E. Spiritual

10. *In 1996, the surgeon general's report* **Physical Activity and Health** *was published. Which one of the following statements is true according to this report?*

    A. More than 60% of American adults are not regularly physically active.
    B. Physical activity rises dramatically during adolescence.
    C. Significant health benefits can be obtained by walking 10–15 minutes, 3 days per week.
    D. Physical activity does not reduce the risk of premature mortality from colon cancer.
    E. Physical activity has no relationship to mental health.

11. *Which major goal listed is included within the* **Healthy People 2010 Health for All** *framework?*

    A. Increase the lifespan
    B. Decrease infectious disease
    C. Improve environmental health
    D. Decrease chronic disease
    E. Increase quality and years of healthy life

12. *The* **Healthy People 2010** *objective for prevalence of obesity is:*

    A. <30 **B.** <15 **C.** <75 **D.** <50 **E.** <10

13. *There are several ways to measure quality of life, including years of healthy life. How many years of healthy life does the average American experience?*

    A. 77 **B.** 64 **C.** 55 **D.** 83 **E.** 47

14. *Individual behaviors and environmental factors are responsible for about ____% of all premature deaths in the United States.*

    A. 70 **B.** 50 **C.** 100 **D.** 25 **E.** 80

15. *What is the* **Healthy People 2010** *objective for reducing the proportion of adults who engage in no leisure-time physical activity?*

    A. 5 **B.** 12 **C.** 33 **D.** 20 **E.** 8

16. *Complete this* **Healthy People 2010** *objective: Increase to at least ____% the proportion of trips made by walking (adults).*

    A. 25 **B.** 10 **C.** 75 **D.** 60 **E.** 50

17. *In 1998–1999, 46% of worksites with 50 or more employees offered physical activity and/or fitness programs at the worksites or through their health plans. What is the* **Healthy People 2010** *objective?*

    A. 50% **B.** 100% **C.** 75% **D.** 10% **E.** 45%

18. *According to the National College Health Risk Behavior Survey, less than ____ in 10 college students participate in aerobic activities that make them sweat and breathe hard for at least 20 minutes on three or more days each week.*

    A. 1 **B.** 2 **C.** 3 **D.** 4 **E.** 5

19. *Adults cite 10 common barriers for not adopting more physically active lifestyles. Which barrier listed below is not on this list?*

    A. Do not have enough time to exercise
    B. Find it inconvenient to exercise
    C. Find exercise boring
    D. Poor health
    E. Lack confidence in their ability to be physically active

20. *Chronic disease accounts for about ____ of all deaths today.*

    A. Two thirds **B.** One fourth
    C. One third **D.** One half
    E. Three fourths

21. *Which statement regarding physical activity in America is true?*

    A. Those with lower incomes and less education tend to exercise more often.
    B. Thirty-eight percent of Americans report essentially sedentary lifestyles.
    C. Physical inactivity decreases with increase in age.
    D. For all ages, inactivity is higher among men than women.
    E. Inactivity is higher among whites than African Americans.

22. *About 1 in ____ American adults are performing physical activities that enhance muscular strength and endurance two or more days per week.*

    A. 10 **B.** 2 **C.** 4 **D.** 20 **E.** 5

23. *The percentage of high school students attending physical education classes daily during the 1990s ____.*

    A. Dropped **B.** Increased **C.** Stayed the same

Answers

1. D	**9.** C	**17.** C
2. E	**10.** A	**18.** D
3. B	**11.** E	**19.** D
4. A	**12.** B	**20.** A
5. E	**13.** B	**21.** B
6. A	**14.** A	**22.** E
7. C	**15.** D	**23.** A
8. B	**16.** A	

REFERENCES

1. Breslow L. From disease prevention to health promotion. *JAMA* 281:1030–1033, 1999.
2. O'Donnell M P. Definition of health promotion: Part II: Levels of programs. *Am J Health Promotion* 1(2):6–9, 1986.
3. Office of the Assistant Secretary for Health and Surgeon General. *Healthy People: The Surgeon General's Report on Health Promotion and Disease Prevention.* DHEW (PHS) Publication No. 79-55071. Washington, DC: U.S. Government Printing Office, 1979.
4. Department of Health and Human Services. *Promoting Health/Preventing Disease: Objectives for the Nation.* Washington, DC: U.S. Government Printing Office, Fall 1980.
5. Public Health Service, U.S. Department of Health and Human Services. *Healthy People 2000: National Health Promotion and Disease Prevention Objectives.* DHHS Publication No. (PHS) 91-50212. Washington, DC: U.S. Government Printing Office, 1991.
6. U.S. Department of Health and Human Services. *Healthy People 2010.* Washington, DC: January 2000. www.health.gov/healthypeople/.
7. U.S. Department of Health and Human Services. *Physical Activity and Health: A Report of the Surgeon General.* Atlanta, GA: U.S. Department of Health and Human Services, Centers for Disease Control and Prevention, National Center for Chronic Disease Prevention and Health Promotion, 1996.
8. Wharton JC. *Crusaders for Fitness: The History of American Health Reformers.* Princeton, NJ: Princeton University Press, 1982.
9. Spears B, Swanson RA. *History of Sports and Physical Activity in the United States.* Dubuque, IA: W.C. Brown Co., 1978.
10. Rice EA, Hutchinson JL, Lee M. *A Brief History of Physical Education.* New York: The Ronald Press Co., 1958.
11. Pate RR. A new definition of youth fitness. *Physician Sportsmed* 11:77–83, 1983.
12. Kraus H, Hirschland RP. Muscular fitness and health. *JAMA,* 17–19, December, 1953. See also: Kraus H, Hirschland RP. Minimum muscular fitness tests in school children. *Res Q Am Assoc Health Phys Educ* 25:178–188, 1954.
13. Bowerman WJ, Harris WE. *Jogging.* New York: Grosset & Dunlap, 1967, 1977.
14. Cooper KH. *Aerobics.* New York: Bantam Books, Inc., 1968.
15. Cooper KH. *The New Aerobics.* New York: M. Evans and Company, Inc., 1970.
16. Cooper KH. *The Aerobics Way.* New York: M. Evans and Company, Inc., 1977.
17. Cooper M, Cooper KH. *Aerobics for Women.* New York: M. Evans and Co., Inc., 1972.
18. Higdon H. Running after 40. *Runner's World,* August 1978, p. 36.
19. Henderson J. *Long Slow Distance: The Humane Way to Train.* Mountain View, CA: World Publications, 1969.
20. Ullyot J. *Women's Running.* Mountain View, CA: World Publications, 1976.
21. Sheehan GA. *Dr. Sheehan on Running.* Mountain View, CA: World Publications, 1976.
22. Fixx IF. *The Complete Book of Running.* New York: Random House, 1977.
23. Garrick JG, Requa RK. Aerobic dance: A review. *Sports Med* 6:169–179, 1988.
24. Amend PC. Health clubs: A new resource for health promotion. *Med Exerc Nutr Health* 2:170–176, 1993.
25. Sol N, Foster C. *ACSM's Health/Fitness Facility Standards and Guidelines.* Champaign, IL: Human Kinetics, 1992.
26. Tharrett SJ, Peterson JA. *ACSM's Health/Fitness Facility Standards and Guidelines* (2nd ed.). Champaign, IL: Human Kinetics, 1997.
27. National Center for Health Statistics. Summary health statistics for U.S. adults: National Health Interview Survey, 2002. *Vital and Health Statistics,* Series 10, No. 222. Hyattsville, MD: USDHHS, 2004.
28. National Center for Health Statistics. Health behaviors of adults: United States, 1999–2001. *Vital and Health Statistics,* Series 10, No. 219. Hyattsville, MD: USDHSS, 2004.
29. Brownson RC, Jones DA, Pratt M, Blanton C, Heath GW. Measuring physical activity with the behavioral risk factor surveillance system. *Med Sci Sports Exerc* 32:1913–1918, 2000.
30. Crespo CJ, Ainsworth BE, Ketayian SJ, Heath GW, Smit E. Prevalence of physical inactivity and its relation to social class in U.S. adults: Results from the Third National Health and Nutrition Examination Survey, 1988–1994. *Med Sci Sports Exerc* 31:1821–1827, 1999.
31. Centers for Disease Control and Prevention. Prevalence of no leisure-time physical activity—35 states and the District of Columbia, 1988–2002. *MMWR* 53:82–86, 2004.
32. Office of Disease Prevention and Health Promotion, Public Health Service. Summary of findings from National Children and Youth Fitness Study. *JOPERD,* January 1985.
33. Youth Physical Fitness in 1985. *The President's Council on Physical Fitness and Sports School Population Fitness Survey.* President's Council on Physical Fitness and Sports, 450 Fifth St., NW, Suite 7103, Washington, DC 20001, 1985.
34. Ross JG, Pate RR, Delpy LA, Gold RS, Svilar M. New health-related fitness norms. *JOPERD,* November/December 1987, 66–77.
35. Pate RR, Ross JG. Factors associated with health-related fitness. *JOPERD,* November/December 1987, 93–96.

36. Ross JG, Pate RR. The National Children and Youth Fitness Study II: A summary of findings. *JOPERD,* November/December 1987, 51–56, 57–62.

37. Centers for Disease Control and Prevention. Participation in high school physical education—United States, 1991–2003. *MMWR* 53:844–847. 2004.

38. Centers for Disease Control and Prevention. Physical activity among children aged 9–13 years—United States, 2002. *MMWR* 52:785–788, 2003.

39. A Report to the President from the Secretary of Health and Human Services and the Secretary of Education. *Promoting Better Health for Young People Through Physical Activity and Sports.* Fall, 2000. http://www.cdc.gov/.

40. Trudeau F, Laurencelle L, Tremblay J, Rajic M, Shephard RJ. Daily primary school physical education: effects on physical activity during adult life. *Med Sci Sports Exerc* 31:111–117, 1999.

41. Casperson CJ, Pereira MA, Curran KM. Changes in physical activity patterns in the United States, by sex and cross-sectional age. *Med Sci Sports Exerc* 32:1601–1609, 2000.

42. Centers for Disease Control and Prevention. Guidelines for school and community programs to promote lifelong physical activity among young people. *MMWR* 46(No. RR-6): 1–35, 1997.

43. U.S. Department of Health and Human Services, Public Health Service. *1992 National Survey of Worksite Health Promotion Activities.* Washington, DC: U.S. Government Printing Office, 1993. Published also in: *Am J Health Promotion* 7(6):452–463, 1993.

44. Erfurt JC, Foote A, Heirich MA, Brock BM. *The Wellness Outreach at Work Program: A Step-by-Step Guide.* NIH Publication No. 95-3043, August 1995.

45. Goetzel RZ, Kahr TY, Aldana SG, Kenny GM. An evaluation of Duke University's Live for Life health promotion program and its impact on employee health. *Am J Health Promotion* 10:340–342, 1996.

46. Wilson MG. A comprehensive review of the effects of worksite health promotion on health-related outcomes: An update. *Am J Health Promotion* 11:107–108, 1996.

47. Riedel JE, Lynch W, Baase C, Hymel P, Peterson KW. The effect of disease prevention and health promotion on workplace productivity: A literature review. *Am J Health Promotion* 15:iii–v, 2001.

48. Shephard RJ. A critical analysis of worksite fitness programs and their postulated economic benefits. *Med Sci Sports Exerc* 24:354–370, 1992.

49. Pelletier KR. A review and analysis of the clinical and cost-effectiveness studies of comprehensive health promotion and disease management programs at the worksite: 1995–1998 update (IV). *Am J Health Promotion* 13:333–345, 1999.

50. Office of Disease Prevention and Health Promotion. Worksite programs target health and cost benefits. *Prevention Report,* August/September 1994.

51. Powell KE, Blair SN. The public health burdens of sedentary living habits: Theoretical but realistic estimates. *Med Sci Sports Exerc* 26:851-856, 1994.

52. U.S. Department of Health and Human Services, Public Health Service, Centers for Disease Control and Prevention. *Promoting Physical Activity: A Guide for Community Action.* Champaign, IL: Human Kinetics, 1999.

53. King AC. Community and public health approaches to the promotion of physical activity. *Med Sci Sports Exerc* 26:1405–1412, 1994.

54. Pate RR, Pratt M, Blair SN, et al. Physical activity and public health: A recommendation from the Centers for Disease Control and Prevention and the American College of Sports Medicine. *JAMA* 273:402–407, 1995.

PHYSICAL FITNESS ACTIVITY 1.1

What Is Your Personal Exercise Program?

This chapter fully described the exercise habits of Americans. The National Health Interview Survey (NHIS) by the National Center for Health Statistics is presently one of the best data sources for this type of information. Data from NHIS have been collected continuously since 1957.

In this Physical Fitness Activity, you will be answering questions on exercise taken directly from the NHIS section on Health Promotion and Disease Prevention. Fill in the blanks in the table on the next page, and then summarize your exercise program by answering the following questions.

Physical Fitness Activity Questions

1. Summarize your answers to the NHIS questionnaire by filling in the following:

a. What was your average frequency per week of exercise during the past 2 weeks? *Note:* Count only the sessions where intensity was high or moderate.

_____ average frequency/week

Note: Total the number of times in past 2 weeks and divide by 2. For example, if you jogged 2 times in the past 2 weeks, biked 2 times, and played soccer once, your average frequency per week would be 5 divided by 2, or 2.5 times/week.

b. What was your average *duration per exercise session in minutes* (from part **a**)?

_____ average duration per exercise session (in minutes)

Note: Total the number of minutes spent in exercise during the past 2 weeks, and divide that by the number of exercise sessions. For example, if the jogging sessions lasted 15 minutes each, the biking sessions 30 minutes each, and soccer 40 minutes, the average duration per exercise session in minutes would be 130 min/5 = 26 minutes per session *Note:* Only include sessions from part **a**.

2. How do you compare with ACSM standards?

The American College of Sports Medicine recommends that people exercise at least three times per week, for at least 20 to 30 minutes, at moderate-to-high intensity levels (at least 50% maximal oxygen capacity) (see Chapter 8).

Did you exercise:

Yes	No	
____	____	3 or more times/week?
____	____	20 or more minutes/session?
____	____	At moderate or high heart rate/breathing levels for each session?

National Health Interview Survey, 1990
Health Promotion and Disease Prevention Supplement

A In the past two weeks, have you done any of the following exercises, sports, or physically active hobbies?			B How many times in the past two weeks did you [play/go/do] (*activity in A*)?	C On average, about how many minutes did you actually spend (*activity in A*) on each occasion?	D What usually happened to your heart rate or breathing when you undertook (*activity in A*)? Did you have a small, moderate, or large increase, or no increase at all in your heart rate or breathing?			
	Yes	No	Times	Minutes	Small	Moderate	Large	None
1. Walking for exercise								
2. Jogging or running								
3. Hiking								
4. Gardening/yard work								
5. Aerobic dancing								
6. Other dancing								
7. Calisthenics								
8. Golf								
9. Tennis								
10. Bowling								
11. Biking								
12. Swimming								
13. Weight lifting								
14. Basketball								
15. Baseball								
16. Football								
17. Soccer								
18. Volleyball								
19. Handball/racquetball								
20. Skating								
21. Skiing								
22. Any other type of exercise not mentioned here								
____________________ List here								

PHYSICAL FITNESS ACTIVITY 1.2

Using the Internet to Explore Health and Fitness

In this Physical Fitness Activity, choose an Internet site that deals with health, physical fitness, or *Healthy People 2010* goals; explore the site and print out a topic that updates information presented in this chapter. Prepare a 1- to 3-minute oral report for the students in your class.

Health and Fitness Websites (also see Box 1.1)

- American Alliance for Health, Physical Education, Recreation, and Dance *(www.aahperd.org)*
- American College of Sports Medicine *(www.acsm.org)*
- CDC National Center for Chronic Disease Prevention and Health Promotion *(www.cdc.gov/nccdphp/)*
- President's Council on Physical Fitness and Sports *(www.fitness.gov/)*

Lack of regular physical activity claims about 250,000 lives per year in this country. In this information age, trends show that more people are taking up sedentary lifestyles. Public health, medical, and mental-health professionals recognize the vital importance of physical activity and fitness for the general population.

The lead agency for this high-priority area is the President's Council on Physical Fitness and Sports (PCPFS). The CDC serves as the science advisor. These two agencies posted *Physical Activity and Health: A Report of the Surgeon General* online even before it was published in hard copy. PCPFS also has available an online text version of *How to Celebrate National Physical Fitness and Sports Month.* Within CDC, the National Center for Chronic Disease Prevention and Health Promotion (NCCDPHP) lists online its study of physical inactivity and cardiovascular health and chronic conditions. NCCDPHP and the ACSM collaborated on and helped disseminate online a recommendation that every adult should accumulate 30 minutes or more of daily moderate-intensity physical activity.

Consortium member ACSM provides electronic abstracts of its journal, *Medicine and Science in Sports and Exercise,* for its users. ACSM also features an online version of the NIH Consensus Development Conference Statement on Physical Activity and Cardiovascular Health.

The American Alliance for Health, Physical Education, Recreation, and Dance site features research, information on its national convention, and "Physical Best at a Glance."

Healthy People 2010 Websites

The following agencies have assumed responsibility for the Healthy People 2010 priority areas indicated:

Centers for Disease Control and Prevention

(www.cdc.gov)

- Clinical preventive services
- Diabetes and other chronic disabling conditions
- Educational and community-based programs
- Environmental health
- HIV infection
- Immunizations and infectious diseases

- Occupational safety and health
- Oral health
- Tobacco use and addiction
- Sexually transmitted diseases
- Surveillance and data systems
- Unintentional injuries
- Violent and abusive behavior

Food and Drug Administration
(www.fda.gov)

- Food and drug safety
- Nutrition

Health Resources and Services Administration
(www.hrsa.gov)

- Clinical preventive services
- Educational and community-based programs
- Maternal and infant health

National Institutes of Health
(www.nih.gov)

- Cancer
- Diabetes and other chronic disabling conditions
- Environmental health
- Heart disease and stroke
- Mental health and mental disorders
- Nutrition
- Oral health

Office of Population Affairs
(www.hhs.gov/opa/)

- Family planning

President's Council on Physical Fitness and Sports
(www.fitness.gov/)

- Physical activity and fitness

Substance Abuse and Mental Health Services Administration
(www.samhsa.gov)

- Mental health and mental disorders

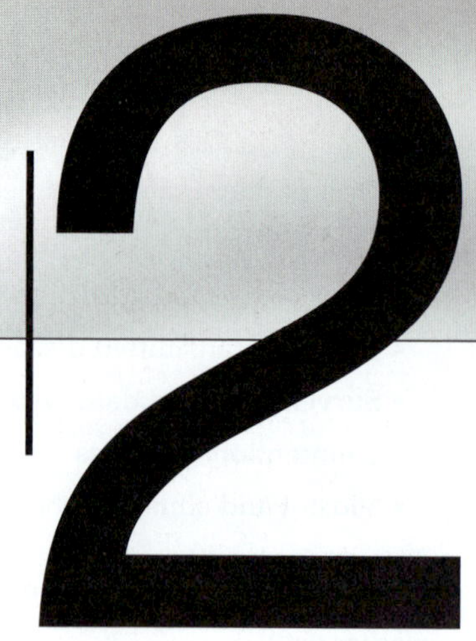

Physical Fitness Defined

Over the years, I have come to look upon physical fitness as the trunk of a tree that supports the many branches which represent all the activities that make life worth living: intellectual life, spiritual life, occupation, love life and social activities.

—Thomas Kirk Cureton, Jr.

Although many definitions of physical fitness have been proposed, there still is much disagreement among physical educators and exercise scientists as to its real meaning. During the first half of the twentieth century, for example, muscular strength was emphasized by many fitness leaders as the primary goal of an exercise program. During the 1970s and 1980s, the pendulum swung the other way toward a focus on cardiorespiratory fitness through aerobic activity. Today, there is more of a focus on health-related physical fitness.

Among physical educators, a furious debate has raged since the late 1800s as to whether youth fitness programs should stress the development of skills important for athletic ability (e.g., hand–eye coordination, agility, balance, speed) or attributes that some researchers feel are more important to health (e.g., cardiorespiratory endurance, optimal body composition, flexibility). (See the Sports Medicine Insight at the end of this chapter). Since the mid-1980s, several organizations have attempted to redefine physical fitness and exercise in light of modern evidence and understanding. This chapter discusses the contemporary definitions of physical fitness terms important to sport and exercise science. Box 2.1 summarizes the definitions of key terms that are explored in this chapter and other chapters of this book.

PHYSICAL ACTIVITY

Physical activity has been defined as any bodily movement produced by skeletal muscles, that results in energy expenditure.[1–3] The energy expenditure can be measured in kilocalories (kcal) or kilojoules (kJ). One kcal is equivalent to 4.184 kJ. In this book, we also use the term *Calories* to denote kcals. One banana, for example, provides about 100 Calories, approximately the amount of energy expended in running a mile.

Everyone performs physical activity in order to sustain life. The amount, however, varies considerably from one individual to another, based on personal lifestyles and other factors. A compendium of physical activities has been developed to provide researchers and practitioners with an estimation of the energy cost for a wide variety of human physical activities. This comprehensive table is available in Appendix E of this book.[4]

Measurement of physical activity is difficult, and researchers have utilized a wide array of methods. Over 50 different measures have been described and can be classified into four general categories:[2]

- *Calorimetry*—direct heat exchange (in an insulated chamber or suit), or indirect measurement through measurement of oxygen consumption and carbon-dioxide production
- *Physiological markers*—heart rate monitoring and use of doubly labeled water (DLW)
- *Mechanical and electronic motion detectors*—pedometers, in-shoe step counters, electronic motion sensors, and accelerometers
- *Occupational and leisure-time survey instruments*—job classification, activity diaries or records, and physical activity recall questionnaires

Box 2.1

Glossary of Terms

The following are key terms related to physical fitness. Review this list, as needed, to investigate terms used in this chapter and throughout the book.

aerobic training: Training that improves the efficiency of the aerobic energy-producing systems and that can improve cardiorespiratory endurance.

agility: A skill-related component of physical fitness that relates to the ability to rapidly change the position of the entire body in space, with speed and accuracy.

anaerobic training: Training that improves the efficiency of the anaerobic energy-producing systems and that can increase muscular strength and tolerance for acid–base imbalances during high-intensity effort.

balance: A skill-related component of physical fitness that relates to the maintenance of equilibrium while either stationary or in motion.

body composition: A health-related component of physical fitness that relates to the relative amounts of muscle, fat, bone, and other vital body tissues.

calorimetry: Methods used to calculate the rate and quantity of energy expenditure when the body is at rest and during physical exertion.

- **direct calorimetry:** A method that gauges the body's rate and quantity of energy production by direct measurement of the body's heat production; the method uses a *calorimeter,* which is a chamber that measures the heat expended by the body.
- **indirect calorimetry:** A method of estimating energy expenditure by measuring respiratory gases; given that the amount of O_2 and CO_2 exchanged in the lungs normally equals that used and released by body tissues, caloric expenditure can be measured by CO_2 production and O_2 consumption.

cardiorespiratory endurance (cardiorespiratory fitness): A health-related component of physical fitness that relates to the ability of the circulatory and respiratory systems to supply oxygen during sustained physical activity.

coordination: A skill-related component of physical fitness that relates to the ability to use the senses, such as sight and hearing, together with body parts, in performing motor tasks smoothly and accurately.

detraining: Changes the body undergoes in response to a reduction or cessation of regular physical training.

endurance training and endurance activities: Repetitive aerobic use of large muscles (e.g., walking, bicycling, swimming).

exercise (exercise training): Planned, structured, and repetitive bodily movement done to improve or maintain one or more components of physical fitness.

flexibility: A health-related component of physical fitness that relates to the range of motion available at a joint.

kilocalorie (kcal): A measurement of energy: 1 kilocalorie = 1 Calorie = 4,184 joules = 4.184 kilojoules.

kilojoule (kjoule or kJ): A measurement of energy: 4.184 kilojoules = 4,184 joules = 1 Calorie = 1 kilocalorie.

maximal heart rate (HR_{max}): The highest heart rate value attainable during an all-out effort to the point of exhaustion.

maximal heart rate reserve: The difference between maximal heart rate and resting heart rate.

maximal oxygen uptake ($\dot{V}O_{2max}$): The maximal capacity for oxygen consumption by the body during maximal exertion; also known as aerobic power, maximal oxygen consumption, and cardiorespiratory endurance capacity.

metabolic equivalent (MET): A unit used to estimate the metabolic cost (oxygen consumption) of physical activity, 1 MET equals the resting metabolic rate of approximately 3.5 ml O_2 per kilogram of body weight per minute.

muscular endurance: The ability of the muscle to continue to perform without fatigue.

physical activity: Bodily movement that is produced by the contraction of skeletal muscle and that substantially increases energy expenditure.

physical fitness: A set of attributes that people have or achieve, which relates to the ability to perform physical activity.

power: A skill-related component of physical fitness that relates to the rate at which one can perform work.

rating of perceived exertion (RPE): A person's subjective assessment of how hard he or she is working; the Borg scale is a numerical scale for rating perceived exertion.

reaction time: A skill-related component of physical fitness that relates to the time elapsed between a stimulus and the beginning of the reaction to it.

resistance training: Training designed to increase strength, power, and muscle endurance.

resting heart rate: The heart rate at rest, averaging 60 to 80 beats per minute.

retraining: Recovery of conditioning after a period of inactivity.

speed: A skill-related component of physical fitness relating to the ability to perform a movement within a short period of time.

strength: The ability of the muscle to exert force.

training heart rate (THR): A heart rate goal established by using the heart rate equivalent to a selected training level (percentage of $\dot{V}O_{2max}$). For example, if a training level of 75% $\dot{V}O_{2max}$ is desired, the $\dot{V}O_{2max}$ at 75% is determined and the heart rate corresponding to this $\dot{V}O_2$ is selected as the THR.

Source: U.S. Department of Health and Human Services. *Physical Activity and Health: A Report of the Surgeon General.* Atlanta, GA: U.S. Department of Health and Human Services, Centers for Disease Control and Prevention, National Center for Chronic Disease Prevention and Health Promotion, 1996.

Questionnaire methods are currently the most popular and practical approaches for large groups of individuals. A collection of physical activity questionnaires for health-related research has been published.[5]

Calorimetry and DLW can provide accurate measurements of average daily energy expenditure under controlled laboratory conditions for small groups of subjects. Measurement of energy expenditure away from the laboratory has been enhanced with the development of light metabolic units that can be worn on the chest[6] (see Figure 2.1). DLW is an effective but expensive method for measuring energy expenditure in free-living humans.[7] Briefly, the DLW method requires that the subject ingest a dose of water containing both the isotope deuterium ($^2H_2$) and the stable oxygen isotope ^{18}O (as $^2H_2{}^{18}O$). The technique is safe because the isotopes employed are naturally occurring rather than radioactive. Subjects provide urine, blood, or saliva samples before and three hours after ingestion, as well as each day for several days. Through use of mass spectrometers, energy expenditure is calculated by measuring the difference in the rate of loss between the two isotope labels (which is related to carbon dioxide production and through calculation to oxygen consumption).

EXERCISE

Exercise is not synonymous with physical activity.[1–3] It is a subcategory of physical activity. Exercise is physical activity that is planned, structured, repetitive, and purposive, in the sense that improvement or maintenance of physical fitness is an objective.[3] Virtually all conditioning and many sports activities are considered exercise because they are generally performed to improve or maintain physical fitness. Household and occupational tasks are usually accomplished with little regard to physical fitness. However, a person can structure work and home tasks in a more active form and thus build up physical fitness at the same time the tasks are accomplished. Many people find this more motivating than "running in circles" for exercise.

A COMPREHENSIVE APPROACH TO PHYSICAL FITNESS

During the boom years of the aerobic movement in the 1970s and 1980s, development of cardiorespiratory fitness was emphasized, often to the detriment of musculoskeletal fitness. Although this was a much needed reform from the undue preoccupation with muscular strength and size, which had dominated since the late 1800s, most fitness experts today believe in a more balanced approach to all the components of fitness.[8–13] The focus today is on a comprehensive approach to physical fitness in which three major components—cardiorespiratory fitness, body composition, and musculoskeletal fitness (comprising flexibility, muscular strength, and muscular endurance)—are given equal attention (see Figure 2.2).

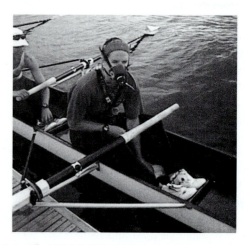

Figure 2.1 The K4b2 (COSMED Ltd., Rome, Italy) is a fully portable breath-by-breath pulmonary gas exchange system for measuring energy expenditure away from the lab.

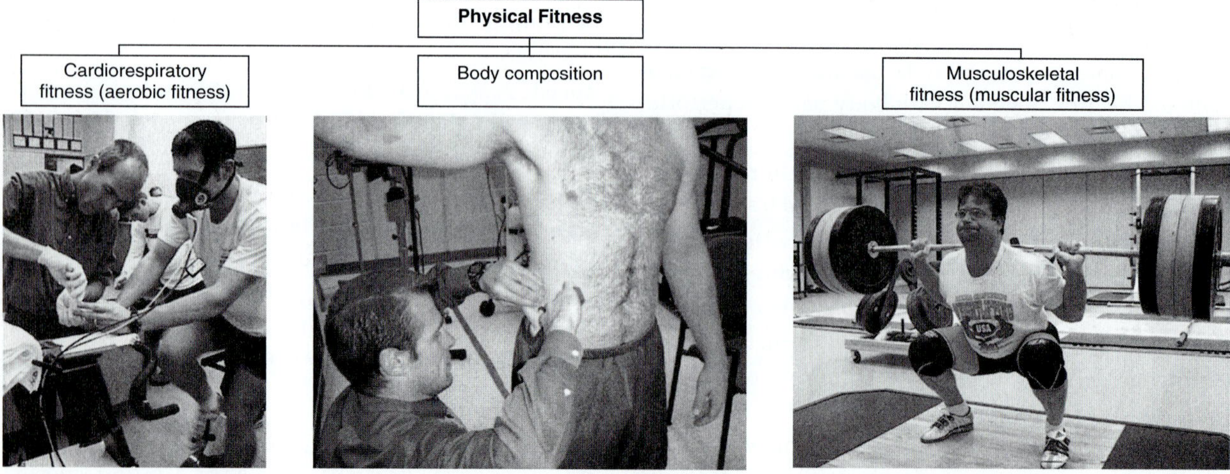

Figure 2.2 The focus today is on a balanced approach to health-related physical fitness, with due attention given to body composition and aerobic and muscular fitness.

The Meaning of Physical Fitness

Several organizations have submitted philosophical definitions of physical fitness. The World Health Organization in 1971, for example, has defined it simply as "the ability to perform muscular work satisfactorily."[14] The Centers for Disease Control and Prevention sponsored a workshop in 1985, bringing together a group of experts who concluded that physical fitness "is a set of attributes that people have or achieve that relates to the ability to perform physical activity."[3] The American College of Sports Medicine in 1990 proposed that "fitness is the ability to perform moderate to vigorous levels of physical activity without undue fatigue and the capability of maintaining such ability throughout life."[15]

The President's Council on Physical Fitness and Sports in 1971 offered one of the more widely used definitions, describing physical fitness as the "ability to carry out daily tasks with vigor and alertness, without undue fatigue and with ample energy to enjoy leisure-time pursuits and to meet unforeseen emergencies."[16] Dr. H. Harrison Clarke wrote that "physical fitness is the ability to last, to bear up, to withstand stress, and to persevere under difficult circumstances where an unfit person would give up. Physical fitness is the opposite to being fatigued from ordinary efforts, to lacking the energy to enter zestfully into life's activities, and to becoming exhausted from unexpected, demanding physical exertion. . . . It is a positive quality, extending on a scale from death to 'abundant life.' "[17]

In 1996, the surgeon general's report *Physical Activity and Health* adopted the 1985 definition of physical fitness proposed by the CDC, and most other organizations have followed suit.[1,3,8,11]

All of these definitions place an emphasis on having vigor and energy to perform work and exercise. Vigor and energy are not easily measured, however, and physical fitness experts have debated for more than a century the important measurable components of physical fitness.[17,18]

The most frequently cited components fall into two groups, one related to health and the other related to athletic skills.[3,11,12,18] Figure 2.3 summarizes the components of health- and skill-related fitness, with examples of the continuum of physical activities that represent each group.

It is felt by some researchers that while the elements of skill-related fitness are important for participation in various dual and team sports, they have little significance for the day-to-day tasks of Americans or for their general health.[3,18] On the other hand, individuals who engage in regular physical activity to develop cardiorespiratory endurance, musculoskeletal fitness, and optimal body fat levels appear to improve their basic energy levels and place themselves at lower risk for the common diseases of our time, including heart disease, cancer, diabetes, osteoporosis, and other chronic disorders.[2]

Athletes who excel in throwing a ball or swinging a golf club should understand that they may not have optimal levels of body fat or cardiorespiratory fitness, and as a consequence may be at higher risk for chronic disease. Also, even though individuals may possess poor coordination, they can still be physically fit and healthy by engaging regularly in aerobic and musculoskeletal exercise. Of course, there are athletes who by the nature of their sport (e.g., soccer or basketball) would be rated high in both the health- and skill-related elements.

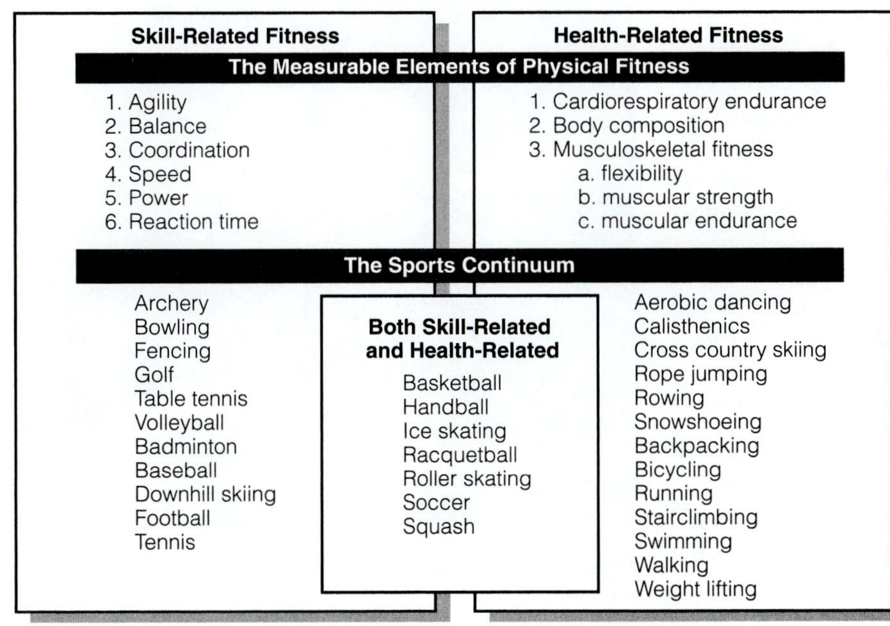

Figure 2.3 Most physical activities exist on a continuum between health- and skill-related fitness. Source: Adapted from Caspersen CJ, Powell KE, Christenson GM. Physical activity, exercise, and physical fitness: Definitions and distinctions for health-related research. *Public Health Rep* 100:126–131, 1985.

Among the general population, many individuals would rather play sports while getting fit than engage in "pure" fitness activities such as running, swimming, or using indoor exercise equipment. Fitness leaders need to individualize their recommendations to fit the goals and interests of their clients, realizing that many need the socialization and "fun" of sports to participate regularly in exercise.

The skill-related components of physical fitness have been defined as follows:[1,3]

Agility—the ability to rapidly change the position of the entire body in space, with speed and accuracy

Balance—the maintenance of equilibrium while stationary or in motion

Coordination—the ability to use the senses, such as sight and hearing, together with body parts, in performing motor tasks smoothly and accurately

Speed—the ability to perform a movement within a short period of time

Power—the rate at which a person can perform work (strength over time)

Reaction time—the time elapsed between a stimulus and the beginning of the reaction to it

The trend today in public policy recommendations is to emphasize the development of the health-related fitness elements, and to push for their prominence in school, worksite, and community programs.[1,2,3,13,19] Exercise testing batteries have been developed for children and adults to ensure that each of the health-related fitness elements is measured, followed by appropriate counseling to improve areas that may be deficient.[13,20–26]

The Elements of Health-Related Physical Fitness

Each of the components of health-related physical fitness can be measured separately from the others, and specific exercises may be applied to the development of each component.[11] In other words, the degree to which each of the five health-related components of physical fitness is developed in any one particular individual can vary widely. For example, a person may be strong but lack flexibility or may have good cardiorespiratory endurance but lack muscular strength. To develop "total" physical fitness for health, each of the components (cardiorespiratory endurance, body composition, and musculoskeletal fitness) must be tested separately and then included within the exercise prescription.

Cardiorespiratory Endurance

Cardiorespiratory endurance or *aerobic fitness* can be defined as the ability of the circulatory and respiratory systems to supply oxygen during sustained physical activity.[1,3,27,28] According to the American College of Sports Medicine, cardiorespiratory endurance is considered health related because low levels have been consistently linked with markedly increased risk of premature death from all causes, especially heart disease.[11]

For many people, being in good shape means having good cardiorespiratory endurance, exemplified by such feats as being able to run, cycle, and swim for prolonged periods of time (see Figure 2.4). High levels of cardiorespiratory endurance indicate a high physical work capacity, which is the ability to release relatively high amounts of energy over an extended period of time. To many fitness leaders, cardiorespiratory endurance is the most important of the health-related physical fitness components.

The laboratory test generally regarded as the best measure of cardiorespiratory endurance is the direct measurement of oxygen uptake during maximal, graded exercise. The exercise is usually performed using a bicycle ergometer or treadmill, which allows the progressive increase in workload from light to exhaustive (maximal) exercise. However, laboratory measurement of $\dot{V}O_{2max}$ is expensive, time-consuming, and requires highly trained personnel and therefore is not practical for mass testing situations or the testing of most patients on a day-to-day basis.

Various tests to estimate $\dot{V}O_{2max}$ have been developed as substitutes. These include field tests, stair-climbing tests, submaximal bicycle tests, and maximal treadmill and cycle ergometer tests. These tests are described in detail in Chapter 4.

Based on existing evidence concerning exercise prescription for the enhancement of health and cardiorespiratory fit-

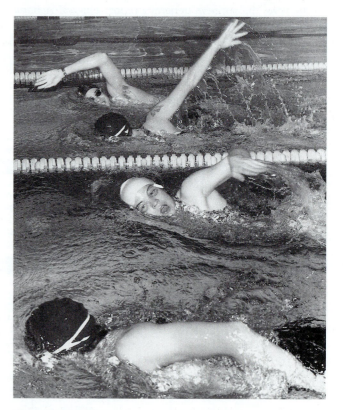

Figure 2.4 Cardiorepiratory endurance can be defined as the ability to continue or persist in strenuous tasks involving large muscle groups for extended periods of time. Swimming is one example.

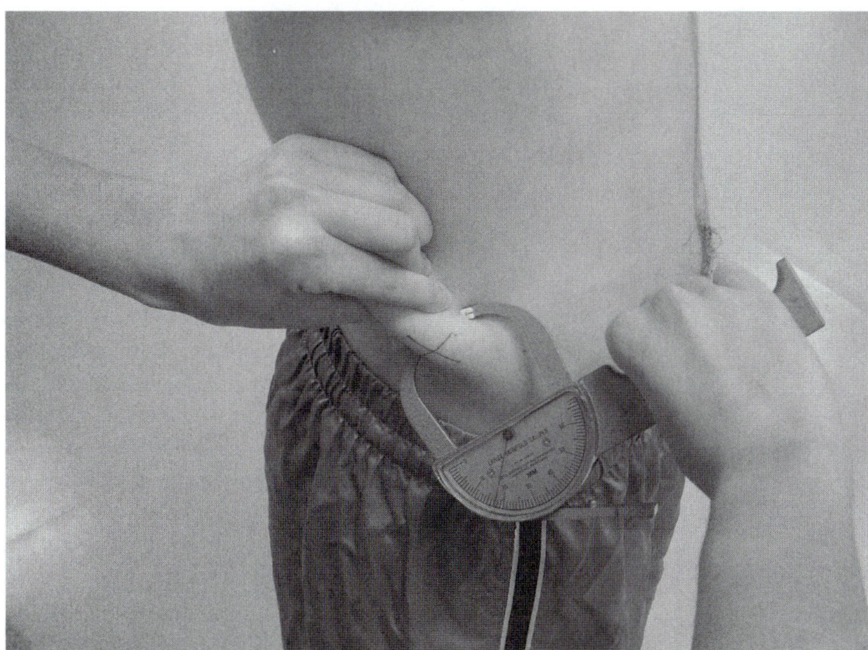

Figure 2.5 *Body composition* is the body's relative amounts of fat and lean body tissue, or fat-free mass (muscle, bone, water). Chapter 5 reviews procedures for measuring body fat through the use of skinfold calipers.

ness, the American College of Sports Medicine has recommended that large-muscle-group activity corresponding to either 40–85% $\dot{V}O_{2max}$ or 55–90% of maximal heart rate be engaged in for 20–60 minutes, three to five days a week.[11]

This recommendation has been subjected to a great deal of scrutiny since the late 1980s. In general, there is a growing consensus that when development of fitness is the major concern, higher intensity and longer, continuous duration of aerobic effort is required; when improvement of health is the goal, lower-intensity physical activity spread throughout the day appears sufficient. The CDC and ACSM recommend that every U.S. adult accumulate 30 minutes or more of moderate-intensity physical activity on most, preferably all, days of the week.[1,11] Exercise prescription is discussed in Chapter 8.

Body Composition

Body composition refers to the body's relative amounts of fat and lean body tissue or fat-free mass (e.g., muscle, bone, water).[1–3] Body weight can be subdivided simply into two components: fat weight (the weight of fat tissue) and fat-free weight (the weight of the remaining lean tissue). *Percent body fat,* the percentage of total weight represented by fat weight, is the preferred index used to evaluate a person's body composition. Obesity is defined as an excessive accumulation of fat weight. Men have optimal body fat levels when the percent of body fat is 15% or less; they are considered obese when the body fat percentage is 25% and higher. The optimal body fat level for women is 23% or less, and they are considered obese when their body fat percentage is 33% or higher (see Chapter 5).

Interest in measurement of body composition has grown tremendously since the mid-1970s, largely because of its relationship to both sports performance and health. Elite athletes, individuals seeking to reach or maintain optimal body weight, and patients in hospitals have all benefited from the increased popularity and accuracy of body composition measurement.

Research to establish ways of determining body composition through indirect methods began during the 1940s. Since then, a wide variety of methods have been developed. The most precise measure for assessing body composition using the two-compartment model is hydrostatic (underwater) weighing, although skinfold testing is the method of choice for many physical educators and exercise scientists (see Figure 2.5). When conducted appropriately, estimation of percent body fat from skinfold measurements correlates well with hydrostatic weighing ($r > .80$). Chapter 5 deals with these methods, as well as some newer techniques for determining body composition.

Musculoskeletal Fitness

Musculoskeletal fitness or muscular fitness has three components: flexibility, muscular strength, and muscular endurance.

1. *Flexibility* is the functional capacity of the joints to move through a full range of movement.[1–3,11] Flexibility is specific to each joint of the body. Muscles, ligaments, and tendons largely determine the amount of movement possible at each joint (see Figure 2.6).
2. *Muscular strength* relates to the ability of the muscle to exert force. In other words, it is the maximal one-effort force that can be exerted against a resistance, or the maximum amount of force that one can generate in an isolated movement of a single muscle group.[1–3,11] The stronger the individual the greater the amount of force that can be generated. Lifting heavy weights maximally once or twice, or exerting maximal force when gripping a hand dynamometer,

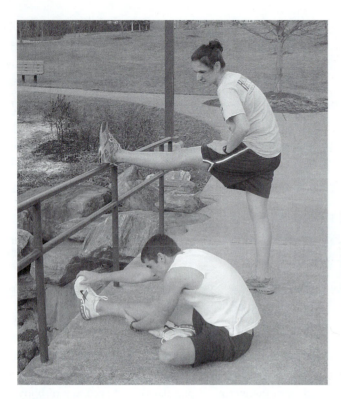

Figure 2.6 *Flexibility* is defined as the functional capacity of the joints to move through a full range of movement.

provides measurements of muscular strength (see Figure 2.7).

3. *Muscular endurance* relates to the muscle's ability to continue to perform without fatigue.[1–3,11] In other words, it is the ability of the muscles to apply a submaximal force repeatedly or to sustain a submaximal muscular contraction for a certain period of time. Common muscular-endurance exercises are sit-ups, push-ups, chin-ups, or lifting weights 10–15 times in succession (see Figure 2.8).

Elaborate and expensive musculoskeletal fitness testing equipment is available, and books have been written describing the sophisticated testing that can be done with it.[28] For most people, however, simple and inexpensive musculoskeletal fitness tests such as the sit-and-reach flexibility test, push-ups, sit-ups, pull-ups, and various weight-lifting measures are available with extensive norms.[20–25] These are described in Chapter 6. Most of the health-related benefits of musculoskeletal fitness have focused on the contribution of abdominal muscle strength and endurance and lower back–hamstring flexibility for the prevention of low-back pain, a topic also explored in Chapter 6. Muscular fitness is also important in reducing the loss of muscle size and strength leading to frailty in old age (see Chapter 15).

Chapter 8 deals with conditioning principles to improve musculoskeletal fitness. The American College of Sports Medicine recommends that static stretching exercises be sustained for 10–30 seconds and then repeated three to four times, at least two to three times per week, to develop flexibility.[11] It is also recommended that an active aerobic warm-up precede vigorous stretching exercises.

For the development of muscular strength and endurance, the American College of Sports Medicine recommends a minimum of one set of 8–12 repetitions of 8–10 exercises that condition the major muscle groups at least 2 to 3 days per week.[11] Optimal gains in strength are provided by three sets of five to seven repetitions of a weight-resistance exercise.

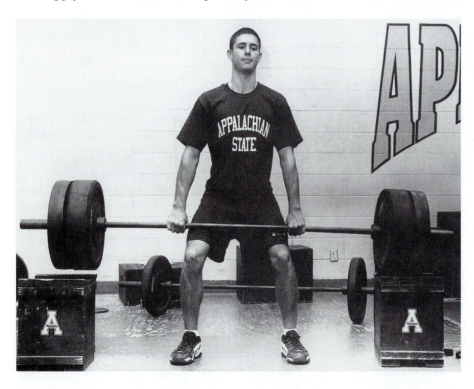

Figure 2.7 *Strength* relates to the ability of the muscle to exert force.

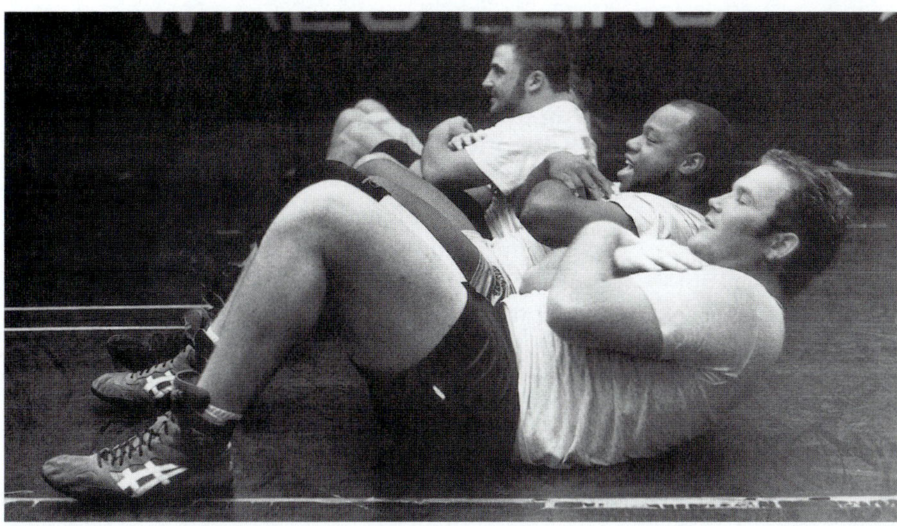

Figure 2.8 *Muscular endurance* relates to the muscle's ability to continue to perform without fatigue.

SPORTS MEDICINE INSIGHT

Physical Fitness in Children and Youth: The Role of Physical Education

The American College of Sports Medicine developed physical activity recommendations for school-aged youths.[29] Here are key statements from this landmark publication:

- School-age youths should participate daily in 60 minutes or more of moderate to vigorous physical activity (see Figure 2.9). The activity should be developmentally appropriate, involve variety, and be enjoyable. For youths who have been physically inactive, an incremental approach to the 60-minute goal is recommended. Increasing activity by 10% per week, an approach used in athletic training, appears to be acceptable and achievable. Experience shows that attempting to achieve too much too rapidly is often counterproductive and may lead to injury.

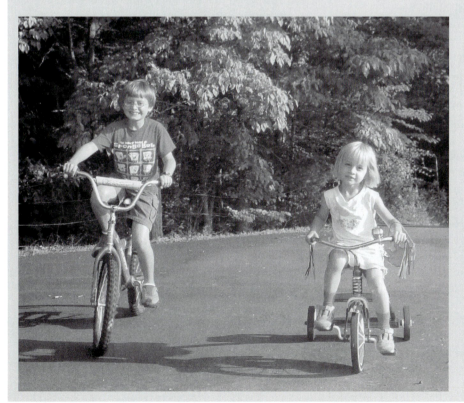

Figure 2.9 School-aged youths need at least 60 minutes of physical activity a day, which can take the form of play.

(continued)

SPORTS MEDICINE INSIGHT *(continued)*

Physical Fitness in Children and Youth: The Role of Physical Education

- There is good evidence that this amount of physical activity is associated with improved musculoskeletal health, body composition, and cardiovascular health. Although more research is needed, physical activity by school-aged youths has some benefits on lipids and lipoproteins, blood pressure, self-concept, anxiety and depression symptoms, and academic performance.
- Types and contexts of activities are variable and change with age during childhood and adolescence. Activities of children aged 6 to 9 years are largely anaerobic (as in nonsustained activities of games such as "tag"), and they help the child learn basic and more specialized motor skills. As children move into the pubertal transition (about age 10–14 years, earlier in girls than in boys), these skills are incorporated into a variety of individual and group activities and many organized sports. Mature structure and function are approached or attained in late adolescence (age 15–18 years), thus physical activity programs can be more structured.
- Physical inactivity is a strong contributor to overweight. Sedentary activities such as excessive television viewing, computer use, video games, and telephone conversations should be discouraged. Reducing sedentary behaviors to less than 2 hours per day is important to health and to increasing physical activity.
- The recommended 60 minutes or more of physical activity can be achieved in a cumulative manner in school during physical education, recess, intramural sports, and before- and after-school programs. Youth need daily quality physical education from kindergarten through grade 12. Both physical education and recess afford the opportunity to achieve this goal without any evidence of compromising academic performance.
- Opportunities to influence youth participation in physical activities are readily available at home and school, as well as in community and health-care settings. Parents and caregivers have the responsibility to ensure that children have the opportunity to explore and learn through movement activities and to be physically active. Communities, organizations, and institutions within communities likewise have a responsibility to provide children with opportunities for and access to safe physical activities, and with qualified adult leaders. Health-care providers should assess physical activity patterns and counsel patients and families about appropriate amounts of physical activity and its health benefits. Although time in the office setting is limited, it is recommended that physicians should be a strong advocate of a physically active lifestyle for youths—at home, in schools, and in communities.

In 1997, the CDC released guidelines urging schools and communities to encourage physical activity among young people so that they will continue to engage in physical activity in adulthood and obtain the health benefits of physical activity throughout life.[30] The CDC provided guidelines about 10 aspects of school and community programs, including these on the importance of physical education:

- Establish policies that promote enjoyable, lifelong physical activity among young people (e.g., require comprehensive and daily physical education for students in kindergarten through grade 12).
- Implement physical education curricula and instruction that emphasize enjoyable participation in physical activity and that help students develop the knowledge, attitudes, motor skills, behavioral skills, and confidence needed to adopt and maintain physically active lifestyles (e.g., emphasize skills for lifetime physical activities such as dance, strength training, jogging, swimming, bicycling, cross-country skiing, walking, and hiking rather than those for competitive sports).

According to the CDC, "School and community programs that promote regular physical activity among young people could be among the most effective strategies for reducing the public health burden of chronic diseases associated with sedentary lifestyles. Programs that provide students with the knowledge, attitudes, motor skills, behavioral skills, and confidence to participate in physical activity may establish active lifestyles among young people that continue into and throughout their adult lives."[30]

Despite the emphasis on the need for quality physical education programs by the ACSM, CDC, and the

(continued)

SPORTS MEDICINE INSIGHT *(continued)*

Physical Fitness in Children and Youth: The Role of Physical Education

Surgeon General's Office,[1,10,29–31] available data indicate that physical activity levels begin to decline as children approach their teenage years and continue to decline throughout adolescence and even more strongly during young adulthood. Unfortunately, most U.S. students do not participate in daily physical education, and the proportion of students with daily physical education has been declining over time.[31] Only 17% of middle/junior high schools and 2% of high schools required physical education 5 days per week each year. The majority of high school students take physical education for only 1 year between 9th and 12th grades. Among U.S. high school students, nearly half (45%) do not play on any sports teams during the year, nearly half (44%) are not even enrolled in a physical education class, and only 29% attend daily physical education classes.[31] *Healthy People 2010* includes objectives for increasing the percentage of schools offering, and the percentage of students participating in, daily physical education classes (see Chapter 1).

In 2000, the Secretary of Health and Human Services and the Secretary of Education released their report, "Promoting Better Health for Young People Through Physical Activity and Sports."[31] Ten strategies were described to promote lifelong participation in enjoyable and safe physical activity and sports (these were listed in Chapter 1). These focused on the roles of families, school and after-school programs, youth sports and recreation programs, community environments, and the media. Several of the strategies emphasized the important role of physical education:

- Help all children, from pre-kindergarten through grade 12, to receive quality, daily physical education. Help all schools to have certified physical education specialists; appropriate class sizes; and the facilities, equipment, and supplies needed to deliver quality, daily physical education.
- Publicize and disseminate tools to help schools improve their physical education and other physical activity programs.
- Implement an ongoing media campaign to promote physical education as an important component of a quality education and long-term health.

In this report, physical education was placed at the core of a comprehensive approach to promoting physical activity through schools, and the underlying rationale included these arguments:[31]

- Physical education helps students develop the knowledge, attitudes, skills, behaviors, and confidence needed to be physically active for life, while providing an opportunity for students to be active during the school day.
- Leading professionals in the field of physical education have developed a new kind of physical education that is fundamentally different from the stereotypical "roll out the balls and play" classes of decades past that featured little meaningful instruction and lots of humiliation for students who were not athletically coordinated. Professional associations, academic experts, and many teachers across the country are promoting and implementing quality physical education programs that emphasize participation in lifelong physical activity by all students.
- The emphasis today is on keeping all students active for most of the class period; building students' confidence in their physical abilities; influencing moral development by providing students with opportunities to assume leadership, cooperate with others, and accept responsibility for their own behavior; and having fun.
- Qualified and appropriately trained physical education teachers are the most essential ingredient of a quality physical education program. Unfortunately, many schools do not have qualified professionals teaching physical education.
- The large class sizes with which physical educators are often confronted are a key barrier to the implementation of quality physical education. Physical education should have the same class sizes as other subjects.
- Perhaps the most urgently needed tool that has not yet been developed is a standardized assessment of student performance in physical education. Such a tool would measure achievement in knowledge, motor skills, and self-management skills.

SUMMARY

1. *Physical activity, exercise,* and *physical fitness* are terms that describe different concepts. Physical activity is defined as any bodily movement produced by skeletal muscles that results in energy expenditure.
2. Exercise is a subcategory of physical activity and is planned, structured, repetitive, and purposive, in the sense that improvement or maintenance of physical fitness is an objective.
3. Several organizations have proposed definitions of physical fitness, most of them emphasizing attributes that people have or achieve, that relate to the ability to perform physical activity.
4. The measurable elements of physical fitness fall into two groups: skill-related fitness and health-related fitness. The former includes agility, balance, coordination, speed, power, and reaction time. The latter includes cardiorespiratory endurance, body composition, and musculoskeletal fitness, which includes flexibility, muscular strength, and muscular endurance.

Review Questions

1. ***Based on the information of this chapter, which activity listed scores highest in the development of all five of the measurable elements of health-related physical fitness?***

   A. Badminton **B.** Running
   C. Bowling **D.** Rowing
   E. Baseball

2. ***____ is physical activity that is planned for purposes of improving health.***

   A. Physical fitness **B.** Exercise
   C. Work **D.** Aerobics

3. ***Musculoskeletal fitness has three components, including flexibility, muscular strength, and ____.***

   A. Cardiovascular endurance
   B. Muscular endurance
   C. Agility
   D. Coordination
   E. Speed

4. ***____ has been defined as any bodily movement produced by skeletal muscles that results in energy expenditure.***

   A. Flexibility **B.** Physical activity
   C. Muscular endurance **D.** Power
   E. Body composition

5. ***Which one is* not *a measurable element of health-related physical fitness?***

   A. Flexibility
   B. Cardiorespiratory endurance
   C. Muscular endurance
   D. Coordination
   E. Body composition

6. ***The CDC and ACSM recommend that every U.S. adult accumulate ____ minutes or more of moderate-intensity physical activity on most, preferably all, days of the week.***

   A. 10 **B.** 15 **C.** 20 **D.** 30 **E.** 45

7. ***____ relates to the rate at which one can perform work (strength over time).***

   A. Reaction time **B.** Power
   C. Agility **D.** Flexibility
   E. Cardiorespiratory endurance

8. ***Body composition refers to the body's relative amounts of fat and ____.***

   A. Fat free mass **B.** Muscle
   C. Bone **D.** Total body weight
   E. Body water weight

9. ***____ is the maximal one-effort force that can be exerted against a resistance.***

   A. Flexibility **B.** Muscular endurance
   C. Muscular strength **D.** Agility
   E. Coordination

10. ***____ is the functional capacity of the joints to move through a full range of movement.***

    A. Flexibility **B.** Muscular endurance
    C. Muscular strength **D.** Agility
    E. Coordination

11. ***Who has defined physical fitness as "the ability to perform moderate to vigorous levels of physical activity without undue fatigue and the capability of maintaining such ability throughout life"?***

    A. World Health Organization
    B. Centers for Disease Control and Prevention
    C. Dr. Kenneth H. Cooper
    D. American College of Sports Medicine
    E. President's Council on Physical Fitness and Sports

12. ***For the development of muscular strength and endurance, the ACSM recommends a minimum of one set of 8–12 repetitions of ____ exercises that condition the major muscle groups at least two to three days per week.***

    A. 8–10 **B.** 4–5 **C.** 15–20 **D.** 12–17 **E.** 2–3

13. ***The ACSM recommends that static stretching exercises be sustained for 10–30 seconds and then repeated three to four times, at least ____ times per week, to develop flexibility.***

A. 1–2 **B.** 2–3 **C.** 3–4 **D.** 4–5 **E.** 5–7

Answers

1. D	**8.** A
2. B	**9.** C
3. B	**10.** A
4. B	**11.** D
5. D	**12.** A
6. D	**13.** B
7. B	

REFERENCES

1. U.S. Department of Health and Human Services. *Physical Activity and Health: A Report of the Surgeon General.* Atlanta, GA: U.S. Department of Health and Human Services, Centers for Disease Control and Prevention, National Center for Chronic Disease Prevention and Health Promotion, 1996.
2. Bouchard C, Shephard R J, Stephens T. *Physical Activity, Fitness, and Health: International Proceedings and Consensus Statement.* Champaign, IL: Human Kinetics, 1994.
3. Caspersen CJ, Powell KE, Christenson GM. Physical activity, exercise and physical fitness: Definitions and distinctions for health-related research. *Public Health Rep* 100:120–131, 1985.
4. Ainsworth BE, Haskell WL, Whitt MC, Irwin ML, Swartz AM, Strath SJ, O'Brien WL, Bassett DR, Schmitz KH, Emplaincourt PO, Jacobs DR, Leon AS. Compendium of physical activities: An update of activity codes and MET intensities. *Med Sci Sports Exerc* 32(suppl):S498–S516, 2000.
5. Kriska AM, Caspersen CJ. A collection of physical activity questionnaires for health-related research. *Med Sci Sports Exerc* 29(suppl):S1–S205, 1997.
6. Duffield R, Dawson B, Pinnington HC, Wong P. Accuracy and reliability of a Cosmed K4b2 portable gas system. *J Sci Med Sport* 7:11–22, 2004.
7. Speakman JR. The history and theory of the doubly labeled water technique. *Am J Clin Nutr* 68(suppl):932S–938S, 1998.
8. Corbin CB, Pangrazi RP, Franks BD. Definitions: Health, Fitness, and Physical Activity. *President's Council on Physical Fitness and Sports Research Digest,* Series 3, No. 9, March 2000.
9. American College of Sports Medicine. *ACSM's Resource Manual for Guidelines for Exercise Testing and Prescription* (4th ed.). Philadelphia: Lippincott William & Wilkins, 2001.
10. U.S. Department of Health and Human Services, Public Health Service, Centers for Disease Control and Prevention. *Promoting Physical Activity: A Guide for Community Action.* Champaign, IL: Human Kinetics, 1999.
11. American College of Sports Medicine. *ACSM's Guidelines for Exercise Testing and Prescription* (6th ed.). Philadelphia: Lippincott Williams & Wilkins, 2000.
12. Nieman DC. The exercise test as a component of the total fitness evaluation. *Prim Care* 28:119–135, 2001.
13. Canadian Society for Exercise Physiology. *The Canadian Physical Activity, Fitness & Lifestyle Appraisal.* Ottawa, Ontario: Canadian Society for Exercise Physiology, 1996.
14. Anderson KL, Shephard RJ, Denolin H, et al. *Fundamentals of Exercise Testing.* Geneva: World Health Organization, 1971.
15. American College of Sports Medicine. The recommended quantity and quality of exercise for developing and maintaining cardiorespiratory and muscular fitness in healthy adults. *Med Sci Sports Exerc* 22:265–274, 1990.
16. President's Council on Physical Fitness and Sports. *Physical Fitness Research Digest* (Series 1, No. 1). Washington, DC, President's Council on Physical Fitness and Sports, 1971.
17. Clarke HH. *Application of Measurement to Health and Physical Education.* Englewood Cliffs, NJ: Prentice-Hall, Inc., 1967.
18. Pate RR. A new definition of youth fitness. *Physician Sportsmed* 11:77–83, 1983.
19. U.S. Department of Health and Human Services. *Healthy People 2010.* Washington, DC: January 2000. http://www.health.gov/healthypeople/.
20. The Cooper Institute for Aerobics Research. *The FITNESSGRAM Test Administration Manual.* Champaign, IL: Human Kinetics, 1999.
21. Golding LA, Myers CR, Sinning WE. *The Y's Way to Physical Fitness* (3rd ed.). Champaign, IL: Human Kinetics, 1989.
22. American Alliance for Health, Physical Education, Recreation and Dance. *Physical Best Activity Guide—Elementary and Secondary Levels.* Champaign, IL: Human Kinetics, 1999.
23. Cooper Institute for Aerobics Research. *The Strength Connection.* Dallas: Cooper Institute for Aerobics Research, 1990.
24. American College of Sports Medicine. *ACSM Fitness Book* (2nd ed.). Champaign, IL: Human Kinetics, 1998.
25. President's Council on Physical Fitness and Sports. *Get Fit: A Handbook for Youth Ages 6–17.* Washington, DC: President's Council on Physical Fitness and Sports, 1999.
26. Winnick JP, Short FX. *The Brockport Physical Fitness Test Manual.* Champaign, IL: Human Kinetics, 1999.
27. Baranowski T, Bouchard C, Bar Or O, et al. Assessment, prevalence, and cardiovascular benefits of physical activity and fitness in youth. *Med. Sci Sports Exerc* 24(suppl 6):S237–S246, 1992.
28. Heyward VH. *Advanced Fitness Assessment and Exercise Prescription* (3rd ed.). Champaign, IL: Human Kinetics, 1998.
29. American College of Sports Medicine. Physical activity recommendations for school-aged youth. *Med Sci Sports Exerc*: (in press).
30. Centers for Disease Control and Prevention. Guidelines for school and community programs to promote lifelong physical activity among young people. *MMWR* 46(No. RR-6):1–35, 1997.
31. A Report to the President from the Secretary of Health and Human Services and the Secretary of Education. *Promoting Better Health for Young People Through Physical Activity and Sports.* Fall 2000. http://www.cdc.gov/.

PHYSICAL FITNESS ACTIVITY 2.1

Ranking Activities by Health-Related Value

As discussed in this chapter, there are five measurable elements of health-related fitness:

Cardiorespiratory endurance
Body composition
Musculoskeletal fitness } **Flexibility**, **Muscular endurance**, **Muscular strength**

Sports and other forms of physical activity vary in their capacity to develop each component. In this Physical Fitness Activity, you will be ranking different sports and exercises in terms of their capacity to promote such development, using a 5-point scale for each of the five health-related fitness components. Answer the questions to the best of your ability, and then *compare* your answers in a group session with your teacher or your local fitness expert.

Rate each physical activity or sport in terms of its capacity to develop each of the five health-related components: 1 = not at all; 2 = somewhat or just a little bit; 3 = moderately; 4 = strongly; 5 = very strongly. Then answer the following question.

What five activities received the highest total score (add the five component scores for each activity)?

#1 Overall activity ____________________

#2 Overall activity ____________________

#3 Overall activity ____________________

#4 Overall activity ____________________

#5 Overall activity ____________________

Physical Activity—Recreational	Cardiorespiratory Endurance	Body Composition	Flexibility	Muscular Endurance	Muscular Strength	Total
Archery						
Backpacking						
Badminton						
Basketball						
Nongame						
Game play						
Bicycling						
Pleasure						
15 mph						
Bowling						
Calisthenics						
Canoeing, rowing, kayaking						
Dancing						
Social and square						
Aerobic						
Fencing						
Fishing						
Bank, boat, or ice						
Stream, wading						
Football (touch)						

Physical Activity—Recreational	Cardiorespiratory Endurance	Body Composition	Flexibility	Muscular Endurance	Muscular Strength	Total
Golf						
Power cart						
Walking, with bag						
Handball						
Hiking, cross-country						
Horseback riding						
Paddleball, racquetball						
Rope jumping						
Running						
12 min per mile						
6 min per mile						
Sailing						
Scuba diving						
Skating						
Ice						
Roller						
Skiing, snow						
Downhill						
Cross-country						
Skiing, water						
Sledding, tobogganing						
Snowshoeing						
Soccer						
Squash						
Stair climbing						
Swimming						
Table tennis						
Tennis						
Volleyball						
Walking briskly						
Weight training, circuit						
Physical Activity—Nonrecreational						
Bricklaying, plastering						
Digging ditches						
Shoveling light earth						
Splitting wood						

part II

Screening and Testing

chapter 3

Testing Concepts

All facilities offering exercise equipment or services should conduct a cardiovascular screening of all new members and/or prospective users.
—ACSM/AHA, 1998

Much has been learned about exercise and health during the past 40 years since the fitness movement first began. In general, exercise has been found to be both safe and beneficial for most people. However, there are some individuals that can suffer ill health from exercise. There's probably not a single fitness enthusiast in America who has not read the reports of famous athletes dying on basketball courts, runners found dead with their running shoes on, executives discovered slumped over their treadmills, or middle-aged men suffering heart attacks while shoveling snow.

Whether exercise is beneficial or hazardous to the heart depends on who the person is. For most people, regular exercise reduces the risk of heart disease by about one half compared to those who are physically inactive (see Chapter 10 and Figure 3.1). However, for those who are at high risk for heart disease to begin with, vigorous exercise bouts can trigger fatal heart attacks. About 6 out of 100,000 middle-aged men die during or after exercise each year.[1] Studies show that these victims tend to be men who were sedentary, over age 35 years, already had heart disease or were at high risk for it, and then exercised too hard for their fitness levels (see Chapter 16).[1,2] And for patients with heart disease, the incidence of a heart attack or death during exercise is 10 times that of otherwise healthy individuals.[1]

Also of concern is congenital cardiovascular disease, now the major cause of athletic death in high school and college. In one study of 158 athletes who died young (average age 17) and in their prime, 134 of them had heart or blood vessel defects that were present at birth.[3] Most common was hypertrophic cardiomyopathy, a thickening of the heart's main pumping muscle. In other words, when a

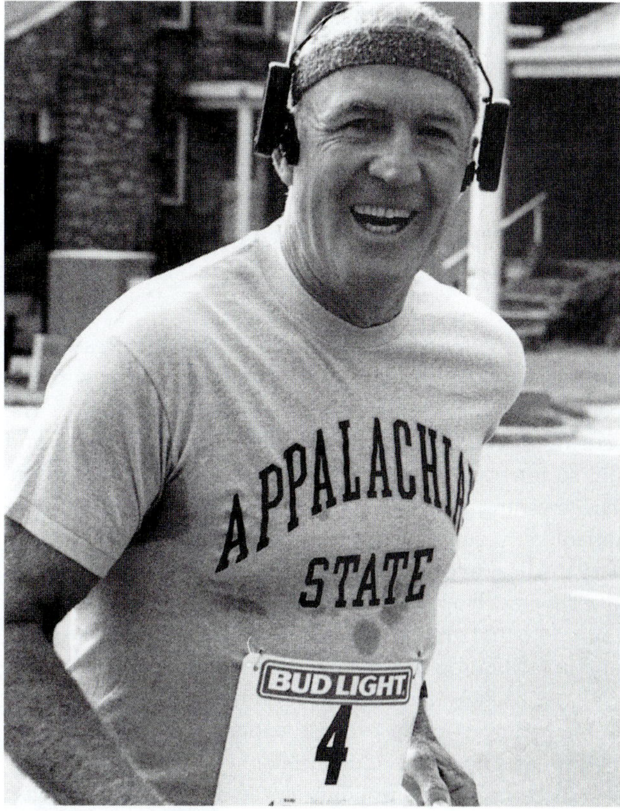

Figure 3.1 For most people, regular exercise reduces the risk of heart disease by about one half compared to those who are physically inactive.

young athlete dies during or shortly after exercise, it is most often due to a birth defect of the cardiovascular system.[1–3]

Health screening is a vital process of first identifying individuals at high risk for exercise-induced heart problems and then referring them to appropriate medical care.[1,2] Despite the proven benefits of screening, efforts to screen new members at enrollment into health/fitness facilities are limited and inconsistent.[1]

Efforts to promote physical activity will result in increasing numbers of individuals with and without risk of heart disease joining health/fitness facilities and community exercise programs. Surveys reveal that 50% of health/fitness facility members are older than 35 years, and the fastest growing segments are middle-aged and elderly participants.[1] According to the American Heart Association, more than one fourth of all Americans have some form of cardiovascular disease (including high blood pressure), and the prevalence rises with age.[4] To ensure safe exercise participation, it is essential that people with underlying cardiovascular disease be identified before they initiate exercise programs.

The first half of this chapter focuses on guidelines health and fitness professionals can use to help protect participants when initiating exercise or athletic programs and emphasizes several key issues:

1. Always obtain a medical history or pre-exercise health risk appraisal on each participant.
2. Stratify individuals according to their disease risk.
3. Refer high-risk individuals to a health-care provider for medical evaluation and a graded exercise test.

PREPARTICIPATION HEALTH SCREENING

All facilities offering exercise equipment or services should conduct preparticipation health screening of all new members and/or prospective users, regardless of age.[1,2,5] The screening procedure should be simple, easy to perform, and not so intensive that it serves to discourage participation. The screening questionnaires should be interpreted and documented by qualified staff to limit the number of unnecessary medical referrals and avoid barriers to participation.

The health appraisal questionnaire is useful in classifying a potential exercise participant according to disease risk and in facilitating the exercise prescription process. In general, the background information obtained from the questionnaire improves the exercise leader's ability to adjust the program to meet individual needs.

There are many questionnaires available for pre-exercise screening (see Physical Fitness Activity 3.2 for a comprehensive questionnaire). A comprehensive medical/health questionnaire should include the following:[2]

- Medical diagnoses
- Previous physical examination findings
- History of symptoms
- Recent illness, hospitalization, new medical diagnoses, or surgical procedures
- Orthopedic problems
- Medication use and drug allergies
- Lifestyle habits
- Exercise history
- Work history
- Family history of disease

When testing large numbers of individuals in a short period of time, or in most health/fitness facility settings, a shorter, simpler medical/health questionnaire is preferable. A brief, self-administered medical questionnaire called the *Physical Activity Readiness Questionnaire* (PAR-Q) has been used very successfully (see Figure 3.2).[6–8] The PAR-Q was designed in the 1970s by Canadian researchers and used in conjunction with the Canadian fitness testing program. After years of successful use and a revision in 1994, the PAR-Q is now recognized by experts as a safe pre-exercise screening measure for those who plan to engage in low-to-moderate (but not vigorous) exercise training.[7] Participants are directed to contact their personal physician if they answer "yes" to one or more questions.

In 1998, the American College of Sports Medicine (ACSM) and the American Heart Association (AHA) published a slightly more complex questionnaire than the PAR-Q[1] (see Physical Fitness Activity 3.1). The ACSM/AHA questionnaire uses history, symptoms, and risk factors to direct an individual to either initiate an exercise program or contact his or her physician. Persons at higher risk are directed to seek facilities providing appropriate levels of staff supervision. The questionnaire takes only a few minutes to complete, identifies high-risk participants, documents the results of screening, educates the consumer, and encourages and fosters appropriate use of the health-care system.

The ACSM recommends that all individuals interested in participating in organized exercise programs be evaluated for heart disease risk factors, using guidelines from the National Cholesterol Education Program.[2] These include the following seven risk factors (which should not be viewed as an all-inclusive list, but are used by the ACSM for counting risk factors prior to risk stratification):

- *Family history.* Myocardial infarction, coronary revascularization, or sudden death before 55 years of age in father or other male first-degree relative or before 65 years of age in mother or other female first-degree relative.
- *Cigarette smoking.* Current cigarette smoker or those who have quit within the previous 6 months.
- *Hypertension.* Systolic blood pressure (BP) of ≥140 mm Hg or diastolic BP ≥90 mm Hg, confirmed by

Physical Activity Readiness Questionnaire-PAR-Q (revised 1994)

PAR-Q & YOU

(A Questionnaire for People Aged 15 to 69)

Regular physical activity is fun and healthy, and increasingly more people are starting to become more active every day. Being more active is very safe for most people. However, some people should check with their doctor before they start becoming much more physically active.

If you are planning to become much more physically active than you are now, start by answering the seven questions in the box below. If you are between the ages of 15 and 69, the PAR-Q will tell you if you should check with your doctor before you start. If you are over 69 years of age, and you are not used to being very active, check with your doctor.

Common sense is your best guide when you answer these questions. Please read the questions carefully and answer each one honestly: check YES or NO.

YES	NO	
☐	☐	1. Has your doctor ever said that you have a heart condition *and* that you should only do physical activity recommended by a doctor?
☐	☐	2. Do you feel pain in your chest when you do physical activity?
☐	☐	3. In the past month, have you had chest pain when you were not doing physical activity?
☐	☐	4. Do you lose your balance because of dizziness or do you ever lose consciousness?
☐	☐	5. Do you have a bone or joint problem that could be made worse by a change in your physical activity?
☐	☐	6. Is your doctor currently prescribing drugs (for example, water pills) for your blood pressure or heart condition?
☐	☐	7. Do you know of *any other reason* why you should not do physical activity?

If you answered

YES to one or more questions

Talk with your doctor by phone or in person BEFORE you start becoming much more physically active or BEFORE you have a fitness appraisal. Tell your doctor about the PAR-Q and which questions you answered YES.

- You may be able to do any activity you want—as long as you start slowly and build up gradually. Or, you may need to restrict your activities to those which are safe for you. Talk with your doctor about the kinds of activities you wish to participate in and follow his/her advice.
- Find out which community programs are safe and helpful for you.

NO to all questions

If you answered NO honestly to *all* PAR-Q questions, you can be reasonably sure that you can:

- start becoming much more physically active—begin slowly and build up gradually. This is the safest and easiest way to go.
- take part in the fitness appraisal—this is an excellent way to determine your basic fitness so that you can plan the best way for you to live actively.

DELAY BECOMING MUCH MORE ACTIVE:

- If you are not feeling well because of a temporary illness such as a cold or a fever—wait until you feel better; or
- If you are or may be pregnant—talk to your doctor before you start becoming more active.

Please note: If your health changes so that you then answer YES to any of the above questions, tell your fitness or health professional. Ask whether you should change your physical activity plan.

Informed Use of the PAR-Q: The Canadian Society for Exercise Physiology, Health Canada, and their agents assume no liability for persons who undertake physical activity, and if in doubt after completing this questionnaire, consult your doctor prior to physical activity.

You are encouraged to copy the PAR-Q but only if you use the entire form.

Note: If the PAR-Q is being given to a person before he or she participates in a physical activity program or a fitness appraisal, this section may be used for legal or administrative purposes.

I have read, understood and completed this questionnaire. Any questions I had were answered to my full satisfaction.

NAME ______________________

SIGNATURE ______________________ DATE ______________________

SIGNATURE OF PARENT ______________________ WITNESS ______________________
or GUARDIAN (for participants under the age of majority)

Supported by: Health Canada Santé Canada

Reprinted from the 1994 revised version of the Physical Activity Readiness Questionnaire (PAR-Q and YOU). The PAR-Q and YOU is a copyrighted, pre-exercise screen owned by the Canadian Society for Exercise Physiology.

Figure 3.2 The Physical Activity Readiness Questionnaire (PAR-Q) offers an easy, brief evaluation of an individual's readiness to exercise before the individual starts an exercise program.

measurements on at least two separate occasions, or on antihypertensive medication.

- *Dyslipidemia.* Total serum cholesterol of >200 mg/dl or high-density lipoprotein cholesterol of <40 mg/dl, or on lipid-lowering medication. If low-density lipoprotein cholesterol is available, use >130 mg/dl rather than the total cholesterol of <200 mg/dl. If the high-density lipoprotein cholesterol is >60 mg/dl subtract one risk factor from the sum of positive risk factors (negative risk factor).
- *Impaired fasting glucose.* Fasting blood glucose of ≥100 mg/dl, confirmed by measurements on at least two separate occasions.
- *Obesity.* Body mass index of ≥30 kg/m^2, or waist girth of >102 cm for men and >88 cm for women, or waist/hip ratio ≥0.95 for men and ≥0.86 for women.
- *Sedentary lifestyle.* Persons not participating in a regular exercise program or not meeting the minimal physical activity recommendations from the U.S. Office of the Surgeon General's report—accumulating 30 minutes or more of moderate physical activity on most days of the week.

The ACSM also recommends that preparticipation questionnaires include the following list of major signs or symptoms suggestive of cardiovascular and pulmonary disease:[2]

- Pain, discomfort (or other anginal equivalent) in the chest, neck, jaw, arms, or other areas that may be due to ischemia
- Shortness of breath at rest or with mild exertion
- Dizziness or syncope
- Orthopnea (discomfort in breathing which is brought on or aggravated by lying flat) or paroxysmal nocturnal dyspnea (acute difficulty in breathing appearing suddenly at night, usually waking the patient after an hour or two of sleep)
- Ankle edema
- Palpitations (forcible or irregular pulsation of the heart perceptible to the individual, usually with an increase in frequency or force, with or without irregularity in rhythm) or tachycardia (rapid beating of the heart, typically over 100 beats per minute at rest)
- Intermittent claudication (a condition caused by lack of blood flow and oxygen to the leg muscles, characterized by attacks of lameness and pain, brought on by walking)
- Known heart murmur
- Unusual fatigue or shortness of breath with usual activities

USING SCREENING RESULTS FOR RISK STRATIFICATION

Once symptom and risk factor screening has been conducted using questionnaires, the individual considering exercise testing and prescription should be stratified according to disease risk. Stratification according to disease risk is important for several reasons:

- To identify those in need of referral to a health-care provider for more extensive medical evaluation
- To ensure the safety of exercise testing and participation
- To determine the appropriate type of exercise test or program

The ACSM recommends using these risk stratification levels:[2]

- *Low risk.* Men <45 and women <55 years of age who are asymptomatic and meet no more than one risk factor threshold.
- *Moderate risk.* Men ≥45 and women ≥55 years of age or those who meet the threshold for two or more risk factors.
- *High risk.* Individuals with one or more signs or symptoms or with known cardiovascular, pulmonary, or metabolic disease including diabetes mellitus.

Once individuals have been stratified according to risk, decisions can be made regarding the need for medical examination and exercise testing. The depth of the medical or physical examination for any individual considering an exercise program depends on the disease risk stratification. When a medical evaluation or recommendation is advised or required, written and active communication by the exercise staff with the individual's personal physician is strongly recommended. The form shown in Boxes 3.1 and 3.2 can be used for this referral.[1]

Current medical examination and exercise testing is not necessary for low-risk individuals or those at moderate risk desiring to initiate a moderate-intensity exercise program (40–60% maximal oxygen uptake), but are recommended for high-risk individuals and those at moderate risk desiring to initiate a vigorous exercise program (>60% maximal oxygen uptake) and for high-risk individuals desiring to initiate a moderate exercise program.[1,2] During exercise testing, physician supervision is only recommended for high-risk individuals undergoing submaximal or maximal tests, and those at moderate risk undergoing maximal tests. Although the pre-exercise and testing guidelines are less rigorous for those at low risk, exercise testing still provides valuable information for establishing a safe and effective exercise prescription[2] (see Figure 3.3). A comprehensive physical fitness testing

Box 3.1

Sample Physician Referral Form*

Dear Dr. ______________________________________,

Your patient ________________________ would like to begin a program of exercise and/or sports activity at

____

(Name of health/fitness facility)

After reviewing his/her responses to our cardiovascular screening questionnaire, we would appreciate your medical opinion and recommendations concerning his/her participation in exercise/sports activity. Please provide the following information and return this form to:

____

(Name)

____

(Address)

____

(Telephone, fax)

1. Are there specific concerns or conditions our staff should be aware of before this individual engages in exercise/sports activity at our facility? Yes/No If yes, please specify:

   ____

2. If this individual has completed an exercise test, please provide the following:
   a. Date of test: ____________________
   b. A copy of the final exercise test report and interpretation
   c. Your specific recommendations for exercise training, including heart rate limits during exercise:

   ____

3. Please provide the following information so that we may contact you if we have any further questions:

   ____ I AGREE to the participation of this individual in exercise/sports activity at your health/fitness facility.

   ____ I DO NOT AGREE that this individual is a candidate to exercise at your health/fitness facility because:

   ____

Physician's signature ____

Physician's name ____

Address ____

Telephone/Fax ____

Thank you for your help.

Must be accompanied by a medical release form.

Source: American College of Sports Medicine and American Heart Association. Recommendations for cardiovascular screening, staffing, and emergency policies at health/fitness facilities. *Med Sci Sports Exerc* 30:1009–1018, 1998. Used with permission.

battery is recommended with body composition, aerobic fitness, and muscular fitness tests to help plan a total fitness exercise program.[2]

In general, most individuals, except for those with known serious disease, can begin a moderate exercise program such as walking without a medical evaluation or graded exercise test. Whenever people are in doubt about their own personal health and safety while exercising, a medical evaluation is recommended. Diagnostic exercise testing is not recommended as a routine screening procedure in adults who have no evidence of heart disease (See Figure 3.4). As emphasized earlier in this chapter, risk of serious medical complications during exercise is low unless an individual is at high risk for cardiovascular disease. The celebrated exercise physiologist Dr. Per Olaf Astrand has emphasized that

Box 3.2

Sample Authorization for Release of Medical Information

1. I hereby authorize ______________________ to release the following information from the medical record of:

____
(*Patient's name*)

____
(*Address*)

______________________ ______________________
(*Telephone*) (*Date of birth*)

2. Information to be released (*if specific treatment dates are not indicated, information from the most recent visit will be released*):

____ Exercise test

____ Most recent history and physical exam

____ Most recent clinic visit

____ Consultations

____ Laboratory results (specify) ______________________

____ Other (specify) ______________________

3. Information to be released to:

Name of person/organization ______________________

Address ______________________

Telephone ______________________

4. Purpose of disclosure information: ______________________

5. I do not give permission for disclosure or redisclosure of this information other than that specified above.

6. I request that this consent become invalid 90 days from the date I sign it or ______________________.

I understand that this consent can be revoked at any time except to the extent that disclosure made in good faith has already occurred in reliance of this consent.

7. Patient's signature ______________________ Date ____________

Witness ______________________
(*Please print*)

Signature ______________________

Source: American College of Sports Medicine and American Heart Association. Recommendations for cardiovascular screening, staffing, and emergency policies at health/fitness facilities. *Med Sci Sports Exerc* 30:1009–1018, 1998. Used with permission.

Anyone who is in doubt about the condition of his health should consult his physician. But as a general rule, moderate activity is less harmful to the health than inactivity. You could also put it this way: A medical examination is more urgent for those who plan to remain inactive than for those who intend to get into good physical shape.

Contraindications for Exercise and Exercise Testing

Although most people in the United States can safely undergo exercise testing and prescription, there are some who should not exercise. The risks for such people outweigh the benefits. The ACSM has established contraindications for exercise and exercise testing in out-of-hospital settings.[2] A

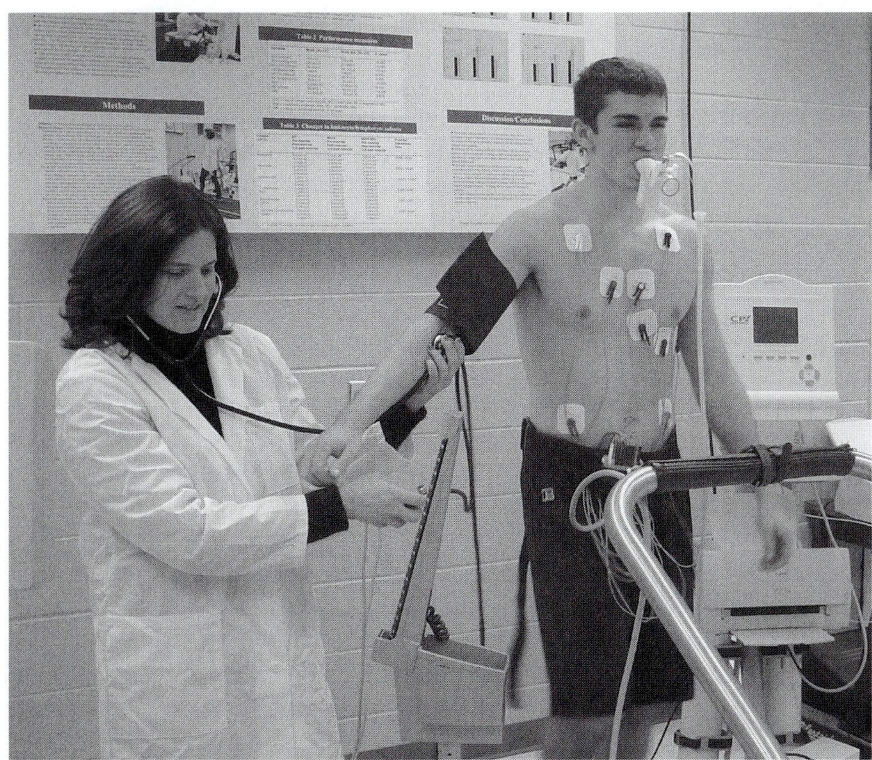

Figure 3.3 For people of all ages, information from the maximal graded exercise test is valuable in establishing an effective and safe exercise prescription.

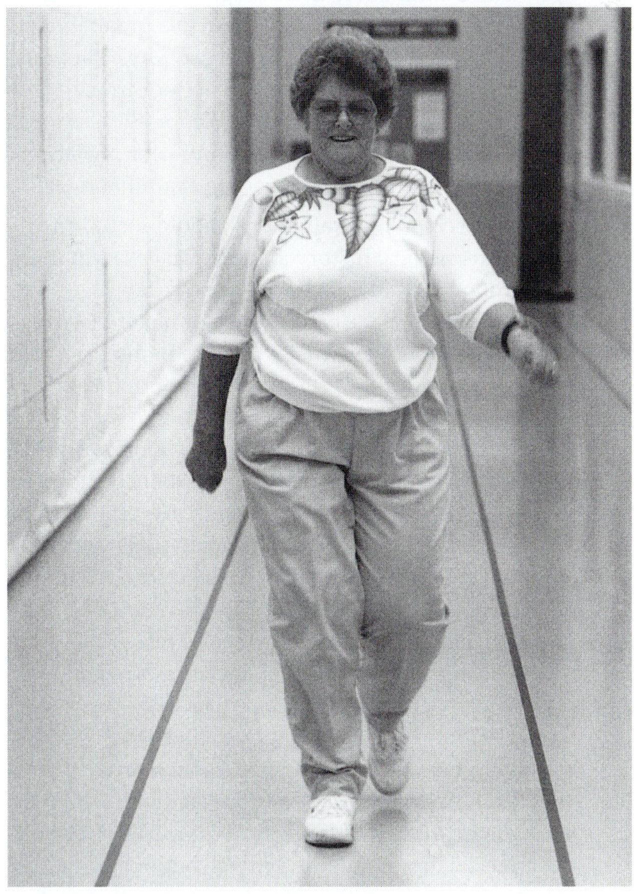

Figure 3.4 For individuals at increased risk without symptoms, an exercise test or medical evaluation may not be necessary if moderate exercise is undertaken gradually, with appropriate guidance.

contraindication means that most experts would agree that it is inadvisable for the individual to be exercise tested or to engage in active exercise. These contraindications should be diagnosed only by medical doctors. The exercise leader should draw the attention of the attending physician to this ACSM contraindication listing (summarized in Table 3.1).

CARDIOVASCULAR SCREENING OF COMPETITIVE ATHLETES

An average of 12–20 athletes, most of them high school students, die suddenly each year from congenital heart defects that are not detected during normal physical examinations.[9–15] About a third of the cases of sudden cardiac death are caused by a congenital heart defect called hypertrophic cardiomyopathy (thickened heart muscle), with the next most frequent cause being congenital coronary anomalies.

In the United States, there are nearly 10–12 million scholastic athletes. Although most states require a regular physical once every 1 or 2 years for these athletes, the cost for the more sensitive tests (e.g., two-dimensional echocardiography) that would detect heart defects ranges from $400 to $2,000 a screening. However, even with echocardiography, some athletes are incorrectly classified (e.g., false-positive or false-negative).[9]

The sudden death of a young athlete is tragic, but the financial, ethical, medical, and legal issues involved in preparticipation screening have created huge barriers. In 1996, the AHA published a consensus statement on

TABLE 3.1 Contraindications to Exercise Testing

Absolute

- A recent significant change in the resting ECG suggesting significant ischemia, recent myocardial infarction (within 2 days) or other acute cardiac event
- Unstable angina
- Uncontrolled cardiac arrhythmias causing symptoms or hemodynamic compromise
- Severe symptomatic aortic stenosis
- Uncontrolled symptomatic heart failure
- Acute pulmonary embolus or pulmonary infarction
- Acute myocarditis or pericarditis
- Suspected or known dissecting aneurysm
- Acute systemic infection accompanied by fever, body aches, or swollen lymph glands

Relative*

- Left main coronary stenosis
- Moderate stenotic valvular heart disease
- Electrolyte abnormalities (e.g., hypokalemia, hypomagnesemia)
- Severe arterial hypertension (i.e., systolic BP of >200 mm Hg and/or a diastolic BP of >110 mm Hg) at rest
- Tachyarrhythmias or bradyarrhythmias
- Hypertrophic cardiomyopathy and other forms of outflow tract obstruction
- Neuromuscular, musculoskeletal, or rheumatoid disorders that are exacerbated by exercise
- High-degree atrioventricular block
- Ventricular aneurysm
- Uncontrolled metabolic disease (e.g., diabetes, thyrotoxicosis, or myxedema)
- Chronic infectious disease (e.g., mononucleosis, hepatitis, AIDS)
- Mental or physical impairment leading to inability to exercise adequately.

*Relative contraindications can be superseded if benefits outweigh risks of exercise. In some instances, these individuals can be exercised with caution and/or using low-level end points, especially if they are asymptomatic at rest.

Source: American College of Sports Medicine. *ACSM's Guidelines for Graded Exercise Testing and Prescription* (7th ed.). Philadelphia: Lippincott Williams & Wilkins, 2006. (Used with permission.)

this issue from a panel of experts.[9] Here are the key recommendations:

1. "The AHA recommends that some form of preparticipation cardiovascular screening for high school and collegiate athletes is justifiable and compelling, based on ethical, legal, and medical grounds."[9] Although such tests as 12-lead electrocardiography, echocardiography, or graded exercise testing improve detection of cardiovascular disease in large populations of young or older athletes, the AHA expert panel concluded that "it is not prudent to recommend routine use" of these tests because of practical and cost-efficiency considerations.
2. "Consequently, we conclude that a complete and careful personal and family history and physical examination designed to identify (or raise suspicion of) those cardiovascular lesions known to cause sudden death or disease progression in young athletes is the best available and most practical approach to screening populations of competitive sports participants, regardless of age. Such cardiovascular screening is an obtainable objective and should be mandatory for all athletes. We recommend that both a history and a physical examination be performed before participation in organized high school (grades 9 through 12) and collegiate sports. Screening should then be repeated every 2 years. In intervening years an interim history should be obtained."[9] The AHA panel emphasized that because states vary so much in their screening standards and procedures, "we also recommend developing a national standard for preparticipation medical evaluations."
3. "We strongly recommend that athletic screening be performed by a healthcare worker with the requisite training, medical skills, and background to reliably obtain a detailed cardiovascular history, perform a physical examination, and recognize heart disease."[9] The AHA panel urged that "while it is preferable that such an individual be a licensed physician, this may not always be feasible, and under certain circumstances it may be acceptable for an appropriately trained registered nurse or physician assistant to perform the screening examination."
4. "Athletic screening evaluations should include a complete medical history and physical examination, including brachial artery blood pressure measurement."[9] The cardiovascular history (with input from both the athletes and the parents) should include key questions designed to determine (1) prior occurrence of exertional chest pain/discomfort or syncope/near-syncope, as well as excessive, unexpected, and unexplained shortness of breath or fatigue associated with exercise; (2) past detection of a heart murmur or increased systemic blood pressure; and (3) family history of premature death (sudden or otherwise), or significant disability from cardiovascular disease in close relative(s) younger than 50 years old or specific knowledge of the occurrence of certain conditions (e.g., hypertrophic cardiomyopathy, dilated cardiomyopathy, long QT syndrome, Marfan syndrome, or clinically important arrhythmias).

   The cardiovascular physical examination should emphasize (but not necessarily be limited to) (1) precordial auscultation in both the supine and standing positions to identify, in particular, heart murmurs consistent with dynamic left ventricular outflow obstruction; (2) assessment of the femoral artery pulses to exclude coarctation of the aorta; (3) search for and recognition of any of the physical stigmata of Marfan syndrome; and (4) brachial blood pressure measurement in the sitting position. When cardiovascular abnormalities are identified or suspected, the athlete should be referred to a cardiovascular specialist for further evaluation or confirmation. See Box 3.3 for a sample form that can be used for the preparticipation physical evaluation.[14]

INFORMED CONSENT

Like it or not, we live in an increasingly litigious society. Today's exercise program director, recreation administrator, or exercise testing program director is much more likely to be sued than his or her predecessors. In general, legal claims against exercise professionals are based on either alleged violations of contract law or tort principles.[2,5] A legal contract is a promise or performance bargained for and given in exchange for another. Most tort claims affecting the exercise professional are based on allegations of either negligence or malpractice, and commonly involve the following:[2,16–20]

- Failure to monitor an exercise test properly
- Failure to evaluate physical impairments competently
- Failure to prescribe a safe exercise intensity or program
- Failure to provide appropriate supervision
- Rendition of advice later construed to represent medical diagnosis
- Failure to refer participants to physician
- Failure to respond adequately to an untoward event
- Failure to disclose certain information in the informed-consent process

By law, any subject, patient, or client who is exposed to possible physical, psychological, or social injury must give informed consent prior to participation in a program.[2,5] *Informed consent* can be defined as the knowing consent of an individual or that person's legally authorized representative, with free power of choice and the absence of undue inducement or any element of force, fraud, deceit, duress, or other form of constraint or coercion.

The subject should read the informed-consent form and then sign it in the presence of a witness, indicating that the document has been read and consent given to participation under the described conditions. The consent form should be written so as to be easily understood by each participant, in the language in which the person is fluent.

Separate forms should be used for diagnostic exercise testing and for the exercise program itself (see Figures 3.5 and 3.6 for sample forms). No sample form should be adopted unless approved by local legal counsel. The following items should be included in the informed-consent form:[2,5]

1. A general statement of the background of the program and objectives
2. A fair explanation of the procedures to be followed
3. A description of any and all risks attendant to the procedures
4. A description of the benefits that can reasonably be expected
5. An offer to answer any of the subject's queries
6. An instruction that the subject, client, or patient is free to withdraw consent and to discontinue participation in the program at any time without prejudice to the person
7. An instruction that in the case of questionnaires and interviews, the participant is free to refuse to answer specific items or questions
8. An explanation of the procedures to be taken to ensure the confidentiality of the information derived from the participant

While it should be understood that execution of an informed-consent form does not protect the exercise or medical director from legal action, if the program is in accordance with established guidelines and run by a qualified staff, and the participant voluntarily assumes risk as outlined in the consent form, the possibility of legal action is minimized.[2,5]

HEALTH/FITNESS FACILITY STANDARDS AND GUIDELINES

In 1997, the ACSM established six standards and nearly 500 guidelines for health/fitness facilities, which have had a rather dramatic effect on the industry.[5,20] These standards should be regarded as a benchmark of competency that probably will be used in a court of law to assess performance and service.[20] In its 211-page book, the ACSM has provided an extensive list of guidelines for physical plant safety, effective signage, organizational structure and professional staffing, user screening, emergency and safety procedures, external grounds, the control desk, laundry room, locker rooms, fitness testing and wellness areas, exercise classrooms, pool areas, and specialty areas (e.g., the spa, physical therapy area, climbing walls).[5]

ACSM has established "user screening" guidelines given by the ACSM for health/fitness facilities. Preactivity screening should be conducted for all users of health/fitness facilities using ACSM guidelines. Informed consent should also be obtained (Figures 3.5 and 3.6). In regard to staffing, the ACSM has recommended that "each person who has supervisory responsibility for a physical activity program or area at a facility must have demonstrable professional competence in that physical activity program or area."[5] The ACSM defines demonstrable professional competence as "some combination of education and professional experience that would be recognized by

Box 3.3

Sample Preparticipation Physical Evaluation Form

Preparticipation Physical Evaluation

Date of examination ____________
Name ____________ Sex ______ Age ______ Date of birth ____________
Grade ______ School ____________ Sport(s) ____________
Address ____________ Phone ____________
Personal physician ____________
In case of emergency, contact:
Name ____________ Relationship ____________ Phone (H) ____________ (W) ____________

Explain "Yes" answers below

Circle questions you don't know the answers to. **Yes** **No**

1. Has a doctor ever denied or restricted your participation in sports for any reason? ☐ ☐
2. Do you have an ongoing medical condition (like diabetes or asthma)? ☐ ☐
3. Are you currently taking any prescription or nonprescription (over-the-counter) medicines or pills? ☐ ☐
4. Do you have allergies to medicines, pollens, foods, or stinging insects? ☐ ☐
5. Have you ever passed out or nearly passed out DURING exercise? ☐ ☐
6. Have you ever passed out or nearly passed out AFTER exercise? ☐ ☐
7. Have you ever had discomfort, pain, or pressure in your chest during exercise? ☐ ☐
8. Does your heart race or skip beats during exercise? ☐ ☐
9. Has a doctor ever told you that you have (check all that apply):
   ☐ High blood pressure ☐ A heart murmur
   ☐ High cholesterol ☐ A heart infection
10. Has a doctor ever ordered a test for your heart? (for example, ECG, echocardiogram) ☐ ☐
11. Has anyone in your family died for no apparent reason? ☐ ☐
12. Does anyone in your family have a heart problem? ☐ ☐
13. Has any family member or relative died of heart problems or of sudden death before age 50? ☐ ☐
14. Does anyone in your family have Marfan syndrome? ☐ ☐
15. Have you ever spent the night in a hospital? ☐ ☐
16. Have you ever had surgery? ☐ ☐
17. Have you ever had an injury, like a sprain, muscle or ligament tear, or tendinitis, that caused you to miss a practice or game? If yes, circle affected area below: ☐ ☐
18. Have you had any broken or fractured bones or dislocated joints? If yes, circle below: ☐ ☐
19. Have you had a bone or joint injury that required x-rays, MRI, CT, surgery, injections, rehabilitation, physical therapy, a brace, a cast, or crutches? If yes, circle below: ☐ ☐

Head	Neck	Shoulder	Upper arm	Elbow	Forearm	Hand/ fingers	Chest
Upper back	Lower back	Hip	Thigh	Knee	Calf/ shin	Ankle	Foot/ toes

20. Have you ever had a stress fracture? ☐ ☐
21. Have you been told that you have or have had an x-ray for atlantoaxial (neck) instability? ☐ ☐
22. Do you regularly use a brace or assistive device? ☐ ☐
23. Has a doctor ever told you that you have asthma or allergies? ☐ ☐

Yes **No**

24. Do you cough, wheeze, or have difficulty breathing during or after exercise? ☐ ☐
25. Is there anyone in your family who has asthma? ☐ ☐
26. Have you ever used an inhaler or taken asthma medicine? ☐ ☐
27. Were you born without or are you missing a kidney, an eye, a testicle, or any other organ? ☐ ☐
28. Have you had infectious mononucleosis (mono) within the last month? ☐ ☐
29. Do you have any rashes, pressure sores, or other skin problems? ☐ ☐
30. Have you had a herpes skin infection? ☐ ☐
31. Have you ever had a head injury or concussion? ☐ ☐
32. Have you been hit in the head and been confused or lost your memory? ☐ ☐
33. Have you ever had a seizure? ☐ ☐
34. Do you have headaches with exercise? ☐ ☐
35. Have you ever had numbness, tingling, or weakness in your arms or legs after being hit or falling? ☐ ☐
36. Have you ever been unable to move your arms or legs after being hit or falling? ☐ ☐
37. When exercising in the heat, do you have severe muscle cramps or become ill? ☐ ☐
38. Has a doctor told you that you or someone in your family has sickle cell trait or sickle cell disease? ☐ ☐
39. Have you had any problems with your eyes or vision? ☐ ☐
40. Do you wear glasses or contact lenses? ☐ ☐
41. Do you wear protective eyewear, such as goggles or a face shield? ☐ ☐
42. Are you happy with your weight? ☐ ☐
43. Are you trying to gain or lose weight? ☐ ☐
44. Has anyone recommended you change your weight or eating habits? ☐ ☐
45. Do you limit or carefully control what you eat? ☐ ☐
46. Do you have any concerns that you would like to discuss with a doctor? ☐ ☐

FEMALES ONLY

47. Have you ever had a menstrual period? ☐ ☐
48. How old were you when you had your first menstrual period? ______
49. How many periods have you had in the last 12 months? ______

Explain "Yes" answers here: ____________

____
____
____
____
____
____

I hereby state that, to the best of my knowledge, my answers to the above questions are complete and correct.

Signature of athlete ____________ Signature of parent/guardian ____________ Date ______

(continued)

Box 3.3

Sample Preparticipation Physical Evaluation Form *(continued)*

Preparticipation Physical Evaluation

Name ______________________________ Date of birth ______________

Height ______ Weight ______ % Body fat (optional) ______ Pulse ______ Blood pressure ___/___ (___/___, ___/___)

Vision R 20/ ______ L 20/ ______ Corrected: Y N Pupils: Equal ______ Unequal ______

Follow-Up Questions on More Sensitive Issues	**Yes**	**No**
1. Do you feel stressed out or under a lot of pressure?	☐	☐
2. Do you ever feel so sad or hopeless that you stop doing some of your usual activities for more than a few days?	☐	☐
3. Do you feel safe?	☐	☐
4. Have you ever tried cigarette smoking, even 1 or 2 puffs? Do you currently smoke?	☐	☐
5. During the past 30 days, did you use chewing tobacco, snuff, or dip?	☐	☐
6. During the past 30 days, have you had at least 1 drink of alcohol?	☐	☐
7. Have you ever taken steroid pills or shots without a doctor's prescription?	☐	☐
8. Have you ever taken any supplements to help you gain or lose weight or improve your performance?	☐	☐
9. Questions from the Youth Risk Behavior Survey (http://www.cdc.gov/HealthYouth/yrbs/index.htm) on guns, seatbelts, unprotected sex, domestic violence, drugs, etc.		

Notes: ______________________________

	Normal	Abnormal Findings	Initials*
MEDICAL			
Appearance			
Eyes/ears/nose/throat			
Hearing			
Lymph nodes			
Heart			
Murmurs			
Pulses			
Lungs			
Abdomen			
Genitourinary (males only)†			
Skin			
MUSCULOSKELETAL			
Neck			
Back			
Shoulder/arm			
Elbow/forearm			
Wrist/hand/fingers			
Hip/thigh			
Knee			
Leg/ankle			
Foot/toes			

*Multiple-examiner set-up only.

†Having a third party present is recommended for the genitourinary examination.

Notes: ______________________________

Name of physician (print/type) ______________________ **Date** __________

Address ______________________ **Phone** __________

Signature of physician ______________________, **MD or DO**

Source: Reprinted from the Preparticipation Evaluation (monograph) Third Edition. Leawood, Kansas: American Academy of Family Physicians, American Academy of Pediatrics, American College of Sports Medicine (ACSM), American Medical Society for Sports Medicine, American Orthopaedic Society for Sports Medicine, American Osteopathic Academy of Sports Medicine, Phys Sportsmed © 2005 The McGraw-Hill Companies.

Testing Objectives: I understand that the tests that are about to be administered to me are for the purpose of determining my physical fitness status, including heart, lung, and blood vessel capacities for whole body activity, body composition (ratio of body fat to muscle, bone, and water), muscular endurance and strength, and joint flexibility.

Explanation of Procedures: I understand that the tests that I will undergo will be performed on a treadmill, bicycle, or steps. The tests are designed to increase the demands on the heart, lung, and blood vessel system. This increase in effort will continue until exhaustion or other symptoms prohibit further exercise. During the test, heart rate, blood pressure, and electrocardiographic data will be periodically measured. Body composition will be determined through use of skinfolds or underwater weighing to determine levels of body fat versus fat-free weight. Muscular endurance and strength will be determined through the use of body calisthenics and/or equipment. The sit-and-reach test will be used to determine the flexibility of the hip joint.

Description of Potential Risks: I understand that there exists the possibility that certain abnormal changes may occur during the testing. These changes could include abnormal heart beats, abnormal blood pressure response, various muscle and joint strains or injuries, and in rare instances, heart attack. Professional care throughout the entire testing process should provide appropriate precaution against such problems.

Benefits to Be Expected: I understand that the results of these tests will aid in determining my physical fitness status and in determining potential health hazards. These results will facilitate a better individualized exercise prescription.

I have read the foregoing information and understand it. Questions concerning these procedures have been answered to my satisfaction. I also understand that I am free to deny answering any questions during the evaluation process, or to withdraw consent and discontinue participating in any procedures. I have also been informed that the information derived from these tests is confidential and will not be disclosed to anyone other than my physician or others who are involved in my care or exercise prescription, without my permission. However, I am in agreement that information from these tests not identifiable to me can be used for research purposes.

Participant's Signature ______________________________ Date ________________

Witness Signature ___________________________________ Date ________________

Figure 3.5 Consent to graded exercise testing and other physical fitness tests.

General Statement of Program Objectives and Procedures: I understand that this physical fitness program may include exercises to build the cardiorespiratory system (heart and lungs), the musculoskeletal system (muscle endurance and strength, and flexibility), and to improve body composition (decrease of body fat in individuals needing to lose fat, with an increase in weight of muscle and bone). Exercises may include aerobic activities (treadmill walking/running, bicycle riding, rowing machine exercise, group aerobic activity, swimming, and other such activities), calisthenics, and weight lifting to improve muscular strength and endurance, and flexibility exercises to improve joint range of motion.

Description of Potential Risks: I understand that the reaction of the heart, lung, and blood vessel system to such exercise cannot always be predicted with accuracy. I know there is a risk of certain abnormal changes occurring during or following exercise, which may include abnormalities of blood pressure or heart rate, ineffective functioning of the heart, and in rare instances, heart attacks. Use of the weight-lifting equipment , and engaging in heavy body calesthenics, can lead to musculoskeletal strains, pain, and injury if adequate warm-up, gradual progression, and safety procedures are not followed. Safety procedures are listed on the wall of the fitness facility. In addition, trained staff members will be supervising during all times to help ensure that these risks are minimized. The staff members are trained in CPR and first aid and regularly practice emergency procedures. Equipment is inspected and maintained on a regular basis.

Description of Potential Benefits: I understand that a program of regular exercise for the heart and lungs, muscles, and joints has many associated benefits. These may include a decrease in body fat, improvement in blood fats and blood pressure, improvement in psychological function, and a decrease in risk of heart disease.

I have read the foregoing information and understand it. Any questions that may have occurred to me have been answered to my satisfaction. I understand that I am free to withdraw from this program without prejudice at any time I desire. I am also free to decline answering specific items or questions during interviews or when filling out questionnaires. The information that is obtained will be treated as privileged and confidential and will not be released or revealed to any person other than my physician without my express written consent. The information obtained, however, may be used for a statistical or scientific purpose with my right of privacy retained.

Signature of Participant ______________________________ Date______________

Signature of Witness ________________________________ Date _____________

Figure 3.6 Consent for physical fitness programs.

both the industry and the public at large as representing a relatively high level of competence and credibility."[5] Within the health and fitness industry, an indication of professional competence for four different program areas includes the following:

1. *Fitness director.* Four-year college education in a health- or fitness-related field or substantially equivalent work experience; certification from a nationally recognized association or organization in the health and fitness industry; CPR certification and first-aid training; 1 year or more of work experience in the fitness field
2. *Aerobics coordinator; physical activity instructor.* Two-year college education in a health- or fitness-related field or substantially equivalent work experience; certification from a nationally recognized association or organization in the health and fitness industry; CPR certification and first-aid training
3. *Aquatics director.* Certification in advanced lifesaving; certification in water-safety instruction; at least 1 year of work experience in aquatics; pool-operation training; CPR certification and first-aid training
4. *Fitness testing staff.* Four-year college education in a health- or fitness-related field or related exercise-science field; current professional certification from a nationally recognized association or organization in the health and fitness industry; CPR certification and first-aid training

(See the Sports Medicine Insight and Box 3.4, at the end of this chapter, for more information on professional certification.)

All health/fitness facilities must be prepared to handle situations that arise unexpectedly and must have a comprehensive emergency plan that provides guidelines for the staff. Emergency plan guidelines, according to the ACSM, include the following:[5]

1. Provisions for physical access to all areas of the facility, as well as a plan for the handling and disposition of bystanders
2. Provisions for documenting all events to provide a basis for the orderly evaluation of a situation after it occurs and the subsequent follow-up actions that may be taken
3. Provisions for securing and using specific protocols and emergency supplies, including the development of a written emergency plan, listing specific steps that the staff should perform to satisfy the basic emergency goals
4. Provisions in an emergency plan for contact and interaction with a predetermined community emergency resource

CONCEPTS AND PURPOSES IN PHYSICAL FITNESS TESTING

Reduced to its simplest terms, the function of measurement is to determine status.[2,22–24] Ideally, status should be determined before individualized exercise counseling is conducted. The information from the physical fitness testing can be used along with the medical test information to better meet the individual's needs.

When conducting physical fitness tests, several important test criteria should be considered:[22–24]

1. *Validity.* Refers to the degree to which the test measures what it was designed to measure; a valid test is one that measures accurately what it is used to measure.
2. *Reliability.* Deals with how consistently a certain element is measured by the particular test; concerned with the repeatability of the test. If a person is measured two separate times by the same tester or by two different people, the results should be close to the same.
3. *Norms.* Represent the achievement level of a particular group to which the measured scores can be compared; norms provide a useful basis for interpretation and evaluation of test results.
4. *Economy.* Refers to ease of administration, the use of inexpensive equipment, the limitation of time needed to administer the test, and the simplicity of the test so that the person taking it can easily understand the purpose and results.

So in other words, a good physical fitness test accurately measures what it is supposed to measure, can be consistently used by different people, produces results that can be compared to a data set, and is relatively inexpensive, simple, and easy to administer.

In a complete physical fitness program, testing of participants before, during, and after participation is important for several reasons:[2,22–24]

1. To assess current fitness levels (both strengths and weaknesses)
2. To identify special needs for individualized counseling
3. To evaluate progress
4. To motivate and educate

Test results are best viewed as a means to an end, not as an end in themselves. In other words, the testing process should be used to help individuals know more about themselves so that appropriate health and fitness goals can be established. Expensive, elaborate, and lengthy testing is seldom needed (except in research) and can be distractive (Figure 3.7). Scores on the various items of the simple and inexpensive test batteries noted at the end of this chapter are adequate to identify the strengths and weaknesses of

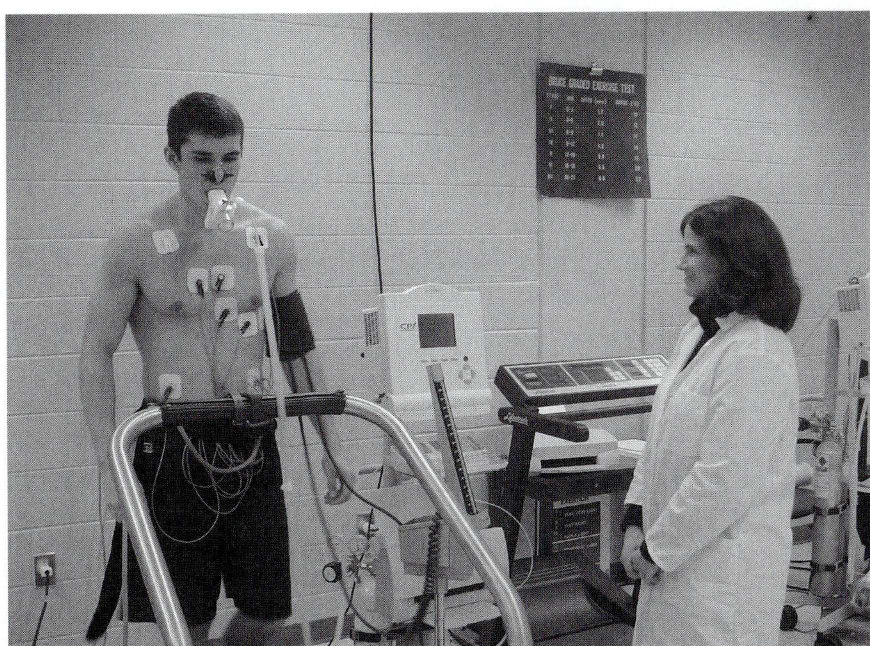

Figure 3.7 Expensive and elaborate testing such as direct measurement of $\dot{V}O_{2max}$ during graded exercise testing is seldom needed for the average fitness participant.

participants, so that special attention can be given to individualized goals and objectives. If anything, it is better to undertest than overtest so that more time and attention can be given to counseling and guiding each participant through the exercise program.

PHYSICAL FITNESS TESTING BATTERIES

The very process of administering a fitness test draws attention to what is considered worthy of special attention in a person's lifestyle. The test results can therefore be used to educate, motivate, and stimulate interest in exercise and other health-related topics.

Recommended Order for Fitness-Evaluation Tests

The evaluation procedure has a recommended order for both safety and efficiency. In general, it is best for the participant to fill out the medical/health status questionnaire at home before coming to the testing center. The testing batteries listed at the end of this chapter usually take only about 1 hour.

Precise instructions should be given to the participants before they come to the testing site. In general they should come in exercise attire (and bring a swimsuit if necessary); avoid eating or drinking for 3 hours before the test; avoid alcohol, tobacco, and coffee for at least 3 hours before the test; avoid exercise the day of the test; try to get a good night's sleep; and bring the medical/health status questionnaire.

If blood is to be analyzed, alcohol consumption and vigorous exercise should be avoided for 24 hours beforehand, and a 12-hour fast is recommended. Diabetics should be allowed to keep their dietary habits and injections of insulin as regular as possible. According to the ACSM, patients should continue their medication regimen on their usual schedule so that the exercise test responses will be consistent with responses expected during exercise training.[2]

The organization of the testing session is important. It should begin with the quiet, resting tests (heart rate, blood pressure, blood drawing, all after a 5-minute rest). Body composition measures should follow next, and then the graded exercise test for cardiorespiratory endurance. Finally, the musculoskeletal tests should be given.

If musculoskeletal tests precede the graded exercise test, the heart rate can be elevated, giving false information on fitness status, especially when submaximal tests are conducted.

Immediate feedback and counseling should follow the testing. Follow-up evaluations should be conducted after 3–6 months, after 1 year of training, and yearly thereafter.[2,22–24]

Health-Related Fitness Testing Batteries

The YMCA, Canadian Society for Exercise Physiology, American Fitness Alliance, and President's Council on Physical Fitness and Sports have each developed physical fitness testing batteries that follow the recommended criteria of testing outlined in this chapter. They are valid, reliable, and economical, and they have sound norms. In addition, most follow a comprehensive health-related fitness approach, testing each of the five components.[25]

The norms for the various tests within these batteries are found in Appendix A. Descriptions of how to conduct the tests are found in the following chapters of this book. A brief outline of each testing battery is listed in this section.

YMCA

The YMCA physical fitness testing battery for adults is administered in the following order:[26]

- Standing height
- Weight
- Resting heart rate
- Resting blood pressure
- Skinfold tests for men and women (at three or four sites)
- Submaximal cycle test for cardiorespiratory endurance; 3-minute step test for mass testing
- Sit-and-reach test (for flexibility)
- Bench-press test (35 pounds, women; 80 pounds, men) at a rate of 30 times per minute for muscular endurance and strength
- Timed (1 minute) sit-ups for abdominal muscular endurance; or abdominal curl-ups

The YMCA also has a testing manual for youths:[27]

- Skinfolds (triceps and calf)
- Run (1 mile)
- Sit-and-reach test (for flexibility)
- Modified pull-ups
- Curl-ups (40 maximum)

Canadian Physical Activity, Fitness & Lifestyle Appraisal (CPAFLA)

In 1981, the Canada Fitness Survey was initiated and funded by Fitness and Amateur Sport in Canada.[7] A major objective of the survey was to provide reliable statistics on physical activity patterns and fitness levels of the Canadian population. The survey sample consisted of 11,884 households that had been identified by Statistics Canada and that were located in urban and rural areas of each province. Members of these households, 15,519 between the ages of 7 and 69, undertook the Canadian Standardized Test of Fitness; this was the largest and most comprehensive study of physical activity and fitness ever undertaken. In 1996 and 2003, these data were repackaged by the Canadian Society for Exercise Physiology as the "Canadian Physical Activity, Fitness & Lifestyle Appraisal" (CPAFLA).[7] (See Appendix A for norms.) The CPAFLA is administered in the following order (after pretest screening using the PAR-Q and a consent form):[7]

- Resting heart rate
- Resting blood pressure
- Standing height
- Body mass (weight)
- Waist girth
- Skinfolds (triceps, biceps, subscapular, iliac crest, medial calf)
- Canadian aerobic fitness step test
- Grip strength (right and left hands)
- Push-ups
- Trunk-forward flexion
- Partial curl-ups
- Vertical jump

AAHPERD: Health-Related Fitness Test for College Students

AAHPERD released the results of its testing program for college students in 1985.[28] The study population consisted of 5,158 young adults in colleges from all geographic regions of the United States. The data for the study were collected under the supervision of 24 coinvestigators. The test items in order are as follows (see Appendix A for norms):

- Two-site skinfold test (triceps and subscapular)
- Mile run or 9-minute run for cardiorespiratory endurance
- Sit-and-reach test for flexibility
- Timed (1 minute) sit-ups for abdominal muscular endurance

FITNESSGRAM®

FITNESSGRAM® is a youth fitness testing system developed by the Cooper Institute for Aerobics Research and now a part of the testing program of the American Fitness Alliance.[29–32] The test items are health related and use criterion-referenced standards for each age and sex group. These standards are thought to represent minimum levels of performance that most often correlate with health. Physical Best is a companion product to FITNESSGRAM®, and is the educational component of a comprehensive health-related physical fitness education program sponsored by the American Fitness Alliance (AAHPERD, The Cooper Institute, and Human Kinetics).[29–32]

Recommended test items of the FITNESSGRAM® include:

- Aerobic capacity (select one)

  The pacer. A 20-meter progressive, multistage shuttle run set to music

  One-mile walk/run.

  Walk test. Available for secondary students

- Body composition (select one)

  Percent body fat. Calculated from triceps and calf skinfold measurements

  Body mass index. Calculated from height and weight

- Muscle strength, endurance, and flexibility

  Abdominal strength. Curl-up test

  Trunk extensor strength and flexibility. Trunk lift

  Upper Body Strength (select one). 90-degree push-up, pull-up, flexed arm hang, modified pull-up

  Flexibility (select one). Back-saver sit-and-reach, shoulder stretch

The Brockport Physical Fitness Test is a health-related test developed specifically for youths with physical and mental disabilities.[33] Go to the American Fitness Alliance Internet site for more information: www.americanfitness.net

The President's Challenge

The President's Council on Physical Fitness and Sports School Population Fitness Survey was conducted in 1985. Data were collected to assess the physical fitness status of American public school children ages 6–17. A four-stage probability sample was designed to select approximately 19,200 boys and girls from 57 school districts and 187 schools.

Data from this survey provide the norms for the current Presidential Physical Fitness Award Program, or "President's Challenge" (about 3 million awards distributed each year).[34] The test battery consists of five required items:

1. *Curl-ups.* A test of muscular endurance: Perform for 1 minute, knees bent, arms crossed, hands on opposite shoulders, and feet anchored by a partner. Partial curl-ups are allowed as an option to curl-ups (knees bent, feet not anchored, reach fingertips to knees every 3 seconds).
2. *Shuttle run.* A total-body coordination test, with parallel lines marked 30 feet apart, and the students timed as they race to pick up two blocks from the distant line and run them to the starting line.
3. *One-mile run/walk.* To measure heart/lung endurance by the fastest time to cover a 1-mile distance. Alternative distances for younger children are 1/4 mile for those aged 6–9 years old.
4. *Pull-ups.* To measure upper-body strength and endurance by maximum number of pull-ups completed using either an overhand or underhand grasp of the bar. Right-angle push-ups are an optional test to pull-ups, with the body lowered until there is a 90-degree angle at the elbows, with the body and legs straight. The flexed-arm hang is another alternative test to pull-ups, with the student assuming an overhand or underhand grasp, chin above the bar, and holding this position as long as possible.
5. *V-sit reach.* To measure flexibility of the lower back and hamstrings by reaching forward in the V position, and legs held flat by a partner. The sit-and-reach test can be used as an option to the V-sit reach, using a specially constructed flexibility box.

Young people, ages 6–17, can receive one of four awards as part of the President's Challenge:

1. *Presidential Physical Fitness Award.* Score at or above the 85th percentile on all five items.
2. *National Physical Fitness Award.* Score at or above the 50th percentile on all five items.
3. *Participant Physical Fitness Award.* Attempt all five items but score below the 50th percentile on one or more of them.
4. *Health Fitness Award.* Test scores meet or exceed the specified health criteria on each of these five items—partial curl-ups, 1-mile run (or distance option), V-sit reach (or sit-and-reach), right-angle push-ups (or pull-ups), and body mass index (derived from height and weight).

SPORTS MEDICINE INSIGHT

Certification for Health and Fitness Professionals

Certification provides health/fitness professionals with public recognition of their knowledge, technical skills, and experience in their particular field. It certifies that the individual is qualified to practice in accordance with the standards deemed to be essential by the certifying body.[35,36] See Box 3.4 for a listing of organizations that provide certifications for the health/fitness industry.

The most prestigious health and fitness certification program is conducted by the American College of Sports Medicine (ACSM). This Sports Medicine Insight provides a description of the ACSM's certification program. This textbook was written to help individuals prepare for the ACSM Health/Fitness Instructor certification written and practical exams.

(continued)

SPORTS MEDICINE INSIGHT *(continued)*

Certification for Health and Fitness Professionals

ABOUT THE AMERICAN COLLEGE OF SPORTS MEDICINE

The American College of Sports Medicine has more than 20,000 international, national, and regional chapter members. The ACSM is the largest, most respected sports medicine and exercise science organization in the world.

The ACSM's mission statement reflects this goal: "The American College of Sports Medicine promotes and integrates scientific research, education, and practical applications of sports medicine and exercise science to maintain and enhance physical performance, fitness, health, and quality of life" (see www.acsm.org).

The ACSM was founded in 1954. Since that time, members have applied their knowledge, training, and dedication in sports medicine and exercise science to promote healthier lifestyles for people around the globe. Working in a wide range of medical specialties, allied health professions, and scientific disciplines, members are committed to the diagnosis, treatment, and prevention of sports-related injuries and the advancement of the science of exercise.

ACSM Certification and Registry Programs

ACSM credentialing provides the best measure of competence of sports medicine and health and fitness professionals for clients and employers. It is the most rigorous in the industry, requiring the highest level of knowledge and skill and establishing the standard for all other certifications.

ACSM Certified Personal Trainer™

The ACSM Certified Personal Trainer™ (cPT) is a fitness professional involved in developing and implementing an individualized approach to exercise leadership in healthy populations and/or those individuals with medical clearance to exercise. Using a variety of teaching techniques, the cPT is proficient in leading and demonstrating safe and effective methods of exercise by applying the fundamental principles of exercise science. The cPT is proficient in writing appropriate exercise recommendations, leading and demonstrating safe and effective methods of exercise, and motivating individuals to begin and to continue with their healthy behaviors.

The written exam is delivered in a computer-based testing format at an authorized Pearson VUE testing center. The exam contains approximately 125–150 multiple-choice questions based on KSAs (knowledge, skills, and abilities) distributed across the nine content areas.

Minimum requirements include a high school diploma or equivalent *and* a current adult CPR certification that has a practical skills examination component (such as the American Heart Association or the American Red Cross).

Recommended competencies include: (1) Demonstrate competence in the KSAs required of the cPT as listed in the upcoming new edition of *ACSM's Guidelines for Exercise Testing and Prescription.*[2] (2) Have adequate knowledge of and skill in risk factor and health status identification, fitness appraisal, and exercise prescription. (3) Demonstrate ability to incorporate suitable and innovative activities that will improve an individual's functional capacity. (4) Demonstrate the ability to effectively educate and/or communicate with individuals regarding lifestyle modification.

ACSM Health/Fitness Instructor®

The ACSM Health/Fitness Instructor® (HFI) is a professional qualified to assess, design, and implement individual and group exercise and fitness programs for apparently healthy individuals and individuals with controlled disease. The HFI is skilled in evaluating health behaviors and risk factors, conducting fitness assessments, writing appropriate exercise prescriptions, and motivating individuals to modify negative health habits and maintain positive lifestyle behaviors for health promotion. The HFI certification provides professionals with recognition of their practical experience and demonstrated competence as leaders of health and fitness programs in the university, corporate, commercial, or community settings in which their clients participate in health-promotion and fitness-related activities.

Minimum requirements include: (1) have an associate's degree or a bachelor's degree in a health-related field from a regionally accredited college or university (one is eligible to sit for the exam if the candidate is in the last term or semester of the degree program), *and* (2) possess current Adult CPR certification that has a practical skills examination component (such as the American Heart Association or the American Red Cross).

Recommended competencies include: (1) Demonstrate competence in the KSAs required of the HFI and ACSM Group Exercise Leader® as listed in *ACSM's Guidelines for Exercise Testing and Prescription.*[2] (2) Have work-related experience within the health and fitness field.

(continued)

SPORTS MEDICINE INSIGHT *(continued)*

Certification for Health and Fitness Professionals

(3) Have adequate knowledge of and skill in risk factor and health status identification, fitness appraisal, and exercise prescription. (4) Demonstrate ability to incorporate suitable and innovative activities that will improve an individual's functional capacity. (5) Demonstrate the ability to effectively educate and/or communicate with individuals regarding lifestyle modification. (6) Have knowledge of exercise science including kinesiology, functional anatomy, exercise physiology, nutrition, program administration, psychology, and injury prevention.

A 2-day workshop may be conducted in conjunction with the HFI certification examination. Workshops are neither a prerequisite for certification nor are they intended to provide the full experience and knowledge necessary for the successful completion of the examination. Workshops provide both a review of the KSAs of the HFI and a forum for the acquisition of new knowledge and skills.

Participants should have prior experience and competence in monitoring heart rate (HR) and blood pressure (BP) both at rest and during exercise. BP training sessions are typically available from the local chapter of the American Heart Association. Experience in leading an exercise class, basic counseling skills, and knowledge of functional anatomy and exercise physiology are also expected before attendance.

The practical exam consists of three 20-minute stations and evaluates knowledge, skills, and abilities in body composition and flexibility assessment and demonstration, strength and conditioning exercise demonstration, and cardiovascular fitness assessment using a cycle ergometer.

ACSM Exercise Specialist®

The Exercise Specialist® (ES) is a health-care professional certified by the ACSM to deliver a variety of exercise assessment, training, rehabilitation, risk-factor identification, and lifestyle management services to individuals with or at risk for cardiovascular, pulmonary, and metabolic disease(s). These services are typically delivered in cardiovascular/pulmonary rehabilitation programs, physicians' offices, or medical fitness centers. The ACSM Exercise Specialist® is also competent to provide exercise-related consulting for research, public health, and other clinical and nonclinical services and programs.

Minimum requirements include a bachelor's degree in an allied health field from a regionally accredited college or university, 600 hours of practical experience in a clinical exercise program (e.g., cardiac/ pulmonary rehabilitation programs; exercise testing; exercise prescription; electrocardiography; patient education and counseling; disease management of cardiac, pulmonary, and metabolic diseases; and emergency management), and current certification as a Basic Life Support Provider or CPR for the Professional Rescuer (available through the American Heart Association or the American Red Cross).

Recommended competencies include: (1) Demonstrate competence in the KSAs as listed in *ACSM's Guidelines for Exercise Testing and Prescription.*[2] (2) Have knowledge of functional anatomy, exercise physiology, pathophysiology, electrocardiography, human behavior/psychology, gerontology, graded exercise testing for healthy and diseased populations, exercise supervision/leadership, patient counseling, and emergency procedures related to exercise testing and training situations.

The workshop offered for the ES requires a certain degree of job knowledge and training in cardiopulmonary rehabilitation, exercise testing, exercise prescription, and program development for workshop participation. The program content of the ES workshop is based on a basic knowledge of exercise physiology, pathophysiology, pharmacology, electrocardiography, exercise program leadership, and counseling. The workshop serves as a review and supplements the background experience of the well-prepared participant. It is not intended to independently prepare a candidate for ES certification.

In the practical examination, each station is scored using a checklist format that contains expected or appropriate actions for each clinical problem. An overall rating of the candidate's organizational skills, techniques, and interpersonal skills contributes to the candidate's final score. The clinical problems tested include various cardiovascular, pulmonary, metabolic, and musculoskeletal conditions seen in both inpatient and outpatient settings. (See www.acsm.org for details.)

ACSM Registered Clinical Exercise Physiologist®

The Clinical Exercise Physiologist works in the application of exercise and physical activity for those clinical and pathological situations where it has been shown to provide therapeutic or functional benefit. Patients for whom services are appropriate may include, but are not limited to, those with cardiovascular, pulmonary, metabolic, immunological, inflammatory, orthopedic, and neuromuscular diseases and conditions. This list will be modified as indications and procedures of application are further developed and mature. Furthermore, the Clinical Exercise Physiologist applies exercise principles to groups such as geriatric, pediatric, or obstetric populations, and to society as a whole in preventive

(continued)

SPORTS MEDICINE INSIGHT *(continued)*

Certification for Health and Fitness Professionals

activities. The Clinical Exercise Physiologist performs exercise evaluation, exercise prescription, exercise supervision, exercise education, and exercise outcome evaluation. The practice of Clinical Exercise Physiologists should be restricted to clients who are referred by and are under the continued care of a licensed physician.

Information and Exam Registration The ACSM Registered Clinical Exercise Physiologist (RCEP) is an allied health professional who works with persons with chronic diseases and conditions for which exercise has been shown to be beneficial. The RCEP performs health, physical activity, and fitness assessments, and prescribes exercise and physical activity primarily in hospitals or other health-provider settings. The RCEP has met at least the minimum standards set by the ACSM for education, training, and experience, and has demonstrated sufficient mastery of knowledge and abilities as determined by the RCEP Board.

Minimum requirements include a master's degree in exercise science, exercise physiology, or kinesiology from a regionally accredited college or university, current certification as a Basic Life Support Provider or CPR for the Professional Rescuer (available through the American Heart Association or the American Red Cross), and 600 clinical hours with experience in each of the clinical practice areas (may be completed as part of a formal degree program in exercise physiology). (See www.acsm.org for details.)

The RCEP is an allied health professional who uses exercise and physical activity to assess and treat patients at risk of or with chronic diseases or conditions for which exercise has been shown to provide therapeutic and/or functional benefit. Patients for whom RCEP services are appropriate may include, but are not limited to, persons with cardiovascular, pulmonary, metabolic, cancerous, immunologic, inflammatory, orthopedic, musculoskeletal, neuromuscular, gynecological, and obstetrical diseases and conditions. The RCEP provides scientific, evidence-based primary and secondary preventative and rehabilitative exercise and physical activity services to populations ranging from children to older adults. The RCEP performs exercise screening, exercise testing, exercise prescription, exercise and physical activity counseling, exercise supervision, exercise and health education/promotion, and evaluation of exercise and physical activity outcome measures. The RCEP works individually and as part of an interdisciplinary team in clinical, community, and public health settings. The practice and supervision of the RCEP is guided by published professional guidelines, standards, and applicable state and federal regulations. The practice of clinical exercise physiology is restricted to patients who are referred by and are under the care of a licensed physician.

Box 3.4

Prominent Certifying Organizations in the Health/Fitness Industry

Three criteria are often used to judge whether one is qualified to assist someone on basic health, wellness, and exercise-related issues:[35,36]

1. Formal academic preparation
2. Professional experience
3. Professional certification

Many organizations offer some form of certification for health and fitness professionals. A list of the more prominent certifying organizations is presented here. Certification is recommended to gain a competitive advantage in the hiring process and to stay abreast of issues related to health and fitness.

Aerobics and Fitness Association of America (AFAA). Offers numerous types of certification (www.afaa.com).

American College of Sports Medicine (ACSM). Offers four certifications: personal trainer, health/fitness instructor exercise specialist, and registered clinical exercise physiologist (www.acsm.org).

American Council on Exercise (ACE). Offers four types of certification: group fitness, personal trainer, lifestyle and weight-management consultant, and clinical exercise specialist (www.acefitness.org).

International Sports Sciences Association (ISSA). Offers numerous types of certification (www.fitnesseducation.com).

National Dance-Exercise Instructor's Training Association (NDEITA). Offers certification for aerobics instructors and personal trainers (www.ndeita.com).

National Federation of Professional Trainers (NFPT). Offers certification in personal training (www.nfpt.com).

National Strength and Conditioning Association (NSCA). Offers certification for two groups: strength and conditioning professionals and personal trainers (www.nsca-lift.org).

Young Men's Christian Association (YMCA). Offers numerous certifications (www.ymca.net).

SUMMARY

1. For those who are at high risk for heart disease to begin with, vigorous exercise bouts can trigger fatal heart attacks. These victims tend to be men who were sedentary, over age 35 years, already had heart disease or were at high risk for it, and then exercised too hard for their fitness levels.
2. Health screening is a vital process in first identifying individuals at high risk for exercise-induced heart problems, and then referring them to appropriate medical care.
3. All facilities offering exercise equipment or services should conduct a health and cardiovascular screening of all new members and/or prospective users, regardless of age.
4. Several types of health appraisal questionnaires are available including a comprehensive medical/health questionnaire, the Physical Activity Readiness Questionnaire (PAR-Q), and the 1998 ACSM/AHA questionnaire.
5. When a medical evaluation or recommendation is advised or required, written and active communication by the exercise staff with the individual's personal physician is strongly recommended.
6. The ACSM recommends that the information gathered from the screening process be used to stratify participants into one of three risk strata: low risk, moderate risk, high risk. The ACSM and AHA recommend that participants be classified into one of three risk strata: apparently healthy (class A-1), persons at increased risk (classes A-2 and A-3), or persons with known cardiovascular disease (classes B, C, and D).
7. The depth of the medical or physical examination for any individual considering an exercise program depends on the disease risk stratification.
8. The AHA recommends that some form of preparticipation cardiovascular screening for high school and collegiate athletes is justifiable and compelling, based on ethical, legal, and medical grounds.
9. We live in an increasingly litigious society. Proper informed-consent forms and the adoption of appropriate strategies for reducing liability exposure are needed.
10. The function of measurement is to determine health and fitness status. Tests should be valid, reliable, have sound norms, and be economical in terms of money, time, and testing expertise.
11. Physical fitness tests have several purposes, including assessment of status, identification of special needs, evaluation of progress, and motivation.
12. Evaluation procedures should follow a certain order for both safety and efficiency.
13. The YMCA, Canadian Society for Exercise Physiology, American Fitness Alliance, and President's Council on Physical Fitness and Sports have developed health-related physical fitness testing batteries.

Review Questions

1. ***About ____ out of 100,000 middle-aged men die during or after exercise each year.***

   A. 6 **B.** 20 **C.** 50 **D.** 78 **E.** 97

2. ***The major cause of athletic death in high school and college each year is***

   A. Major injury
   B. Congenital cardiovascular disease
   C. Ischemic heart disease
   D. Exercise-induced stroke
   E. Cocaine-related cerebral hemorrhage

3. ***If a male 40 years of age smokes 20 cigarettes per day, has normal blood pressure, and a father who died at age 48 of a heart attack, the American College of Sports Medicine would classify that individual as:***

   A. Low risk **B.** Moderate risk **C.** High risk

4. ***Which symptom listed below is* not *suggestive of heart, lung, or metabolic disease?***

   A. Pain or discomfort in the chest or surrounding areas
   B. Headache after exercise
   C. Unaccustomed shortness of breath
   D. Dizziness or fainting
   E. Severe pain in leg muscles during walking

5. ***The American College of Sports Medicine recommends that all apparently healthy females over the threshold age of ____ years take a maximal graded exercise test before starting a vigorous exercise program.***

   A. 25 **B.** 35 **C.** 40 **D.** 55 **E.** 60

6. ***Which individual(s) described below should have a medical exam and graded exercise test prior to starting a moderate walking program?***

   A. A 60-year-old obese and sedentary woman with no symptoms of heart disease
   B. A 40-year-old male who smokes and has chest pain and difficulty breathing after climbing stairs
   C. A 55-year-old sedentary female with high blood pressure
   D. A 22-year-old male student with a father who died at age 50 from a heart attack
   E. All of the above

7. *Which risk factor listed below is **not** on the American College of Sports Medicine's list for classifying individuals prior to exercise?*

   A. Serum cholesterol > 200 mg/dl
   B. HDL cholesterol ≤ 45 mg/dl
   C. Body mass index ≥ 30 kg/m^2
   D. Systolic BP ≥ 140 or diastolic BP ≥ 90 mm Hg
   E. Family history of heart disease in parents or siblings prior to age 55 for males and age 65 for females

8. ____ *deals with how consistently a certain element is measured by a particular test, in other words, the repeatability of the test.*

   A. Validity **B.** Reliability **C.** Economy

9. *Class B in the ACSM/AHA risk stratification scheme includes which one of the following individuals?*

   A. Cardiovascular disease patient at low risk
   B. Cardiovascular disease patient at moderate-to-high risk
   C. Men >45 and women >55 years of age, no symptoms of disease, apparently healthy with no known disease, two or more cardiovascular risk factors
   D. Men <45 and women <55 years of age, no symptoms of disease, apparently healthy with no known disease, no cardiovascular risk factors

10. *Moderate exercise, according to the ACSM, is defined as less than or equal to a threshold of ____% $\dot{V}O_{2max}$*

    A. 80 **B.** 40 **C.** 60 **D.** 30 **E.** 75

11. *Individuals at moderate risk, according to the American College of Sports Medicine, are those with ____ or more major coronary risk factors.*

    A. 1 **B.** 2 **C.** 3 **D.** 4 **E.** 5

12. *When administering a physical fitness testing battery, body composition measures should come before graded exercise testing for cardiorespiratory endurance.*

    A. True **B.** False

13. *Physician supervision is recommended during exercise testing for*

    A. A low-risk male who is undergoing maximal testing
    B. A moderate-risk female who is undergoing maximal testing
    C. An individual at moderate risk undergoing submaximal testing
    D. A low-risk, 57-year-old male who is undergoing submaximal testing

14. *How many risk factors does a 55-year-old male have, according to the ACSM, if he has no family history of heart disease, does not smoke, has a blood pressure of 134/84 mm Hg, a serum cholesterol of 244 mg/dl, a sedentary lifestyle, and a body mass index of 32 kg/m^2?*

    A. 1 **B.** 2 **C.** 3 **D.** 4 **E.** 5

15. *About 12–20 athletes, most of them high school students, die suddenly each year from congenital heart defects. About a third of the cases of sudden cardiac death are caused by a congenital heart defect called*

    A. Myocardial infarction
    B. Stroke
    C. Echocardiography
    D. Hypertrophic cardiomyopathy
    E. Ischemia

Answers

1. A
2. B
3. B
4. B
5. D
6. B
7. B
8. B
9. A
10. C
11. B
12. A
13. B
14. C
15. D

REFERENCES

1. American College of Sports Medicine and American Heart Association. Recommendations for cardiovascular screening, staffing, and emergency policies at health/fitness facilities. *Med Sci Sports Exerc* 30:1009–1018, 1998.
2. American College of Sports Medicine. *ACSM's Guidelines for Graded Exercise Testing and Prescription* (7th ed.). Philadelphia: Lippincott Williams & Wilkins, 2006.
3. Maron BJ, Shirani J, Poliac LC, Mathenge R, Roberts WC, Mueller FO. Sudden death in young competitive athletes: Clinical, demographic, and pathological profiles. *JAMA* 276:199–204, 1996.
4. American Heart Association. *Heart Disease and Stroke Statistics—2005 update.* Dallas: American Heart Association, 2004.
5. Tharrett SJ, Peterson JA. *ACSM's Health/Fitness Facility Standards and Guidelines* (2nd ed.). Champaign, IL: Human Kinetics, 1997.
6. Shephard RJ, Thomas S, Weller I. The Canadian Home Fitness Test: 1991 update. *Sports Med* 11:358–366, 1991.
7. Canadian Society for Exercise Physiology. *The Canadian Physical Activity, Fitness & Lifestyle Appraisal.* Ottawa, Ontario: Canadian Society for Exercise Physiology, 1996; 2nd ed., 1998; 3rd ed., 2003 (www.csep.ca).
8. Cardinal BJ, Esters J, Cardinal MK. Evaluation of the revised physical activity readiness questionnaire in older adults. *Med Sci Sports Exerc* 28:468–472, 1996.
9. American Heart Association. Cardiovascular preparticipation screening of competitive athletes. *Circulation* 94:850–856, 1996.
10. Cantwell JD. Preparticipation physical evaluation: Getting to the heart of the matter. *Med Sci Sports Exerc* 30(suppl): S341–S344, 1998.

11. Corrado D, Basso C, Schiavon M, Thiene G. Screening for hypertrophic cardiomyopathy in young athletes. *N Engl J Med* 339:364–369, 1998.
12. Lyznicki JM, Nielsen NH, Schneider JF. Cardiovascular screening of student athletes. *Am Family Phys* 62:765–774, 2000.
13. Maron BJ, Gohman TE, Aeppli D. Prevalence of sudden cardiac death during competitive sports activities in Minnesota high school athletes. *J Am Coll Cardiol* 32:1881–1884, 1998.
14. Matheson GO. *Preparticipation Physical Evaluation* (3rd ed.). Minneapolis: McGraw-Hill, 2005.
15. Maron BJ, Douglas PS, Graham TP, Nishimura RA, Thompson PD. Task Force 1: Preparticipation screening and diagnosis of cardiovascular disease in athletes. *J Am Coll Cardiol* 45:1322–1326, 2005.
16. Cotton DJ, Cotton MB. *Legal Aspects of Waivers in Sport, Recreation, and Fitness Activities.* Canton, OH: PRC Publishing, Inc., 1997.
17. Eickhoff-Shemek JM, Whife CJ. The legal aspects: Internet personal training and/or coaching. What are the legal issues? Part I. *ACSM's Health and Fitness Journal* 8(3):25–26, 2004.
18. Eickhoff-Shemek JM, Forbes FS. Waivers are usually worth the effort. *ACSM's Health and Fitness Journal* 3(4):24–30, 1999.
19. Eickhoff-Shemek JM, Deja K. Four steps to minimize legal liability in exercise programs. *ACSM's Health and Fitness Journal* 4(4):13–18, 2000.
20. Napolitano F. The ACSM health/fitness facility standards. *ACSM's Health and Fitness Journal* 3(1):38–39 and 3(5):38–39, 1999.
21. Fletcher GF, Balady G, Froelicher VF, Hartley LH, Haskell WL, Pollock ML. Exercise standards: A statement for healthcare professionals from the American Heart Association. *Circulation* 91:580–615, 1995.
22. Maud PJ, Foster C. *Physiological Assessment of Human Fitness.* Champaign, IL: Human Kinetics, 1995.
23. Clarke HH. *Application of Measurement to Health and Physical Education.* Englewood Cliffs; NJ: Prentice-Hall, Inc., 1967.
24. Johnson BL, Nelson JK. *Practical Measurements for Evaluation in Physical Education.* Minneapolis: Burgess Publishing Co., 1979.
25. Nieman DC. The exercise test as a component of the total fitness evaluation. *Prim Care* 28:119–135, 2001.
26. Golding LH. *YMCA Fitness Testing and Assessment Manual.* (4th ed.). Champaign, IL: Human Kinetics, 2000.
27. Franks B. *YMCA Youth Fitness Test Manual.* Champaign, IL: Human Kinetics, 1989.
28. Pate RR. *Norms for College Students: Health Related Physical Fitness Test.* Reston, VA: American Alliance for Health, Physical Education, Recreation, and Dance, 1985.
29. National Association for Sport and Physical Education. *Physical Best Activity Guide—Elementary Level.* Champaign, IL: Human Kinetics, 2004.
30. National Association for Sport and Physical Education. *Physical Best Activity Guide—Middle and High School Levels.* Champaign, IL: Human Kinetics, 2004.
31. American Alliance for Health, Physical Education, Recreation and Dance. *Physical Education for Lifelong Fitness: The Physical Best Teacher's Guide.* Champaign, IL: Human Kinetics, 1999.
32. The Cooper Institute. *Fitnessgram/Actvitygram Test Administration Manual.* Champaign, IL: Human Kinetics, 2004.
33. Winnick JP, Short FX. *The Brockport Physical Fitness Test Kit.* Champaign, IL: Human Kinetics, 1999.
34. President's Council on Physical Fitness and Sports. *Get Fit: A Handbook for Youth Ages 6–17.* Washington, DC: President's Council on Physical Fitness and Sports, 2001 (www.presidentschallenge.org).
35. Peterson JA, Bryant CX, Stevenson R. Making professional certification work for your facility. *Fitness Management,* July 1996, 36–38.
36. Keteyian SJ. ACSM's personal trainer certification hits the ground running. *ACSM's Health and Fitness Journal* 9(2):28–29, 2005.

PHYSICAL FITNESS ACTIVITY 3.1

Are You Ready to Exercise?

Name ____

Age __________

Sex ____ M ____ F

1. Turn to the questionnaire on the following page and carefully answer all of the questions.

2. Based on your questionnaire responses, in what ACSM category would you put yourself (see text 1)?

_____ Low risk

_____ Moderate risk

_____ High risk

3. Based on your ACSM category, and whether you plan to exercise moderately or vigorously, what guidelines for exercise testing and participation apply to you?

____

____

____

____

____

4. Do you need a medical exam and diagnostic exercise test prior to starting your exercise program?

_____ Yes

_____ No

AHA/ACSM Preparticipation Screening Questionnaire (AHA/ACSM, 1998)[1]

Assess Your Health Needs by Marking All *true* Statements

History

You have had:

- ☐ A heart attack
- ☐ Heart surgery
- ☐ Cardiac catheterization
- ☐ Coronary angioplasty (PTCA)
- ☐ Pacemaker/implantable cardiac
- ☐ Defibrillator/rhythm disturbance
- ☐ Heart valve disease
- ☐ Heart failure
- ☐ Heart transplantation
- ☐ Congenital heart disease

Other health issues:

- ☐ You have diabetes.
- ☐ You have asthma or other lung disease.
- ☐ You have burning or cramping sensation in your lower legs when walking short distance.
- ☐ You have musculoskeletal problems that limit your physical activity.
- ☐ You have concerns about the safety of exercise.
- ☐ You take prescription medication(s).
- ☐ You are pregnant.

Symptoms

- ☐ You experience chest discomfort with exertion.
- ☐ You experience unreasonable breathlessness.
- ☐ You experience dizziness, fainting, blackouts.
- ☐ You take heart medications.

Recommendations

If you marked any of the statements in this section, consult your health-care provider before engaging in exercise. You may need to use a facility with a **medically qualified staff.**

Cardiovascular risk factors

- ☐ You are a man older than 45 years.
- ☐ You are a woman older than 55 years or you have had a hysterectomy or you are postmenopausal.
- ☐ You smoke or quit smoking within the previous 6 months.
- ☐ Your blood pressure is greater than 140/90 mm Hg.
- ☐ You don't know your blood pressure.
- ☐ You take blood pressure medication.
- ☐ Your blood cholesterol level is > 200 mg/dl.
- ☐ You don't know your cholesterol level.
- ☐ You have a blood relative who had a heart attack before age 55 (father/brother) or 65 (mother/sister).
- ☐ You are diabetic or take medicine to control your blood sugar.
- ☐ You are physically inactive (i.e., you get less than 30 minutes of physical activity on at least 3 days/week).
- ☐ You are more than 20 pounds overweight.

If you marked two or more of the statements in this section, you should consult your health-care provider before engaging in exercise. You might benefit by using a facility with a **professionally qualified exercise staff** to guide your exercise program.

- ☐ None of the above is true.

You should be able to exercise safely without consulting your health-care provider in almost any facility that meets your exercise program needs.

 PHYSICAL FITNESS ACTIVITY 3.2

Medical/Health Questionnaire

According to the American College of Sports Medicine, a medical examination and clinical exercise test is recommended prior to (1) moderate or vigorous exercise training for those at high risk for disease, and (2) vigorous exercise training for moderate-risk individuals. The ACSM recommends that the pretest medical history be thorough and include 11 components: medical diagnoses, previous physical examination findings, history of symptoms, recent illness, hospitalization or surgical procedures, orthopedic problems, medication use and drug allergies, lifestyle habits, exercise history, work history, and family history of disease. The following medical and health questionnaire meets these criteria and can be used to gain a useful history on clients at fitness-testing facilities located in worksites, hospitals, and universities. In this activity, select a faculty member or member of the community that you feel would benefit from this process. Have the person answer the questions in the medical questionnaire, and then summarize important findings in the following blanks.

1. Symptoms or signs of disease: ____________________

____

____

____

2. Chronic disease risk factors: ____________________

____

____

____

3. Personal and family medical history: ____________________

____

____

____

4. Medications: ____________________

____

____

____

5. Summary of lifestyle habits: ____________________

____

____

____

Medical/Health Questionnaire

Personal Information

Today's Date ___________________ Please print your name ___________________________________

How old are you? ________ years Sex ❑ Male; ❑ Female

Please circle the highest grade in school you have completed:

Elementary school	1	2	3	4	5	6	7	8
High school	9	10	11	12				
College/Postgrad	13	14	15	16	17	18	19	20+

What is your marital status? ❑ Single; ❑ Married; ❑ Widowed; ❑ Divorced/Separated

Race or ethnic background:

❑ White, not of Hispanic origin ❑ American Indian/Alaskan native ❑ Asian
❑ Black, not of Hispanic origin ❑ Pacific Islander ❑ Hispanic

What is your job or occupation? Check the one that applies to the greatest percentage of your time.

❑ Health professional ❑ Disabled, unable to work ❑ Service
❑ Manager, educator, professional ❑ Operator, fabricator, laborer ❑ Unemployed
❑ Skilled crafts ❑ Homemaker ❑ Student
❑ Technical, sales, support ❑ Retired ❑ Other

Symptoms or Signs Suggestive of Disease

Place a check in the box if your answer is "yes."

❑ **1.** Have you experienced unusual pain or discomfort in your chest, neck, jaw, arms, or other areas that may be due to heart problems?

❑ **2.** Have you experienced unusual fatigue or shortness of breath at rest, during usual activities, or during mild-to-moderate exercise (e.g., climbing stairs carrying groceries, brisk walking, cycling)?

❑ **3.** Have you had any problems with dizziness or fainting?

❑ **4.** When you stand up, or sometimes during the night while you are sleeping, do you have difficulty breathing?

❑ **5.** Do you suffer from swelling of the ankles (ankle edema)?

❑ **6.** Have you experienced an unusual and rapid throbbing or fluttering of the heart?

❑ **7.** Have you experienced severe pain in your leg muscles during walking?

❑ **8.** Has a doctor told you that you have a heart murmur?

Chronic Disease Risk Factors

Place a check in the box if your answer is "yes."

❑ **9.** Are you a male over age 45 years, or a female over age 55 years, or a female who has experienced premature menopause and is not on estrogen replacement therapy?

❑ **10.** Has your father or brother had a heart attack or died suddenly of heart disease before age 55 years; has your mother or sister experienced these heart problems before age 65 years?

❑ **11.** Are you a current cigarette smoker?

❑ **12.** Has a doctor told you that you have high blood pressure (more than 140/90 mm Hg), or are you on medication to control your blood pressure?

❑ **13.** Is your total serum cholesterol greater than 240 mg/dl, or has a doctor told you that your cholesterol is at a high-risk level?

❑ **14.** Do you have diabetes mellitus?

❑ **15.** Are you physically inactive and sedentary (little physical activity on the job or during leisure time)?

❑ **16.** During the past year, would you say that you experienced enough stress, strain, and pressure to have a significant effect on your health?

❑ **17.** Do you eat foods nearly every day that are high in fat and cholesterol such as fatty meats, cheese, fried foods, butter, whole milk, or eggs?

❑ **18.** Do you tend to avoid foods that are high in fiber such as whole-grain breads and cereals, fresh fruits, or vegetables?

❑ **19.** Do you weigh 30 or more pounds more than you should?

❑ **20.** Do you average more than two alcoholic drinks each day?

Medical History

21. Please check which of the following conditions you have had or now have. Also check medical conditions in your family (father, mother, brother[s], or sister[s]). Check as many as apply.

Personal	Family	Medical Condition
❑	❑	Coronary heart disease, heart attack, coronary artery surgery
❑	❑	Angina
❑	❑	High blood pressure
❑	❑	Peripheral vascular disease
❑	❑	Phlebitis or emboli
❑	❑	Other heart problems (specify: ______________________)
❑	❑	Lung cancer
❑	❑	Breast cancer
❑	❑	Prostate cancer
❑	❑	Colorectal cancer (bowel cancer)
❑	❑	Skin cancer
❑	❑	Other cancer (specify: ____________________________)
❑	❑	Stroke
❑	❑	Chronic obstructive pulmonary disease (emphysema)
❑	❑	Pneumonia
❑	❑	Asthma
❑	❑	Bronchitis
❑	❑	Diabetes mellitus
❑	❑	Thyroid problems
❑	❑	Kidney disease
❑	❑	Liver disease (cirrhosis of the liver)
❑	❑	Hepatitis
❑	❑	Gallstones/gallbladder disease
❑	❑	Osteoporosis
❑	❑	Arthritis
❑	❑	Gout
❑	❑	Anemia (low iron)
❑	❑	Bone fracture
❑	❑	Major injury to foot, leg, knee, hip, or shoulder
❑	❑	Major injury to back or neck
❑	❑	Stomach/duodenal ulcer
❑	❑	Rectal growth or bleeding
❑	❑	Cataracts
❑	❑	Glaucoma
❑	❑	Hearing loss
❑	❑	Depression
❑	❑	High anxiety, phobias
❑	❑	Substance abuse problems (alcohol, other drugs, etc.)
❑	❑	Eating disorders (anorexia, bulimia)
❑	❑	Problems with menstruation

❑ ❑ Hysterectomy

❑ ❑ Sleeping problems

❑ ❑ Allergies

❑ ❑ Any other health problems (please specify, and include information on any recent illnesses, hospitalizations, or surgical procedures):

____

____

22. Please check any of the following medications you currently take regularly. Also give the name of the medication.

	Medication	Name of Medication
❑	Heart medicine	______________
❑	Blood pressure medicine	______________
❑	Blood cholesterol medicine	______________
❑	Hormones	______________
❑	Birth control pills	______________
❑	Medicine for breathing/lungs	______________
❑	Insulin	______________
❑	Other medicine for diabetes	______________
❑	Arthritis medicine	______________
❑	Medicine for depression	______________
❑	Medicine for anxiety	______________
❑	Thyroid medicine	______________
❑	Medicine for ulcers	______________
❑	Painkiller medicine	______________
❑	Allergy medicine	______________
❑	Other (please specify)	______________

Physical Fitness, Physical Activity/Exercise

23. In general, compared to other persons your age, rate how physically fit you are:

1❑ 2❑ 3❑ 4❑ 5❑ 6❑ 7❑ 8❑ 9❑ 10❑

Not at all physically fit — Somewhat physically fit — Extremely physically fit

24. Outside of your normal work or daily responsibilities, how often do you engage in exercise that at least moderately increases your breathing and heart rate and makes you sweat, for at least 20 minutes (such as brisk walking, cycling, swimming, jogging, aerobic dance, stair climbing, rowing, basketball, racquetball, vigorous yard work).

❑ 5 or more times per week ❑ 3–4 times per week ❑ 1–2 times per week

❑ Less than 1 time per week ❑ Seldom or never

25. How much hard physical work is required on your job?

❑ A great deal ❑ A moderate amount ❑ A little ❑ None

26. How long have you exercised or played sports regularly?

❑ I do not exercise regularly ❑ Less than 1 year ❑ 1–2 years

❑ 2–5 years ❑ 5–10 years ❑ More than 10 years

Diet

27. On average, how many servings of fruit do you eat per day? (One serving = 1 medium apple, banana, orange, etc.; ½ cup of chopped, cooked, or canned fruit; ¾ cup of fruit juice.)

❑ None ❑ 1 ❑ 2 ❑ 3 ❑ 4 or more

28. On average, how many servings of vegetables do you eat per day? (One serving = ½ cup cooked or chopped raw, 1 cup raw leafy, ¾ cup of vegetable juice.)

❑ None ❑ 1–2 ❑ 3 ❑ 4 ❑ 5 or more

29. On average, how many servings of bread, cereal, rice, or pasta do you eat per day? (One serving = 1 slice of bread, 1 ounce of ready to-eat cereal, ½ cup of cooked cereal, rice, or pasta.)

❑ None ❑ 1–3 ❑ 4–6 ❑ 7–9 ❑ 10 or more

30. When you use grain and cereal products, do you emphasize:

❑ Whole grain, high fiber ❑ Mixture of whole grain and refined ❑ Refined, low fiber

31. On average, how many servings of red meat (not lean) do you eat per day (One serving = 2–3 ounces of steak, roast beef, lamb, pork chops, ham, burgers, etc.)

❑ None ❑ 1 ❑ 2 ❑ 3 ❑ 4 or more

32. On average, how many servings of fish, poultry, lean meat, cooked dry beans, peanut butter, or nuts do you eat per day? (One serving = 2–3 ounces of meat, ½ cup of cooked dry beans, 2 tablespoons of peanut butter, or ⅓ cup of nuts.)

❑ None ❑ 1 ❑ 2 ❑ 3 ❑ 4 or more

33. On average, how many servings of dairy products do you eat per day? (One serving = 1 cup of milk or yogurt, 1.5 ounces of natural cheese, 2 ounces of processed cheese.)

❑ None ❑ 1 ❑ 2 ❑ 3 ❑ 4 or more

34. When you use dairy products, do you emphasize

❑ Regular ❑ Low fat ❑ Nonfat

35. How would you characterize your intake of fats and oils (e.g., regular salad dressings, butter or margarine, mayonnaise, vegetable oils)?

❑ High ❑ Moderate ❑ Low

Body Weight

36. How tall are you (without shoes)? ______ feet ______ inches

37. How much do you weigh (minimal clothing and without shoes)? ______ pounds

38. What is the most you have ever weighed? ______ pounds

39. Are you *now* trying to

❑ Lose weight ❑ Gain weight ❑ Stay about the same ❑ Not trying to do anything

Psychological Health

40. How have you been feeling in general during the past month?

❑ In excellent spirits ❑ In very good spirits
❑ In good spirits mostly ❑ I've been up and down in spirits a lot
❑ In low spirits mostly ❑ In very low spirits

41. During the past month, would you say that you experienced ____ stress?

❑ A lot of ❑ Moderate ❑ Relatively little ❑ Almost no

42. In the past year, how much effect has stress had on your health?

❑ A lot ❑ Some ❑ Hardly any or none

43. On average, how many hours of sleep do you get in a 24-hour period?

❑ Less than 5 ❑ 5–6.9 ❑ 7–9 ❑ More than 9

Substance Use

44. Have you smoked at least 100 cigarettes in your entire life?

❑ Yes ❑ No

45. How would you describe your cigarette smoking habits?

❑ Never smoked

❑ Used to smoke

How many years has it been since you smoked? ____ years

❑ Still smoke

How many cigarettes a day do you smoke on average? ____ cigarettes/day

46. How many alcoholic drinks do you consume? (A "drink" is a glass of wine, a wine cooler, a bottle/can of beer, a shot glass of liquor, or a mixed drink.)

❑ Never use alcohol ❑ Less than 1 per week ❑ 1–6 per week

❑ 1 per day ❑ 2–3 per day ❑ More than 3 per day

Occupational Health

47. Please describe your main job duties.

____

____

	All of the time	Most of the time	Some of the time	Rarely or never
48. After a day's work, do you often have pain or stiffness that lasts for more than 3 hours?	❑	❑	❑	❑
49. How often does your work entail repetitive pushing and pulling movements or lifting while bending or twisting, leading to back pain?	❑	❑	❑	❑

chapter 4

Cardiorespiratory Fitness

Cardiorespiratory fitness is considered health-related because (a) low levels of cardiorespiratory fitness have been associated with a markedly increased risk of premature death from all causes and specifically from cardiovascular disease, (b) increases in cardiorespiratory fitness are associated with a reduction in death from all causes, and (c) high levels of cardiorespiratory fitness are associated with higher levels of habitual physical activity, which are, in turn, associated with many health benefits.

—American College of Sports Medicine[1]

The laboratory test generally regarded as the best measure of heart and lung endurance is the direct measurement of oxygen uptake during maximal exercise.[1–4] The exercise is usually performed using a bicycle ergometer or treadmill, which allows the progressive increase in workload from light-to-exhaustive (maximal) exercise. The amount of oxygen consumed during the exercise test is measured using various methods (douglas bag collection of expired air, mixing box and gas-flow meter, or computerized metabolic carts).[5] (See Figure 4.1.) New portable metabolic systems that can be strapped to the chest have been developed, which should revolutionize measurement of oxygen consumption outside of laboratory settings.[6] Measurement of $\dot{V}O_{2max}$ should be specific to the sport practiced by the individual being tested because of the very unique muscular, circulatory, and metabolic adaptations that occur.

Maximal oxygen uptake ($\dot{V}O_{2max}$) is defined as the greatest rate at which oxygen can be consumed during exercise or the maximal rate at which oxygen can be taken up, distributed, and used by the body during physical activity.[5] ("$\dot{V}$" is the volume used per minute, "O_2" is oxygen, and "max" represents maximal exercise conditions.[1–5])

$\dot{V}O_{2max}$ is usually expressed in terms of milliliters of oxygen consumed per kilogram of body weight per minute ($ml \cdot kg^{-1} \cdot min^{-1}$). By factoring in body weight, it becomes possible to compare the $\dot{V}O_{2max}$ of people of varying size in different environments. It should be noted that expressing $\dot{V}O_{2max}$ in $ml \cdot kg^{-1} \cdot min^{-1}$ may unfairly underestimate the aerobic fitness of individuals with large amounts of body fat.[7]

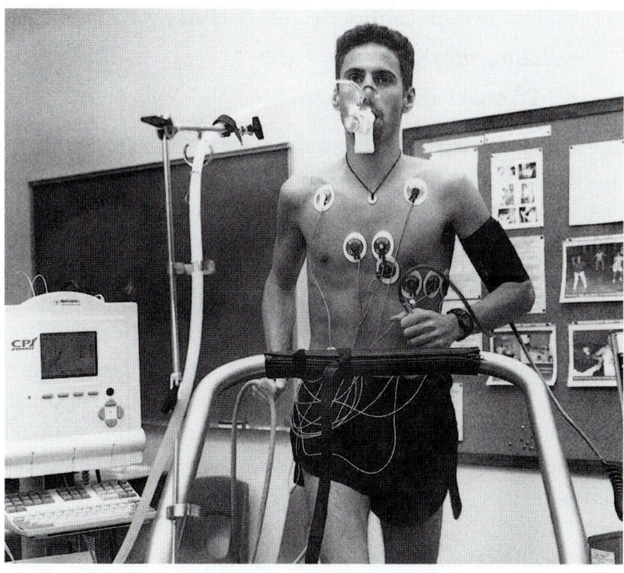

Figure 4.1 $\dot{V}O_{2max}$ is best measured in the laboratory during a maximal exercise test in which the oxygen consumed is measured by a computerized metabolic cart.

A high level of $\dot{V}O_{2max}$ depends on the proper functioning of three important systems in the body:

1. The *respiratory system,* which takes up oxygen from the air in the lungs and transports it into the blood
2. The *cardiovascular system,* which pumps and distributes the oxygen-laden blood throughout the body

3. The *musculoskeletal system,* which uses the oxygen to convert stored carbohydrates and fats into adenosine triphosphate (ATP) for muscle contraction and heat production[5]

In the laboratory, several criteria are used to determine whether an individual's true $\dot{V}O_{2max}$ has been achieved:[8,9]

- Oxygen consumption plateaus during the last minutes of a graded exercise test (defined as a rise of less than 2 ml $\cdot$ kg$^{-1}\cdot$ min^{-1} between the final test stages).
- The *respiratory exchange ratio* (RER) (ratio of the volume of carbon dioxide produced to the volume of oxygen consumed) increases to 1.15 or higher.
- The subject's heart rate increases to within 10 beats of the age-predicted maximum (maximum heart rate is estimated by subtracting the age from 220).
- Blood lactate levels rise above 8 mmol/liter.

Laboratory measurement of $\dot{V}O_{2max}$ is expensive and time-consuming, requires highly trained personnel, and therefore is not practical for most testing situations. Various formulas and tests have been developed as substitutes and are the focus of this chapter:

- Nonexercise test $\dot{V}O_{2max}$ prediction equations
- Field tests of cardiorespiratory endurance
- Submaximal laboratory tests
- Maximal laboratory tests

It is assumed that before these tests are conducted, the preliminary considerations outlined in the previous chapter have been attended to (medical/health status questionnaire, consent form, and for those at high risk, a physical examination by a physician, treadmill test, and possibly a blood lipid analysis). It is also assumed that the order outlined for each testing battery is followed, with subjects following the appropriate pretest preparation routine (abstention from food, tobacco, alcohol, and caffeine for 3 hours, proper hydration, comfortable exercise clothes, adequate sleep, and avoidance of exercise the day of the test).

RESTING AND EXERCISE BLOOD PRESSURE AND HEART RATE DETERMINATION

When conducting a bicycle or treadmill test, the tester should include heart rate, blood pressure, and electrocardiogram (ECG) monitoring on all high risk individuals. The test can then be used for determination of both cardiorespiratory fitness and potential health problems such as high blood pressure and heart disease (as diagnosed by a physician). Although blood pressure and ECG monitoring is not necessary when testing apparently healthy subjects, some testing facilities do it as an extra precaution.

TABLE 4.1 Classification of Blood Pressure for Adults

BP Classification	SBP mm Hg	DBP mm Hg
Normal	< 120	and < 80
Prehypertension	120–139	or 80–89
Stage 1 hypertension	140–159	or 90–99
Stage 2 hypertension	≥ 160	or ≥ 100

Source: National High Blood Pressure Education Program. *The Seventh Report of the Joint National Committee on Detection, Evaluation, and Treatment of High Blood Pressure.* National Heart, Lung, and Blood Institute, National Institutes of Health, NIH Publication No. 04-5230. Bethesda, MD: National Institutes of Health, 2003.

Resting Blood Pressure

Blood pressure is the force of blood against the walls of the arteries and veins created by the heart as it pumps blood to every part of the body. *Hypertension* is simply a condition in which the blood pressure is chronically elevated above optimal levels. The Joint National Committee on Detection, Evaluation, and Treatment of High Blood Pressure has established blood pressure classifications[10] (see Table 4.1).

Hypertension is diagnosed for adults when *diastolic* measurements (blood pressure when the heart is resting) on at least two separate visits average 90 mm Hg or higher, or *systolic* measurements (while the heart is beating) are 140 mm Hg or higher. There are two stages of hypertension, with stage 2 diagnosed when measurements are equal to or greater than 160/100 mm Hg. Prehypertension (120–139/80–89) is included as a separate category because this is now considered to be a risk factor for future hypertension and cardiovascular disease.[10] Recommended follow-up testing procedures for hypertension are given in Table 4.2.

As many as 65 million people in the United States have hypertension.[10] Prevalence increases with age and is higher among blacks than whites[11] (see Figure 4.2). (See Chapter 10 for more information on hypertension.) Healthcare professionals are urged to measure blood pressure at each patient visit.

To take the resting blood pressure, a sphygmomanometer and a stethoscope are needed.[12–14] The *sphygmomanometer* consists of an inflatable compression bag enclosed in an unyielding covering called the cuff, plus an inflating bulb, a manometer from which the pressure is read, and a controlled exhaust valve to deflate the system. The *stethoscope* is made of rubber tubing attached to a device that amplifies the sounds of blood passing through the blood vessels (see Figure 4.3). This equipment can be obtained in most drug stores for about $30, though more expensive blood pressure equipment is available.

Those taking blood pressure should be trained by qualified instructors. For each patient, blood pressure should be measured two or three times until consistency is achieved. A single blood pressure reading does not provide an accurate measure.[12–14] Several blood pressure readings by different observers, or on different occasions by the same ob-

TABLE 4.2 Recommendations for Follow-Up Based on Initial Blood Pressure Measurements for Adults Without Acute End Organ Damage

Initial Blood Pressure, mm Hg*	Follow-Up Recommended†
Normal	Recheck in 2 years
Prehypertension	Recheck in 1 year‡
Stage 1 hypertension	Confirm within 2 months‡
Stage 2 hypertension	Evaluate or refer to source of care within 1 month. For those with higher pressures (e.g., > 180/110 mm Hg), evaluate and treat immediately or within 1 week depending on clinical situation and complications.

*If systolic and diastolic categories are different, follow recommendations for shorter time follow-up (e.g., 160/86 mm Hg should be evaluated or referred to source of care within 1 month).
†Modify the scheduling of follow-up according to reliable information about past BP measurements, other cardiovascular risk factors, or target organ disease.
‡Provide advice about lifestyle medications.

Source: National High Blood Pressure Education Program. *The Seventh Report of the Joint National Committee on Detection, Evaluation, and Treatment of High Blood Pressure.* National Heart, Lung, and Blood Institute, National Institutes of Health, NIH Publication No. 04-5230. Bethesda, MD: National Institutes of Health, 2003.

server, are recommended to check the validity of initially high values. See Physical Fitness Activity 4.4.

For best results in taking blood pressure:[12–14]

- Measurements should be taken with a mercury-stand sphygmomanometer, a recently calibrated aneroid manometer, or a validated electronic device. Aneroid and electronic devices should be checked against a mercury manometer at least once a year.
- Two or more readings should be taken 30–60 seconds apart, and averaged. If the first two readings differ by more than 5 mm Hg, additional readings should be obtained.
- Take the measurement in a quiet room with the temperature approximately 70–74° Fahrenheit (21–23° C).
- Having the upper arm bare makes it easier to adjust the cuff.
- With older people, because of potential arterial obstructions it is best to take readings on both arms. If the pressures differ by more than 10 mm Hg, obtain simultaneous readings in the two arms and thereafter use the arm with the higher pressure.

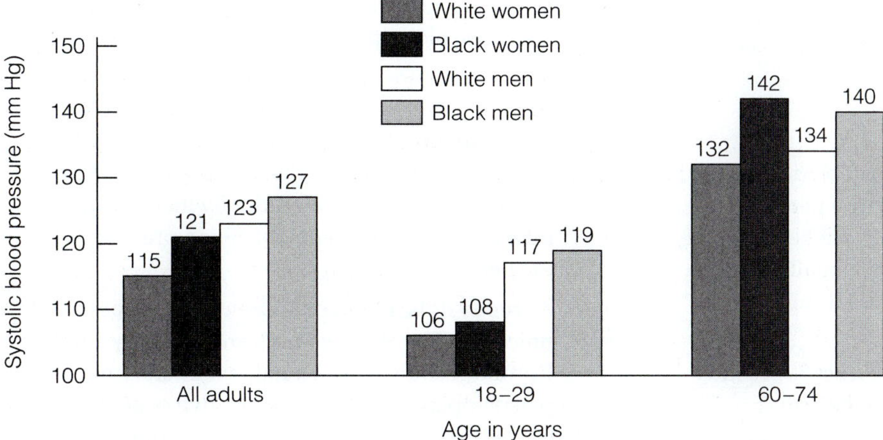

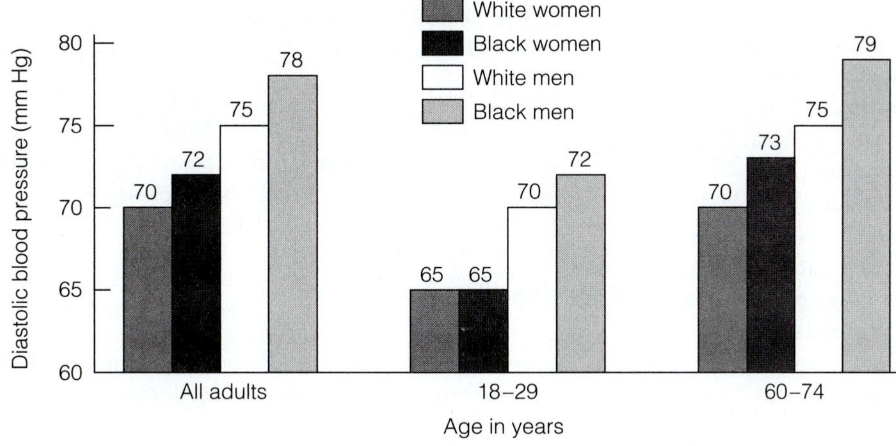

Figure 4.2 Mean systolic (top) and diastolic (bottom) blood pressure by race, sex, and age. The average blood pressure in the United States varies among subgroups, being higher in blacks versus whites and older versus younger adults. Source: National Health and Nutrition Examination Survey III, 1988–1991.[11]

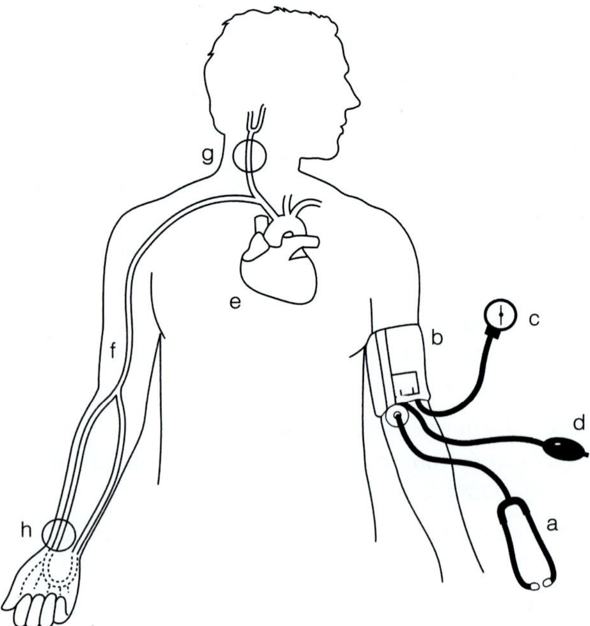

Figure 4.3 Blood pressure is taken with a stethoscope (a) and sphygmomanometer, which consists of an inflatable cuff (b) connected by rubber tubes to a monometer, which measures pressure in millimeters of mercury (c), and a rubber bulb that regulates air during the measurements (d). Blood pressure is the force of blood against the walls of the arteries and veins created by the heart (e) as it pumps. The blood pressure cuff fits over the brachial artery (f). The upper circle (g) represents the common carotid artery, and the lower circle (h) the radial artery, for sensing the heart rate.

- Use the proper size cuff. The rubber bladder should encircle at least 80% of the arm. If the person's arm is large, the adult normal size cuff will be too small (making the reading larger than it actually should be) and the "obese" size bladder is strongly recommended.
- Between determinations, allow at least 30 seconds for normal circulation to return to the arm.
- The subject should be comfortably seated with the arm straight (just slightly flexed), palm up, and the whole forearm supported at heart level on a smooth surface.
- Anxiety, emotional turmoil, food in the stomach, bladder distension, climate variation, exertion, and pain all may influence blood pressure, and when possible, should be controlled or avoided. Heavy exercise or eating should be avoided, and the individual being tested should sit quietly for at least 5 minutes before the test. The tested person should also avoid smoking or ingesting caffeine for at least 30 to 60 minutes prior to measurement. If the individual is on medication for hypertension, the time since the prior dose should be noted (it may be useful to take readings at the end of a dosing interval).
- Place the cuff (deflated) with the lower margin about 1 inch above the inner elbow crease (antecubital space). The rubber bag should be over the brachial artery (in the inner part of the upper arm; see Figure 4.3).
- Place the earpieces of the stethoscope into the ear canals, angled forward to fit snugly. For resting blood pressures, switch the stethoscope head to the bell, or low-frequency, position.
- The stethoscope should be applied lightly just above and medial to the antecubital space (but make sure that the head makes contact with the skin around its entire circumference). Excessive pressure on the stethoscope head can erroneously lower diastolic readings. The stethoscope should not touch clothing, the cuff, or the cuff tubing (to avoid unnecessary rubbing sounds). The tubing should come from the top of the cuff to avoid interference.
- With the stethoscope in place, the pressure should be raised 20–30 mm Hg above the point at which the pulse sound disappears. (Listen carefully through the stethoscope as the cuff bladder is inflated. The pressure will close off the blood flow in the brachial artery, causing the pulse sound to stop.)
- The pressure should be slowly released at a rate of 2 mm Hg per second or heart beat. Do not go slower than this, however, because it can cause pain and also raise blood pressure.
- As the pressure is released, the blood pressure sounds (the *Korotkoff sounds*) become audible and pass through several phases. Phase 1 (the systolic pressure) is marked by the appearance of faint, clear tapping sounds, which gradually increase in intensity. This represents the blood pressure when the heart is contracting.
- A true systolic blood pressure cannot be obtained unless the Korotkoff sounds are relatively sharp. Korotkoff sounds can be made louder by having the person open and clench the fist five or six times while the arm is raised and then starting over again.
- To obtain the diastolic blood pressure the following rules should be followed:

  At rest. Diastolic blood pressure equals the disappearance of the pulse sound (also called the fifth sound).

  During exercise testing. Sometimes the disappearance of sound drops all the way to zero. Therefore, the point at which there is an abrupt muffling sound (fourth phase) should be used for the diastolic blood pressure.

Exercise Blood Pressure

Blood pressure should be taken at least every 3 minutes during exercise testing on the treadmill or bicycle (see Figure 4.4).

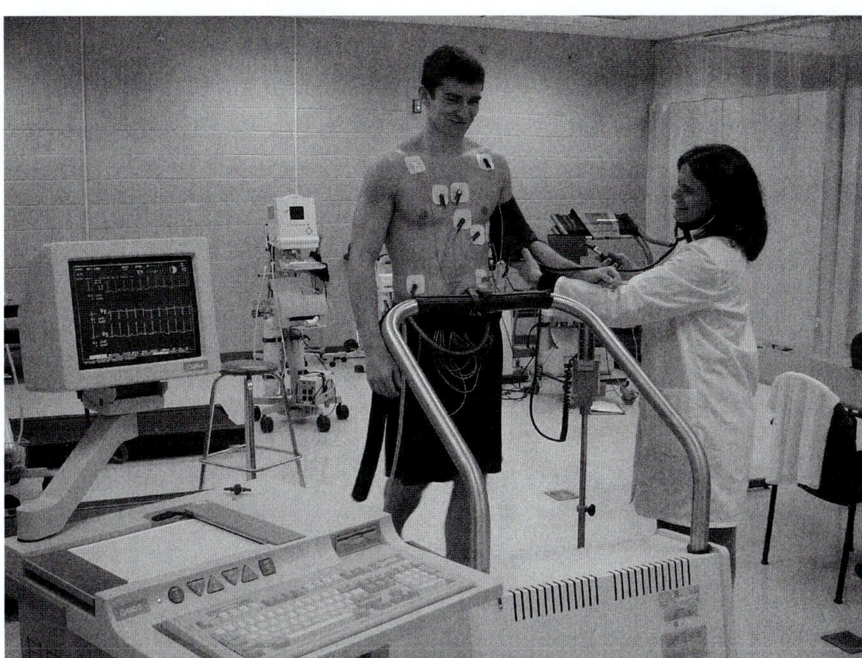

Figure 4.4 Blood pressure determination during exercise is a difficult skill and requires considerable experience. Korotkoff sounds are easier to hear if the tubes are not allowed to rub or bump the subject or the treadmill. The stethoscope head should be attached to the subject's arm. The manometer should be at the level of the subject's heart.

Several important principles should be followed when taking blood pressure readings during exercise:[15,16]

- If the exercise stages are 3 minutes long (as in the Bruce treadmill protocol, for example), blood pressure readings should be taken at 2 minutes and 15 seconds into each stage. The cuff should be taped onto the person being tested for the entire test, but the inflating bulb should be removed between readings.
- It is best to stand on a stool and have the person being tested raise his or her arm to heart level while you support it. The subject's arm should be relaxed and not grasping a treadmill or cycle bar. If you are using a mercury-stand sphygmomanometer, the mercury column should be elevated to the person's heart level.
- Taking blood pressure during exercise is somewhat difficult because of the noise. It is best to raise the cuff pressure quickly until pulse sounds disappear and then, because the heart rate is higher than at rest, let the cuff pressure fall 5-6 mm Hg per second. Try to focus only on the pulse sounds through the stethoscope and keep the various tubes from flapping and rubbing against objects. Keep ambient noise in the testing room to a minimum. If you can't hear the pulse sounds, it may be necessary to stop the test for 15 seconds for a quick blood pressure determination.
- During exertion, the diastolic reading stays basically the same as the resting diastolic, whereas the systolic rises linearly with the increase in workload (see Figure 4.5).
- Peak exercise blood pressures vary according to age and gender[17] (see Figure 4.6).

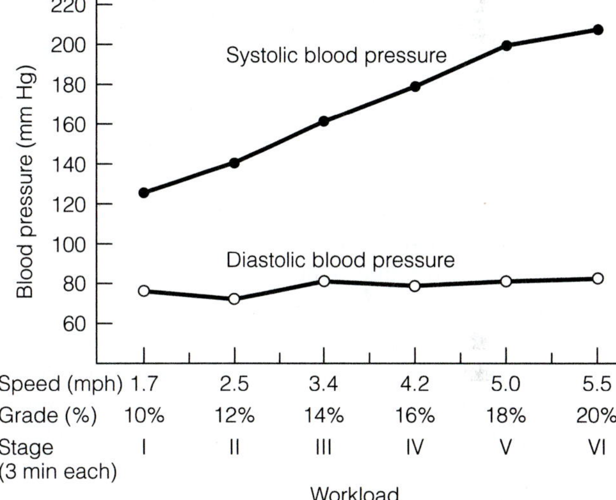

Figure 4.5 Pattern of systolic and diastolic blood pressures during graded exercise testing.

- If the systolic rises above 260 mm Hg, or the diastolic rises above 115 mm Hg, the test should be terminated.[1,18] The test should also be stopped if the systolic blood pressure drops ≥10 mm Hg from baseline with increasing workload.
- During recovery, blood pressure should be taken every 2 to 3 minutes.

Resting Heart Rate

The resting heart rate can be obtained through *auscultation* (using the bell of the stethoscope), *palpation* (feeling the pulse with your fingers), or ECG recordings. When taking

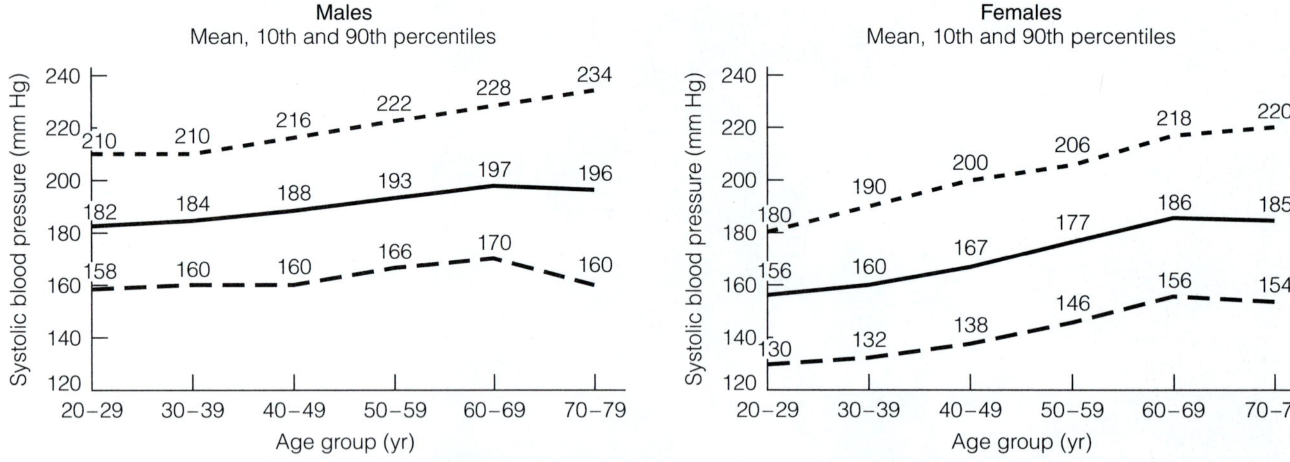

Figure 4.6 Peak exercise systolic blood pressures are higher in men than women, and they increase with advancing age. Data are from 7,863 male and 2,406 female apparently healthy people (Bruce treadmill max test). Source: Daida H, et al. *Mayo Clin Proc* 71:445–452, 1996.

heart rate by auscultation, the bell of the stethoscope is placed to the left of the sternum, just above the level of the nipple. The heartbeats (lub-dub) can be counted for 30 seconds and then multiplied by 2 to obtain beats per minute (bpm).

In using palpation techniques, the pulse is best determined during rest, at the radial artery (lateral aspect of the palm side of the wrist, in line with the base of the thumb) (see Figure 4.3). The tip of the middle and index fingers should be used (not the thumb, which has a pulse of its own). Start the stopwatch simultaneously with the pulse beat. Count the first beat as zero. Continue counting for 30 seconds and then multiply by 2 to get the total heartbeats per minute. See Physical Fitness Activity 4.3 at the end of the chapter.

During exercise, the carotid artery is easier to palpate because it is bigger than the radial (see Figure 4.3). When palpating the carotid (in the neck just lateral to the larynx), heavy pressure should not be applied because pressure receptors (baroreceptors) in the carotid arteries can detect the pressure and cause a reflex slowing of the heart rate.

The heart rate is a variable that fluctuates widely and easily, due to the same factors that influence blood pressure. Resting heart rate is best determined upon awakening, and averaged from measurements taken on at least three separate mornings. Lower heart rates are usually (but not always) indicative of a heart conditioned by exercise training—a heart able to push out more blood with each beat (having a larger stroke volume) and therefore needing fewer beats (see Appendix A, Table 21). Accordingly, the resting heart rate usually drops with regular exercise, decreasing approximately one beat every 1 or 2 weeks for the first 10 to 20 weeks of the program. Some of the best endurance athletes in the world have resting heart rates as low as 30–45 bpm. For example, Miguel Indurain, one of the best cyclists in history, had a resting heart rate of 28 bpm. Women have slightly higher resting pulse rates than men, while age appears to have little effect.[19] Resting pulse rates are also slightly higher in the fall and winter than in spring and summer, and higher in smokers versus nonsmokers.

Exercise Heart Rate

Heart rate during exercise is best determined through the use of an *electrocardiogram* (ECG), a record of the electrical activity of the heart. Several methods are used:

- Using a heart rate ruler, count two or three R waves (depending on the ruler) from the reference arrow, and then read the heart rate from the ruler (see Figure 4.7).
- Counting the number of larger squares between R waves and dividing into 300 (for example, if two large blocks are between R waves, then the heart rate is 300/2 or 150 bpm).
- Counting the number of millimeters between four R waves and dividing into 6,000 (for example, if 40 mm separate four R waves, then the heart rate is 6,000/40, or 150 bpm).

Figure 4.8 shows a form for practicing ECG heart rate determination.

Another method involves auscultation with the stethoscope. The blood pressure cuff can be filled, the systolic blood pressure taken, and then midway between the systolic and diastolic blood pressures (usually around 100 to 110 mm Hg), the release of pressure can be stopped and the pulse counted through the stethoscope for 10 seconds. (Often, the pulse sounds are very loud when this method is used.) The pressure can then be released for diastolic blood pressure determination.

Several types of heart rate measuring devices have been developed. Heart rate monitors using chest electrodes are very accurate, stable, and functional. A telemetry device

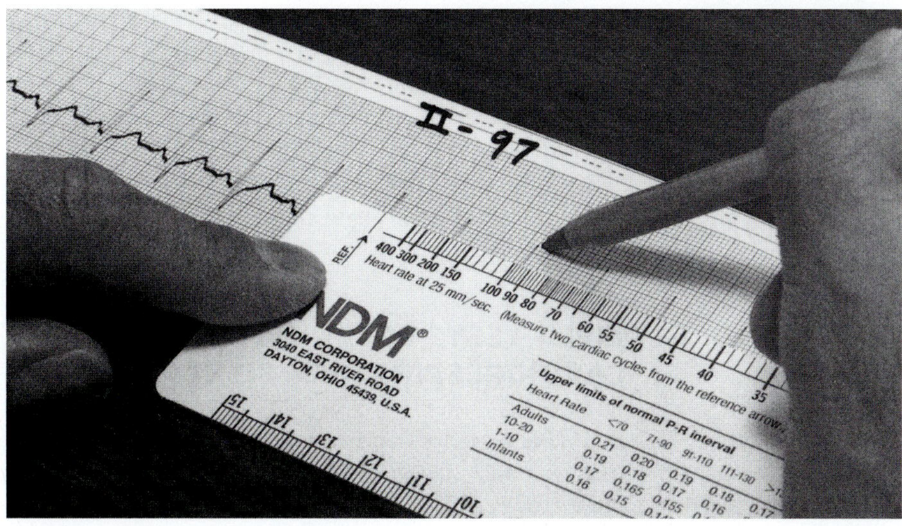

Figure 4.7 The heart rate can be determined from an ECG recording by using a heart rate ruler. With this particular ruler, heart rate is determined by reading the ruler after counting two heart rate cycles to the right of the reference arrow.

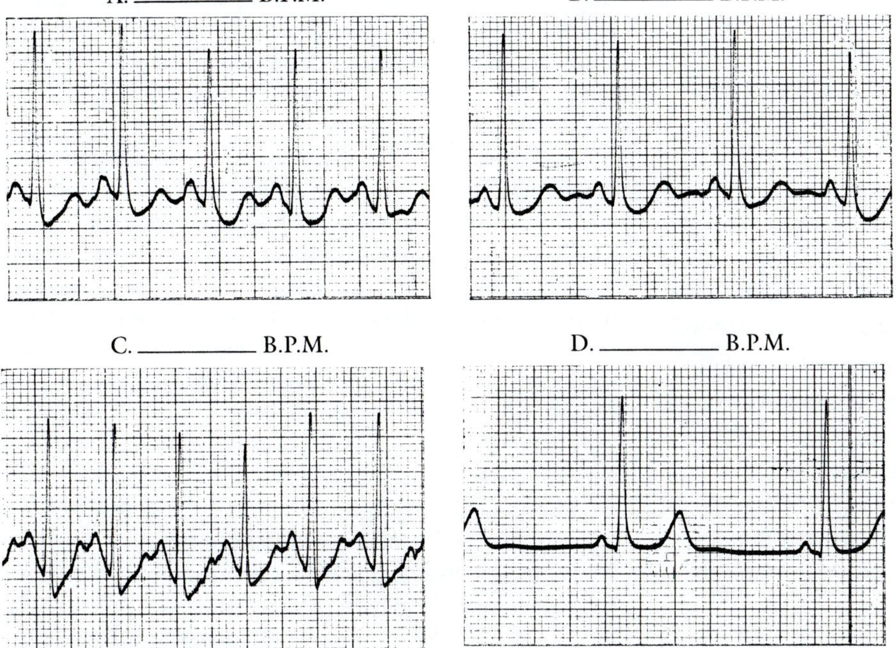

Quick Method–Number of squares between R waves divided into 300 gives the rate per minute.
Use of Ruler–Be sure to count the appropriate number of R waves from the reference point.

Figure 4.8 Use this form to practice heart rate determination from ECG recording strips. Practice each of the three methods described in this section (ECG ruler, large-square method, four-R method).

with permanent electrodes is attached to the chest, with the heart rate signal sent to a receiver worn on the wrist. Heart rate and elapsed time are displayed (the heart rate is updated every 5 seconds). These heart rate monitors can now be purchased for as little as $50. Heart rate monitors using photocells to measure the opacity of blood flow (earlobe or fingertip) are not recommended.

NONEXERCISE TEST $\dot{V}O_{2max}$ PREDICTION EQUATIONS

Direct measurement of $\dot{V}O_{2max}$ with computerized metabolic carts is the most valid and reliable marker of cardiorespiratory fitness. However, the time, expense, and technical supervision required have made laboratory measurements of $\dot{V}O_{2max}$ impractical for large populations involved in epidemiological studies of exercise and disease. Several researchers have developed regression equations that predict $\dot{V}O_{2max}$ using nonexercise test variables such as age, gender, body composition, and level of physical activity.[20–25] Although these prediction equations are not as accurate as laboratory testing of $\dot{V}O_{2max}$, they do allow researchers to broadly classify people as having poor, average, or good cardiorespiratory fitness.

One of the most commonly used nonexercise prediction equations for $\dot{V}O_{2max}$ was developed by researchers at the University of Houston, using age, physical activity status, and percent body fat or body mass index (BMI).[20] See Physical Fitness Activity 4.5 at the end of the chapter. The percent body fat equation is slightly more accurate than the BMI equation. Physical activity is rated from the subject's exercise habits, using the following code:

1. Does not participate regularly in programmed recreation, sport, or physical activity.

   0 points: Avoids walking or exertion (e.g., always uses elevator, drives whenever possible instead of walking)

   1 point: Walks for pleasure, routinely uses stairs, occasionally exercises sufficiently to cause heavy breathing or perspiration

2. Participates regularly in recreation or work requiring modest physical activity, such as golf, horseback riding, calisthenics, gymnastics, table tennis, bowling, weight lifting, or yard work:

   2 points: 10–60 minutes per week

   3 points: More than 1 hour per week

3. Participates regularly in heavy physical exercise (such as running or jogging, swimming, cycling, rowing, skipping rope, running in place) or engages in vigorous aerobic activity (such as tennis, basketball, or handball).

   4 points: Runs less than 1 mile per week or spends less than 30 minutes per week in comparable physical activity

   5 points: Runs 1–5 miles per week or spends 30–60 minutes per week in comparable physical activity

   6 points: Runs 5–10 miles per week or spends 1–3 hours per week in comparable physical activity

   7 points: Runs more than 10 miles per week or spends more than 3 hours per week in comparable physical activity

The physical activity rating (PA−R) is used in the following equations to estimate $\dot{V}O_{2max}$ in $ml \cdot kg^{-1} \cdot min^{-1}$:[20]

- % fat model

$(r = 0.81, SEE = 5.35\ ml \cdot kg^{-1} \cdot min^{-1})^*$

$$\dot{V}O_{2max}\ ml \cdot kg^{-1} \cdot min^{-1} = 50.513 + 1.589\ (PA-R) - 0.289\ (age) - 0.552(\%\ fat) + 5.863\ (gender)$$

[gender = 0 for female, 1 for male]

- BMI model

$(r = 0.783, SEE = 5.70\ ml \cdot kg^{-1} \cdot min^{-1})$

$$\dot{V}O_{2max}\ ml \cdot kg^{-1} \cdot min^{-1} = 56.363 + 1.921\ (PA-R) - 0.381\ (age) - 0.754\ (BMI) + 10.987\ (gender)$$

[gender = 0 for female, 1 for male]

*r = correlation coefficient
SEE = standard error of estimate

For example, the estimated $\dot{V}O_{2max}$ for a 45-year-old woman with 25% body fat and a physical activity rating of 5 would be

$$\dot{V}O_{2max} = 50.513 + (1.589 \times 5) - (0.289 \times 45) - (0.552 \times 25) + (5.863 \times 0) = 31.7\ ml \cdot kg^{-1} \cdot min^{-1}$$

FIELD TESTS FOR CARDIORESPIRATORY FITNESS

A number of performance tests such as maximal endurance runs on a track have been devised and validated for testing large groups in field situations.[26–41] These tests are practical, inexpensive, less time-consuming than laboratory tests, easy to administer for large groups, and quite accurate when properly conducted. Although outdoor cycling and pool swimming tests have been developed for estimating $\dot{V}O_{2max}$, they do not appear to be as valid as running tests.[30–32]

Endurance runs should be of 1 mile or greater to test the aerobic system. For ease of administration, the 1-mile and 1.5-mile runs are most commonly used. Various set-timed runs such as the 12-minute run are hard to administer because exact distance determination is difficult. With the 1-mile or 1.5-mile runs, those being tested run the set distance around a track (or exactly measured course) while their time is measured (see Figure 4.9). The objective is to cover the distance in the shortest possible time.[26] The effort should be maximal and only made by those properly motivated and experienced in running.

The 1-mile run is used in several fitness test batteries (see Chapter 3). Norms are found in Appendix A (Tables 9, 10, 17, 18, 20). Researchers from the University of Georgia have developed a generalized equation for prediction of $\dot{V}O_{2max}$ in $ml \cdot kg^{-1} \cdot min^{-1}$ for males and females between the ages of 8 and 25.[26] The equation is based on a total sample of 490 males and 263 females and has a standard error of estimate of $4.8\ ml \cdot kg^{-1} \cdot min^{-1}$, giving it an accuracy that is as good as or better than that of most other field methods for estimating $\dot{V}O_{2max}$ in children and adults. The regression equation for prediction of $\dot{V}O_{2max}$ from the 1-mile run time (MRT) is

$$\dot{V}O_{2max}\ ml \cdot kg^{-1} \cdot min^{-1} = (-8.41 \times MRT) + (0.34 \times MRT^2) + (0.21 \times age \times gender) - (0.84 \times BMI) + 108.94$$

[MRT = mile run time in minutes; gender = 0 for females, 1 for males; BMI = body mass index, kg/m^2]

For example, if a 15-year-old can run a mile in 6.5 minutes and has a BMI of 21, the equation would estimate a $\dot{V}O_{2max}$ of $54.2\ ml \cdot kg^{-1} \cdot min^{-1}$:

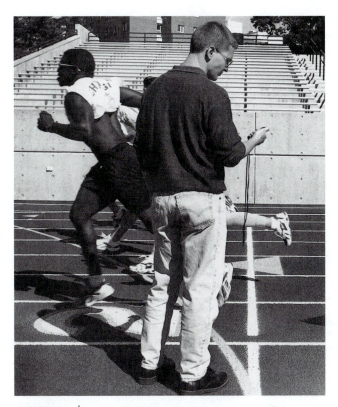

Figure 4.9 $\dot{V}O_{2max}$ can be estimated quite accurately from the time taken to run 1 mile as fast as possible. This test is recommended only for those who are apparently healthy and accustomed to running.

$$(-8.41 \times 6.5) + (0.34 \times 6.5^2) + (0.21 \times 15 \times 1) - (0.84 \times 21) + 108.94 = 54.2 \text{ ml} \cdot \text{kg}^{-1} \cdot \text{min}^{-1}$$

Normative data for the 1.5-mile run are found in Table 4.3 and Appendix A, Table 23. $\dot{V}O_{2max}$ can be estimated from the 1.5-mile run for college students using the following equation:[28]

$$\dot{V}O_{2max} (\text{ml} \cdot \text{kg}^{-1} \cdot \text{min}^{-1}) = 88.02 + (3.716 \times \text{gender}) - (0.1656 \times \text{kg}) - (2.767 \times \text{time})$$

[gender = 0 for female, 1 for male; kg = body weight; time = total run time in minutes]

For example, if a 70-kg male can run 1.5 miles in 9 minutes, his estimated $\dot{V}O_{2max}$ would be

$$55.2 \text{ ml} \cdot \text{kg}^{-1} \cdot \text{min}^{-1} = [88.02 + (3.716 \times 1) - (0.1656 \times 70) - (2.767 \times 9)]$$

Equations have also been developed to predict $\dot{V}O_{2max}$ from ability to run other distances at maximal speed.[35] Table 4.4 summarizes these equations for various racing distances. Notice that the correlations of calculated values of $\dot{V}O_{2max}$ with actual measured $\dot{V}O_{2\,max}$ are very high (0.88 to 0.98).

TABLE 4.3 Norms for the 1.5-Mile Run Test (for People Between the Ages of 17 and 35)

Fitness Category	Time: Ages 17–25	Time: Ages 26–35
Superior		
Males	< 8:30	< 9:30
Females	< 10:30	< 11:30
Excellent		
Males	8:30–9:29	9:30–10:29
Females	10:30–11:49	11:30–12:49
Good		
Males	9:30–10:29	10:30–11:29
Females	11:50–13:09	12:50–14:09
Moderate		
Males	10:30–11:29	11:30–12:29
Females	13:10–14:29	14:10–15:29
Fair		
Males	11:30–12:29	12:30–13:29
Females	14:30–15:49	15:30–16:49
Poor		
Males	> 12:20	> 13:29
Females	> 15:49	> 16:49

Note: Before taking this running test, it is highly recommended that the student or individual be "moderately fit." Sedentary people should first start an exercise program and slowly build up to 20 minutes of running, 3 days per week, before taking this test.

Source: Draper DO, Jones GL. The 1.5 mile run revisited—An update in women's times. *JOPERD*, September 1990, 78–80. Reprinted with permission. *JOPERD* is a publication of the American Alliance for Health, Physical Education, Recreation and Dance, 1990 Association Drive, Reston, VA 20191.

These equations assume that the person being tested has run the distance at maximum speed. The average running speed is computed in kilometers per hour (kmh), and the equation is used to calculate the $\dot{V}O_{2max}$ in METs.

One *MET* is equal to the resting oxygen consumption of the reference average human, which equals 3.5 ml · kg^{-1} · min^{-1}. To get $\dot{V}O_{2max}$, the number of METs is multiplied by 3.5 ml · kg^{-1} · min^{-1}. (See example in Table 4.4.)

Table 4.5 summarizes calculations from the equations in Table 4.4. Equivalent relationships between $\dot{V}O_{2max}$ and running performance for races ranging from 1.5 km to 42.195 km (marathon) are given. Notice, for example, that running a mile in 6:01 demands the same $\dot{V}O_{2max}$ (56 ml · kg^{-1} · min^{-1}) as running the 5 km in 21:23, the 10 km in 46:17, or the marathon in 3:49:28.

The maximal endurance run tests are only for the healthy (ACSM "apparently healthy" category). Cooper suggests that the 1.5-mile run test should not be taken unless the subject can already jog nonstop for 15 minutes.[32] In addition, there always should be proper warm-up of slow jogging and calisthenics. After the test, there should be an adequate "warm-down" or "cool-down," with several minutes of walking, followed by flexibility exercises.

TABLE 4.4 Estimation of $\dot{V}O_{2max}$ from Average Running Speed During Racing

Racing Distance (km)	Equation to Calculate $\dot{V}O_{2max}$	Correlation
1.5	METs = 2.4388 + (0.8343 × kmh)	0.95
1.6093 (mile)	METs = 2.5043 + (0.8400 × kmh)	0.95
3	METs = 2.9226 + (0.8900 × kmh)	0.98
5	METs = 3.1747 + (0.9139 × kmh)	0.98
10	METs = 4.7226 + (0.8698 × kmh)	0.88
42.195 (marathon)	METs = 6.9021 + (0.8246 × kmh)	0.85

Note: kmh = average racing speed in competition in kilometers per hour. 1 MET = 3.5 $ml \cdot kg^{-1} \cdot min^{-1}$. To calculate total oxygen power, multiply number of METs times 3.5 $ml \cdot kg^{-1} \cdot min^{-1}$. For example, if you can run a 5-km race in 18:30 (which is 16.2 kmh, calculated by multiplying the number of kilometers in the race by 60, and then dividing by the race time in decimal form [5 × 60]/18.5 = 16.2 kmh), using the preceding equation, $\dot{V}O_{2max}$ in METs is equal to

METs = 3.1747 + (0.9139 × 16.2) = 18 METs

$\dot{V}O_{2max}$ in $ml \cdot kg^{-1} \cdot min^{-1}$ = 18 METs × 3.5 $ml \cdot kg^{-1} \cdot min^{-1}$. = 63 $ml \cdot kg^{-1} \cdot min^{-1}$

Source: Tokmakidis SP, Léger L, Mercier D, Péronnet F, Thibault G. New approaches to predict $\dot{V}O_{2max}$ and endurance from running performance. *J Sports Med* 27:401–409, 1987.

TABLE 4.5 Equivalent Performances for Various Distances

$\dot{V}O_{2max}$ ($ml \cdot kg^{-1} \cdot min^{-1}$)	Performance Time for Various Distances (hours:minutes:seconds)				
	1.5 km	1 mile	5 km	10 km	42.2 km
28	13:30	14:46	56:49	2:39:14	31:41:25
31.5	11:27	12:29	47:04	2:02:00	16:35:05
35	9:56	10:49	40:10	1:38:53	11:13:52
38.5	8:46	9:33	35:02	1:23:08	8:29:26
42	7:51	8:33	31:04	1:11:43	6:49:30
45.5	7:07	7:44	27:54	1:03:03	5:42:21
49	6:30	7:03	25:20	0:56:15	4:54:07
52.5	5:59	6:29	23:11	0:50:47	4:17:48
56	5:32	6:01	21:23	0:46:17	3:49:28
59.5	5:09	5:36	19:50	0:42:30	3:26:44
63	4:50	5:14	18:30	0:39:33	3:08:06
66.5	4:32	4:55	17:20	0:36:33	2:52:34
70	4:17	4:38	16:18	0:34:10	2:39:23
73.5	4:03	4:23	15:23	0:32:12	2:28:05
77	3:50	4:09	14:34	0:30:12	2:18:16
80.5	3:39	3:57	13:50	0:28:33	2:09:41
84	3:29	3:46	13:10	0:27:04	2:02:06
87.5	3:20	3:36	12:34	0:25:44	1:55:21

Source: Tokmakidis SP, Léger L, Mercier D, Péronnet F, Thibault G. New approaches to predict $\dot{V}O_{2max}$ and endurance from running performance. *J Sports Med* 27:401–409, 1987.

A 1-mile walk test is available for testing a wide variety of people.[37] Walking is safer than running and more easily performed by most Americans. Three hundred and forty-three males and females, 30 to 69 years of age, were tested using a 1-mile walk test. They walked a mile as fast as possible, performing the test a minimum of two times, with heart rates monitored. They then were given a treadmill $\dot{V}O_{2max}$ test, and the 1-mile walk results correlated very highly with actual measured $\dot{V}O_2$ (r = .93).

The following equation was developed to determine $\dot{V}O_{2max}$ from 1-mile walk test results:[37]

$$\begin{aligned}\dot{V}O_{2max}\,(L \cdot min^{-1}) &\\ = 6.9652 &+ (0.0091 \times \text{body weight, lb}) \\ &- (0.0257 \times \text{age}) + (0.5955 \times \text{gender}) \\ &- (0.2240 \times \text{mile walk time in minutes}) \\ &- (0.0115 \times \text{ending heart rate})\end{aligned}$$

For example, if a male subject weighs 150 lb, is 30 years old, and can walk 1 mile in 12 minutes with an ending heart rate of 120 beats $\cdot$ min^{-1} (gender, 1 = male, 0 = female):

$$\dot{V}O_{2max} = 6.9652 + (0.0091 \times 150 \text{ lb}) - (0.0257 \times 30) + (0.5955 \times 1) - (0.2240 \times 12 \text{ min}) - (0.0115 \times 120 \text{ bpm})$$

$$= 4.09 \text{ liters of oxygen per minute } (L \cdot min^{-1})$$

To change the $\dot{V}O_{2max}$ units from liters per minute to milliliters per kilogram body weight (in order to use fitness classification tables), first multiply 4.09 $\cdot$ min^{-1} by 1000 to get milliliters (4.09 $L \cdot ml \cdot min^{-1} \times 1000 = 4090\ ml \cdot min^{-1}$). Next divide the body weight (lb) by 2.2046 to get kilograms (150 lb/2.2046 lb/kg = 68.04 kg. Next divide the $\dot{V}O_{2max}$ by body weight (4090 $ml \cdot min^{-1}$/68.04 kg = 60.1 $ml \cdot kg^{-1} \cdot min^{-1}$). Using the $\dot{V}O_{2max}$ norms in Appendix A (Table 24), this 30-year-old male would be classified as being in "athletic" cardiorespiratory shape. The original 1-mile walk equation has been adapted for college students because it overpredicts $\dot{V}O_{2max}$ by 16–23%.[34] This equation is recommended for college students. See Physical Fitness Activity 4.6 at the end of the chapter.

$\dot{V}O_{2max}$ $ml \cdot kg^{-1} \cdot min^{-1}$ = 88.768 + (8.892 × gender with M=1, F=0) − (0.0957 × weight in pounds) − (1.4537 × walk time in minutes) − (0.1194 × ending heart rate).

For example, a college female weighing 128 lb and able to walk 1 mile in 13 minutes with an ending heart rate of 133 bpm would have this estimated $\dot{V}O_{2max}$:

$$\dot{V}O_{2max} = 88.768 + (8.892 \times 0) - (0.0957 \times 128) - (1.4537 \times 13.0) - (0.1194 \times 133) = 41.7\ ml \cdot kg^{-1} \cdot min^{-1}$$

The 1-mile walk test has been shown to be valid for elderly subjects if they are accustomed to walking.[41, 42] This test can be administered outdoors on a track or indoors on a treadmill and will give similar results.[38]

A 1-mile track jog test has been developed for college students.[28] Although the mile run is commonly used to measure cardiorespiratory fitness in the college setting, there is considerable dissatisfaction with it because students dislike the maximum effort required. In the 1-mile track jog test, students self-select a steady, comfortable pace (recommended total mile times are greater than 8 minutes for males and 9 minutes for females, with an ending heart rate of less than 180 bpm). After jogging the mile at the same pace throughout, the ending time and heart rate are recorded, with $\dot{V}O_{2max}$ estimated using this equation:[28]

$$\dot{V}O_{2max}\ (ml \cdot kg^{-1} \cdot min^{-1}) = 100.5 + (8.344 \times \text{gender}) - (0.1636 \times \text{kg}) - (1.438 \times \text{time}) - (0.1928 \times \text{bpm})$$

[gender = 0 for female, 1 for male; kg = body weight; time = mile jog time; bpm = ending heart rate]

For example, if a female college student weighing 60 kg jogs a mile in 10 minutes with an ending heart rate of 150 bpm, her $\dot{V}O_{2max}$ would be

$$47.4\ ml \cdot kg^{-1} \cdot min^{-1} = [100.5 + (8.344 \times 0) - (0.1636 \times 60) - (1.438 \times 10) - (0.1928 \times 150)]$$

Using Table 24 in Appendix A, her fitness level would be rated "good." This formula has been shown to correlate highly (r=.87) with directly measured $\dot{V}O_{2max}$.

SUBMAXIMAL LABORATORY TESTS

During submaximal testing, physiological responses (usually heart rate) to exercise are measured. The workload is usually fixed—for example, a particular grade and speed on a treadmill, a fixed rate and resistance on a cycle *ergometer* (an apparatus for measuring the amount of work performed), or a fixed rate of stepping and fixed height of bench in a step test. Usually heart rate is measured during and at the end of such exercise.

On the other hand, the physiological response may be fixed and the exercise required to reach the response measured (e.g., work required to reach a heart rate of 170 bpm). The reasoning underlying both types of submaximal tests is that the person with the higher $\dot{V}O_{2max}$ is able to accomplish a given amount of exercise with less effort (or more exercise at a particular heart rate).[43]

The submaximal exercise test makes three assumptions:[3,5,43–45]

1. That a linear relationship exists between heart rate, oxygen uptake, and workload
2. That the maximum heart rate at a given age is uniform
3. That the mechanical efficiency (oxygen uptake at a given workload) is the same for everyone

These assumptions are not entirely accurate, however, and can result in a 10–20% error in estimating $\dot{V}O_{2max}$. Figure 4.10 shows that in most submaximal tests, heart rates at submaximal workloads are plotted, then extrapolated to an estimated maximum heart rate level, and then further extrapolated to an average oxygen consumption. These extrapolations can result in substantial error.

The *maximum heart rate* is the fastest heart rate that can be measured when the individual is brought to total exhaustion during a graded exercise test. A formula has been developed to represent the average maximum heart rate in humans:

$$\text{Maximum heart rate} = 220 - \text{age}$$

The maximum heart rate varies substantially among different people of the same age, however. (One standard

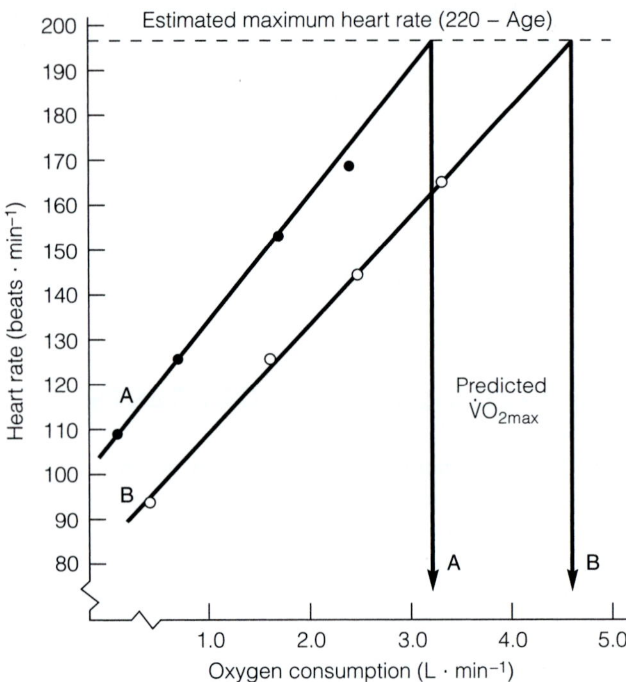

Figure 4.10 In most submaximal tests, heart rates at submaximal workloads are plotted (A or B), then extrapolated to an estimated maximum heart rate level, and then further extrapolated to an estimated workload that has been associated with an average oxygen consumption. These extrapolations can result in substantial error. Source: McArdle WO, Katch FI, Katch VL. *Exercise Physiology: Energy, Nutrition, and Human Performance.* Philadelphia: Lea & Febiger, 1991.

deviation is ± 12 bpm, which means that two thirds of the population varies an average of plus-or-minus 12 heart beats from the average.) (See Chapter 8 for other equations used to estimate maximum heart rate.) If the line connecting submaximal heart rates is extrapolated to an average maximum heart rate level that is really 12 beats lower than the real maximum heart rate in an individual, the final extrapolation to the workload and estimated oxygen consumption will underestimate the true cardiorespiratory fitness of the individual (see Figure 4.10).

Oxygen uptake at any given workload can vary 15% among different people.[44,45] In other words, people vary in the amount of oxygen they require to perform a certain exercise workload. Some are more efficient than others, and thus the average oxygen consumption associated with a given workload may differ significantly from one person to another.

For these reasons, $\dot{V}O_{2max}$ predicted by submaximal stress tests tends to be overestimated for those who are highly trained (who respond with a low heart rate to a given workload and are mechanically efficient), and underestimated for the untrained (those with a high heart rate for a given workload, who are also inefficient).

Nonetheless, submaximal exercise testing has its place in cardiorespiratory fitness determination.[1,43] Sometimes large populations are required to be tested, and the time, equipment, and skill needed to measure $\dot{V}O_{2max}$ are prohibitive. The measurement of $\dot{V}O_{2max}$ through maximal testing requires an all-out physical effort. For some people, such effort can be hazardous and at the very least often requires medical supervision and evaluation. Also, maximal testing, while definitely the most accurate way to determine fitness status, requires a high level of motivation. Submaximal exercise testing, though not as valid, can still give a somewhat accurate picture of fitness status without the expense, risk, and hard effort.

Step Tests

Prior to the widespread use of treadmills and cycle ergometers for exercise testing, maximal step-testing protocols were recommended by the American Heart Association.[46,47] However, adjustable steps were required and the extreme up and down stepping action for fit subjects made measurement of heart rate and blood pressure extremely difficult. Maximal step testing constitutes a safety hazard for some subjects and is no longer a recommended protocol for estimation of aerobic fitness. Submaximal step-test protocols however, have been developed for estimation of aerobic fitness and $\dot{V}O_{2max}$, the two most common ones being the modified Canadian Aerobic Fitness Test (mCAFT) and the YMCA 3-minute step test.

The Modified Canadian Aerobic Fitness Test

The modified Canadian Aerobic Fitness Test (mCAFT) is a practical, fairly accurate, inexpensive, and fun way to determine cardiorespiratory endurance.[48–52]

The original CAFT was developed in the mid-1970s, when the Canadian government suggested that many Canadians would be motivated to increase their habitual exercise if there were a simple exercise test that indicated their current physical condition.[49]

The CAFT was designed using double steps each 8 inches high and wide, as in a domestic staircase. The double step is climbed to an age- and sex-specific rhythm set by a cassette tape. Fitness is assessed from test duration and the radial or carotid pulse count immediately following exercise.

Since the 1970s, the CAFT has been used by millions worldwide, with the only reported complications being a very small number of minor muscle pulls (caused by stumbling) and very rare episodes of dizziness or transient loss of consciousness (arising from preexisting conditions).[48,49] The test has been well received and has achieved its primary objective of stimulating an interest in endurance exercise.

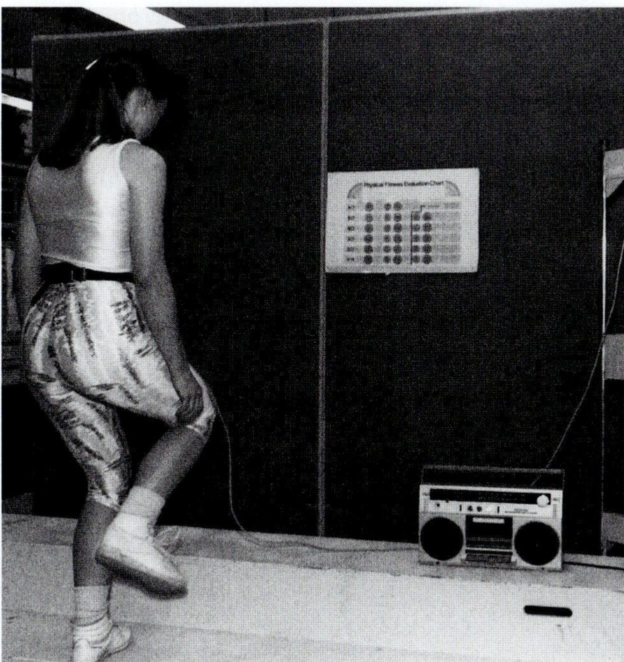

Figure 4.11 The modified Canadian Aerobic Fitness Test is a step test performed on two 8-inch (20.3-cm) steps.

Using the CAFT with an electrocardiogram or chest heart rate monitor for heart rate determination gives a closer approximation of aerobic fitness than the Astrand–Rhyming bicycle test.[50] A properly administered mCAFT, with postexercise heart rate accurately recorded, offers a convenient submaximum tool for evaluating cardiorespiratory fitness, particularly in such settings as employee fitness programs.[52] With the relatively high correlation with directly measured maximum oxygen uptake, it provides a means of accurately testing large populations without sophisticated equipment.[48]

The Canadian Physical Activity Fitness & Lifestyle Appraisal (CPAFLA), which includes all the instructions on how to take the mCAFT test, plus the cassette tape and other fitness materials, can be obtained from the Internet site of the Canadian Society for Exercise Physiology: *www.csep.ca.*

The mCAFT is a modified step test performed on two 8-inch (20.3-cm) steps (see Figure 4.11). Based on the age of the person being tested, the tape is set at a certain stepping tempo. The person then steps up and down the steps at the given rate for 3 minutes. The cassette gives instructions and time signals as to when to start and stop exercising and how to measure the postexercise heart rate.

Table 4.6a gives the stepping cadence for the modified CAFT.[52] After an initial stepping level is chosen according to the age group (Table 4.6b), subjects step for 3 minutes on the double steps in time to the musical tape or metronome, set at the proper cadence. Subjects step at progressively higher cadences until they reach a ceiling heart rate (85% of

TABLE 4.6a Stepping Cadences for Men and Women Performing the Modified Canadian Aerobic Fitness Test (mCAFT)

	Cadence (steps/min)	
Exercise Level	Males	Females
1	66	66
2	84	84
3	102	102
4	114	114
5	132	120
6	144	132
7	118*	144
8	132*	118*

*All exercise levels use two 8-inch (20.3-cm) steps except for levels 7 and 8 in men, and 8 in women, which use a single 16-inch step. The double-step exercise levels use a six-step cycle, whereas for single-step levels there are four steps per cycle.

TABLE 4.6b Starting Levels for Performing the mCAFT in Each Gender and Age Group[30]

	Starting Level	
Age Group (yr)	Males	Females
15–19	4	3
20–29	4	3
30–39	3	3
40–49	3	2
50–59	2	1
60–69	1	1

TABLE 4.6c Oxygen Cost in $ml \cdot kg^{-1} \cdot min^{-1}$ for Stages of the mCAFT

Stage	Males	Females
1	15.9	15.9
2	18.0	18.0
3	22.0	22.0
4	24.5	24.5
5	29.5	26.3
6	33.6	29.5
7	36.2	33.6
8	40.1	36.2

Source: The Canadian Physical Activity, Fitness & Lifestyle Approach: CSEP-Health & Fitness Program's Health-Related Appraisal and Counseling Strategy, 3rd Edition © 2003. Reprinted with permission of the Canadian Society for Exercise Physiology.

age-predicted maximum heart rate) or the end of level 8. Notice from Table 4.6a that a single 16-inch step is used during the highest exercise levels to provide a suitable intensity for the very fit. Some people need a bit of coaching to get used to the rhythm of the beat. The stepping procedure for the double step follows a six-count format:

1. Right foot on the first step
2. Left foot on top of the second step
3. Right foot on top of the second step along with the left
4. Left foot down to the first step
5. Right foot down to the floor
6. Left foot down to the floor along with the right

For the highest exercise levels (7 and 8 for men, 8 for women), a four-step cycle is used on the single 16-inch step.

The pulse is taken immediately after each 3-minute stepping exercise level, while the participant stands motionless. If the pulse is low enough (below 85% of maximum heart rate), another 3-minute stepping exercise is undertaken at a faster rate, with the process continuing until the ceiling heart rate or top exercise level is reached.

The mCAFT should not be taken after a large meal, after performing vigorous exercise, after using alcohol, coffee or tobacco, or in hot rooms. Once the mCAFT has been completed, an aerobic fitness score should be established, using the following equation:[52]

$$\text{Aerobic fitness score} = 10[17.2 + (1.29 \times O_2 \text{ cost}) - (0.09 \times \text{kg}) - (0.18 \times \text{age})]$$

The oxygen cost for the different stages of the mCAFT are given in Table 4.6c. For example, if a male subject 35 years of age and weighing 70 kg (154 lb) begins stepping at stage 4 and completes stages 5, 6, and 7 (oxygen cost of 36.2 L/min) before reaching his heart rate ceiling of 157 bpm (85% of maximum heart rate), then the aerobic fitness score would be

$$\begin{aligned}\text{Aerobic fitness score} &= 10[17.2 + (1.29 \times 36.2) - (0.09 \times 70) - (0.18 \times 35)]\\ &= 513\end{aligned}$$

Table 4.7 summarizes the classification system used by CPAFLA for the mCAFT.[52] An aerobic fitness score of 513 for a 35-year-old male is classified as "excellent" (an aerobic fitness level that is generally associated with optimal health benefits). The mCAFT step test should be discontinued if subjects begin to stagger, complain of dizziness, extreme leg pain, nausea or chest pain, or if they show facial pallor.

The YMCA 3-Minute Step Test

The YMCA uses the 3-minute step test for mass testing of participants. (See norms, Appendix A, Table 22).[53]

TABLE 4.7 Health Benefit Zone from Aerobic Fitness Score

Zone	Males	Females
Age 15–19		
Excellent	574+	490+
Very Good	524–573	437–489
Good	488–523	395–436
Fair	436–487	368–394
Needs improvement	<436	<368
Age 20–29		
Excellent	556+	472+
Very Good	506–555	420–471
Good	472–505	378–419
Fair	416–471	350–377
Needs improvement	<416	<350
Age 30–39		
Excellent	488+	454+
Very Good	454–487	401–453
Good	401–453	360–400
Fair	337–400	330–359
Needs improvement	<337	<330
Age 40–49		
Excellent	470+	400+
Very Good	427–469	351–399
Good	355–426	319–350
Fair	319–354	271–318
Needs improvement	<319	<271
Age 50–59		
Excellent	418+	366+
Very Good	365–417	340–365
Good	301–364	310–339
Fair	260–300	246–309
Needs improvement	<260	<246
Age 60–69		
Excellent	384+	358+
Very Good	328–383	328–357
Good	287–327	296–327
Fair	235–286	235–295
Needs improvement	<235	<235

Source: The Canadian Physical Activity, Fitness & Lifestyle Approach: CSEP-Health & Fitness Program's Health-Related Appraisal and Counseling Strategy, 3rd Edition © 2003. Reprinted with permission of the Canadian Society for Exercise Physiology.

The equipment involved includes a 12-inch high, sturdy bench; a metronome set at 96 bpm (four clicks of the metronome equals one cycle, up 1,2, down 3,4), which should be properly calibrated with a wrist watch; a timing clock for the 3-minute stepping exercise and 1-minute recovery; and preferably a stethoscope to count the pulse rate.[53]

It is important to first demonstrate the stepping technique to the person to be tested (four counts—right foot up onto the bench on 1, left foot up on 2, right foot down to the floor on 3, and left foot down on 4). The exerciser should have some preliminary practice and should be well rested with no prior exercise of any kind.

The test involves stepping up and down at the 24-steps-per-minute rate for 3 minutes, and then immediately sitting down. Within 5 seconds the tester should be counting the pulse with the stethoscope and should *count for 1 full minute.* The person being tested can take her or his own pulse at the same time by palpating the radial artery, providing a double check of the count. The 1-minute count limit reflects the heart's ability to recover quickly, with a low versus high count reflecting better fitness.

The total 1-minute postexercise heart rate is the score for the test and should be recorded. It can be affected by many factors other than fitness, such as emotion, tiredness, prior exercise, resting and maximum heart rates that differ from population averages, and miscounting.

Other Step Tests

McArdle and colleagues have devised a step test (the Queens College Step Test) for college students to predict $\dot{V}O_{2max}$.[54] Subjects step at a rate of 22 steps per minute (females) or 24 steps per minute (males) for 3 minutes. The bench height is 16.25 inches (about the height of a gymnasium bleacher). After exercise, the subject remains standing, waits 5 seconds, and takes a 15-second heart rate count. See Physical Fitness Activity 4.7 at the end of the chapter. The $\dot{V}O_{2max}$ ($ml \cdot kg^{-1} \cdot min^{-1}$) is predicted using this equation:

Males

$$\text{Predicted } \dot{V}O_{2max} = 111.33 - (0.42 \times \text{heart rate})$$

Females

$$\text{Predicted } \dot{V}O_{2max} = 65.81 - (0.1847 \times \text{heart rate})$$

The standard error of prediction using the equation is within plus or minus 16% of the actual $\dot{V}O_{2max}$ and is considered suitable for mass testing.[54]

There are additional step tests described in the literature. The Harvard Step Test is for young men, who step 30 times per minute for 5 minutes on a 20-inch bench. A description of the test is given by Brouha.[55] There is also the Astrand–Rhyming nomogram, which may be used to predict $\dot{V}O_{2max}$ from postexercise heart rate and body weight during bench stepping. The subject steps at a rate of 22.5 steps per minute for 5 minutes. The bench height is 33 cm for women and 40 cm for men. The postexercise heart rate is obtained by counting the number of beats between 15 and 30 seconds immediately after exercise (then multiplying by 4).[56]

Box 4.1

Stepping Ergometry and MET-Energy Calculations

Each MET is equal to 3.5 ml of oxygen per kilogram of body weight per minute ($3.5\ ml \cdot kg^{-1} \cdot min^{-1}$). Total oxygen uptake can thus be determined by multiplying the MET value by $3.5\ ml \cdot kg^{-1} \cdot min^{-1}$. The equations are based on submaximal, steady-state exercise; thus, caution should be taken in extrapolating to $\dot{V}O_{2max}$ (data may overpredict $\dot{V}O_{2max}$ by 1 to 2 METs).

The equation for stepping ergometry is

$$\dot{V}O_2\ ml \cdot kg \cdot min = 0.2\ (\text{stepping rate}) + 1.33 \cdot 1.8\ (\text{step height})\ (\text{stepping rate}) + 3.5$$

where stepping rate is in $steps \cdot min^{-1}$, and step height is in meters (1 inch = 0.0254 m). For example, if a participant steps at 20 $steps \cdot min^{-1}$ on an 8-inch step (0.2032 m), then $\dot{V}O_2$ is

$$\begin{aligned}\dot{V}O_2\ ml \cdot kg^{-1} \cdot min^{-1} &= (0.2 \cdot 20) + (1.33 \cdot 1.8 \cdot 0.2032\ m \cdot 20) + 3.5 \\ &= 17.23\ ml \cdot kg^{-1} \cdot min^{-1}\end{aligned}$$

or 4.9 METS

Because 1 MET = $1\ kcal \cdot kg^{-1} \cdot hour^{-1}$, energy expenditure in $kcal \cdot min^{-1}$ can be determined by multiplying the MET value by the body weight of the person in kilograms, and then dividing by 60 minutes per hour. For example, for a person weighing 65 kg,

$$\begin{aligned}5\ \text{METs} &= 5\ kcal \cdot kg^{-1} \cdot hour^{-1} \\ &= 5\ kcal \cdot kg^{-1} \cdot hour^{-1} \times 65\ kg \cdot hour^{-1} \\ &= 325\ kcal \cdot hour^{-1}\end{aligned}$$

or $5.4\ kcal \cdot min^{-1}$

ACSM Bench-Stepping Equation

The American College of Sports Medicine has published an equation for estimating the energy expenditure for stepping in terms of METs[1,18] (see Box 4.1). To use this and other ACSM metabolic equations, two units must be understood: METs and $kcal \cdot min^{-1}$. As explained earlier, 1 MET is equal to $3.5\ ml \cdot kg^{-1} \cdot min^{-1}$ or the oxygen consumption during rest. One MET is also equal to $1\ kcal \cdot kg^{-1} \cdot hour^{-1}$. Thus the energy expenditure in $kcal \cdot min^{-1}$ can be determined by multiplying the MET value of the exercise by the body weight of the person tested in kilograms and then dividing by 60 (minutes per hour). (See Box 4.1. See also Physical Fitness Activity 4.1 at the end of this chapter.)

Treadmill Submaximal Laboratory Tests

Submaximal testing is conducted not only on steps but also with the treadmill. Submaximal testing on treadmills can use a cutoff point based on a predetermined heart rate—for example, 85% of the predicted heart rate range.

There are limitations, however, when using the test heart rate as a single measure of fitness. Heart rate does not always correlate closely with $\dot{V}O_2$ and is often affected by emotional state, environmental noise, stress, age, and previous meal and beverage intake. For these reasons several submaximal treadmill tests have been developed using multiple regression techniques to estimate $\dot{V}O_{2max}$ from measured factors.[57–63] One submaximal treadmill test was developed and cross-validated on males and females spanning a wide range of age and fitness levels.[57] In this test a brisk walking pace, ranging from 2.0–4.5 mph and eliciting a heart rate within 50–70% of age-predicted maximum, should be established during a 4-minute warm-up at 0% grade. This should be followed by a second 4-minute stage in which the speed remains the same, but the treadmill is raised to a 5% grade. The ending heart rate should be measured and used in the following equation to estimate $\dot{V}O_{2max}$:

$$\begin{aligned}\dot{V}O_{2max} &= 15.1 + (21.8 \times \text{speed}) \\ &-(0.327 \times \text{heart rate}) - (0.263 \times \text{speed} \times \text{age}) \\ &+(0.00504 \times \text{heart rate} \times \text{age}) + (5.98 \times \text{gender})\end{aligned}$$

[speed is treadmill speed in mph; gender = 0 for females, 1 for males]

For example, if a 45-year-old male walks at 3.0 mph up a 5% grade at a heart rate of 145 bpm, his $\dot{V}O_{2max}$ would be estimated as

$$\begin{aligned}\dot{V}O_{2max} &= 15.1 + (21.8 \times 3\text{ mph}) \\ &-(0.327 \times 145\text{ bpm}) - (0.263 \times 3\text{ mph} \times 45\text{ yr}) \\ &+(0.00504 \times 145\text{ bpm} \times 45\text{ yr}) + (5.98 \times 1) \\ &= 36.4\text{ ml} \cdot \text{kg}^{-1} \cdot \text{min}^{-1}\end{aligned}$$

This equation is fairly valid; 68% of the time, values are within $\pm 4.85\text{ ml} \cdot \text{kg} - 1 \cdot \text{min}^{-1}$ of actual $\dot{V}O_{2max}$.[57]

Cycle Ergometer Submaximal Laboratory Tests

Before discussing submaximal cycle ergometer tests, a comparison of the advantages and disadvantages of treadmills versus bicycles is helpful (see Box 4.2). The most commonly used submaximal cycle ergometer tests include the multistage physical work capacity test developed by Sjostrand[64] and a single-stage test by Astrand and Rhyming.[56] Both tests assume that because heart rate and $\dot{V}O_2$ are linearly related over a broad range, the submaximal heart rate at a certain workload can predict $\dot{V}O_{2max}$. The YMCA has adopted these tests for use in its nationwide testing program.[53]

Box 4.2

Treadmills versus Cycle Ergometers

In general both treadmills and cycle ergometers have their place in exercise testing facilities.

Advantages of Treadmills

1. Walking, jogging, and running are the most natural forms of locomotion. Most Americans are unaccustomed to bicycling (the treadmill was invented in the United States, the cycle ergometer in Europe).
2. In general, subjects reach higher $\dot{V}O_{2max}$ values during treadmill tests than they do with the cycle. $\dot{V}O_{2max}$ is usually 5–25% lower with cycle tests than with treadmill tests, depending on the participant's conditioning and leg strength. Only elite cyclists can achieve $\dot{V}O_{2max}$ values on cycles that equal treadmill values.

Disadvantages of Treadmills

1. Treadmills are more expensive than most cycle ergometers.
2. The treadmill is less portable than the cycle, requires more space, is heavy, and makes more noise.
3. The power (workload) of the treadmill cannot be measured directly in $\text{kg} \cdot \text{m} \cdot \text{min}^{-1}$ or watts, so it must be calculated.
4. The workload on the treadmill depends on body weight. In longitudinal studies with body weight changes, the workload changes. The body weight has a much smaller effect on cycle ergometer performance.
5. The danger of a fall is greater while running on a treadmill than while cycling on the cycle ergometer.
6. Measurement of heart rate and blood pressure is more difficult when a person is exercising on a treadmill than when on a cycle.

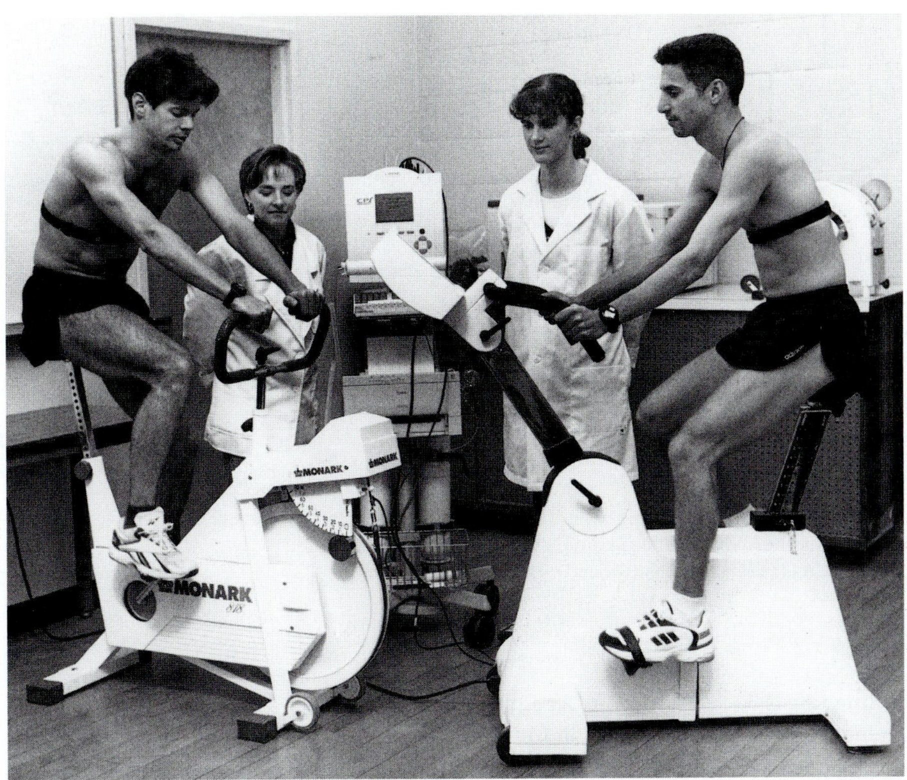

Figure 4.12 Mechanically braked cycle ergometers such as the Monark model pictured here have a front flywheel braked by a belt running around the rim attached to a weighted pendulum. The workload is adjusted by tightening or loosening the brake belt. The pedaling rate has to be maintained by the exerciser in time to a metronome. Good mechanically braked models cost between $750 and $1,000. The electronically braked ergometer uses an electromagnetic braking force to adjust the workload. The resistance is variable in relation to the pedaling rate, so that a constant work output in watts is maintained. However, electronically braked ergometers cost over $2,500.

A Description of Cycle Ergometers

A few facts on cycle ergometers include the following:[53]

- There are two major types of bicycle ergometers—mechanically braked and electronically braked (see Figure 4.12). The mechanically braked cycle ergometers are very accurate in workload adjustment and are not as expensive as the electronic versions. The mechanically braked cycle ergometers have a front flywheel braked by a belt running around the rim, attached to a weighted pendulum. The workload is adjusted by tightening or loosening the brake belt. The pedaling rate has to be maintained by the person being tested, in time to a metronome. The electronically braked ergometers use an electromagnetic braking force to adjust the workload (the resistance is variable in relation to the pedaling rate, so that a constant work output in watts is maintained). (*Note:* Because of the high expense of the electronically braked ergometer the rest of this discussion focuses on mechanically braked cycle ergometers.)
- The mechanically braked cycle ergometer should be accurate, easily calibrated, have constant torque, and have a range of 0–2,100 $\text{kg} \cdot \text{m} \cdot \text{min}^{-1}$. Several ergometers meet these specifications. (See the equipment list in Appendix B.)
- The calibration of the cycle should always be checked before testing. If using the Monark, be sure the red line on the pendulum weight is reading 0 on the workload scale. An adjusting wing nut easily corrects malalignments. The calibration of the cycle itself is done precisely at the factory, and unless the adjusting screw on the pendulum weight has been tampered with, there is seldom a need for recalibration. The calibration can be checked by hanging a known 2- or 4-kg weight on the part of the strap that moves the pendulum weight. The pendulum weight should read exactly 2 or 4 kg. If the numbers don't agree, the adjusting screw on the pendulum weight should be adjusted.
- The seat height of the ergometer should be set to the leg length of the rider. With the pedal in its lowest position if the heel of the foot is put onto the pedal, the leg should be straight. When the ball of the foot is put onto the pedal (as should be done during cycling), a slight bend of the leg at the knee should be apparent.
- The workload on the Monark or other mechanically braked bicycles is usually expressed in *kilogram-meters per minute* ($\text{kg} \cdot \text{m} \cdot \text{min}^{-1}$) or in *watts* (1 watt = 6 $\text{kg} \cdot \text{m} \cdot \text{min}^{-1}$). The equation $W = F \times D$ (W = work in $\text{kg} \cdot \text{m} \cdot \text{min}^{-1}$; F = force or resistance in kilograms; D=distance traveled by the flywheel rim per pedal revolution) applies to the Monark cycle ergometers. On a Monark, the flywheel travels 6 meters per pedal revolution. If the resistance is set with the front handwheel knob (which sets the weighted pendulum at 1 kilopond or 1 kilogram, 2 kiloponds, etc.), the workload is easily

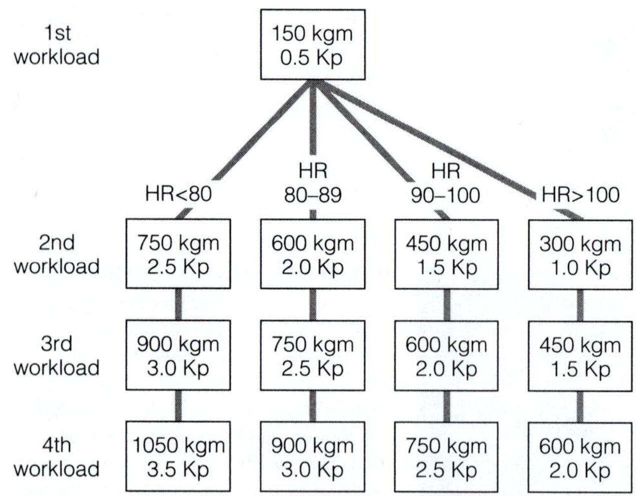

Directions:

1. Set the first workload at 150 kgm/min (0.5 Kp).
2. If the HR in the third minute is
   - less than (<) 80, set the second load at 750 kgm (2.5 Kp);
   - 80 to 89, set the second load at 600 kgm (2.0 Kp);
   - 90 to 100, set the second load at 450 kgm (1.5 Kp);
   - greater than (>) 100, set the second load at 300 kgm (1.0 Kp)
3. Set the third and fourth (if required) loads according to the loads in the columns below the second loads.

Figure 4.13 Guide to setting workloads for males on the YMCA's submaximal cycle ergometer test.
Source: Reprinted and adapted with permission of the YMCA of the USA, 101 N. Wacker Drive, Chicago, IL 60606.

figured out. If, for example, the cycling rate is 50 revolutions per minute (rpm) with the weighted pendulum set at 2 kg, then the workload is

$$\begin{aligned} \text{Work} &= 2\ \text{kg} \times 6\ \text{m} \cdot \text{rpm}^{-1} \times 50\ \text{rpm} \\ &= 600\ \text{kg} \cdot \text{m} \cdot \text{min}^{-1} (100\ \text{watts}) \end{aligned}$$

The YMCA Submaximal Cycle Test

Following is a step-by-step approach in conducting the YMCA's popular submaximal cycle ergometer test:[53]

- For the YMCA test set the metronome at 100 bpm, for a rate of 50 rpm (one beat for each foot down). Let the person being tested get used to the cadence, warming up for about 3 to 5 minutes.
- Next, set the workload, using Figure 4.13. The initial workload is set at 150 kg · m · min^{-1}.

  The person cycles at the first workload for 3 minutes, then stops, with the heart rate counted immediately, using either a stethoscope for 10 seconds (and then multiplying by 6) or a heart rate monitor. If there is doubt as to the accuracy of the heart rate, let the subject cycle another minute at the same workload and try again. The objective is to get a steady-state heart rate at this particular workload.
- Check Figure 4.13 to decide on the next workload setting. Workloads are adjusted on the basis of heart rate response.
- Regularly check the workload setting on the cycle ergometer during each workload period. As the friction belt gets hot, the workload creeps upward, so continual readjustment during the early stages is necessary.
- Again check the pulse after 3 or 4 minutes of cycling at the new workload. Determine the steady state pulse rate, and check Figure 4.13 to determine the third and final workload. (*Note:* If the first workload produced a heart rate greater than 110 bpm, the third workload is not necessary.)
- Throughout the test, watch for exertional intolerance or other signs of undue fatigue or unusual response. Explain to the participant that the rating of perceived exertion should be between 3 and 5 on the Borg scale[65] (see Figure 4.14).
- The objective of the YMCA submaximal bicycle test is to obtain two heart rates between 110 and 150 bpm. There is a linear relationship between heart rate and workload between these two rates for most people. When the heart rate is less than 110, many external stimuli can affect the rate (talking, laughter, nervousness). Once the heart rate climbs between 110 and 150, external stimuli should no longer affect the rate and there is a linear relationship. If the heart rate climbs above 150, the relationship becomes curvilinear. So the objective of this test is to obtain two heart rates between 110 and 150 bpm (steady state) at two different workloads to establish linearity between heart rate and workload for the person being tested.
- To establish the line, two points are needed. It is important that the heart rates taken be true steady-state values. To ensure this, it is better to let participants cycle beyond 3 minutes, especially during the second workload (the heart rate takes longer to plateau when the workload is harder).
- Once the test is completed, the two steady-state heart rates should be plotted against the respective

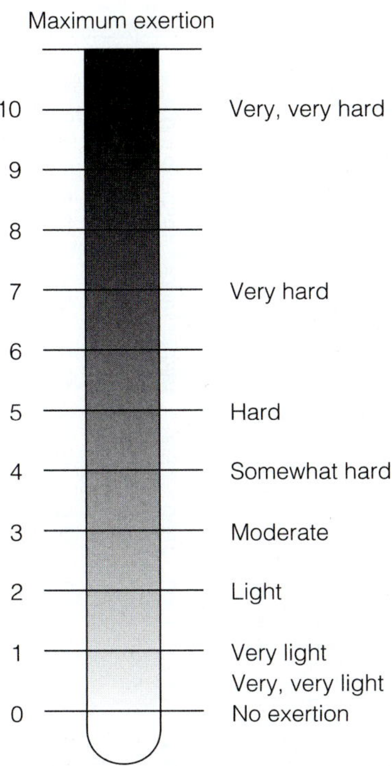

Figure 4.14 Borg scale rating of perceived exertion. During exercise heart rates of 110–115, exercise for most people will feel "3—Moderate" to "5—Hard." If the exercise feels harder than this, the workload should be reassessed. Source: Noble B, Borg GAV, Jacobs I, Ceci R, Kaiser P. A category ratio perceived exertion scale: Relationship to blood and muscle lactates and heart rate. *Med Sci Sports Exerc* 15:523–528, 1983.

workload in Figure 4.15. A straight line is drawn through the two points and extended to that participant's predicted maximal heart rate (220 − age). The point at which the diagonal line intersects the horizontal predicted maximal heart rate line represents the maximal working capacity for that participant. A perpendicular line should be dropped from this point to the baseline where the maximal physical workload capacity can be read in $kg \cdot m \cdot min^{-1}$.

- The maximal physical workload capacity in $kg \cdot m \cdot min^{-1}$ can then be used to predict a person's maximum oxygen uptake. These values are listed at the bottom of the graph. Use the norms in Appendix A (Tables 23 and 24) for interpretation. Remember that these results are predictions or estimates, not direct measurements, and are thus open to error (but usually within 15% of the actual value).

Cycling Equations

The American College of Sports Medicine has developed a formula to estimate the MET cost of leg and arm ergometry.[1] Box 4.3 describes the use of the formulas.

An equation has also been developed for estimating $\dot{V}O_2$ during outdoor bicycling on a level surface.[66]

$$\dot{V}O_2(L \cdot min^{-1}) = -4.5 + (0.17 \times \text{rider kmh}) + (0.052 \times \text{wind kmh}) + (0.022 \times \text{weight, kg})$$

For example, if a 70-kg bicyclist is cycling at 30 kmh (kilometers per hour) with no headwind in his face, his oxygen consumption would be

$$\dot{V}O_2 = -4.5 + (0.17 \times 30) + (0.052 \times 0) + (0.022 \times 70) = 2.14\ L \cdot min^{-1}$$

$$\text{or} \quad 30.6\ ml \cdot kg^{-1} \cdot min^{-1}[(2.14/70) \times 1{,}000]$$

Drafting (riding closely behind another cyclist) reduces the oxygen consumption by 18–39% depending on speed and the formation and number of riders being drafted.[66]

MAXIMAL LABORATORY TESTS

The graded exercise test (GXT) to exhaustion, with ECG monitoring, is considered the best substitute for the gold-standard test (direct $\dot{V}O_{2max}$ determination). This diagnostic functional capacity test is mandatory for all people in the high-risk category who want to start an exercise program.[1]

The maximal graded exercise test (usually done with a treadmill or cycle ergometer) with ECG serves several purposes:[1,67]

- To diagnose overt or latent heart disease
- To evaluate cardiorespiratory functional capacity (heart and lung endurance)
- To evaluate responses to conditioning or cardiac-rehabilitation programs
- To increase individual motivation for entering and adhering to exercise programs

Maximal Graded Exercise Treadmill Test Protocols

When deciding on a test modality the treadmill should be considered for most individuals because it tends to produce the best test outcomes. For example, among one group of triathletes, $\dot{V}O_{2max}$ from tethered swimming or cycle ergometry was 13–18% and 3–6% lower respectively, than values obtained from treadmill running.[68]

Figures 4.16 and 4.17 describe the most commonly used maximal treadmill protocols.[69–71] There are many other protocols, many of which have been developed for cardiac patients or athletes.[71] For example, in the Naughton protocol high-risk patients first go through a 4-minute warm-up, with the speed then set at 2 mph and the grade increased 3.5% every 2 minutes until maximal effort is reached.[72] In

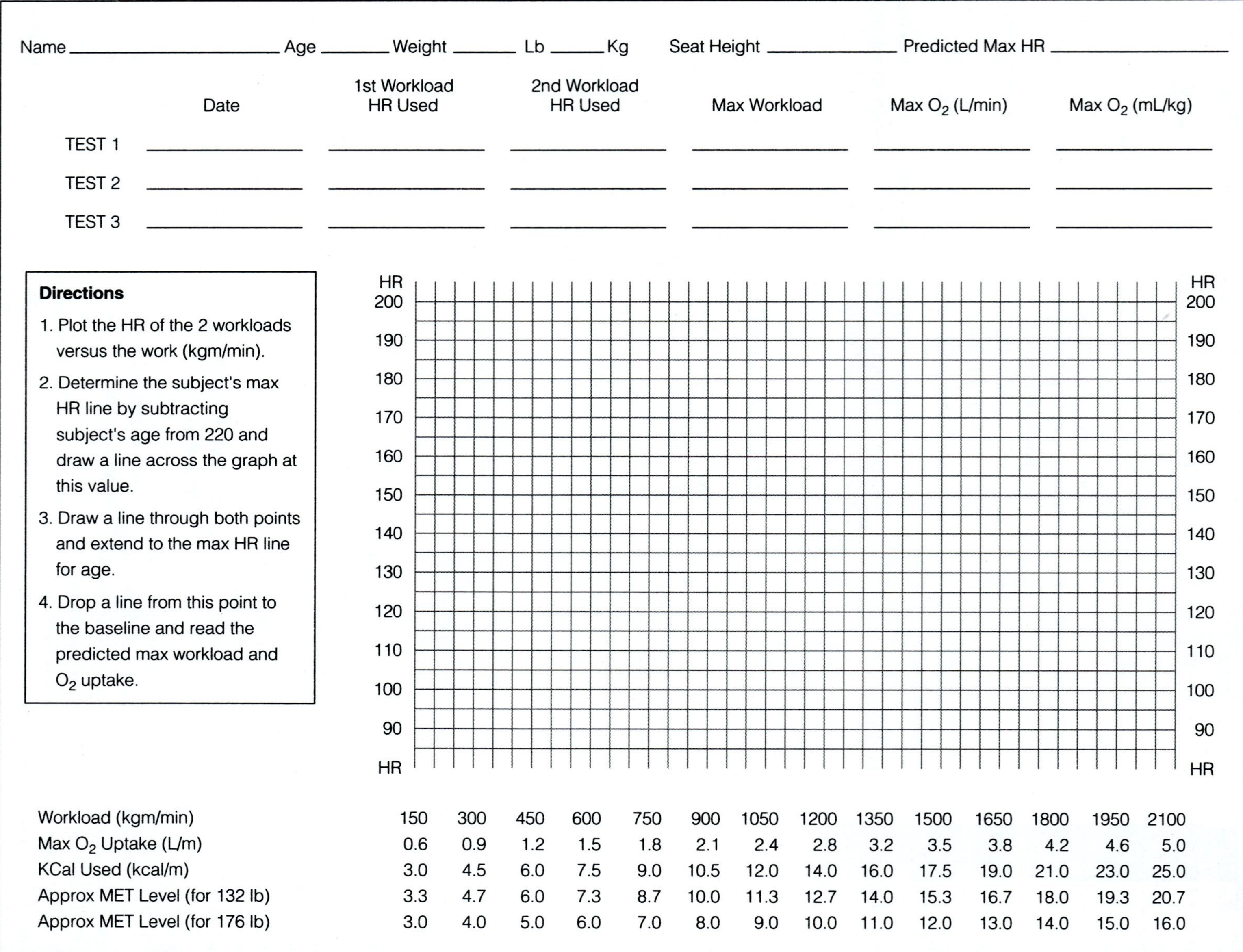

Name ____________ Age ______ Weight ______ Lb ______ Kg Seat Height ____________ Predicted Max HR ____________

	Date	1st Workload HR Used	2nd Workload HR Used	Max Workload	Max O_2 (L/min)	Max O_2 (mL/kg)
TEST 1						
TEST 2						
TEST 3						

Directions

1. Plot the HR of the 2 workloads versus the work (kgm/min).
2. Determine the subject's max HR line by subtracting subject's age from 220 and draw a line across the graph at this value.
3. Draw a line through both points and extend to the max HR line for age.
4. Drop a line from this point to the baseline and read the predicted max workload and O_2 uptake.

Workload (kgm/min)	150	300	450	600	750	900	1050	1200	1350	1500	1650	1800	1950	2100
Max O_2 Uptake (L/m)	0.6	0.9	1.2	1.5	1.8	2.1	2.4	2.8	3.2	3.5	3.8	4.2	4.6	5.0
KCal Used (kcal/m)	3.0	4.5	6.0	7.5	9.0	10.5	12.0	14.0	16.0	17.5	19.0	21.0	23.0	25.0
Approx MET Level (for 132 lb)	3.3	4.7	6.0	7.3	8.7	10.0	11.3	12.7	14.0	15.3	16.7	18.0	19.3	20.7
Approx MET Level (for 176 lb)	3.0	4.0	5.0	6.0	7.0	8.0	9.0	10.0	11.0	12.0	13.0	14.0	15.0	16.0

Figure 4.15 Graph for determining $\dot{V}O_{2max}$ from submaximal heart rates obtained during the YMCA's submaximal cycle test. Source: Reprinted and adapted with permission of the YMCA of the USA, 101 N. Wacker Drive, Chicago, IL 60606.

Box 4.3

Estimated Oxygen Demand Formula for Leg and Arm Ergometry[9]

The ACSM formula for estimating oxygen demands for leg ergometer exercise is

$$\dot{V}O_2\ \text{ml} \cdot \text{kg}^{-1} \cdot \text{min}^{-1} = \frac{\text{kg} \cdot \text{m} \cdot \text{min}^{-1} \times 1.8}{\text{kg} + 7} + 7$$

For example, if a 70-kg man cycles at a work rate of 900 kg · m · min^{-1}, the $\dot{V}O_2$ in ml · kg^{-1} · min^{-1} = [900 kg · m · min^{-1} 1.8)/kg + 7 = 30.14 ml · kg^{-1} · min^{-1} or 8.6 METs.

The ACSM formula for estimating oxygen demands for arm erogometry is

$$\dot{V}O_2\ \text{ml} \cdot \text{kg}^{-1} \cdot \text{min}^{-1} = \frac{\text{kg} \cdot \text{m} \cdot \text{min}^{-1} \times 3}{\text{kg} + 35} + 3.5$$

For example if a 70-kg man performs arm ergometry at 450 kg·m·min^{-1}, then

$\dot{V}O_2$ m · kg^{-1} · m^{-1} = 450 kg · m · min^{-1} × 3
70 + 3.5 = 22.8 ml · kg^{-1} · m^{-1}
or 6.5 METs

the Costill and Fox protocol for the athlete, following a 10-minute warm-up, the speed is set at 8.9 mph, with the grade increasing 2% every 2 minutes until exhaustion.[73] Of the treadmill protocols, the Bruce (Figure 4.16) is by far the most popular, followed by the Balke (Figure 4.17). The Bruce has relatively large, abrupt increases in workload every 3 minutes (8.5 ml · kg^{-1} · min^{-1} each stage), and some have criticized the test for this. Nonetheless, excellent maximal data can be obtained and because the test is so widely used, there is an abundance of comparative data. (See Appendix A, Table 23.)

The main criticism of the Balke test is its duration (nearly twice as long as the Bruce). In testing large numbers of people, the length of time needed for the Balke makes its use prohibitive. Ken Cooper uses the Balke protocol at the Aerobics Center in Dallas because he feels the Balke allows for a more gradual warm-up and is therefore safer.[32] The Balke is basically an uphill walking test, whereas the Bruce starts out as an uphill walking test and then in stage 4 becomes an uphill running test.

In general, $\dot{V}O_{2max}$ can be estimated accurately from performance time on the treadmill (see Figure 4.18). Maximal treadmill tests using performance time show very high correlations with laboratory-determined $\dot{V}O_{2max}$.[71] Thus,

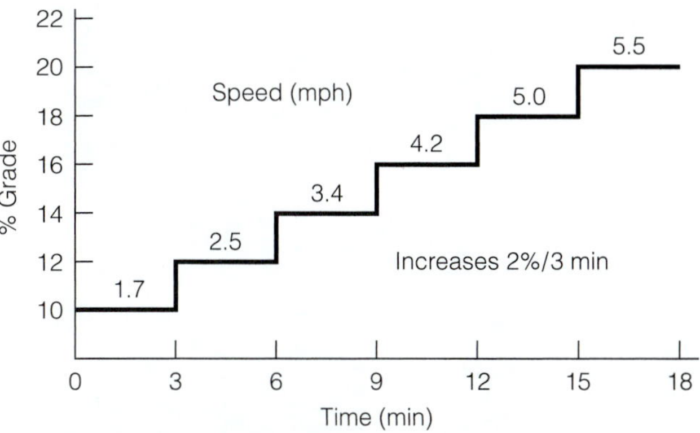

Figure 4.16 The Bruce maximal graded exercise test protocol. Source: Bruce RA, Kusumi F, Hosmer D. Maximal oxygen intake and nomographic assessment of functional aerobic impairment in cardiovascular disease. *Am Heart J* 85:546–562, 1973.

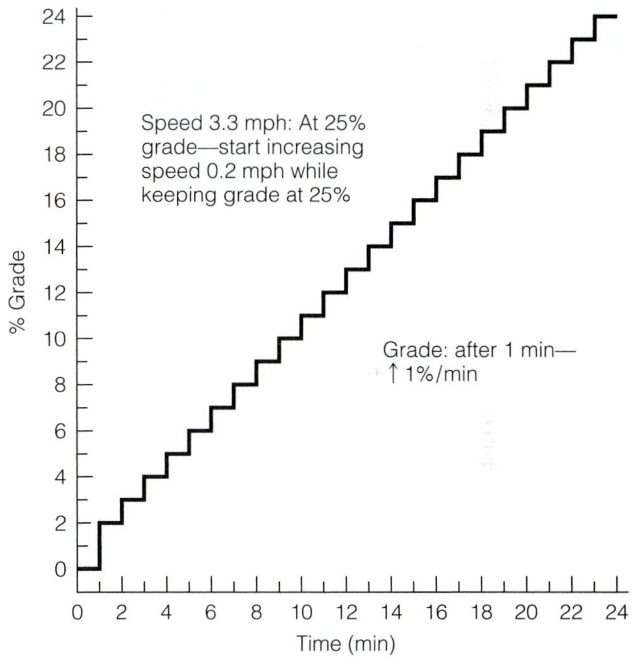

Figure 4.17 The Balke maximal graded exercise test protocol. Source: Balke B, Ware RW. An experimental study of "physical fitness" of Air Force personnel. *U.S. Armed Forces Medical Journal* 10(6):675–688, 1959.

actual measurement of $\dot{V}O_{2max}$ is not always necessary if the person is taken to a "true max," which means

- The person is allowed to practice one time before the maximal test to become "habituated" to the treadmill.
- Testers give verbal support to urge on the subject until exhaustion is reached.
- When the subject is "maxed out," there is no additional increase in heart rate despite an increase

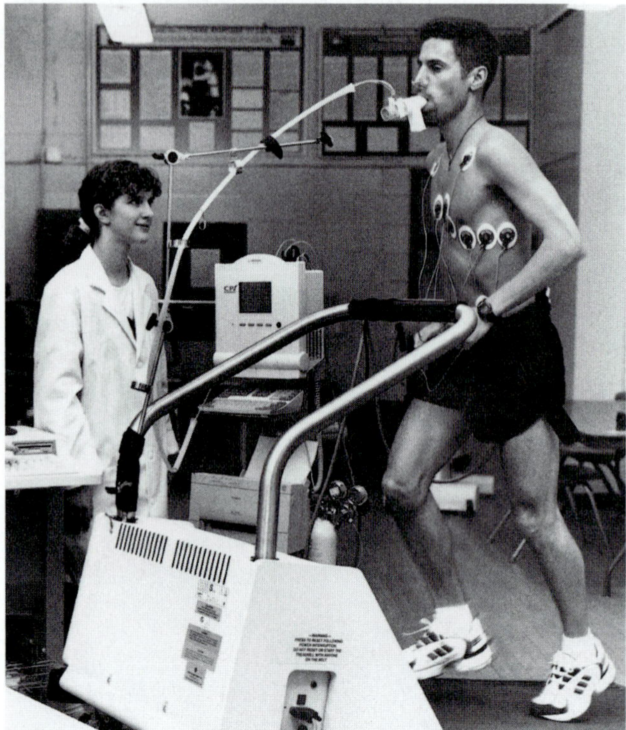

Figure 4.18 $\dot{V}O_{2max}$ can be estimated accurately from performance time on the treadmill if the subject is taken to a "true max" and does *not* hold on to the treadmill bar.

in workload, signs of exertional intolerance (fatigue staggering, inability to keep up with the workload, facial pallor), and a maximal rating of perceived exertion is given (Figure 4.14).

- During the test, the subject is not allowed to hold on to the treadmill bar, except for the tips of two fingers, to maintain balance when needed.[74]

To ensure valid and reliable $\dot{V}O_{2max}$ values, the testing protocol should be very specific to the type of exercise the person is accustomed to. The laboratory environment should be 20–23°C, 50% humidity, and if follow-up testing is conducted, tests should be repeated at the same time of the day, using the exact same procedures.[75] Practical procedures for administering a maximal graded exercise treadmill test include the following:

- Pretest

  Ensure that all equipment is in good working order (and calibrated) and that supplies are in place.

  Review the medical/health questionnaire, have the participant read and sign the consent form, and ensure appropriate physician supervision.

  For high-risk subjects, obtain a 12-lead resting ECG in supine and exercise postures (otherwise, attach a heart rate monitor for heart rate measurement).

  Obtain blood pressure measurements in the supine and exercise postures.

  Review the treadmill test procedures and have the participant practice walking on the treadmill (and ensure that he or she can exercise without hanging on the bar).

- Exercise

  Take heart rate/ECG measurements during the last 15 seconds of every stage and at peak exercise (educate the participate to give a warning prior to grabbing the bar when they feel they no longer can continue).

  Take blood pressure measurement during the last minute of each stage (if systolic blood pressure does not change or decreases between stages, verify immediately).

  Take the rating of perceived exertion (RPE) at the end of each stage. Observe and record symptoms reported by the participant.

  Ensure that stage changes are made on time, with the treadmill adjusted to the exact speed and grade.

  Urge the participant to exercise as long as possible (and ensure safety by putting a hand behind the participant's back). When the subject is maxed out, note the time exactly, obtain the maximum heart rate and blood pressure, and slow down the treadmill to stage 1.

- Posttest

  Obtain heart rate/ECG and blood pressure measurements every 1–2 minutes for at least 5 minutes to allow any exercise induced changes to return to baseline.

  Continue to record symptoms reported by the participant.

Treadmill Equations for Predicting $\dot{V}O_{2max}$

When the participant is allowed to exercise to maximal capacity in this way, $\dot{V}O_{2max}$ can be estimated very precisely. Appendix A (Table 23) contains a table that accurately estimates $\dot{V}O_{2max}$ based on length of time until exhaustion with the Bruce or Balke protocol.[76] Appendix A (Tables 24 and 25) also contains norms for classifying $\dot{V}O_{2max}$.

Formulas have been developed for predicting $\dot{V}O_{2max}$ from maximal treadmill tests.[3,70,77,78] These are summarized in Table 4.8. The critical measurement is time to exhaustion with subjects not holding onto the bar or being aided in any way.

TABLE 4.8 Equations for Estimating $\dot{V}O_{2max}$ from Maximal Treadmill Tests

Protocol	Equation
Bruce[78]	$\dot{V}O_{2max}$ (ml · kg^{-1} · min^{-1})=14.76 − (1.379 × time) + (0.451 × time^2) − (0.012 × time^3)
Balke[77]	$\dot{V}O_{2max}$ (ml · kg^{-1} · min^{-1})=11.12 + (1.51 × time)

Box 4.4

ACSM Energy Requirements Formulas*

The American College of Sports Medicine formulas for these data are as follows:

Walking

$$\dot{V}O_2\ ml \cdot kg^{-1} \cdot min^{-1} = speed\ m \cdot min^{-1} \times 0.1\ ml \cdot kg^{-1} \cdot min^{-1}/m \cdot min^{-1} + 3.5\ ml \cdot kg^{-1} \cdot min^{-1}$$

Example: For a walking speed of 80 m · min^{-1} (3 mph):

$$\dot{V}O_2 = 80\ m \cdot min^{-1} \times 0.1\ ml \cdot kg^{-1} \cdot min^{-1}/m \cdot min^{-1} + 3.5\ ml \cdot kg^{-1} \cdot min^{-1} = 11.5\ ml \cdot kg^{-1} \cdot min^{-1} \quad (METs = 11.5/3.5 = 3.3)$$

Graded Walking

Use the preceding equation plus:

$$\dot{V}O_2\ ml \cdot kg^{-1} \cdot min^{-1} = percent\ grade \times speed\ m \cdot min^{-1} \times 1.8\ ml \cdot kg \cdot min^{-1}/m \cdot min^{-1}$$

Example: If a person walks at 80 m · min^{-1} up a 13% grade, then $\dot{V}O_2$ is equal to 11.5 ml · kg^{-1} · min^{-1} (see above) plus:

$$0.13 \times 80\ m \cdot min^{-1} \times 1.8\ ml \cdot kg \cdot min^{-1}/m \cdot min^{-1} = 18.72$$

$$\dot{V}O_2 = 11.5 + 18.72 = 30.22\ ml \cdot kg^{-1} \cdot min^{-1}\ (8.64\ METs)$$

Jogging and Running (speeds over 5 mph)

$$\dot{V}O_2\ ml \cdot kg^{-1} \cdot min^{-1} = speed\ m \cdot min^{-1} \times 0.2\ ml \cdot kg^{-1} \cdot min^{-1}/m \cdot min^{-1} + 3.5\ ml \cdot kg^{-1} \cdot min^{-1}$$

Example: For a running speed of 200 m · min^{-1} (7.5 mph):

$$\dot{V}O_2\ ml \cdot kg^{-1} \cdot min^{-1} = 200\ m \cdot min^{-1} \times 0.2\ ml \cdot kg^{-1} \cdot min^{-1}/m \cdot min^{-1} + 3.5\ ml \cdot kg^{-1} \cdot min^{-1} = 43.5 \quad (METs = 43.5/3.5 = 12.4)$$

Note: For speeds in units of kmh, the MET requirement is approximately equal to the speed (10 kmh = 10 METs; 16 kmh = 16 METs).

Inclined Running

Use the equation for running, plus:

$$\text{On treadmill: } \dot{V}O_2\ ml \cdot kg^{-1} \cdot min^{-1} = speed\ in\ m \cdot min^{-1} \times percent\ grade \times 0.9\ ml \cdot kg \cdot min^{-1}/m \cdot min^{-1}$$

*1 mph = 26.8 m · min^{-1} = 1.6 km · hour^{-1}

Maximal Treadmill Test for College Students

A maximal treadmill graded exercise test for college students has been developed by researchers at Arizona State University, which (a) allows the participant to select a comfortable walking-jogging speed, (b) is time-efficient, and (c) is relatively accurate in estimating $\dot{V}O_{2max}$.[78] The test protocol is as follows:

- *Stage 1.* Participant walks up a 5% grade at a self-selected, brisk pace for 3 minutes.
- *Stage 2.* Participant has the option to either continue walking briskly on a 5% grade, or self-select a comfortable jogging pace on a 0% grade for 3 minutes. The first two stages are considered a warm-up.
- *Stages 3 to maximum.* Starting at 0% grade, increase treadmill grade by 1.5% each minute while keeping the speed constant until participants are unable to continue despite verbal encouragement. Note ending speed in miles per hour (mph) and the final treadmill percent grade that the participant is able to sustain for close to 1 minute.

$\dot{V}O_{2max}$ in ml · kg^{-1} · min^{-1} is estimated from this formula:[79]

$$\dot{V}O_{2max}\ ml \cdot kg^{-1} \cdot min^{-1} = 4.702 - (0.0924 \times kg) + (6.191 \times mph) + (1.311 \times \%\ grade) + (2.674 \times gender)$$

For gender, males are given 1, females 0. For example, if a 70-kg male chooses a jogging speed of 5.4 mph, and is maxed out after the treadmill grade reaches 10%, the estimated $\dot{V}O_{2max}$ is

$$4.702 - (0.0924 \times 70) + (6.191 \times 5.4) + (1.311 \times 10) + (2.674 \times 1) = 47.4\ ml \cdot kg^{-1} \cdot min^{-1}$$

The standard error of estimate is 2.1ml · kg^{-1} · min^{-1}.

ACSM Equations for Estimating $\dot{V}O_2$ for Walking and Running

The American College of Sports Medicine has developed steady-state $\dot{V}O_2$ formulas for running outdoors and on the treadmill, and also for walking (see Box 4.4).[1] The formula for graded treadmill exercise has been validated with a

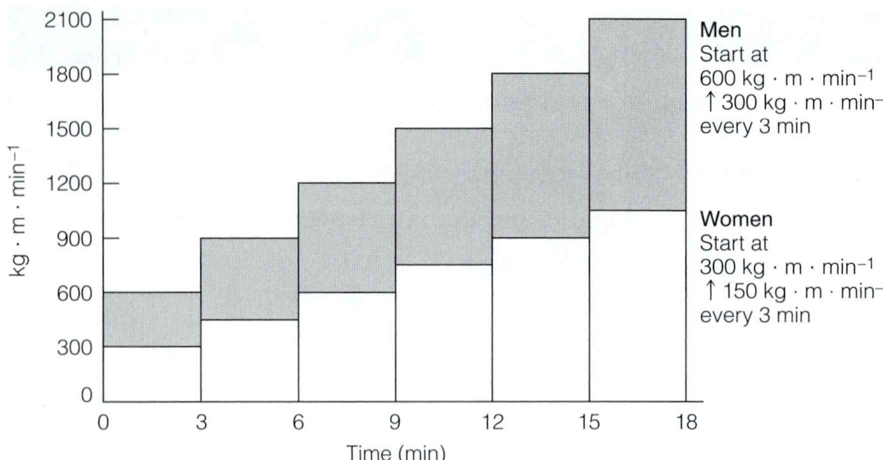

Figure 4.19 The Astrand maximal graded cycle exercise test protocol. The metronome should be set at 100, with a cycling rate of 50 rpm (one foot down with each click of the metronome). With the pedaling speed at 50 rpm, 300 kg · m/min is achieved with the cycle ergometer belt tension set at 1 kg, 600 kg · m/min at 21 kg, 900 kg · m/min at 3 kg, etc. Source: Astrand PO. *Work Tests with the Bicycle Ergometer.* Varberg, Sweden: AB Cykelfabriken Monark, 1965.

large number of people and found to be accurate for adults.[1] Once again, these data are *steady-state* values, which means that if they are used to predict $\dot{V}O_{2max}$ data 2–4 minutes from the end point should be used. *Note:* 1 mph = 26.8 m · min^{-1} = 1.6 kmh.

Maximal Graded Exercise Cycle Test Protocols

There are two recommended maximal graded exercise cycle test protocols: the Astrand and the Storer–Davis.[80,81]

The Astrand Maximal Cycle Protocol

For the Astrand maximal cycle test, the initial workload is 300 kg·m·min^{-1} (50 watts) (1 kp at 50 rpm) for women, and 600 kg·m·min^{-1} (100 watts) (2 kp at 50 rpm) for men[80] (see Figure 4.19). After 2 minutes at this initial workload the workload is increased every 2 to 3 minutes in increments of 150 kg·m·min^{-1} (= 25 watts, or ½ kp) for women, and 300 kg·m·min^{-1} (50 watts, or 1 kp) for men. The test is continued until the participant is exhausted or can no longer maintain the pedaling frequency of 50 rpm. A metronome should be used, with the tester carefully ensuring that the proper cadence is maintained.

The $\dot{V}O_{2max}$ for most people (except for elite cyclists) will be lower when derived from the maximal cycle test than when derived from the Bruce's treadmill protocol.

Caution should be used with estimating $\dot{V}O_{2max}$ from the ACSM cycle formula. The ACSM cycle formula assumes that a steady state has been achieved, and for the normal population, it has been shown that $\dot{V}O_2$ often plateaus 1 to 3 minutes before the test is completed (if the participant is taken to a true max). Steady-state $\dot{V}O_2$ tables will thus overpredict $\dot{V}O_{2max}$, unless steady-state values 2 to 4 minutes from the end point are used. In addition, the ACSM formulas may not be accurate for workloads over 200 watts. For people with high fitness levels, direct measurement of $\dot{V}O_{2max}$ is necessary.

The Storer–Davis Maximal Cycle Protocol

The Storer–Davis equation was developed to make maximal cycle ergometer testing more practical and accurate and to provide a valid method for estimating $\dot{V}O_{2max}$. This equation was developed after testing 115 males and 116 females ages 20 to 70.[81] After a 4-minute warm-up at 0 watts, the workload is increased by 15 watts/min, with a recommended rate of 60 rpm. On a mechanically braked ergometer, the kp setting should be increased ¼ kp each minute (see Figure 4.20).

The equation uses the final workload in watts:

Males

$$\dot{V}O_{2max}\ (\text{ml} \cdot \text{min}^{-1}) = (10.51 \times \text{watts}) + (6.35 \times \text{kg}) - (10.49 \times \text{age}) + 519.3\ \text{ml} \cdot \text{min}^{-1}$$

Females

$$\dot{V}O_{2max}\ (\text{ml} \cdot \text{min}^{-1}) = (9.39 \times \text{watts}) + (7.7 \times \text{kg}) - (5.88 \times \text{age}) + 136.7\ \text{ml} \cdot \text{min}^{-1}$$

For males, the correlation with measured oxygen consumption is very high (r = .94). The standard error of estimate (SEE) is low for both males (± 212 ml · min^{-1}) and females (± 145 ml · min^{-1}) (r = .93). This equation has been validated for use with adolescents.[82]

The Wingate Anaerobic Test

The maximal treadmill and cycle protocols described thus far test cardiorespiratory capacity. A different type of test has been developed to test maximal anaerobic power. *Anaerobic power* is the ability to exercise for a short time at high power levels and is important for various sports where sprinting and power movements are common (e.g., football).

The Wingate Anaerobic Test (WAnT) was developed during the 1970s at the Department of Research and Sport

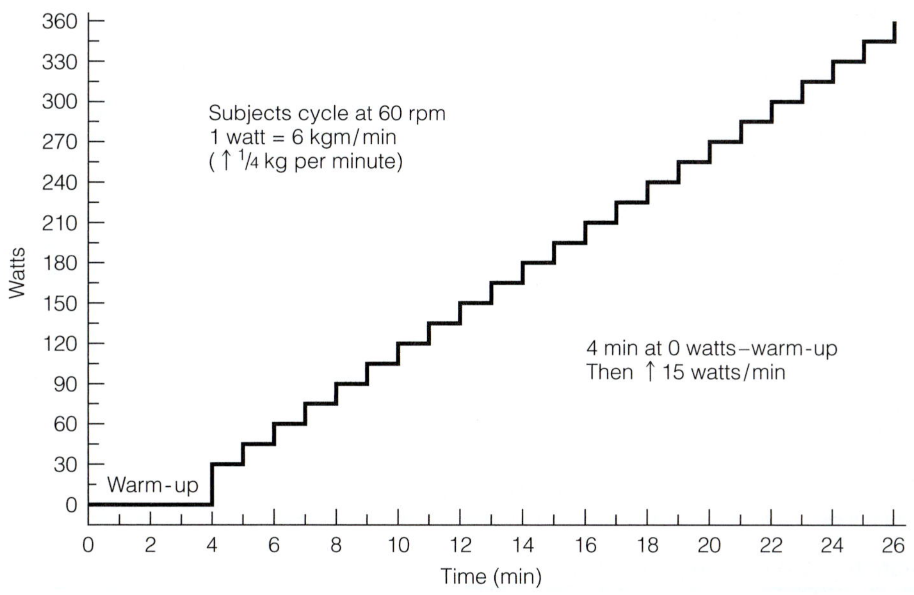

Figure 4.20 The Storer–Davis maximal cycle protocol. In the protocol, subjects cycle for 4 min at 0 watts to warm up. The workload is then increased 15 watts per minute, at a recommended rate of 60 rpm. On a mechanically braked ergometer, the kg setting should be increased ¼ kg each minute. Source: Storer TW, Davis JA, Caiozzo VJ. Accurate prediction of $\dot{V}O_{2max}$ in cycle ergometry. *Med Sci Sports Exerc* 22:704–712, 1990.

Medicine of the Wingate Institute for Physical Education and Sport in Israel.[83,84] The impetus for the development of the WAnT was the lack of interest in anaerobic performance as a component of fitness, and the scarcity of appropriate easily administered laboratory tests. Various other tests for anaerobic power and capacity have been promoted at various times, including the vertical jump, the Margaria step–running test, high-velocity treadmill running, and leg extensor force, but none of them have achieved the prominence and acceptance of the WAnT.

The WAnT requires pedaling or arm cranking on a cycle ergometer for 30 seconds at maximal speed against a constant force (with 5 minutes of both warm-up and cool-down recommended).[83,84] Power in watts is determined by counting pedal revolutions (watts = kp × rpm) or by using computerized equipment (Figure 4.21).[85]

Three indices are measured: (1) peak power (the highest mechanical power in watts elicited during the test, usually within the first 5 seconds); (2) mean power (the average power sustained throughout the 30-second period); (3) rate of fatigue (peak power minus the lowest power, divided by the peak power).

A predetermined force is used to ensure that a supramaximal effort is given. As a general guideline, with the Monark ergometer, a force of 0.090 kp/kg body weight should be used with adult nonathletes and of 0.100 kp/kg with adult athletes. The Monark cycle ergometer, however, is limited to athletes weighing less than 95 kg unless it is mechanically adapted. The use of toe stirrups increases performance by 5–12%. Some tentative norms have been developed[83] (see Table 4.9).

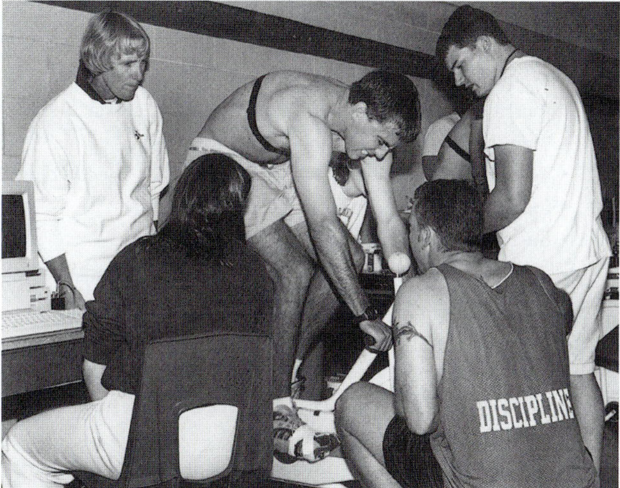

Figure 4.21 The Wingate Anaerobic Test requires pedaling for 30 seconds at maximal speed against a constant force. Verbal encouragement is recommended throughout the test.

When to Terminate the Maximal GXT-ECG Test

As emphasized in Chapter 3, maximal exercise testing, with precautions, is a relatively safe procedure.[1] The risk of death in clinical exercise laboratories is less than 0.01%, and the risk of acute heart attack during or immediately after an exercise test is ≤ 0.04% .[1] The risk of a complication requiring hospitalization is ≤ 0.2% .[1] The death rate is even lower in preventive medicine clinics, suggesting that the rate of complications during exercise testing is higher in coronary-prone individuals. Some individuals should not take a maximal GXT (see Table 3.1 in Chapter 3).

To safely conduct a maximal GXT-ECG test, various criteria should be carefully adhered to, and emergency drugs and equipment, along with an attending physician, should be available.[1]

In a maximum graded exercise stress test, the exercise usually continues until the participant voluntarily terminates the test because of exhaustion. Occasionally, for safety

TABLE 4.9 Young Adult (Ages 18–25) Norms for the Wingate Anaerobic Test

	Males		Females	
Classification	Peak Power (watts/kg)	Mean Power (watts/kg)	Peak Power (watts/kg)	Mean Power (watts/kg)
Very poor	5.4–6.8	5.1–6.0	6.3–7.3	4.3–4.9
Poor	6.8–7.5	6.0–6.4	7.3–7.8	4.9–5.2
Below average	7.5–8.2	6.4–6.9	7.8–8.3	5.2–5.5
Average	8.2–8.8	6.9–7.3	8.3–8.8	5.5–5.8
Good	8.8–9.5	7.3–7.7	8.8–9.3	5.8–6.1
Very good	9.5–10.2	7.7–8.2	9.3–9.8	6.1–6.4
Excellent	10.2–11.6	8.2–9.0	9.8–10.8	6.4–7.0
Elite sprinters/jumpers	11.0–12.2	8.5–9.5		
Elite rowers	11.2–12.2	9.9–10.9		

Source: Data from Inbar O, Bar-Or O, Skinner JS. *The Wingate Anaerobic Test.* Champaign, IL: Human Kinetics, 1996.

TABLE 4.10 Indications for Terminating Exercise Testing

Absolute Indications

- Drop in systolic blood pressure of ≥ 10 mm Hg from baseline blood pressure despite an increase in workload, when accompanied by other evidence of ischemia
- Moderate to severe angina
- Increasing nervous system symptoms (e.g., ataxia, dizziness, or near syncope)
- Signs of poor perfusion (cyanosis or pallor)
- Technical difficulties monitoring the ECG or systolic blood pressure
- Subject's desire to stop
- Sustained ventricular tachycardia
- ST elevation (≥ 1.0 mm) in leads without diagnostic Q waves (other than V_1 or VR)

Relative Indications

- Drop in systolic blood pressure of ≥ 10 mm Hg from baseline blood pressure despite an increase in workload, in the absence of other evidence of ischemia
- ST or QRS changes such as excessive ST depression (>2 mm horizontal or downsloping ST segment depression) or marked axis shift (see source below)
- Arrhythmias other than sustained ventricular tachycardia, including multifocal PVCs, triplets of PVCs, supraventricular tachycardia; heart block, or bradyarrhythmias
- Fatigue, shortness of breath, wheezing, leg cramps, or claudication
- Development of bundle-branch block or intraventricular conduction delay that cannot be distinguished from ventricular tachycardia
- Increasing chest pain
- Hypertensive response*

*Systolic blood pressure of more than 250 mm Hg and/or a diastolic blood pressure of more than 115 mm Hg.

Source: American College of Sports Medicine. *ACSM's Guidelines for Graded Exercise Testing and Prescription* (7th ed.). Philadelphia: Lippincott Williams & Wilkins, 2006. Used with permission.

reasons, the test may have to be terminated prior to the point of maximal exercise. General indications for test termination—those that do not rely on physician involvement or ECG monitoring—are listed below. More specific termination criteria for clinical or diagnostic testing are provided in Table 4.10 (and require physician interpretation). General indications for stopping an exercise test in low-risk adults include:[1]

- Onset of angina or angina-like pains (severe constricting pain in the chest, often radiating from the center of the chest to a shoulder [usually left] and down the arm, due to lack of blood flow and oxygen to the heart muscle usually because of coronary heart disease)
- Significant drop (20 mm Hg) in systolic blood pressure or a failure of the systolic blood pressure to rise with an increase in exercise intensity
- Excessive rise in blood pressure (systolic blood pressure rises above 260 mm Hg, or the diastolic blood pressure rises above 115 mm Hg)

- Signs of poor perfusion: light-headedness, confusion, ataxia, pallor, cyanosis, nausea, or cold and clammy skin
- Failure of heart rate to increase with increased exercise intensity
- Noticeable change in heart rhythm
- Subject requests to stop
- Physical or verbal manifestations of severe fatigue
- Failure of the testing equipment

Emergency Procedures

The American College of Sports Medicine advises the following:[1]

- All personnel involved with exercise testing and supervision should be trained in basic cardiopulmonary resuscitation (CPR) and preferably advanced cardiac life support (ACLS).
- There should be at least one, and preferably two, licensed and trained ACLS personnel and a physician immediately available at all times when maximal sign- or symptom-limited exercise testing is performed.
- Telephone plans should be established and posted. Regular rehearsal of emergency plans and scenarios should be conducted and documented.
- Regular drills should be conducted at least quarterly for all personnel.
    - A specific person or persons should be assigned to the regular maintenance of the emergency equipment and to the regular surveillance of all pharmacologic substances.
    - Records should be kept documenting the function of emergency equipment such as defibrillator, oxygen supply, and suction. In addition, expiration dates for pharmacologic agents and other supportive supplies should be kept.
    - Hospital emergency departments and other sources of support should be advised as to the exercise testing lab location as well as the usual times of operation.

Personnel

It is advised that ACSM-certified personnel administer the graded exercise test (see Chapter 3). When low-risk, young adult participants are being tested, a physician need not be in attendance (but a qualified physician should be the overall director of any testing program and should be consulted concerning protocols and emergency procedures). When testing people classified as high risk, the test should be physician supervised.[1]

SPORTS MEDICINE INSIGHT

Administering the Electrocardiogram

Learning to interpret the electrocardiogram (ECG) takes special training under the guidance of experienced health professionals. Nevertheless, many experts feel that health and fitness leaders should be familiar with basic ECG principles. In addition, treadmill or cycle ergometer operators are expected to be able to know when abnormal ECG patterns appear on the oscilloscope (and to call the attending physician, or if necessary terminate the test). The following description should be reviewed with an instructor familiar with ECG interpretation.

THE ECG

The *ECG* presents a visible record of the heart's electrical activity, by means of a stylus that traces the activity on a continuously moving strip of special heat-sensitive paper.[86] All heartbeats appear as a similar pattern, equally spaced, and consist of three major units (see Figure 4.22):

- *P wave* (transmission of electrical impulse through the atria)
- *QRS complex* (impulse through the ventricles)
- *T wave* (electrical recovery or repolarization of the ventricles)

Heart cells are charged or *polarized* in the resting state (negative ions inside the cell, positive outside), but when electrically stimulated, they depolarize (positive ions go inside the heart cell, negative ions go outside) and contract. Thus, when the heart is stimulated, a wave of depolarization passes through the heart (an advancing wave of positive charges within the cells). As the positive wave of depolarization within the heart cells moves toward a positive skin electrode, there is a positive upward deflection recorded on the ECG.

(continued)

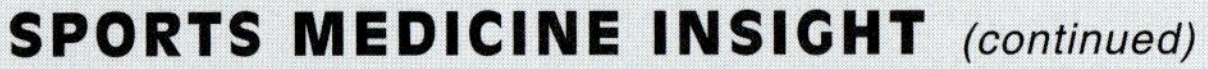

SPORTS MEDICINE INSIGHT *(continued)*

Administering the Electrocardiogram

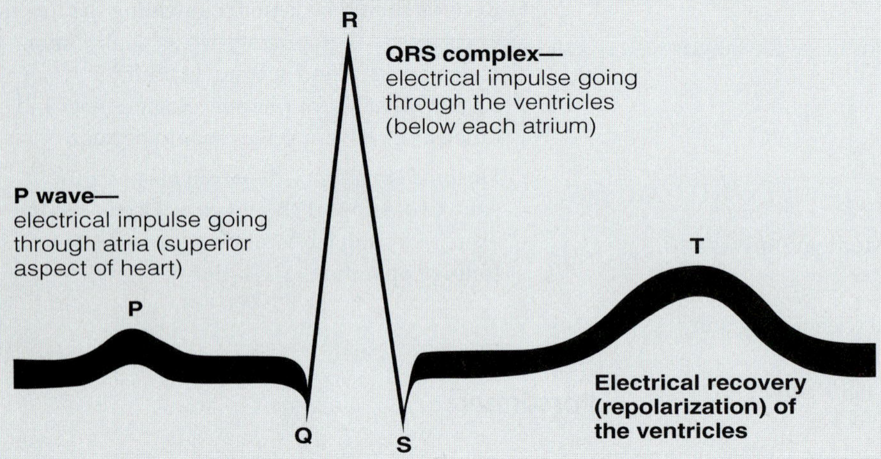

Figure 4.22 Normal single heartbeat. All heartbeats consist of three major units, the P wave, the QRS complex, and the T wave, which represent the transmission of electrical impulses through the heart.

The P wave (atrial wave) begins in the *sinoatrial* (SA) node (the normal physiological pacemaker) located near the top of the atrium. The impulse reaches the *atrioventricular* (AV) node located in the superior aspect of the ventricles. There is a 1⁄10-second pause, allowing blood to enter the ventricles from the contracting atria (see Figure 4.23).

The QRS complex (ventricular wave) begins in the AV node. After the 1⁄10-second pause, the AV node is stimulated, initiating an electrical impulse that starts down the AV bundle, called the *bundle of HIS* into the *bundle branches* and finally into the *Purkinje fibers.* The neuromuscular conduction system of the ventricles is composed of specialized nervous material that transmits the electrical impulse from the AV node into the ventricular heart cells.

The ECG is recorded on ruled paper. The smallest divisions are 1-millimeter squares. On the horizontal line, 1 small block represents 0.04 second (1 large block of 5 small blocks is 0.20 second). On the vertical axis, 1 small block represents 1⁄10 of a millivolt (10 small blocks vertically or 2 large blocks is 1 millivolt) (see Figure 4.24).

The standard ECG is composed of 12 separate leads:

Limb leads: Lead 1, Lead 2, Lead 3

Augmented unipolar leads: aVR, aVL, aVF

Chest leads: $V_1, V_2, V_3, V_4, V_5, V_6$

An *ECG lead* is a pair of electrodes placed on the body and connected to an ECG recorder. An axis is an imaginary line connecting the two electrodes. The electrodes for the three limb leads are placed on the right arm, left arm, and left leg. The ground electrode is placed on the right leg. This is electronically equivalent to placing the electrodes at the two shoulders and the symphysis pubis. From these three electrodes (plus the ground), the ECG recorder can make certain electrodes positive and others negative to produce six leads (1, 2, 3, aVR, aVL, aVF) (see Figure 4.25).

It is not the purpose of this book to give details on how to interpret the ECG. The exercise technician can administer the resting 12-lead ECG, but a qualified physician (especially cardiologists and internists) should interpret the results.[67] The resting 12-lead ECG should be administered to high-risk patients before the treadmill ECG to help screen out those with various contraindications to exercise.

EXERCISE TEST ELECTRODE PLACEMENT

The diagnostic GXT should be performed with a multiple-lead electrocardiographic system. The best possible GXT-ECG test is one in which all 12 leads are monitored. The *Mason-Likar* 12-lead exercise ECG system should be used, in which the six precordial electrodes are placed in

(continued)

SPORTS MEDICINE INSIGHT *(continued)*

Administering the Electrocardiogram

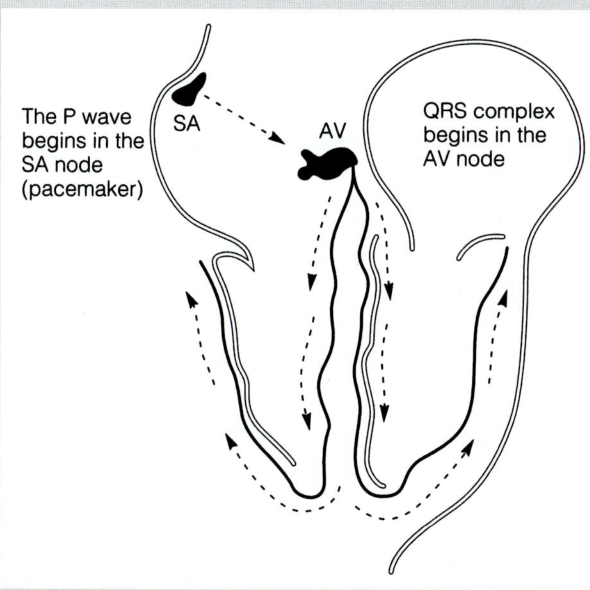

Figure 4.23 Normal electrical pathway. The P wave (atrial wave) begins in the SA node (normal physiological pacemaker) located near the top of the atrium. The QRS complex (ventricular wave) begins in the AV node.

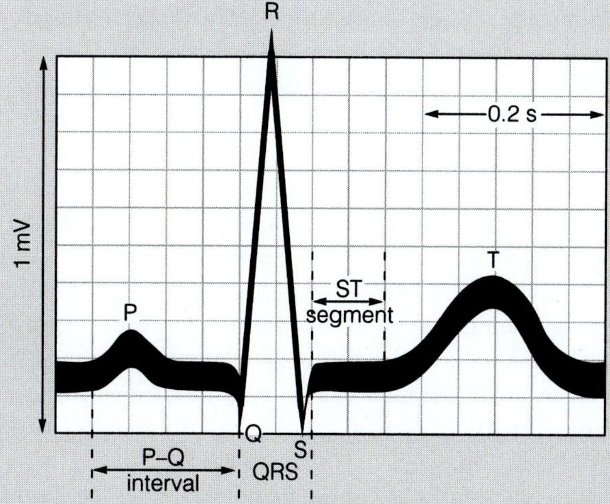

Figure 4.24 On the horizontal line, one small block represents 0.04 second or 1 millimeter. One large block of five small blocks is 0.20 second. On the vertical axis, one small block represents 1⁄10 of a millivolt. Ten small blocks vertically or two large blocks is 1 millivolt.

Standard or bipolar limb leads	*Electrodes connected*	*Marketing code*
Lead 1	LA & RA	·
Lead 2	LL & RA	· ·
Lead 3	LL & LA	· · ·
Augmented unipolar limb leads		
aVR	RA & (LA-LL)	—
aVL	LA & (RA-LL)	— —
aVF	LL (RA-LA)	— — —
Chest or precordial leads		
V	C & (LA-RA-LL)	(see data on right)

Recommended positions for multiple chest leads
(Line art illustration of chest positions)

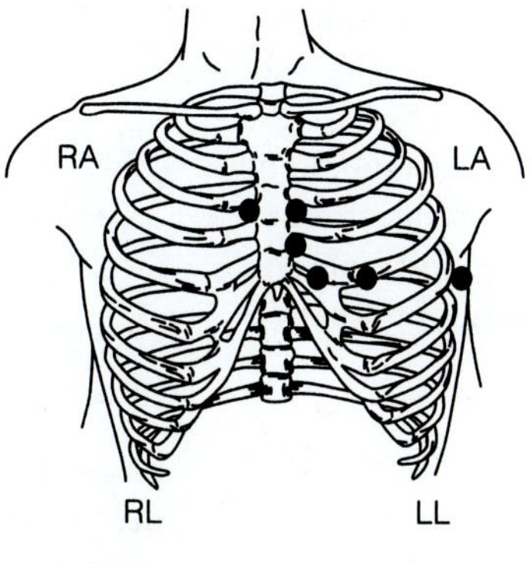

RA LA RL LL

Lead	Position	Code
V_1	Fourth intercostal space at right margin of sternum	— ·
V_2	Fourth intercostal space at left margin of sternum	— · ·
V_3	Midway between position 2 and position 4	— · · ·
V_4	Fifth intercostal space at junction of left midclavicular line	— · · · ·
V_5	At horizontal level of position 4 at left anterior axillary line	— · · · · ·
V_6	At horizontal level of position 4 at left midaxillary line	— · · · · · ·

Figure 4.25 Ten electrode positions form 12 leads for the routine electrocardiogram. Electrodes should be placed in the exact anatomical position noted so that the physician can compare the ECG with appropriate standards.

(continued)

SPORTS MEDICINE INSIGHT *(continued)*

Administering the Electrocardiogram

their usual positions: the right and left arm electrodes are placed on the shoulders at the distal ends of the clavicles; and the right and left leg electrodes are positioned at the base of the torso, just medial to the anterior iliac crests[1,87] (see Figure 4.25).

However, the majority of abnormal ECG responses to exercise can be picked up by lead V_5 alone. When only V_5 is monitored, the CM5 electrode placement system is generally used, in which the second electrode (the negative) is placed on the top third of the sternum (RA electrode), and the third electrode (the ground) is placed on the right side of the chest in the V_5 position (RL electrode).[1,87] The V_5 electrode (LA) is put in its normal position.

All leads should be continuously monitored by oscilloscope and recordings taken at the end of each minute of exercise or when significant ECG changes or abnormalities are noted on the screen. During recovery, this should continue every 1 to 2 minutes for the 8-minute postexercise test.

During the early part of the recovery period, the participant should exercise at low intensity (2 mph, 0% grade on the treadmill). The ECG and blood pressure should be recorded every 1 to 2 minutes for at least 8 minutes of recovery (or longer if there are abnormalities). The participant should not be allowed to stand still or sit still immediately following the exercise test. After approximately 2 minutes of cool-down, the subject can sit down and continue to move her or his feet for several more minutes. Disposable electrodes (available for about 25 cents each) stick on the body very well despite the accumulation of sweat, and they conduct the electrical impulses from the body to the ECG with little or no movement-artifact interference. Proper skin preparation is essential for the best ECG recordings. The resistance of the skin should be lowered by first cleansing thoroughly with an alcohol saturated gauze pad and then removing the superficial layer of the skin by rubbing vigorously. Shaving of the skin is not necessary.

BASIC PRINCIPLES IN ARRHYTHMIA DETERMINATION

An *arrhythmia* is any disturbance of rate, rhythm, or conduction of electrical impulses in the heart. The following criteria should be systematically analyzed for each ECG strip (while watching the oscilloscope), until the ability to pick out abnormal ECGs becomes automatic.

1. *R to R intervals.* Evenly spaced (maximum allowable difference between R waves is 3 small squares)
2. *P waves.*
   a. Within the 3 × 3 small square box
   b. Positive
   c. Same consistent, rounded shape
3. *P-R interval.* 3 to 5 small squares (0.12 to 0.20 second)
4. *P to QRS ratio.* Always 1:1 ratio
5. *QRS duration.* Less than 2½ small squares (0.10 second)

The exercise technician should be (a) able to monitor the screen and pick out any abnormal PQRST wave complex, and (b) alert to call the supervising physician for an interpretation. However, the exercise technician does not necessarily need to know how to interpret abnormal ECGs during exercise. (One of the most common ECG abnormalities during the exercise test is the premature ventricular contraction [PVC]). (See Figure 4.26 for examples of PVCs.)

One of the major purposes in giving a treadmill ECG stress test is to load the heart muscle beyond normal demands to see whether any obstruction to blood flow in the coronary arteries can be picked up on the ECG.[1] During the maximal exercise test coronary blood flow increases fivefold. If the coronary blood vessel is restricted approximately two thirds, the ST segment of the PQRST wave complex may be depressed.

ST segment depression is determined if all the following criteria are present (see Figure 4.26 for examples):

- 1 mm or more depressed (below baseline)
- At least 0.08 second (2 small squares) in length
- Flat or downsloping
- Three or more consecutive complexes

When ST segment depression is recorded, this is a "positive" test for coronary heart disease (CHD). When ST segment depression is not present, the test is called "negative."

The supervising physician should know that the specificity, sensitivity, and diagnostic accuracy of the test can vary considerably according to the prevalence of

(continued)

SPORTS MEDICINE INSIGHT *(continued)*

Administering the Electrocardiogram

CHD in the population being tested (Bayes theorem) and according to criteria used.[1,87] Ischemic chest pain induced by the exercise test is strongly predictive of CHD and is even more predictive with ST segment depression.[1,87] Severity of CHD is also related to the time of appearance of ST segment depression, with changes occurring early translating to a poor prognosis and increased risk of multivessel disease. The probability and severity of CHD are also directly related to the amount of ST segment depression and the downslope.

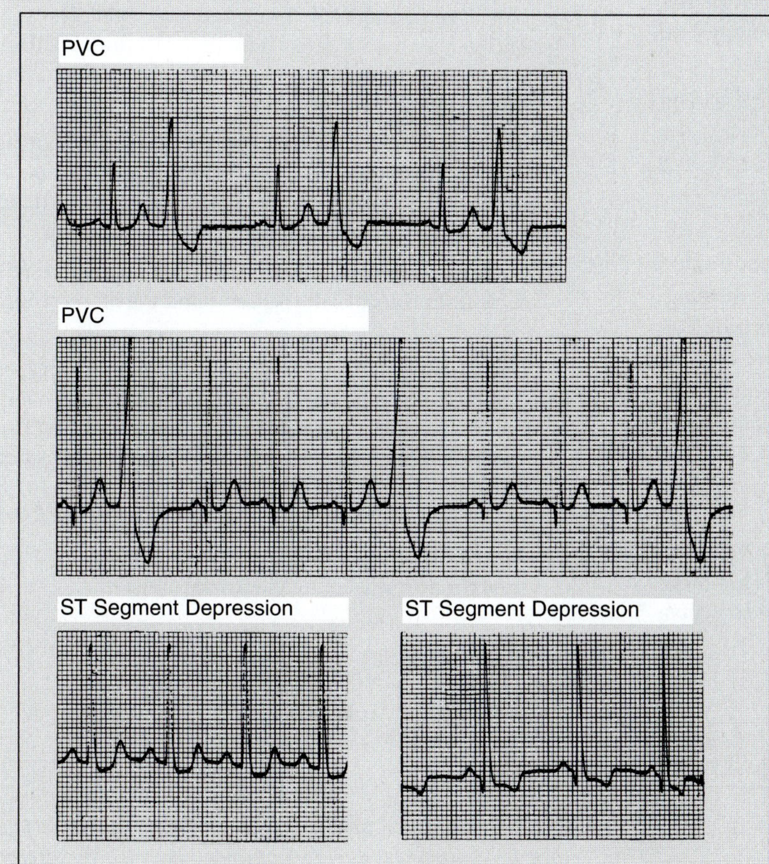

Figure 4.26 One of the most common arrhythmias is the premature ventricular contraction (PVC). ST segment depression may occur when coronary blood vessels are partially restricted, decreasing blood flow during exercise.

SUMMARY

1. While the direct measurement of $\dot{V}O_{2max}$ is the best estimate of heart and lung endurance, for various practical reasons, other tests have been developed as substitutes. These include field tests (mainly running tests), step tests (YMCA 3-minute step test, Canadian Home Fitness Step Test), submaximal laboratory tests (YMCA submaximal cycle test), and maximal laboratory tests (both cycle and treadmill).
2. This chapter provided a detailed description of these tests. Maximal treadmill testing with ECG is explained in detail because of its great value in diagnosing overt or latent heart disease, evaluating cardiorespiratory functional capacity, evaluating responses to conditioning or cardiac rehabilitation programs, and increasing individual motivation for entering and adhering to exercise programs.
3. Resting and exercise blood pressure and heart rate determination are reviewed. The diagnosis of adult hypertension is confirmed when the average of two or more measurements on at least two separate visits are 140/90 mm Hg or higher.

4. Principles for taking blood pressure measurements are listed. At rest, diastolic blood pressure equals the disappearance of the pulse sound (fifth Korotkoff sound).
5. Heart rate can be determined through several methods including the use of heart rate rulers, auscultation with a stethoscope, and heart rate monitors.
6. A number of performance tests, such as maximal endurance runs on a track, have been devised for testing large groups in field situations. Equations for predicting $\dot{V}O_{2max}$ from one's ability to run various distances at maximal speed have been developed. A 1-mile walk test has been developed to more safely test adults.
7. Both maximal and submaximal step tests have been developed for predicting $\dot{V}O_{2max}$. Of these, the Canadian Aerobic Fitness Test and the YMCA's 3-minute step test have been most widely used.
8. The American College of Sports Medicine has developed equations for predicting oxygen consumption during bench stepping, cycling, walking, and running. Two important terms are used by the American College of Sports Medicine in its equations and calculations—METs and $kcal \cdot min^{-1}$. One MET is equal to 3.5 $ml \cdot kg^{-1} \cdot min^{-1}$, or the oxygen consumption during rest. One MET is also equal to 1 $kcal \cdot kg^{-1} \cdot hour^{-1}$.
9. Both treadmill and cycle ergometers are used in testing cardiorespiratory fitness. In the United States, most facilities use treadmills for exercise testing because walking, jogging, and running are more familiar to Americans, who generally are unaccustomed to cycling. In addition, most people reach higher $\dot{V}O_{2max}$ values during treadmill tests than they do with the cycle.
10. A complete description of cycle ergometers is presented. The workload on the Monark or other mechanically braked cycles is usually expressed in kilogram-meters per minute ($kg \cdot m \cdot min^{-1}$) or in watts (1 watt = 6 $kg \cdot m \cdot min^{-1}$). Work = kg setting $\times$ 6 $m \cdot rpm^{-1} \times rpm = kg \cdot m \cdot min^{-1}$.
11. One of the best submaximal cycle protocols is the one used by the YMCA in its testing program. The objective of the YMCA submaximal cycle test is to obtain two heart rates between 110 and 150 bpm and then extrapolate these to an estimated maximal oxygen consumption.
12. The most commonly used maximal treadmill protocols are the Bruce and the Balke. $\dot{V}O_{2max}$ can be estimated accurately from performance time to exhaustion during these protocols.
13. There are two recommended maximal graded exercise cycle test protocols: the Astrand and the Storer–Davis.
14. The maximal treadmill and cycle protocols described herein test maximal cardiorespiratory capacity. A different type of test, the Wingate Anaerobic Test (WAnT), has been developed to test maximal anaerobic power. The WAnT requires pedaling or arm cranking on a cycle ergometer for 30 seconds at maximal speed against a constant force.
15. The Sports Medicine Insight reviewed basic principles for administering electrocardiograms.

Review Questions

1. *One MET represents*

   A. Resting oxygen consumption
   B. Oxygen consumption during running
   C. Oxygen consumption during walking
   D. Maximal oxygen consumption

2. ***Hypertension is diagnosed for adults when the average of two or more diastolic blood pressure measurements on at least two separate visits is ____ mm Hg or higher, and/or the systolic measurements are ____ mm Hg or higher.***

   A. 110/60　B. 140/90
   C. 120/80　D. 160/100
   E. 180/110

3. ***The pressure in the artery when the heart is resting is called the***

   A. Systolic pressure
   B. Diastolic pressure

4. ***$\dot{V}O_{2max}$ is defined as the greatest rate at which oxygen can be consumed during maximal exercise conditions and is usually expressed in terms of***

   A. $ml \cdot kg^{-1} \cdot min^{-1}$　B. $mg \cdot min^{-1}$
   C. $ml \cdot kg^{-1}$　D. $g \cdot kg^{-1}$
   E. None of these

5. ***During a graded exercise test on a treadmill, the systolic blood pressure in healthy participants***

   A. Increases　B. Stays the same　C. Decreases

6. ***Resting oxygen consumption is ____ $ml \cdot kg^{-1} \cdot min^{-1}$ in the average human.***

   A. 11.5　B. 3.5　C. 50　D. 245　E. 75

7. ***Which fitness test uses a 1-minute recovery heart rate to determine fitness classification?***

   A. Canadian Aerobic Fitness Test
   B. YMCA 3-minute step test

C. 1.5-mile run test
D. Bruce treadmill test

8. *Which maximal treadmill test protocol has a larger workload increase per stage?*

A. Bruce B. Balke

9. *A diastolic blood pressure of 84 mm Hg is classified as*

A. Normal B. Prehypertension
C. Optimal D. Stage 1 hypertension
E. Stage 2 hypertension

10. *If the blood pressure is less than 145/95 mm Hg, it should be rechecked within*

A. 2 months B. 6 months
C. 1 year D. 2 years

11. *During exercise testing, the ____ Korotkoff sound should be used for systolic blood pressure.*

A. Second B. Third
C. First D. Fifth
E. Fourth

12. *If 50 mm separate 4 R waves, the heart rate is*

A. 100 B. 120 C. 150 D. 200 E. 250

13. *Which submaximal test uses two 8-inch steps?*

A. Canadian Aerobic Fitness Test
B. YMCA 3-minute step test
C. Katch and McArdle step test

14. *On a cycle ergometer such as the Monark, 10 watts equal ____ $kg \cdot m \cdot min^{-1}$.*

A. 10 B. 20 C. 30 D. 40 E. 60

15. *On a cycle ergometer such as the Monark, if a client cycles at 60 rpm at a setting of 2 kp, the workload is ____ $kg{\cdot}m{\cdot}min^{-1}$.*

A. 120 B. 2,000 C. 30 D. 520 E. 720

16. *The Wingate test measures*

A. Aerobic power B. Muscular endurance
C. Anaerobic power

17. *Which one of the following is* **not** *a criteria for exercise test termination during those that do not rely on physician involvement or ECG monitoring?*

A. Subject asks to stop
B. Significant drop in systolic BP
C. Diastolic BP that rises above 90 mm Hg
D. Onset of angina
E. Signs of poor perfusion, including light-headedness, confusion, ataxia, cyanosis

18. *If a 60-kg man runs 9 mph for 45 minutes, how many kilocalories will he expend?*

A. 750 B. 857 C. 1,142 D. 665 E. 443

19. *If a 70-kg man is expending 10 METs during exercise, how many kilocalories per minute is this?*

A. 11.7 B. 4.8 C. 8.8 D. 6.2 E. 13.3

20. *If a 60-kg woman is cycling at a work rate of 900 $kg \cdot m \cdot min^{-1}$, the energy expenditure in METs is*

A. 9.7 B. 16.2 C. 7.9 D. 15.3 E. 11.4

21. *If a person walks at 3.5 mph, what is the energy expenditure in METs?*

A. 2.3 B. 3.7 C. 5.3 D. 3.0 E. 6.9

22. *If a 50-kg man is expending 10 METs during exercise, how many kilocalories per hour is this?*

A. 500 B. 600
C. 650 D. 750
E. None of these

23. *Which one of the following is* **not** *a criterion used to determine whether an individual's true $\dot{V}O_{2max}$ has been achieved?*

A. Oxygen consumption plateaus during the last minutes of a graded exercise test.
B. Respiratory exchange ratio increases to 1.0 or higher.
C. Subject's heart rate increases to within 10 beats of the age-predicted maximum.
D. Blood lactate levels rise above 8 mmol/liter.

24. *The 1-mile walk equation does* **not** *use which one of the following measurements or factors?*

A. Ending heart rate B. Total walk time
C. Body weight D. Gender
E. Body mass index

25. *The Wingate anaerobic test requires pedaling on a cycle ergometer for ____ seconds.*

A. 30 B. 60 C. 10 D. 5 E. 120

Answers

1. A	5. A	9. B	13. A	17. C	21. B	25. A
2. B	6. B	10. A	14. E	18. D	22. A	
3. B	7. B	11. C	15. E	19. A	23. B	
4. A	8. A	12. B	16. C	20. A	24. E	

REFERENCES

1. American College of Sports Medicine. *ACSM's Guidelines for Graded Exercise Testing and Prescription* (6th ed.). Philadelphia: Lippincott Williams & Wilkins, 2000; 7th ed., 2006.
2. Wilmore JH, Costill DL. *Physiology of Sport and Exercise.* Champaign, IL: Human Kinetics, 2004.
3. Maud PJ, Foster C. *Physiological Assessment of Human Fitness.* Champaign, IL: Human Kinetics 1995.
4. Bassett DR, Howley ET. Maximal oxygen uptake: "Classical" versus "contemporary" viewpoints. *Med Sci Sports Exerc* 29:591–603, 1997.
5. American College of Sports Medicine. *Resource Manual for Guidelines for Exercise Testing and Prescription* (5th ed.). Philadelphia: Lippincott William & Wilkins, 2006.
6. Doyon KH, Perrey S, Abe D, Hughson RL. Field testing of $\dot{V}O_{2peak}$ in cross-country skiers with portable breath-by-breath system. *Can J Appl Physiol* 26:1–11, 2001.
7. Vanderburgh PM, Katch FI. Ratio scaling of $\dot{V}O_{2max}$ penalizes women with larger percent body fat, not lean body mass. *Med Sci Sports Exerc* 28:1204–1208, 1996.
8. Howley ET, Bassett DR, Welch HG. Criteria for maximal oxygen uptake: Review and commentary. *Med Sci Sports Exerc* 27:1292–1301, 1995.
9. Duncan GE, Howley ET, Johnson BN. Applicability of $\dot{V}O_{2max}$ criteria: Discontinuous versus continuous protocols. *Med Sci Sports Exerc* 29:273–278, 1997.
10. National High Blood Pressure Education Program. *The Seventh Report of the Joint National Committee on Detection, Evaluation, and Treatment of High Blood Pressure.* National Heart, Lung, and Blood Institute, National Institutes of Health, NIH Publication No. 04-5230. Bethesda, MD: National Institutes of Health, 2003.
11. Hajjar I, Kotchen TA. Trends in prevalence, awareness, treatment, and control of hypertension in the United States, 1988–2000. *JAMA* 290:199–206, 2003.
12. American Society of Hypertension Public Policy Position Paper. Recommendations for routine blood pressure measurement by indirect cuff sphygmomanometry. *Am J Hypertension* 5:207–209, 1992.
13. Reeves RA. Does this patient have hypertension? How to measure blood pressure. *JAMA* 273:1211–1218, 1995.
14. Perloff D, Grim C, Flack J, et al. Human blood pressure determination by sphygmomanometry. *Circulation* 88:2460–2470, 1993.
15. Griffin SE, Robergs RA, Heyward VH. Blood pressure measurement during exercise: A review. *Med Sci Sports Exerc* 29:149–159, 1997.
16. Lightfoot JT, Tuller B, Williams DF. Ambient noise interferes with auscultatory blood pressure measurement during exercise. *Med Sci Sports Exerc* 28:502–508, 1996.
17. Daida H, Allison TG, Squires RW, Miller TD, Gau GT. Peak exercise blood pressure stratified by age and gender in apparently healthy subjects. *Mayo Clinic Proc* 71:445–452, 1996.
18. Scott AL, Brozic A, Myers J, Ignaszewski A. Exercise stress testing: An overview of current guidelines. *Sports Med* 27:285–312, 1999.
19. Gillum RF. Epidemiology of resting pulse rate of persons ages 25–74: Data from NHANES 1971–74. *Pub Health Rep* 107:193–201, 1992.
20. Jackson AS, Blair SN, Mahar MT, Wier LT, Ross RM, Stuteville JE. Prediction of functional aerobic capacity without exercise testing. *Med Sci Sports Exerc* 22:863–870, 1990.
21. Matthews CE, Heil DP, Freedson PS, Pastides H. Classification of cardiorespiratory fitness without exercise testing. *Med Sci Sports Exerc* 31:486–493, 1999.
22. Williford HN, Scharff-Olson M, Wang N, Blessing DL, Smith FH, Duey WJ. Cross-validation of non-exercise predictions of $\dot{V}O_{2peak}$ in women. *Med Sci Sports Exerc* 28:926–930, 1996.
23. Whaley MH, Kaminsky LA, Dwyer GB, Getchell LH. Failure of predicted $\dot{V}O_{2peak}$ to discriminate physical fitness in epidemiological studies. *Med Sci Sports Exerc* 27:85–91, 1995.
24. George JD, Stone WJ, Burkett LN. Non-exercise $\dot{V}O_{2max}$ estimation for physically active college students. *Med Sci Sports Exerc* 29:415–423, 1997.
25. Cardinal BJ. Predicting cardiorespiratory fitness without exercise testing in epidemiologic studies: A concurrent validity study. *J Epidemiol* 6:31–35, 1996.
26. Cureton KJ, Sloniger MA, O'Bannon JP, Black DM, McCormack WP. A generalized equation for prediction of $\dot{V}O_{2peak}$ from 1-mile run/walk performance. *Med Sci Sports Exerc* 27:445–451, 1995.
27. Draper DO, Jones GL. The 1.5-mile run revisited: An update in women's times. *JOPERD,* September 1990, 78–80.
28. George JD, Vehrs PR, Allsen PE, Fellingham GW, Fisher AG. $\dot{V}O_{2max}$ estimation from a submaximal 1-mile track jog for fit college-age individuals. *Med Sci Sports Exerc* 25:401–406, 1993.
29. American Alliance for Health, Physical Education, Recreation and Dance. *AAHPERD Norms for College Students: Health Related Physical Fitness Test.* Reston, VA: American Alliance for Health, Physical Education, Recreation and Dance, 1985.
30. Conley DS, Cureton KJ, Hinson BT, Higbie EJ, Weyand PG. Validation of the 12-minute swim as a field test of peak aerobic power in young women. *Res Quart Exerc Sport* 63:153–161, 1992.
31. Conley DS, Cureton KJ, Dengel DR, Weyand PG. Validation of the 12-minute swim as a field test of peak aerobic power in young men. *Med Sci Sports Exerc* 23:766–773, 1991.
32. Cooper KH. *The Aerobics Way.* New York: M. Evans and Co., 1977.
33. Zwiren LD, Freedson PS, Ward A, Wilke S, Rippe JM. Estimation of $\dot{V}O_{2max}$: A comparative analysis of five exercise tests. *Res Quart Exerc Sport* 62:73–78, 1991.
34. Dolgener FA, Hensley LD, Marsh JJ, Fjelstul JK. Validation of the Rockport Fitness Walking Test in college males and females. *Res Quart Exerc Sport* 65:152–158, 1994.
35. Tokmakidis SP, Leger L, Mercier D, Peronnet F, Thibault G. New approaches to predict $\dot{V}O_{2max}$ and endurance from running performance. *J Sports Med* 27:401–409, 1987.
36. Laukkanen POR, Pasanen M, Tyry T, Vuori I. A 2-km walking test for assessing the cardiorespiratory fitness of healthy adults. *Int J Sports Med* 12:356–362, 1991.
37. Kline GM, Porcari JP, Hintermeister R, Freedson PS, Ward A, McCarron RF, Ross J, Rippe JM. Estimation of $\dot{V}O_{2max}$ from a one-mile track walk, gender, age, and body weight. *Med Sci Sports Exerc* 19:253–259, 1987.
38. Widrick J, Ward A, Ebbeling C, Clemente E, Rippe JM. Treadmill validation of an over-ground walking test to predict peak oxygen consumption. *Eur J Appl Physiol* 64:304–308, 1992.
39. George JD, Fellingham GW, Fisher AG. A modified version of the Rockport Fitness Walking Test for college men and women. *Res Quart Exerc Sport* 69:205–209, 1998.
40. Grant S, Corbett K, Amjad AM, Wilson J, Aitchison T. A comparison of methods of predicting maximum oxygen uptake. *Br J Sports Med* 29:147–152, 1995.
41. Fenstermaker KI, Plowman SA, Looney MA. Validation of the Rockport Fitness Walking Test in females 65 years and older. *Res Quart Exerc Sport* 63:322–327, 1992.
42. Warren BJ, Dotson RG, Nieman DC, Butterworth DE. Validation of a one-mile walk test in elderly women. *J Aging Phys Act* 1:13–21, 1993.

43. Montoye HJ, Ayen T, Washbum RA. The estimation of $\dot{V}O_{2max}$ from maximal and sub-maximal measurements in males, age 10–39. *Res Quart Exerc Sport* 57:250–253, 1986.

44. Cavanagh PR, Kram R. The efficiency of human movement: A statement of the problem. *Med Sci Sport Exerc* 17:30–308, 1985.

45. Thomas SG, Weller IMR, Cox MH. Sources of variation in oxygen consumption during a stepping task. *Med Sci Sports Exerc* 25:139–144, 1993.

46. Nagle FS, Balke B, Naughton JP. Gradational step tests for assessing work capacity. *J Appl Physiol* 20:745–748, 1965.

47. Ellestad MH, Blomqvist CG, Naughton JP. Standards for adults exercise testing laboratories. *Circulation* 59:421A–430A, 1979.

48. Shephard RJ, Thomas S, Weller I. The Canadian Home Fitness Test: 1991 update. *Sports Med* 11:358–366, 1991.

49. Shephard RJ. Current status of the step test in field evaluations of aerobic fitness: The Canadian Home Fitness Test and its analogues. *Sports Med Training Rehab* 6:29–41, 1995.

50. Jette M, Mongeon J, Shephard RJ. Demonstration of a training response by the Canadian Home Fitness Test. *Eur J Appl Physiol* 49:143–150, 1982.

51. Weller IM, Thomas SG, Gledhill N, Paterson D, Quinney A. A study to validate the modified Canadian Aerobic Fitness Test. *Can J Appl Physiol* 20:211–221, 1995.

52. Canadian Society for Exercise Physiology. *The Canadian Physical Activity Fitness & Lifestyle Appraisal.* Ottawa, Ontario: Canadian Society for Exercise Physiology, 1996; 2nd ed., 1998; 3rd ed., 2003 (www.csep.ca).

53. Golding LA, Myers CR, Sinning WE. *Y's Way to Physical Fitness: The Complete Guide to Fitness Testing and Instruction* (3rd ed.). Chicago: YMCA of the USA, 1989.

54. McArdle WD, Katch FI, Katch VL. *Exercise Physiology: Energy, Nutrition, and Human Performance.* Philadelphia: Lea & Febiger, 1991.

55. Brouha L. The step test: A simple method of measuring physical fitness for muscular work in young men. *Res Quart Exerc Sport* 14:31–36, 1943.

56. Astrand PO, Rhyming I. A nomogram for calculation of aerobic capacity (physical fitness) from pulse rate during submaximal work. *J Appl Physiol* 7:218–221, 1954.

57. Ebbeling CB, Ward A, Puleo EM, Widrick J, Rippe JM. Development of a single-stage submaximal treadmill walking test. *Med Sci Sports Exerc* 23:966–973, 1991.

58. Foster C, Crowe AJ, Daines E. Predicting functional capacity during treadmill testing independent of exercise protocol. *Med Sci Sports Exerc* 28:752–756, 1996.

59. George JD, Vehrs PR, Allsen PE, Fellingham GW, Fisher AG. Development of a submaximal treadmill jogging test for fit college-aged individuals. *Med Sci Sports Exerc* 25:643–647, 1993.

60. Hermiston RT, Faulkner JA. Prediction of maximal oxygen uptake by a stepwise regression technique. *J Appl Physiol* 30:833–837, 1971.

61. Metz KF, Alexander JF. Estimation of maximal oxygen intake from submaximal work parameters. *Res Ouart Exerc Sport* 42:187–193, 1971.

62. Town GP, Golding LA. Treadmill test to predict maximum aerobic capacity. *J Phy Ed* 74:6–8, 1977.

63. Wilmore JH, Roby FB, Stanforth PR. Ratings of perceived exertion, heart rate, and treadmill speed in the prediction of maximal oxygen uptake during submaximal treadmill exercise. *J Cardio Rehab* 5:540–546, 1985.

64. Sjostrand T. Changes in respiratory organs of workmen at an ore melting works. *Acta Med Scand* (suppl) 196:687–695, 1947.

65. Noble B, Borg GAV, Jacobs I, Ceci R, Kaiser P. A category ratio perceived exertion scale: Relationship to blood and muscle lactates and heart rate. *Med Sci Sports Exerc* 15:523–528, 1983.

66. McCole SD, Claney K, Conte JC, Anderson R, Hagberg JM. Energy expenditure during bicycling. *J Appl Physiol* 68:748–753, 1990.

67. Gibbons RJ, Balady GJ, Beasley JW, et al. ACC/AHA guidelines for exercise testing: Executive summary. A report of the American College of Cardiology/American Heart Association Task Force on Practice Guidelines (Committee on Exercise Testing). *Circulation* 96:345–354, 1997.

68. O'Toole ML, Douglas PS, Hiller WDB. Applied physiology of a triathlon. *Sports Med* 8:201–225, 1989.

69. Bruce RA, Kusumi F, Hosmer D. Maximal oxygen intake and nomographic assessment of functional aerobic impairment in cardiovascular disease. *Am Heart J* 85:546–562, 1973.

70. Balke B, Ware RW. An experimental study of "physical fitness" of Air Force personnel. *U.S. Armed Forces Med J* 10(6):675–688, 1959.

71. Heyward VH. *Advanced Fitness Assessment & Exercise Prescription* (3rd ed.). Champaign, IL: Human Kinetics Books, 1998.

72. Naughton J, Balke B, Nagle F. Refinement in methods of evaluation and physical conditioning before and after myocardial infarction. *Am J Cardiol* 14:837–842, 1964.

73. Costill DL, Fox EL. Energetics of marathon running. *Med Sci Sports Exerc* 1:81–86, 1969.

74. Manfre MJ, Yu GH, Varma AA, Mallis GI, Kearney K, Karageorgia MA. The effect of limited handrail support on total treadmill time and the prediction of $\dot{V}O_{2max}$. *Clin Cardiol* 17:445–450, 1994.

75. McConnell TR. Practical considerations in the testing of $\dot{V}O_{2max}$ in runners. *Sports Med* 5:57–68, 1988.

76. Pollock ML, Wilmore JH, Fox SM. *Exercise in Health and Disease.* Philadelphia: WB Saunders Co., 1984.

77. Froelicher VF, Lancaster MC. The prediction of maximal oxygen consumption from a continuous exercise treadmill protocol. *Am Heart J* 87:445–450, 1974.

78. Foster C, Jackson AS, Pollock ML, Taylor MM, Hare J, Sennett SM, Rod JL, Sarwar M, Schmidt DH. Generalized equations for predicting functional capacity from treadmill performance. *Am Heart J* 108:1229–1234, 1984.

79. George JD. Alternative approach to maximal exercise testing and $\dot{V}O_{2max}$ prediction in college students. *Res Quart Exerc Sport* 67:452–457, 1996.

80. Åstrand PO. *Work Tests with the Bicycle Ergometer.* Varberg, Sweden: AB Cykelfabriken Monark, 1965.

81. Storer TW, Davis JA, Caiozzo VJ. Accurate prediction of $\dot{V}O_{2max}$ in cycle ergometry. *Med Sci Sports Exerc* 22:704–712, 1990.

82. Jung AP, Nieman DC, Kernodle MW. Prediction of maximal aerobic power in adolescents from cycle ergometry. *Pediatr Exerc Sci* 13:167–172, 2001.

83. Inbar O, Bar-Or O, Skinner JS. *The Wingate Anaerobic Test.* Champaign, IL: Human Kinetics, 1996.

84. Bar-Or O. The Wingate anaerobic test: An update on methodology reliability, and validity. *Sports Med* 4:381–394, 1987.

85. Mcklin RC, O'Bryant HS, Zehnbauer TM, Collins MA. A computerized method for assessing anaerobic power and work capacity using maximal cycle ergometry. *J Appl Sports Sci Res* 4:135–140, 1990.

86. Dubin D. *Rapid Interpretation of EKGs.* Tampa: Cover Publishing Co., 1974.

87. Evans CH. *Exercise Testing: Current Applications for Patient Management.* Philadelphia: W.B. Saunders Co., 1994.

PHYSICAL FITNESS ACTIVITY 4.1

Practical Use of the ACSM Equations

The American College of Sports Medicine equations presented in this chapter are highly useful for health and fitness instructors. However, the use of these equations can be initially confusing to some students. It is highly recommended that prospective instructors practice using the equations many times over, applying them to varying situations to gain a full understanding of them. In the ACSM Health/Fitness Instructor Certification program, the ACSM equations are an integral part of the process.

Here are some sample questions to help you learn how to use the equations. Correct answers are noted with an asterisk (*). Consult your instructor to help clarify use of the equations. However, all the information you need to solve these problems is in this chapter.

1. If a person is cycling at 60 rpm with the bicycle ergometer set at 2 kp, the workload in watts is
   a. 200
   b. *120
   c. 150
   d. 180
   e. None of the above
2. If a 60-kg man runs 9 mph for 45 minutes, how many kilocalories will he expend?
   a. 750
   b. 857
   c. 1142
   d. *665
   e. 443
3. If a 100-kg man is expending 5 METs during exercise, how many kilocalories/min is this?
   a. 7.5
   b. 4.8
   c. 5.8
   d. 6.2
   e. *8.3
4. If a 60-kg woman is cycling at a work rate of 600 $kg \cdot m \cdot min^{-1}$, the energy expenditure in METs is
   a. *7.1
   b. 6.2
   c. 8.0
   d. 5.3
   e. 4.0
5. If a person walks at 5.0 mph, what is the energy expenditure in METs?
   a. 2.3
   b. *4.8
   c. 5.3
   d. 3.0
   e. 6.9

6. If the person in question 5 is a male weighing 70 kg, how many kilocalories would he burn if he walked for 30 minutes?

   a. 100
   b. 284
   c. 154
   d. *168
   e. 220

7. The oxygen cost of running on the level at 300 meters/min would be about

   a. 6 METs
   b. 8 METs
   c. 10.5 METs
   d. 12.5 METs
   e. *18.1 METs

8. If a person is cycling at 50 rpm with the cycle ergometer set at 4 kp, the workload in $kg \cdot m \cdot min^{-1}$ is

   a. 200
   b. *1,200
   c. 1,500
   d. 2,200
   e. None of the above

9. If a 50-kg man is expending 10 METs during exercise, how many kilocalories per hour is this?

   a. *500
   b. 600
   c. 650
   d. 750
   e. None of the above

10. If a 72-kg man is cycling at a work rate of $kg \cdot m \cdot min^{-1}$, the energy expenditure in $ml \cdot kg^{-1} \cdot min^{-1}$ is

    a. 15
    b. *22
    c. 34
    d. 48
    e. None of the above

11. If an 80-kg person walks at 2.0 mph, how many kilocalories will be expended after 2 hours?

    a. *405
    b. 502
    c. 609
    d. 650
    e. None of the above

12. The oxygen cost in $ml \cdot kg^{-1} \cdot min^{-1}$ of running on the level at 8 mph would be

    a. 34.2
    b. *46.4
    c. 53.9
    d. 56.7

e. 65.0

Questions 13 to 18 apply to Mr. Smith's graded exercise test on a cycle ergometer (3-minute stages, 80 rpm). This was conducted without a physician present because Mr. Smith is an athlete training for national competition, is 22 years old, weighs 65 kg, and is apparently healthy.

Stage	Work Rate (watts)	Heart Rate	Blood Pressure	RPE
1	50	100	125/70	2
2	100	135	140/72	3
3	150	150	150/70	4
4	200	164	160/73	5
5	250	178	172/70	6
6	300	190	185/73	8
7	350	200	190/72	9
8	400	205	195/75	10

13. The final workload in kilogram-meters per minute is approximately
    a. 1,200
    b. *2,400
    c. 1,500
    d. 3,500
    e. None of the above
14. What was the final approximate "kg" setting (if the test was conducted on a Monark mechanically braked cycle)?
    a. *5.0
    b. 3.5
    c. 4.4
    d. 6.4
    e. None of the above
15. What was the energy expenditure in METs during stage 7 (assume he reached close to a steady state)?
    a. 15.6
    b. 17.4
    c. *18.6
    d. 20.2
    e. None of the above
16. What is his energy expenditure in kcal $\cdot$ min^{-1} during stage 5?
    a. *15.0
    b. 10.4
    c. 11.5
    d. 8.6

e. None of the above

17. What is his energy expenditure in METs during stage 3?

a. 5.4

b. *9.1

c. 9.5

d. 10.8

e. 12.4

18. What is his energy expenditure in L · min during stage 6?

a. *3.70

b. 4.23

c. 5.67

d. 5.80

e. None of the above

PHYSICAL FITNESS ACTIVITY 4.2

Cardiorespiratory Endurance Testing

In this chapter, detailed information is given for several tests of cardiorespiratory endurance ($\dot{V}O_{2max}$), including the following:

- 1-mile run
- YMCA 3-minute step test
- Canadian Aerobic Fitness Test
- YMCA submaximal cycle test
- Storer–Davis maximal cycle test
- Bruce maximal treadmill test

Under the supervision of your instructor or a local fitness center director, using the directions outlined in the chapter and the norms outlined in Appendix A, take each of these six tests and fill in the cardiorespiratory test worksheet. Be sure to follow the precautions outlined in this chapter. If you are not categorized as "low risk" using the ACSM guidelines, these tests should not be taken unless under the direct supervision of a physician (see Chapter 3).

After taking these tests, answer the following questions.

1. Did the estimated $\dot{V}O_{2max}$ vary widely for the six different tests? (Define "widely" as more than 25% from the Bruce treadmill maximal test result.)
   a. Yes
   b. No
2. If you answered "yes" on question 1, list at least five reasons as to why you feel $\dot{V}O_{2max}$ varied so widely.
   a. ______________________________
   b. ______________________________
   c. ______________________________
   d. ______________________________
   e. ______________________________

Assessment of Cardiorespiratory Endurance Testing

Test	Your Score	Classification
1-mile run		
YMCA 3-minute step test		
Canadian Aerobic Fitness Test		
YMCA submaximal cycle test		
Storer–Davis maximal cycle test		
Bruce maximal treadmill test		

Note: Record all scores in $ml \cdot kg^{-1} \cdot min^{-1}$, except for the YMCA 3-minute step test. Use $\dot{V}O_{2max}$ norms from Appendix A for classification. For the 1-mile run, use the estimating equation from Table 4.4. For the YMCA 3-minute step test, record 60-second recovery pulse, and then use norms in Appendix A (Table 22). For the Canadian Aerobic Fitness Test, use the aerobic fitness score described in the text. For the YMCA submaximal cycle test, use Figure 4.15. For the Storer–Davis maximal cycle test, use equations from text. For the Bruce maximal treadmill, use the equation described in Table 4.8.

PHYSICAL FITNESS ACTIVITY 4.3

Measurement of Your Resting Heart Rate

As emphasized in the text, a low resting heart rate usually indicates a heart conditioned by regular aerobic exercise. Some people have a low resting heart rate due to various genetic factors, but they can still lower their resting heart rates through exercise training.

Many factors can increase the resting heart rate to levels that are higher than normal (see chapter discussion). To rule out these factors, the resting heart rate is best measured a few minutes after awakening when seated on the edge of the bed. In this Physical Fitness Activity, you will take your resting heart rate, using the artery in your wrist or neck, three mornings in a row after getting out of bed. Put three fingers at the base of your thumb on the bottom of your wrist to count the heartbeats for 1 full minute using the radial artery, or three fingers on either side of your voice box on the neck (carotid artery). Do not press too hard.

Record these values in the blanks below, average them, and then using Table 21 in Appendix A, classify your resting heart rate from the YMCA norms.

Resting Heart Rate Measurements:

First morning: ____________ beats per minute

Second morning: ____________ beats per minute

Third morning: ____________ beats per minute

Average resting heart rate: ____________ beats per minute

Classification

(Table 21, Appendix A) ____________

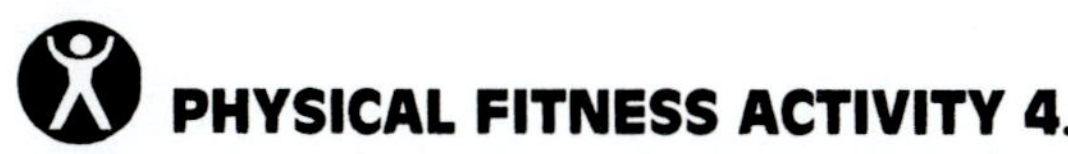

PHYSICAL FITNESS ACTIVITY 4.4

Measurement of Your Resting Blood Pressure

Follow the procedures summarized in the text. Sit quietly for at least 5 minutes before having your blood pressure measured. Be totally relaxed. The same factors that raise the resting heart rate can elevate the blood pressure (stress and anxiety, food in the stomach, a full bladder, pain, extreme hot or cold, tobacco use, caffeine, and certain kinds of medications). Ideally, two measurements should be taken on two separate days. If this is not practical, have your blood pressure measured twice during the class session, and then average. Use Table 4.1 to classify your blood pressure.

Resting Blood Pressure Measurements:

First reading: ____________ mm Hg

Second reading: ____________ mm Hg

Average resting blood pressure: ____________ mm Hg

Classification (Table 4.1) ____________

PHYSICAL FITNESS ACTIVITY 4.5

Estimation of $\dot{V}O_{2max}$ Using an Equation

Low levels of cardiorespiratory fitness have been linked to most of the leading causes of death, including heart disease, stroke, cancer, and diabetes. Direct measurement of cardiorespiratory fitness or $\dot{V}O_{2max}$ is expensive and requires trained technicians and medical supervision. There has been much interest in developing simple methods of estimating $\dot{V}O_{2max}$, especially for large groups of people. One method that is gaining widespread acceptance is the use of an estimating equation that factors in several personal characteristics including age, gender, height, weight, and physical activity habits.

Use the equation below to estimate your $\dot{V}O_{2max}$. You will need a calculator. Calculate your body mass index (BMI) from Figure 5.11. It should be emphasized that this equation provides a "ballpark" estimate of your $\dot{V}O_{2max}$, and that other methods, especially running and walking tests, are preferred. Once you estimate your $\dot{V}O_{2max}$, use Table 24 in Appendix A to obtain your classification.

Equation for Estimating $\dot{V}O_{2max}$

$\dot{V}O_{2max}$ $ml \cdot kg^{-1} \cdot min^{-1}$ = ______________ ______________
Classification (Table 24, Appendix A)

56.363 − (________ × 0.381)
age

− (____________ × 0.754)
Body mass index

+ (______________________ × 1.921)
physical activity rating, 0 to 7*

+ 10.987 (if you are a male) or 0 (if you are a female)

Example: Calculate $\dot{V}O_{2max}$ in $ml \cdot kg^{-1} \cdot min^{-1}$ for a 20-year-old female college student who is 5 foot, 5 inches tall (65 inches), weighs 130 pounds, and swims laps 45 minutes each week.

$\dot{V}O_{2max}$ $ml \cdot kg^{-1} \cdot min^{-1}$ = 42.0 Average
Classification (Table 24, Appendix A)

56.363 − 20 × 0.381)
age

− (21.7 × 0.754)
Body mass index

+ (5 × 1.921)
physical activity rating, 0 to 7*

+ 0 (female)

*Pick a physical activity rating that best fits your typical habits:

I. Does not participate regularly in programmed recreation sport or physical activity.
   - **0 points:** Avoids walking or exertion (e.g., always uses elevator, drives whenever possible instead of walking)
   - **1 point:** Walks for pleasure, routinely uses stairs, occasionally exercises sufficiently to cause heavy breathing or perspiration.

II. Participates regularly in recreation or work requiring modest physical activity, such as golf, horseback riding, calisthenics, gymnastics, table tennis, bowling, weight lifting, or yard work.
   - **2 points:** 10 to 60 minutes per week.
   - **3 points:** Over 1 hour per week.

III. Participates regularly in heavy physical exercise (such as running or jogging, swimming, cycling, rowing, skipping rope, running in place) or engages in vigorous aerobic-type activity (such as tennis, basketball, or handball).
   - **4 points:** Runs less than 1 mile per week or spends less than 30 minutes per week in comparable physical activity.
   - **5 points:** Runs 1 to 5 miles per week or spends 30 to 60 minutes per week in comparable physical activity.
   - **6 points:** Runs 5 to 10 miles per week or spends 1 to 3 hours per week in comparable physical activity.
   - **7 points:** Runs over 10 miles per week or spends over 3 hours per week in comparable physical activity.

PHYSICAL FITNESS ACTIVITY 4.6

The 1-Mile Walk Test

To take the test, walk a mile around a track or measured course as fast as possible, measure the total walking time, and then take the heart rate just after finishing.
This equation is recommended for college students:

$\dot{V}O_{2max}$ ml · kg^{-1} · min^{-1} = 88.768 + (8.892 × ________________ (gender with M=1, F=0)

− (0.0957 × ________________ (weight in pounds)

− (1.4537 × ________________ (walk time in minutes in decimal format)

− (0.1194 × ________________ (ending exercise heart rate)

For example, a college female weighing 128 pounds and able to walk 1 mile in 13 minutes with an ending heart rate of 133 beats per minute would have this estimated $\dot{V}O_{2max}$: 88.768 + (8.892 × 0) − (0.0957 × 128) − (1.4537 × 13.0) − (0.1194 × 133) = 41.7 ml · kg^{-1} · min^{-1}.

One-mile walking time:	________________	minutes
Ending heart rate:	________________	beats per minute
Fitness rating (from Table 24, Appendix A)	________________	

PHYSICAL FITNESS ACTIVITY 4.7

A Step Test for College Students

As explained in the text, in this step test, the heart rate is taken for 15 seconds after stepping up and down on a 16.25-inch bench for 3 minutes at a rate of 24 steps per minute for men and 22 for women, and is then applied to the equations listed below to determine $\dot{V}O_{2max}$. Overweight individuals and those with medical problems or leg injuries should not take this test.

1. The step test requires a stopwatch, metronome, and stepping bench (16.25 inches high, typical of most gymnasium bleachers). The metronome should be set at 96 beats per minute for men and 88 beats per minute for women. Practice stepping to a four-step cadence (up with the right foot, up with the left foot, down with the right foot, down with the left foot) to ensure 24 complete step-ups per minute for men and 22 step-ups per minute for women.
2. Begin the test and perform the step-ups for exactly 3 minutes.
3. After stepping, remain standing, wait 5 seconds, and then count the heart rate at the wrist or neck for 15 seconds.
4. Convert the 15-second pulse count into beats per minute by multiplying by 4.
5. Use these equations and to estimate $\dot{V}O_{2max}$, and Table 24, Appendix A to classify your fitness status.

MALES: Predicted $\dot{V}O_{2max}$ = 111.33 − (0.42 × heart rate in bpm)

FEMALES: Predicted $\dot{V}O_{2max}$ = 65.81 − (0.1847 × heart rate in bpm)

15-second pulse count after stepping:	______________	beats
Convert heart rate to beats per minute	______________	beats/minute
Estimated $\dot{V}O_{2max}$ from equations	______________	$ml \cdot kg^{-1} \cdot min^{-1}$
$\dot{V}O_{2max}$ classification	______________	
(from Table 24, Appendix A)		

chapter 5

Body Composition

Fat is a chronic preoccupation of much of the adult population, though possibly for different reasons in different places. In most parts of the world, fat is regarded as aesthetically undesirable when it becomes superficially evident. There is the more compelling reason for concern over excess fat for its adverse influence on longevity and, more specifically, on the degenerative diseases.

—Dr. William E. Siri, 1956

BODY COMPOSITION TERMINOLOGY

Interest in measurement of body composition has grown tremendously since the early 1970s when the modern-day fitness movement began. Elite athletes, people involved with weight-management programs, and patients in hospitals have all benefited from the increased popularity and accuracy of body composition measurement.[1–3]

There are several important reasons for measuring body composition:

- *To assess the decrease in body fat weight that occurs in response to a weight-management program.* About 100 million American adults are overweight, with the highest rates found among the poor and minority groups (see Chapter 13). Body composition measurement throughout the entire weight-loss process helps people make informed decisions about their diet and exercise programs.
- *To help athletes determine the best body composition for performance.* Most athletes are very concerned with body composition. In some sports such as wrestling, gymnastics, ballet dancing, bodybuilding, and distance running, athletes attempt to reach the lowest body fat levels possible. In other sports such as weight lifting, football, baseball, and rowing, a large fat-free mass is paramount. Accurate body composition measurement is critical to guide athletes as they seek the optimal level of fat and fat-free mass associated with their sport.
- *To monitor fat and fat-free weight in patients with disease.* High body fat is an important risk factor for some diseases (e.g., heart disease, certain types of cancer, diabetes, and high blood pressure). Low muscle and bone mass predicts future development of osteoporosis. Thus body composition measurement serves an important role in the prevention of chronic disease.
- *To track long-term changes that occur in body fat and fat-free mass with aging.* Body fat doubles between the ages of 20 and 65 years. Often, during middle age, extra fat is gained around the stomach and trunk areas, which is especially harmful to long-term health. Muscular strength in most people is maintained to about 45 years of age, but then falls by about 5–10% per decade thereafter. In older people, muscle weakness may decrease the ability to accomplish the common activities of daily living, leading to dependency on others. Body composition measurement throughout the life cycle helps people prepare for the changes that occur late in life.

Research to establish ways of determining body composition through indirect methods began during the 1940s. Since then, a wide variety of methods have been developed. These methods are described here, with emphasis on the most practical techniques.

Most body composition analyses are based on seeing the body as consisting of two separate components: fat and fat-free.[3] Thus, *body composition* is often defined as the ratio of fat to fat-free mass. Common terms used in the study of body composition include those defined in Table 5.1.[1]

TABLE 5.1 Glossary of Terms Used in Body Composition Measurement

Android obesity	Upper-body obesity, with fat accumulation in the trunk and abdomen. Associated with a high risk for obesity-related health problems.
Bioelectrical impedance	A method of determining body composition by passing a harmless current through the body, measuring electrical impedance, and estimating body composition through use of equations.
Body composition	The proportions of fat, muscle, and bone making up the body; usually expressed as percent of body fat.
Body mass index (BMI)	A calculation of body weight and height indices for determining degree of obesity. The most common formula for body mass index is body weight in kilograms divided by height in meters squared, and is also called the Quetelet index.
Body type	Also called somatype, refers to the build of the body as determined by genetics. The mesomorphic body type is athletic, with heavy bone and muscle mass; the ectomorphic body type is thin, linear, and lean, with low amounts of bone and muscle mass; the endomorphic body type is heavy, big, and soft, with large amounts of both fat-free and fat mass.
DEXA	The acronym for dual-energy x-ray absorptiometry, which is a method for estimating body composition. It uses a low radiation dose to measure bone mineral mass, fat mass, and nonbone fat-free mass (a three-component model).
Fat-free mass	All fat-free tissues in the body, including water, muscle, bone, connective tissue, and internal organs. Also called fat-free weight or lean body weight. Estimated by subtracting the fat mass from total body weight.
Fat mass	All the fat in the body; fats that can be extracted from the fat tissues and other tissues in the body. Also called fat weight. Estimated by multiplying the percent body fat by the total body weight.
Frame size	Refers to small, medium, or large skeletal mass; usually estimated through use of the elbow breadth.
Gynoid obesity	Lower-body obesity, with fat accumulation in the hips and thighs.
Height–weight indices	Formulas that use height and weight to estimate underweight, normal weight, overweight, and obesity.
Height–weight tables	Tables that provide a healthy weight range for a given height.
Hips circumference	The largest circumference of the buttocks-hips area while the person is standing.
Ideal body weight	The healthiest body weight taking into account fat-free mass and fat mass. Calculated by dividing the fat-free mass by 100% minus desired percent body fat.
Obesity	An excessive amount of total body fat for a given body weight.
Percent body fat	Also called relative body fat; fat mass expressed as a percentage of total body mass.
Reference body weight	The midpoint weight of the weight range for a given height.
Relative body weight	The body weight divided by the midpoint value of the recommended weight range.
Skinfold caliper	A special caliper that gives millimeter measurements of skinfolds.
Skinfold measurements	The most widely used method for determining body fat percent; calipers are used to measure the thickness of a double fold of skin at various sites.
Stadiometer	A vertical ruler mounted on a wall with a horizontal headboard to measure height.
Total body density	The total body mass expressed relative to total body volume.
Underwater weighing	A method of determining body composition by weighing the individual underwater. In this procedure, whole-body density is calculated from body volume, and then body density is converted to percent body fat through use of equations.
Waist circumference	The smallest waist circumference below the rib cage and above the belly button, while standing with abdominal muscles relaxed (not pulled in). Also called the abdominal circumference.
Waist-to-hip ratio (WHR)	The ratio of waist and hip circumferences.

To study body composition, the body mass is subdivided into two or more components. The classic two-component model divides the body mass into fat and fat-free mass (see Figure 5.1a). The *fat mass* contains all extractable lipids, and the *fat-free mass* includes water, protein, and mineral components (see Figure 5.1b). In 1963, Brozek and colleagues dissected three white male cadavers and measured the density of body fat at 0.901 grams per cubic centimeter (g/cc) and the density of the fat-free mass as 1.10 g/cc. The Brozek et al.[4] equation estimated percent body fat as follows:

$$\text{Percent body fat} = [(4.57/\text{body density}) - 4.142] \times 100$$

This was similar to an equation published 2 years earlier by Siri:[5]

$$\text{Percent body fat} = [(4.95/\text{body density}) - 4.50] \times 100$$

Since the 1960s, these two formulas have been used to estimate percent body fat from the body density obtained from hydrostatic or underwater weighing, once considered the gold standard method. (This method of measuring body composition is described in detail later on in this chapter.) However, recent technological advances for measuring water (isotope dilution), mineral (dual-energy x-ray absorptiometry [DEXA]), and protein (neutron activation analysis) have shown that the fat-free mass varies widely among groups because of age, sex, ethnicity, level of body fatness, and physical activity level. Because the fat-free mass varies among people, the two-component model equations of Brozek et al.[4] and Siri[5] can either under- or overestimate the actual percent of body fat. Table 5.2 summarizes the fat-free mass densities recently measured for different groups of

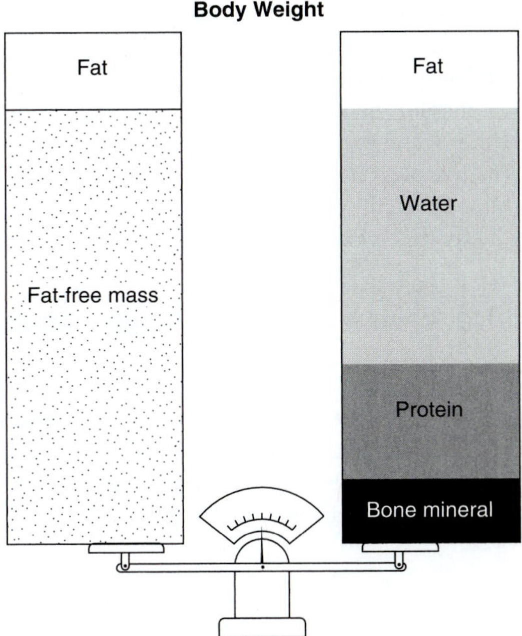

Figure 5.1a There are two body composition models currently in use: the two-component model (fat-free mass and fat) and the four-component model (bone mineral, protein, water, and fat).

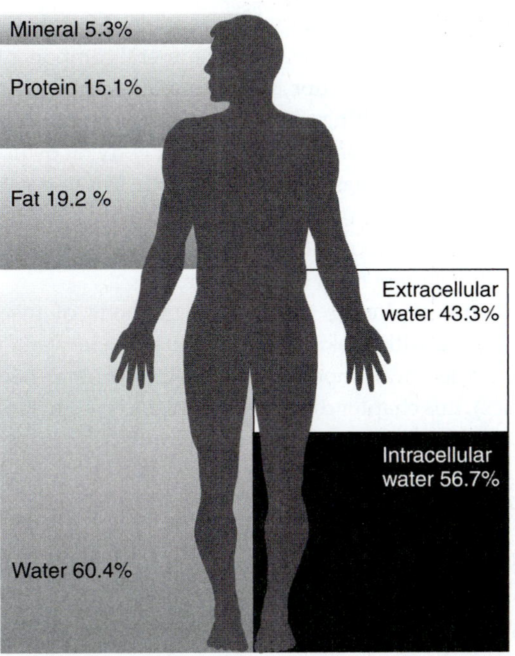

Figure 5.1b Body composition on the molecular level for the 70-kg reference man. The reference man is about 60% water, with the rest composed of fat, bone mineral, and protein.

TABLE 5.2 Population-Specific Fat-Free Mass Density and Formulas for Conversion of Body Density to Percent Body Fat

Population	Age (yr)	Gender	Fat-Free Mass Density (g/cc)	Percent Fat Formula*
White	7–12	Male	1.084	(5.30/Db) – 4.89
		Female	1.082	(5.35/Db) – 4.95
	13–16	Male	1.094	(5.07/Db) – 4.64
		Female	1.093	(5.10/Db) – 4.66
	17–19	Male	1.098	(4.99/Db) – 4.55
		Female	1.095	(5.05/Db) – 4.62
	20–80	Male	1.10	(4.95/Db) – 4.50
		Female	1.097	(5.01/Db) – 4.57
Black	18–32	Male	1.113	(4.37/Db) – 3.93
	24–79	Female	1.106	(4.85/Db) – 4.39
American Indian	18–60	Female	1.108	(4.81/Db) – 4.34
Hispanic	20–40	Female	1.105	(4.87/Db) – 4.41
Japanese native	18–48	Male	1.099	(4.97/Db) – 4.52
	18–48	Female	1.111	(4.76/Db) – 4.28
	61–78	Male	1.105	(4.87/Db) – 4.41
	61–78	Female	1.100	(4.95/Db) – 4.50
Obese	17–62	Female	1.098	(5.00/Db) – 4.56
Anorexic	15–30	Female	1.087	(5.26/Db) – 4.83

*Db = density of body.

Source: Data from: Evaluation of body composition: Current issues. *Sports Med* 22:146–156, 1996. Heyward VH, Stolarczyk LM. *Applied Body Composition Assessment*. Champaign, IL: Human Kinetics, 1996.

people, using multicomponent models that take into account variations in the water and mineral components.[1] For these various subgroups, the estimated body density from underwater weighing, skinfold equations, and bioelectrical equations can be converted to percent body fat by using the conversion formulas listed in Table 5.2. These population-specific conversion formulas were calculated by Heyward, using multicomponent model estimates of fat-free mass density obtained from the literature.[1]

Before exploring the various methods of measuring body composition (skinfold techniques, underwater weighing, bioelectrical impedance, DEXA, and other new techniques), this chapter discusses height and weight tables and the use of various height-to-weight ratios.

HEIGHT AND WEIGHT MEASUREMENTS

Weight measurement alone cannot accurately determine the body fat status of a person (see Figure 5.2). Weight measurement does not differentiate between fat-free mass and fat mass. In other words, some people with *mesomorphic* or athletic, muscular body types (such as bodybuilders) can have normal or low body fat even though they are overweight according to standard charts. Some people who are *ectomorphic* (or lean, thin, and linear) with low amounts of fat-free mass can be underweight according to the weight charts and extremely low in body fat as well (endurance athlete). The *endomorphic* (heavy, big, soft) individual is overweight from large amounts of both fat-free and fat mass (e.g., football lineman).[2]

Figure 5.3 summarizes the effect of body type (or somatype) on fat mass and body weight. Body type is strongly affected by genetics with little influence from lifestyle and exercises habits. Most people are a mixture of the three body types, with tendencies toward one. Only 5% of the population are "pure" ectomorphs or "pure" mesomorphs. Because total body weight is so strongly related to somatype, body composition (i.e., the ratio of fat to fat-free mass) is a much better indication of ideal body weight than is the total weight obtained from stepping on a weight scale.

This chapter emphasizes skinfold measurements and underwater weighing in assessing body composition prior to estimation of ideal body weight. Because of the widespread use of height–weight tables, however, a brief review of this methodology is given first.

Historical Review of Height–Weight Tables

Since the 1940s, tables have been developed by the Metropolitan Life Insurance Company for "ideal" and "desirable" weights.[6–9] They were derived from the 1959 Build and Blood Pressure Study, based on the combined experience of 26 life insurance companies in the United States and Canada

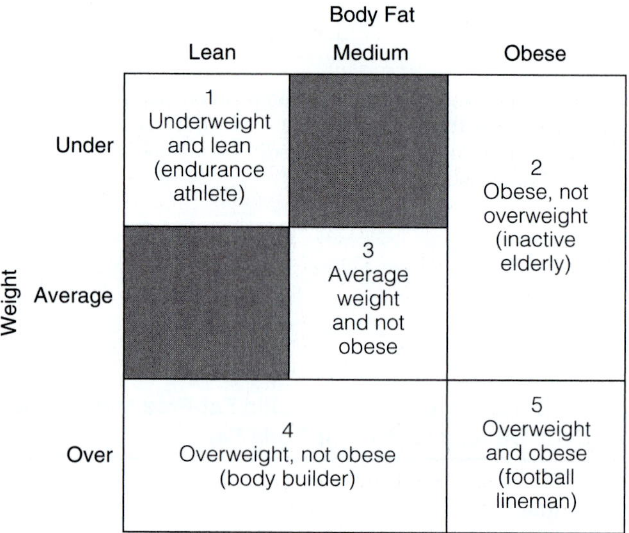

Figure 5.2 The relationship among three categories of body weight and body fat can be described in five different ways. Weight measurement alone cannot accurately determine the body fat status of a person.

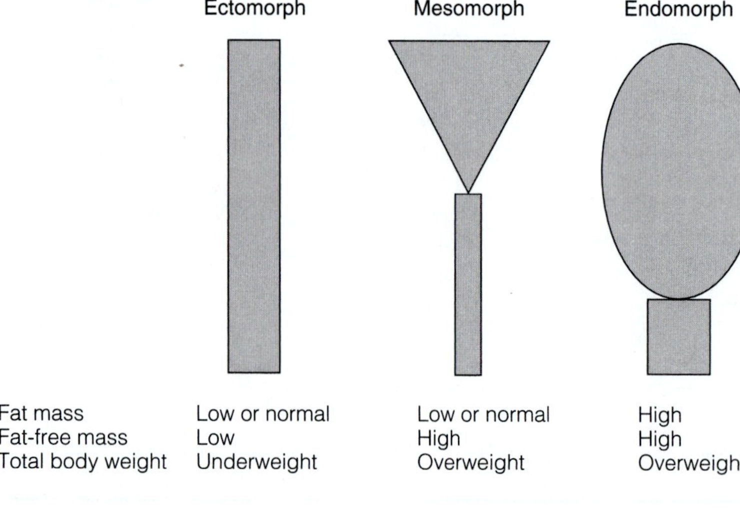

Figure 5.3 Somatypes. Body type or somatype has a strong influence on total body weight.

from 1935 to 1954, involving observation of nearly 5 million insured people for periods of up to 20 years. Height and weight were measured with street shoes and indoor clothing. The study excluded those with heart disease, cancer, or diabetes. In the resulting 1959 Metropolitan Life Insurance Co. "Desirable Weights for Men and Women," "desirable weights" were those associated with the lowest mortality.[7]

These 1959 tables set forth weight ranges for small-, medium-, and large-frame men and women of differing heights. Unfortunately, the method of determining frame size was not given.[6,8]

On March 1, 1983, the Metropolitan Life Insurance Company issued new height–weight tables derived from the 1979 Build Study[8] (see Table 5.3). It utilized data from 25 insurance companies reporting the U.S. and Canadian mortality experience from 1954 to 1972 for more than 4 million insured, again excluding applicants with major diseases.

In these tables, weights associated with lowest mortality are no longer called "desirable" or "ideal." A method for determining *frame size* by utilizing elbow breadth measurement was included (see Table 5.4). These frame size measurements were based on the National Health and Nutrition Examination Survey (NHANES I and II) data and devised so that 50% of the population fell within the medium-frame area, 25% within the small-frame area, and 25% within the large-frame area.[10]

There are several considerations to bear in mind in using the 1983 weight tables.[7–10]

- The 1983 weight tables present weight ranges that are 2–13% higher than the 1959 tables.[7,8] These upward revisions, however, are not uniformly distributed throughout the height categories; the largest increases are for the shorter men and women.
- The tables are based on specific populations that are not representative of the whole population. The data for the 1983 tables were drawn from people who were able to purchase nongroup insurance (excluding those who purchased group insurance) and who were 25–59 years of age (excluding the elderly). Thus insurees were predominantly white, middle-class adults. Blacks, Asians, and low-income and other population groups were not represented proportionally. Also, people with serious chronic diseases or acute illnesses were not included.
- No consideration was made for cigarette smoking. Cigarette smoking is associated with lower weight and shorter life span. Including smokers in the data thus skewed the "ideal weights" upward.[11]
- The height–weight tables were based on the lowest mortality and did not take into account the health problems often associated with obesity. Such disease conditions as cardiovascular disease, cancer, hypertension, high blood cholesterol levels, and many other health problems are more prevalent among the obese. For these reasons, the American Heart Association and others have urged the populace to use the weight tables as a "mere gross estimate."[7]
- Only initial weights were used in the determination of ideal weight. People taking out insurance policies

TABLE 5.3 1983 Metropolitan Height–Weight Tables

(In Pounds by Height and Frame in Indoor Clothing, Men—5 lb, 1-Inch Heel; Women—3 lb, 1-Inch Heel)

Men				Women			
	Frame				Frame		
Height (in)	Small	Medium	Large	Height (in)	Small	Medium	Large
62	128–134	131–141	138–150	58	102–111	109–121	118–131
63	130–136	133–143	140–153	59	103–113	111–123	120–134
64	132–138	135–145	142–156	60	104–115	113–126	122–137
65	134–140	137–148	144–160	61	106–118	115–129	125–140
66	136–142	139–151	146–164	62	108–121	118–132	128–143
67	138–145	142–154	149–168	63	111–124	121–135	131–147
68	140–148	145–157	152–172	64	114–127	124–138	135–151
69	142–151	148–160	155–176	65	117–130	127–141	137–155
70	144–154	151–163	158–180	66	120–133	130–144	140–159
71	146–157	154–166	161–184	67	123–136	133–147	143–163
72	149–160	157–170	164–188	68	126–139	136–150	146–167
73	152–164	160–174	168–192	69	129–142	139–153	149–170
74	155–168	164–178	172–197	70	132–145	142–156	152–173
75	158–172	167–182	176–202	71	135–148	145–159	155–176
76	162–176	171–187	181–207	72	138–151	148–162	158–179

Source: Data from the Metropolitan Life Insurance Company, New York.

TABLE 5.4 Height and Elbow Breadth

		Elbow Breadth (in)		
	Height (in, no shoes)	**Small Frame**	**Medium Frame**	**Large Frame**
Men	61–62	<2½	2½–2⅞	>2⅞
	63–66	<2⅝	2⅝–2⅞	>2⅞
	67–70	<2¾	2¾–3	>3
	71–74	<2¾	2¾–3⅛	>3⅛
	75	<2⅞	2⅞–3¼	>3¼
Women	57–58	<2¼	2¼–2½	>2½
	59–62	<2¼	2¼–2½	>2½
	63–66	<2⅜	2⅜–2⅝	>2⅝
	67–70	<2⅜	2⅜–2⅝	>2⅝
	71	<2½	2½–2¾	>2¾

Note: Tables adapted to represent height without shoes. To measure the elbow breadth, extend the arm, and then bend the forearm upward at a 90-degree angle, fingers straight up, palm turned toward the body. Measure with a sliding caliper the width between the two prominent bones on either side of the elbow (measure the widest point). Make sure that the arm is positioned correctly and that the upper arm is parallel to the ground.

Source: Data from Metropolitan Life Insurance Company, New York.

had their weights measured, but no further data were collected on weight or development of disease after the policy was initially purchased. If weight changed between issuance of the policy and death, this was not taken into account.[7]

- Finally, weight tables do not provide information on actual body composition. As stated previously, what really matters is the quality of the weight, not the quantity. "Ideal body weight" is not ideal for everyone at a given height because of bone and muscle differences. Thus, height–weight tables are merely gross estimates, and other methods, such as anthropometric measures, should be used to refine the estimate of proper weight.

In 1990, the U.S. Department of Agriculture (USDA) published a new table of "Suggested Weight for Adults."[12] There were two unique features of the USDA table:

1. One weight range was given for *both* men and women.
2. A separate weight range for a given height was listed for people 35 years and over. Men or any individuals with more muscle and bone than normal were urged to use the upper end of the weight range for their height.

It was the second feature that caused the most controversy among scientists because older people were allowed to be 10–18 pounds heavier than their younger counterparts.[13,14] While some researchers felt that this amount of weight gain after age 35 was normal and posed no risk to health, others felt that risk of coronary heart disease, hypertension, diabetes, and other obesity-related diseases was increased.

Researchers from the Framingham Heart Study and the Harvard Medical School were foremost in urging that the weight tables be changed.[14] There was a growing consensus that "the present standards are too permissive," and that there is "no biological rationale for recommending that people increase their weight as they grow older."[14]

In response to these concerns, the Dietary Guidelines Advisory Committee of the USDA submitted an updated height–weight table in 1995 (Table 5.5).[15] The updated table listed one healthy weight range for a given height for men and women of all ages. In the words of the committee, "The health risks due to excess weight appear to be the same for older adults as for younger adults. Based on published data, there appears to be no justification for the establishment of a cut point that increases with age."[15] Weight ranges were given in the table "because people of the same height may have equal amounts of body fat but different amounts of muscle and bone. However, the ranges do not mean that it is healthy to gain weight, even within the same weight range. The higher weights in the healthiest weight range apply to people with more muscle and bone."[15] The *Dietary Guidelines for Americans, 2000 and 2005,* dropped the height–weight table and recommended use of the body mass index (see section entitled "Body Mass Index"). Nearly all health and medical organizations use the body mass index to classify adults, and use of the height–weight tables is no longer advocated.

Relative Weight

Obesity has been defined as being 20% or more overweight, using the concept of relative weight. *Relative weight* uses the ratio or percentage of actual weight to desirable weight. Most researchers use as the point of reference the midpoint value of the weight range for the subject's height. A man who is 70 inches tall and weighs 180 pounds, for example, would have the following relative weight, using the midpoint value of the range given in the 1995 USDA tables (Table 5.5).

TABLE 5.5 1995 USDA Healthy Weight Ranges for Men and Women

Height (no shoes)	Weight (lb) (without clothes)
4′10″	91–119
4′11″	94–124
5′0″	97–128
5′1″	101–132
5′2″	104–137
5′3″	107–141
5′4″	111–146
5′5″	114–150
5′6″	118–155
5′7″	121–160
5′8″	125–164
5′9″	129–169
5′10″	132–174
5′11″	136–179
6′0″	140–184
6′1″	144–189
6′2″	148–195
6′3″	152–200
6′4″	156–205
6′5″	160–211
6′6″	164–216

Source: USDA. *1995 Dietary Guidelines for Americans.*

$$\text{Relative weight} = \left(\frac{\text{body weight}}{\text{midpoint value of weight range}}\right) \times 100$$

$$= \left(\frac{180}{153}\right) \times 100 = 117.6\%$$

In other words, this person is 17.6% overweight. Standards for relative weight are given in Table 5.6. As with any value taken from a height–weight table, these standards can be inaccurate for people with higher than normal amounts of muscle and bone. Use of relative weight was common in large epidemiological studies prior to 1980, but since then, most investigators have shifted to the body mass index.

Measuring Body Weight

Body weight should be measured on a physician's balance-beam scale, with minimal clothing, preferably shorts and light T-shirt, and no shoes, or better yet, a disposable paper gown[16] (see Figure 5.4). The beam scale should have movable weights, with the scale readable from both sides. Balance-beam scales are available from various companies.

The scale should be positioned on a level, solid floor (not carpet), so that the measurer can stand behind the beam, facing the person being measured, and can move the beam weights without reaching around. The scale should be calibrated each time before use by putting the beam weight on zero, and seeing whether the beam scale balances out. If not, a screwdriver can be used on the movable tare weight to adjust the beam weight. The weight should be read to the nearest 0.25 pound.

TABLE 5.6 Standards for Relative Weight

<90%	Underweight
90–110%	Desirable
111–119%	Overweight
120–139%	Mild obesity
140–199%	Moderate obesity
≧200%	Severe obesity

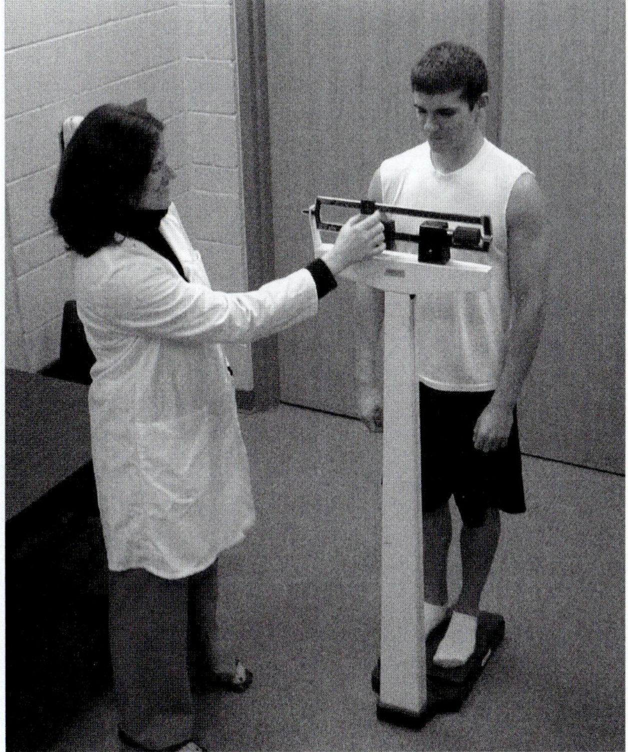

Figure 5.4 Body weight should be measured on a physician's balance-beam scale, with minimal clothing.

If the objective is to assess changes in weight, great care should be taken to repeat measurement of weight under the same conditions and at the same time of day.[17] The weight of an average adult varies approximately 4 to 5 pounds (2 kg) within a day.

Growth charts are a basic screening tool for assessing the nutritional status and general well-being of infants, children, and adolescents.[17,18] Data from five national health examination surveys collected from 1963 to 1994 and five supplementary data sources were combined to establish an analytic growth chart data set.[18] Growth charts showing weight-for-age percentiles for boys and girls, ages 2–20 years, are shown in Figures 5.5 and 5.6.

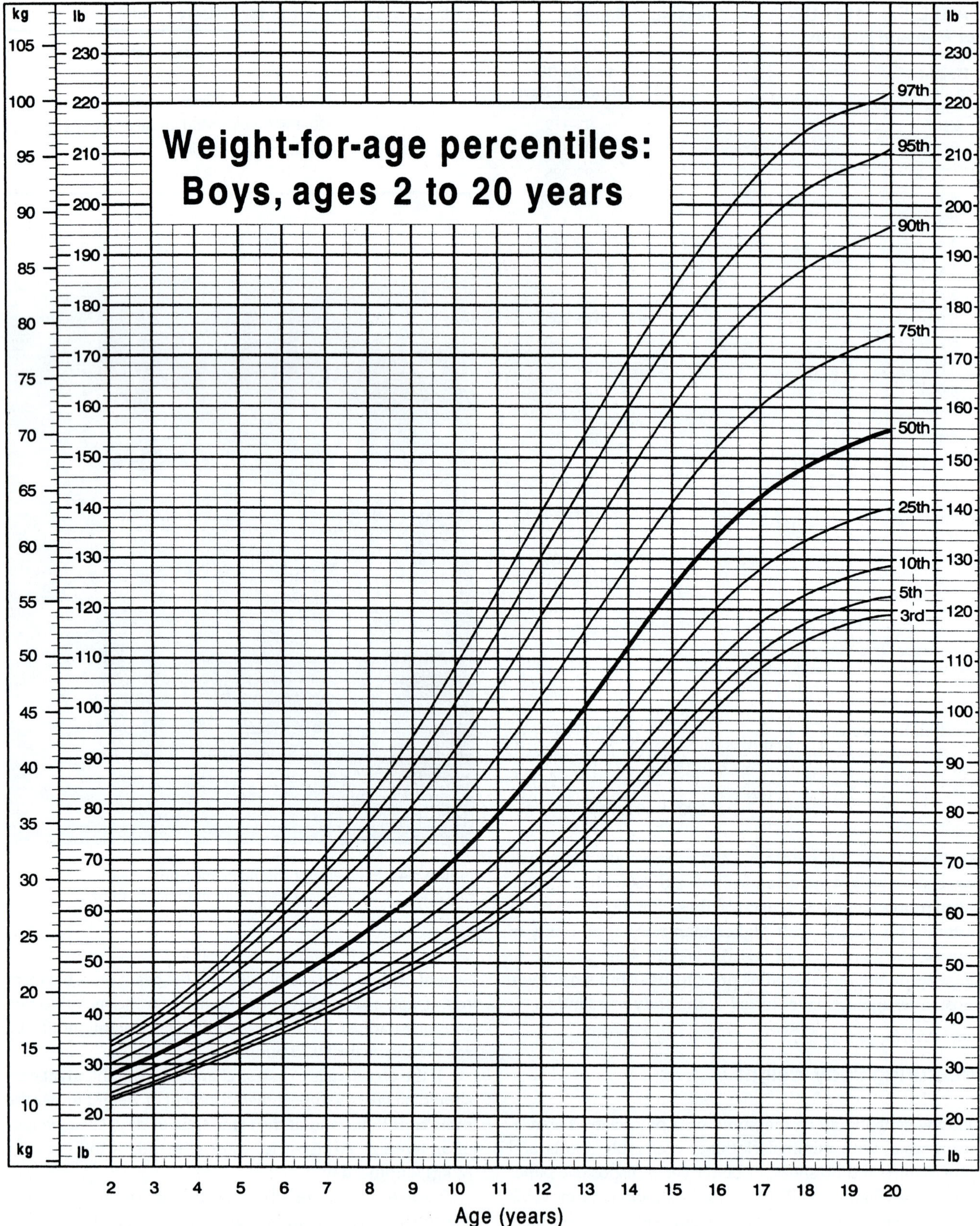

Figure 5.5 Weight-to-age percentiles for boys aged 2–20 years, CDC growth charts: United States.
Source: Developed by the National Center for Health Statistics in collaboration with the National Center for Chronic Disease Prevention and Health Promotion (2000).

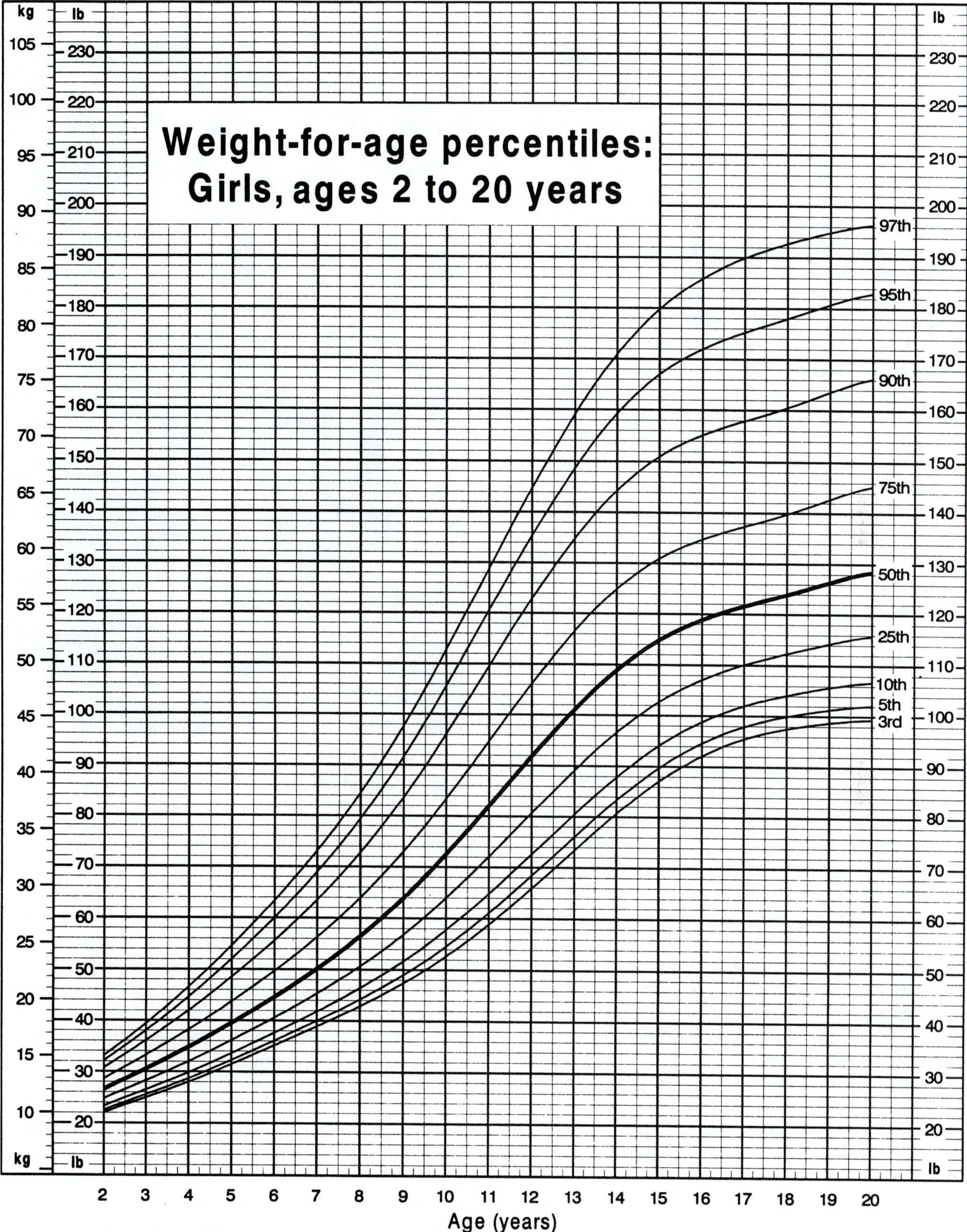

Figure 5.6 Weight-to-age percentiles for girls aged 2–20 years, CDC growth charts: United States.
Source: Developed by the National Center for Health Statistics in collaboration with the National Center for Chronic Disease Prevention and Health Promotion (2000).

Measuring Height

The measurement of height (or stature) requires a vertical ruler with a horizontal headboard that can be brought into contact with the highest point on the head.[16] The headboard and ruler taken together are called a *stadiometer*.

When measuring height, have the person stand without shoes, heels together, back as straight as possible, heels, buttocks, shoulders, and head touching the wall, and looking straight ahead. Weight should be distributed evenly on both feet, arms hanging freely by the sides of the body. Just before measurement, the person being measured should inhale deeply and hold the breath while the headboard is brought onto the highest point on the head, with sufficient pressure to compress the hair.[16,17] Fixed and portable stadiometers are available from various companies.

If a professional stadiometer is not available, a ruler should be affixed to the wall, and a right-angle measuring block (such as a clipboard on edge) used, measuring straight back from the crown of the head. A wall should be chosen that does not have a baseboard, and a floor without a carpet should be used (see Figure 5.7). Measurement of height while standing on a physician balance-beam scale is *not* recommended—it invites substantial error.

Growth charts showing stature-for-age percentiles for boys and girls ages 2–20 years are shown in Figures 5.8 and 5.9.[18]

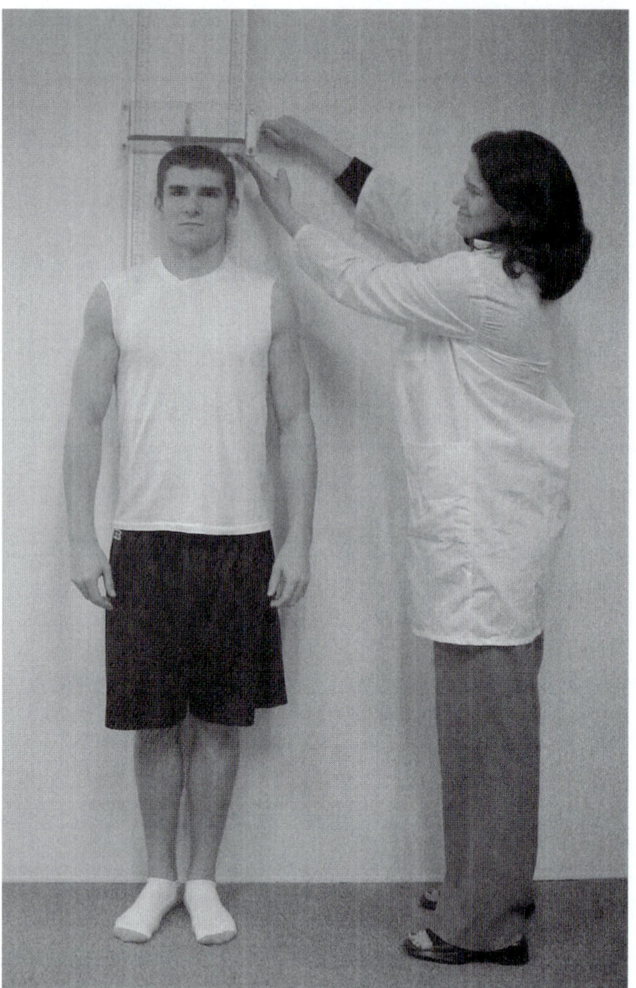

Figure 5.7 Height should be measured while standing erect, with heels, buttocks, back of shoulders, and head touching the vertical ruler. A right-angle object should be brought into contact with the highest point on the head after a deep inhalation and holding of breath.

Measuring Frame Size

As discussed previously, frame size is most commonly determined by measuring the width of the elbow. Other measures have been proposed as estimates of frame size, including bony chest diameter and wrist circumference, but national norms are not yet available for these measurements.[19]

When measuring the width of the elbow, the person being measured should stand erect, with the right arm extended forward perpendicular to the body. The arm is then flexed until the elbow forms a 90-degree angle, with fingers up, palm facing inward[19] (see Figure 5.10). The measurer should first feel for the widest bony width of the elbow, and put the caliper heads at those points.

A sliding caliper should be used[17,19] (Figure 5.10), with pressure firm enough to compress soft tissue over the bone. Table 5.4 summarizes how the data are used to determine frame size. Sliding calipers are available from various companies.

Body Mass Index

A commonly used measure of obesity is the *body mass index* (BMI).[20,21] A number of body mass indices have been developed, all derived from body weight and height measurements. The more popular BMIs include the weight–height ratio W/H, Quetelet index W/H^2, and Khosla–Lowe index W/H^3. These indices represent different attempts to adjust body weight for height to derive a height-free measure of obesity.[21] These BMIs are widely used in large population studies because of their simplicity of measurement and calculation and their low cost.

The *Quetelet index* or kg/m^2 (body weight in kilograms, divided by height in meters squared) is the most widely accepted BMI. This measure was an attempt by the nineteenth-century mathematician Lambert Adolphe Jacques Quetelet to describe the relation between body weight and stature in humans. Studies have shown that the Quetelet index correlates rather well (r = .70) with actual measurement of body fat from hydrostatic weighing.[1–3] However, the standard error of estimate (SEE) is 5% body

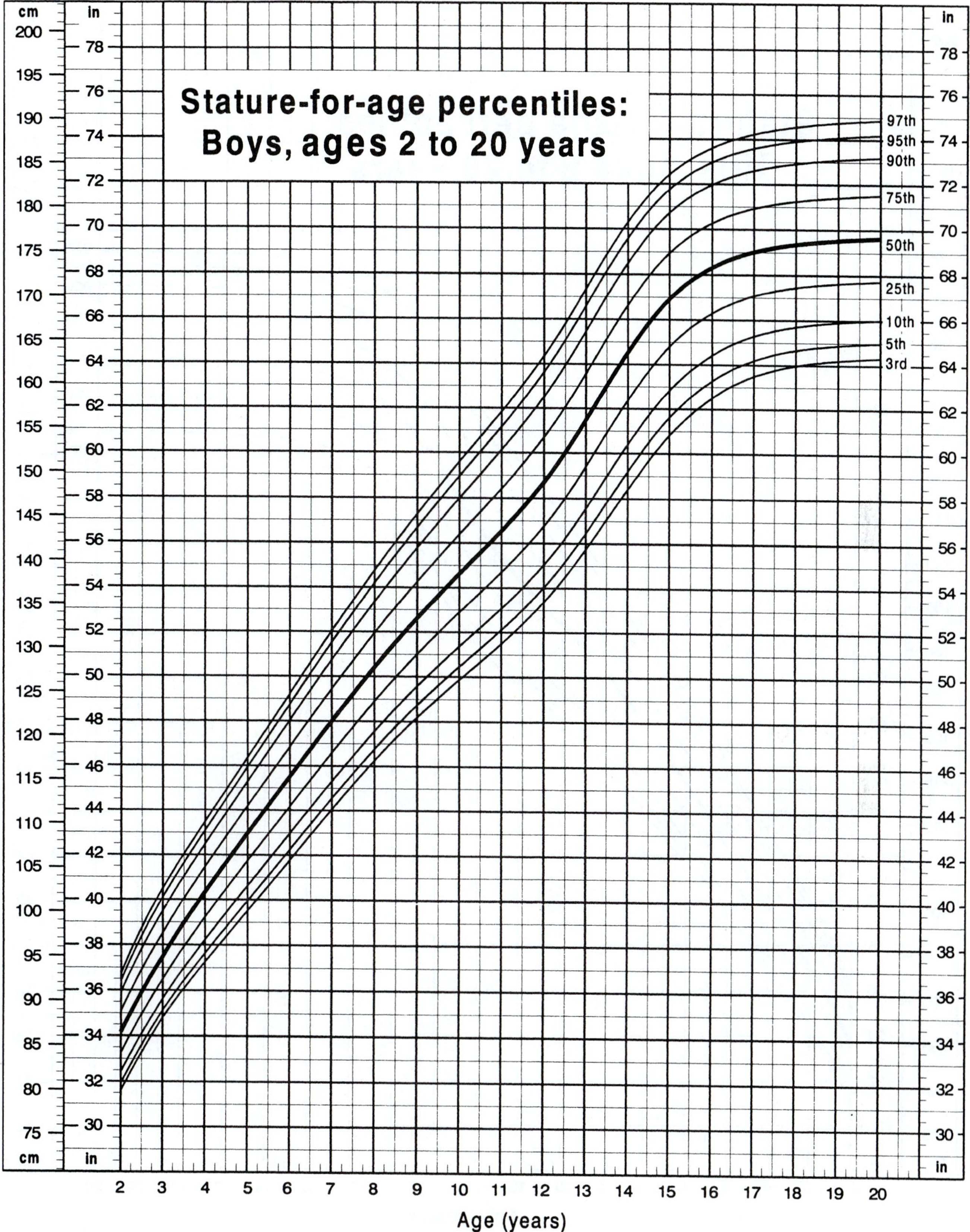

Figure 5.8 Stature-for-age percentiles for boys aged 2–20 years, CDC growth charts: United States.
Source: Developed by the National Center for Health Statistics in collaboration with the National Center for Chronic Disease Prevention and Health Promotion (2000).

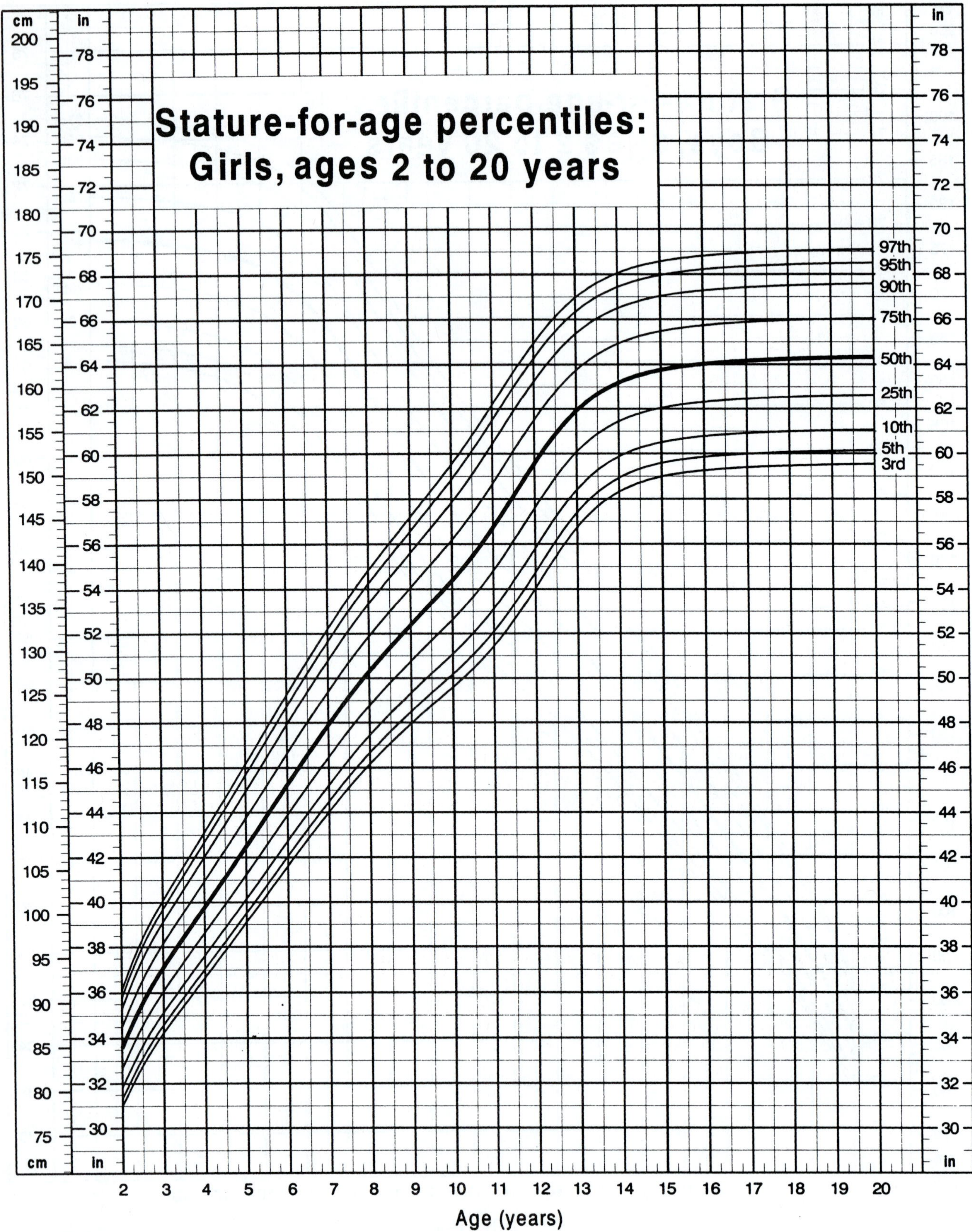

Figure 5.9 Stature-for-age percentiles for girls aged 2–20 years, CDC growth charts: United States.
Source: Developed by the National Center for Health Statistics in collaboration with the National Center for Chronic Disease Prevention and Health Promotion (2000).

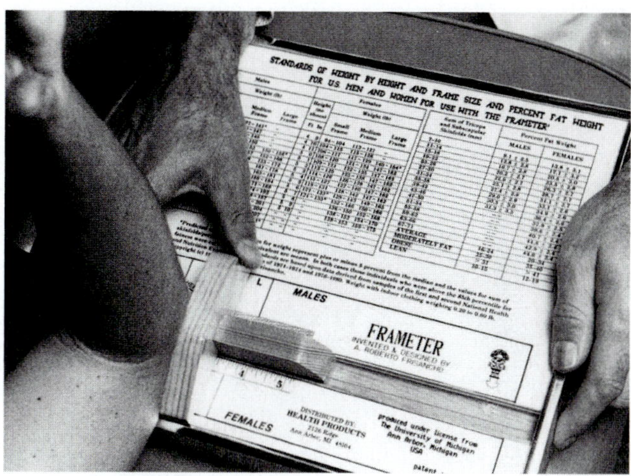

Figure 5.10 The elbow breadth measurement is used for determining frame size. With the arm in this position, the sliding caliper is used to measure the widest point at the elbow.

fat, which means that if a person is 15% fat, the Quetelet index would predict a percent body fat ranging from 10 to 20% two thirds of the time.[1–3] Table 5.7 summarizes the relationship between BMI and percent body fat in adult males and females for three age groups.

The following example can be used to learn how to calculate the Quetelet index. For example, a man weighing 154 pounds (or 70 kilograms—divide weight in pounds by 2.2), standing 68 inches tall (or 1.727 meters tall—multiply height in inches by 0.0254) has a Quetelet index of

$$\text{Quetelet index} = \frac{70 \text{ kg}}{(1.727 \text{ m})^2} = \frac{70}{2.98} = 23.5 \text{ kg/m}^2$$

Another simpler method uses this formula:

$$\text{Quetelet index} = (\text{pounds/inches}^2) \times 704.5$$

Using our subject:

$$(154/68^2) \times 704.5 = 23.5 \text{ kg/m}^2$$

Figure 5.11 makes calculation of the Quetelet index easy, through use of a nomogram. Table 5.8 allows calculation of the BMI by choosing a body weight at a given height. Figure 5.12 depicts the average Quetelet index for American males and females in BMI in 1960–1962 and 1999–2002. Notice the substantial increase during this 40-year period.[21] Figures 5.13 and 5.14 show BMI-for-age percentiles for boys and girls, ages 2–20.[18]

Several systems for classification of overweight and obesity using BMI have been recommended during the past 25 years. In 1998, the National Heart, Lung, and Blood Institute's (NHLBI) Obesity Education Initiative published guidelines that are now widely followed by most health professionals (see Table 5.9).[22] Overweight is here defined as a BMI of 25–29.9 kg/m^2 and obesity as a BMI of ≥ 30 kg/m^2. According to the NHLBI, a more accurate measure of total body fat is achieved using BMI than relying on weight alone. BMI also has an advantage over relative weight (e.g., based on the Metropolitan Life Insurance Tables). Ideal body weight tables were developed primarily from white, higher-socioeconomic-status populations and have not been documented to accurately reflect body fat content in the public at large. In addition, separate tables are required for men and women (whereas, the same BMI standards are used for both genders). BMI is a practical indicator of the severity of obesity, can be calculated from tables or nomograms, and is a direct calculation based on height and weight. In general, calculation of BMI is simple, rapid, and inexpensive. An International Obesity Task Force has concluded

TABLE 5.7 Relationship between Body Mass Index and Percent Body Fat in Adult Males and Females

Age	Increased Risk (BMI < 18.5)	Healthy (BMI 18.5–24.9)	Increased Risk (BMI 25–29.9)	High Risk (BMI 30+)
		Adult Males		
20–39	≤7.9%	8–19%	20–24%	≥25%
40–59	≤10.9%	11–21%	22–27%	≥28%
60–79	≤12.9%	13–24%	25–29%	≥30%
		Adult Female		
20–39	≤20.9%	21–32%	33–38%	≥39%
40–59	≤22.9%	23–33%	34–39%	≥40%
60–79	≤23.9%	24–35%	36–41%	≥42%

Source: Data from Gallagher D, Heymsfield SB, Heo M, Jebb SA, Murgatroyd PR, and Sakamoto Y. Healthy percentage body fat ranges: An approach for developing guidelines based on body mass index. *Am J Clin Nutr* 72:694–701, 2000. See also the "body fat lab" at Shape Up America!: *www.shapeup.org*.

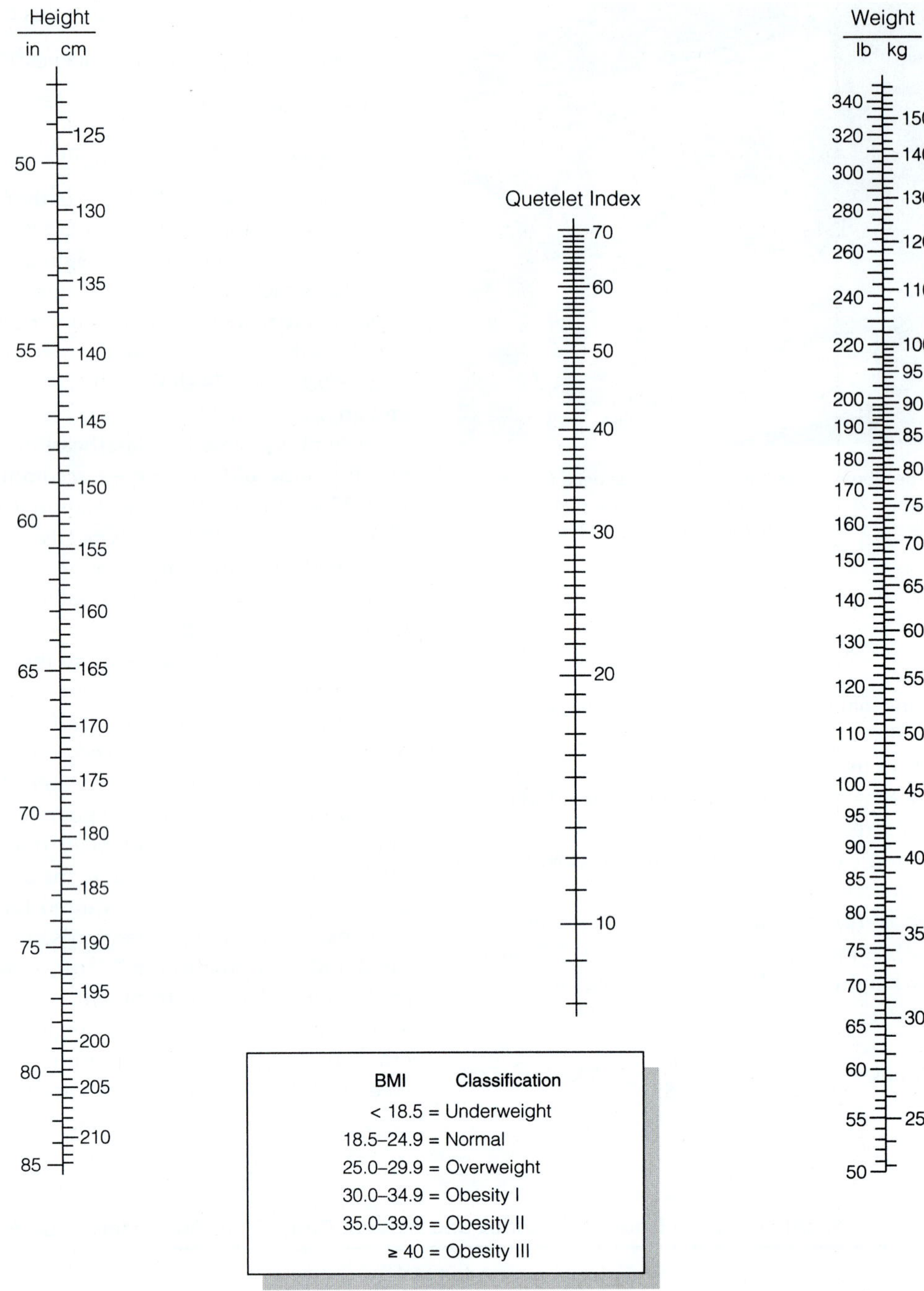

BMI	Classification
< 18.5	= Underweight
18.5–24.9	= Normal
25.0–29.9	= Overweight
30.0–34.9	= Obesity I
35.0–39.9	= Obesity II
≥ 40	= Obesity III

Figure 5.11 The Quetelet index (kg/m^2) is calculated from this nomogram by reading the central scale after a straight edge is placed between height and body weight.

TABLE 5.8 Body Mass Index Table

Directions: First find your height (no shoes), next locate your body weight at that height, and then find your BMI (top row).

	Healthy Weight						Overweight					Obese											Very Obese													
BMI	**19**	**20**	**21**	**22**	**23**	**24**	**25**	**26**	**27**	**28**	**29**	**30**	**31**	**32**	**33**	**34**	**35**	**36**	**37**	**38**	**39**	**40**	**41**	**42**	**43**	**44**	**45**	**46**	**47**	**48**	**49**	**50**	**51**	**52**	**53**	**54**
Height (in)																	**Body Weight (lb)**																			
58	91	96	100	105	110	115	119	124	129	134	138	143	148	153	158	162	167	172	177	181	186	191	196	201	205	210	215	220	224	229	234	239	244	248	253	258
59	94	99	104	109	114	119	124	128	133	138	143	148	153	158	163	168	173	178	183	188	193	198	203	208	212	217	222	227	232	237	242	247	252	257	262	267
60	97	102	107	112	118	123	128	133	138	143	148	153	158	163	168	174	179	184	189	194	199	204	209	215	220	225	230	235	240	245	250	255	261	266	271	276
61	100	106	111	116	122	127	132	137	143	148	153	158	164	169	174	180	185	190	195	201	206	211	217	222	227	232	238	243	248	254	259	264	269	275	280	285
62	104	109	115	120	126	131	136	142	147	153	158	164	169	175	180	186	191	196	202	207	213	218	224	229	235	240	246	251	256	262	267	273	278	284	289	295
63	107	113	118	124	130	135	141	146	152	158	163	169	175	180	186	191	197	203	208	214	220	225	231	237	242	248	254	259	265	270	278	282	287	293	299	304
64	110	116	122	128	134	140	145	151	157	163	169	174	180	186	192	197	204	209	215	221	227	232	238	244	250	256	262	267	273	279	285	291	296	302	308	314
65	114	120	126	132	138	144	150	156	162	168	174	180	186	192	198	204	210	216	222	228	234	240	246	252	258	264	270	276	282	288	294	300	306	312	318	324
66	118	124	130	136	142	148	155	161	167	173	179	186	192	198	204	210	216	223	229	235	241	247	253	260	266	272	278	284	291	297	303	309	315	322	328	334
67	121	127	134	140	146	153	159	166	172	178	185	191	198	204	211	217	223	230	236	242	249	255	261	268	274	280	287	293	299	306	312	319	325	331	338	344
68	125	131	138	144	151	158	164	171	177	184	190	197	203	210	216	223	230	236	243	249	256	262	269	276	282	289	295	302	308	315	322	328	335	341	348	354
69	128	135	142	149	155	162	169	176	182	189	196	203	209	216	223	230	236	243	250	257	263	270	277	284	291	297	304	311	318	324	331	338	345	351	358	365
70	132	139	146	153	160	167	174	181	188	195	202	209	216	222	229	236	243	250	257	264	271	278	285	292	299	306	313	320	327	334	341	348	355	362	369	376
71	136	143	150	157	165	172	179	186	193	200	208	215	222	229	236	243	250	257	265	272	279	286	293	301	308	315	322	329	338	343	351	358	365	372	379	386
72	140	147	154	162	169	177	184	191	199	206	213	221	228	235	242	250	258	265	272	279	287	294	302	309	316	324	331	338	346	353	361	368	375	383	390	397
73	144	151	159	166	174	182	189	197	204	212	219	227	235	242	250	257	265	272	280	288	295	302	310	318	325	333	340	348	355	363	371	378	386	393	401	408
74	148	155	163	171	179	186	194	202	210	218	225	233	241	249	256	264	272	280	287	295	303	311	319	326	334	342	350	358	365	373	381	389	396	404	412	420
75	152	160	168	176	184	192	200	208	216	224	232	240	248	256	264	272	279	287	295	303	311	319	327	335	343	351	359	367	375	383	391	399	407	415	423	431
76	156	164	172	180	189	197	205	213	221	230	238	246	254	263	271	279	287	295	304	312	320	328	336	344	353	361	369	377	385	394	402	410	418	426	435	443

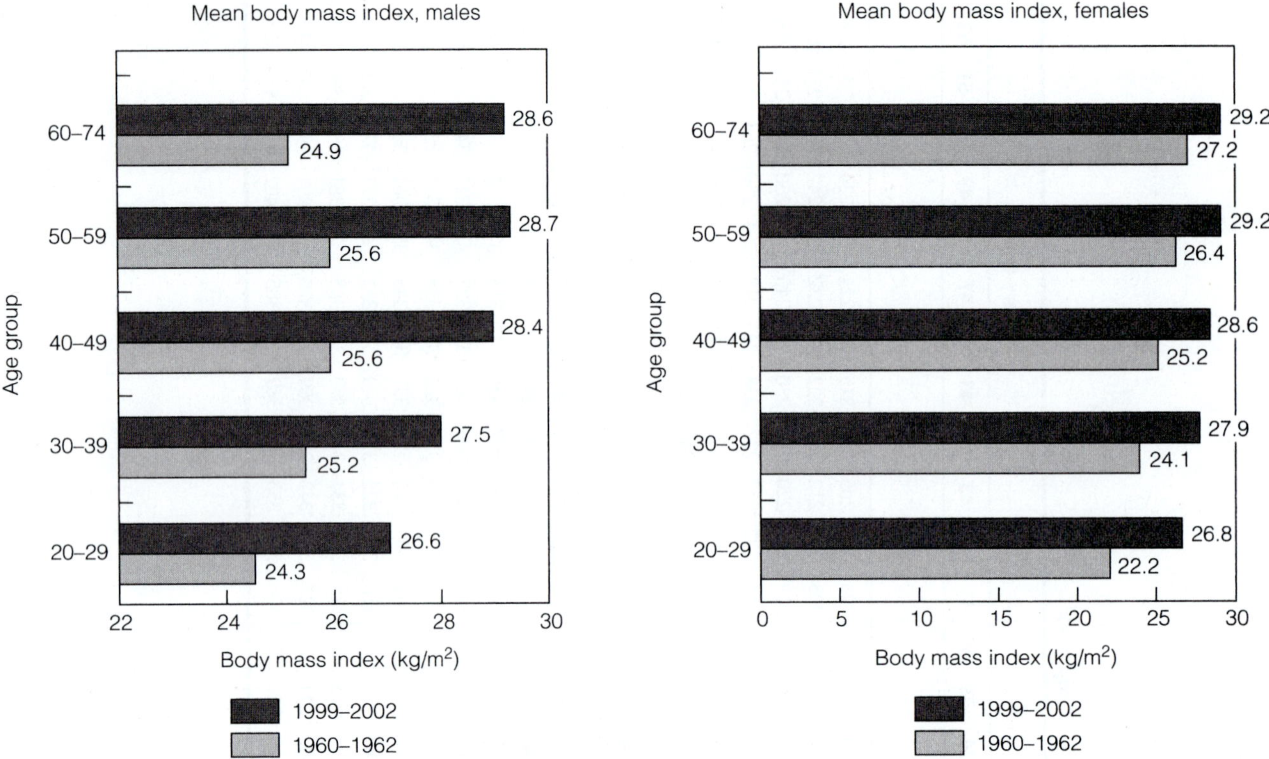

Figure 5.12 The average body mass index (kg/m^2) of American males (left) and females (right) has increased substantially since 1960-1962.[21]

that the NHLBI classification scheme is a reasonable measure with which to assess fatness in children and adolescents.[23]

Limitations of using BMI to classify individuals into categories of normal, overweight, or obese must be recognized.[22] For example, BMI overestimates body fat in persons who are very muscular, can underestimate body fat in persons who have lost muscle mass (e.g., the elderly) or in patients with edema, and gives a high BMI to very short persons (under 5 feet) that may not reflect fatness. Health professionals should use clinical judgment in adapting for these limitations and use other body composition methods to refine classification.

The basis for the NHLBI BMI classification scheme stems from epidemiologic studies that relate relative BMI to risk of morbidity and mortality.[22] For example, relative risk for cardiovascular disease increases in a graded fashion with increasing BMI. The relation between BMI and disease risk, however, varies among individuals and different populations. Therefore, the BMI classification must be viewed as a broad generalization. The NHLBI recommends the use of the waist circumference with BMI to classify disease risk (see Table 5.9). Although waist circumference and BMI are interrelated, waist circumference provides an independent prediction of risk over and above that of BMI. Waist circumference measurement is particularly useful in individuals who are categorized as normal or overweight on the BMI scale. At BMIs greater than or equal to 35, waist circumference has little added predictive power of disease risk beyond that of BMI. It is therefore not necessary to measure waist circumference in individuals with BMIs of 35 and higher. Instructions on measurement of the waist circumference are given later in this chapter. The *Dietary Guidelines for Americans* includes a simple scheme for following the NHLBI recommendations[24] (See Box 5.1).

SKINFOLD MEASUREMENTS

Although the BMI provides important information regarding the link between obesity and personal health, it provides an imprecise indication of percent body fat (see Table 5.7). Estimation of fat-free mass and percent body fat can be conducted using a wide variety of techniques, but the most widely used and practical method is based on skinfold measurements.[1–3,25–32]

Skinfold measurements can be taken quickly and easily at little expense, both within the laboratory and during field testing (e.g., health fairs). A certain amount of skill is necessary to identify the skinfold sites and then measure them accurately for all types of individuals. For this reason, initial attempts should be made under the guidance of a skilled class instructor or a qualified health professional until reliable and valid results can be obtained. Human Kinetics provides materials and videotapes for training (www.humankinetics.com).

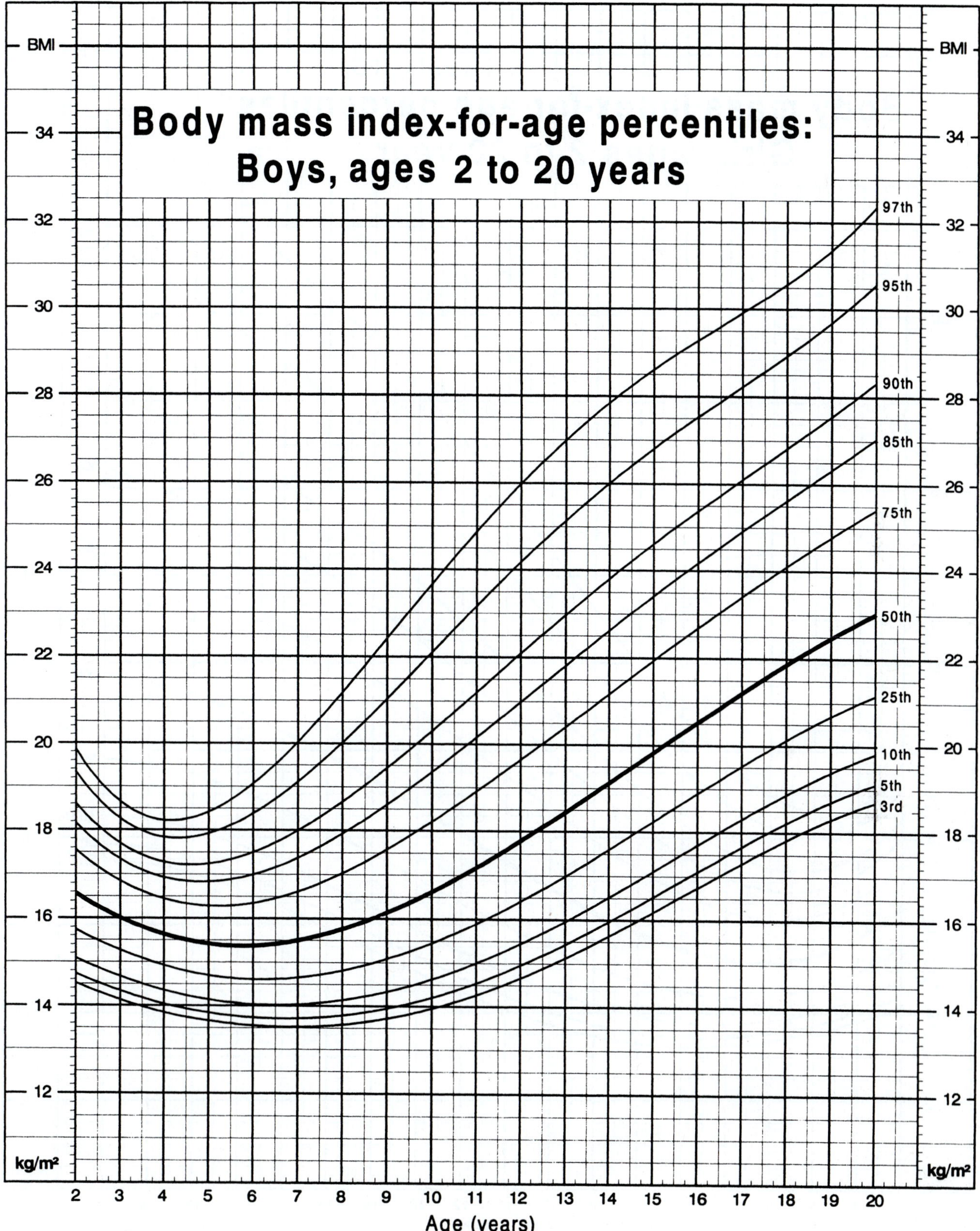

Figure 5.13 Body mass index-for-age percentiles for boys aged 2–20 years, CDC growth charts: United States.
Source: Developed by the National Center for Health Statistics in collaboration with the National Center for Chronic Disease Prevention and Health Promotion (2000).

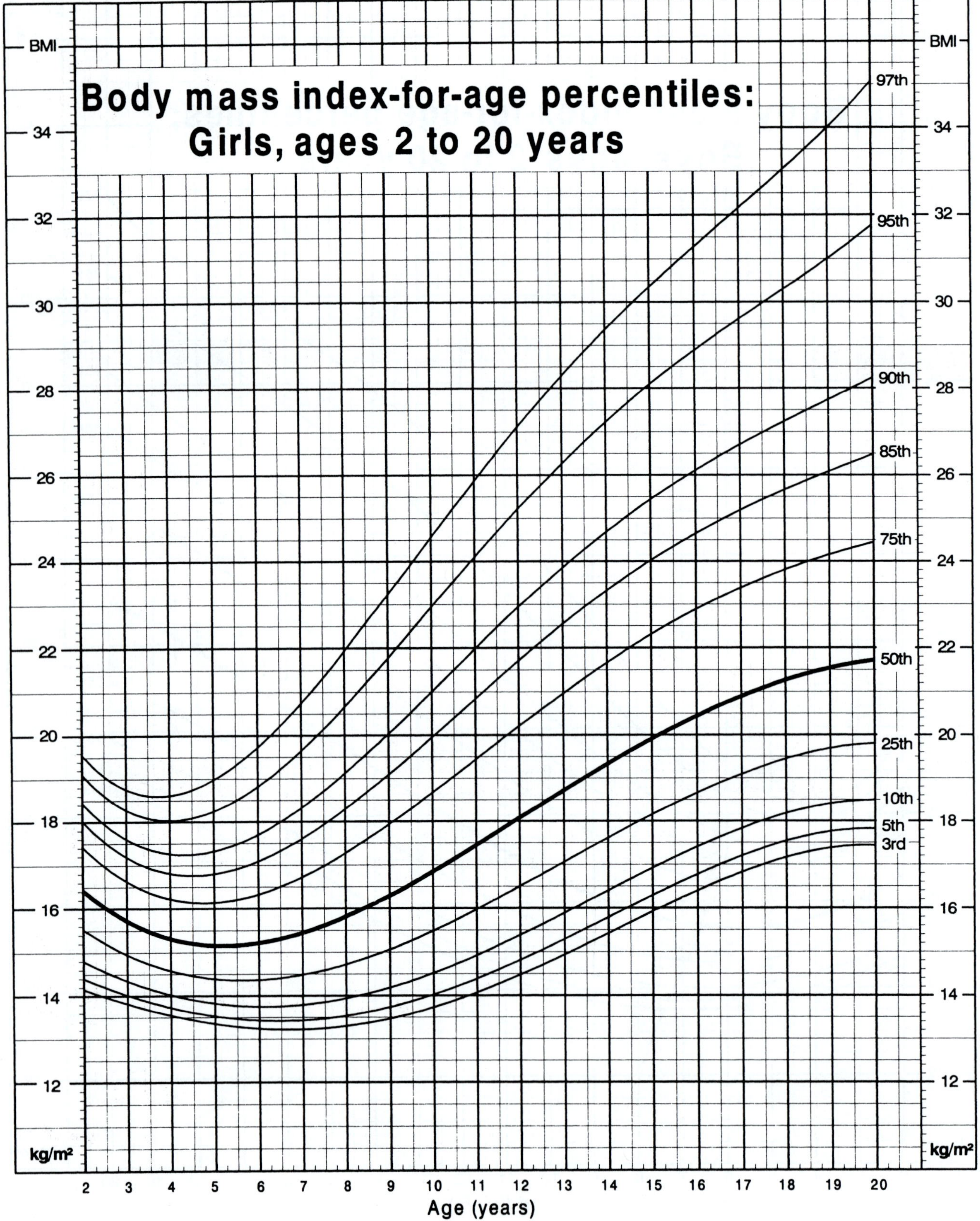

Figure 5.14 Body mass index-for-age percentiles for girls aged 2–20 years, CDC growth charts: United States. Source: Developed by the National Center for Health Statistics in collaboration with the National Center for Chronic Disease Prevention and Health Promotion (2000).

TABLE 5.9 Disease Risk Associated with Body Mass Index and Waist Circumference

Classification	Obesity Class	BMI (kg/m²)	Disease Risk Relative to Normal Weight and Waist Circumference* Men ≤40 in Women ≤35 in	>40 in >35 in
Underweight		<18.5		
Normal		18.5–24.9		
Overweight		25.0–29.9	Increased	High
Obesity	I	30.0–34.9	High	Very high
	II	35.0–39.9	Very high	Very high
Extreme obesity	III	≥40	Extremely high	Extremely high

*Disease risk for type 2 diabetes, hypertension, and cardiovascular disease.

Source: NHLBI Obesity Education Initiative Expert Panel (1998). *Clinical Guidelines on the Identification, Evaluation, and Treatment of Overweight and Obesity in Adults.* National Heart, Lung, and Blood Institute: www.nhlbi.nih.gov/nhlbi/.

Box 5.1

BMI, Waist Circumference, and Disease Risk Factors

How to Evaluate Your Weight (Adults)

1. Weigh yourself and have your height measured. Find your BMI category in the chart. The higher your BMI category, the greater the risk for health problems.
2. Measure around your waist, just above your hip bones, while standing. Health risks increase as waist measurement increases, particularly if waist is greater than 35 inches for women or 40 inches for men. Excess abdominal fat may place you at greater risk of health problems, even if your BMI is about right.
3. Refer to the list below to find out how many other risk factors you have.

The higher your BMI and waist measurement, and the more risk factors you have, the more you are likely to benefit from weight loss.

Find Out Your Other Risk Factors for Chronic Disease

The more of these risk factors you have, the more you are likely to benefit from weight loss if you are overweight or obese.

- Do you have a personal or family history of heart disease?
- Are you a male older than 45 years or a postmenopausal female?
- Do you smoke cigarettes?
- Do you have a sedentary lifestyle?
- Has your doctor told you that you have any of the following?
  - — High blood pressure
  - — Abnormal blood lipids (high LDL cholesterol, low HDL cholesterol, high triglycerides)
  - — Diabetes

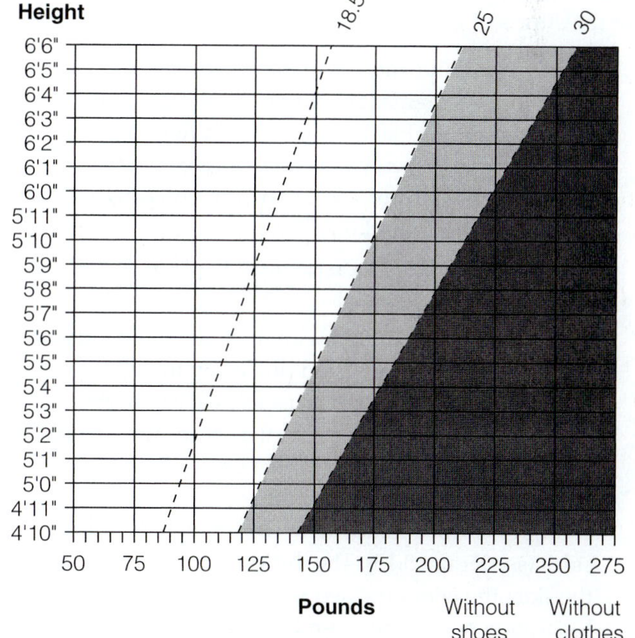

Directions: Find your weight on the bottom of the graph. Go straight up from that point until you come to the line that matches your height. Then look to find your weight group.

☐ **Healthy Weight** BMI from 18.5 up to 25 refers to healthy weight.

Overweight BMI from 25 up to 30 refers to overweight.

Obese BMI 30 or higher refers to obesity. Obese persons are also overweight.

Source: Report of the Dietary Guidelines Advisory Committee on the Dietary Guidelines for Americans, 2000.

When performed correctly, skinfold measures provide an estimate of percent body fat that has a high correlation ($r \geq .80$) with underwater weighing, DEXA, and other body composition testing standards.[1–3,25,26] The keys to accurate skinfold testing are locating and marking the specific sites where the calipers will be placed and then applying the calipers correctly to measure the sites. Specific rules and procedures should be followed during skinfold testing to minimize misclassification of individuals during counseling.

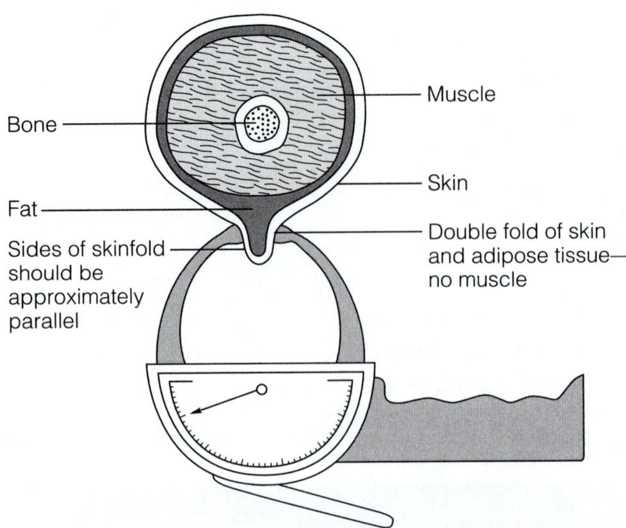

Figure 5.15 The double fold of skin and subcutaneous adipose tissue grasped by the thumb and index finger of the left hand should be large enough to form approximately parallel sides. Care should be taken to elevate only skin and adipose tissue. Source: Lee RD, Nieman DC. *Nutritional Assessment*. Copyright © 1993 The McGraw-Hill Companies. All rights reserved. Used with permission.

Rules for Taking Skinfolds

Researchers in the United States (including those performing large national surveys of the U.S. population that form the basis for normative data worldwide) take skinfold measurements on the right side of the body.[24] European investigators, on the other hand, tend to take measurements on the left side of the body. Most research, however, reveals that it matters little on which side measurements are taken.[26] Students in the United States should be taught to take all skinfold measurements on the right side, to coincide with the efforts of U.S. researchers.

1. As a general rule, those with little experience in skinfold measurement should mark the site to be measured with a black felt pen. Use a flexible steel tape with sites when you need to locate a body midpoint. With experience, however, you can locate the sites without marking.[26]
2. Feel the site prior to measurement to prepare yourself and the subject.
3. Firmly grasp the skinfold with the thumb and index finger of your left hand, and pull away from the subject's body. While this is usually easy with thin people, it is much harder with the obese and can be somewhat uncomfortable for the person being tested. The amount of tissue pinched up must be enough to form a fold with approximately parallel sides (see Figure 5.15). The thicker the fat layer under the skin, the wider the necessary fold (and the more separation needed between thumb and index finger).
4. Hold the caliper in your right hand, perpendicular to the skinfold and with the skinfold dial facing up and easily readable. Place the caliper heads ¼–½ inch away from the fingers holding the skinfold, so that the pressure of the caliper will not be affected.
5. Do not place the skinfold caliper too deep into the skinfold or too far away on the tip of the skinfold. Try to visualize where a true double fold of skin thickness is, and place the caliper heads there. It is good practice to position the caliper arms one at a time—first the fixed arm on one side, and then the lever arm on the other.
6. Read the dial approximately 4 seconds after the pressure from your hand has been released on the lever arm of the caliper jaw.
7. Take a minimum of two measurements at each site. Measurements should be at least 15 seconds apart, to allow the skinfold site to return to normal. If consecutive measurements vary by more than 10%, take more until there is consistency.
8. Maintain the pressure with the thumb and forefinger throughout each measurement.
9. When measuring the obese, it may be impossible to elevate a skinfold with parallel sides, particularly over the abdomen (see Figure 5.16). In this situation, try using both hands to pull the skinfold away, while a partner attempts to measure the width. If the skinfold is too wide for the calipers, you will have to use underwater weighing or another technique.
10. Do not take measurements when the subject's skin is moist because there is a tendency to grasp extra skin, obtaining inaccurately large values. Also do not take measurements immediately after exercise or when the person being measured is overheated because the shift of body fluid to the skin will inflate normal skinfold size.
11. It takes practice to be able to grasp the same amount of skinfold consistently at the same location every time. Accuracy can be tested by having several technicians take the same measurements and compare results. It may take up to 20–50 practice sessions to become proficient.

Calipers should be accurately calibrated and have a constant pressure of 10 g/mm^2 throughout the full measurement range[1,3,26,32] (see Figure 5.17). Box 5.2 provides a summary of the major skinfold calipers and their approximate prices.

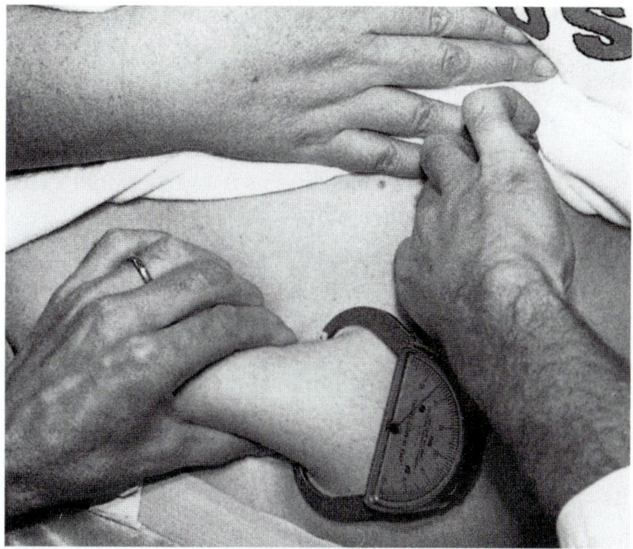

Figure 5.16 Skinfold measurement is very difficult with obese subjects, and experience is required to know just where the caliper heads should be placed.

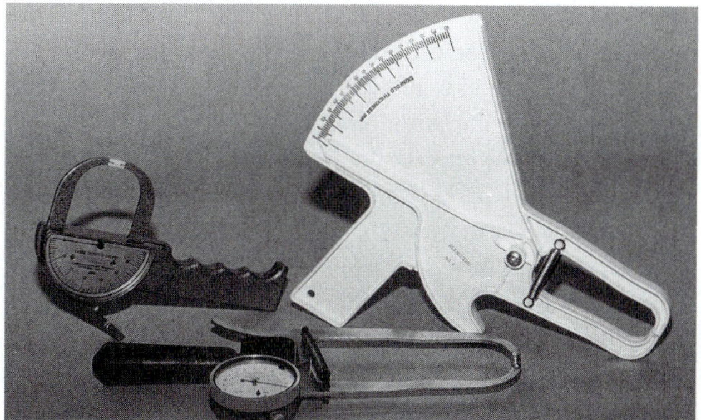

Figure 5.17 Pictured are the Lange, Harpenden, and Slim Guide skinfold calipers.

Box 5.2

Description of Skinfold Calipers

The following is a brief description of the major types of skinfold calipers, listed in order of decreasing retail price.

1. *Harpenden.* This has been a standard research caliper for many years. Some skinfold equations in use today are based on studies done using the Harpenden. It is accurate to within ± 0.2 mm. Some researchers have provided data that the Harpenden skinfold calipers provide smaller values when compared to the Lange skinfold calipers. $485
2. *Skyndex 1.* This unique caliper has a built-in computer, that calculates and displays percent body fat directly on its LCD (liquid-crystal display) digital readout, thus eliminating the necessity to add the skinfold readings and compute the percent body fat from formulas or tables. It is available with Durnin, Jackson–Pollock, and Slaughter–Lohman formulas. Only one program is in each caliper, and the desired formula needs to be specified when ordering. $450
3. *Skyndex 11.* This is basically the same as the Skyndex 1, except that it does not have the built-in computer. It has an easy-to-read digital readout and a "hold" feature. When the user is satisfied with the reading, the hold button can be pushed, and this will lock the reading on the digital display until it can be written down. A second push on the hold button returns the caliper to "0." $240
4. *Lange.* This is the best selling of the high-priced calipers. Jackson–Pollock skinfold data were obtained using the Lange skinfold calipers. It has been manufactured since 1962 and is widely used in schools, colleges, fitness centers, etc. $300
5. *Baseline or Jamar or TEC.* This is a copy of the Lange but is made in Korea and sold under several different names. It appears to be identical to the Lange, even to the paint color. However, its internal quality is not as high, and repair has been reported to be a problem. $195
6. *Slim Guide.* This is much lower priced than any of the aforementioned calipers yet will produce results that are almost as accurate. This is the only low-cost caliper accurate enough to be used for professional measurements and is the most widely used professional caliper. Its primary disadvantage is that it does not look professional. The caliper is easy to use, with convenient pistol grip and trigger. It is very durable. $30
7. *Fat-O-Meter.* A low-priced economy caliper. The caliper is small and lightweight and can be conveniently carried in a pocket. Although not as accurate as other calipers, it will provide reasonable estimates of body fat if correct procedures are carefully followed. $18

Each of these calipers is available through Creative Health Products, www.chponline.com.

The accuracy of skinfold measurements can be reduced by many factors, including measurement at the wrong sites, inconsistencies among different calipers and testers, and the use of inconsistent equations.[26] However, when testers practice together and take care to standardize their testing procedures, inconsistencies among testers can usually be held under 1%. The largest source of error is the nonstandardization of site selection.[1–3,26]

Eight skinfold sites are described here next. They are in accordance with the Airlie Consensus Conference that resulted in the publication of the *Anthropometric Standardization Reference Manual*.[26] The Jackson–Pollock equations are commonly used to estimate fat-free mass and fat mass from three to seven skinfold measurements.[25] The skinfold sites used by Jackson and Pollock vary slightly from the recommendations of the Airlie Consensus Conference, and these differences will be noted below. The American College of Sports Medicine uses the Jackson–Pollock skinfold site descriptions, and individuals studying for certification exams should understand differences between the two systems of skinfold testing.[33]

To reduce error, skinfold sites should be precisely determined and verified by a trained instructor before measurement. The measurements should be made carefully, in a quiet room, and without undue haste. (Figures 5.18 to 5.27 depict the correct site marking and method of measurement for each site.)

- *Chest.* The chest or pectoral skinfold is measured using a skinfold with its long axis directed to the nipple. The skinfold is picked up just next to the anterior axillary fold (front of armpit line; see Figure 5.18). The measurement is taken ½ inch from the fingers. The site is approximately 1 inch from the anterior axillary line toward the nipple. The measurement is the same for both men and women. In the Jackson–Pollock procedures, the chest/pectoral skinfold site is one half the distance between the anterior axillary line and the nipple for men, and one third of this distance for women.[25]
- *Abdomen.* A horizontal fold is picked up slightly more than 1 inch (3 cm) to the side of and ½ inch below the naval (see Figure 5.19). The Jackson–Pollock procedure uses a vertical fold 2 cm to the right of the umbilicus.[25]
- *Thigh.* Pick up a vertical fold on the front of the thigh, midway between the hip (inguinal crease) and the nearest border of the patella or kneecap (see Figures 5.20 and 5.21). The person being tested should first flex the hip to make it easier to locate the inguinal crease. Be sure to pick a spot on the hip crease that is exactly above the midpoint of the front of the thigh. The closest border of the kneecap should be located while the knee is extended. When measuring the thigh skinfold, the

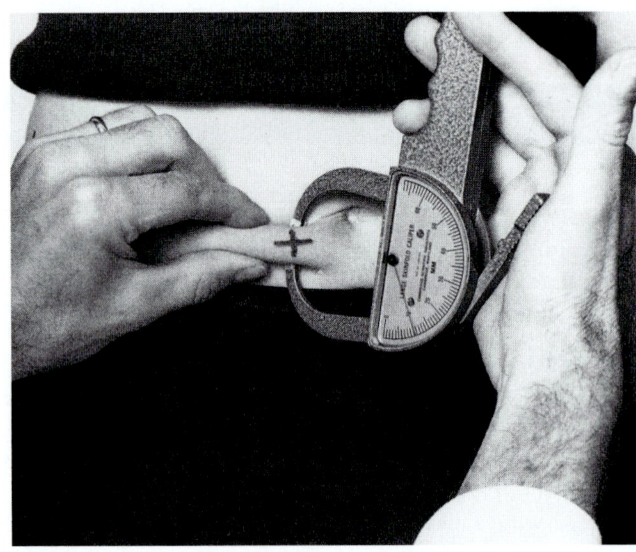

Figure 5.19 Measurement of the abdominal skinfold.

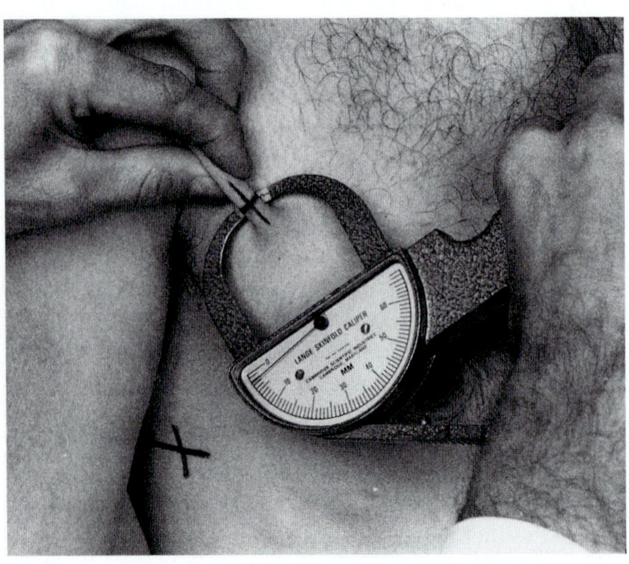

Figure 5.18 Measurement of the chest or pectoral skinfold.

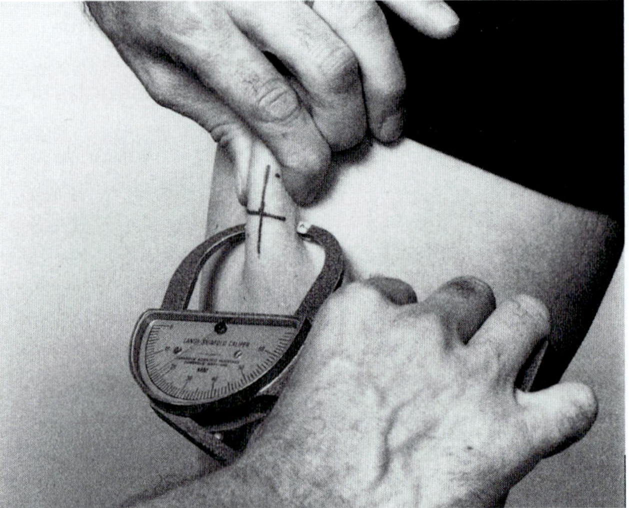

Figure 5.20 Measurement of the thigh skinfold.

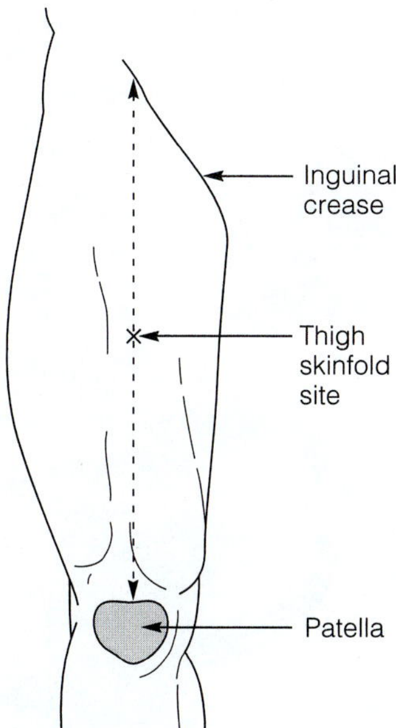

Figure 5.21 The thigh skinfold site lies along the anterior midline of the thigh halfway between the inguinal crease and the proximal border of the patella. Source: Lee RD, Nieman DC. *Nutritional Assessment.* Copyright © The McGraw-Hill Companies. All rights reserved. Used with permission.

body weight should be shifted to the other foot while the leg on the side of the measurement is relaxed, with the knee slightly flexed and the foot flat on the floor.

- *Triceps.* Measure a vertical fold on the rear midline of the upper arm, halfway between the lateral projection of the acromion process of the scapula (bump on back side of shoulder) and the inferior part of the olecranon process (the elbow; see Figure 5.22a and b). The site should first be marked by measuring the distance between the lateral projection of the acromial process and the lower border of the olecranon process of the ulna, using a tape measure, with the elbow flexed to 90 degrees. The midpoint is marked on the lateral side of the arm. The skinfold is measured with the arm hanging loosely at the side. The measurer stands behind the person being measured and picks up the skinfold site on the back of the arm, with the thumb and index finger directed down toward the feet. The triceps skinfold is picked up with the left thumb and index finger, approximately ½ inch above the marked level where the tips of the caliper are applied.
- *Suprailiac.* Measure a diagonal fold above the crest of the ilium at the spot where an imaginary line would come down from the midaxillary line (see Figures 5.23 and 5.24). The person being measured should stand erect, with feet together. The arms should hang by the sides but can be moved slightly to improve access to the site. A diagonal fold should be grasped just to the rear of the midaxillary line, following the natural cleavage lines of the skin. The skinfold caliper jaws should be applied about ½ inch from the fingers. In the Jackson–Pollock procedure, a diagonal fold is taken with the natural angle of the iliac crest at the anterior axillary line immediately superior to the iliac crest.[25]
- *Midaxillary.* Measure a horizontal fold on the midaxillary line at the level of the xiphi-sternal junction (bottom of the sternum, where the xiphoid process begins; see Figure 5.25). The arm of the person being measured can be moved slightly backward during measurement to allow easy access to the site. In the Jackson–Pollock procedure, a vertical fold is used at this site.[25]

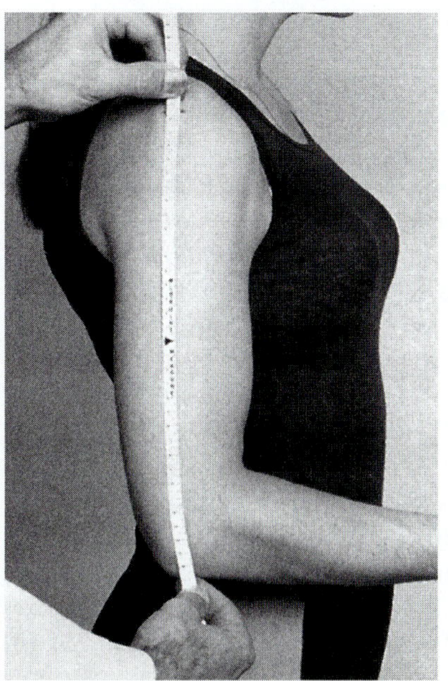

(a)

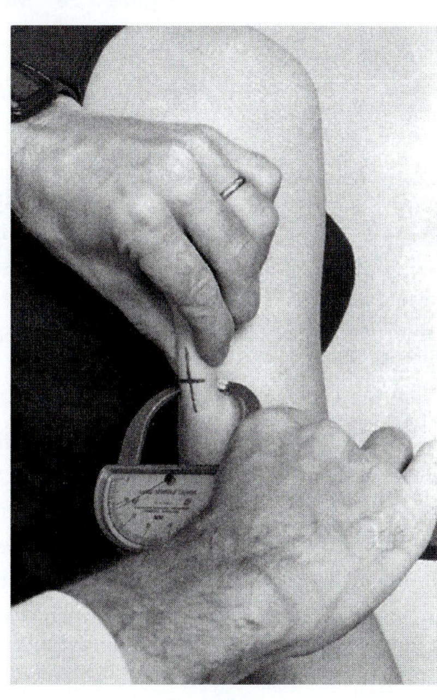

(b)

Figure 5.22 Measurement of the triceps skinfold.

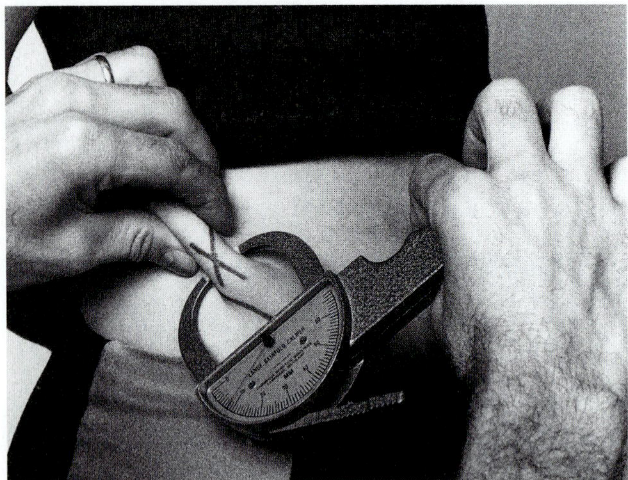

Figure 5.23 Measurement of the suprailiac skinfold.

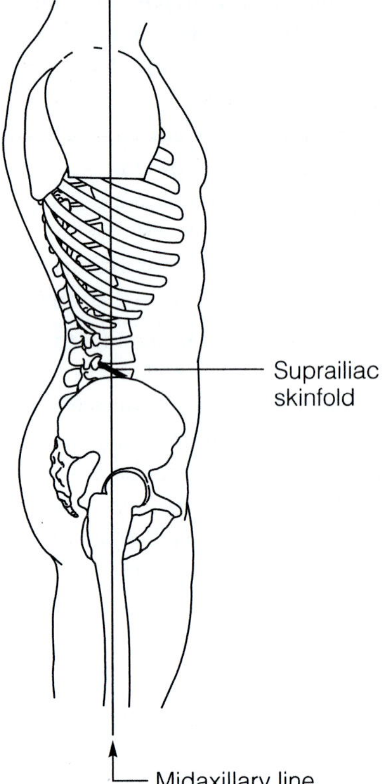

Figure 5.24 The suprailiac skinfold is measured just above the iliac crest at the midaxillary line. The long axis of the skinfold follows the natural cleavage lines of the skin.
Source: Lee RD, Nieman DC. *Nutritional Assessment*.

- *Subscapular.* The site is just below the lowest angle of the scapula (see Figure 5.26). A fold is taken on a diagonal line directed at a 45-degree angle toward the right side. To locate the site, the measurer should feel for the bottom of the scapula. In some cases, it helps to place the arm of the person being measured behind his or her back.

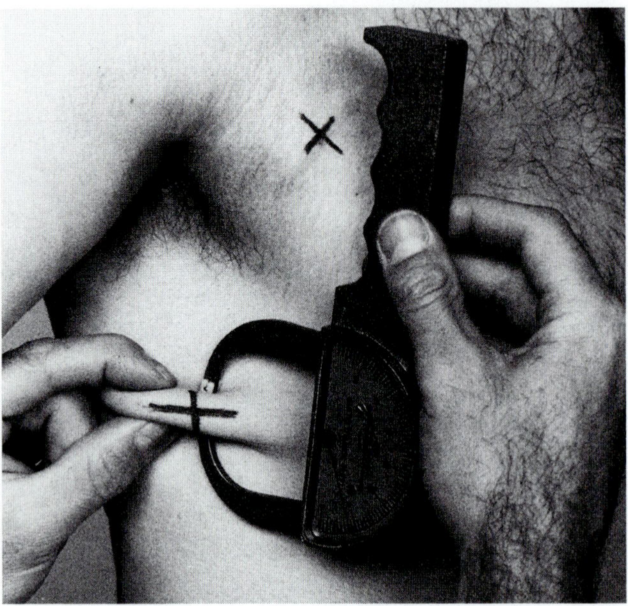

Figure 5.25 Measurement of the midaxillary skinfold.

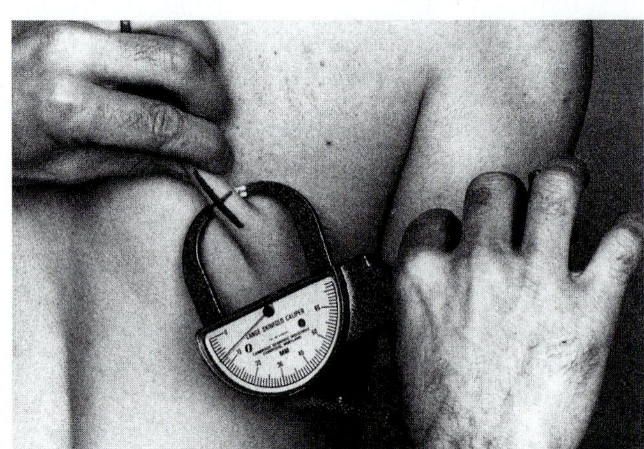

Figure 5.26 Measurement of the subscapular skinfold.

- *Medial calf.* For the measurement of the medial calf skinfold, the person being measured sits with his or her right knee flexed to about 90 degrees, sole of the foot on the floor. The level of the maximum calf circumference is marked on the inside (medial) of the calf (see Figure 5.27). Facing from the front, the measurer raises a vertical skinfold and measures at the marked site.

One-Site Skinfold Test

The triceps skinfold site has been used most often in large population group studies. The average triceps skinfold thicknesses (in millimeters) for various age groups are given in Figure 5.28. The data were derived from the National Health and Examination Survey (NHANES) for 1999–2002.[21] (See Appendix A, Table 27.)

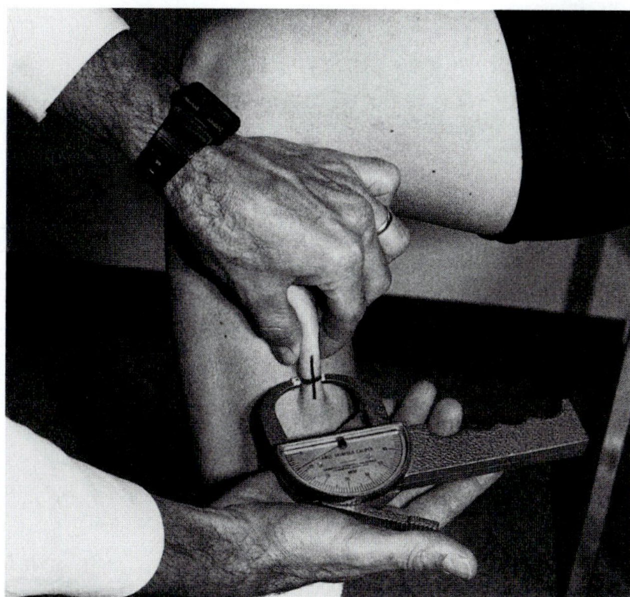

Figure 5.27 Measurement of the medial calf skinfold.

Care should be taken when classifying obesity with the use of just one skinfold site. No equations for body fat estimation have been developed using just the triceps skinfold, and individual values must therefore be compared to tables developed from national norms. Some people have a higher proportion of their body fat distributed on the backs of their upper arms than others, which could lead to an overestimation of their degree of obesity. Therefore, the single-site skinfold test should only be used as a rough approximation of obesity.

Two-Site Skinfold Test for Children, Youths, and College-Age Adults

The two-site skinfold test, using the triceps and subscapular sites, is the most commonly used body composition test for young people ages 6–22.[1,3,26,34–38] Norms utilizing the sum of triceps and subscapula or triceps and medial calf skinfolds have been developed and are found in Appendix A (Tables 1, 2, 11–13) and in Figures 5.29 and 5.30.[34–36]

The choice of the triceps and subscapular sites over other commonly measured sites (medial calf, abdomen, suprailiac, thigh, etc.) was originally made for several reasons:[3,36]

- Correlations between these sites and other measures of body fat have been consistently among the highest in many studies.
- These sites are more reliably and objectively measured than most other sites.
- There are available national norms for these sites.

Some parents of school-age children are concerned that the modesty of their children is infringed upon when the physical educator raises the shirt of the child to gain access to the subscapular site. The medial calf skinfold site is more easily accessible, and studies have found it to be valid and reliable.[3,36]

Unfortunately, many public school physical educators do not support skinfold testing, often because they feel inadequately trained to conduct it or to interpret results accurately.[37]

Teachers are also encouraged to attend workshops where training is offered on the skinfold-measurement technique. It is recommended that skinfold measurements be taken for all children at least once a year, with records kept to track children from year to year.

Equations to estimate percent body fat of children and youths from the sum of triceps and calf skinfolds are as follows:[3]

Males 6–17 years

% body fat = (0.735 × sum of skinfolds) + 1.0

Females 6–17 years

% body fat = (0.1610 × sum of skinfolds) + 5.0

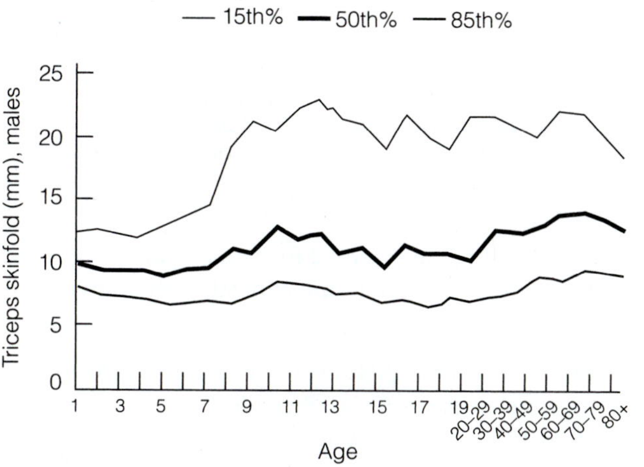

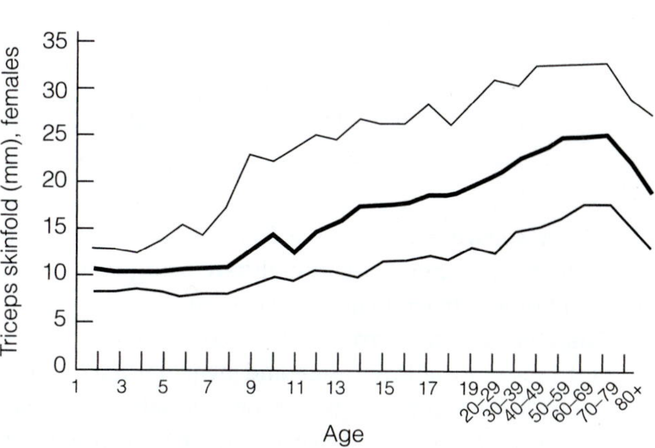

Figure 5.28 Average triceps skinfold of American males (left) and females (right). The area around the mean represents the fifteenth and eighty-fifth percentiles of a national sample of individuals of all ages.[21]
Source: CDH, NCHS. Advance Data 361, July 7, 2005.

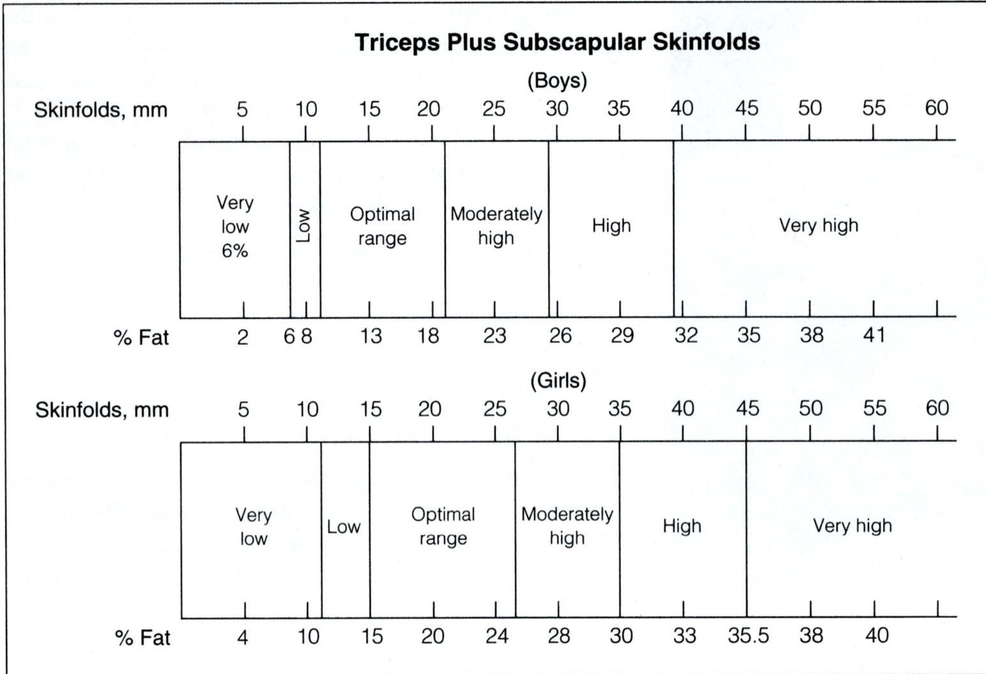

Figure 5.29 Body fat standards for children and youths (ages 6–17) using the triceps and subscapular skinfolds. Source: Lohman TG. The use of skinfold to estimate body fatness on children and youth. *JOPERD*, November/December 1987, 98–102. Reprinted with permission from the *Journal of Physical Education, Recreation & Dance*, a publication of the American Alliance for Health, Physical Education, Recreation, and Dance, 1900 Association Drive, Reston, VA 22091.

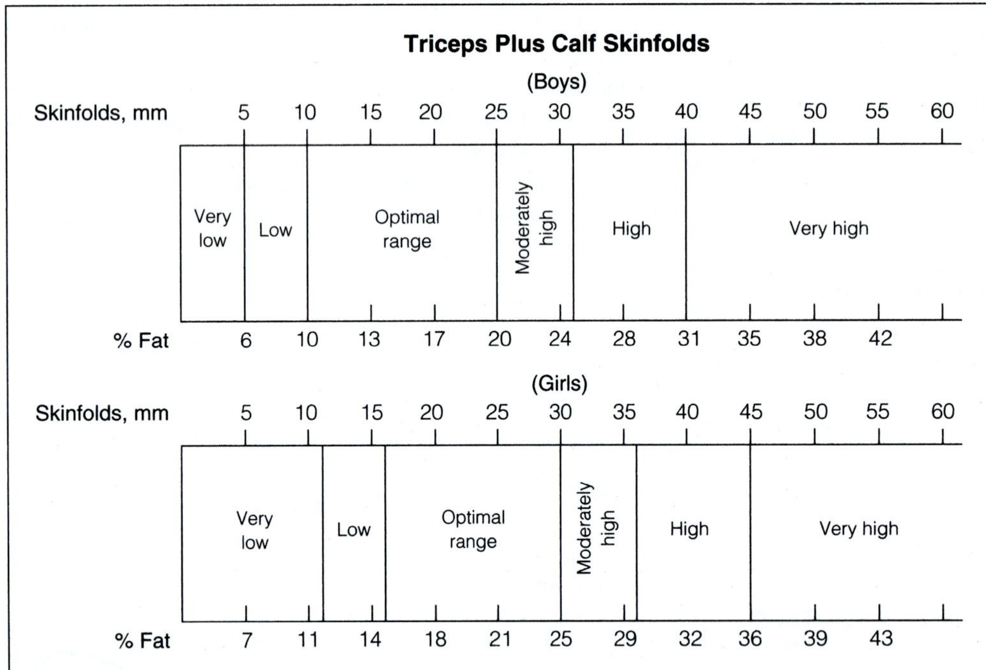

Figure 5.30 Body fat standards for children and youths (ages 6–17) using the triceps and medial calf skinfolds. Source: Lohman TG. The use of skinfold to estimate body fatness on children and youth. *JOPERD*, November/December 1987, 98–102. Reprinted with permission from the *Journal of Physical Education, Recreation & Dance*, a publication of the American Alliance for Health, Physical Education, Recreation, and Dance, 1900 Association Drive, Reston, VA 22091.

Computer software is available from Human Kinetics to calculate body composition of children, using these equations and others (www.humankinetics.com).

There is some concern that these equations underpredict fat mass in the low range and overpredict fat mass for the mid- to higher range.[38] A new equation has been developed and cross-validated using DEXA as the reference method.[38] This equation uses body weight (kilograms), two skinfold measures (triceps and abdomen), ethnicity (1 for Caucasian and 2 for African American), and gender (1 for male and 2 for female), and has potential for widespread use in the clinical evaluation of children ages 4–11:

Fat mass (kg) = (0.308 × body weight) + (0.230 × triceps skinfold) + (0.641 × gender) + (0.857 × ethnicity) + (0.053 × abdomen skinfold) − 7.62

For example, if an 8-year-old male Caucasian child weighs 27 kg, with a triceps skinfold of 10 mm and an abdominal skinfold of 15 mm:

Fat mass (kg) = (0.308 × 27 kg) + (0.230 × 10 mm) + (0.641 × 1) + (0.857 × 1) + (0.053 × 15 mm) − 7.62 = 5.3

To get body fat percent, divide the fat mass (5.3 kg) by total body mass (27 kg) and multiply by 100: $(5.3/27) \times 100 = 19.6\%$. Figures 5.29 and 5.30 indicate that this male child would be classified into the high end of the "optimal range" for body fat.

Multiple Skinfold Tests for Adults

Since 1951, a large number of body composition regression equations using anthropometric techniques (skinfold measurements and circumference and diameter measures) have been published.[25] Most of these equations have been developed for specific types of people (athletes or young men or elderly women, etc.) and are thus limited to the groups they were developed for.[25]

The more recent trend has been to develop generalized rather than population-specific equations. These equations have been developed using regression models that take into account data from many different research projects. The main advantage is that one generalized equation replaces several population-specific equations without a loss in prediction accuracy for a wide range of people.[25]

Jackson and Pollock have published generalized equations for adult men and women[25,39,40] (see Table 5.10). The three-site equations utilizing triceps, suprailiac, and abdomen skinfolds for adult females, and chest, abdomen, and thigh skinfolds for adult males have been most widely used.

Notice that the equations in Table 5.10 predict either percent body fat or body density. The body density formulas require an additional step to estimate percent body fat, using the formulas summarized earlier in this chapter in Table 5.2. For ease of determination, a nomogram has been developed to calculate percent body fat using age and the sum of three skinfolds for both men and women[41] (see Figure 5.31).[25]

The nomogram is based on the three-site skinfold equations listed in Table 5.10, which use the chest, abdomen, and thigh sites for males, and the triceps, suprailiac, and thigh skinfolds for women. However, this nomogram is based on the Brozek equation, which is applicable only for white male and female adults.

Table 5.11 summarizes equations from Durnin and Womersley,[42] which have been used by many researchers, and

TABLE 5.10 Generalized Body Composition Equations

Males

7-Site Formula

Body density = 1.11200000 − 0.00043499 *(sum of seven skinfolds)* + 0.00000055 *(sum of seven skinfolds)*^{2} − 0.00028826 *(age)*
(chest, midaxillary, triceps, subscapular, abdomen, suprailiac, thigh)

4-Site Formula

Percent body fat = 0.29288 *(sum of four skinfolds)* − 0.0005 *(sum of four skinfolds)*^{2} + 0.15845 *(age)* − 5.76377
(abdomen, suprailiac, tricep, thigh)

3-Site Formula

Body density = 1.1093800 − 0.0008267 *(sum of three skinfolds)* + 0.0000016 *(sum of three skinfolds)*^{2} − 0.0002574 *(age)*
(chest, abdomen, thigh)

Body density = 1.1125025 − 0.0013125 *(sum of three skinfolds)* + 0.0000055 *(sum of three skinfolds)*^{2} − 0.0002440 *(age)*
(chest, triceps, subscapular)

Percent body fat = 0.39287 *(sum of three skinfolds)*−0.00105 *(sum of three skinfolds)*^{2} + 0.15772 *(age)* − 5.18845
(abdomen, suprailiac, triceps)

Females

7-Site Formula

Body density = 1.0970 − 0.00046971 *(sum of seven skinfolds)* + 0.00000056 *(sum of seven skinfolds)*^{2} − 0.00012828 *(age)*
(chest, midaxillary, triceps, subscapular, abdomen, suprailiac, thigh)

4-Site Formula

Percent body fat = 0.29669 *(sum of four skinfolds)* − 0.00043 *(sum of four skinfolds)*^{2} + 0.02963 *(age)* − 1.4072
(abdomen, suprailiac, tricep, thigh)

3-Site Formula

Percent body fat = 0.41563 *(sum of three skinfolds)* − 0.00112 *(sum of three skinfolds)*^{2} + 0.03661 *(age)* + 4.03653
(triceps, abdomen, suprailiac)

Body density =1.0994921 − 0.0009929 *(sum of three skinfolds)* + 0.0000023 *(sum of three skinfolds)*^{2} − 0.0001392 *(age)*
(triceps, suprailiac, thigh)

Note: The researchers who developed these equations used vertical instead of horizontal skinfolds at the abdominal and midaxillary sites.

Sources: Jackson AS, Pollock ML. Practical assessment of body composition. *Phys Sportsmed* 13:76–90, 1985. Golding LA, Myers CR, Sinning WE. *The Y's Way to Physical Fitness* (3rd ed.), 1989. Champaign, IL: Human Kinetics, Inc.

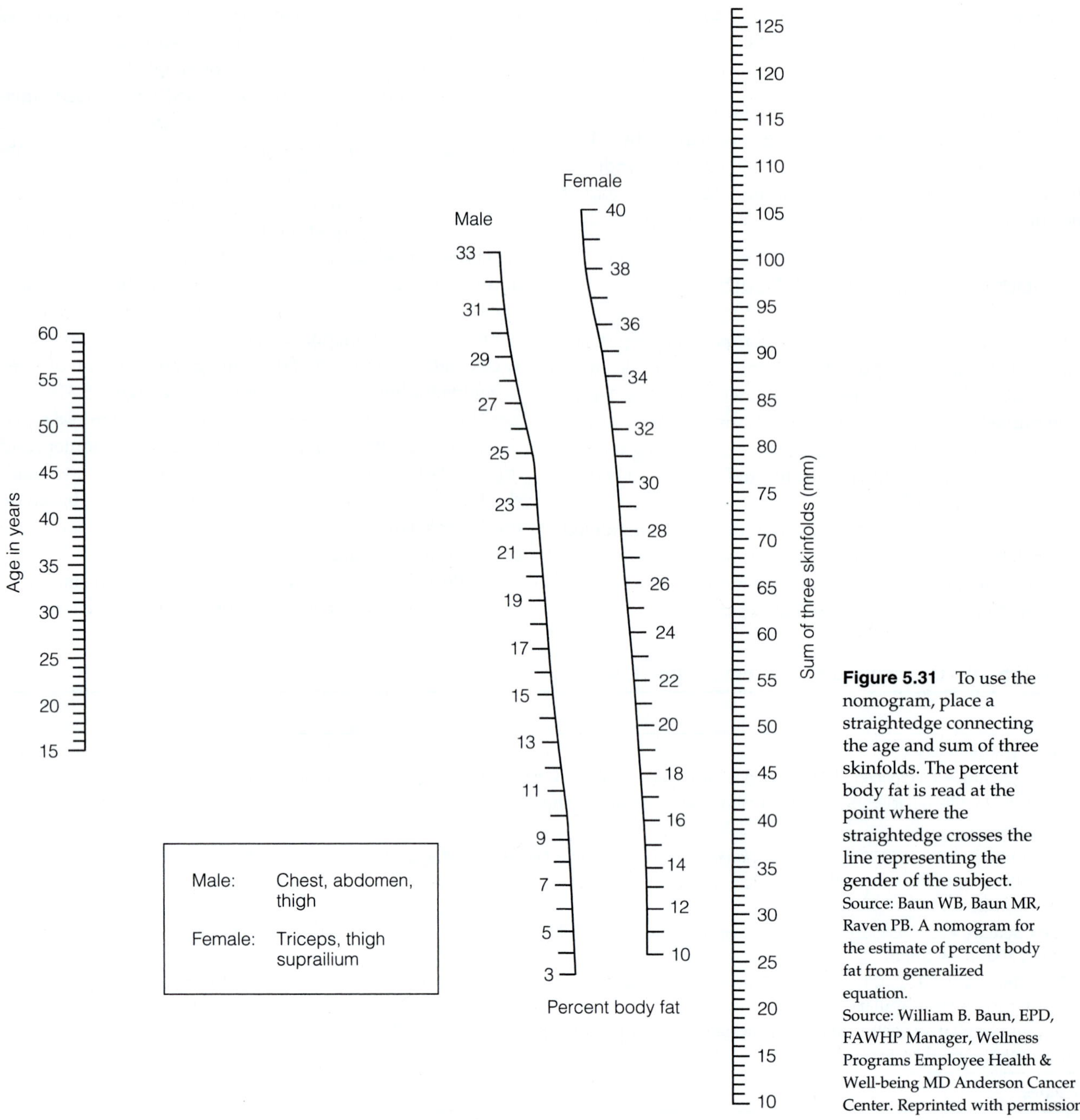

Figure 5.31 To use the nomogram, place a straightedge connecting the age and sum of three skinfolds. The percent body fat is read at the point where the straightedge crosses the line representing the gender of the subject.
Source: Baun WB, Baun MR, Raven PB. A nomogram for the estimate of percent body fat from generalized equation.
Source: William B. Baun, EPD, FAWHP Manager, Wellness Programs Employee Health & Well-being MD Anderson Cancer Center. Reprinted with permission.

TABLE 5.11 Calculation* of Body Density According to the Method of Durnin and Womersley

Equations for Men		Equations for Women	
Age range		**Age range**	
17–19	$D = 1.1620 - 0.0630 \times (\log \Sigma)$	17–19	$D = 1.1549 - 0.0678 \times (\log \Sigma)$
20–29	$D = 1.1631 - 0.0632 \times (\log \Sigma)$	20–29	$D = 1.1599 - 0.0717 \times (\log \Sigma)$
30–39	$D = 1.1422 - 0.0544 \times (\log \Sigma)$	30–39	$D = 1.1423 - 0.0632 \times (\log \Sigma)$
40–49	$D = 1.1620 - 0.0700 \times (\log \Sigma)$	40–49	$D = 1.1333 - 0.0612 \times (\log \Sigma)$
50+	$D = 1.1715 - 0.0779 \times (\log \Sigma)$	50+	$D = 1.1339 - 0.0645 \times (\log \Sigma)$

*Based on four skinfolds: biceps, triceps, subscapula, and suprailiac. Sum and calculate logarithm.

Note: To calculate percent body fat, use the percent fat equations summarized in Table 5.2.

Source: Durnin JVGA, Womersley J. Body fat assessment from total body density and its estimation from skinfold thickness: Measurements on 481 men and women aged 16 to 72 years. *Br J Nutr* 32:77–97, 1974.

which vary according to the age of the subject. The equations are based on the logarithm of the sum of four skinfolds (biceps, triceps, subscapular, and suprailiac). The biceps skinfold is defined as a vertical fold on the anterior aspect of the upper arm, directly opposite the triceps skinfold site.

Table 5.2 summarizes age- and sex-specific constants for conversion of body density (derived from equations in Table 5.10) to percent body fat in children and youths.[1] These constants are necessary, in that the density of the fat-free mass is lower in children than in adults, because of less bone mineral and more water, proportionately. Thus, use of "adult" skinfold equations (Table 5.10) to predict body density generally *overestimates* percent body fat in children and youths.[43] To determine percent body fat from body density for an 11-year-old boy, using the fat-free mass density of 1.084, the equation would be (Table 5.2)

$$\%\text{ body fat} = \left(\frac{5.30}{\text{body density}} - 4.89\right) \times 100$$

A sample skinfold testing form is outlined in Figure 5.32. In making the calculations for fat, lean body weight (fat-free mass), and ideal body weight, the following formulas should be used:

$$\text{Pounds of fat} = \text{total weight} \times \%\text{ body fat}$$

$$\text{Lean body weight} = \text{total weight} - \text{fat weight}$$

$$\text{Ideal body weight} = \frac{\text{present lean body weight}}{100\% - \text{desired fat}\%}$$

For example, if a subject weighs 200 pounds, has 25% body fat, and desires to have 15% body fat,

$$\text{Body fat} = 200 \times 0.25 = 50\text{ lb}$$

$$\text{Lean body weight} = 200 - 50 = 150\text{ lb}$$

$$\text{Ideal body weight} = \frac{150}{0.85} = 176\text{ lb}$$

The ideal weight formula assumes that the lean body weight stays the same during weight loss. Excess body

Skinfold Measurements

Name ____________________ Date __________

Age ________ Sex ________ Height ________ Weight ________

MEASUREMENTS (mm)

________	Chest	________	Suprailiac
________	Abdominal	________	Midaxillary
________	Thigh	________	Subscapular
________	Triceps	________	Medial Calf

CALCULATIONS
(Use appropriate formula)

________ Total skinfolds (mm)

________ Body fat percent

________ Pounds of fat
(Total wt × body fat %)

________ Pounds of lean body weight
(Total wt – fat wt)

________ Classification
(see norms)

________ Ideal body weight
[LBW / (100% – desired fat %)]

Figure 5.32 A sample worksheet for body composition calculations for skinfold measures.

weight, however, has been determined to be 75% body fat and 25% lean body weight (fat-free mass). For some people, therefore, a reduction in lean body weight is actually desirable and should be represented in the equation by subtracting 25% of the excess weight (e.g., 25% of 12 excess pounds, or 3 pounds) from the present lean body weight.

Norms for body fat are listed in Table 5.12. Athletes involved in sports where the body weight is supported, such as canoeing, kayaking, and swimming, tend to have higher body fat values than athletes involved in sports such as running, which are very anaerobic (sprinting) or very aerobic (marathoning).[44,45] An extensive listing of the relative body fat of male and female athletes from a variety of sports is given in Appendix A, Table 28.

It is important to recognize that every measurement method has defined sources of error. Researchers have estimated that the standard error of estimate (SEE) for percent body fat when using the underwater weighing technique (with residual volume measured accurately) is 2.7%.[1,3] Generalized equations using skinfolds add only about 1% to this measurement error.[3] In other words, if on the basis of the seven-site skinfold equation a person is calculated to have 15% body fat, two thirds of the time the actual percent body fat will range within ±4% of that estimated 15% (11–19% body fat).

TABLE 5.12 Body Fat Ranges for Ages 18 and Older

Classification	Male	Female
Unhealthy range (too low)	5% and below	8% and below
Acceptable range (lower end)	6–15%	9–23%
Acceptable range (higher end)	16–24%	24–31%
Unhealthy range (too high)	25% and above	32% and above

	Average Body Fat Ranges for Elite Athletes*	
	Males	**Females**
Endurance athletes	**4–15%**	**12–26%**
Long-distance runners	4–14%	12–20%
Swimmers	5–14%	14–26%
Cross-country skiers	7–14%	15–23%
Canoers/rowers	6–15%	14–24%
Athletes in sports that emphasize leanness	**4–10%**	**10–19%**
Wrestlers	4–10%	
Gymnasts	4–10%	10–19%
Body builders	4–10%	10–17%
Team/dual sport athletes	**7–21%**	**18–27%**
Basketball players	7–11%	18–27%
Baseball players	11–15%	
Football players	9–21%	
Volleyball players	9–15%	20–25%
Tennis players	14–17%	19–22%
Power athletes	**5–20%**	**17–30%**
Shot-putters/discus throwers	15–20%	23–30%
Weight lifters	8–16%	
Sprinters	5–17%	17–21%

*Body fat ranges represent the average for national and international class athletes for a particular sport but do not encompass extreme values sometimes measured.

Sources: Lohman TG. *Advances in Body Composition Assessment: Current Issues in Exercise Science,* Monograph Number 3. Champaign, IL: Human Kinetics, 1992. Wilmore JH. Design issues and alternatives in assessing physical fitness among apparently healthy adults in a health examination survey of the general population. In National Center for Health Statistics, Drury TF (ed.). *Assessing Physical Fitness and Physical Activity in Population-Based Surveys.* DHHS Pub. No. (PHS) 89-1253. Public Health Service. Washington, DC: U.S. Government Printing Office, 1989.

UNDERWATER WEIGHING

The most widely used laboratory procedure for measuring body density is *underwater weighing.* In this procedure, whole-body density is calculated from body volume, according to Archimedes' principle of displacement, which states that an object submerged in water is buoyed up by the weight of the water displaced.[1,3]

The protocol requires weighing a person underwater, as well as on land. The densities of bone and muscle tissues are higher than that of water, while fat is less dense than water. Thus a person with more bone and muscle mass will weigh more in water and thus have a higher body density and lower percentage of body fat.

By using a standard formula, the volume of the body is calculated and the individual's body density determined. From body density, percent body fat can be calculated using the formulas described in Table 5.2.

To determine body density from underwater weighing, the following equation has been developed:[1,3]

$$\text{Body density} = \frac{Wa}{(Wa - Ww)/Dw - (RV + 100 \text{ ml})}$$

(Wa = body weight out of water; Ww = in water; Dw = density of water; RV = volume. 100 ml is the estimated air volume of the gastrointestinal tract.)

Equipment

The equipment is simple and relatively inexpensive (see Figure 5.33). In some new systems, the chair seat rests on load cells that are directly connected to a computer for instant analysis and feedback (but these systems are expensive and are no more accurate when used by experienced technicians). The scale and chair can be suspended from a diving board or an overhead beam into a pool, small tank, or hot tub that is 4–5 feet deep. The water should be warm enough to be comfortable (85–92°F) and undisturbed by wind or the motions of other people during the time of the test. The water should be filtered and chlorinated. Use a 9-kilogram autopsy scale with 15–25 gram divisions.

The chair can be constructed of ¾- to 1-inch plastic pipe, which can be cut and assembled easily. The direct cost is only about $30 in materials (the plastic pipe and glue). Figure 5.33 gives an example of one type of underwater weighing chair. A simple cradle can also be used.[1]

The back height of the chair in Figure 5.33 is 24 inches, the width 32 inches. Other joints and dimensions need not be precise and can be estimated from the figure. It is important that the chair be assembled so that the person being weighed can sit underwater with legs slightly bent and the water at shoulder level. Very small or large people will have to adapt their sitting position.

Holes should be drilled in the plastic pipe to avoid air entrapment. The chair should be weighed down with skin-diving weights or barbell weights to ensure that the weight of the chair underwater (tare weight) is at least 3 kg for normal-weight people being weighed and 4–6 kg for obese people.

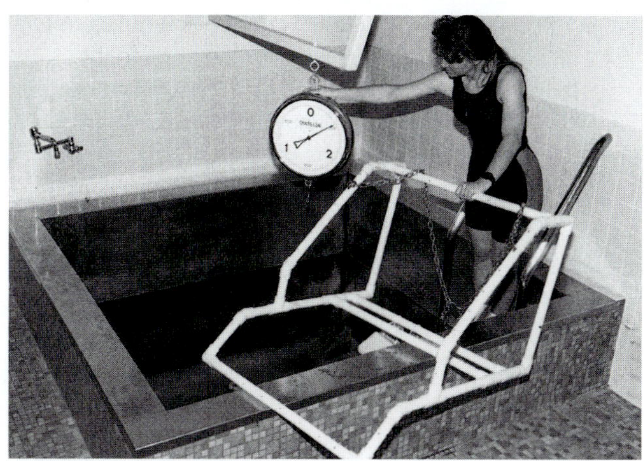

Figure 5.33 Equipment for underwater weighing includes a tank of sufficient size and shape for total human submersion, an accurate scale for measuring weight with 15–25 gram divisions, a method of measuring water temperature so that water density can be corrected, and a chair that has been weighted to prevent flotation.

Procedures

1. *Obtain basic data* (name, date, age, sex, height). The form in Figure 5.34 can be used to record these data.

Body Composition Worksheet

Name____________________ Date__________

Age________ Sex________ Height (shoes off)__________

SKINFOLDS (mm)

Male		Female	
________	Chest	Suprailiac	________
________	Abdominal	Midaxillary	________
________	Thigh	Subscapular	________
________	TOTAL		________

HYDROSTATIC MEASUREMENTS

______ Body weight in air (pounds)
______ Net body weight in water (kg) (subtract tare from gross weight)
    ______ Gross weight in water (kg)
    ______ Tare weight (weight of appartus – kg)
______ H_2O density (see norms) ______ ______ ______
______ Residual volume (L) ______ ______ ______
______ (use equation or measure directly) (take 4–6 determinations until steady)

CALCULATIONS

______ Body fat % = (495/density) – 450

$$\text{Density} = \text{dry wt.}/\left[\left(\frac{\text{dry wt.} - \text{net underwater wt.}}{\text{Density water}}\right) - (\text{RV} + 100\text{ml})\right]$$

______ Fat weight (pounds) (dry body weight × fat %)
______ Lean body weight (pounds) (dry body weight – fat weight)
______ Fat % classification (see norms)

RECOMMENDATIONS

______ Estimated ideal weight weight [LBW/(100% – desired fat %)]
    ________ ________ ________
______ Pounds of fat you need to lose
______ Pounds of lean body weight you need to gain

Figure 5.34 Body composition worksheet.

The person being weighed should be wearing only a swimsuit and have an opportunity to go to the bathroom before being weighed. The person should not eat or smoke for 2–3 hours before the test and should try to avoid foods that can cause excessive amounts of intestinal gas. Care should be taken to expel any trapped air from the swimsuit.

2. *Take skinfolds.* Because some people have difficulty in blowing out all the air from their lungs underwater, it is a good idea to have skinfold data to help verify the results.
3. *Give basic instructions.*
   a. *How to sit in chair.* Sit in the chair with seat on the back bars, feet on the forward bar in the corners, legs slightly bent, hands gripping the lower side bars (see Figure 5.35).
   b. *Underwater position.* After making a full exhalation of air from the lungs, slowly lean forward until the head is underwater. Continue to press all air out of the lungs. When all air is out, count for 5–7 seconds, then come up (see Figure 5.36). The test will be repeated 4–10 times until a consistent reading is obtained.

   Note: When the person goes under water, keep one hand on the scale to steady it. Try to keep the water as calm as possible to get a good reading on the scale needle. The person being weighed should be as still as possible underwater during the 5–7 second count.
4. *Record the consistent underwater weight.* The underwater weight should be recorded as the "gross weight in water (kg)," and then the tare weight (weight of chair apparatus alone) should be subtracted from it to obtain the "net body weight in water." It is important to be exact in determining the gross underwater weight. A 100-gram error can result in close to a 1% body fat error.

   Many testers have trouble with the oscillations of the scale needle. To minimize this, use a small tank, keep the water as calm as possible, and teach the person being tested to move as slowly as possible. Testers should practice reading the scale with known weights attached.
5. *Determine the water density.* Measure the temperature of the water, and then consult Table 5.13 for the water density.
6. *Determine the residual volume.* The residual volume is the amount of air left in the lungs after a maximal expiration. The residual volume can be measured or estimated. Measurement of residual volume can be conducted using nitrogen washout, helium dilution, or oxygen dilution. Measurement of residual volume can take place while the person being weighed is inside or outside the tank.[1–3,46–48] When

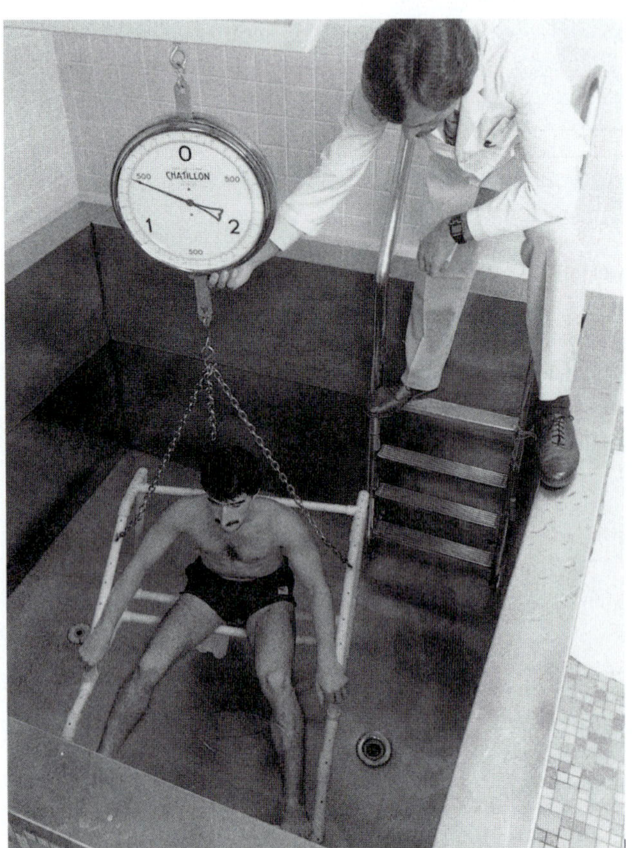

Figure 5.35 The position of the person being weighed, before underwater weighing.

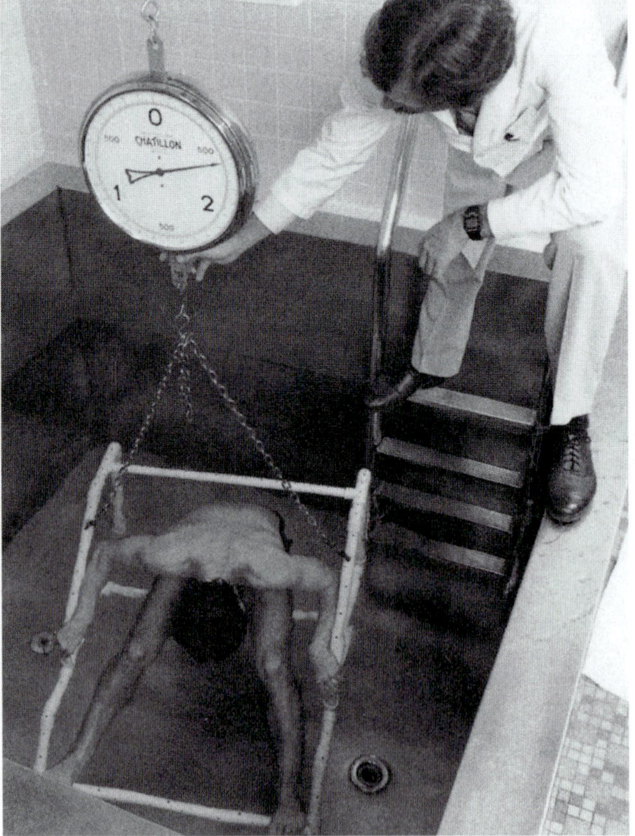

Figure 5.36 The position of the person being weighed, during underwater weighing.

TABLE 5.13 Density of Water at Different Temperatures

Water Temp (°C)	Density H_2O	Water Temp (°C)	Density H_2O
23.0	0.9975412	31.0	0.9953450
24.0	0.9972994	32.0	0.9950302
25.0	0.9970480	33.0	0.994734
26.0	0.9967870	34.0	0.9947071
27.0	0.9965166	35.0	0.9940359
28.0	0.9962371	36.0	0.9936883
29.0	0.9959486	37.0	0.9933328
30.0	0.9956511		

Source: Handbook of Chemistry and Physics, 86th edition, © 2005. Reprinted by permission of Routledge/Taylor & Francis, LLC.

possible, it is desirable to measure residual volume when the subject is in the tank, but this is not always practical with some modern automated equipment.

Whenever possible, residual volume should be measured directly. When residual volume is estimated, hydrostatically determined percent body fat is no more accurate than when measured with skinfolds because of the large amount of error in residual volume estimation formulas.[46]

When necessary, the following formulas can be used to estimate residual volume (RV) in liters:[49]

Males

$$RV = (0.017 \times \text{age in years}) + (0.06858 \times \text{height in inches}) - 3.447$$

Females

$$RV = (0.009 \times \text{age in years}) + (0.08128 \times \text{height in inches}) - 3.9$$

7. *Calculate percent body fat.* Following is an example of how to use the formula:

$$\text{Body density} = \frac{\text{body weight}}{\text{body volume}}$$

$$\text{Body volume} = \left(\frac{\text{body wt kg} - \text{underwater wt kg}}{\text{density of } H_2O}\right) - (\text{RV} + 100 \text{ ml})$$

$$\text{Relative fat\%} = \left(\frac{495}{\text{density}}\right) - 450$$

$$\text{Fat weight} = \text{body weight} \times \text{relative fat percent}$$

$$\text{Lean weight} = \text{body weight} - \text{fat weight}$$

$$\text{Ideal weight} = \frac{\text{present lean body weight}}{(100\% - \text{desired fat\%})}$$

Example: Male, 18 years of age, weighs 180 lb (81.8 kg), has a net underwater weight of 3.8 kg. Estimated RV is 1.660 (adding 100 ml for gastrointestinal trapped = 1.760), based on his height of 70 inches, age, and sex. The density of the water is 0.995678 based on a water temperature of 30°C.

$$\text{Body volume} = \left(\frac{81.8 - 3.8}{0.995678}\right) - 1.760 = 76.579$$

$$\text{Body density} = \frac{81.8}{76.579} = 1.0682$$

$$\text{Relative fat\%}^* = \left(\frac{495}{1.0682}\right) - 450 = 13.4\%$$

$$\text{Fat weight} = (180 \text{ lb} \times 0.134) = 24.1 \text{ lb}$$

$$\text{Lean body weight} = 180 - 24.1 = 155.9$$

Ideal weight if the person wants to get to 10% body fat (often for athletic reasons)

$$= \frac{155.9}{(100\% - 10\%)} = \frac{155.9}{0.9}$$

$$= 173.2 \text{ lb} \quad (\text{needs to lose 9 lb fat})$$

BIOELECTRICAL IMPEDANCE

Many publications are available for evaluating the effectiveness of bioelectrical impedance analysis (BIA) (impedance plethysmography).[1–3,50–65] BIA was developed in the 1960s and has emerged as one of the most popular methods for estimating relative body fat. A harmless 50-kHz current (800 microamps maximum) is generated and passed through the person being measured (see Figure 5.37). The measurement of electrical impedance is detected as the resistance to electrical current. Electrical impedance is greatest in fat tissue (14–22% water) because the conductive pathway is directly related to the percentage of water (which is greatest in the fat-free tissue, averaging 73%).

The total body water can be detected, therefore, as shifts in total body impedance. Total body water is accurately measured using bioelectrical impedance analysis from the following equation:[3]

Total body water (kg) =

$$0.593 \times \left(\frac{\text{height, cm}^2}{\text{whole} - \text{body resistance, ohm}}\right) + (0.065 \times \text{body weight, kg})$$

For example, a person weighing 70 kg and standing 170 cm tall, with a 470-ohm resistance (measured through bioelectrical impedance) would have a total body water of 41.0 kg or 58.6% of total body weight.

There is a wide variety of BIA equations available for predicting fat-free mass and percent body fat. Table 5.14 summarizes several of them that have been developed for specific population groups.[1] In general, it is best not to use the fat-free mass and percent body fat estimates obtained

*This is the Siri equation, which applies only to white male and female adults. See Table 5.2 to choose the appropriate formula for other individuals.

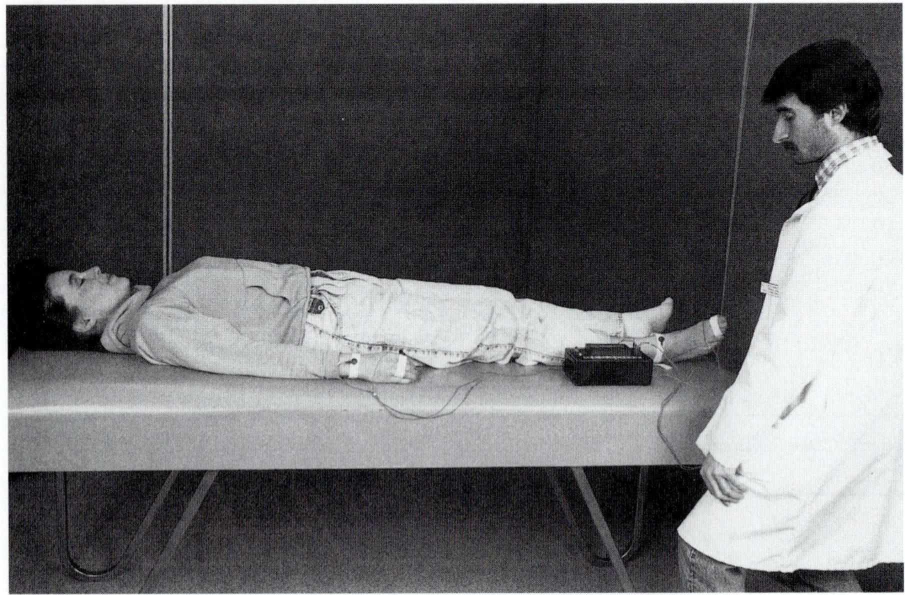

Figure 5.37 Bioelectrical impedance procedures are relatively simple. The person lies on a table with limbs not touching his or her body. Electrodes are placed on the right hand and right foot, and a harmless 50-kHz current (800 microamps maximum) is passed through him or her. The measurement of electrical conductance (or impedance) is detected as the resistance to electrical current.

TABLE 5.14 BIA Prediction Equations for Specific Populations

Population	Equation
White, boys and girls, 6–10 years	TBW (1)* = 0.593 (HT^2/R) + 0.065 (BW) + 0.04
White, boys and girls, 10–19 years	FFM (kg) = 0.61 (HT^2/R) + 0.25 (BW) + 1.31
Women, 18–29 years	FFM (kg) = 0.4764 (HT^2/R) + 0.295 (BW) + 5.49
Women, 30–49 years	FFM (kg) = 0.493 (HT^2/R) + 0.141 (BW) + 11.59
Women, 50–70 years	FFM (kg) = 0.474 (HT^2/R) + 0.180 (BW) + 7.3
Women, 65–94 years	FFM (kg) = 0.28 (HT^2/R) + 0.27 (BW) + 0.31 (thigh C) − 1.732
Men, 18–29 years	FFM (kg) = 0.485 (HT^2) + 0.338 (BW) + 5.32
Men, 17–62 years, <20% body fat	FFM (kg) = 0.00066360 (HT^2/R) + 0.02117 (R) + 0.62854 (BW) − 0.12380 (age) + 9.33285
Men, 17–62 years, ≥20% body fat	FFM (kg) = 0.00088580 (HT^2) + 0.2999 (R) + 0.42688 (BW) − 0.07002 (age) + 14.52435
Men, 50–70 years	FFM (kg) = 0.600 (HT^2/R) + 0.186 (BW) + 0.226 (X_c) - 10.9
Men, 65–94 years	FFM (kg) = 0.28 (HT^2/R) + 0.27 (BW) + 0.31 (thigh C) − 2.768

*To convert TBW to FFM, use the following age–gender hydration constants:

Boys		*Girls*
5–6 years FFM (kg) = TBW/0.77		5–6 years FFM (kg) = TBW/0.78
7–8 years FFM (kg) =TBW/0.768		7–8 years FFM (kg) = TBW/0.776
9–10 years FFM (kg) = TBW/0.762		9–10 years FFM (kg) = TBW/0.77

Note: FFM = fat-free mass; TBW = total body weight (kg); BW = body weight (kg); HT = height (cm); R = resistance (ohms); X_c = reactance; thigh C = thigh circumference (cm).

Source: Data from: Heyward VH, Stolarczyk LM. *Applied Body Composition Assessment.* Champaign, IL: Human Kinetics, 1996.

directly from the BIA analyzer unless the equations are known to apply directly to the subjects being measured.[1]

There are several sources of measurement error with the BIA method, which need to be controlled as much as possible to improve accuracy and reliability:[1,3,57]

> *Instrumentation.* BIA analyzers differ greatly from one company to another and can be a source of substantial error. To control for this error, the same instrument should be used when monitoring body composition changes in clients (and research subjects) over time.
>
> *Subject and environmental factors.* The client's state of hydration can greatly affect the BIA process. Factors such as eating, drinking, voiding of fluids, and exercising can affect hydration state and therefore introduce error. Cool, ambient temperatures cause a drop in skin temperature that results in an underestimation of fat-free mass. Client and environmental guidelines prior to BIA measurements include the following:
>
> 1. No eating or drinking within 4 hours of the test
> 2. No exercise within 12 hours of the test
> 3. Urinate within 30 minutes of the test

4. No alcohol consumption within 48 hours of the test
5. No diuretic medications within 7 days of the test
6. No testing of female clients who perceive they are retaining water during that stage of their menstrual cycle
7. BIA measurements made in a room with normal ambient temperature

Technician skill. The BIA technician should ensure that the client is lying in a supine position with arms and legs comfortably apart, at about a 45-degree angle to each other (see Figure 5.37). BIA measures are taken on the right side of the body. Electrodes need to be correctly positioned at the wrist and ankle, according to manufacturer guidelines. The sensor (proximal) electrodes should be placed on the dorsal surface of the wrist so that the upper border of the electrode bisects the head of the ulna and placed on the dorsal surface of the ankle so that the upper border of the electrode bisects the medial and lateral malleoli. The source (distal) electrodes should be placed at the base of the second or third metacarpal–phalangeal joints of the hand and foot. There should be at least 5 centimeters between the proximal and distal electrodes. A new leg-to-leg BIA system, combined with a digital scale that employs stainless-steel pressure-contact foot-pad electrodes for standing impedance and body weight measurements, has been developed by the Tanita Corporation (see Figure 5.38).[58–61] This system has been found to perform as well as the conventional arm-to-leg gel-electrode BIA system but is much quicker and easier to use. A hand-held, arm-to-arm bioimpedance analyzer has also been shown to be valid in estimating body composition (Omron Body Logic Body Fat Analyzer, Omron Healthcare, Vernon Hills, IL).[65]

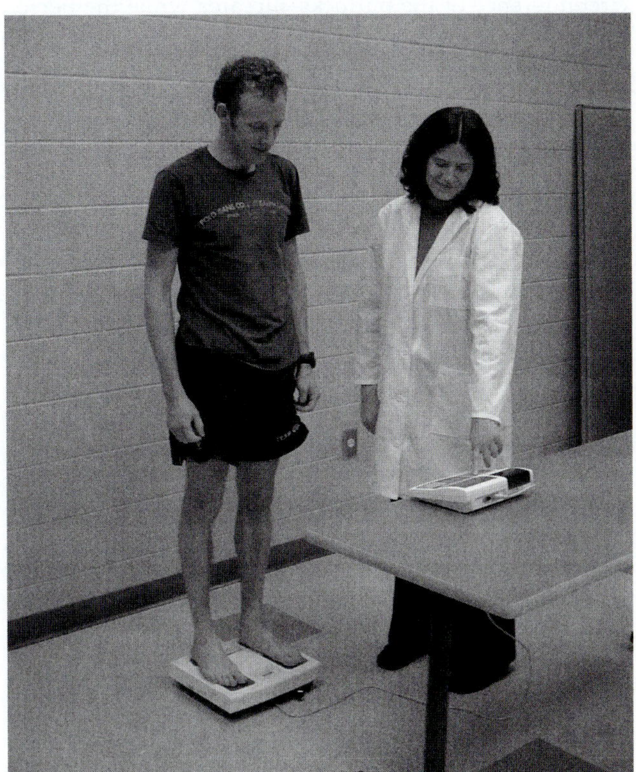

Figure 5.38 The Tanita Corporation has developed a BIA system using stainless-steel pressure-contact foot-pad electrodes.

When the appropriate BIA equation is used and the sources of measurement error are controlled, estimation of fat-free mass and relative body fat through the BIA method has been found to have about the same accuracy as the skinfold method. The BIA method, however, may be more preferable in some settings than the skinfold method because it does not require a high degree of technician skill, and it is more comfortable and less intrusive. There is still debate over whether BIA accurately predicts changes in body composition during a weight-loss program.[59,61–64] Published studies are mixed, with some supporting the accuracy of BIA in detecting fat-free mass and body composition changes, while others claim there is substantial over- or underestimation when compared to the underwater weighing method.

NEAR-INFRARED LIGHT INTERACTANCE

Near-infrared (NIR) light interactance has been used by the USDA since the 1960s to measure the protein, fat, and water content of agricultural products.[1] In 1984, researchers first applied this technology to study human body composition. During the late 1980s, a commercial NIR analyzer was developed (the FUTREX-5000) and marketed as a fast, accurate, and easy method for analyzing human body composition.

The FUTREX-5000 emits near-infrared light at two frequencies (938 nm and 948 nm) into the biceps area of the dominant arm. At these frequencies, body fat absorbs the light, while the lean body mass reflects the light. A light wand measures the amount of light emitted and reflected back, providing an estimate of the distribution of body fat and fat-free mass in the biceps area. FUTREX Inc. claims that research has shown that taking measurements of other anatomical sites does not significantly improve the accuracy of the estimation of relative body fat.

There are several advantages in using the FUTREX-5000 over other methods of estimating body fat percentage: fasting is not required, there is no need for disrobing, measurements can be made before or after exercise, there is no need for voiding, and women can take measurements during any day of the menstrual cycle.

However, numerous researchers have reported unacceptable prediction errors (SEE = 3.7–6.3% body fat).[1–3,66–68] The manufacturer's equation—which incorporates body weight, height, gender, exercise level, and optical density measurements—has been found to systematically underestimate body fat percentage by as much as 2–10% with the underestimation especially apparent with obese clients. At this time, most experts recommend that more research is needed to substantiate the validity, accuracy, and applicability of the NIR method for body composition assessment.[1–3]

TOPOGRAPHY OF THE HUMAN BODY

The male *android* (or apple shape) type of obesity is characterized by a predominance of body fat in the upper half of the body. In contrast, the female *gynoid* (or pear shape) form of obesity is characterized by excess body fat in the lower half of the body, especially the hips, buttocks, and thighs (see Figure 5.39). The third type of obesity is the intermediate form, characterized by both upper- and lower-body fat predominance.

The male type of obesity, which can occur in both genders, is associated with many of the health problems of obesity, including hypertension, high serum cholesterol levels, cardiovascular disease, and diabetes.[69]

Many different methods have been used to estimate android obesity, including the waist-to-hip circumference ratio, various skinfold ratios (e.g., subscapular-to-triceps ratio and trunk-to-peripheral skinfold ratios), and sophisticated imaging techniques such as computed tomography (CT) or DEXA, or magnetic resonance imaging (MRI).[3] These imaging techniques (see the Sports Medicine Insight at end of the chapter) allow a precise measurement of the amount of deep abdominal or visceral fat, versus subcutaneous fat.

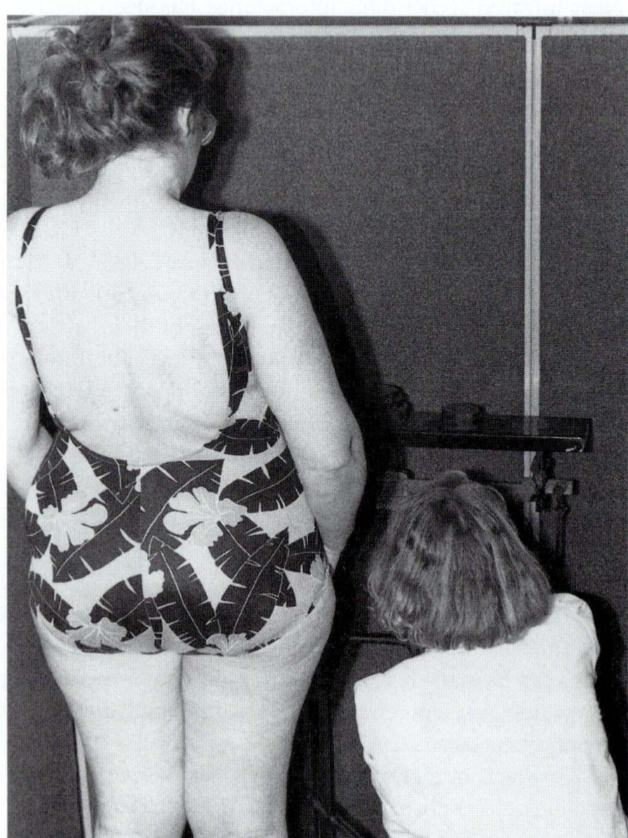

Figure 5.39 This subject has gynoid obesity, characterized by excess body fat in the lower half of the body.

It is the visceral fat that appears to be most strongly related to various negative health consequences; these cells release and take in fat more readily than other cells (e.g., fat cells in the gluteal and femoral regions), which leads to increased risk of disease. Abdominal fat cells release their fatty acids straight to the liver, which appears to be a factor in the increased risk of metabolic disorders.

Some researchers have found that the *ratio of waist-to-hip circumference* (WHR) is a simple and convenient method of determining the type of obesity present. Circumferences should be measured while wearing only nonrestrictive briefs or underwear, or a light smock over the underwear.

Waist or abdominal circumference is defined as the smallest waist circumference below the rib cage and above the umbilicus, while standing with abdominal muscles relaxed (not pulled in).[26] (See Figure 5.40.) The measurer faces the person being measured and places an inelastic tape in a horizontal plane, at the level of the natural waist (the narrowest part of the torso, as seen from the rear). If there appears to be no "smallest" area around the waist, the measurement should be made at the level of the navel.

Hip or gluteal circumference is defined as the largest circumference of the buttocks–hip area while the person is standing[26] (see Figure 5.40). The measurer should squat at the person's side to see where the buttocks circumference is the greatest, and should place an inelastic tape around the buttocks and hips in a horizontal plane at that point, without compressing the skin. An assistant is needed to help position the tape on the opposite side of the body.

The WHR is calculated by dividing the waist circumference by the hip circumference. For example, the idealized beauty contest female with a waist of 24 inches and hips of 36 inches would have a WHR of 0.67. In one study of 44,820 women who were members of TOPS Clubs, Inc. (Take Off Pounds Sensibly), the WHR varied between 0.39 and 1.45.[70] Women with higher WHRs were at greater risk for diabetes, hypertension, gallbladder disease, and oligomenorrhea (irregular menses).

More research is needed to establish precise norms for the WHR. At present, the risk of disease increases steeply when the WHR of men rises above 0.9, and of women, above 0.8.[69]

The WHR has been criticized for misclassifying people, due to factors unrelated to visceral fat, including frame size and gluteal muscle mass.[71,72] There is good evidence that the waist circumference alone correlates highly with visceral fat and is associated with increased risk of disease.[71,73] In 1998, the National Heart, Lung, and

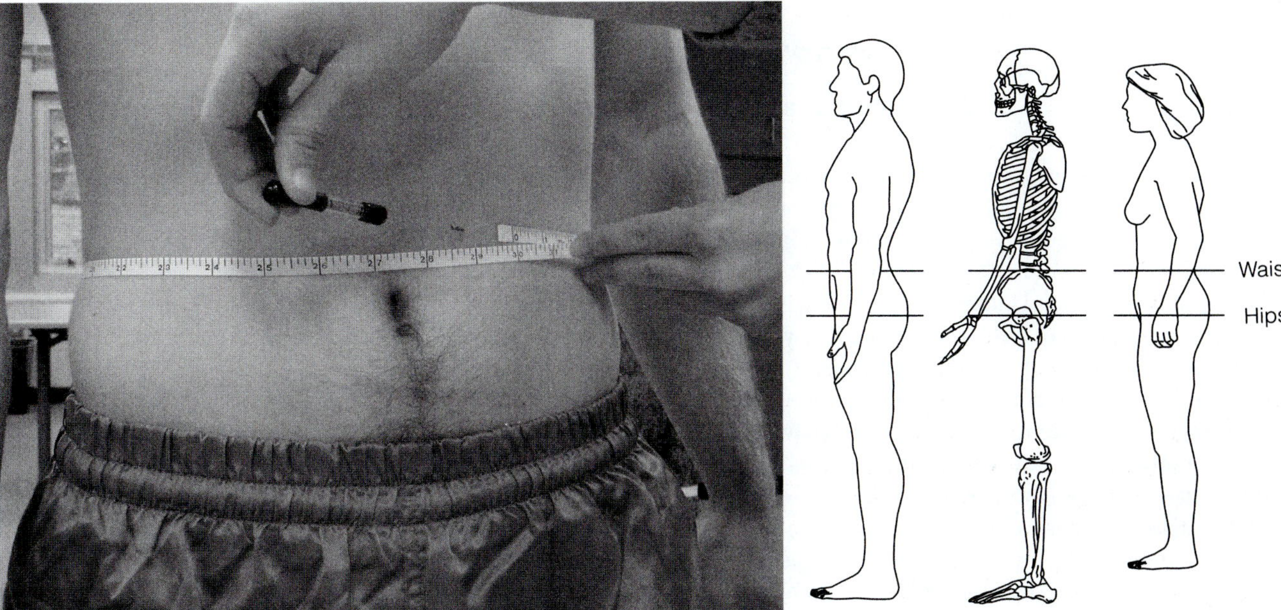

Figure 5.40 Location of the waist and hip circumferences.

Blood Institute (NHLBI) expert panel on obesity concluded that the waist circumference was more highly associated with disease risk than the WHR.[22] As summarized in Table 5.9, a high waist circumference (defined as >40 inches in men and >35 inches in women) combined with a BMI >25 predicts increased disease risk. At BMIs ≥35, waist circumference has little added predictive power of disease risk beyond that of BMI.

Various prediction equations have been developed to estimate body fat levels of military personnel.[1,74] These equations use various combinations of body weight, height, neck, abdomen, hip, thigh, arm, forearm, and wrist circumferences to predict either fat-free mass or percent body fat. However, these prediction equations have yielded large and unacceptable errors (SEE = 3.7–5.2% body fat).[1] Most experts do not recommend the use of these anthropometry equations in determining to dismiss personnel from the armed services when their body fat percentage exceeds military standards.[1,74]

One equation for predicting body composition of men from girth measurements has been developed and has a relatively low SEE of 3.6%.[75] The regression equation is as follows:

$$\begin{aligned}\%\ \text{body fat} &\\ &= -47.371817 + (0.57914807 \times \text{abdomen})\\ &\quad + (0.25189114 \times \text{hips}) + (0.21366088 \times \text{iliac})\\ &\quad - (0.35595404 \times \text{weight kg})\end{aligned}$$

The abdomen and hip circumferences were described earlier in this section. The iliac circumference is taken between the abdomen and hip circumference levels, at the iliac crest.

Table 5.15 presents a comparison of various methods of determining body composition.

TABLE 5.15 Comparison among Body Composition Methods: Cost, Ease of Use, and Accuracy in Estimating Body Fat

Method	Cost	Ease of Use	Accuracy
Quetelet index	Low	Easy	Low
Three- to seven-site skinfold tests	Low	Moderate	Moderate
Hydrostatic weighing	Moderate	Difficult	High
Bioelectrical impedance	Moderate	Easy	Moderate
TOBEC (total body electrical conductivity)	Very high	Easy	High
DEXA	High	Easy	High
Computed tomography	Very high	Difficult	Moderate
Near-infrared light interactance	Moderate	Easy	Moderate
Magnetic resonance imaging	Very high	Difficult	Moderate

Sources: See References 1–3.

SPORTS MEDICINE INSIGHT

Other Methods of Determining Body Composition

This chapter has reviewed some of the more practical and standard methods for determining body composition. Underwater weighing requires relatively expensive equipment and direct measurement of residual volume for optimum accuracy. Underwater weighing is impractical for some groups of individuals including young children, the elderly, and diseased patients. In contrast, Quetelet's index is a simple and practical measurement of degree of overweight, but it is insensitive to individuals with low or high amounts of muscle and bone. Skinfold measurements can give an accurate assessment of body fat levels when conducted by experienced health professionals. Bioelectrical impedance analysis and near-infrared interactance (FUTREX-5000) are highly convenient methods but have limitations for certain types of individuals. For regional fat distribution, calculations using waist and hip circumferences are useful, but they do not accurately assess the deep abdominal fat.

Table 5.16 summarizes the relative costs, ease of use, and accuracy of these and other techniques. This section reviews several of the newer and more promising methods for assessing body fat.

DEXA

The advent of dual-energy x-ray absorptiometry (DEXA) in 1987 has created much excitement among body composition researchers because this method allows simultaneous measurement of bone mineral, fat, and nonbone lean tissue.[1–3,76–82] DEXA is safe (low radiation dose) and quick (6–10 minutes), requires virtually no cooperation from the subject, and makes study of the elderly, young, and diseased much easier than with other methods (see Figure 5.41).

Manufacturers of DEXA machines have designed software that allows personnel with minimal training to operate the scanners. Most studies have concluded that DEXA is a precise method and correlates highly with results from underwater weighing or multicomponent models.[31,76–82]

DEXA uses a stable x-ray generator and two energy levels as the radiation source. A series of transverse scans are made of the subject, from head to toe, at 1-cm intervals, with bone mineral and soft tissue composition determined from the differential attenuation of the two energy photon beams. After passing through the subject, the attenuated beam is detected by a sodium-iodide detector. DEXA is based on a three-component model of composition (bone, fat, and lean soft tissue) and can therefore provide accurate assessments of fat and lean tissue in individuals with below- and above-average bone mineral.

DEXA does have several limitations that preclude its use as a criterion in body fat comparison studies. The DEXA method is dependent on geometric models and the assumption of constant hydration in fat-free soft tissues.[31] Severely obese individuals cannot be tested with DEXA. DEXA machines do not always give

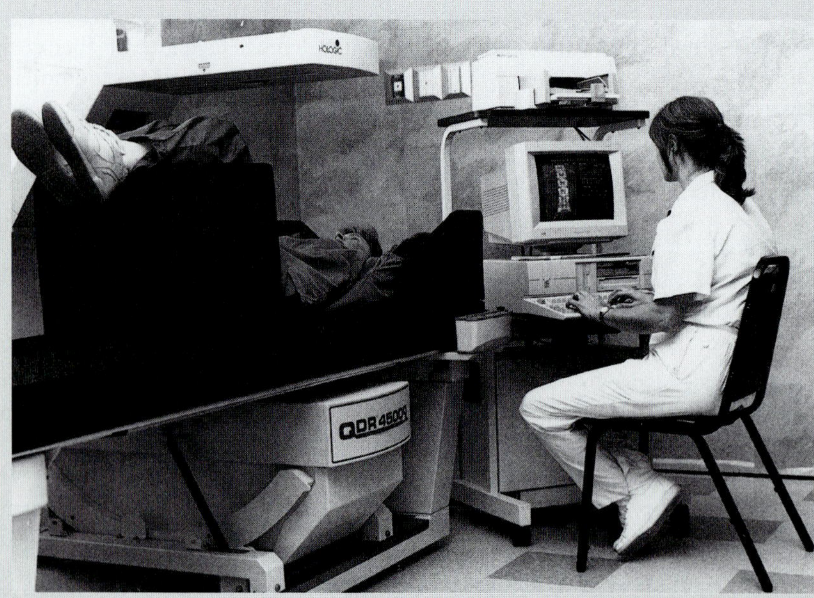

Figure 5.41 Originally developed for assessing bone mineral, recent technology has enabled estimates of fat and lean tissue via DEXA.

(continued)

SPORTS MEDICINE INSIGHT *(continued)*

Other Methods of Determining Body Composition

the same results.[81,82] Further research is needed to refine the equations used in the DEXA machines using data from four- to six-compartment body composition models.[31]

MAGNETIC RESONANCE IMAGING (MRI)

The accurate determination of total body fat, both internal and subcutaneous, is an important health issue. Internal fat, in particular, visceral fat, is a critical factor in disease development, especially diabetes mellitus, hypertension, and coronary heart disease. Computed tomography provides accurate measurements of internal and subcutaneous fat deposits, but a fundamental drawback of the method is exposure to ionizing radiation, making whole body fat measurements, especially for serial studies, impractical. MRI is an alternative technique for measurement of body fat deposits and has been validated in phantoms, animals, and human cadavers.[83–87] For a simple but accurate determination of the mass of abdominal adipose tissue, one MRI slice at the level between the second and third lumbar vertebrae gives a high and consistent predictive value for abdominal fat.

In MRI, the hydrogen nuclei of water and lipid molecules are excited by electromagnetic radiation in the presence of a magnetic field, resulting in a detectable signal, which is measured. The amount of water and lipid, and their freedom of motion, define the signal size, permitting discrimination between these tissues.

Subjects lie in the magnet, with arms placed above the head. For the entire body, transverse slices (10 mm thickness) are acquired every 50 mm, from head to toe. Computers outline edges of the body and areas of adipose and nonfatty tissues, and calculate volumes. MRI uses no ionizing radiation and is therefore safe for all types of individuals.

High-quality images of the body tissues are provided, allowing study of the amount and distribution of fat. MRI is relatively rapid (about 30 minutes), and subjects need only lie still. Drawbacks of the method are its restricted availability and high cost. Its greatest usefulness may be for measurement of visceral fat distribution.

TOTAL BODY ELECTRICAL CONDUCTIVITY (TOBEC)

Lean tissues conduct electricity much better than fat does. TOBEC operates on the principle that an object placed in an electromagnetic field will perturb the field, and the degree of perturbation depends on the quantity of conducting material (primarily electrolytes in lean body mass). Since 1971, the lean tissues of farm animals have been measured by putting them in a box that emits electrical impulses and measures responses.

The TOBEC system for human use consists of a large solenoid coil into which the person being measured is slid on a stretcher. The coil (driven by a 5-MHz radio frequency current) induces a current within the person's body in proportion to the mass of the conductive tissues. The instrument measures 10 total body conductivity readings in about 10 seconds. Studies show a very high correlation with hydrostatic weighing ($r = .93$).[88–90] TOBEC has also been found to be very sensitive to small changes in lean body mass and total body water. The major limitation of this technique is the high cost of the equipment.

COMPUTED TOMOGRAPHY (CT)

With this method, a computed tomography (CT) scanner is used to produce a cross-sectional image of the distribution of x-ray transmission. The person being measured is placed next to an x-ray tube, which directs a collimated beam of x-ray photons toward a scintillation detector.

Computed tomography can readily distinguish adipose tissue from adjacent skin, muscles, bones, vascular structures, and intra-abdominal and pelvic organs because fat transmits poorly. The cross-sectional CT images can be obtained at any level within the body. Computed tomography can thus noninvasively quantify body fat distribution at various sites—particularly useful is CT's ability to give a ratio of intra-abdominal to extra-abdominal fat.[91–94] The potential for using CT in assessing body composition is limited by problems of radiation exposure, high cost, and low availability.

AIR DISPLACEMENT PLETHYSMOGRAPHY

A new air displacement plethysmograph, referred to as the BOD POD® Body Composition System (Life Measurement, Inc., Concord, CA) has been developed to measure human body composition.[95–102] (see Figure 5.42). The system determines body volume through an air-displacement method. A volume-perturbing element (movable diaphragm) is mounted on the wall separating

(continued)

SPORTS MEDICINE INSIGHT *(continued)*

Other Methods of Determining Body Composition

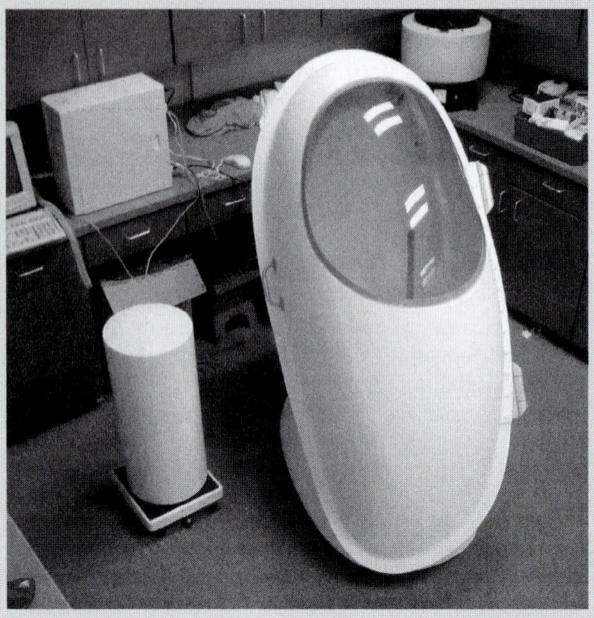

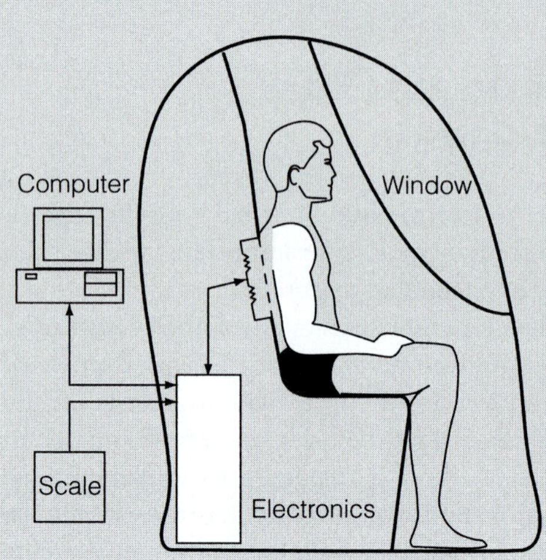

Figure 5.42 The air-displacement plethysmograph for measuring body composition.

the front and rear chambers of the dual-chambered plethysmograph. When this diaphragm is oscillated under computer control, it produces complementary volume perturbations in the two chambers (equal in magnitude but opposite in sign). These volume perturbations produce very small pressure fluctuations that are analyzed to yield chamber air volume. The process is repeated with the subject inside the chamber. Body volume must be corrected for thoracic gas volume (quantity of air in the lungs during normal tidal breathing), and this can be estimated or directly measured through the BOD POD. The BOD POD utilizes the inverse relationship between pressure *(P)* and volume *(V)* to determine body volume. Once body volume is determined, the principles of densitometry are used to determine body composition from body density (body = body mass/body volume). The BOB POD uses the same two-component model as underwater weighing, but is based on air displacement rather than water immersion. The majority of studies have shown that air-displacement plethysmography is an accurate and suitable alternative to underwater weighing, but with the same limitations of two-component compared to multicomponent models.[95–102]

This new method has several advantages over hydrostatic weighing, in that it is quick (about 5 minutes), relatively simple to operate, and can accommodate special populations such as the obese, the elderly, and the disabled. Limited demands are made on the subjects, and instructions are minimal. The BOD POD is mobile, so it can be moved from one location to another. Minimal training is needed to operate the BOD POD, due to the menu-driven software and the small number of tasks required to reliably and accurately operate the system.

SUMMARY

1. This chapter discussed the various methods of measuring obesity, starting with the least precise and progressing toward the more accurate (weight tables, body mass index, skinfolds, underwater weighing). The chapter ended with a brief discussion of some of the newer laboratory methods of evaluating body composition.
2. In general, when considering validity, reliability, economy, and good norms, skinfold tests are probably most practical and useful. With proper training and practice, testers can learn to assess body composition quickly and accurately. However, careful selection of specific anatomic sites and observance of rules for measuring are important.
3. Height–weight tables only provide a rough estimate of ideal weight. Frame size can be determined by measuring the width of the elbow. Use of the Quetelet index (kg/m^2) produces a higher correlation with actual body composition than does use of the height–weight tables.

4. Underwater weighing remains the laboratory standard, but the time, expense, and expertise needed is prohibitive for many clinical settings.
5. More research is needed to develop some of the newer techniques. Bioelectrical impedance is a convenient, safe, accurate, and rapid method of body composition analysis.
6. Fat distribution on the body has been shown to be an important predictor of the health consequences of obesity. A number of the researchers have found that the waist circumference is an accurate and convenient method for determining type of obesity.

Review Questions

A female client weighs 135 pounds, is 66 inches tall, and is measured to be 20% fat. Answer Questions 1 to 6 based on this information.

1. ***What is her fat weight?***

   A. 40 **B.** 50 **C.** 70 **D.** 27

2. ***What is her fat-free mass (lean body weight)?***

   A. 135 **B.** 108 **C.** 100 **D.** 162

3. ***If your client wants to reduce her body fat to 17% (for athletic reasons), what would her ideal weight be? (Assume fat-free mass stays the same.)***

   A. 100 **B.** 150 **C.** 120 **D.** 130 **E.** 135

4. ***What is her Quetelet index?***

   A. 21.8 **B.** 24.5 **C.** 22.3 **D.** 20.1 **E.** 28.9

5. ***How would you classify this client based on her Quetelet index?***

   A. Underweight **B.** Obese, class 1
   C. Normal **D.** Obese, class 2
   E. Obese, class 3

6. ***How would you classify this client based on body fat percent?***

   A. Unhealthy, too low
   B. Unhealthy, too high
   C. Acceptable range (lower end)
   D. Acceptable range (higher end)

7. ***If a male client has 7% body fat with a Quetelet index of 19 kg/m^2, he probably looks like***

   A. An elite distance runner
   B. A football linebacker
   C. An average college student
   D. A ballet dancer

8. ***Which body composition technique would provide the best information regarding body composition?***

   A. Height–weight tables
   B. Quetelet index
   C. Underwater weighing
   D. Seven-site skinfolds
   E. Bioelectrical impedance

9. ***Frame size is typically estimated by measuring the***

   A. Width of the elbow
   B. Circumference of the ankle
   C. Width of the hips
   D. Circumference of the wrist

10. ***When the waist circumference rises above a threshold of ____ in a woman, this is an indication of elevated disease risk.***

    A. 27 **B.** 35 **C.** 40 **D.** 30 **E.** 24

11. ***A Quetelet index below a threshold of ____ is considered underweight.***

    A. 13 **B.** 20 **C.** 18.5 **D.** 40 **E.** 25

12. ***The body composition of a male is considered to be at an unhealthy range, too low, when body fat percentage falls below a threshold of ____%.***

    A. 5 **B.** 12 **C.** 9 **D.** 16 **E.** 20

13. ***Which skinfold site is measured using a horizontal skinfold (Airlie Consensus Conference method)?***

    A. Thigh **B.** Abdomen
    C. Triceps **D.** Suprailiac
    E. Chest

14. ***The two-site skinfold test (triceps and medial calf/subscapular) is recommended especially for***

    A. Elderly adults **B.** Infants
    C. Middle-age adults **D.** Children/youths

15. ***The four-compartment model for body composition measurement is based on protein, bone mineral, fat, and ____.***

    A. Skeletal muscle **B.** Fat-free mass
    C. Skeleton **D.** Water
    E. Blood

16. *The athletic, muscular body build is called*

A. Mesomorphic
B. Endomorphic
C. Ectomorphic

17. *A stadiometer is used for measuring*

A. Weight B. Stature
C. Body composition D. Skinfolds
E. Frame size

18. *Which skinfold site is measured on an imaginary line coming down from the midaxillary line?*

A. Thigh B. Abdomen
C. Triceps D. Suprailiac
E. Chest

19. *What is the relative weight of a 30-year-old female who weighs 200 pounds, is 65 inches tall, and has a medium frame?*

A. 219 B. 178 C. 53.7 D. 1.06 E. 151

20. *Based on the textbook, how would you rank the woman in Question 19?*

A. Underweight B. Overweight
C. Mildly obese D. Moderately obese
E. Severely obese

Answer Questions 21–26 based on these measurements from your subject, Linda (use the nomogram from the textbook):

Age: 25
Weight: 160 pounds
Height: 65 inches
Frame size: medium (2.5 inches, elbow breadth)
Triceps skinfold: 30 mm
Suprailiac skinfold: 25 mm
Thigh skinfold: 45 mm

21. *What is her Quetelet index or body mass index?*

A. 27 B. 37 C. 21 D. 31 E. 25

22. *What is her body fat percent (to nearest whole number)?*

A. 30 B. 23 C. 25 D. 45 E. 35

23. *What is her fat weight?*

A. 35 B. 42 C. 56 D. 70 E. 50

24. *What is her fat-free mass or lean body weight?*

A. 104 B. 95 C. 125 D. 112 E. 123

25. *How would you classify Linda's fat percentage?*

A. Unhealthy range, too low
B. Acceptable range, lower end
C. Acceptable range, higher end
D. Unhealthy range, too high

26. *If Linda wants to have 22% body fat, what is her ideal weight?*

A. 145 B. 133 C. 138 D. 120 E. 153

27. *Which rule for taking skinfolds listed here is* **not** *correct?*

A. At least two measurements taken 15 seconds apart are recommended for each site.
B. The goal is to pull away the skinfold so that a fold with approximately parallel sides is formed.
C. The dial should be read 10 seconds after releasing the lever arm of the caliper.
D. Measurements should not be taken when the skin is hot or moist.

28. *The equation, [(495/body density) − 450], is used to determine*

A. Body mass index B. Relative weight
C. Percent body fat D. Ideal body weight

29. *To conduct the underwater weighing test to determine body density, which one of the following is* **not** *needed?*

A. Residual volume B. Tare weight
C. Dry land weight of subject D. Water density
E. Age of subject

30. *Fat-free mass is about ____% water.*

A. 40 B. 50 C. 73 D. 81 E. 90

31. *The ____ type of obesity is characterized by a predominance of body fat in the upper half of the body.*

A. Android B. Gynoid

32. *Total body mass expressed relative to total body volume equals*

A. Total body density B. Relative body fat
C. Fat-free mass D. Fat mass
E. Obesity

33. *Which body composition technique measures total body volume?*
A. Air displacement plethysmography
B. Underwater weighing
C. TOBEC
D. DEXA
E. MRI

Answers

1. D	**9.** A	**17.** B	**26.** B
2. B	**10.** B	**18.** D	**27.** C
3. D	**11.** C	**19.** E	**28.** C
4. A	**12.** A	**20.** D	**29.** E
5. C	**13.** B	**21.** A	**30.** C
6. C	**14.** D	**22.** E	**31.** A
7. A	**15.** D	**23.** C	**32.** A
8. C	**16.** A	**24.** A	**33.** A
		25. D	

REFERENCES

1. Heyward VH, Wagner DR. *Applied Body Composition Assessment.* Champaign, IL: Human Kinetics, 2004.
2. Heymsfield SB. *Human Body Composition.* Champaign, IL: Human Kinetics, 2005.
3. Lohman TG. *Advances in Body Composition Assessment: Current Issues in Exercise Science, Monograph Number 3.* Champaign, IL: Human Kinetics, 1992.
4. Brozek J, Grande F, Anderson IT, Kemp A. Densiometric analysis of body composition: Revision of some quantitative assumptions. *Ann New York Academy Sciences* 110:113–140, 1963.
5. Siri WE. Body composition from fluid spaces and density: Analysis of methods. In Brozek J, Henschel A (eds.). *Techniques for Measuring Body Composition.* Washington, DC: National Academy of Sciences, 1961.
6. Weigley ES. Average? Ideal? Desirable? A brief overview of height–weight tables in the United States. *J Am Diet Assoc* 84:417, 1984.
7. Robinette-Weiss N. The Metropolitan Height–Weight Tables: Perspectives for use. *J Am Diet Assoc* 84:1480–1481, 1984.
8. Abraham S. Height–weight tables: Their sources and development. *Clin Consult Nutr Support* 3:5-8, 1983. Reprinted in Shils ME, Young VR. *Modern Nutrition in Health and Disease.* Philadelphia: Lea & Febiger, 1988, pp. 1509–1513.
9. Simopoulos AP. Obesity and body weight standards. *Annu Rev Public Health* 7:481–492, 1986.
10. National Institutes of Health. Consensus development conference statement. Health implications of obesity. *Ann Intern Med* 103:981–1077, 1985.
11. Garrison RJ. Cigarette smoking as a confounder of the relationship between relative weight and long term mortality. *JAMA* 249:2199–2203, 1983.
12. U.S. Department of Agriculture, U.S. Department of Health and Human Services. *Nutrition and Your Health: Dietary Guidelines for Americans* (3rd ed.). Washington, DC: U.S. Government Printing Office, 1990.
13. Willett WC, Stampfer M, Manson J, Van Itallie T. New weight guidelines for Americans: Justified or injudicious? *Am J Clin Nutr* 53:1102–1103, 1991.
14. Marwick C. Obesity experts say less weight still best. *JAMA* 269:2617–2618, 1993.
15. U.S. Department of Agriculture, Agricultural Research Service, Dietary Guidelines Advisory Committee, 1995. *Report of the Dietary Guidelines Advisory Committee on the Dietary Guidelines for Americans, 1995, to the Secretary of Health and Human Services and the Secretary of Agriculture.* Washington, DC: Author, 1995.
16. Gordon CC, Chumlea WC, Roche AF. Stature, recumbent length, and weight. In Lohman TG, Roche AF, Martorell R (eds.). *Anthropometric Standardization Reference Manual.* Champaign, IL: Human Kinetics, 1988.
17. Frisancho AR. *Anthropometric Standards for the Assessment of Growth and Nutritional Status.* Ann Arbor: The University of Michigan Press, 1990.
18. Kuczmarski RJ, Ogden CL, Grummer-Strawn LM, et al. CDC growth charts: United States. *Advance Data from Vital and Health Statistics,* No. 314. Hyattsville, MD: National Center for Health Statistics, 2000. (See also http://www.cdc.gov/growthcharts.)
19. Himes JH, Frisancho RA. Estimating frame size. In Lohman TG, Roche AF, Martorell R (eds.). *Anthropometric Standardization Reference Manual.* Champaign, IL: Human Kinetics, 1988.
20. Gallagher D, Heymsfield SB, Heo M, Jebb SA, Murgatroyd PR, Sakamoto Y. Healthy percentage body fat ranges: An approach for developing guidelines based on body mass index. *Am J Clin Nutr* 72:694–701, 2000. (See also the "body fat lab" at Shape Up America!: www.shapeup.org.)
21. Ogden CL, Fryar CD, Carroll MD, Flegal KM. Mean body weight, height, and body mass index, United States 1960–2002. *Advance Data* 347:1–20, 2004. See also McDowell MA, Fryar CD, Hirsch R, Ogden CKL. Anthropometric reference data for children and adults: U.S. population, 1999–2002. *Advance Data* 36:1–32, 2005.
22. Expert Panel on the Identification, Evaluation, and Treatment of Overweight and Obesity in Adults. Executive Summary. *Arch Intern Med* 158:1855–1867, 1998.
23. Dietz WH, Bellizzi MC. Introduction: The use of body mass index to assess obesity in children. *Am J Clin Nutr* 70(suppl):123S–125S, 1999.
24. U.S. Department of Agriculture, U.S. Department of Health and Human Services. Nutrition and Your Health: Dietary Guidelines for Americans. Home and Garden Bulletin, No. 232 (5th ed.), 2000.
25. Jackson AS, Pollock ML. Practical assessment of body composition. *Phys Sportsmed* 13:76–90, 1985.
26. Lohman TG, Roche AF, Martorell R. *Anthropometric Standardization Reference Manual.* Champaign, IL: Human Kinetics, 1988.
27. Heyward VH. Practical body composition assessment for children, adults, and older adults. *Int J Sport Nutr* 8:285–307, 1998.
28. Wagner DR, Heyward VH. Techniques of body composition assessment: A review of laboratory and field methods. *Res Q Exerc Sport* 70:135–149, 1999.
29. Ellis KJ. Selected body composition methods can be used in field studies. *J Nutr* 131:1589S–1595S, 2001.

30. Heymsfield SB, Nunez C, Testolin C, Gallagher D. Anthropometry and methods of body composition measurement for research and field application in the elderly. *Eur J Clin Nutr* 54:S26–S32, 2000.
31. Wang ZM, Deurenberg P, Guo SS, Pietrobelli A, Wang J, Pierson RN, Heymsfield SB. Six-compartment body composition model: Inter-method comparison of total body fat measurement. *Int J Obesity* 22:329–337, 1998.
32. Cataldo D, Heyward VH. Pinch an inch: A comparison of several high-quality and plastic skinfold calipers. *ACSM's Health & Fitness Journal*, 4(3):12–16, May/June 2000.
33. American College of Sports Medicine. *ACSM's Guidelines for Graded Exercise Testing and Prescription* (6th ed.). Philadelphia: Lippincott Williams & Wilkins, 2000.
34. Public Health Service. Summary of findings from National Children and Youth Fitness Study. *JOPHER*, January 1985, pp. 44–90.
35. Ross JG, Pate RR, Delpy LA, Gold RS, Svilar M. New health-related fitness norms. *JOPERD*, November–December 1987, pp. 66–70.
36. Lohman TG. The use of skinfold to estimate body fatness on children and youth. *JOPERD*, November–December 1987, pp. 98–102.
37. Riley JH. A critique of skinfold tests from the public school level. *JOPERD*, October 1990, pp. 71–73.
38. Dezenberg CV, Nagy TR, Gower BA, Johnson R, Goran MI. Predicting body composition from anthropometry in pre-adolescent children. *Int J Obesity* 23:253–259, 1999.
39. Jackson AS, Pollock ML, Ward A. Generalized equations for predicting body density of women. *Med Sci Sport Exerc* 12:175–182, 1980.
40. Jackson AS, Pollock ML. Generalized equations for predicting body density of men. *Br J Nutr* 40:497–504, 1978.
41. Baun WB, Baun MR, Raven PB. A nomogram for the estimate of percent body fat from generalized equation. *Res Q Exerc Sport* 52:380–384, 1981.
42. Durnin JVGA, Womersley J. Body fat assessment from total body density and its estimation from skinfold thickness: Measurements on 481 men and women aged 16 to 72 years. *Br J Nutr* 32:77–97, 1974.
43. Lohman TG. Applicability of body composition techniques and constants for children and youth. *Ex Sport Sci Rev* 14:325–357, 1986.
44. Fleck SJ. Body composition of elite American athletes. *Am J Sports Med* 11:398, 1983.
45. Wilmore JH. Design issues and alternatives in assessing physical fitness among apparently healthy adults in a health examination survey of the general population. In National Center for Health Statistics, Drury TF (ed.). *Assessing Physical Fitness and Physical Activity in Population-Based Surveys*. DHHS Pub. No. (PHS) 89-1253. Public Health Service. Washington, DC: U.S. Government Printing Office, 1989.
46. Morrow JR, Jackson AS, Bradley PW, Hartung GH. Accuracy of measured and predicted residual lung volume on body density measurement. *Med Sci Sports Exerc* 18:647–652, 1986.
47. Van der Ploeg GE, Gunn SM, Withers RT, Modra AC, Crockett AJ. Comparison of two hydrodensitometric methods for estimating percent body fat. *J Appl Physiol* 88:1175–1180, 2000.
48. Nelson AG, Stuart DW, Fisher AG. The effect of hydrostatic weighing protocols on body density measurement. *Med Sci Sports Exerc* 17:246, 1985.
49. Goldman HI, Becklake MR. Respiratory function tests. *Am Rev Tuberc Pulm Dis* 79:457–467, 1959.
50. Lockner DW, Heyward VH, Griffin SE, Marques MB, Stolarczyk LM, Wagner DR. Cross-validation of modified fatness-specific bioelectrical impedance equations. *Int J Sport Nutr* 9:48–59, 1999.
51. Bumgartner RN, Ross R, Heymsfield SB. Does adipose tissue influence bioelectric impedance in obese men and women? *J Appl Physiol* 84:257–262, 1998.
52. Biaggi RR, Vollman MW, Nies MA, Brener CE, Flakoll PJ, Levenhagen DK, Sun M, Karabulut Z, Chen KY. Comparison of air-displacement plethysmography with hydrostatic weighing and bioelectrical impedance analysis for the assessment of body composition in healthy adults. *Am J Clin Nutr* 69:898–903, 1999.
53. Stolarczyk LM, Heyward VH, Van Loan MD, Hicks VL, Wilson WL, Reano LM. The fatness-specific bioelectrical impedance analysis equations of Segal et al: Are they generalizable and practical? *Am J Clin Nutr* 66:8–17, 1997.
54. Heymsfield SB, Wang ZM, Visser M, Gallagher D, Pierson RN. Techniques used in the measurement of body composition: An overview with emphasis on bioelectrical impedance analysis. *Am J Clin Nutr* 64(suppl):478S–484S, 1996.
55. Kyle UG, Bosaeus I, DeLorenzo AD, et al. Bioelectrical impedance analysis—Part I: Review of principles and methods. *Clin Nutr* 23:1226–1243, 2004.
56. Houtkooper LB, Lohman TG, Going SB, Howell WH. Why bioelectrical impedance analysis should be used for estimating adiposity. *Am J Clin Nutr* 64(suppl):436S–448S, 1996.
57. NIH. Bioelectrical impedance analysis in body composition measurement: National Institutes of Health Technology Assessment Conference Statement. *Am J Clin Nutr* 64(suppl):524S–532S, 1996.
58. Nunez C, Gallagher D, Visser M, Pi-Sunyer FX, Wang Z, Heymsfield SB: Bioimpedance analysis: Evaluation of leg-to-leg system based on pressure contact foot-pad electrodes. *Med Sci Sports Exerc* 29:524–531, 1997.
59. Utter AC, Nieman DC, Ward AN, Butterworth DE. Use of the leg-to-leg bioelectrical impedance method in assessing body-composition change in obese women. *Am J Clin Nutr* 69:603–607, 1999.
60. Tyrrell VJ, Richards G, Hofman P, Gillies GF, Robinson E, Cutfield WS. Foot-to-foot bioelectrical impedance analysis: A valuable tool for the measurement of body composition in children. *Int J Obes Relat Metab Disord* 25:273–278, 2001.
61. Powell LA, Nieman DC, Melby C, Cureton K, Schmidt D, Howley ET, Costello C, Hill JO, Mault JR, Alexander H, Stewart DJ. Assessment of body composition change in a community-based weight management program. *J Am Coll Nutr* 20:26–31, 2001.
62. Evans EM, Saunders MJ, Spano MA, Arngrimmson SA, Lewis RD, Cureton KJ. Body-composition changes with diet and exercise in obese women: A comparison of estimates from clinical methods and a 4-component model. *Am J Clin Nutr* 70:5–12, 1999.
63. Carella MJ, Rodgers CD, Anderson D, Gossain VV. Serial measurements of body composition in obese subjects during a very-low-energy diet (VLED) comparing bioelectrical impedance with hydrodensitometry. *Obes Res* 5:250–256, 1997.
64. Hendel HW, Gotfredsen A, Hojgaard L, Andersen T, Hilsted J. Change in fat-free mass assessed by bioelectrical impedance, total body potassium and dual x-ray absorptiometry during prolonged weight loss. *Scand J Clin Lab Invest* 56:671–679, 1996.
65. Gibson AL, Heyward VH, Mermier CM. Predictive accuracy of Omron® Body Logic Analyzer in estimating relative body fat in adults. *Int J Sport Nutr Exerc Metab* 10:216–227, 2000.
66. Heyward VH. Evaluation of body composition: Current issues. *Sports Med* 22:146–156, 1996.
67. McLean KP, Skinner JS. Validity of Futrex-5000 for body composition determination. *Med Sci Sports Exerc* 24:253–258, 1992.

68. Heyward VH, Cook KL, Hicks VL, et al. Predictive accuracy of three field methods for estimating relative body fatness of nonobese and obese women. *Int J Sport Nutr* 2:75–86, 1992.

69. Van Itallie TB. Topography of body fat: Relationship to risk of cardiovascular and other diseases. In Lohman TG, Roche AF, Martorell R (eds.). *Anthropometric Standardization Reference Manual.* Champaign, IL: Human Kinetics, 1988.

70. Rimm AA, Hartz AJ, Fischer ME. A weight shape index for assessing risk of disease in 44,820 women. *J Clin Epidemiol* 41:459–465, 1988.

71. Lemieux S, Prud'homme D, Bouchard C, Tremblay A, Despres J-P. A single threshold value of waist girth identifies normal-weight and overweight subjects with excess visceral adipose tissue. *Am J Clin Nutr* 64:685–693, 1996.

72. Taylor RW, Keil D, Gold EJ, Williams SM, Goulding A. Body mass index, waist girth, and waist-to-hip ratio as indexes of total and regional adiposity in women: Evaluation using receiver operating characteristic curves. *Am J Clin Nutr* 67:44–49, 1998.

73. Zhu S, Heymsfield SB, Toyoshima H, Wang Z, Pietrobelli, Heshka S. Race-ethnicity-specific waist circumference cutoffs for identifying cardiovascular disease risk factors. *Am J Clin Nutr* 81:409–415, 2005.

74. Bathalon GP, Hughes VA, Campbell WW, Fiatarone MA, Evans WJ. Military body fat standards and equations applied to middle-aged women. *Med Sci Sports Exerc* 27:1079–1085, 1995.

75. Tran ZV, Weltman A. Predicting body composition of men from girth measurements. *Human Biol* 60:167–175, 1988.

76. Houtkooper LB, Going SB, Sproul J, Blew RM, Lohman TG. Comparison of methods for assessing body-composition changes over 1 y in postmenopausal women. *Am J Clin Nutr* 72:401–406, 2000.

77. Salamone LM, Fuerst T, Visser M, Kern M, Lang T, Dockrell M, Cauley JA, Nevitt M, Tylavsky F, Lohman TG. Measurement of fat mass using DEXA: A validation study in elderly adults. *J Appl Physiol* 89:345–352, 2000.

78. Plank LD, Dual-energy x-ray absorptiometry and body composition. *Curr Opin Clin Nutr Metab Care* 8:305–309, 2005.

79. Van Loan MD. Is dual-energy x-ray absorptiometry ready for prime time in the clinical evaluation of body composition? *Am J Clin Nutr* 68:1155–1156, 1998.

80. Clasey JL, Hartman ML, Kanaley J, Wideman L, Teates CD, Bouchard C, Weltman A. Body composition by DEXA in older adults: Accuracy and influence of scan mode. *Med Sci Sports Exerc* 29:560–567, 1997.

81. Modlesky CM, Evans EM, Millard-Stafford ML, Collins MA, Lewis RD, Cureton KJ. Impact of bone mineral estimates on percent fat estimates from a four-component model. *Med Sci Sports Exerc* 31:1861–1868, 1999.

82. Lantz H, Samuelson G, Bratteby LE, Mallmin H, Sjöström L. Differences in whole body measurements by DXA-scanning using two Lunar DPX-L machines. *Int J Obesity* 23:764–770, 1999.

83. Thomas EL, Saeed N, Hajnal JV, Brynes A, Goldstone AP, Frost G, Bell JD. Magnetic resonance imaging of total body fat. *J Appl Physiol* 85:1778–1785, 1998.

84. Ross R, Shaw KD, Rissanen J, Martel Y, deGuise J, Avruch L. Sex differences in lean and adipose tissue distribution by magnetic resonance imaging: Anthropometric relationships. *Am J Clin Nutr* 59:1277–1285, 1994.

85. Kamel EG, McNeill G, Han TS, Smith FW, Avenell A, Davidson L, Tothill P. Measurement of abdominal fat by magnetic resonance imaging, dual-energy x-ray absorptiometry and anthropometry in non-obese men and women. *Int J Obesity* 23:686–692, 1999.

86. Abate N, Garg A, Coleman R, Grundy SM, Peshock RM. Prediction of total subcutaneous abdominal, intraperitoneal, and retroperitoneal adipose tissue masses in men by a single axial magnetic resonance imaging slice. *Am J Clin Nutr* 65:403–408, 1997.

87. Ross R., Advances in the application of imaging methods in applied and clinical physiology. *Acta Diabetol* 40(suppl I):545–550, 2003.

88. Van Loan MD, Belko AZ, Mayclin PL, Barbieri TF. Use of total-body electrical conductivity for monitoring body composition changes during weight reduction. *Am J Clin Nutr* 46:5–8, 1987.

89. Cochran WJ, Wong WW, Fiorotto ML, et al. Total body water estimated by measuring total-body electrical conductivity. *Am J Clin Nutr* 48:946–950, 1988.

90. De Bruin NC, van Velthoven KAM, Stijnen T, Juttmann RE, Degenhart HJ, Visser HKA. Body fat and fat-free mass in infants: New and classic anthropometric indexes and prediction equations compared with total-body electrical conductivity. *Am J Clin Nutr* 61:1195–1205, 1995.

91. Grauer WO. Quantification of body fat distribution in the abdomen using computed tomography. *Am J Clin Nutr* 39:631–637, 1984.

92. Jensen MD, Kanaley JA, Reed JE, Sheedy PF. Measurement of abdominal and visceral fat with computed tomography and dual-energy x-ray absorptiometry. *Am J Clin Nutr* 61:274–278, 1995.

93. Wang Z-M, Gallagher D, Nelson ME, Matthews DE, Heymsfield SB. Total-body skeletal muscle mass: Evaluation of 24-h urinary creatinine excretion by computerized axial tomography. *Am J Clin Nutr* 63:863–869, 1996.

94. Orphanidou C, McCargar L, Birmingham L, Mathieson J, Goldner E. Accuracy of subcutaneous fat measurement: Comparison of skinfold calipers, ultrasound, and computed tomography. *J Am Diet Assoc* 94:855–858, 1994.

95. Ballard TP, FaFara L, Vukovich MD. Comparison of Bod Pod® and DXA in female collegiate athletes. *Med Sci Sports Exerc* 36:731–735, 2004

96. Wagner DR, Heyward VH, Gibson AL. Validation of air displacement plethysmography for assessing body composition. *Med Sci Sports Exerc* 32:1339–1344, 2000.

97. Fields DA, Hunger GR, Goran MI. Validation of the BOD POD with hydrostatic weighing: Influence of body clothing. *Int J Obes Relat Metab Disord* 24:200–205, 2000.

98. Fields DA, Goran MI. Body composition techniques and the four-compartment model in children. *J Appl Physiol* 89:613–620, 2000.

99. Nunez C, Kovera AJ, Pietrobelli A, Heshka S, Horlick M, Kehayias JJ, Wang Z, Heymsfield SB. Body composition in children and adults by air displacement plethysmography. *Eur J Clin Nutr* 53:382–387, 1999.

100. Koda M, Ando F, Niino N, Tsuzuku S, Shimokata H. Comparison between the air displacement method and dual energy x-ray absorptiometry for estimation of body fat. *J Epidemiol* 10(1 suppl):S82–S89, 2000.

101. McCrory MA, Mole PA, Gomez TD, Dewey KG, Bernauer EM. Body composition by air-displacement plethysmography by using predicted and measured thoracic gas volumes. *J Appl Physiol* 84:1475–1479, 1998.

102. Sardinha LB, Lohman TG, Teixeira PJ, Guedes DP, Going SB. Comparison of air displacement plethysmography with dual-energy x-ray absorptiometry and 3 field methods for estimating body composition in middle-aged men. *Am J Clin Nutr* 68:786–793, 1998.

PHYSICAL FITNESS ACTIVITY 5.1

Measurement of Body Composition

In this activity, you will be measuring the body composition of at least one individual, using several different methods. It is highly recommended that you duplicate the worksheet from this activity and measure three or more individuals.

The body composition methods for this activity have been fully described in this chapter, and you should review each description before administering the test. Ideally, you should first learn the techniques while in a class laboratory under experienced supervision. Misclassification of the body composition status of an individual can lead to undue anxiety.

Body Composition Measurement

Name ______________________ Date ______________

Age __________ Sex __________ Height __________ Weight ______________

Skinfolds and BIA Measurements

______________ Chest ______________ Suprailiac

______________ Abdominal ______________ Midaxillary

______________ Thigh ______________ Subscapular

______________ Triceps ______________ Total (mm)

______________ Impedance (BIA)

Hydrostatic Measurements

______________ Net weight in water (kg) (Gross wt = ______________)

(Tare wt = ______________)

____

______________ ______________

______________ ______________

______________ Water density

______________ Residual volume (L) (measured)

Client and environmental guidelines prior to BIA measurements include the following:

- ❑ 1. No eating or drinking within 4 hours of the test.
- ❑ 2. No exercise within 12 hours of the test.
- ❑ 3. Urinate within 30 minutes of the test.
- ❑ 4. No alcohol consumption within 48 hours of the test.
- ❑ 5. No diuretic medications within 7 days of the test.
- ❑ 6. No testing of female clients who perceive they are retaining water during that stage of their menstrual cycle.
- ❑ 7. BIA measurements should be made in a room with normal ambient temperature.

Calculations		*Classification*
____________	Frame size (mm)	____________
____________	Body mass index (kg/m^2)	____________
____________	Relative weight (%)	____________
____________	Skinfold body fat %	____________
____________	BIA body fat %	____________
____________	Hydrostatic body fat %	____________
____________	Fat weight (lb) (*total weight* × *fat%*)	____________
____________	Fat-free weight (lb) (*total weight* − *fat weight*)	
____________	Ideal body weight (lb) [*fat-free weight*/(*100%* − *desired fat%*)]	

Body Composition Classification Tables

1995 USDA Healthy Weight Ranges

Height (no shoes)	Frame (mm) (medium)		Weight (lb) (without clothes)	
	M	F	Range	Midpoint
4′10″		57–64	91–119	105
4′11″		57–64	94–124	109
5′0″		57–64	97–128	112.5
5′1″	64–73	57–64	101–132	116.5
5′2″	64–73	57–64	104–137	120.5
5′3″	67–73	60–67	107–141	124
5′4″	67–73	60–67	111–146	128.5
5′5″	67–73	60–67	114–150	132
5′6″	67–73	60–67	118–155	136.5
5′7″	70–76	60–67	121–160	140.5
5′8″	70–76	60–67	125–164	144.5
5′9″	70–76	60–67	129–169	149
5′10″	70–76	60–67	132–174	153
5′11″	70–79	64–70	136–179	157.5
6′0″	70–79	64–70	140–184	162
6′1″	70–79	64–70	144–189	166.5
6′2″	70–79	64–70	148–195	171.5
6′3″	73–83	64–70	152–200	176
6′4″	73–83		156–205	180.5
6′5″	73–83		160–211	185.5
6′6″	73–83		164–216	190

Weight ranges are for men and women. People with low muscle and bone mass should use low end of weight range, and vice versa. For same size, values below the range are rated "small" and above, "large."

Percent Body Fat Norms

Classification	Male	Female
Unhealthy range (too low)	≤5%	≤8%
Acceptable range (lower end)	6–15%	9–23%
Acceptable range (higher end)	16–24%	24–31%
Unhealthy range (too high)	≥25%	≥32%

Body Mass Index Norms (M & F)

Underweight	<18.5 kg/m^2
Normal	18.5–24.9 kg/m^2
Overweight	25–29.9 kg/m^2
Obesity I	30–34.9 kg/m^2
Obesity II	35–39.9 kg/m^2
Obesity III	≥40 kg/m^2

Relative Body Weight Norms (M & F)

Underweight	<90%
Desirable	90–110%
Overweight	111–119%
Mild obesity	120–139%
Moderate obesity	140–199%
Severe obesity	>200%

PHYSICAL FITNESS ACTIVITY 5.2

Case Study: Providing Body Composition Counseling for a Female Track and Field Athlete

The track and field coach refers a female collegiate shot-put athlete to your body composition lab for testing. She is 70 inches tall, weighs 245 pounds, has a waist circumference of 37 inches, a BMI of 35.2, and a percent body fat of 32% (determined by underwater weighing). Although this athlete has been very successful in competition, the body composition data indicates she is at very high disease risk if she continues to carry this fat mass throughout adulthood (see Table 5.9). What advice would you give this athlete and her coach?

____

____

____

____

____

Author comments: Coaches often feel that field athletes must carry a lot of weight to be successful. However, this female athlete is carrying too much fat mass (both from athletic and health perspectives). This athlete should attempt to decrease her fat mass while increasing her fat-free mass through proper dietary habits and resistance training. Once her competitive days are over, she should attain a healthy BMI and waist circumference to ensure long-term health.

chapter 6

Musculoskeletal Fitness

That which is used develops. That which is not used wastes away.
—Hippocrates

MUSCULAR FITNESS

More than 600 muscles are used by humans to work, play sports, and accomplish daily tasks. (See Appendix C for a summary of the major muscles of the body.) Skeletal muscle is the body's most abundant tissue, making up about 23% of a female's body weight and 40% of a male's. Millions of tiny protein filaments within the muscle work together to contract and pull on tendons and other tissues to create movement around joints. (See Box 6.1 for definitions of words commonly used in musculoskeletal fitness.)

Skeletal muscles are very responsive to use and disuse. Those that are forcefully exercised become larger, a phenomenon called muscular hypertrophy. On the other hand, a muscle that is not used will atrophy or decrease in size and strength and become inflexible. Good muscular fitness depends on the development of three basic components:

1. *Muscular strength.* The maximal one-effort force that can be exerted against a resistance
2. *Muscular endurance.* The ability of the muscles to apply a submaximal force repeatedly or to sustain a muscular contraction for a certain period of time
3. *Flexibility.* The functional capacity of the joints to move through a full range of movement

The purpose of this chapter is to describe the various types of tests that measure each of these three elements, concentrating on the tests that were outlined in the testing batteries at the end of Chapter 3.

Elaborate and expensive musculoskeletal fitness testing equipment is available, and many books have been written describing it, including the use of isokinetic equipment for testing muscular strength and endurance.[1–3] The purpose of both this book and this chapter, however, is to concentrate more on the physical fitness tests that are widely available, inexpensive (yet valid and reliable), and health-related.

HEALTH-RELATED BENEFITS OF MUSCULOSKELETAL FITNESS

Systems of resistance training for developing muscular strength and endurance are reviewed in Chapter 8. In this chapter, we discuss some of the benefits of musculoskeletal fitness, as well as means for enhancing it. The American College of Sports Medicine,[4] the American Heart Association,[5] and the surgeon general's report on physical activity and health[6] have each acknowledged the importance of strength training as a key component of physical fitness and quality of life (especially in old age). These organizations have recommended performing one set of 8–12 repetitions of 8–10 exercises two to three times per week, for persons under 50–60 years of age and the same regimen using 10–15 repetitions for persons over 50–60 years of age.[4–7] This is a basic program, however, and greater gains in muscular strength and power can be experienced using a higher intensity (fewer repetitions with greater weight) with multiple sets.[8,9]

Box 6.1

Glossary of Terms Used in Musculoskeletal Fitness

ballistic flexibility: The ability to engage in bobbing, bouncing, rebounding, and rhythmic motions.

connective tissues: The structural or framework tissues of the body (e.g., ligaments, tendons, and fibrous sheaths).

dynamic flexibility: The ability to engage in slow, rhythmic movements throughout the full range of joint motion.

flexibility: The capacity of the joints to move through a full range of movement.

ligaments: A band or sheath of fibrous tissue connecting two or more bones.

lordosis: A forward pelvis tilt (curvature in the lower back), often caused by weak abdominal muscles and inflexible posterior thigh and lower back muscles.

low-back pain: Pain in the lower back, ranging from a dull annoyance to a chronic, crippling disability.

muscular atrophy: A decrease in muscle bulk and size due to lack of use.

muscular endurance: The ability of the muscles to repeat a submaximal effort repeatedly.

muscular hypertrophy: An increase in muscle bulk and size due to training.

muscular strength: The maximum one-effort force that can be generated against a resistance.

one-repetition maximum (1-RM): The greatest weight that can be lifted once.

osteoporosis: A loss of bone mass, associated with an increased risk of fracture.

skeletal muscle: Muscle connected to bone; the body's most abundant tissue.

spine: The bony vertebral column; composed of 24 vertebrae.

static flexibility: The ability to hold a stretched position.

tendons: Fibrous cords or bands of variable length that connect a muscle with its bony attachment.

Development of muscular strength and endurance has been associated with several important health-related benefits, including increased bone density and connective tissue strength, lean body mass and muscle strength, anaerobic power and capacity, and self-esteem.[7–11] Between the ages of 30 and 70, muscle mass and strength decrease by an average of 30%, much of this due to inactivity. The weakness and frailty of old age is often attributed to this loss of muscular strength and has been shown in several studies to be in part reversible through resistance training.[11–16]

Although there are some indications that high-volume resistance training may lead to reduced resting heart rate and blood pressure, improvements in the blood lipid profile and insulin sensitivity, and an increase in aerobic power, results of studies have been inconclusive, with reported changes small at best when compared to aerobic endurance training (see Table 6.1).[7,10,16–20]

Oxygen uptake during heavy resistance exercise using large muscle groups seldom exceeds 60% of maximal aerobic power, even though heart rates of up to 170 beats per minute and blood pressures exceeding 400/300 mm Hg have been recorded during the last repetitions of a set to volitional fatigue. Most studies have shown that during weight training exercise at a measured percent heart rate maximum, the aerobic demand or percent $\dot{V}O_{2max}$ is less than for endurance exercise. While mean heart rates are usually between 60% and 100% of maximum during weight lifting, oxygen consumption averages 35–60% of aerobic power.[9]

Although the mechanism underlying the higher heart rate of weight training exercise compared to endurance exercise at the same oxygen consumption is unknown, it may be related in part to enhanced sympathetic activity. The net result is that skeletal muscle oxidative capacity in resistance-trained individuals is lacking and aerobic power is not enhanced to a significant degree (Table 6.1).[7]

The American College of Sports Medicine (ACSM) maintains that "optimal musculoskeletal function requires that an adequate range of motion be maintained in all joints. Of particular importance is maintenance of flexibility in the lower back and posterior thigh regions. Lack of flexibility in this area may be associated with an increased risk for development of chronic lower back pain."[21] The ACSM recommends that static stretching be engaged in at least 2–3 days per week, that an active warm-up precede vigorous stretching, and that each session involve at least four repetitions of each stretching exercise, sustained for 10 to 30 seconds.[15–21]

Many potential benefits have been linked to flexibility, but limited data exist to support these claims. See Chapter 8 for a discussion.[22–24]

PREVENTION AND TREATMENT OF LOW-BACK PAIN

Low-back pain is a common ailment among modern-day men and women.[25–32] At some point in their lives, 60–80% of all Americans and Europeans will experience a bout of low-back pain, ranging from a dull, annoying ache to intense and prolonged pain. After headaches, low-back pain is the second most common ailment in the United States and is topped only by colds and flus in time lost from work. Next to arthritis, low-back pain is the most frequently reported disability.

TABLE 6.1 Health and Fitness Benefits of Aerobic Compared to Strength Training

Variable	Aerobic Exercise	Resistance Exercise
Resting blood pressure	↓↓	↔↓
Serum HDL cholesterol	↑↑	↔↑
Insulin sensitivity	↑↑	↑
Percent body fat	↓↓	↓
Bone mineral density	↑	↑↑↑
Strength	↔↑	↑↑↑
Physical function in old age	↑↑	↑↑↑
$\dot{V}O_{2max}$	↑↑↑	↔↑

Number of arrows refers to strength of scientific evidence, with three arrows indicating conclusive evidence.

↑ increased
↓ decreased
↔ no change

Source: Pollock ML, Vincent ML. Resistance training for health. *The President's Council on Physical Fitness and Sports Research Digest* (Series 2, No. 8). December 1996.

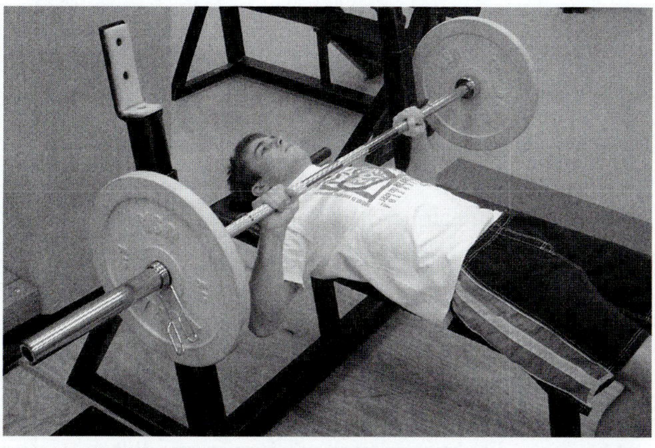

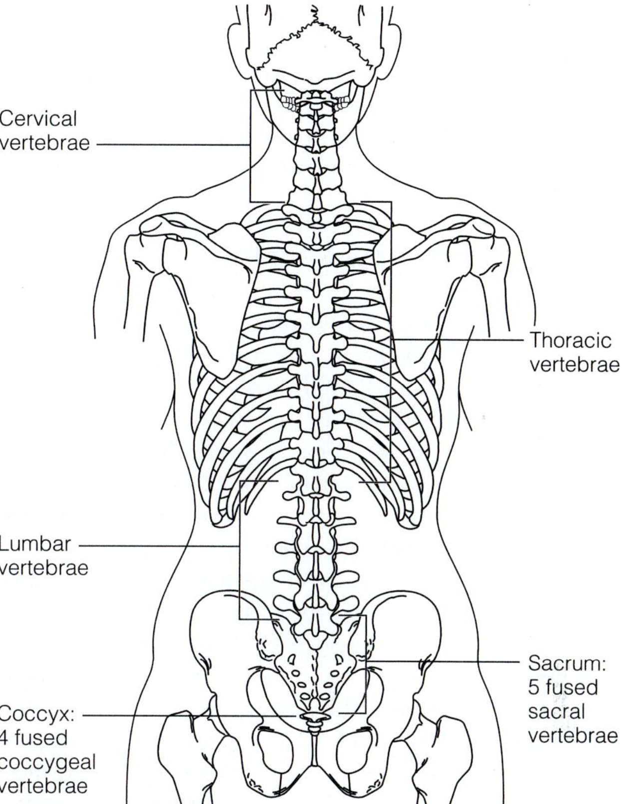

Figure 6.1 The human spine is made up of 24 vertebrae divided into five distinct regions. Low-back pain is most commonly experienced at the L4–L5 lumbar segment.[18,22]

A nationwide government survey revealed that back pain lasting for at least a week is reported by 18% of the working population each year.[30] Of these, about half attributed the cause of the back pain to a work-related activity or injury, with the proportion much higher among workers in farming, forestry, or fishing occupations. This problem is not unique to the civilian population, in that back pain accounts for at least 20% of all medical discharges from the U.S. Army.

Low-back pain commonly affects people in their most productive years, resulting in a substantial economic cost to society. When all the costs connected with low-back pain are added up—job absenteeism, medical and legal fees, social security disability payments, worker's compensation, long-term disability insurance—the bill to business, industry, and the government has been estimated to range from 50–100 billion dollars per year.[29]

Males and females appear to be affected equally, with most cases of low-back pain occurring between the ages of 25 and 60 years, with a peak at about 40 years of age.[25] The first attack often occurs early in life, however, with up to one third of adolescents reporting they have experienced at least one bout of low-back pain.[33] A 25-year study of schoolchildren in Denmark showed that low-back pain during the growth period is an important risk factor for low-back pain later in life.[34] Because of this, preventive measures should start within elementary schools.

Fortunately, most low-back pain is self-limiting.[25–27] Without treatment, 60% of back pain sufferers go back to work within a week, and nearly 90% return within 6 weeks. A significant proportion (at least one third) of those experiencing low-back pain once have recurrent episodes. Pain remains for up to 5–10% of patients, creating a chronic condition. About 70–90% of the total costs related to back pain are borne by these patients. Data from the National Health Interview Survey indicate that 32 adults per 1,000 population experience activity limitation due to chronic back conditions, with this rate being substantially higher among the poor (77/1000) and those with low education (54/1000).[32]

The spine is composed of 24 vertebrae, 23 discs, 31 pairs of spinal nerves, 140 attaching muscles, plus a large number of ligaments and tendons (see Figure 6.1). Though humans are born with 33 separate vertebrae (the bones that form the spine), by adulthood, most people have only 24. The 9 vertebrae at the base of the spine grow together. Of these, 5 form the sacrum, while the lowest 4 form the coccyx. Seven cervical vertebrae (C1 to C7) support and provide movement for the head, while 12 thoracic vertebrae (T1 to T12) join with and are supported by the ribs. The 5 lumbar vertebrae (L1 to L5) are most frequently involved in back pain because they carry most of the body's stress. Anatomically, the term *low-back-pain syndrome* is applied to pain experienced in the lumbosacral region (L1 to S1 vertebrae). The most commonly indicated site of low-back pain is the L4–L5 lumbar segment.

Risk Factors for Low-Back Pain

Multiple risk factors for low-back pain have been reported.[25–28, 32–43] (See Box 6.2 for a self-quiz for estimating risk of low-back pain.)[35] Many cases of low-back pain appear to be due to unusual stresses on the muscles and ligaments that support the spine of susceptible individuals. When the body is in poor shape, for example, weak spinal and abdominal muscles may be unable to support the spine properly during certain types of lifting or physical activities.

Nonetheless, even hardy occupational workers or athletes who exercise beyond their tolerance are susceptible. Rowers, triathletes, professional golfers and tennis players, wrestlers, and gymnasts, for example, have all been reported to have high rates of back injury (up to 30% in golfers and football players, for example).[44–46] Among athletes, back pain and degenerative changes of the spine later on in life are most prevalent among those who experience extreme loading and twisting as a regular part of their training (e.g., weight lifters, track and field power athletes, and gymnasts).[45] Jobs that involve bending and twisting, or lifting heavy objects repeatedly—especially when the loads are beyond a worker's strength—are a chief cause of low-back pain.[39,41]

Certain occupations—such as truck or bus driving, fire fighting, or nursing—are particularly hard on the back.[39] The truck driver, for example, sits for long periods of time in a vibrating truck and then often helps to unload the truck, lifting and straining at the end of the day. This explains why truck driving ranks first in worker's compensation cases for low-back pain. Firefighters also have a high incidence of low-back pain, which has been related to such high-risk activities as operating charged water hoses, climbing ladders, breaking windows, and lifting heavy objects.[47]

In general, for all workers, occupational risk factors include heavy lifting; lifting with bending and twisting motions; pushing and pulling; slipping, tripping, or falling; and long periods of sitting or driving, especially with vibrations. Individual risk factors may include obesity, smoking, poor posture, psychological stress and anxiety, minimal physical activity level, and reduced degree of muscular strength and joint flexibility.[33–43]

Prevention of low-back pain has typically involved several recommendations:[25–28, 32–43]

- Exercise regularly to strengthen back and abdominal muscles.
- Lose weight, if necessary, to lessen strain on the back. Most studies have shown that obese people are at greater risk for developing low-back pain.
- Avoid smoking. Studies have consistently shown that smokers have a risk of low-back pain 1.5 to 2.5 times that of nonsmokers.
- Lift by bending at the knees, rather than the waist, using leg muscles to do most of the work.
- Receive objects from others or from platforms near to the body, and avoid twisting or bending at the waist while handling or transferring the objects.
- Avoid sitting, standing, or working in any one position for too long.
- Maintain a correct posture (sit with shoulders back and feet flat on the floor, or on a footstool or chair rung. Stand with head and chest high, neck straight, stomach and buttocks held in, and pelvis forward). See Physical Fitness Activity 6.1 for more on posture.

Box 6.2

A Self-Quiz for Estimating Risk of Low-Back Pain

Take the following quiz to evaluate your own risk for low-back pain.

1. _____ Am I overweight?
2. _____ Does my stomach stick out?
3. _____ Do I smoke, especially heavily?
4. _____ Does my work require a lot of sitting, especially without breaks?
5. _____ Is my chair at work comfortable?
6. _____ Does my work entail repetitive pushing and pulling movements or lifting while bending or twisting? (This applies whether you're working at home, in an office, in a warehouse, or outdoors.)
7. _____ Does my work require me to use power tools or heavy moving equipment or to drive a lot?
8. _____ Is my bed comfortable?
9. _____ Do I stand in one place a lot when I work, at home or on the job?
10. _____ Do I slouch most of the time?
11. _____ Is my car seat comfortable for me?
12. _____ Do I engage in any kind of exercise or sport regularly?
13. _____ Does stress in my daily life make my back pain worse?
14. _____ Do I get enough calcium in my diet, especially if I'm over 50?

Source: YMCA of the USA. *YMCA Healthy Back Book.* Champaign, IL: Human Kinetics, 1994. Used with permission of the YMCA of the USA, 101 N. Wacker Drive, Chicago, IL 60606.

- Use a comfortable, supportive seat while driving.
- Use a firm mattress, and sleep either on the side, with knees drawn up, or on the back, with a pillow under bent knees.
- Try to reduce emotional stress that causes muscle tension.
- Be thoroughly warmed up before engaging in vigorous exercise or sports.
- Undergo a gradual progression when attempting to improve strength or athletic ability.

Education is the most common back pain prevention strategy used in industry. There are many different types of programs, including comprehensive "back school" programs, which provide information on how the back works, preferred lifting techniques, optimal posture, exercises to prevent back pain, and management of stress and pain.

Despite the numerous causes and risk factors that have been related to low-back pain, most attention has been directed toward viewing low-back pain as a by-product of deficient musculoskeletal fitness.[25] Many researchers feel that the combination of a weak back and a back-straining occupation greatly increases the risk of low-back pain. In particular, emphasis has been placed on the relationship of low-back pain to weak abdominal and back muscles, and poor flexibility of lower back and hamstring muscle groups. Low-back pain has been described as a disease of the sedentary lifestyle, and most fitness testing batteries from professional organizations include some version of a sit-up to evaluate abdominal strength and endurance and the sit-and-reach test to evaluate low-back and hamstring flexibility.

Theoretically, weak muscles that are easily fatigued cannot support the spine in proper alignment. When standing, weak abdominals and inflexible posterior thigh muscles allow the pelvis to tilt forward, causing a curvature in the lower back (called *lordosis*). This places increased stress on the spine and a greater load on other muscles, leading to their fatigue. The tight hamstring muscles and lower back muscles, combined with the weak abdominals, can lead to the low-back pain syndrome (see Figure 6.2).

A study in Japan, for example, showed that subjects with a prior history of low-back pain had weaker trunk muscle strength and a "generalized muscular weakness" when compared to those who had not experienced low-back pain.[48] A study of youths in Finland found that a low level of physical activity and decreased spinal and abdominal muscle strength characterized those who developed low-back pain.[49] Many other studies have reported that low-back-pain patients have low trunk muscle strength, reducing support and stabilization of the spine.[25,26,37]

The evidence is far from conclusive, however, that poor musculoskeletal fitness predicts low-back pain among the general population.[50–54] For example, in one study of 119 nurses, performance on fitness and back-related isometric strength tests did not effectively predict low-back pain during an 18-month period.[50] A 10-year study of 654 people in

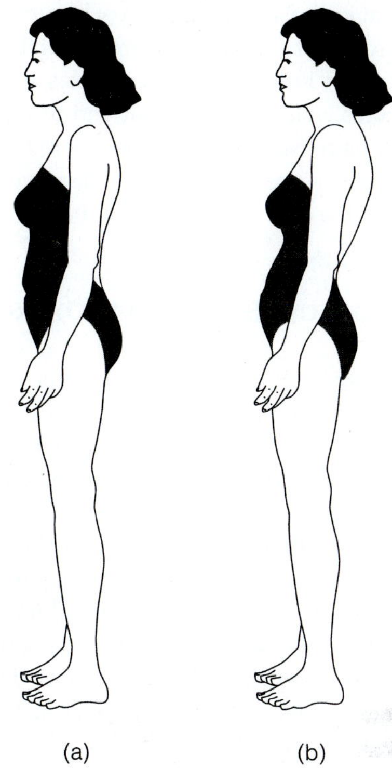

Figure 6.2 Good posture and poor posture with a forward tilt of the pelvis. See Physical Fitness Activity 6.1 for more on posture.

Finland failed to demonstrate any relationship between muscle function at baseline and the development of low-back pain.[52] In both adolescents and adults, flexibility measurements have been reported to have a low predictive value for low-back pain.[51,55] Regarding prevention, most experts feel that (a) exercise interventions may be mildly protective against back pain, but (b) evidence is limited to support the contention that exercises to strengthen back or abdominal muscles and to improve overall fitness can decrease the incidence and duration of low-back pain episodes. For example, in a randomized controlled trial of 402 subjects with weak abdominal muscles, instruction on abdominal muscle strength exercise failed to lower low-back-pain episodes during a 2-year period.[54] However, as the researchers noted, compliance with the exercise program was poor, highlighting the major challenge in all low-back-pain prevention programs.

There is some indication, however, that low levels of musculoskeletal fitness are predictive of recurrent low-back pain.[25] In other words, when an individual of any age suffers a low-back problem and then, as a reaction, engages in very little exercise, the likelihood of further episodes is enhanced. This can set up a vicious cycle, leading to chronic back problems.

For years, the 1-minute timed bent-knee sit-up has been used for measurement of abdominal strength and endurance, while the sit-and-reach test has been touted as a measure of low-back and hamstring flexibility. Unfortunately, there is no evidence that people who score low on both tests are at increased risk of low-back pain in the future. Andrew Jackson, working with researchers at the Cooper Institute for Aerobics Research in Dallas, Texas, studied the effect of low scores on the sit-up and sit-and-reach tests on future low-back pain: Nearly 3,000 adults were followed for 6 years—those who scored low on these tests were not at increased risk for the development of low-back pain.[56]

Treatment of Low-Back Pain with Exercise

Treatment of low-back pain has proven to be complex and frustrating.[28] The optimal management of low-back pain is still under debate.[57–70] Many nonsurgical treatments are available for patients with low-back pain, but few have been proven effective or clearly superior to others.

Nonsurgical treatments include physical therapy (with exercise), strict and extended bed rest, trigger-point injections, spinal manipulation, epidural steroid injections, conventional traction, corsets, and transcutaneous electrical stimulation. Many treatments have been added to the list of ineffective treatments, with little guidance as to the clearly effective ones.[28]

Physical therapy with exercise is recommended by physicians more than any other nonsurgical treatment for low-back pain (both acute and chronic),[71] yet, according to most experts, the role of exercise in treatment of low-back pain remains controversial. One review, for example, reported that only one of four well-designed studies has found a positive effect of exercise therapy in low-back-pain patients.[69] Another systematic review of randomized controlled trials using exercise therapy for treatment of low-back pain concluded there is little good evidence that specific exercises are effective for acute low-back pain, but may be helpful for patients with chronic low-back pain to increase return to normal daily activities and work.[59] In one of the earliest studies, Kraus and Raab used musculoskeletal exercises to treat 3,000 adult patients with chronic and acute back pain, and they reported "good" improvement in 65% and "fair" improvement in 26% of the patients, while only 9.2% had "poor" improvement.[67] In this study, however, no control group was used for determining whether patients engaging in no exercise at all would have experienced similar improvement.

Some researchers advocate an intensive back-muscle-strengthening exercise program to treat low-back pain.[64,65] Patients cannot exercise strenuously at first, but after various pain control measures are initiated, patients are gradually progressed through an increasingly difficult series of resistance exercises to improve back muscle strength. In one study of 105 low-back-pain patients in Denmark, 30 sessions of intense back extensor exercises, over a 3-month period, led to significant improvement, relative to groups exercising less intensely.[64] Other studies have shown that lumbar extension strength training over a 2- to 3-month period is associated with decreased low-back and leg pain and an improved ability to perform daily activities.[57] Some researchers have urged that strengthening the entire trunk area over an extended period of time is critical to treating low-back pain.[70, 72, 73] This approach, however, is not accepted by all low-back-pain experts, and it is time consuming and costly, requiring trained staff and hospital resources.

A study of 186 civil workers who sought treatment for acute low-back pain in Helsinki, Finland, has provided some of the best data to date regarding the relative merits of bed rest, exercise, and ordinary activity in the treatment of acute back pain.[70] The patients were randomized to one of three groups: bed rest (for 2 days), exercise (back extension and side bending movements), and normal activity (continue normal daily routines within the limits permitted by the back pain).

As shown in Figure 6.3, after 3 weeks, those patients who maintained normal activities were significantly better off than those who had either rested in bed or exercised. Their back pain was less intense and did not last as long, and they had missed fewer days on the job and felt better able to work. Recovery was slowest for the bed-rest patients. The researchers concluded that avoiding bed rest and maintaining ordinary activity, as tolerated, led to the most rapid recovery.

Most experts now feel that low-back pain should be treated as a benign, self-limiting condition that usually requires little medical intervention.[28] In a large study of close to 1,000 patients in Norway, researchers reported that light and normal activity combined with information and instruction designed to increase activity and reduce fear associated with the condition had a significantly better effect on sickness leave than did ordinary medical practice.[68]

This conclusion is similar to that reached by a panel of 23 experts sponsored by the U.S. Agency for Health Care Policy and Research, which reviewed nearly 4,000 studies on back pain. Among the agency's recommendations:[28]

- Engage in low-stress activities such as walking, biking, or swimming during the first 2 weeks after symptoms begin, even if the activities make the symptoms a little worse. "The most important goal," the panel concludes, "is to return to your normal activities as soon as it is safe."

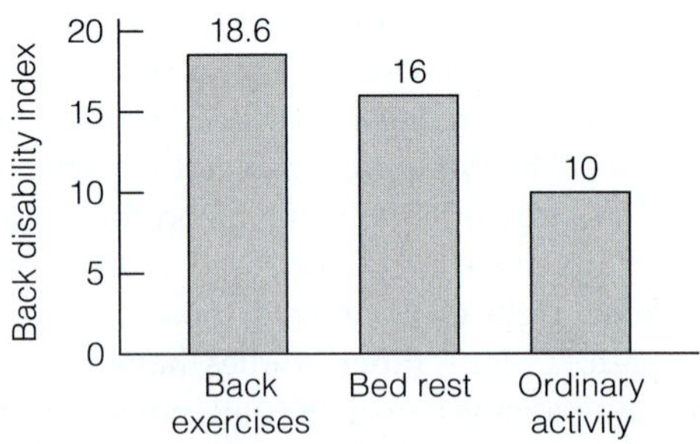

Figure 6.3 Treatment of acute low-back pain: Ordinary activity is superior to bed rest or back exercises. In this study of Finnish civil workers, those who maintained normal activities had better recovery from low-back pain than did those resting in bed or engaging in back exercises.
Source: Data from Malmivaara A, Häkkinen U, Aro T, et al. The treatment of acute low back pain: Bed rest, exercises, or ordinary activity? *N Engl J Med* 332:351–355, 1995.

- Bed rest usually is not necessary and should not last longer than 2–4 days. More than 4 days of rest can weaken muscles and delay recovery.
- Nonprescription pain relievers such as aspirin and ibuprofen work as well as prescription painkillers and muscle relaxants and cause fewer side effects.
- Among treatments not recommended, due to lack of evidence that they work, are traction, acupuncture, massage, ultrasound, and transcutaneous electrical nerve stimulation.
- Diagnostic tests such as x-rays and CT scans are rarely useful during the first month of symptoms, so they should be avoided during that time.
- Surgery helps only 1 in 100 people with acute low-back problems. It should be done during the first 3 months of symptoms only when a serious underlying condition, such as a fracture or a dislocation, is suspected.
- Spinal manipulation by a chiropractor or other therapist can be helpful when symptoms begin, but patients should be reevaluated if they have not improved after 4 weeks of treatment.

TESTS FOR MUSCULAR ENDURANCE AND STRENGTH

Although low-back pain has prompted great interest in abdominal, back, and thigh muscle strength, fitness instructors must maintain interest in all muscle groups. Because muscular strength and endurance are specific to each muscle group,[1] no single test can be used to evaluate total body muscle strength and endurance. It is recommended that the selected strength and endurance battery include measures for the upper body, midbody, and lower body.

In this chapter, the emphasis is on field tests for musculoskeletal fitness used in physical fitness testing batteries described in Chapter 3.[74–77]

Abdominal Tests: Bent-Knee Sit-Ups and Partial Curl-Ups

Abdominal exercises are used for a variety of reasons, including improved posture and appearance, enhanced sports performance, and the prevention and treatment of low-back pain. As discussed earlier in this chapter, although abdominal and back strength have been linked to diminished low-back pain, the data are far from consistent. The Sports Medicine Insight at the end of this chapter summarizes current understanding regarding the appropriate exercises for abdominal fitness.

During the 1950s and 1960s, straight-leg sit-ups were commonly used in physical fitness testing batteries for children and youths.[78–85] After concerns were raised about lower-back strain and the reliance on hip flexor muscles during the straight-leg sit-up, the bent-leg sit-up test (knees bent to 90 degrees) with the hands clenched behind the neck became the test of choice during the 1970s and 1980s. However, researchers soon reported that stress was still placed on the lower back, due to anterior pelvic tilt, and that the hip flexor muscles became dominant in the late stage of the test after the spine had been fully flexed by the abdominal muscles.[80–83] Support at the feet while performing the sit-up was found to increase hip flexor activity and decrease rectus abdominis muscular activity.

Nonetheless, some testing batteries still use the bent-knee sit-up but alter the position of the hands. Partial curl-ups (also called "abdominal crunches" or "half sit-ups"), in which the spine is flexed less than 30 degrees, do not cause strong recruitment of the hip flexor muscles and appear to place less strain on the lower back.[79,84] Performing the partial curl-up with the feet unsupported and the knees flexed has been reported to maximize abdominal muscle activity.

To perform the 1-minute bent-knee sit-up with the arms crossed over the chest, follow these instructions (see Figure 6.4):[74]

- Start on the back, with knees flexed, feet on floor, with the heels 12–18 inches from the buttocks.

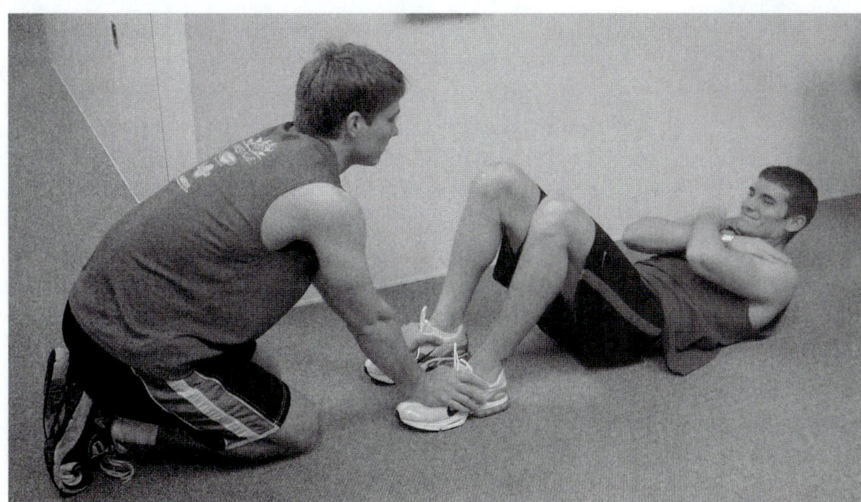

Figure 6.4 The 1-minute timed bent-knee sit-up test. The purpose of this test is to evaluate abdominal muscle strength and endurance.

- The arms are crossed on the chest, with the hands on the opposite shoulders. The arms must be folded across and flat against the chest.
- The feet are held by the partner, to keep them firmly on the ground.
- During the sit-up, arm contact with the chest must be maintained. This is critically important. Another important rule is that the buttocks must remain on the mat, no more than 18 inches from the heels.
- In the up position, the elbow and forearm must touch the thighs (without the arms pulling away from the chest).
- In the down position, the midback makes contact with the floor.
- The number of correctly executed sit-ups performed in 60 seconds is the score. See Appendix A for norms for all age groups (Tables 5, 6, 15, 20, 34). Figure 6.5 represents normative data from the Canadian Fitness Survey.

The protocol used for the partial curl-up test in the Canadian Physical Activity, Fitness & Lifestyle Appraisal program is as follows (see Figure 6.6):[74]

- Apply masking tape and string across a gym mat in two parallel lines, 10 cm apart.
- The individual to be tested should lie in a supine position, with the head resting on the mat, arms straight and fully extended at the sides and parallel to the trunk, palms of the hands in contact with the mat, and the middle fingertip of both hands at the 0 mark line. The knees should be bent at a 90-degree angle. The heels must stay in contact with the mat, and the test is performed with the shoes on.
- Set a metronome to a cadence of 50 beats per minute. The subject performs as many consecutive

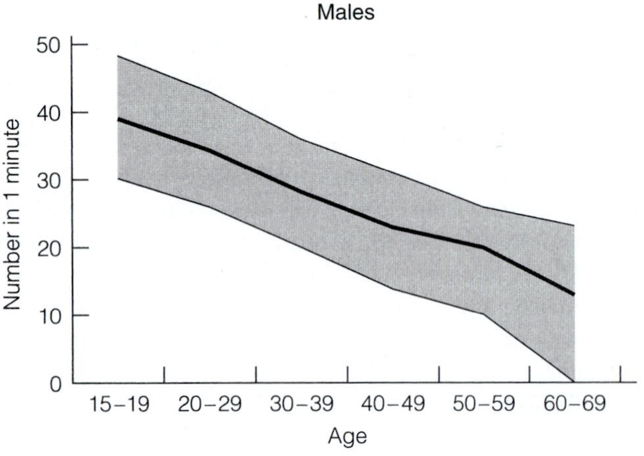

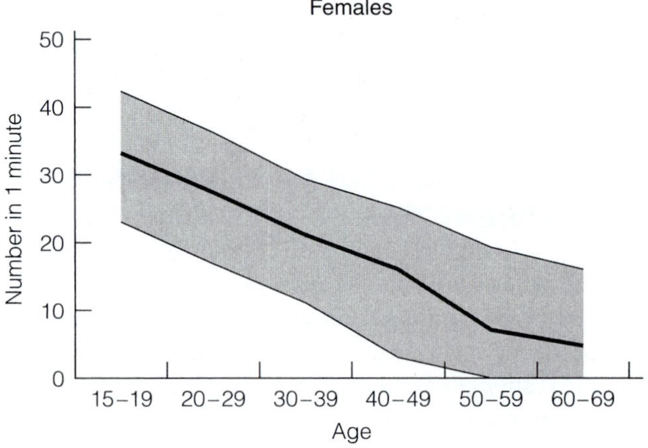

Figure 6.5 Normative data (15th, 50th, and 85th percentiles) from Canada on the 1-minute timed sit-ups in males (left) and females (right).[74] Source: Data based on the Canada Fitness Survey, 1981.

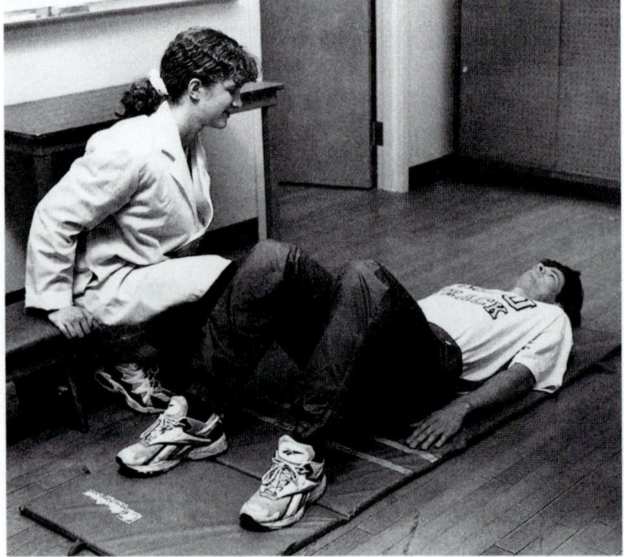

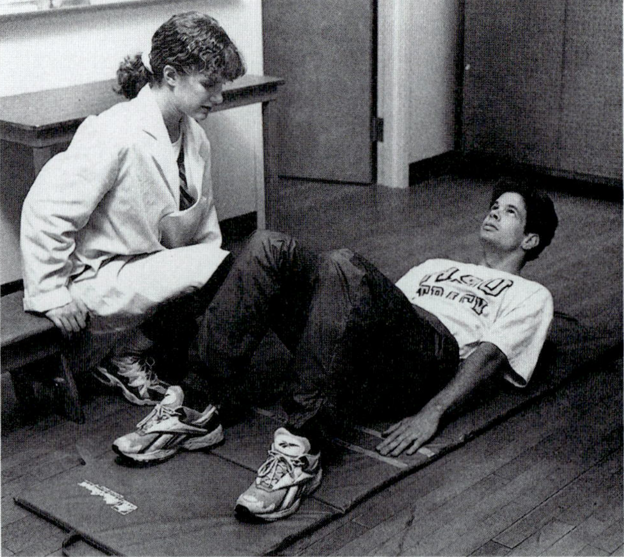

Figure 6.6 The partial curl-up test should be conducted with the feet unsupported.

curl-ups as possible, without pausing, at a rate of 25 per minute. The test is terminated after 1 minute. During each curl-up, the upper spine should be curled up so that the middle fingertips of both hands reach the 10-cm mark. During the curl-up the palms and heels must remain in contact with the mat. Anchoring of the feet is not permitted. On the return, the shoulder blades and head must contact the mat, and the fingertips of both hands must touch the 0 mark. The movement is performed in a slow, controlled manner at a rate of 25 per minute.

- The test is terminated before 1 minute if subjects experience undue discomfort, are unable to maintain the required cadence, or are unable to maintain the proper curl-up technique (e.g., heels come off the floor) over two consecutive repetitions, despite cautions by the test supervisor.

Norms for the Canadian partial curl-up test appear in Table 31 of Appendix A. FITNESSGRAM® standards for the partial curl-up are in Table 19 of Appendix A.[74] The FITNESSGRAM® partial curl-up protocol is slightly different from that of the Canadian test.[76] The parallel strips on the mat are placed 3 inches apart for grades kindergarten through 4, and 4½ inches apart for older children and youths. The knees are at a 140-degree angle, and the curl-up is performed at a cadence of 20 per minute. The student continues without pausing until the technique can no longer be followed or 75 curl-ups have been conducted.

Pull-Ups

The purpose of this test is to measure the muscular strength and endurance of the arms and shoulder girdle.[86]

The Traditional Pull-Up

The traditional pull-up requires the following procedures (see Figure 6.7):

- The person being tested starts in a hanging position, with arms straight, hands in an *overhand* position (palms away).
- The body is pulled upward until the chin is over the bar.
- After each pull-up, the person returns to a fully extended hanging position.
- Swinging and snap-up movements are to be avoided.
- A partner should hold an extended arm across the front of the person's thighs to prevent swinging. The knees should stay straight during the entire test.
- The score is the total number of pull-ups until exhaustion. (See norms in Appendix A, Tables 3, 4, 18, 19, 38.)

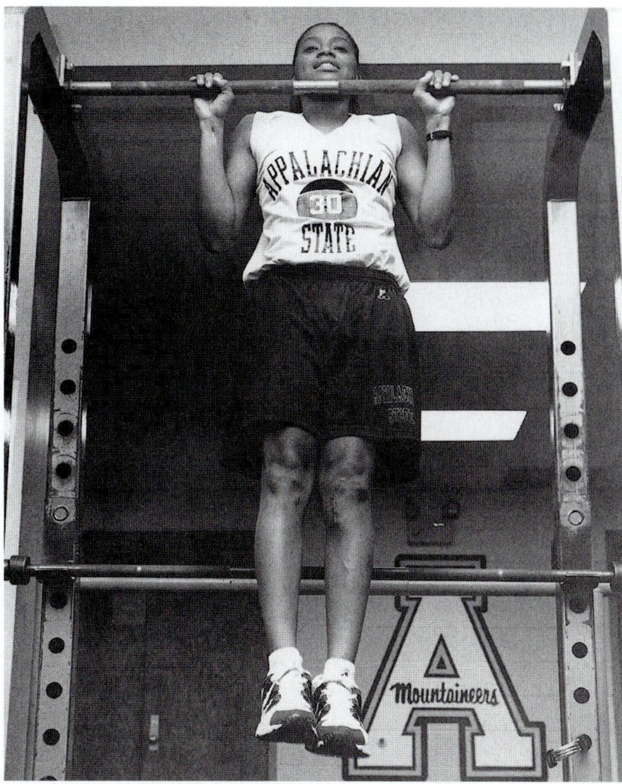

Figure 6.7 Traditional pull-ups. The purpose of this test is to measure the muscular strength and endurance of the arms and shoulder girdle in pulling the body upward.

The Modified Pull-Up

Experience has revealed certain problems with the traditional pull-up and the flexed-arm hang.[87–90] Performance is markedly affected by body weight, and a large proportion of children are incapable of doing even one pull-up.

In 1985, the President's Council on Physical Fitness and the Sports School Population Fitness Survey revealed that 70% of all girls (ages 6–17) tested could not do more than one pull-up, with 55% not being able to do even one.[91] Forty percent of boys ages 6–12 could not do more than one pull-up, and 25% could not do any. Fifty-five percent of all girls could not hold their chins over a raised bar for more than 10 seconds. Forty-five percent of boys 6–14 could not hold their chins over a raised bar for more than 10 seconds.

A better test of upper-body muscular strength and endurance may be a modification of the traditional pull-up. This modified pull-up was used in the National Children and Youth Fitness Study II for children ages 6–9, but it can be used for all age groups.[87,89] In the FITNESSGRAM® testing program, the modified pull-up test is recommended for all students, especially those who cannot do one traditional pull-up[76] (see Appendix A, Table 19).

- The subject is positioned on the back, with shoulders directly below a bar that is set at a height 1 or 2 inches beyond reach.
- An elastic band is suspended across the uprights parallel to and 7–8 inches below the bar.

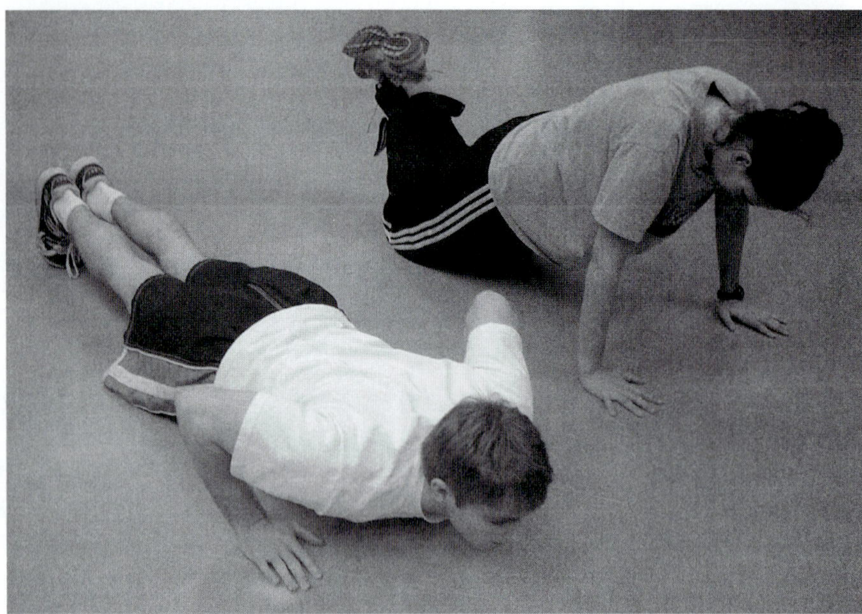

Figure 6.8 Push-ups. The purpose of the push-up test is to assess upper-body (triceps, anterior deltoids, and pectoralis major) muscle strength and endurance.

- In the start position, the subject is suspended holding onto the bar, buttocks off the floor, arms and legs straight, and only heels in contact with the floor.
- The bar is held with an overhand grip (palm away from the body), with thumbs around the bar.
- A pull-up is completed when the chin is hooked over the elastic band. The movement should be accomplished using only the arms, with the body kept rigid and straight. The body is then lowered to starting position and the pull-up repeated as many times as possible.

Flexed-Arm Hang

The purpose of the flexed-arm hang is to assess forearm and upper-arm flexor strength and endurance, and it is included in many fitness testing programs for children and youths.[76,77,91]

- The height of the bar should be adjusted so that it is slightly higher than the subject's standing height.
- The subject (both boys and girls) should use an overhand grip.
- With the assistance of two spotters, the subject is raised to a position with the chin above the bar (not touching), arms flexed, chest close to the bar.
- Spotters then release their support and start a stopwatch, with the subject trying to keep the chin above the bar as long as possible without extraneous body movement.
- The watch is stopped when the chin touches the bar or falls below the level of the bar.
- Total seconds are recorded and can be compared with norms (Appendix A, Table 19).

Push-Ups

The purpose of the push-up test is to assess upper-body (triceps, anterior deltoids, and pectoralis major) muscle strength and endurance and is used in many testing batteries. It is administered differently to males and females in some testing batteries, but not all.[74–77]

Males

- The person being tested assumes the standard position for a push-up, with the body rigid and straight, toes tucked under, and hands approximately shoulder-width apart and straight under the shoulders.
- A partner places a fist on the floor beneath the person's chest, who lowers himself until his chest touches the fist, keeping his back perfectly straight; he then raises himself back up to the starting position (see Figure 6.8).
- The most common performance error is not keeping the back rigid and straight throughout the entire push-up.
- Rest is allowed in the up position only.
- The score is the total number of push-ups to exhaustion. (See norms in Appendix A, Tables 29 and 33.)

Females

- Everything is the same as for the males, except that the test is performed from the bent-knee position (see Figure 6.8). In addition, the person being tested should make sure that her hands are slightly ahead of her shoulders in the up position, so that her

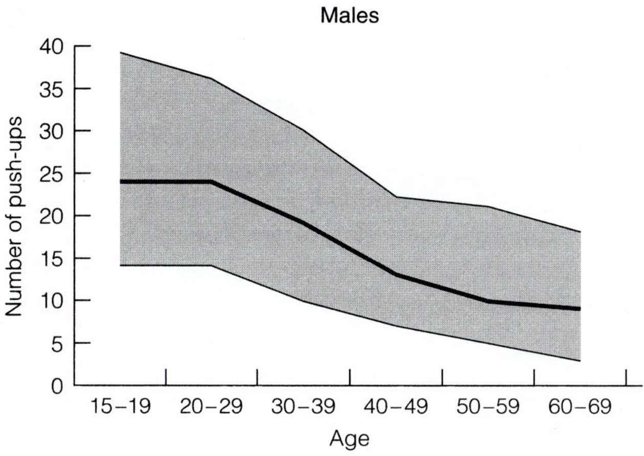

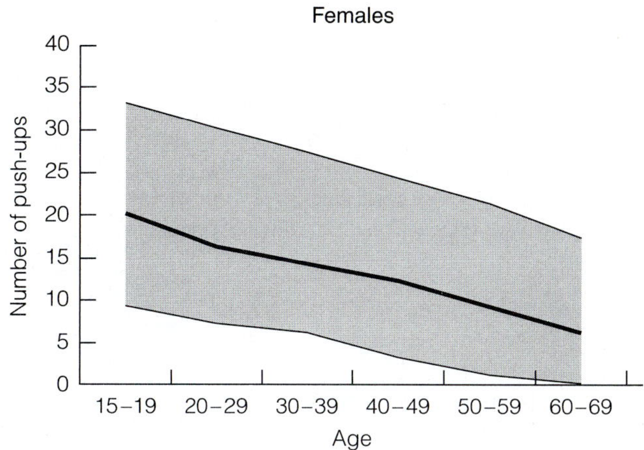

Figure 6.9 Normative data (15th, 50th, and 85th percentiles) from Canada on push-ups for males (left) and females (right).[74] Source: Data based on the Canada Fitness Survey, 1981.

hands are directly under her shoulders in the down position.

- A common error for females also is not keeping the back rigid.
- The score is the total number of push-ups to exhaustion. (See norms in Appendix A, Tables 29 and 33.) Figure 6.9 shows normative data from the Canadian Fitness Survey.[74]

Grip Strength Test with Hand Dynamometer

The grip strength test is used in the Canadian Physical Activity, Fitness & Lifestyle Appraisal program.[74] Both the right and left hands should be measured. (See norms in Appendix A, Table 30.)

The hand-grip *dynamometer* should be adjustable for any hand size.[92] A maximum reading pointer should be available to hold the reading until it is manually reset.

The purpose of the hand-grip dynamometer test is to measure the static strength of the grip squeezing muscles.[92–98] The hand-grip test is easy to administer, relatively inexpensive, portable, and highly reliable. There is some concern, however, that the hand-grip strength test does not correlate well with muscle mass.[98] Hand-grip strength tends to be higher in taller and heavier people.[95]

To perform the test (see Figure 6.10):[92–98]

- The person being tested should first dry and chalk both hands.
- The dynamometer should be adjusted and placed comfortably in the hand to be tested. The second joint of the hand should fit snugly under the handle, which should be gripped between the fingers and the palm at the base of the thumb.

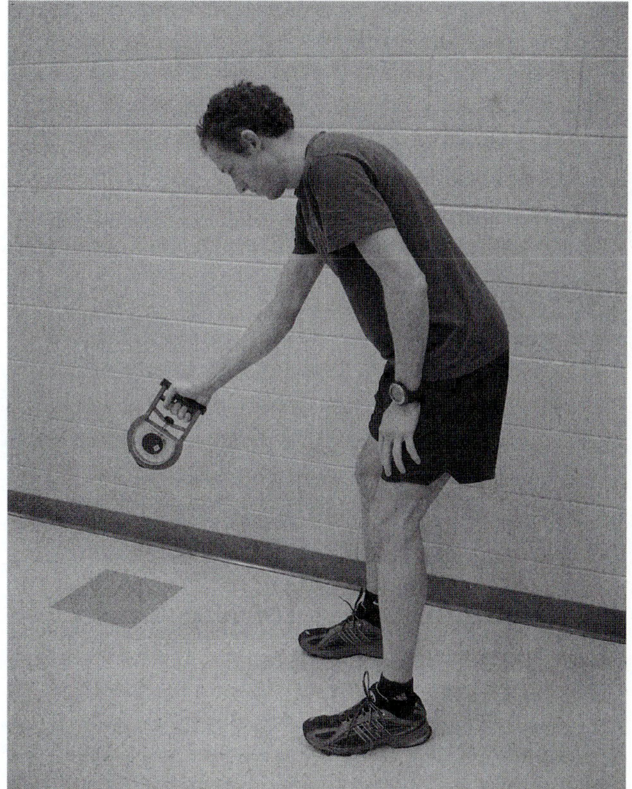

Figure 6.10 Grip strength test with hand dynamometer. Both the right and left hands should be measured. The purpose of the hand-grip dynamometer test is to measure the static strength of the grip-squeezing muscles.

- The person should assume a slightly bent forward position, with the hand to be tested out in front of her or his body. The person's hand and arm should be free of the body, not touching anything. The arm can be slightly bent.
- The test involves an all-out gripping effort for 2–3 seconds. No swinging or pumping of the arm is

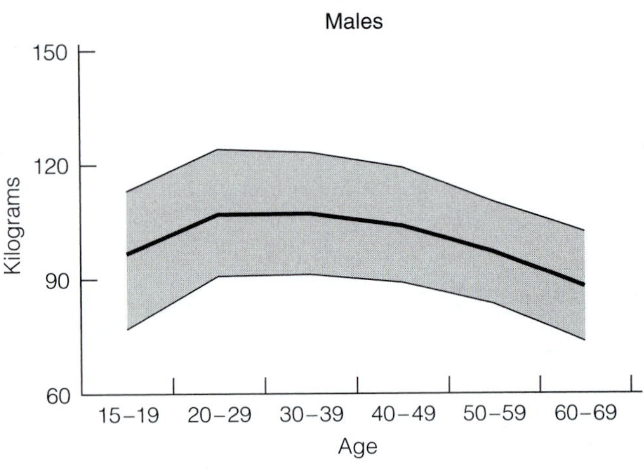

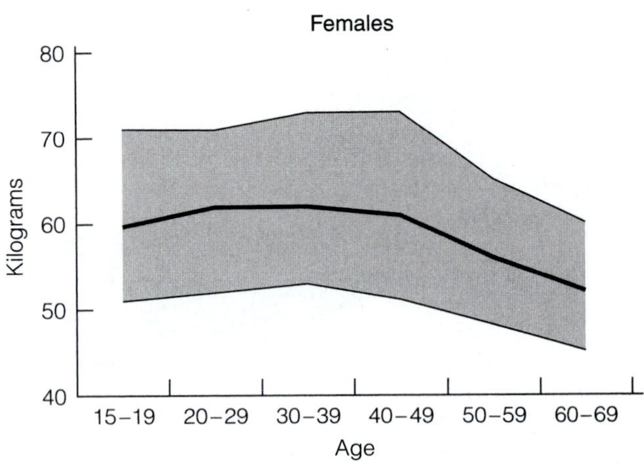

Figure 6.11 Normative data (15th, 50th, and 85th percentiles) from Canada on the grip strength of the right and left hands (combined) for males (left) and females (right).[79] Source: Data based on the Canada Fitness Survey, 1981.

allowed. The dial can be visible for motivational purposes.

- The score is the sum of the test of both hands, based on the best of 2–4 trials for each. The scale is read in kilograms.

Figure 6.11 shows normative data from the Canadian Fitness Survey.[74] Hand-grip strength diminishes with age and has been used as a risk factor for early death and disability.[96,97]

Bench-Press Strength and Endurance Tests

The two bench-press tests discussed in this chapter are the 1-RM test for strength and the YMCA test for muscular endurance.

Bench-Press 1-RM Test for Strength

The muscular strength of the major muscle groups can be measured with the one-repetition maximum test (1-RM) (the greatest weight that can be lifted once for a muscle group).[21,86,99] The objective of the 1-RM bench-press test is to test the strength of the muscles involved in arm extension (triceps, pectoralis major, anterior deltoid).

The test is performed as follows (see Figure 6.12):

- The person being tested should first be allowed to become familiar with the bench-press test by practicing a few lifts with light weights. For the test, the person lies on her or his back on a bench, with arms extended and hands gripping the bar, approximately shoulder-width apart. The bar is lowered until it touches the chest and then is pushed straight up, with maximum effort, until the arms are locked once again. The person breathes in as the weight is being lowered and breathes out during the weight-lifting phase. (This helps to prevent *Valsalva's maneuver*—the high buildup of blood pressure and decrease of blood flow to the brain, owing to the high pressures that are built up in the chest during weight lifting.)
- Free weights can be used with a spotter, but the use of machine weights allows for safer and easier testing sessions, especially when a series of trials is necessary to determine a true 1-RM.
- As many trials are allowed as it takes to achieve a true maximum effort. Each trial requires maximum effort for one repetition. Allow 1–3 minutes between trials.
- The best lifting score is divided by the person's weight, to derive a ratio. (See Appendix A, Table 35 for the norms.) Norms for strength-to-body-weight ratios are also available for the arm curl, lat pull-down, leg press, leg extension, and leg curl.[1] The Cooper Institute for Aerobic Research has published detailed norms for both men and women for the 1-RM bench-press and leg-press tests.[21,75] (See Appendix A, Tables 35 and 36.)

YMCA Bench-Press Test for Muscular Endurance

There are several types of weight-lifting tests used to test muscular endurance. One test of muscular endurance uses a fixed percentage of the person's body weight as the resistance, with the test score being the number of times this weight can be lifted.

Another method uses a fixed percentage (preferably 70%) of 1-RM or absolute strength for the resistance. Good norms have yet to be established, however, for these types of tests. On the basis of limited data, 12–15 repetitions at 70% of 1-RM appear optimal for most people; athletes should aim for 20–25 repetitions.

The YMCA has developed a bench-press test for muscular strength and endurance using an absolute weight. The advantage of this is that for certain occupations (fire fighting, construction, etc.), being able to work with absolute

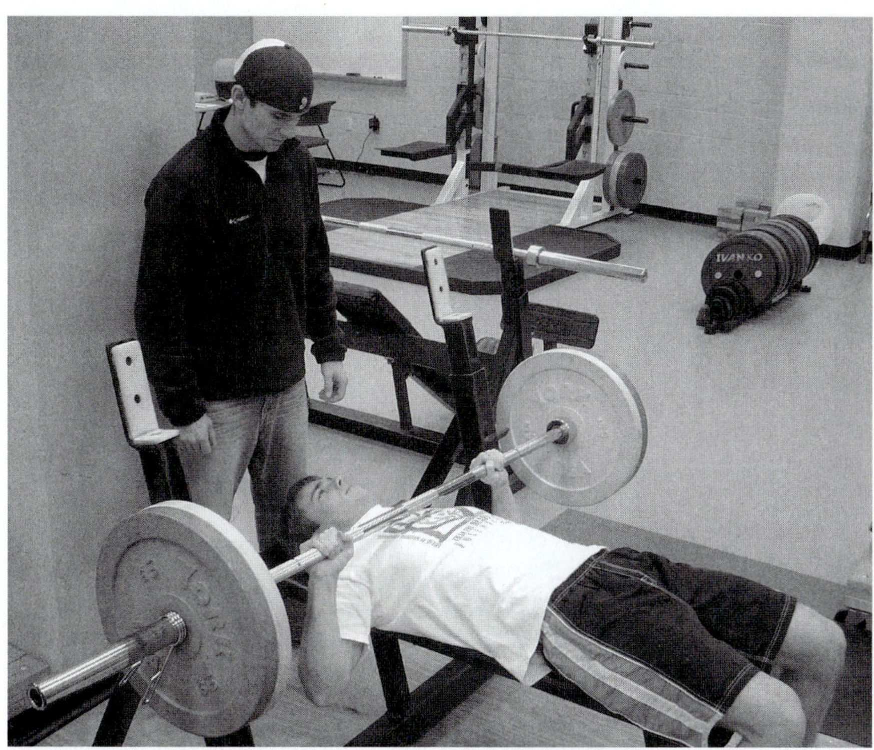

Figure 6.12 Bench-press 1-RM test for strength. Muscular strength can be measured with the one-repetition maximum (1-RM) test.

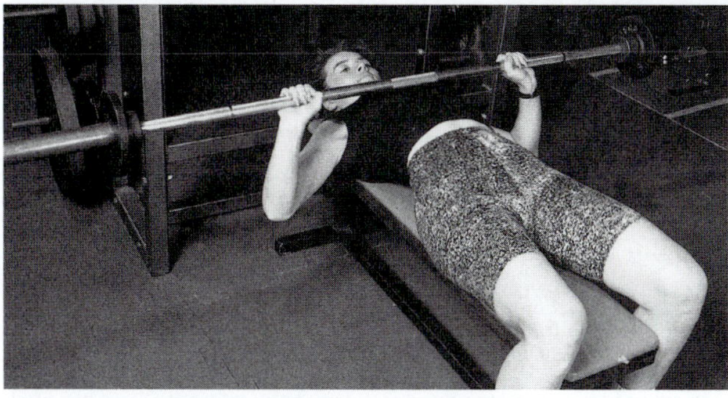

Figure 6.13 YMCA bench-press test for muscular endurance. The YMCA has developed a bench-press test for muscular strength and endurance using an absolute weight (35 pounds for females, 80 pounds for males).

weights is very important. The disadvantage of such a test is that it discriminates against lighter people.

The YMCA bench-press test uses the following steps (see Figure 6.13):[75]

- Use a 35-pound barbell for women and an 80-pound barbell for men.
- Set a metronome for 60 beats per minute.
- The person being tested lies on a bench, with feet on the floor.
- A spotter hands the weight to the person. The down position is the starting position (elbows flexed, hands shoulder-width apart, hands gripping the barbell, palms facing up).
- The person presses the barbell upward using free weights (with careful spotting) to fully extend the elbows. After each extension, the barbell is returned to the original down position, the bar touching the chest. The rhythm is kept by the metronome, each click representing a movement up or down (30 lifts per minute).
- The score is the number of successful repetitions. (See Appendix A, Table 37 for the norms.) The test is terminated when the person is unable to reach full extension of the elbows or breaks cadence and cannot keep up with the rhythm of the metronome. Emphasize *proper breathing technique* (breathe in as weight comes down to chest, breathe out as weight is pushed up).

Parallel-Bar Dips

This test is for measuring the muscular strength and endurance of the arms and shoulder girdle (triceps, deltoid, and pectoralis major and minor).

To perform the test, follow these steps[86] (see Figure 6.14):

- The person being tested should assume a straight-arm support position between parallel bars, with legs straight.
- The body should be lowered until the elbows form a right angle, with the upper arm (humerus) parallel to the floor. The tester should indicate to the person when the proper position is attained.
- The person should then push back up to a straight-arm support and continue the exercise for as many repetitions as possible.

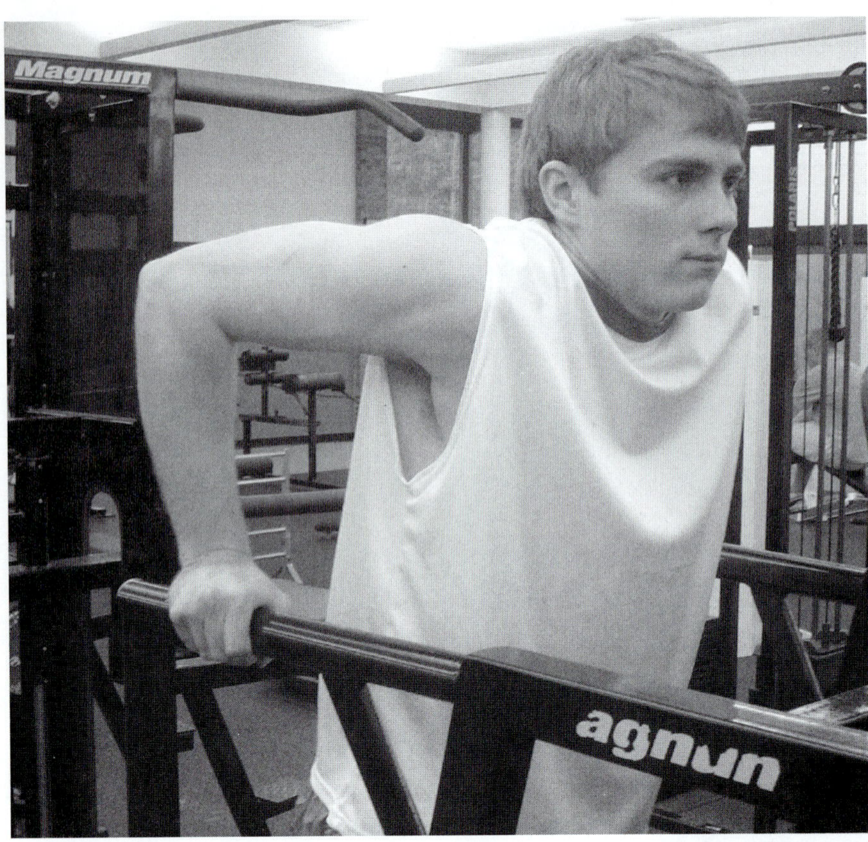

Figure 6.14 Parallel-bar dip. This test is for measuring the muscular strength and endurance of the arms and shoulder girdle (triceps, deltoid, and pectoralis major and minor).

- Rest is permitted in the up position. No swinging or kicking is allowed during the test.
- The score is the total number of bar dips until exhaustion. (Excellent is ≥25; good is 18–24, average is 9–17, fair is 4–8, and poor ≤3) (see Table 39 in Appendix A.)

FLEXIBILITY TESTING

As stated in Chapter 2, flexibility is the capacity of a joint to move fluidly through its full range of motion.[1] The major limitation to joint flexibility is tightness of soft tissue structures (joint capsule, muscles, tendons, ligaments). The muscle is the most important and modifiable structure in terms of improving flexibility.[100]

Flexibility is related to age and physical activity.[100] As a person ages, flexibility decreases, although this is due more to inactivity than to the aging process itself. Exercises to increase flexibility are discussed in Chapter 8.

Nearly all health-related physical fitness testing batteries now use the sit-and-reach test for a measure of flexibility. The sit-and-reach test is singled out because it has been noted in some clinical settings that people with low-back problems often have a restricted range of motion in the hamstring muscles and the lower back.

However, as noted earlier in this chapter, there are limited scientific data to back the assertion that people with poor flexibility are more likely to develop low-back pain in the future.[56] There is also some doubt as to whether the sit-and-reach test (all forms, including the modified test or the "back saver" test using one leg at a time) actually measures lower-back flexibility because studies have concluded it is actually a better measure of hamstring flexibility.[101–106] There probably is no test of flexibility that will discriminate between those who will develop low-back pain and those who will not.[105] Hip joint flexibility, however, is important for sports performance, and for this reason, the sit-and-reach test will probably remain as a component of most fitness test batteries.

Some researchers also feel that subjects with longer arms or shorter legs receive better ratings from the sit-and-reach test than those with shorter arms or longer legs, even though they may not have better lower-back and hamstring flexibility.

A modified sit-and-reach test has been proposed to deal with this problem.[106,107] In the modified protocol, subjects first sit with head, back, and hips against a wall; legs straight; and feet flat against a 12-inch box. While maintaining contact with the wall (including the head), the subject reaches as far forward as possible to determine a zero point and then conducts the typical sit-and-reach test, using this zero point as the reference. Norms for this modified test are available, but the test has not yet been adopted for use in national testing.[107]

Figure 6.15 shows the flexibility testing box that can be purchased or constructed before administering the test. It is 12 inches high and has an overlap in front so that minus readings can be obtained when the person being tested is unable to reach her or his feet. The various testing batteries

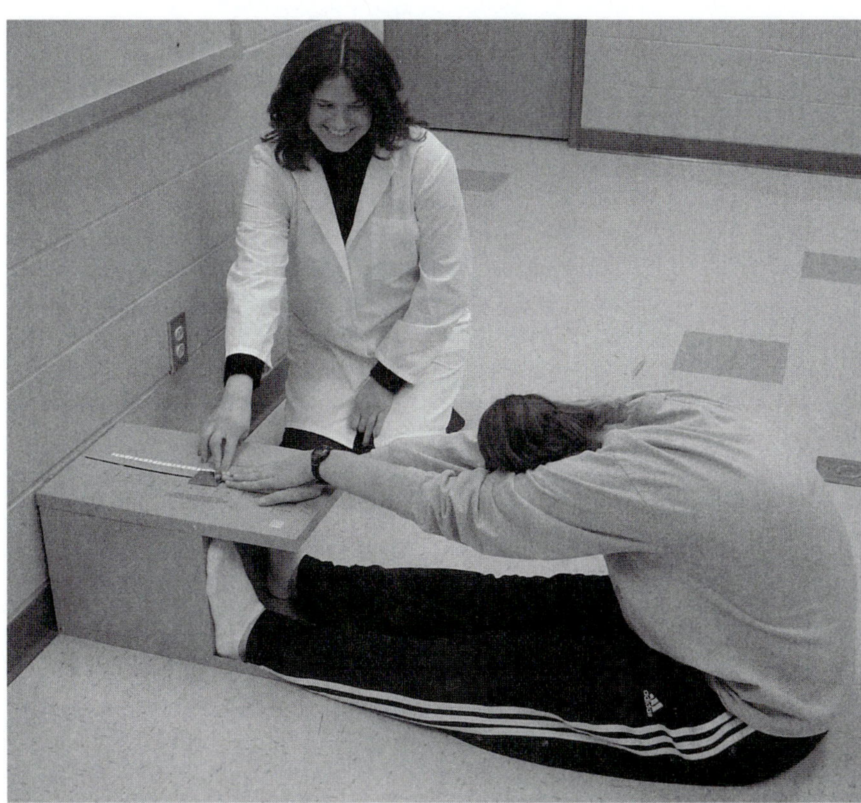

Figure 6.15 The purpose of the sit-and-reach flexibility test is to evaluate the flexibility of the lower back and posterior leg muscles. A flexibility box is required, which is 12 inches high and has an overlap toward the person being tested; it can be purchased or constructed.

use different measuring-scale settings at the footline. For standardization purposes, the footline can be set at zero, with plus or minus readings in inches or centimeters, measured from the zero line. (See norms in Appendix A, Tables 7, 8, 18, 19, 32.)

If a box is not available, a 12-inch bench with a ruler taped onto it can be used.

To perform the sit-and-reach test for flexibility (see Figure 6.15),[74]

- The person being tested should first warm up, using static stretching exercises (discussed in Chapter 8). A brisk walking or cycling warm-up is also advisable (on a treadmill or ergometer, if available). Warm muscles can stretch more safely.
- To start, the person being tested removes her or his shoes and sits facing the flexibility box, with knees fully extended, feet 4 inches apart. The feet should be flat, heels touching, against the end board.
- To perform the test, the arms are extended straight forward, with the hands placed on top of each other, fingertips perfectly even. The person reaches directly forward, palms down, as far as possible along the measuring scale, extending forward maximally four times, and then holds the position of maximum reach for 1–2 seconds.
- The score is the most distant point reached on the fourth trial, measured to the nearest centimeter (or quarter of an inch). The test administrator should remain close to the scale and note the most distant line touched by the fingertips of both hands. If the hands reach unevenly, the test should be readministered. The tester should place one hand lightly on the person's knees to ensure that they remain locked. Figure 6.16 shows normative data from the Canadian Fitness Survey.[74]

Many other methods are used in addition to the sit-and-reach test for measuring flexibility.[1] Flexibility of one joint does not necessarily indicate flexibility in other joints, and there is no general flexibility test for the whole body.[108] Various tests have been devised to measure the range of motion of each major body joint using a goniometer (a protractor-like device with arms that are attached to body segments using the joint as a fulcrum) and Leighton flexometer (360-degree dial with weighted pointer).[1] Other flexibility tests used for the general population include the shoulder rotation test, total body rotation test, and the shoulder flexibility test.[1,76]

Shoulder Flexibility Test

The shoulder joints are used in many different sports movements, work activities, and activities of daily living. To perform the shoulder flexibility test, follow these procedures after warming up:[107]

- Raise one arm, bend the elbow, and reach down across your back as far as possible.

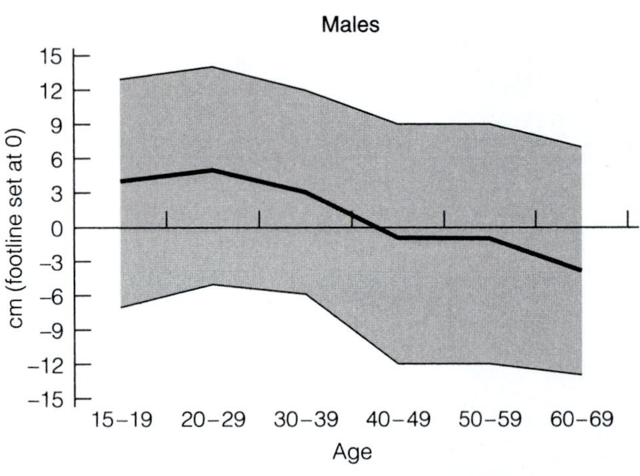

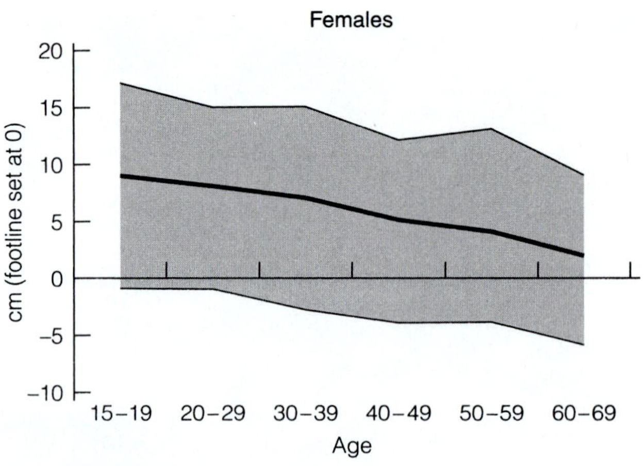

Figure 6.16 Normative data (15th, 50th, and 85th percentiles) from Canada on the sit-and-reach test (in centimeters) for males (left) and females (right).[79] Source: Data based on the Canada Fitness Survey, 1981.

- At the same time, extend the other arm down and then up behind the back, trying to cross the fingers over those of the other hand.
- Measure the distance of finger overlap to the nearest ¼ inch. If the fingers overlap, score as a plus; if they fail to meet, score as a minus.
- Repeat with the arms crossed in the opposite direction. Average the two scores, and use the norms in Physical Fitness Activity 6.2 for classification.

Trunk Rotation Flexibility Test

The trunk rotation flexibility test measures flexibility across several joints of the body. To perform this flexibility test, follow these procedures after warming up:[107]

- Tape two yardsticks to the wall at shoulder height, one right side up and the other upside down. Draw a line on the floor perpendicular to the wall at the 15-inch marks on the rulers.
- Stand with the feet shoulder-width apart, toes on the line, left shoulder to the wall at arm's length (fist closed).
- With the left arm at the side, raise the right arm to shoulder height and rotate the trunk to the right as far as possible, reaching along the yardstick with fist closed and palm down. Reach as far as possible, and then hold the final position for 2 seconds. During the test, the knees should be slightly bent, with the feet always pointing straight ahead and on the toe line.
- A partner should record the distance reached by the knuckle of the little finger to the nearest ¼ inch. Perform the test twice and average the two scores.
- Next perform the test facing the opposite direction using the upside-down yardstick (the greater the rotation, the higher the score). Perform two trials and average. Then average the scores from both directions and use the norms in Physical Fitness Activity 6.2 for classification.

VERTICAL JUMP

The vertical jump is a simple yet effective test for measuring muscular power and has been used as an index of sports training.[9,74] For example, in one large study of 774 Finnish males and females, vertical jumping height was found to be highest in those engaging in a variety of sports, compared to those who practiced aerobic training alone (e.g., running, cycling, or swimming) or who largely avoided all forms of exercise.[109]

The vertical jump test is included in the Canadian Physical Activity, Fitness & Lifestyle Appraisal (CPAFLA), and it can be scored in two ways: as a straight height jumped, and in terms of leg power.[74] In the test, clients take a standing position facing sideways to a wall on which a measuring tape has been attached. Special equipment for measuring vertical jump can also be used, as shown in Figure 6.17. Standing erect with the feet flat on the floor, the client reaches as high as possible on the tape, with the arm and fingers fully extended and the palm toward the wall. This is recorded as the beginning height. Standing about a foot away from the wall, the individual brings the arms downward and backward, while bending the knees to a balanced semisquat position, and then jumps as high as possible, with the arms moving forward and upward. The

TABLE 6.2 Age Group and Gender Classifications for Leg Power (watts) from Vertical Jump

Age	Excellent	Very Good	Good	Fair	Needs Improvement
15–19					
Male	≥4644	4185–4643	3858–4184	3323–3857	≤3322
Female	≥3167	2795–3166	2399–2794	2156–2398	≤2155
20–29					
Male	≥5094	4640–5093	4297–4639	3775–4296	≤3774
Female	≥3250	2804–3249	2478–2803	2271–2477	≤2270
30–39					
Male	≥4860	4389–4859	3967–4388	3485–3966	≤3484
Female	≥3193	2550–3192	2335–2549	2147–2334	≤2146
40–49					
Male	≥4320	3700–4319	3242–3699	2708–3241	≤2707
Female	≥2675	2288–2674	2101–2287	1688–2100	≤1687
50–59					
Male	≥4019	3567–4018	2937–3566	2512–2936	≤2511
Female	≥2559	2161–2558	1701–2160	1386–1700	≤1385
60–69					
Male	≥3764	3291–3763	2843–3290	2383–2842	≤2382
Female	≥2475	1718–2474	1317–1717	1198–1316	≤1197

Source: The Canadian Physical Activity, Fitness & Lifestyle Approach: CSEP's Health & Fitness Program's Health-Related Appraisal and Counselling Strategy, 3rd Edition © 2003. Reprinted with permission of the Canadian Society for Exercise Physiology.

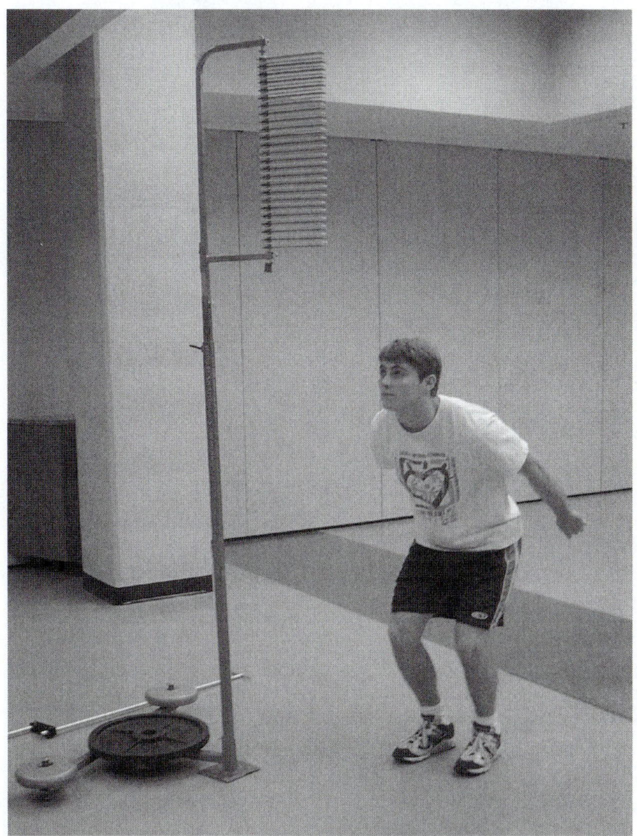

Figure 6.17 The vertical jump is a simple yet effective test for measuring the muscular power of the legs.

tape should be touched at the peak height of the jump with the fingers of the arm facing the wall. Record the highest jump from three trials, with a rest period of 10–15 seconds between trials. Subtract the beginning height from the peak height to determine the height jumped in centimeters.

An equation has been developed for the estimation of peak power from vertical squat jump distance and body mass.[74,110] To reduce variation between individuals the squat jump is recommended, in which subjects assume a bent-knee preparatory position, pause, and then jump vertically as high as possible. Peak power can be estimated from this equation:

$$\text{Peak power (watts)} = (60.7 \times \text{jump height, cm}) + (45.3 \times \text{body mass, kg}) - 2055$$

For example, if an individual that is 45 years old weighing 70 kg can jump 50 cm, then peak power can be estimated as follows:

$$(60.7 \times 50) + (45.3 \times 70) - 2055 = 4151 \text{ watts}$$

Table 6.2 indicates that leg power for this male would be ranked "very good."

In a study of 108 college male and female athletes and nonathletes, males averaged 4535 watts (standard deviation: 731), and females 3052 watts (standard deviation: 588).[110]

SPORTS MEDICINE INSIGHT

Searching for the Safest Abdominal Exercise Challenge

Abdominal exercises are used to improve appearance and posture, develop abdominal strength for sports performance (e.g., gymnastics and wrestling), and prevent and treat low-back pain. A wide variety of abdominal exercises and equipment have been used to maximize abdominal muscle strength and endurance. Concerns, however, have been raised regarding the safety of some abdominal exercises, especially in regard to compressive forces on the lumbar spine. As discussed earlier in this chapter, partial curl-ups (also called "abdominal crunches") have become popular because they appear to optimize abdominal muscle contraction without causing stress to the lower back.

Researchers at the University of Waterloo in Waterloo, Ontario, Canada, have published a series of studies in which they have tried to identify the safer and more effective exercises to train the abdominal muscles.[84,111] Twelve different abdominal exercises have been compared, while abdominal muscular action was measured with electromyographic (EMG) equipment and lumbar spinal compression was measured with specialized equipment. The 12 different abdominal exercises are depicted in Figure 6.18 and can be described as follows.[84]

a. *Straight-leg sit-up.* With the feet anchored and legs straight, and arms positioned with the fingers touching the ears, raise the torso to a vertical position and then return to the starting position.
b. *Bent-leg sit-up.* Similar to the straight-leg sit-up, except that the knees are bent to a 90-degree angle.
c. *Partial curl-up* (with feet anchored). Similar to bent-leg sit-up, except that the arms are straight at the sides of the torso, with the hands flat on the mat, the hands slide forward 10 cm, with the head, shoulders, and torso lifted off the mat.
d. *Partial curl-up* (with feet unanchored). Similar to (c) except that the feet are not anchored.

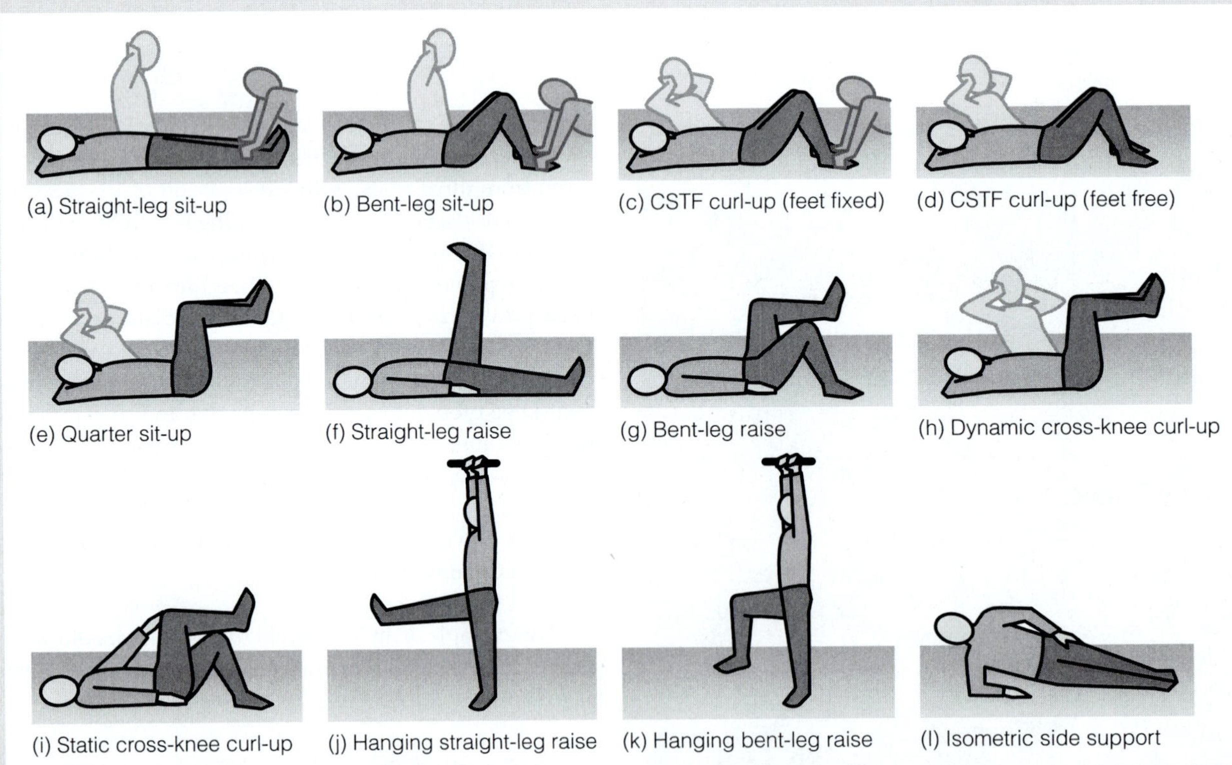

Figure 6.18 Twelve different abdominal exercises (see text for description). Source: Axler CT, McGill SM. Low back loads over a variety of abdominal exercises: Searching for the safest abdominal challenge. *Med Sci Sports Exerc* 29:804–10, 1997.

(continued)

SPORTS MEDICINE INSIGHT *(continued)*

Searching for the Safest Abdominal Exercise Challenge

e. *Quarter sit-up.* Similar to partial curl-up, except that both the knees and the hips are bent at a 90-degree angle (with legs and feet parallel to the ground), and the fingers touch the ears.

f. *Straight-leg raise.* While lying supine, put the hands under the lumbar region, raising both legs to a 90-degree angle off the mat.

g. *Bent-leg raise.* Similar to the straight-leg raise except that the knees are bent at a 90-degree angle, and the bent legs are raised until the hips achieve a 90-degree flexion angle.

h. *Dynamic cross-knee curl-up.* Similar to the quarter sit-up except that the torso is twisted to bring one elbow toward the opposite knee (contact of the elbow to the knee is not recommended).

i. *Static cross-knee curl-up.* Similar to the dynamic cross-knee curl-up except that the hand is brought up and over to the opposite knee and then pushed against the knee for 3 seconds.

j. *Hanging straight-leg raise.* While hanging from the hands on a chin-up bar, lift the straight leg to a horizontal position (avoid pelvic rotation).

k. *Hanging bent-leg raise.* Similar to the hanging straight-leg raise except that the knees are bent to a 90-degree angle.

l. *Isometric side support.* Raise the torso and legs off the mat, supported by only the right foot, right elbow, and right forearm.

The researchers found that no single abdominal exercise best recruited all of the abdominal muscles simultaneously, primarily because the obliques and the rectus abdominis have different functions.[84] Sit-ups with feet unanchored, legs elevated, or twists of the torso did not significantly increase the level of abdominal activity. Contrary to popular belief, no differences in lumbar spine compression or utilization of the hip flexor muscles (psoas) were observed in sit-ups performed with the legs bent versus with the legs straight. No sit-up exercise was considered ideal (defined as high abdominal activity with low lumbar spine compression), although the partial curl-ups came closest. Figure 6.19 shows that it is not possible to recommend just one type of abdominal exercise for all individuals. Several exercises are required to train the entire abdominal muscle area, and different exercises may best suit certain individuals based on their fitness level, training goals, injury history, and other personal characteristics. Several abdominal exercises are not recommended because of their high lumbar compression effects, including the supine straight- or bent-leg raises (f and g), the static cross-knee curl-up (i), and the hanging bent-leg raise (k).

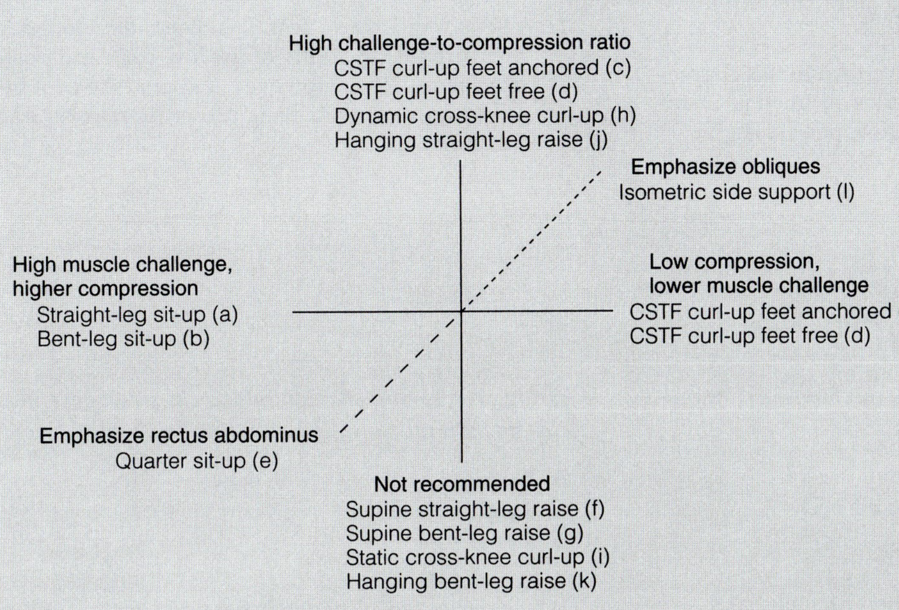

Figure 6.19 Depending on personal fitness goals and characteristics, several different abdominal exercises are recommended to train all of the abdominal muscles. Source: Axler CT, McGill SM. Low back loads over a variety of abdominal exercises: Searching for the safest abdominal challenge. *Med Sci Sports Exerc* 29:804–810, 1997.

SUMMARY

1. This chapter focused on the various musculoskeletal tests that are economical in terms of time, money, and ease of administration, and that are effectively health related. Musculoskeletal testing centers around the flexibility of the lower back and the muscular strength and endurance of the abdominals because of the widespread prevalence of low-back pain in the United States. Although more research is needed, exercises that can improve the musculoskeletal fitness of the lower trunk area in particular may sometimes help in the rehabilitation of low-back pain.
2. At some point in their lives, 60–80% of all Americans and Europeans will experience a bout of low-back pain ranging from a dull, annoying ache to intense and prolonged pain. There are many risk factors for low-back pain. Most low-back pain is due to unusual stresses on the muscles and ligaments that support the spine of people with weak muscles. When the body is in poor shape, weak spinal and abdominal muscles may be unable to support the spine properly during certain types of lifting or physical activities.
3. Prevention of low-back pain is based on recommendations for improving muscular fitness, weight loss, avoidance of smoking, proper lifting techniques, maintenance of proper posture, stress management, and comfortable seats and beds.
4. Recommendations to treat low-back pain are still being debated, but the most important goal is to return to normal activities as soon as it is safe. Bed rest usually isn't necessary and shouldn't last longer than 2–4 days.
5. The musculoskeletal tests described in this chapter are based on the testing batteries outlined in Chapter 3, with the norms listed in Appendix A.
6. The 1-minute timed bent-knee sit-up test has been traditionally used to evaluate abdominal muscle strength and endurance. However, there has been, and still is, dissatisfaction with it. Although research has indicated that the abdominals (spinal flexors) are active during a sit-up, hip flexor muscles are also involved. The use of the hip flexor muscles during the sit-up is potentially harmful to the lower back, especially when the feet are held down. Bending the knees does not appear to avoid this problem. Trunk curling exercises are helpful in increasing the strength and endurance of the abdominal muscles, and a new test using a curl-up motion has been developed.
7. The pull-up is used to measure the muscular strength and endurance of the arms and shoulder girdle. Because many children and youths cannot do a pull-up, a modified pull-up test has been developed.
8. Push-ups are used to assess upper-body muscle strength and endurance; separate tests have been developed for men and women.
9. The grip strength test with the hand dynamometer measures the static strength of the grip-squeezing muscles. However, because strength is specific to each muscle group, it is recommended that additional strength tests be administered.
10. The bench-press exercise can be used for a test either of *strength* (greatest amount of weight that can be lifted just once) or *endurance* (number of successful repetitions using an absolute weight).
11. The sit-and-reach test has been developed to measure the flexibility of the low-back and posterior leg muscles. However, it appears to be a better measure of hamstring rather than lower-back flexibility.

Review Questions

1. *Which one of the following is* **not** *recommended for prevention of low-back pain?*

   A. Lift by bending at the knees, not the waist
   B. Receive heavy objects close to the body
   C. Use a soft sleeping mattress
   D. Avoid cigarette smoking
   E. Exercise regularly to strengthen back and abdominal muscles

2. ***Clinical evidence (but not all research data) points toward lack of flexibility in the lower back and hamstring area combined with relatively weak ____ muscles as an important factor in low-back pain cases.***

   A. Neck **B.** Chest
   C. Thigh **D.** Abdominal
   E. Upper back

3. ***Which one of the following is not a risk factor for low-back pain?***

   A. Obesity
   B. Mental stress and anxiety

C. Sedentary lifestyle
D. Low muscular strength and flexibility
E. High-fat diet

4. *Which test is a measure of flexibility?*

A. One-minute timed sit-ups
B. Hand grip test
C. 1-RM bench-press test
D. Trunk rotation test

5. *____ is the ability of the muscles to apply a submaximal force repeatedly.*

A. Muscular strength B. Muscular endurance
C. Flexibility

6. *Which test is a measure of muscular strength?*

A. One-minute timed, bent-knee sit-ups
B. Pull-ups
C. 1-RM bench press
D. Sit and reach
E. YMCA bench press

7. *The abdominal muscles are spinal ____.*
A. Flexors B. Extensors

8. *What percent of all Americans and Europeans will experience a bout of low-back pain at some point in their lives?*

A. 10–20 B. 25–40
C. 45–60 D. 60–80
E. 85–100

9. *When the abdominals are weak, the pelvis can tilt forward, causing ____, or curvature of the lower back.*

A. Lordosis B. Spina bifida
C. Spina dorsalis D. Spina pedis

10. *There is good evidence that high-volume resistance training compared to aerobic training is associated with which one of the following health/fitness benefits?*
A. Improved function in older age
B. Increased HDL cholesterol
C. Decreased resting blood pressure
D. Decreased percent body fat
E. Increased $\dot{V}O_{2max}$

11. *Oxygen uptake during heavy resistance exercise seldom exceeds a threshold of ____% maximal aerobic power.*

A. 20 B. 33 C. 60 D. 80

12. *Many cases of low-back pain are self-limiting, with ____% of patients back to work within 1 week.*

A. 10 B. 20 C. 35 D. 40 E. 60

13. *The most common site of low-back pain is the ____ segment.*

A. L4–L5 B. T1–T2 C. C1–C2 D. T11–T12

14. *In the Canadian Standardized Test of Fitness, the grip strength test is conducted by measuring*

A. Both the right and left hands, tested separately
B. Both the right and left hands, tested together
C. The right hand alone
D. The left hand alone

15. *The back of the adult is composed of ____ vertebrae.*

A. 15 B. 24 C. 28 D. 32

16. *The YMCA bench-press test for muscular endurance uses a ____-pound bar for women.*

A. 10 B. 25 C. 35 D. 55 E. 80

17. *The peak age for low-back pain is*

A. 15 B. 25 C. 40 D. 65 E. 80

18. *An important low-back pain treatment method according to the U.S. Agency for Health Care Policy and Research is*

A. Bed rest B. Acupuncture
C. Return to normal activities as soon as possible D. Intensive back exercise

19. *Skeletal muscle is the body's most abundant tissue, making up about 23% of a female's body weight and ____% of a male's.*

A. 15 B. 25 C. 40 D. 65 E. 80

20. *Which type of worker is at high risk for low-back pain?*

A. Teacher B. Bus driver
C. Attorney D. Banker
E. Medical doctor

Answers

1. C	11. C
2. D	12. E
3. E	13. A
4. D	14. A
5. B	15. B
6. C	16. C
7. A	17. C
8. D	18. C
9. A	19. C
10. A	20. B

REFERENCES

1. Heyward VH. *Advanced Fitness Assessment and Exercise Prescription* (4th ed.). Champaign, IL: Human Kinetics, 2002.
2. Maud PJ, Foster C. *Physiological Assessment of Human Fitness.* Champaign, IL: Human Kinetics, 1995.
3. Davies GJ. *A Compendium of Isokinetics in Clinical Usage and Rehabilitation Techniques.* (4th ed.). Onalaska, Wisconsin: S & S Publishers, 1992.
4. American College of Sports Medicine, Position Stand. The recommended quantity and quality of exercise for developing and maintaining cardiorespiratory and muscular fitness, and flexibility in healthy adults. *Med Sci Sports Exerc* 30:975–991, 1998.
5. Fletcher GF, Balady G, Froelicher VF, Hartley LH, Haskell WL, Pollock ML. Exercise standards: A statement for healthcare professionals from the American Heart Association. *Circulation* 91:580–615, 1995.
6. U.S. Department of Health and Human Services. *Physical Activity and Health: A Report of the Surgeon General.* Atlanta, GA: U.S. Department of Health and Human Services, Centers for Disease Control and Prevention, National Center for Chronic Disease Prevention and Health Promotion, 1996.
7. Pollock ML, Vincent ML. Resistance training for health. *The President's Council on Physical Fitness and Sports Research Digest.* Series 2, No. 8, December 1996.
8. Fleck SJ, Kraemer WJ. *Designing Resistance Training Programs.* Champaign, IL: Human Kinetics Books, 2003.
9. Baechle TR, Earle RW. *Essentials of Strength Training and Conditioning* (2nd ed.). Champaign, IL: Human Kinetics, 2000.
10. Payne N, Gledhill N, Katzmarzyk PT, Jamnik V, Ferguson S. Health implications of musculoskeletal fitness. *Can J Appl Physiol* 25:114–126, 2000.
11. Kohrt WM, Bloomfield SA, Little KD, Nelson ME, Yingling VR, ACSM. American College of Sports Medicine Position Stand: Physical activity and bone health. *Med Sci Sports Exerc* 36:1985–1990, 2004.
12. Brandon LJ, Gaasch D, Boyette L, Lloyd A. Strength training for older adults: Benefits, guidelines, and adherence. *ACSM's Health & Fitness Journal,* 4(6):12–16, 2000.
13. Brill PA, Macera CA, Davis DR, Blair SN, Gordon N. Muscular strength and physical function. *Med Sci Sports Exerc* 32:412–416, 2000.
14. Hurley BF, Hagberg JM. Optimizing health in older persons: Aerobic or strength training? *Exerc Sport Sci Rev* 26:61–89, 1998.
15. American College of Sports Medicine, Position Stand. Exercise and physical activity for older adults. *Med Sci Sports Exerc* 30:992–1008, 1998.
16. Borst SE. Interventions for sarcopenia and muscle weakness in older people. *Age Aging* 33:548–555, 2004.
17. Pollock ML, Franklin BA, Balady GJ, Chaitman BL, Fleg JL, Fletcher B, Limacher M, Pina IL, Stein RA, Williams M, Bazzarre T. Resistance exercise in individuals with and without cardiovascular disease: Benefits, rationale, safety, and prescription. An advisory from the Committee on Exercise, Rehabilitation, and Prevention, Council on Clinical Cardiology, American Heart Association. *Circulation* 101:828–833, 2000.
18. Tesch PA. Training for bodybuilding. In Komi PV (ed.). *Strength and Power in Sport: The Encyclopaedia of Sports Medicine.* Oxford: Blackwell Scientific Publications, 1992.
19. Fleck SJ. Cardiovascular response to strength training. In Komi PV (ed.). *Strength and Power in Sport: The Encyclopaedia of Sports Medicine.* Oxford: Blackwell Scientific Publications, 1992.
20. Prabhakaran B, Dowling EA, Branch JD, Swain DP, Leutholtz BC. Effect of 14 weeks of resistance training on lipid profile and body fat percentage in premenopausal women. *Br J Sports Med* 33:190–195, 1999.
21. American College of Sports Medicine. *ACSM's Guidelines for Graded Exercise Testing and Prescription* (7th ed.). Philadelphia: Lippincott Williams & Wilkins, 2005.
22. Alter MJ. *Science of Flexibility* (3rd ed.). Champaign, IL: Human Kinetics, 2004.
23. Witvrouw E, Mahieu N, Danneels L, McNair P. Stretching and injury prevention: An obscure relationship. *Sports Med* 34:443–449, 2004.
24. Worrell T, Perrin D, Gansneder B, Gieck J. Comparison of isokinetic strength and flexibility measures between injured and noninjured athletes. *J Orthop Sports Phys Ther* 13:118–125, 1991.
25. Plowman SA. Physical activity, physical fitness, and low back pain. *Exerc Sport Sci Rev* 20:221–242, 1992.
26. Biering-Sorensen F, Bendix T, Jorgensen K, Manniche C, Nielsen H. Physical activity, fitness and back pain. In Bouchard C, Shephard RJ (eds.). *Exercise, Fitness, and Health: A Consensus of Current Knowledge.* Champaign, IL: Human Kinetics, 1994.
27. Deyo RA, Weinstein JN. Low back pain. *N Engl J Med* 344:363–370, 2001.
28. Agency for Health Care Policy and Research. *Clinical Practice Guideline, Acute Low Back Problems in Adults.* Silver Spring, MD: Publications Clearinghouse, 1994.
29. Guo HR, Tanaka S, Halperin WE, Cameron LL. Back pain prevalence in US industry and estimates of lost workdays. *Am J Public Health* 89:1029–1035, 1999.
30. Park C, Wagener D. Health conditions among the currently employed: United States, 1988. National Center for Health Statistics, (PHS) 93-1412. Washington, DC: Government Printing Office, 1993.
31. Lawrence RC, Helmick CG, Arnett FC, Deyo RA, Felson DT, Giannini EH, Heyse SP, Hirsch R, Hochberg MC, Hunder GG, Liang MH, Pillemer SR, Steen VD, Wolfe F. Estimates of the prevalence of arthritis and selected musculoskeletal disorders in the United States. *Arthritis Rheum* 41:778–799, 1998.
32. U.S. Department of Health and Human Services. *Healthy People 2010* (Conference edition, in two volumes). Washington, DC: January 2000. (http://www.health.gov/healthypeople/ or call 1-800-367-4725.)
33. Jones GT, Macfarlane GJ. Epidemiology of low back pain in children and adolescents. *Arch Dis Child* 90:312–316, 2005.
34. Harreby M, Neergaard K, Hesseisoe G, Kjer J. Are radiologic changes in the thoracic and lumbar spine of adolescents risk factors for low back pain in adults? *Spine* 20:2298–2302, 1995.
35. YMCA of the USA. *YMCA Healthy Back Book.* Champaign, IL: Human Kinetics, 1994.
36. Andersson GB. Epidemiological features of chronic low-back pain. *Lancet* 354:581–585, 1999.
37. Takemasa R, Yamamoto H, Tani T. Trunk muscle strength in and effect of trunk muscle exercises for patients with chronic low back pain. *Spine* 20:2522–2530, 1995.
38. Marras WS. Occupational low back disorder causation and control. *Ergonomics* 43:880–902, 2000.
39. Keyserling WM. Workplace risk factors and occupational musculoskeletal disorders, Part 1: A review of biomechanical and psychophysical research on risk factors associated with low-back pain. *AIHAJ* 61:39–50, 2000.
40. Feuerstein M, Berkowitz SM, Huang GD. Predictors of occupational low back disability: Implications for secondary prevention. *J Occup Environ Med* 41:1024–1031, 1999.

41. Kujala UM, Taimela S, Viljanen T, Jutila H, Viitasalo JT, Videman T, Battie MC. Physical loading and performance as predictors of back pain in healthy adults. A 5-year prospective study. *Eur J Appl Physiol* 73:452–458, 1996.

42. van Poppel MN, Hooftman WE, Koes BW. An update of a systematic review of controlled clinical trials on the primary prevention of back pain at the workplace. *Occup Med* (Lond) 54:345–352, 2004.

43. Toda Y, Segal N, Toda T, Morimoto T, Ogawa R. Lean body mass and body fat distribution in participants with chronic low back pain. *Arch Intern Med* 160:3265–3269, 2000.

44. Dreisinger TE, Nelson B. Management of back pain in athletes. *Sports Med* 21:313–319, 1996.

45. Videman T, Sarna S, Battié MC, Koskinen S, Gill K, Paananen H, Gibbons L. The long-term effects of physical loading and exercise lifestyles on back-related symptoms, disability, and spinal pathology among men. *Spine* 20:699–709, 1995.

46. Bono CM. Low-back pain in athletes. *J Bone Joint Surg Am* 86-A(2):382–396, 2004.

47. Nuwayhid IA, Stewart W, Johnson JV. Work activities and the onset of first-time low back pain among New York City firefighters. *Am J Epidemiol* 137:539–548, 1993.

48. Lee J-H, Ooi Y, Nakamura K. Measurement of muscle strength of the trunk and the lower extremities in subjects with history of low back pain. *Spine* 20:1994–1996, 1995.

49. Salminen JJ, Erkinalo M, Laine M, Pentti J. Low back pain in the young: A prospective three-year follow-up study of subjects with and without low back pain. *Spine* 19:2101–2108, 1994.

50. Ready AE, Boreskie SL, Law SA, Russell R. Fitness and lifestyle parameters fail to predict back injuries in nurses. *Can J Appl Physiol* 18:80–90, 1993.

51. Battié MC, Bigos SJ, Fisher LS, et al. The role of spinal flexibility in back pain complaints within industry. *Spine* 15:768–773, 1990.

52. Leino P, Aro S, Hasan J. Trunk muscle function and low back disorders: A ten-year follow-up study. *J Chron Dis* 40:289–296, 1987.

53. McGill SM. Low back stability: From formal description to issues for performance and rehabilitation. *Exerc Sport Sci Rev* 29:26–31, 2001.

54. Helewa A, Goldsmith CH, Lee P, Smythe HA, Forwell L. Does strengthening the abdominal muscles prevent low back pain—a randomized controlled trial. *J Rheumatol* 26:1808–1815, 1999.

55. Kujala UM, Salminen JJ, Taimela S, et al. Subject characteristics and low back pain in young athletes and nonathletes. *Med Sci Sports Exerc* 24:627–632, 1992.

56. Jackson AW, Morrow JR, Brill P, Kohl HW, Gordon NF, Blair SN. Relations of sit-up and sit-and-reach tests to low back pain in adults. *Orthop Sports Phys Ther* 27:22–26, 1998.

57. Carpenter DM, Nelson BW. Low back strengthening for the prevention and treatment of low back pain. *Med Sci Sports Exerc* 31:18–24, 1999.

58. Rainville J, Hartigan C, Martinez E, Limke J, Jouve C, Finno M. Exercise as a treatment for chronic low back pain. *Spine J* 4:106–115, 2004.

59. Van Tulder M, Malmivaara A, Esmail R, Koes B. Exercise therapy for low back pain: A systematic review within the framework of the Cochrane collaboration back review group. *Spine* 25:2784–2796, 2000.

60. Atlas SJ, Deyo RA. Evaluating and managing acute low back pain in the primary care setting. *J Gen Intern Med* 16:120–131, 2001.

61. Casazza BA, Young JL, Herring SA. The role of exercise in the prevention and management of acute low back pain. *Occup Med* 13:47–60, 1998.

62. Indahl A, Haldorsen EH, Holm S, Reikeras O, Ursin H. Five-year follow-up study of a controlled clinical trial using light mobilization and an informative approach to low back pain. *Spine* 23:2625–2630, 1998.

63. Moffett JK, Torgerson D, Bell-Syer S, Jackson D, Llewlyn-Phillips H, Farrin A, Barber J. Randomized controlled trial of exercise for low back pain: Clinical outcomes, costs, and preferences. *BMJ* 319:279–283, 1999.

64. Manniche C, Hesselsoe G, Bentzen L, Christensen I, Lundberg E. Clinical trial of intensive muscle training for chronic low back pain. *Lancet*, December 24/31:1473–1476, 1988.

65. Manniche C, Asmussen K, Lauritsen B, et al. Intensive dynamic back exercises with or without hyperextension in chronic back pain after surgery for lumbar disc protrusion: A clinical trial. *Spine* 18:587–594, 1993.

66. Risch SV, Norvell NK, Pollock ML, Risch ED, et al. Lumbar strengthening in chronic low back pain patients: Physiologic and psychological benefits. *Spine* 18:232–238, 1993.

67. Kraus H, Raab W. *Hypokinetic Disease*. Springfield, IL: Charles C. Thomas, 1961.

68. Indahl A, Velund L, Reikeraas O. Good prognosis for low back pain when left untampered: A randomized clinical trial. *Spine* 20:473–477, 1995.

69. Lahad A, Malter AD, Berg AO, Deyo RA. The effectiveness of four interventions for the prevention of low back pain. *JAMA* 272:1286–1291, 1994.

70. Malmivaara A, Häkkinen U, Aro T, et al. The treatment of acute low back pain: Bed rest, exercises, or ordinary activity? *N Engl J Med* 332:351–355, 1995.

71. Cherkin DC, Deyo RA, Wheeler K, Ciol MA. Physician views about treating low back pain: The results of a national survey. *Spine* 20:1–10, 1995.

72. Nelson BE, O'Reilly E, Miller M. The clinical effects of intensive, specific exercise on chronic low-back pain: A controlled study of 895 consecutive patients with one year follow-up. *Orthopedics* 18:971–981, 1995.

73. Bayramoglu M, Akman MN, Kilinc S, Cetin N, Yavuz N, Ozker R. Isokinetic measurement of trunk muscle strength in women with chronic low-back pain. *Am J Phys Med Rehabil* 80:650-655, 2001.

74. Canadian Society for Exercise Physiology. *The Canadian Physical Activity, Fitness & Lifestyle Appraisal*. Ottawa, Ontario: Author, 1996; 2nd edition, 1998; 3rd edition, 2003. (www.csep.ca.)

75. Golding, LH. *YMCA Fitness Testing and Assessment Manual* (4th ed.). Champaign, IL: Human Kinetics, 2000.

76. *The Cooper Institute Fitnessgram/Activitygram Test Adminsitration Manual*. Champaign, IL: Human Kinetics, 2004.

77. President's Council on Physical Fitness and Sports. *Get Fit: A Handbook for Youth Ages 6–17*. Washington, DC: President's Council on Physical Fitness and Sports, 2001.

78. Jones MA, Stratton G. Muscle function assessment in children. *Acta Paediatr* 89:753–761, 2000.

79. Sparling PB, Millard-Stafford M, Snow TK. Development of a cadence curl-up test for college students. *Res Q Exerc Sport* 68:309–316, 1997.

80. Diener MH, Golding LA, Diener D. Validity and reliability of a one-minute half sit-up test of abdominal strength and endurance. *Sports Med Train Rehab* 6:105–119, 1995.

81. Robertson LD, Magnusdottir H. Evaluation of criteria associated with abdominal fitness testing. *Res Q Exerc Sport* 58:355–359, 1987.

82. Hall GL, Hetzler RK, Perrin D, Weltman A. Relationship of timed sit-up tests to isokinetic abdominal strength. *Res Q Exerc Sport* 63:80–84, 1992.

83. Faulkner RA, Sprigings EJ, McQuarrie A, Bell RD. A partial curl-up protocol for adults based on an analysis of two procedures. *Can J Sport Sci* 14:135–141, 1989.
84. Axler CT, McGill SM. Low back loads over a variety of abdominal exercises: Searching for the safest abdominal challenge. *Med Sci Sports Exerc* 29:804–810, 1997.
85. Alaranta H, Hurri H, Heliovaara M, Soukka A, Harju R. Nondynamometric trunk performance tests: Reliability and normative data. *Scand J Rehabil Med* 26:211–215, 1994.
86. Johnson BL, Nelson JK. *Practical Measurements for Evaluation in Physical Education.* Minneapolis: Burgess Publishing Co., 1979.
87. Pate RR, Ross JG, Baumgartner TA, Sparks RE. The National Children and Youth Fitness Study II. The modified pull-up test. *JOPERD* November/December, 1987, 71–73.
88. Cotten DJ. An analysis of the NCYFS II modified pull-up test. *Res Q Exerc Sport* 61:272–274, 1990.
89. Pate RR, Burgess ML, Woods JA, Ross JG, Baumgartner T. Validity of field tests of upper body muscular strength. *Res Q Exerc Sport* 64:17–24, 1993.
90. Rutherford WJ, Corbin CB. Validation of criterion-referenced standards for tests of arm and shoulder girdle strength and endurance. *Res Q Exerc Sport* 65:110–119, 1994.
91. Reiff GG, Dixon WR, Jacoby D, Ye GX, Spain CC, Hunsicker PA. The President's Council on Physical Fitness and Sports 1985: National School Population Fitness Survey. HHS-Office of the Assistant Secretary for Health, Research Project 282-82-0086, University of Michigan, 1986.
92. Phillips DA, Hornak JE. *Measurement and Evaluation in Physical Education.* New York: John Wiley & Sons, 1979.
93. Larson LA. International Committee for the Standardization of Physical Fitness Tests. *Fitness, Health, and Work Capacity: International Standards for Assessment.* New York: MacMillian Publishing Co., Inc., 1974.
94. Fiutko R. The comparison study of grip strength in male populations of Kuwait and Poland. *J Sports Med* 27:497–500, 1987.
95. Chatterjee S, Chowdhuri BJ. Comparison of grip strength and isometric endurance between the right and left hands of men and their relationship with age and other physical parameters. *J Hum Ergol (Tokyo)* 20:41–50, 1991.
96. Hughes S, Gibbs J, Dunlop D, Edelman P, Singer R, Change RW. Predictors of decline in manual performance in older adults. *J Am Geriatr Soc* 45:905–910, 1997.
97. Laukkanen P, Heikkinen E, Kauppinen M. Muscle strength and mobility as predictors of survival in 75 84-year-old people. *Age Ageing* 24:468–473, 1995.
98. Johnson MJ, Friedl KE, Frykman PN, Moore RJ. Loss of muscle mass is poorly reflected in grip strength performance in healthy young men. *Med Sci Sports Exerc* 26:235–240, 1994.
99. Brzycki M. Strength testing: Predicting a one-rep max from reps-to-fatigue. *JOPERD* January 1993, 88–90.
100. Hein V, Jurimae T. Measurement and evaluation of trunk forward flexibility. *Sports Med Train Rehab* 7:1–6, 1996.
101. Jackson AW, Baker AA. The relationship of the sit and reach test to criterion measures of hamstring and back flexibility in young females. *Res Q Exerc Sport* 57:183–186, 1986.
102. Jackson AW, Langford NJ. The criterion-related validity of the sit and reach test: Replication and extension of previous findings. *Res Q Exerc Sport* 60:384–387, 1989.
103. Magnusson SP, Simonsen EB, Aagaard P, Boesen J, Johannsen F, Kjaer M. Determinants of musculoskeletal flexibility: Viscoelastic properties, cross-sectional area, EMG and stretch tolerance. *Scand J Med Sci Sports* 7:195–202, 1997.
104. Minkler S, Patterson P. The validity of the modified sit-and-reach test in college-age students. *Res Q Exerc Sport* 65:189–192, 1994.
105. Patterson P, Wiksten DL, Ray L, Flanders C, Sanphy D. The validity and reliability of the back saver sit-and-reach test in middle school girls and boys. *Res Q Exerc Sport* 67:448–451, 1996.
106. Hui SSC, Yuen PY. Validity of the modified back-saver sit-and-reach test: A comparison with other protocols. *Med Sci Sports Exerc* 32:1655–1659, 2000.
107. Hoeger WWK, Hoeger SA. *Principles and Labs for Fitness and Wellness.* Belmont, CA: Wadsworth/Thompson Learning, 2004.
108. Shephard RJ, Berridge M, Montelpare W. On the generality of the "sit and reach" test: An analysis of flexibility data for an aging population. *Res Q Exerc Sport* 61:326–330, 1990.
109. Kujala UM, Viljanen T, Taimela S, Viitasalo JT. Physical activity, $\dot{V}O_{2max}$, and jumping height in an urban population. *Med Sci Sports Exerc* 26:889–895, 1994.
110. Sayers SP, Harackiewicz DV, Harman EA, Frykman PN, Rosenstein MT. Cross-validation of three jump power equations. *Med Sci Sports Exerc* 31:572–577, 1999.
111. McGill SM. The mechanics of torso flexion: Sit-ups and standing dynamic flexion maneuvers. *Clin Biochem* 10:184–192, 1995.

PHYSICAL FITNESS ACTIVITY 6.1

Rating Your Posture

Good posture depends on good muscle tone and balance throughout your body and flexible but sturdy joints. There are a number of poor postural habits and practices in standing, sitting, walking, and working which if indulged over the years will cause strain and changes in your postural muscles. Some muscles will lose their tone, while others become shortened and tight. This results in malalignment of the body segments. Habits and practices causing poor posture include sitting and standing with the back curved or slumped, sleeping with a sagging mattress, insufficient sleep and chronic fatigue, general muscle weakness and tightness due to lack of strengthening and stretching exercises, excess body weight, wearing poorly designed shoes, and a poor mental attitude (e.g., lack of self-confidence). See Figure 6.20 for an example of good standing posture.

Use Figure 6.21 to grade your posture. Follow these steps:

- Dress in a swimsuit, with long hair pinned up or away from the ears.
- Breathe deeply and exhale several times to feel relaxed before having your posture checked.
- Stand in front of a mirror. Do not stand too rigidly or too relaxed. With the help of a friend, score your posture using Figure 6.21. Use the posture norms given in the table for classification.

Posture Norms	Points
Perfect posture	80
Good posture	65–79
Fair posture	35–64*
Poor posture	Less than 35*

*Strengthen back and abdominal muscles, and work on hip and neck flexibility.

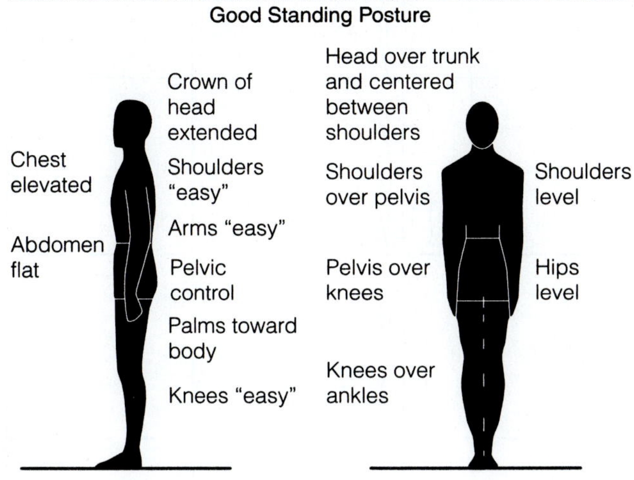

Figure 6.20 Good posture is the correct alignment and balance of the various body segments; the head balanced over the shoulders and trunk, the trunk balanced over the thighs, the thighs balanced over the knees, which are balanced over the feet.

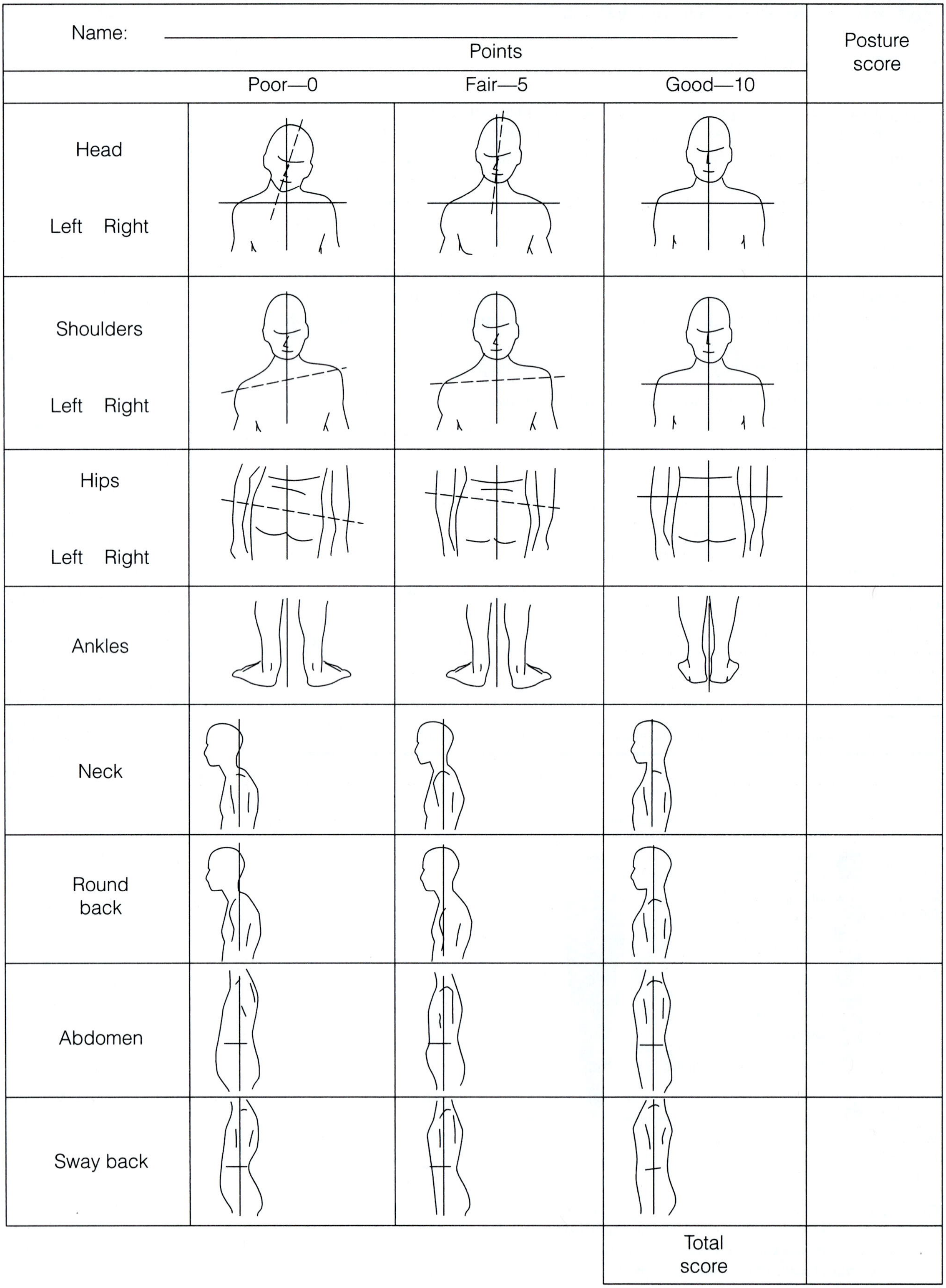

Name: ______________________	Points			Posture score
	Poor—0	Fair—5	Good—10	
Head Left Right				
Shoulders Left Right				
Hips Left Right				
Ankles				
Neck				
Round back				
Abdomen				
Sway back				
			Total score	

Figure 6.21 Worksheet to grade your posture.

PHYSICAL FITNESS ACTIVITY 6.2

Assessment of Muscular Fitness

With the help of your class instructor, take each of the tests of muscular fitness listed below. After taking each test, record your score, and then use the norms in Table 6.3 to classify your results.

Fitness Test	Your Score	Classification
1-min sit-ups		
Partial curl-ups		
Pull-ups		
Parallel bar dips		
Push-ups		
Grip (right and left) strength (kg)		
1-RM bench press (weight ratio)		
Vertical jump (kg · m/second)		
Sit-and-reach test (inches, footline at 0)		
Shoulder flexibility test (inches, average of left and right sides)		
Trunk rotation test (inches, average of left and right sides)		

TABLE 6.3 Norms for Muscular Endurance, Muscular Strength, and Flexibility Tests, College Students*

Fitness Test	Gender	Poor	Below Average	Average	Above Average	Excellent
1-min sit-ups	Male	<33	33–37	38–41	42–47	>47
	Female	<27	27–31	32–35	36–41	>41
Partial curl-ups	Male	<16	16–20	21–22	23–24	25
	Female	<16	16–20	21–22	23–24	25
Pull-ups	Male	<5	5–7	8–11	12–14	>14
	Female	<0	<0	<0	1	>1
Parallel-bar dips	Male	<4	4–8	9–13	14–20	>20
Push-ups	Male	<18	18–22	23–28	29–38	>38
	Female	<17	12–17	18–24	24–32	>32
Grip (right and left) strength (kg)	Male	<84	84–94	95–102	103–112	>112
	Female	<54	54–58	59–63	64–70	>70
1-RM bench press (weight ratio)	Male	<0.77	0.77–0.89	0.90–1.06	1.07–1.19	>1.19
	Female	<0.42	0.42–0.53	0.54–0.58	0.59–0.65	>0.65
Vertical jump (kg · m/second)	Male	<61	61–72	73–87	88–103	>103
	Female	<51	51–57	58–66	67–73	>73
Sit-and-reach test (inches, footline at 0)	Male & female	<−3	−3 to −0.25	0–3.75	4–6.75	≥7
Shoulder flexibility test (inches, average of left and right sides)	Male & female	<−1	−1 to −0.25	0–1.75	2–4.75	≥5
Trunk rotation test (inches, average of left and right sides)	Male & female	<13	13–15.75	16–18.75	19–21.75	≥22

*See text for an explanation of test procedures.

Sources: Adapted from norms in Appendix A of this textbook and these references.[74–77,86,107]

part III

Conditioning for Physical Fitness

chapter 7

The Acute and Chronic Effects of Exercise

In the process of training, the getting wind, as it is called, is largely a gradual increase in the capability of the heart. . . . The large heart of athletes may be due to the prolonged use of their muscles, but no man becomes a great runner or oarsman who has not naturally a capable if not a large heart.

—W. Osler, M.D., 1892[1]

You are reading this textbook, and suddenly you notice black smoke rising from your friend's apartment complex, 1 mile away. If you were to run to your friend's aid, you would notice several immediate changes in body function.

Your breathing rate would quicken, as you take in larger quantities of air with each breath, supplying more vital oxygen to your body. You might observe that your heart is pounding faster as it pumps more blood to your active leg muscles. If your pace is too quick, you may feel a burning sensation in your legs as the lactic acid concentration increases. These sudden, temporary changes in body function caused by exercise are called *acute responses to exercise,* and they disappear shortly after the exercise period is finished.

On the other hand, if you were to run 1 or 2 miles at a hard pace every day, after a few weeks, you might discern some changes in the way your body functioned during both rest and exercise. You might notice that your heart beats more slowly while you sit and study, as well as during your run. The amount of air you breathe in during each mile of your run might decrease, and you might feel less of a burning sensation in your legs. These persistent changes in the structure and function of your body following regular exercise training are called *chronic adaptations to exercise*—changes that enable the body to respond more easily to exercise.

This chapter includes a brief description of the acute and chronic effects of exercise. Only the very basic and important material is covered. For a deeper discussion of exercise physiology, the reader is referred to the excellent textbooks available on this topic.[2–9] In addition, see Appendix C for diagrams of the various body systems and Chapter 9 for a discussion of energy metabolism.

PHYSIOLOGICAL RESPONSES TO ACUTE EXERCISE

The acute responses to exercise are influenced by a number of factors, including the level of training or the fitness status of the participant, ambient temperature and humidity, time of day, sufficiency of sleep, coffee and food intake, use of alcohol and tobacco, menstrual cycle, and general anxiety.[7–10] For example, a person who is anxious about the treadmill test can have higher than normal heart rates during the first and second stages. Those who are fit usually have lower acute responses to certain levels of exercise than those who are unfit. These factors must be considered when interpreting the following discussion of acute effects.

Increase of Heart Rate

Figure 7.1 summarizes several important points relative to the way heart rate responds to increasing levels of exercise, such as during a graded treadmill exercise test (e.g., the Bruce protocol).

- The pre-exercise heart rate may be elevated, owing to the *anticipatory response.* In my own study of nearly 1,000 college students (unpublished data), the average resting heart rate, measured in the student's dorm rooms upon waking for three mornings in a row and then averaged, was 67 beats per minute (bpm). However, when sitting before a treadmill before a maximal graded exercise test, the average

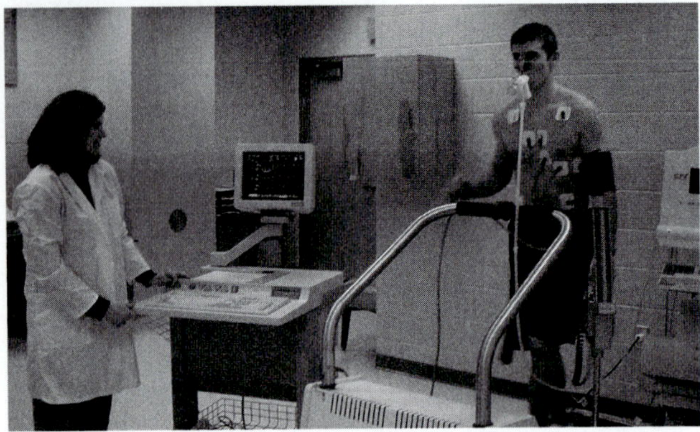

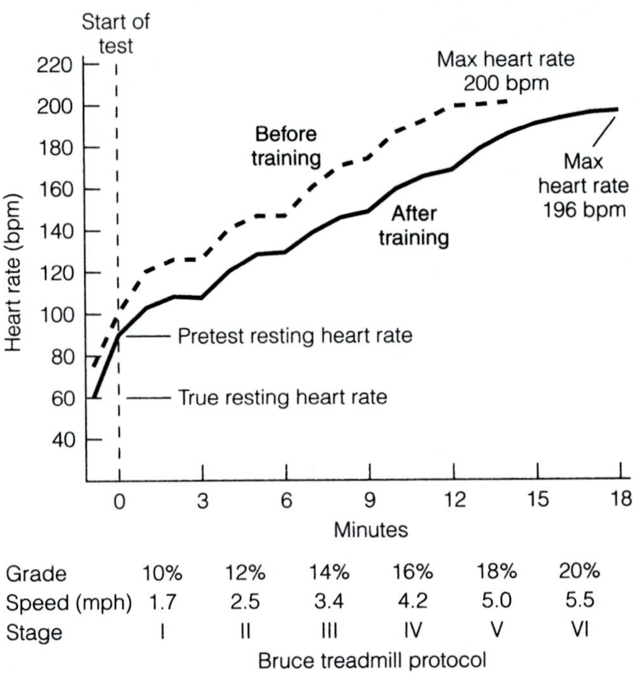

Figure 7.1 Heart rate results during the graded exercise test of a 20-year-old before and after exercise training. Notice that his pretest exercise heart rate is much higher than his true resting heart rate. The exercise heart rate increases in a linear fashion with increase in workload until the maximal heart rate is reached, when it plateaus.

"resting" heart rate of these same students was 95. (This pre-exercise increase is mediated through release of the neurotransmitter norepinephrine from the sympathetic nervous system, and the hormone epinephrine from the adrenal gland.)

- During the graded exercise test, heart rate will increase in direct proportion to the intensity of the exercise. In other words, the heart rate rises in a linear fashion with increasing workload.
- At exhaustion, the rise in heart rate will flatten out. This is called the *maximal heart rate.* When the heart rate increases little if at all after a stage change during a graded exercise test, this is a good indication that the maximal heart rate has been reached.

  The average maximal heart rate is equal to 220 minus the person's age (in years). This equation, however, is the average found in large groups of people. People of a given age vary widely, with a standard deviation of ± 10 to 12 bpm. In other words, the average maximal heart rate for a 20-year-old person is 220 − 20, or 200 bpm. However, two thirds of the people this age vary between 190 and 210 bpm, and 95% vary between 180 and 220 bpm. (See Chapter 8 for a more detailed discussion.)
- At submaximal levels of exercise, when the workload is held steady, the heart rate will increase for 1 to 3 minutes and then level off at a steady-state value. The harder the submaximal workload, the longer the heart rate will take to level off. For example, as you look at Figure 7.1, notice that in Stages 1 and 2, the heart rate plateaus relatively early in the stage, whereas in Stage 5, a more difficult stage, there is little indication of a plateau even after 3 minutes.

Increase of Stroke Volume

The *stroke volume* is the quantity of blood pumped out of the heart per heartbeat.[7] Stroke volume is regulated by several factors, including the amount of venous blood that is returned to the heart, the capacity to enlarge the ventricle, the force of contraction of the heart muscle, arterial pressure, and sympathetic nervous stimulation. Figure 7.2 summarizes several important points regarding the change in stroke volume from rest to exercise exhaustion.

- The change in stroke volume during graded exercise does not follow the pattern of change in the heart rate. Instead of rising linearly with increase in workload, stroke volume increases strongly only up to a workload of 40–60% of $\dot{V}O_{2max}$. Beyond this intensity level, increasing workload brings only small increases in stroke volume.[2,7,8] Highly trained athletes appear capable of increasing their stroke volume after exceeding 40–60% of $\dot{V}O_{2max}$ a bit more than untrained subjects.
- Resting stroke volume values for sedentary people range between 60 and 70 ml of blood per heartbeat. Those who are highly trained may have resting stroke volume values as high as 100–120 ml.[7,8] Submaximal and maximal stroke volumes are also much higher for fit than for sedentary people. Stroke volumes of elite world-class runners have been measured as high as 200 ml per heart beat.[7]
- When changing positions from lying down to standing, there is an immediate drop in the stroke volume because of the influence of gravity and a corresponding increase in heart rate to maintain the flow of blood out of the heart (i.e., cardiac output,

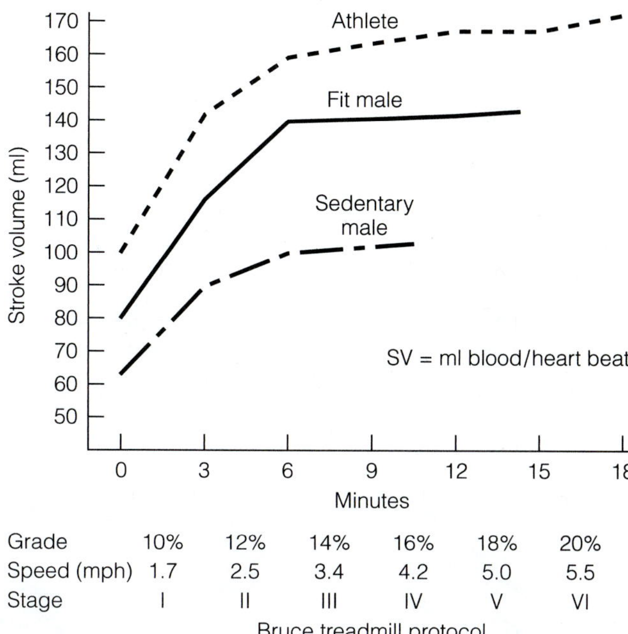

Figure 7.2 Stroke volume represents the amount of blood pumped per beat of the heart. Instead of rising linearly with increase in workload, stroke volume increases strongly up to a workload of 40–60% of $\dot{V}O_{2max}$. There is little change beyond this level, despite increasing workload.

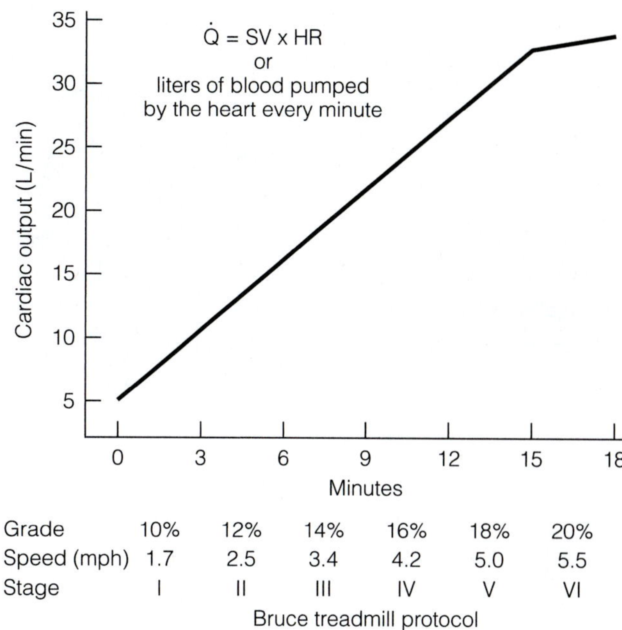

Figure 7.3 Cardiac output ($\dot{Q}$) follows a pattern similar to that of the heart rate. With increasing workload, cardiac output rises linearly and plateaus slightly at exercise exhaustion.

which equals stroke volume times heart rate). When exercise is performed in a horizontal position (as in swimming), the stroke volume is larger, and the heart rate lower than when the same level of upright exercise is performed (as in running). Therefore, heart rate during exercises such as swimming will be lower for a given percentage of $\dot{V}O_{2max}$ than for running. Exercise training heart rates should thus be adjusted downward about 10–15 bpm when exercising in a horizontal position.[10]

Increase in Cardiac Output

Cardiac output (also designated "$\dot{Q}$" by exercise physiologists) is equal to the stroke volume (SV) times the heart rate (HR) ($\dot{Q} = SV \times HR$). In other words, cardiac output represents the quantity of blood pumped out of the heart each minute. At rest, average cardiac output is approximately 5 liters per minute (L/min); it can rise to 20–40 L/min during maximal exercise, the amount depending on individual fitness status and size[7,8] (see Figure 7.3).

Figure 7.3 demonstrates that

- Cardiac output rises linearly with increasing workload and plateaus slightly at exercise exhaustion.
- During the initial stages of exercise, the increase in cardiac output is due to increases in both heart rate and stroke volume. During upright exercise, when the intensity reaches 40–60% of $\dot{V}O_{2max}$, any further increase in cardiac output is due primarily to an increase in heart rate.

Increased Arteriovenous Oxygen Difference

The *arteriovenous oxygen difference* ($a - \bar{v}O_2$) is the difference between the amount of oxygen carried in the arterial blood and the amount in the mixed venous blood. Thus the $a - \bar{v}O_2$ reflects the amount of oxygen extracted by the tissues of the body.[7]

- At rest, the oxygen content of arterial blood is approximately 20 ml of oxygen per 100 ml of blood, compared to an oxygen content of 14 ml/100 ml blood for the mixed venous blood. Thus the resting $a - \bar{v}O_2$ is 6 ml/100 ml blood.
- During very intense exercise, the venous oxygen content can drop to 2–4 ml/100 ml blood. Thus the $a - \bar{v}O_2$ can increase nearly threefold to 16–18 ml/100 ml blood.

Increase in $\dot{V}O_2$

The maximal oxygen uptake $\dot{V}O_{2max}$ can be defined as the "maximal rate at which oxygen can be taken up, distributed, and used by the body in the performance of exercise that utilizes a large muscle mass."[8] In other words, $\dot{V}O_{2max}$ is the

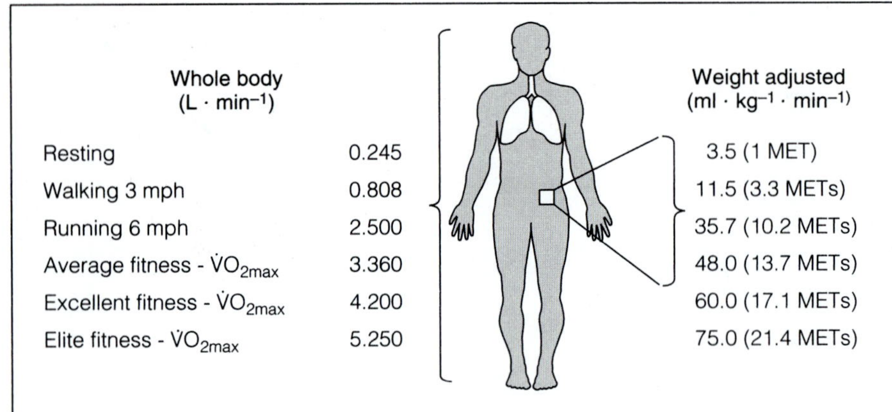

Whole body
(L · min−1)
Weight adjusted
(ml · kg−1 · min−1)
Resting
0.245
3.5 (1 MET)
Walking 3 mph
0.808
11.5 (3.3 METs)
Running 6 mph
2.500
35.7 (10.2 METs)
Average fitness - V̇O2max
3.360
48.0 (13.7 METs)
Excellent fitness - V̇O2max
4.200
60.0 (17.1 METs)
Elite fitness - V̇O2max
5.250
75.0 (21.4 METs)

Figure 7.4 Oxygen consumption ($\dot{V}O_2$) can be expressed in units of $L \cdot min^{-1}$ for the entire body, or in units of $ml \cdot kg^{-1} \cdot min^{-1}$ to represent the oxygen consumption for each kilogram of body weight. The example shows the oxygen consumption in a 70-kg male (25 years old).

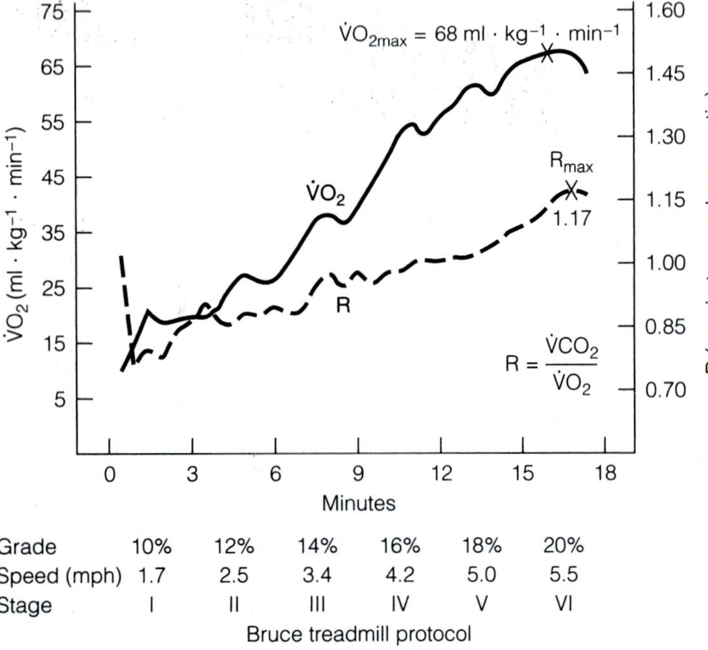

Figure 7.5 With increasing workload, oxygen consumption increases up to the last stage of exercise. At this point, $\dot{V}O_2$ plateaus and is called the $\dot{V}O_{2max}$.

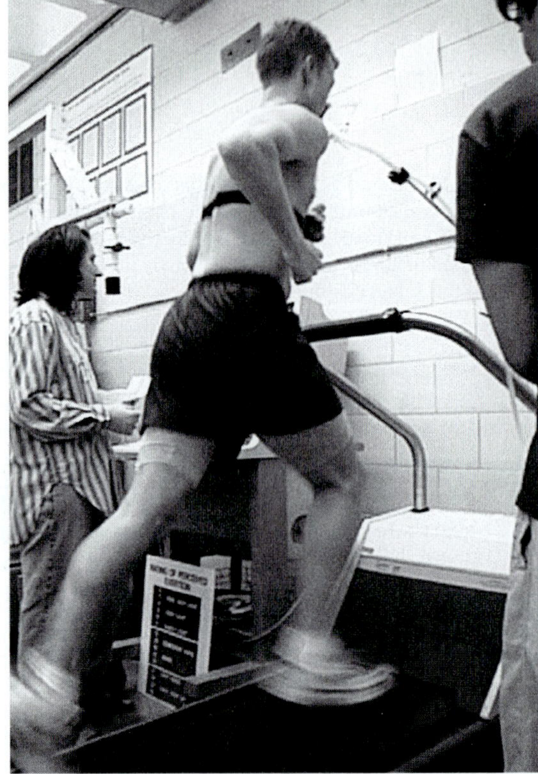

highest rate of oxygen consumption attainable during maximal or exhaustive exercise. $\dot{V}O_{2max}$ is usually expressed in terms of milliliters of oxygen consumed per kilogram of body weight per minute ($ml \cdot kg^{-1} \cdot min^{-1}$). With this allowance for body weight, the $\dot{V}O_{2max}$ of people of varying size and in different environments can be compared. $\dot{V}O_{2max}$ can also be expressed as liters per minute, representing the oxygen consumption of the entire body (see Figure 7.4).

During graded exercise, active muscle tissue needs more and more oxygen to burn the carbohydrates and fats needed for energy production. For every liter of oxygen the body consumes during exercise, approximately 5 kilocalories of energy are produced. Figures 7.5 to 7.7 demonstrate the following:[2,7]

- With increasing workload, oxygen consumption increases up to the last stage of exercise. At this point, $\dot{V}O_2$ plateaus, and is called the $\dot{V}O_{2max}$. If the person being tested is willing to push hard enough, a small decrease in $\dot{V}O_2$ can be seen just prior to exhaustion (as demonstrated in Figure 7.5). Many people, however, do not achieve a true $\dot{V}O_2$ plateau, and for this reason, some exercise physiologists prefer the term "peak $\dot{V}O_2$." $\dot{V}O_{2max}$ values are greatly influenced by size, age, heredity, sex, and level of fitness. (See next section.)
- Figure 7.6 shows that if the cardiac output and a − $\bar{v}O_2$ are known, oxygen consumption can be calculated using the formula, $\dot{V}O_2 = \dot{Q} \times a - \bar{v}O_2$. In other words, if measurement of arterial and mixed venous blood shows that for every liter of blood passing through the tissues, 150 ml of oxygen

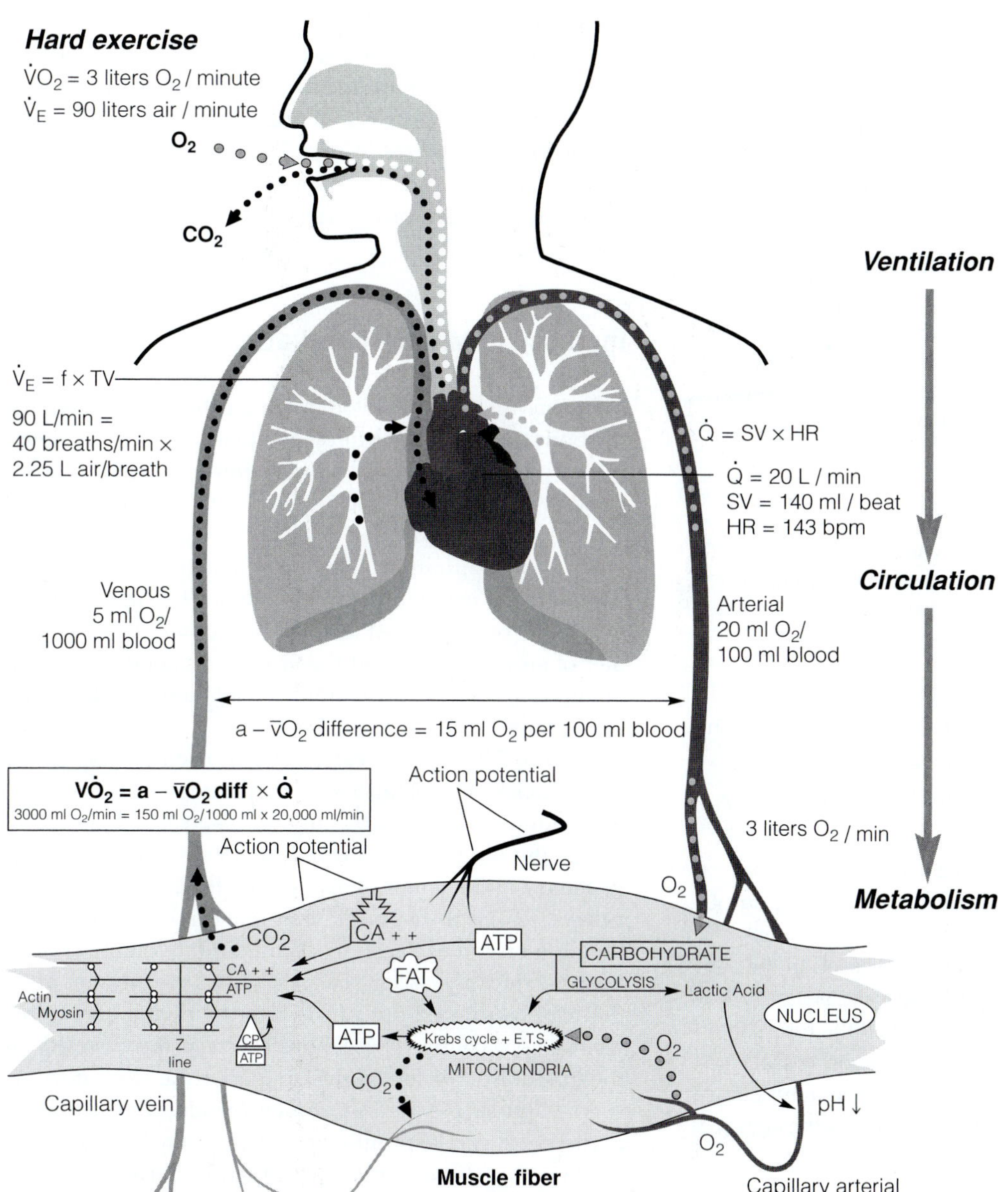

Figure 7.6 A summary of the acute effects of exercise. The body coordinates ventilation, circulation, and metabolism to meet the demands of exercise. If the cardiac output and a $-\ \bar{v}O_2$ are known, oxygen consumption can be calculated using this formula: $\dot{V}O_2 = \dot{Q} \times a - \bar{v}O_2$.

are being consumed, and that 20 liters of blood/minute are passing through those tissues, total oxygen consumption is easily determined by multiplying 150 ml $O_2 \cdot L^{-1}$ by 20 $L \cdot min^{-1}$, which equals 3,000 ml $O_2 \cdot min^{-1}$.

- *Oxygen debt* refers to the volume of oxygen consumed during the recovery period following exercise, in excess of the volume normally consumed at rest (see Figure 7.7). This debt pays back the *oxygen deficit* built up during the initial minutes of exercise, on account of the body adjusting to the exercise, plus other metabolic factors built up during the exercise bout itself.

For example, if you were to start running at a 7-minute-per-mile pace, approximately 3.46 liters of oxygen per minute would be required immediately. However, because your body takes approximately 2 to 3 minutes to adjust to this workload, anaerobic sources of adenosine triphosphate (ATP) (stored ATP and glycolysis) are utilized, building up an oxygen deficit. During recovery, you will breathe harder than during rest, to help restore this deficit and allow your body systems to return to normal.

Increased Systolic BP; Diastolic BP Unchanged

Blood pressure (BP) response during exercise was reviewed in Chapter 4, with an emphasis on accurate measurement (see Figure 4.4). Important concepts include[7]

- The systolic blood pressure increases in direct proportion to the increase in aerobic exercise

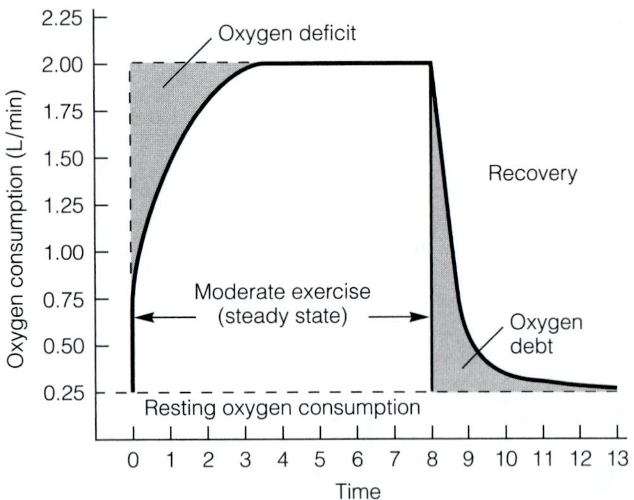

Figure 7.7 *Oxygen debt* refers to the volume of oxygen consumed during the recovery period following exercise, in excess of the volume normally consumed at rest.

intensity, with resting values of 120 mm Hg, often rising to 200 mm Hg or greater at exhaustion.

- The diastolic blood pressure changes little if any during aerobic exercise.
- The exercise-induced increase in systolic blood pressure is related to the increase in cardiac output. The increase in blood pressure would be much higher except that arterial blood vessels in the active muscles dilate, reducing peripheral resistance. *Total peripheral resistance* is the sum of all the forces that oppose blood flow in the body's blood vessel system. During exercise, total peripheral resistance decreases because the blood vessels in the active muscles dilate.
- Cycling with arms (arm ergometry) increases systolic and diastolic blood pressures 15%, compared to cycling with legs. This probably occurs because of the smaller muscle mass in the arms, which offers a greater resistance to blood flow than the larger muscles in the legs.
- Weight lifting or isometric contractions cause large increases in both systolic and diastolic blood pressures. This is discussed in more detail in Chapter 8.
- Some researchers like to report the *mean arterial pressure.* This represents the average pressure exerted by the blood against the inner walls of the arteries. An estimate of mean arterial pressure is obtained by using this equation:[8]

$$\text{Mean arterial pressure} = \tfrac{1}{3}(\text{systolic pressure} - \text{diastolic pressure}) + \text{diastolic pressure}$$

For example, if during Stage 3 of the Bruce treadmill test, the systolic blood pressure is 150 mm Hg and the diastolic blood pressure is 80 mm Hg, then the mean arterial pressure equals one third of the difference between systolic and diastolic blood pressures (0.33×70 mm Hg), or 23 mm Hg, plus the diastolic blood pressure ($23 + 80$), or 103 mm Hg. Maximal exercise mean arterial pressures approximate 130 mm Hg.[8]

Increase in Minute Ventilation

Minute ventilation is the volume of air that is breathed into the body each minute. Minute ventilation is usually determined by measuring the volume of air breathed out or expired ($\dot{V}_E$), and then correcting this for *BTPS,* the volume of air at the temperature and pressure of the body, and 100% water vapor saturation (as in the human lung). The minute ventilation is equal to the tidal volume (TV) times the frequency (f) of breaths. At rest, the *tidal volume* is usually 0.5 liter of air per breath, and the *frequency* is about 12 breaths per minute, resulting in a minute ventilation of 6 liters of air per minute.[7,8]

Figure 7.8 gives the various terms used by respiratory and exercise physiologists when reporting research or clinical findings. The TV is the amount of air breathed into or out of the lung while at rest. The TV usually ranges between 0.4 and 1.0 liter of air per breath. *Inspiratory reserve volume* (IRV) is the amount of air that can be breathed into the lung on top of a resting inspired tidal volume (2.5–3.5 liters). *Expiratory reserve volume* (ERV) is the amount of air that can be pushed out of the lung following an expired resting tidal volume (1.0–1.5 liters). *Residual volume* (RV) is the amount of air left in the lung after the expiratory reserve volume (1–2 liters). *Functional residual capacity* (FRC) is the combined expiratory reserve volume and residual volume. *Forced vital capacity* (FVC) is the total amount of air that can be breathed into the lung on top of the residual volume (usually 3–4 liters for women, 4–5 liters for men). The *total lung capacity* (TLC) represents the total amount of air in the lung.

Figure 7.9 summarizes changes in minute ventilation during graded exercise testing.[3,7,8]

- During graded exercise, minute ventilation increases in a curvilinear pattern from a resting value of $6\ L \cdot min^{-1}$ to $60–120\ L \cdot min^{-1}$ for females and $100–200\ L \cdot min^{-1}$ for males, depending on size and fitness status. Below 50% of $\dot{V}O_{2max}$, minute ventilation increases in a linear fashion with increasing workload. At higher intensities, however, the relationship is curvilinear, with ventilation rising strongly relative to the workload.
- The insert in Figure 7.9 shows that at higher intensities, an increase in minute ventilation is produced primarily from increased breathing rates.

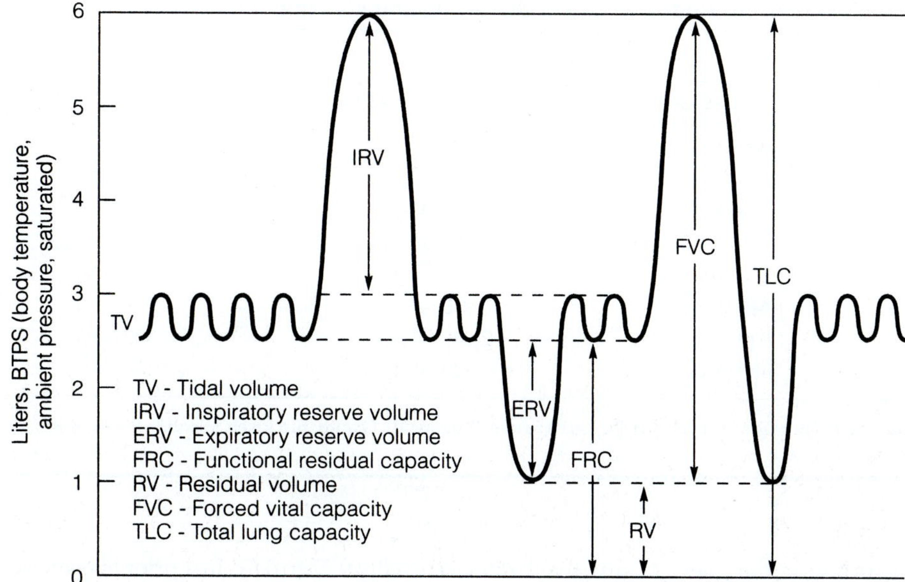

Figure 7.8 Terms used to represent the dynamic lung volumes and capacities.

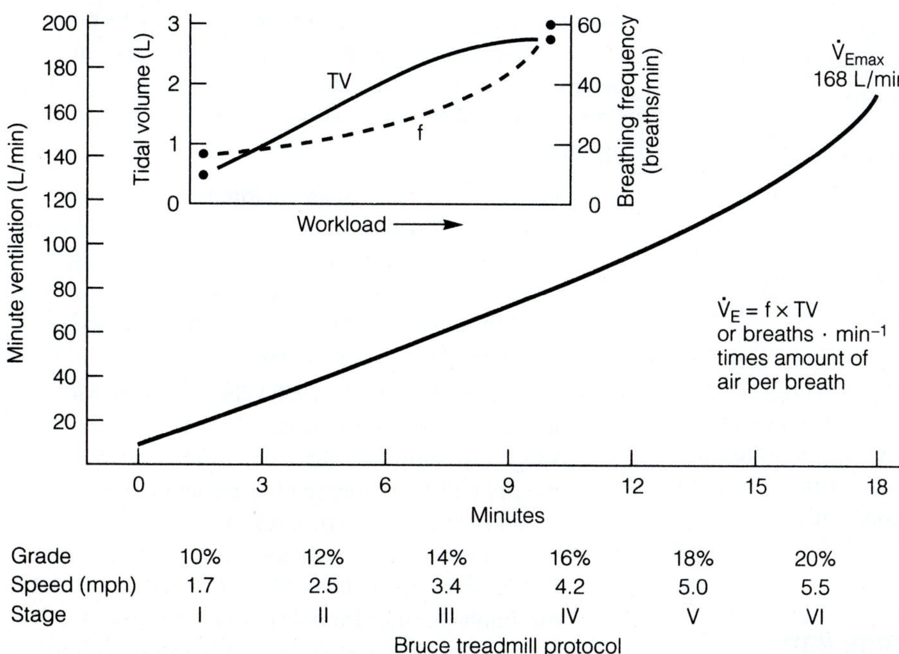

Figure 7.9 Minute ventilation increases in a curvilinear fashion during graded maximal exercise. The frequency of breathing also follows this pattern, while tidal volume plateaus during intense exercise.

The tidal volume tends to plateau at higher intensities.

- During graded exercise, the residual volume increases slightly, with the vital capacity decreasing slightly, keeping the overall total lung volume the same.
- The movement of air in and out of the lung during exercise requires considerable amounts of energy for the respiratory muscles. At rest, the energy cost of ventilation is 1 ml of oxygen per liter of air breathed, or 2% of the total oxygen being consumed at rest. During maximal exercise this can rise to 10%.
- *Lung diffusion* refers to the rate at which gases diffuse from the lung air sacs (*alveoli*) to the blood in the pulmonary capillaries. Diffusion capacity during exercise can increase threefold from a resting value of 25 ml $O_2 \cdot min^{-1} \cdot mm\,Hg^{-1}$ to 75 ml $O_2 \cdot min^{-1} \cdot mm\,Hg^{-1}$ at maximum.

Increased Blood Flow to Active Muscle Areas

- During exercise, blood is redirected away from areas where it is not needed (e.g., organs) and to the

TABLE 7.1 Distribution of Cardiac Output During Rest and Light, Moderate, and Maximal Exercise

	Cardiac Output (ml · min^{-1})			
Vascular Region	**At Rest (6%)**	**Light Exercise (30%)**	**Heavy Exercise (75%)**	**Maximal Exercise (100%)**
Cardiac output	6,000	12,000	24,000	30,000
Cerebral	720 (12%)	720 (6%)	720 (3%)	720 (2%)
Myocardial	240 (4%)	480 (4%)	960 (4%)	1,200 (4%)
Muscle	1,260 (21%)	5,760 (48%)	17,280 (72%)	26,400 (88%)
Renal	1,320 (22%)	1,200 (10%)	720 (3%)	300 (1%)
Hepatosplanchnic	1,560 (26%)	1,440 (12%)	960 (4%)	300 (1%)
Skin	540 (9%)	1,920 (16%)	2,640 (11%)	900 (3%)
Other	360 (6%)	480 (4%)	720 (3%)	180 (<1%)

Source: Data from Shephard RJ, Astrand P-O. *Endurance in Sport: The Encyclopædia of Sports Medicine* (Volume II). Oxford: Blackwell Scientific Publications, 1992.

muscles. At rest, only 21% of the cardiac output goes to the muscles, compared with as much as 88% during exhaustive exercise (see Table 7.1).[2]

- As the body heats up, an increasing amount of blood is directed to the skin, to conduct heat away from the body core. The primary means by which the body loses heat during exercise is through evaporation of sweat on the skin (see Chapter 9). The sweat glands will use fluid from the cells and from the blood to produce the sweat, which can reach 2 to 3 L/h during hard exercise in humid heat. If the sweat rate is high, blood volume will decrease, ultimately to the point of heat injury.
- During endurance exercise, plasma volume shifts to the muscles. During graded exercise testing, 12–16% of the plasma volume leaves the blood and enters the active muscle tissue.[7,9] This plasma volume shift, combined with the fluid loss from sweating, leads to an increase in the thickness of blood called *hemoconcentration.*

Changes in Respiratory Exchange Ratio

During exercise the muscles use oxygen (O_2) to burn carbohydrates and fats, producing carbon dioxide (CO_2) and ATP. Ventilation increases to help bring in more O_2 and to expel CO_2. Exercise physiologists use the *respiratory exchange ratio* (R) to help determine the type of fuel (primarily fat and carbohydrate) being used by the muscles. The respiratory exchange ratio is the ratio between the amount of carbon dioxide produced and the amount of oxygen consumed by the body during exercise ($R = \dot{V}CO_2/\dot{V}O_2$).[7]

The R value will vary, depending on what fuel the muscles are using. When only fats are being used, R = 0.71; when only carbohydrates are being used, R = 1.0.

With hard exercise, the R value approaches 1.0 because carbohydrate is the preferred fuel with heavy exercise. At rest, the R value is usually 0.75 to 0.81. Just prior to exercise, the R value can rise above 1.0, due to pretest anxiety, which causes hyperventilation (which "blows off" CO_2). During recovery, the R value can rise above 1.5, due to the buffering of lactic acid and carbon dioxide production. When R values rise to 1.15 or greater during exercise, this is usually a sign of maximal exertion, with the body relying on anaerobic metabolism.

- Figure 7.5 shows that as the intensity of exercise increases, R increases, meaning that more and more CO_2 is being produced relative to the O_2 being consumed. This indicates that more and more carbohydrate is being used by the muscles as the intensity of exercise increases.
- At rest, the blood pH is 7.4. When the exercise intensity of unconditioned people rises above 50% $\dot{V}O_{2max}$, or above 70–90% for conditioned people, the pH will drop, owing to lactic acid buildup. Blood pH values can drop to 7.0 with maximal exercise; tissue pH levels can drop to 6.5. Blood lactate levels range from 10 mg/100 ml at rest (1.1 millimole per liter [mmol/L] of blood) to 200 mg/100 ml (22 mmol/L of blood) within 5 minutes following exhaustive short-term exercise. Typical lactate values immediately postexercise range from 7.5 to 9.0 mmol/L, with the highest values reached in trained endurance athletes.
- During graded maximal exercise, the *anaerobic threshold* is the point at which blood lactate concentrations start to rise above resting values.[11–14] The anaerobic threshold can be expressed as a percentage of $\dot{V}O_{2max}$. Some of the best athletes in the world have anaerobic thresholds of between 80 and 90% of $\dot{V}O_{2max}$; unfit people average 40–60% of $\dot{V}O_{2max}$.

Although a discussion of the measurement of anaerobic threshold is beyond the scope of this book, Figure 7.10

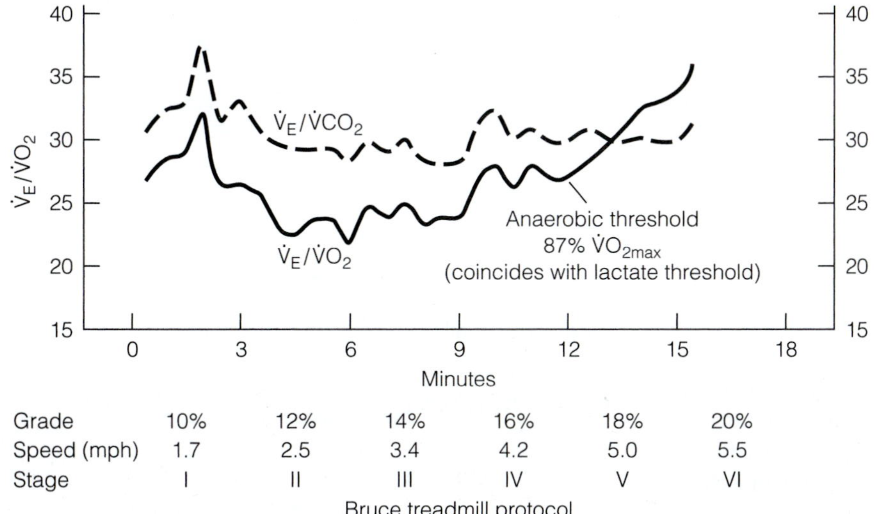

Figure 7.10 Anaerobic threshold in an elite woman masters runner. Anaerobic threshold represents the point at which lactic acid begins to build up in the blood. This can be measured indirectly by looking at the rise in $\dot{V}_E/\dot{V}O_2$ relative to $\dot{V}_E/\dot{V}CO_2$.

shows that anaerobic threshold can be estimated when the ratio of minute ventilation to oxygen consumption ($\dot{V}_E/\dot{V}O_2$) rises sharply, while the ratio of minute ventilation to carbon dioxide consumption ($\dot{V}_E/\dot{V}CO_2$) remains constant.[13,15] Figure 7.10 reflects the measurement of an elite woman masters runner who holds several world records for ultramarathon distances. Her anaerobic threshold of 87% of $\dot{V}O_{2max}$ is very high, thus allowing her to run at an intensity close to her capacity without danger of lactic acid buildup. (See the Sports Medicine Insight at the end of this chapter.)

CHRONIC ADAPTATIONS TO REGULAR EXERCISE

As discussed earlier in this chapter, the persistent changes in the structure and function of the body following regular exercise training are called chronic adaptations to exercise.[2–9]

What quantity of exercise training is necessary to produce chronic adaptations? Do different body systems adapt to exercise training at different rates?

Several of the cardiorespiratory and metabolic responses of exercise adapt very rapidly to exercise training.[16,17] Within the first 1–3 weeks of intensive cardiorespiratory training by young healthy college students, for example (40–60 minutes per session, six sessions per week, 70–90% $\dot{V}O_{2max}$), significant improvements in $\dot{V}O_{2max}$, submaximal exercise heart rate and lactate responses, and ventilation can already be measured. Some adaptations to aerobic exercise, however, take longer. For example, the increase in number of capillaries per muscle fiber may take several months or years.[17]

Interestingly, exercise-induced changes are lost just as rapidly as they are gained. This (the effects of inactivity or detraining) is discussed later in this chapter.

The magnitude of the chronic adaptations of regular exercise training depends on the frequency, intensity, and duration of training, the mode of activity, and the initial fitness status. For example, overweight middle-aged people who have been inactive for many years have the potential for dramatic improvements in cardiorespiratory fitness (e.g., a 100% increase in $\dot{V}O_{2max}$) with weight loss and a few months of regular aerobic exercise. Relatively active college students, on the other hand, can expect smaller improvements (e.g., a 10–20% increase in $\dot{V}O_{2max}$).[2]

Changes That Occur in Skeletal Muscles as a Result of Aerobic Training

Exercise physiologists have had an ongoing debate for several decades regarding the relative importance of "central" versus "peripheral" adaptations to regular cardiorespiratory exercise. Figure 7.6 shows that ventilation and circulation (central elements) work closely with the muscle cells (peripheral elements) to allow physical activity to take place. While most researchers have reported that the circulation, specifically the stroke volume and cardiac output, is the primary limiting factor during intense exercise, some feel that factors within the muscle cells are more important.[18–24] There is a growing consensus that during *acute* intense endurance exercise, the cardiovascular system is limiting (i.e., the ability to deliver oxygen to the muscles), while improvement in $\dot{V}O_{2max}$ with *chronic* exercise training is largely dependent on peripheral changes in the muscles (especially increase in capillary surface area).[18,19]

In response to regular aerobic training, many significant changes take place in the muscle cells.[2–9]

- An increase in *myoglobin* content. (Myoglobin aids in the delivery of oxygen from the blood to the *mitochondria* [organelles in the muscle cell that produce ATP for energy; see Figure 7.6].)

- An increase in the number and size of mitochondria.
- An increase in the concentration of important enzymes in the mitochondria, specifically those of the Krebs cycle and the electron transport system. (These enzymes are involved in the production of ATP from aerobic metabolism.)
- An increase in both the amount of glycogen stored in the muscle and the maximal capacity to oxidize carbohydrates.
- An increased capacity to oxidize fat (from both muscle fat and adipose tissue stores).[25,26] (The trained person thus oxidizes more fat and less carbohydrate during cardiorespiratory exercise [at an absolute workload], which means less glycogen depletion, less lactic acid accumulation, and therefore less muscle fatigue and greater endurance.)
- An increase in the area of slow-twitch fibers. (The *aerobic-type muscle fibers* are called Type I [red, tonic, *slow twitch*]; the *anaerobic-type fibers* are called Type II [white, glycolytic, *fast twitch*]. People vary widely in their proportions of slow-twitch and fast-twitch fibers. This proportion is set at birth and remains constant throughout life.)

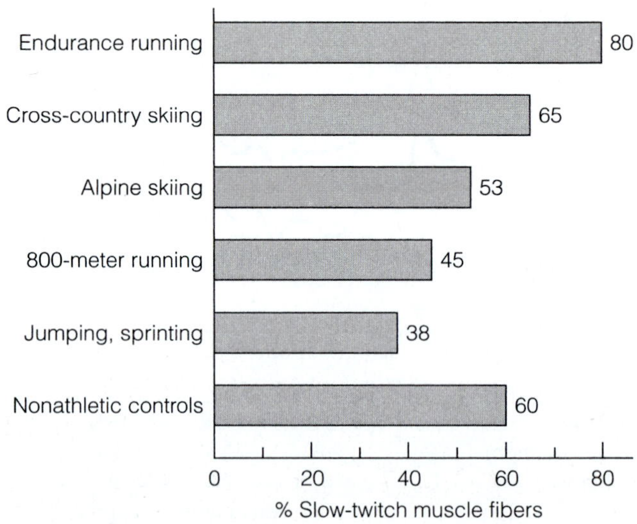

Figure 7.11 Slow-twitch muscle fibers (Type I) among successful endurance competitors. Endurance athletes tend to have a greater proportion of slow-twitch muscle fibers than do jumpers and sprinters. Source: Data from Shepard RJ, Astrand P-O. *Endurance in Sport: The Encyclopedia of Sports Medicine* (Volume II). Oxford: Blackwell Scientific Publications, 1992.

The fast-twitch muscle cells are capable of producing high amounts of ATP through *glycolysis,* a process that does not require oxygen (anaerobic). Fast-twitch muscle cells are important in activities that require sprinting and jumping. Slow-twitch muscle cells generate ATP in the presence of oxygen (aerobically) and have high numbers of mitochondria and a good capillary supply.

Endurance athletes usually have a high proportion of slow-twitch muscle fibers, sprinters a high proportion of fast-twitch muscle fibers. For example, trained endurance athletes average 60–80% slow-twitch fibers, while sprinters average only 35–40% slow-twitch fibers[2] (see Figure 7.11). Blacks have been found to have a higher percentage of fast-twitch fibers than Caucasians, helping to explain why they excel in sports requiring sprinting and jumping.[27]

With regular aerobic training, the size of the slow-twitch fibers can be increased. Some researchers have reported that some fast-twitch muscle cells can be changed into slow-twitch muscle cells through regular aerobic training over a long time period.[28,29] However, fiber transformation appears to be of minor importance, relative to the increase in fiber size.

Major Cardiorespiratory Changes from Exercise Training When at Rest

Several major cardiorespiratory changes at rest follow exercise training:

- An increase in heart size.[1] The size of the left and right ventricular cavities increases, with proportional increases in the thicknesses of the heart muscle walls and septum.[30] These changes occur gradually over months or years of training.[8]
- A decrease in resting heart rate. The resting heart rate decreases approximately one beat per minute for every 1 to 2 weeks of aerobic training for about 10 to 20 weeks. Further decreases are possible if training volume and intensity are increased. Some of the best endurance athletes in the world have resting heart rates below 40 bpm.

In my own study of nearly 1,000 college students (unpublished data), the average college male's resting heart rate decreased from 67 to 60 bpm after 7 weeks of regular aerobic training (5 sessions per week, 30 minutes per session, 70–80% of $\dot{V}O_{2max}$). Female college students on the same program decreased their resting heart rates from 69 to 62 bpm after 7 weeks.

The decrease in resting heart rate is attributable to an increase in *parasympathetic* control (through the vagus nerve, which slows the heart rate).[8] Other aerobic training effects on resting physiologic variables include[7,8]

- An increase in stroke volume, with more blood pumped per beat, with a corresponding decrease in rate. For example, sedentary people have stroke volumes at rest of about 60 ml, whereas those of athletes often measure greater than 100 ml.
- Resting cardiac output. The resting cardiac output stays about the same (about 5 L/min).
- An increase in the total blood volume from about 5 liters in sedentary people to 6 or 7 liters in athletes. The 20–25% increase in blood volume is evident in males and females of all ages.[31–33] Although both plasma volume and hemoglobin increase, the

increase in plasma volume is greater, leading to a slightly decreased *hematocrit,* red blood cell proportion per 100 ml of blood. This increase in the plasma volume is directly linked to the increase in stroke volume. This adaptation is gained after only a few bouts of exercise and is quickly reversed when training ceases.[32]

- An increase in capillary density. Untrained human muscle has about 1.5 to 2.0 capillaries per muscle fiber, whereas elite endurance athletes have two to three times this number.[28,34]

In general, pulmonary function characteristics (total lung capacity, forced vital capacity residual volume) are not changed by training.[35] Some individuals may experience a slight increase in vital capacity and a slight decrease in residual volume.[7] Resting minute ventilation is not affected by training.

Major Cardiorespiratory Changes during Submaximal Exercise

What cardiorespiratory changes during submaximal exercise can be expected following exercise training? Tables 7.2 and 7.3 summarize data from a study conducted on 20 males, of whom 9 were sedentary and 11 were experienced runners.[36] All were tested in the laboratory using the Balke maximal graded exercise test, with cardiorespiratory variables

TABLE 7.2 Differences between Sedentary and Trained Males during a Balke Treadmill Graded Exercise Test (Resting and Maximal Exercise Parameters)

Parameter	Sedentary Males (n = 9)	Trained Males (n = 11)
Age (years)	44.2	42.7
Weight (lb)	185	171
Percent body fat (%)	24.5	12.5
Resting heart rate (bpm)	66.8	52.5
$\dot{V}O_{2max}$ ($ml \cdot kg^{-1} \cdot min^{-1}$)	33.3	54.2
Ventilation, max ($L \cdot min^{-1}$)	119	165
Heart rate, max (bpm)	188	177

Source: Data from Nieman DC, et al. Complement and immunoglobulin levels in athletes and sedentary controls. *Int J Sports Med* 10:124–128, 1989.

TABLE 7.3 Differences between Sedentary versus Trained Males during a Balke Treadmill Graded Exercise Test (Mean [Range])

	Time: Speed: Grade:	5 min 3.3 mph 5%	10 min 3.3 mph 10%	15 min 3.3 mph 15%
VO_2 ($ml \cdot kg^{-1} \cdot min^{-1}$)				
Sedentary males		18.4 (16.0–21.8)	24.8 (22.4–28.2)	32.1 (29.6–34.4)
Trained males		19.7 (17.2–22.8)	26.7 (25.1–30.1)	34.0 (31.3–38.5)
Heart rate (bpm)				
Sedentary males		123 (100–139)	152 (128–175)	177 (164–197)
Trained males		88 (77–96)	107 (98–120)	126 (112–138)
Ventilation ($L \cdot min^{-1}$)				
Sedentary males		42 (35–54)	63 (47–88)	88 (62–106)
Trained males		37 (30–47)	52 (44–64)	66 (57–85)
Respiratory exchange ratio				
Sedentary males		0.95 (0.90–1.09)	1.08 (1.01–1.23)	1.24 (1.12–1.46)
Trained males		0.87 (0.78–1.00)	0.95 (0.87–1.02)	0.99 (0.92–1.06)

Source: Data from Nieman DC, et al. Complement and immunoglobulin levels in athletes and sedentary controls. *Int J Sports Med* 10:124–128, 1989.

measured every 5 minutes to complete exhaustion. During the 3 previous years, the athletes had averaged 42.5 ± 4.0 miles per week of running, with an average personal marathon record of 3.1 ± 0.1 hours.

Maximal oxygen uptake and ventilation were 63% and 39% higher, respectively, for the athletes than for the nonathletes, with percent body fat nearly 50% lower.

Important differences in submaximal exercise parameters between the sedentary and trained males can be summarized as follows:

- There were no significant differences in oxygen consumption during any of the three submaximal workloads. When adjusted for weight changes, training does not appear to decrease oxygen consumption during submaximal exercise. However, among individuals, the amount of oxygen utilized during any given workload can vary widely. Notice in Table 7.3 that oxygen consumption varied 16–36% depending on the workload (see ranges for each workload).
- Heart rates of the trained males were significantly lower than those of the sedentary males. This has been shown by others to be due to a higher stroke volume. The cardiac output at a certain absolute workload does not appear to be affected by exercise training[37] (see also Figures 7.1 and 7.2).
- Ventilation was significantly lower for the trained males than it was for the sedentary males during each stage. They ventilated less air while achieving the same oxygen consumption.

  The trained body is much more efficient in the transport and utilization of oxygen. The $a - \bar{v}O_2$ difference is slightly higher, meaning that the muscle cells are extracting more oxygen. The heightened extraction of oxygen is due to the increased capillary density around each muscle cell.[7,8]
- The respiratory exchange ratio (R) was much lower for the athletes. As discussed earlier, a lower R value indicates that the muscle cells are utilizing more fat and less glycogen for fuel. This decreases the concentration of lactic acid, increasing the anaerobic threshold. This allows one to exercise at a higher intensity without interference from lactic acid. (These benefits result primarily from the exercise-training-induced increase in the number and size of mitochondria.)

Major Cardiorespiratory Changes during Maximal Exercise

During maximal graded exercise testing, subjects are taken to complete exhaustion. What changes during maximal exercise can be expected after regular exercise training? Table 7.2 shows the following differences:

- Training provides a significantly higher maximal aerobic power ($\dot{V}O_{2max}$). This means that a greater amount of oxygen can be consumed during maximal exercise. Figure 7.4 outlines increases in $\dot{V}O_{2max}$ that can be expected in response to increasing levels of training. Figure 7.12 compares $\dot{V}O_{2max}$ among different athletes.[38] Cross-country skiers generally have the highest $\dot{V}O_{2max}$ because almost all the

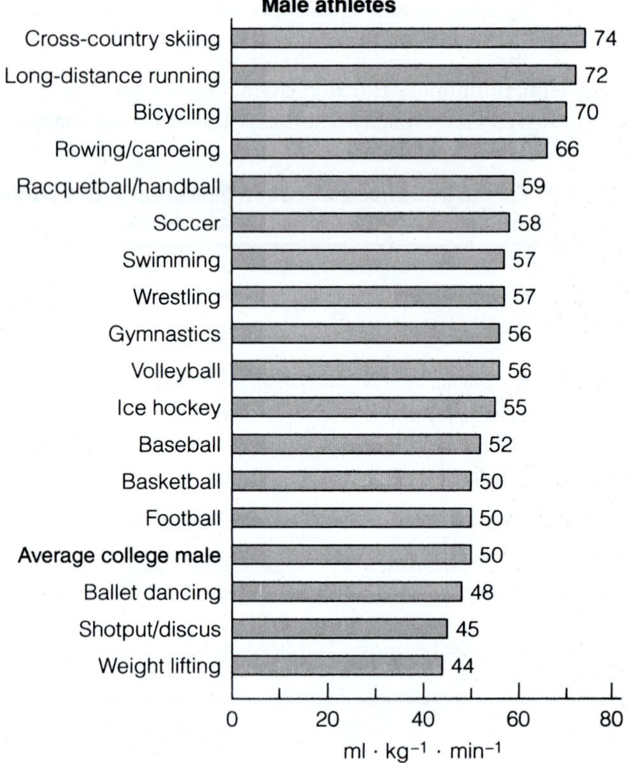

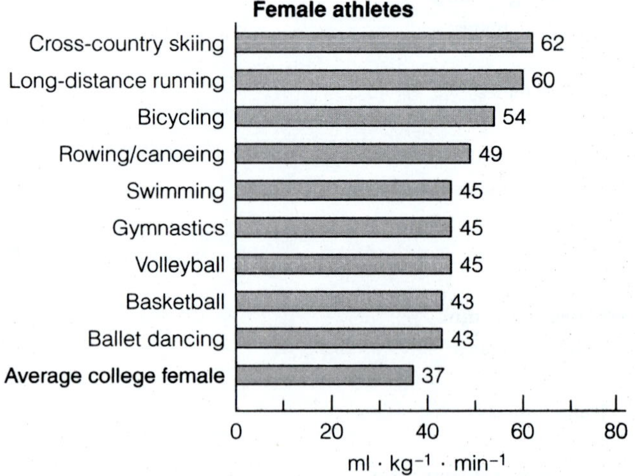

Figure 7.12 Maximal oxygen uptake. Endurance athletes have the highest $\dot{V}O_{2max}$ values for both males and females.
Source: National Center for Health Statistics. Drury EF (ed.), *Assessing Physical Fitness and Physical Activity in Population-Based Surveys.* DHHS Pub. No. (PHS) 89-1253. Public Health Service. Washington, DC: U.S. Government Printing Office, 1989.

major muscle groups in the body are activated.[39] One of the highest $\dot{V}O_{2max}$ values ever measured was in a Scandinavian cross-country skier (93 ml · $kg^{-1} \cdot min^{-1}$).

In my own study of nearly 1,000 college students (unpublished findings), male students had an average $\dot{V}O_{2max}$ of 49.0 ml · $kg^{-1} \cdot min^{-1}$ before and 55.0 ml · $kg^{-1} \cdot min^{-1}$ after 7 weeks of regular aerobic exercise (5 sessions per week, 30 minutes per session, 70–80% of $\dot{V}O_{2max}$). Female college students averaged 36.0 ml · $kg^{-1} \cdot min^{-1}$ before training and 41.0 ml · $kg^{-1} \cdot min^{-1}$ after training.

The 12–14% increase in $\dot{V}O_{2max}$ realized by these young adults after 7 weeks of training is typical.[7] The 36% difference in $\dot{V}O_{2max}$ between genders has also been reported by others.[40] (See section on gender differences.)

- The increase in $\dot{V}O_{2max}$ is primarily attributable to a greater cardiac output and a greater oxygen extraction by the muscle cells. Maximal cardiac output is only about 20 L/min in the untrained, whereas athletes may have maximal outputs ranging between 30 and 40 L/min.[7] Maximal stroke volumes can increase from 100–120 ml/beat to 180–200 ml/beat, and the max $a - \bar{v}O_2$ difference from 14.5 ml/100 ml to 16.0 ml/100 ml.

The major limiting factor to performance according to many studies is cardiac output and the ability to achieve a large stroke volume.[19,22,41] The single biggest difference between endurance-trained and untrained individuals is the size of stroke volume.

- Trained athletes have a higher maximal ventilation. This means that trained people can ventilate more air during maximal exercise. Their maximal tidal volume and frequency are also higher. Large, highly trained endurance athletes such as rowers can have maximal ventilation rates of more than 240 L/min, which are twice the rates of untrained individuals. Lung diffusion capacity also improves with training, meaning that oxygen can diffuse from the lung alveoli to the blood more readily.
- Maximum heart rate usually changes little with training. The maximum heart rate of adults under age 30 may decrease a few beats per minute with exercise training, but more research is needed to establish this relationship.

Other changes that occur during maximal exercise with training include

- An increase of blood flow to the active muscles, with better constriction of blood vessels in inactive areas and vasodilatation in active muscle areas[42]
- An increased ability to tolerate higher lactic acid levels at max

Table 7.4 summarizes the changes in cardiorespiratory parameters that occur during rest, submaximal exercise, and maximal exercise following endurance training. Table 7.5 compares typical values in sedentary, trained, and elite individuals.

Other Physiological Changes with Aerobic Exercise

Other changes that occur in response to regular cardiorespiratory exercise include

- A small decrease in total body fat and a slight increase in lean body weight (see Chapter 11)
- An increase in HDL cholesterol, a decrease in triglycerides, but little or no change in total serum or LDL cholesterol (see Chapter 10)
- A greater ability to exercise in the heat (see Chapter 9)
- An increase in the density and breaking strength of bones, ligaments, and tendons, and an increase in the thickness of cartilage in the joints (see Chapter 15)

TABLE 7.4 Summary of Changes in Cardiorespiratory Parameters with Endurance Training

Cardiovascular Parameter	Resting	Submax Exercise	Maximal Exercise
Oxygen consumption	No change	No change	Increase
Heart rate	Decrease	Decrease	No/slight change
Stroke volume	Increase	Increase	Increase
Cardiac output	No change	No change	Increase
Active muscle blood flow	No change	Increase	Increase
Ventilation	No change	Decrease	Increase
$a - \bar{v}O_2$ difference	No change	Slight increase	Increase
Lactic acid levels	No change	Decrease	Increase

TABLE 7.5 Comparison of Hypothetical Physiological and Body Composition Changes from an Endurance Training Program for a Sedentary, Normal Person and a World-Class Endurance Runner of the Same Age

	Sedentary Normal		
Variable	**Pre-***	**Post-***	**World-Class Athlete**
Cardiovascular			
Resting HR (bpm)	71	59	36
Max HR (bpm)	185	183	174
Resting SV (ml)	65	80	125
Max SV (ml)	120	140	200
Resting $\dot{Q}$ (L/min)	4.6	4.7	4.5
Max $\dot{Q}$ (L/min)	22.2	25.6	34.8
Heart volume (ml)	750	820	1,200
Blood volume (L)	4.7	5.1	6
Resting systolic BP (mm Hg)	135	130	110
Resting diastolic BP (mm Hg)	78	76	70
Respiratory			
Resting $\dot{V}_E$ (L/min)	7	6	6
Max $\dot{V}_E$ (L/min)	110	135	195
Resting F (breaths/min)	14	12	12
Max F (breaths/min)	40	45	55
Resting TV (L/breath)	0.5	0.5	0.5
Max TV (L/breath)	2.75	3.0	3.5
Vital capacity (L)	5.8	6.0	6.2
Residual volume (L)	1.4	1.2	1.2
Metabolic			
$a - \bar{v}O_2$ difference (ml/dL)	6	6	6
Max $a - \bar{v}O_2$ difference (ml/dL)	14.5	15	16
$\dot{V}O_{2max}$ ($ml \cdot kg^{-1} \cdot min^{-1}$)	40.5	49.8	76.7
Max lactate (mmol/L)	7.5	8.5	9
Body composition			
Weight (lb)	175	170	150
Fat weight (lb)	28	21.3	11.3
Lean weight (lb)	147	148.7	138.7
Relative fat (%)	16	12.5	7.5

*= 6-month training program, jogging 3–4 times per week, 30 min/day, at 75% $\dot{V}O_{2max}$. HR = heart rate; SV = stroke volume; $\dot{Q}$ = cardiac output; BP = blood pressure; $\dot{V}_E$ = ventilation; F = frequency; TV = tidal volume.

Source: Wilmore JH, Norton AC. *The Heart and Lungs at Work.* Schiller Park, IL: Beckman Instruments, 1974.

Changes That Occur in Muscles Due to Strength Training

What changes in the skeletal muscle occur in response to strength training (see Figure 7.13)?[43–53] (See Figure 7.14 for an overview of the structure of muscle.)

- Regarding *hypertrophy* (increase in size) of muscle cells, especially the fast-twitch fibers, the fibers of untrained muscle vary considerably in diameter, but strength training brings the smaller muscle fibers up to the size of the larger ones.[4,5] This hypertrophy is caused by an increase in the number and size of myofibrils per muscle cell; increased total protein (especially myosin); and increased amounts and strength of connective, tendinous, and ligamentous tissues. When a pronounced hypertrophy of muscle fibers occurs after high-load, low-repetition resistance training, the capillary density tends to decrease. A training regimen emphasizing moderately high-load, high-repetition exercise as performed by bodybuilders, however, may induce some new capillary growth.[4,5]
- There is growing evidence that training leads to a small increase in the number of muscle cells.

Similarly, there is some support for the theory that extensive weight training may result in some muscle fiber conversions. However, even if hyperplasia and muscle-fiber conversion do take place, the overall effect on the cross-sectional area of the muscle appears to be minor.[44,45,48]

- There is a selective hypertrophy of fast-twitch fibers with an associated increase in the ratio of fast-twitch to slow-twitch muscle fiber area.[4,5] Therefore, people born with a high percentage of fast-twitch fibers can "bulk up" more easily than those with a high percentage of slow-twitch fibers.
- The normal inhibitory nervous impulses from the brain are lessened. During the first 3–5 weeks of strength training, substantial gains in strength occur without concomitant increases in muscle mass.[47,50,51]

The nervous system adapts to regular weight training, resulting in a *disinhibition* of the muscle. With these adaptations, more *motor units* (motor nerve and attached muscle cells) can be activated, and there is a better recruitment pattern and synchronization of motor units. Thus, the increase in strength is not due to an increase in size of muscle cells alone.

- The biochemical changes are small and inconsistent. Traditional weight training programs do not appear to improve either oxidative or glycolytic enzyme activity.[4,5]

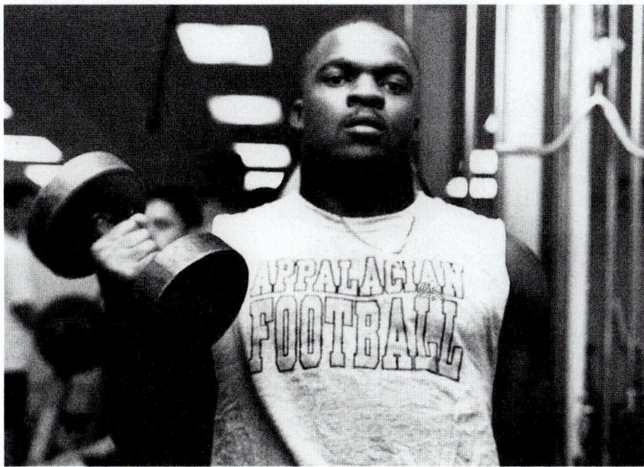

Figure 7.13 Strength training increases the size of muscle fibers and is associated with a better recruitment pattern and synchronization of motor units.

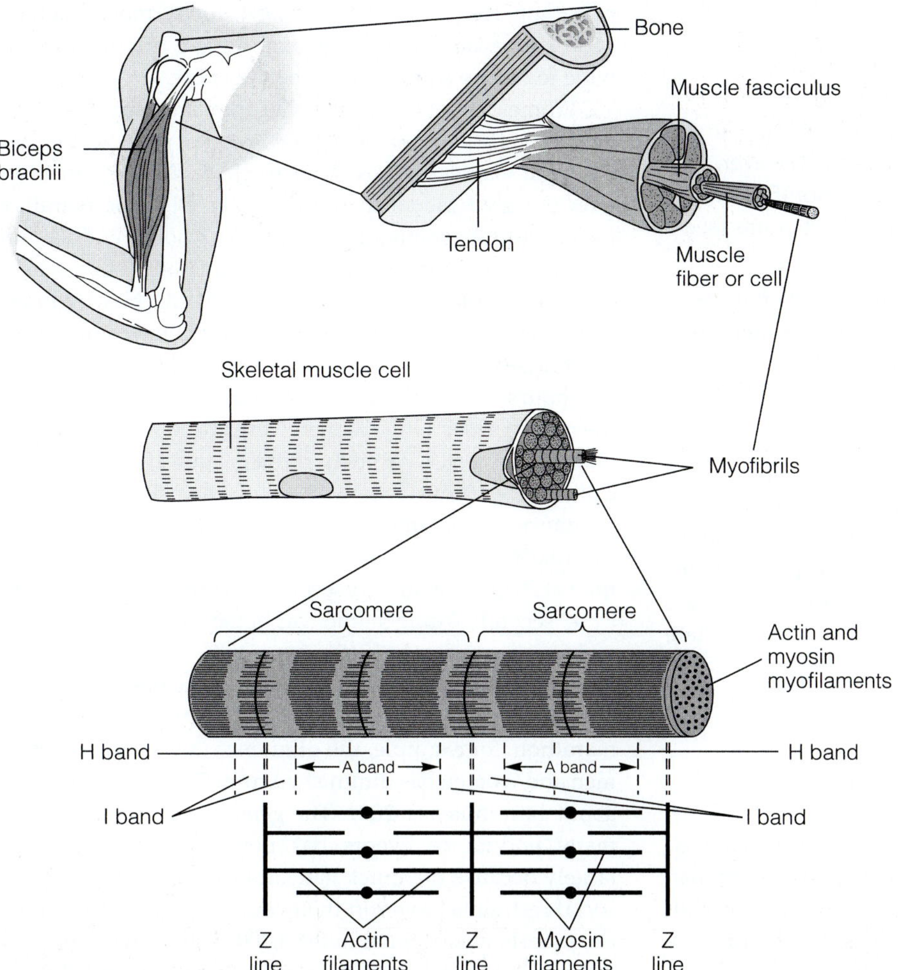

Figure 7.14 The structure of skeletal muscle. *Skeletal muscle* is composed of parallel cells (also called fibers). The number and type of muscle cells (slow twitch) is set at birth. Each muscle cell contains groups of *actin* and *myosin* protein *myofilaments* called *myofibrils.* Skeletal muscle cells have alternating dark and light bands, caused by the overlap of the myosin and actin myofilaments, the basic contractile proteins of skeletal muscle. The smallest functional skeletal muscle subunit capable of contraction is the *sarcomere,* which extends from Z-line to Z-line. Skeletal muscle contraction takes place as the myofilaments slide past each other, and the actin and myosin form and re-form bonds.

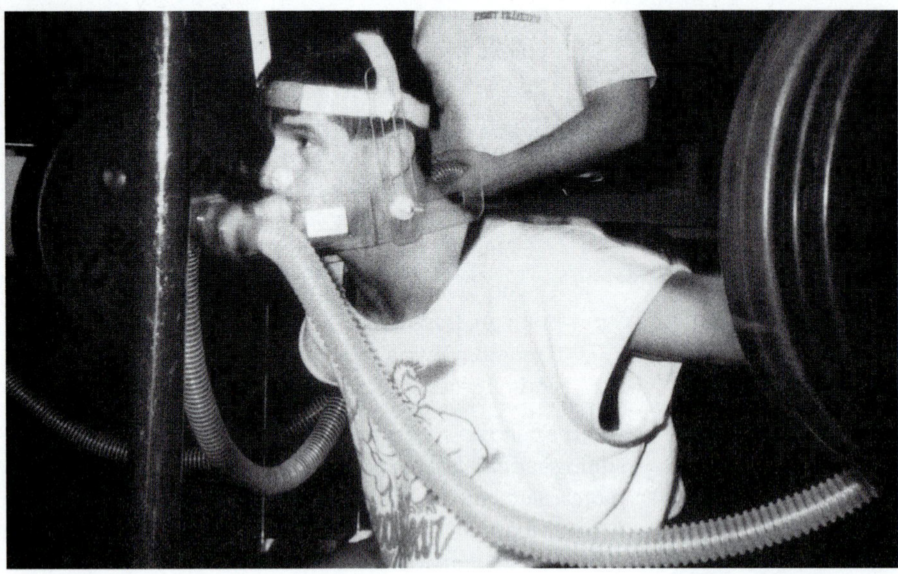

Figure 7.15 Studies show that $\dot{V}O_{2max}$ is not effectively increased by strength training.

- Most studies have shown that weight training programs will increase lean body mass and decrease the percentage of body fat.[50] Weight training programs of 7–24 weeks generally increase the lean body mass by between 0.5 and 3.0%.
- $\dot{V}O_{2max}$ is not effectively increased by strength training programs.[4,5,50,53] There may be small increases in cardiorespiratory fitness after *circuit resistance training* (weight lifting with little pause between a series of different stations). However, these improvements are relatively minor (5–8%) compared to those typical in aerobic programs (see Figure 7.15).
- The heart adapts to the stresses (especially the rise in blood pressure) imposed during weight training by increasing the thickness of the left ventricle wall without an increase in the volume.[4,5]

Interestingly, weight training to increase leg strength has been shown to improve short-term (4–8 min) cycling or running endurance, and long-term cycling, but not long-term running endurance.[52,53] It appears that the increase in leg strength improves endurance performance (despite no improvement in $\dot{V}O_{2max}$) by reducing the rate of fast-twitch fiber recruitment and increasing the lactate threshold.

The Effects of Gender, Age, and Heredity

Do females adapt to regular exercise differently than males? Do middle-aged and elderly people adjust differently than younger adults? Are there special considerations for children and teenagers? How much is the ability to improve $\dot{V}O_{2max}$ due to heredity?

The Influence of Gender

Not long ago, women were thought to be too fragile to compete in athletics. Women were first allowed to participate in the 1912 Olympics, and some events, such as the women's marathon, were only added in 1984. Today, more and more sports are available to women, and there is a push worldwide to ensure equity for women in sport.

Women are also proving that they are capable of feats once thought impossible for the "weaker sex." At the 1984 Olympic Games in Los Angeles, Joan Benoit-Samuelson won the gold medal in the first-ever Olympic marathon race event for women. Her time was 2 hours and 24 minutes, a standard that would have won 11 of the previous 20 men's Olympic marathons. In 1988, Paula Newby-Fraser completed the Hawaiian Ironman triathlon—comprising a 2.4-mile sea swim, a 111-mile cycle ride, and a 26-mile run—in 9 hours and 1 minute, just 30 minutes (6%) slower than the male winner. Only 10 men were ahead of her that year. During the 1990s, women runners and swimmers from China have stunned the world with their dominating performances. For example, Wang Junxia set a world record for the 10,000-meter race in September of 1993 by running a time of 29 minutes and 31 seconds, shattering the old record by 42 seconds. Wang's time was better than the times of all male runners prior to 1949.

The gap between the best men and the best women athletes has shrunk sharply since the early 1970s. In the Boston marathon, for example, the difference in winning times for men and women has diminished from 54 minutes in 1972 to about 14 minutes in 2001. The gender performance gap in many endurance events has now stabilized, however, largely because the quick gains following the loosening of social restraints have run their course. Figure 7.16 summarizes world record times in the 5,000-meter run for men and women. Notice that women started late in racing 5,000 me-

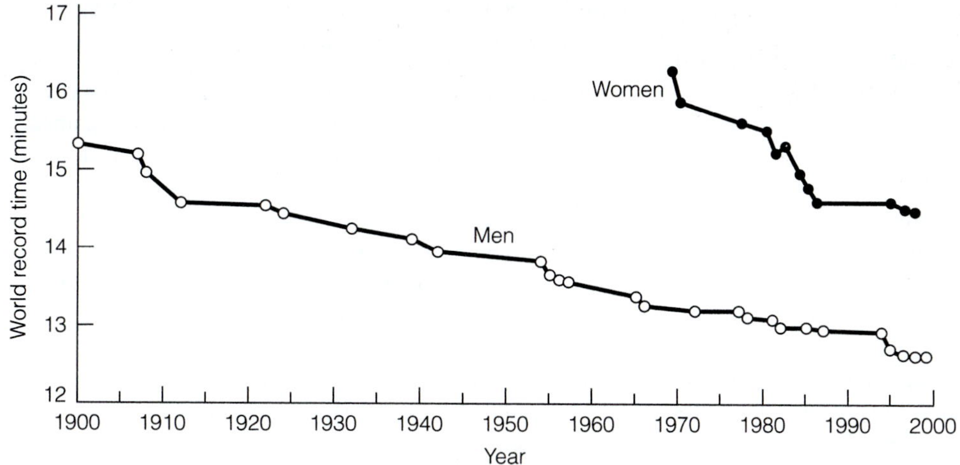

Figure 7.16 Comparison between men and women: progress in the 5,000-meter run. The gender gap in performance has stabilized in the 5,000-meter run and other endurance events.

ters, quickly began to narrow the gender gap, but then stalled during the mid-1980s.

Can women get as fit as men?[6,54–58] At puberty, testosterone secretion in males increases, leading to larger bones and increased muscle mass. In females, estrogen secretion increases, broadening the pelvis, stimulating breast development, and increasing the amount of fat in the thigh and hip areas. These unique sex differences continue into adulthood and largely explain why men and women differ in size, strength, and athletic performance.[6]

When the top female runners in the world are compared with their male counterparts, race times are 9–15% slower over all distances. This gap is not expected to decrease, largely because males and females differ in at least two important areas related to physical fitness.[57]

1. *Heart and lung fitness.* Women have less hemoglobin in their blood than men do, thereby reducing the amount of oxygen that can be delivered to working muscles.[6] Women also tend to have more body fat, less skeletal muscle, and smaller lungs and hearts.[54–57] Together, these factors mean that women have a lower $\dot{V}O_{2max}$ than men (25% lower on average, when comparing nonathletes), and they tend to perform at a lower level in aerobic sports such as running, cycling, swimming, and rowing. When women and men train at the same intensity, duration, and frequency, both show expected improvements in $\dot{V}O_{2max}$. Men, however, usually start and end at higher levels. Elite female athletes have $\dot{V}O_{2max}$ values that exceed those of most men but still fall 8–12% below those of elite male athletes.
2. *Muscle strength and size.* The average woman has about half the upper-body strength of men, and one fourth the lower-body strength.[6] In the weight room, women can experience strength gains with regular training, but increase in muscle size is less than what is seen in most men. Of course, some female bodybuilders have more muscle size and definition than most untrained men. There are few such women, however, and the best female bodybuilders cannot compare in muscle mass to the best male bodybuilders. In general, women have less muscle and more fat than men, and this is an important reason for the gap in performance times between the sexes.[6]

The issue of whether too much exercise can be harmful to women is explored in Chapter 16. For some female athletes, the pressure to keep body weight low and to be successful can lead to heavy training and disordered eating, loss of the menstrual period, and thinning of the bones, a syndrome called the *female athlete triad.*[59]

Do different phases of the menstrual cycle affect a woman's ability to exercise? Although some women report that premenstrual symptoms interfere with ability to exercise, researchers have been unable to link this with actual changes in the body.[6,60] In surveys, between one third and two thirds of female athletes report that their ability to exercise is *not* negatively affected during any phase of the menstrual cycle.[6] Up to one fourth report that performance is hindered during the premenstrual phase and the first few days of menstrual flow, with an improvement during the immediate postmenstrual days. Many women link premenstrual symptoms (PMS) such as fluid retention, weight gain, and mood changes with decreases in ability to exercise.

Scientists have studied whether there are actual physiological explanations for these reports by women athletes. Changes in many body functions do occur throughout the normal menstrual cycle, but researchers have been unable to associate menstrual cycle phase with problems in athletic performance.[60] Also, female athletes report that they can rise above their feelings when necessary to compete, and experts point out that world records have been set during all phases of the menstrual cycle. Joan Benoit-Samuelson's period was due the day of the 1984 Olympic marathon, and she won the gold medal.

The Influence of Age

The influence of the aging process on chronic adaptations to exercise is covered in more detail in Chapter 15. With aging, the ability to engage intensively in physical exercise declines, with a reduction of maximal aerobic power.[61–63] Aerobic power normally decreases 8–10% per decade after 30 years of age. Data suggest that the overall rate of loss is similar for active and inactive people, but that at any given age, the active conserve more function. Most researchers have shown that the cardiorespiratory trainability of the elderly does not differ greatly from that of younger adults when groups are compared on a percentage but not an absolute basis.[61] Between the ages of 30 and 70 years, muscle mass and strength decreased on average about 30%.[43] The aging process appears to account for only a small portion of this loss, with inactivity having the major influence.

Do children and youths respond to aerobic exercise programs in a similar fashion to adults? Most researchers have reported that the cardiorespiratory systems of children and youths respond to regular aerobic exercise in a fashion somewhat similar to that seen in adults.[6,64–70] There are a few differences, however.

Studies have shown that children can improve aerobic fitness after training, but that the increase is less than that found for adults.[64] Several factors may be responsible for this difference: (a) Children often have high aerobic fitness levels to begin with; (b) adults may train more effectively than children; and (c) the bodies of children may lack the ability to adapt and respond fully to regular exercise.

There are some other important differences between children and adults. Children have smaller hearts, lungs, and blood volumes.[6] The heart of a child cannot pump out as much blood per minute of exercise as an adult heart can, resulting in a lower oxygen delivery to the child's working muscles. $\dot{V}O_{2max}$ does not fully develop until late adolescence.

Children have a larger body surface area than adults do, when calculated per unit of body mass.[6] As a result, the smaller the child, the greater is the risk of excessive heat loss. This is particularly important when the child exercises in water, which can draw the body heat from the child very quickly, leading to *hypothermia* (i.e., low body temperature). To prevent hypothermia, children who swim or play in the water should be encouraged to leave the water periodically and to avoid cold lakes and streams.

Children, when compared to adults, have a less well developed sweating capacity.[6] They also produce more heat during activities such as running or vigorous sports play, and they can experience a faster increase in body temperature when dehydrated. These differences put children at risk for heat-related illness during long-term exercise in the heat. Researchers strongly recommend that children drink fluids frequently and avoid excessive exercise in the heat.

In 1993, an international group of experts sponsored by 13 scientific, medical, and governmental organizations submitted guidelines on physical activity for teenagers.[65] Two guidelines were recommended:

1. All adolescents should be physically active nearly every day. The activity can be a part of play, games, sports, work, transportation, recreation, physical education classes, or planned exercise with the family or community. Adolescents should engage in a variety of physical activities, and these should be enjoyable and involve most of the major muscle groups. The experts agreed that this would help reduce the risk of obesity and would promote the development of healthy bones. According to the conference report, "This is consistent with adult recommendations to engage in 30 minutes of daily activities of moderate intensity."[65] Studies show that most adolescents meet this guideline, getting about 60 minutes per day of some type of physical activity, most of this outside of school. Unfortunately, during adolescence, time spent by both girls and boys in physical activity declines, continuing into adulthood.
2. Teenagers should pursue vigorous exercise for 20 minutes or more each session, at least three times a week. Among adolescents, only about two thirds of males and one half of females meet this guideline. Examples of activities that are recommended include brisk walking, jogging, stair climbing, basketball, racquet sports, soccer, dance, swimming laps, skating, weight training, lawn mowing, cross-country skiing, and cycling. The consensus was that the more vigorous exercise should enhance psychological health, increase HDL cholesterol, and increase cardiorespiratory fitness.

Is it safe for children and youths to lift weights?[67–70] For many years, weight training was not recommended for children and adolescents for two reasons: (1) Heavy weight lifting was thought to interfere with bone growth and to promote bone and joint injury; (2) it was claimed that weight training was not effective in children before the time of puberty. Most studies now support weight training as both safe and effective for children and youths.[69] Still, the American Academy of Pediatrics has cautioned that children and adolescents should avoid intensive weight lifting, power lifting, and bodybuilding until they are about 15 years of age.[67] Moderate weight lifting by children should be under adult supervision to decrease the risk of injury. Weight training is recommended two or three times a week for 20 to 30 minutes a session and should be part of an overall comprehensive program designed to increase total fitness.

According to most experts, children can improve strength with appropriate weight training by about 15–30%.[67–70] The rise in strength is not usually related to any measurable increase in muscle size, however. Instead, improvements in nerve and muscle cell interactions occur, augmenting strength.[6,67–70]

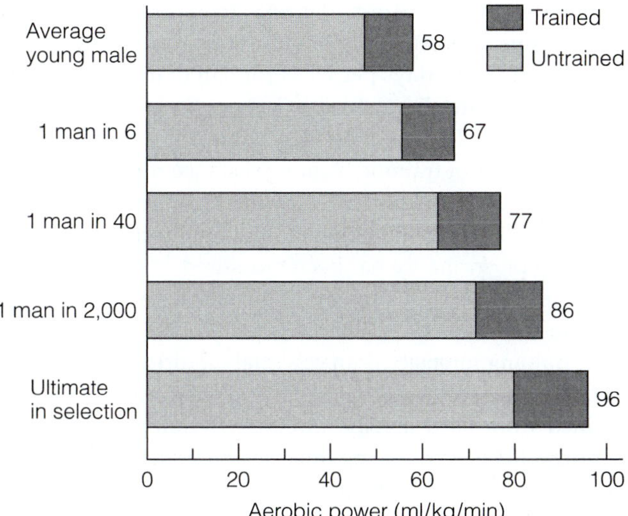

Figure 7.17 Relative importance of inherited athletic selection and rigorous training. Few people are genetically selected for athletic success and a high aerobic power. Even among those selected for a high $\dot{V}O_{2max}$, intense training may improve aerobic power only an additional 20%. Source: Data from Shephard RJ, Astrand P-O. Endurance in Sport: *The Encyclopedia of Sports Medicine* (Volume II). Oxford: Blackwell Scientific Publications, 1992.

The Influence of Heredity

Studies reporting the influence of heredity on aerobic performance have had conflicting results.[71–77] Several twin studies have suggested that $\dot{V}O_{2max}$ and work capacity were almost entirely inherited, whereas others have reported little genetic effect. The best studies now show that 10–40% of the variance in $\dot{V}O_{2max}$, after adjustment for age, sex, and body mass, can be accounted for by family relationships.[71,73]

The sensitivity of physiologic improvement to exercise training is in part dependent on heredity.[72,74–77] There are marked individual differences in responses to exercise training. Age, sex, and race explain little of this variance, while the initial level of phenotype is a major determinant of training response for some traits such as submaximal exercise heart rate and blood pressure but has only a minor effect on others such as $\dot{V}O_{2max}$ and HDL cholesterol.[74–76]

Prior endowment and an adequate training program will produce exceptionally high performance. From a practical point of view, because of heredity, it is almost impossible to accurately predict an individual response to a given training program. Nonetheless, most Olympic winners appear to be genetically selected for their events, and then train long and hard to gain the extra advantage needed for success[2] (see Figure 7.17).

THE EFFECTS OF INACTIVITY

Prolonged inactivity has many detrimental effects on the muscles, bones, and cardiovascular system of the human body.[78–80] Disuse adversely affects all body tissues and all body functions. For example, bed rest leads to a muscle protein loss of 8 grams per day, a bone calcium loss of 1.54 grams per week, a decrease in $\dot{V}O_{2max}$ of 0.8% per day, and a 10–15% decrease in plasma volume within several days.[79,80]

Few humans undergo prolonged bed rest. However, nearly all people have exercised for a certain period of time and then for various reasons reduced or terminated formal exercise while continuing normal day-to-day activities. This period of *detraining* leads to many changes in physiological function.[80–91]

Edward Coyle, from the University of Texas at Austin, has been a leading researcher on the physiological effects of detraining. In one study, Coyle studied the effects of 84 days of no formal exercise on athletes who had been training hard for 10 years.[82,83]

During this long detraining period, the various systems of the body reacted differently. In the first 3 weeks after training ceased, runners quickly lost most of their cardiovascular conditioning, primarily due to a rapid decline in stroke volume. The maximal stroke volume declined 10–14% below the trained level in just 12 days and dropped to a level no different from sedentary controls by the end of the study. $\dot{V}O_{2max}$ declined 7% in the first 21 days and stabilized after 56 days at a level 16% below the trained level. At the end of 8 weeks, the oxidative enzyme levels in the muscles had dropped 40% from the trained levels.

Other researchers have also found that the activities of mitochondrial enzymes are markedly reduced with the cessation of physical training.[84]

Muscle capillarization, however, dropped only 7% below trained levels after 84 days. Although maximal cardiac output and stroke volume declined to untrained levels, $\dot{V}O_{2max}$ levels in the detrained athletes remained 17% above untrained levels, primarily because of an elevation of maximal $a - \bar{v}O_2$ difference.

Eighty-four days of detraining also affected responses to submaximal exercise (74% $\dot{V}O_{2max}$, trained state).[83] Within 8 weeks, most of the negative adaptations occurred, including an 18% increase in oxygen consumption (using the same workload), a 17% increase in heart rate (158 when trained vs. 185 when detrained), a 24% increase in ventilation, a 6% increase in the respiratory exchange ratio, and a 34% increase in the rating of perceived exertion (as measured on the Borg scale). Within 8 weeks, the rise in lactate in response to the same workload was nearly sixfold. Other researchers have shown that running or cycling endurance performance (e.g., running races or cycling time trials) is negatively affected early in the detraining period.[85–88]

Even after detraining for 12 weeks, however, the athletes still had high muscle capillary densities and a mitochondrial enzyme level 50% above that of the sedentary controls. These represent persistent adaptations resulting from many years of hard training and that helped to partially preserve their exercise performance ability.

These studies support the argument that physical activity must be continued on a regular basis if one is to retain the benefits. As noted previously, when athletes detrain after many years of intense training, they display large reductions in cardiorespiratory fitness during the first 12–21 days of inactivity. The decline in stroke volume appears to be largely a result of reduced plasma volume, which also drops 12% within 12–21 days.[81] Interestingly, Coyle has shown that if an athlete who has detrained for 2–4 weeks expands the blood volume back to that of the trained state, using 6% dextran solution in saline, stroke volume and $\dot{V}O_{2max}$ can be increased to within 2–4% of trained values.[80,81]

Researchers have shown that the rise in aerobic power with training is just as rapid as its fall without it. Studies show that most of the improvements in $\dot{V}O_{2max}$ occur within 3 weeks of beginning intense cardiorespiratory training. In addition, once the desired $\dot{V}O_{2max}$ is achieved, it is possible to maintain it by reducing the frequency while maintaining the intensity of training.[92,93]

In one study, 12 participants bicycled and ran for 40 minutes, 6 days per week, following an intensive interval training regimen.[92] After 10 weeks, they continued to train at the same intensity and daily duration, but the frequency was lowered to 2 days per week for half of them, 4 days for the others. After 5 weeks, the $\dot{V}O_{2max}$ in both groups remained at the 25% improved level attained at the end of the first 10 weeks of training. Among distance runners, if training volume is decreased by more than half during a 3-week period while intensity is maintained, no decrement in 5-K running performance has been measured.[85,87]

In other words, it appears to take more energy expenditure to increase $\dot{V}O_{2max}$ than to maintain it. It also appears that training intensity is an essential requirement for maintaining the increased $\dot{V}O_{2max}$ and performance ability gained from hard aerobic training. Detraining also has a strong effect in reducing muscle strength and size.[89–91] Muscular strength returns to control levels within 4–12 weeks of detraining but can be maintained if weight training frequency is just one or two sessions per week.

SPORTS MEDICINE INSIGHT

Factors Affecting Performance

If a group of people are asked to run 10 kilometers or cycle 40 kilometers as fast as possible, would it be possible to predict the top finishers? What factors are most important in cardiorespiratory endurance performance? Three major physiological factors affect cardiorespiratory endurance performance:[94–109]

1. $\dot{V}O_{2max}$
2. Anaerobic threshold
3. Exercise oxygen economy

If a group of people varying widely in activity patterns (sedentary to elite athlete) were examined in the laboratory, $\dot{V}O_{2max}$ would be the most important variable predicting ability to engage in cardiorespiratory endurance events. However, among a homogeneous group of elite endurance athletes, the anaerobic threshold and exercise oxygen economy would be better indicators of performance ability.

Although important, $\dot{V}O_{2max}$ is only one of several factors that determine success in endurance events. There can be a large variation in performance among athletes of equal $\dot{V}O_{2max}$.[94] Relatively low $\dot{V}O_{2max}$ values have been reported among some top-class marathon runners. Derek Clayton, former world-record holder in the marathon (2:08.33), had a $\dot{V}O_{2max}$ of only 66.8 ml · kg^{-1} · min^{-1}, while Frank Shorter, an Olympic gold medalist in the marathon, measured only 72 ml · kg^{-1} · min^{-1}. Kjell Erik Stahl, formerly one of the best master runners in the world, also had a $\dot{V}O_{2max}$ of only 66.8 ml · kg^{-1} · min^{-1}.

Joan Benoit-Samuelson, one of the best female marathon runners in history (2:21), had a $\dot{V}O_{2max}$ of 78 ml · kg^{-1} · min^{-1}, a value much higher than Clayton's, Shorter's, and Stahl's, yet her marathon time was much slower. Obviously, other factors play an important role in cardiorespiratory endurance performance.

Exercise oxygen economy is the oxygen cost of exercise, usually expressed as $\dot{V}O_2$ at a certain running or exercise pace.[104] It is a well-established fact that $\dot{V}O_2$ at a certain workload or running speed can vary considerably among different athletes[94,95,106] (see Figure 7.18). Some of the best

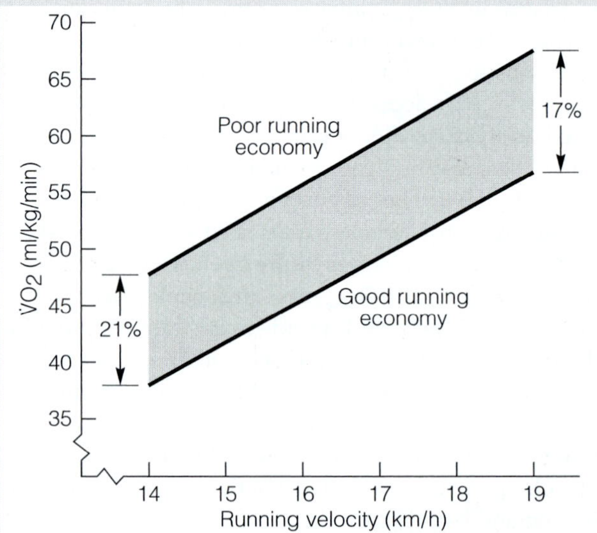

Figure 7.18 Oxygen economy. The shaded area represents the entire range in the oxygen cost of running at different velocities for good and elite runners. Source: Adapted from Sjodin B, Svedenhag H, Brotherhood JR. Applied physiology of marathon running. *Sports Med* 2:83–99, 1985. Data from ADIS Press Limited, Auckland, New Zealand.

(continued)

SPORTS MEDICINE INSIGHT *(continued)*

Factors Affecting Performance

performers have low oxygen requirements at specific running velocities. While it is not possible to explain this variation precisely, biomechanical, physiological, psychological, and biochemical factors probably all play a part. There is good evidence that athletes with a high percentage of slow-twitch fibers have the best exercise oxygen economy.[103,106]

Another important factor influencing athletic performance is the anaerobic threshold. Anaerobic threshold is highly correlated with endurance performance (r = .94 to .98).[11–15,94] If a performer can exercise at a high percentage of $\dot{V}O_{2max}$ before lactic acid builds up in the bloodstream, that capacity provides a great advantage. Such a capacity is built up through long years of training, with an emphasis on interval training (see Figure 7.19).

Other factors, nonphysiological in nature, also play an important role in cardiorespiratory endurance capacity. In one study of 4,358 runners, the most important predictors of 16-K race time, in order, were weekly training distance, age, body mass index, years of regular running, and weekly training frequency.[101] Other studies have also consistently shown weekly training distance to provide the highest correlation with endurance race performance.[94] Although elite athletes often average only 60–65% of $\dot{V}O_{2max}$ intensity during training, most have two or three sessions per week where they run intervals at 5-K and 10-K race pace to improve $\dot{V}O_{2max}$ and the anaerobic threshold.[107,108]

Table 7.6 summarizes the physical and physiological characteristics of different categories of endurance runners.[94]

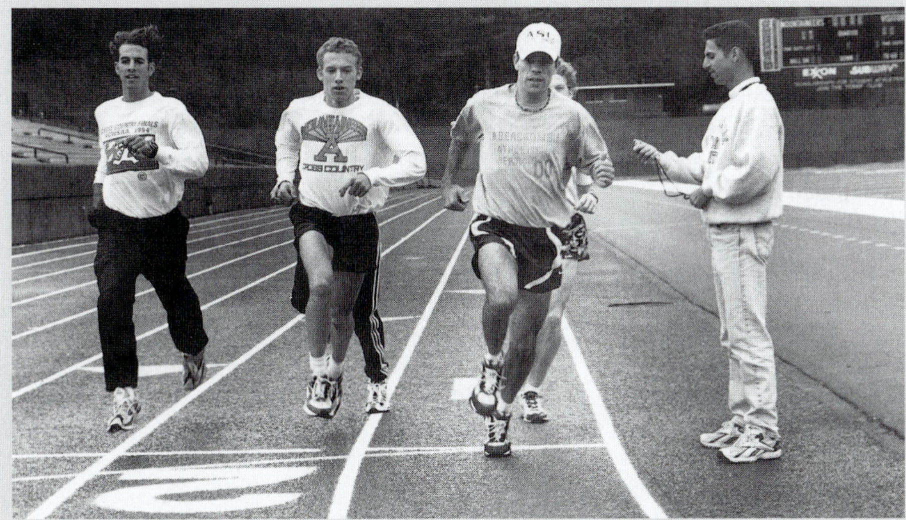

Figure 7.19 The anaerobic threshold is built up through long years of training, with an emphasis on interval training.

TABLE 7.6 Physical and Physiological Characteristics of Different Categories of Endurance Runners

	Elite Runners	Good Runners	Slow Runners
Age (years)	26	30	36
Weight (kg)	66	67	71
Type I fibers (%)	76	64	56
Years of training	7	4	2
Average weekly distance (km)	145	115	57
$\dot{V}O_{2max}$ ($ml \cdot kg^{-1} \cdot min^{-1}$)	72	66	59
$\dot{V}O_2$ at 15 km/h	45	49	51
Lactate threshold*	88	88	85

*Percent $\dot{V}O_{2max}$ when lactic acid is a concentration of 4 mmol/L.

Source: Adapted from Sjodin B, Svedenhag J, Brotherhood JR. Applied physiology of marathon running. *Sports Med* 2:83–99, 1985.

SUMMARY

1. This chapter summarized the acute responses and chronic adaptations that occur with exercise.
2. The acute responses include increases of heart rate, stroke volume, cardiac output, blood flow to active muscles, systolic blood pressure, arteriovenous oxygen difference, ventilation, lung diffusion capacity, oxygen uptake, and a decrease in blood pH and plasma volume (red blood cell count rises).
3. Chronic adaptations include biochemical changes in skeletal muscles (increased myoglobin, mitochondria, enzymes, fuels, slow-twitch fiber area); resting cardiorespiratory changes (increase in heart size, stroke volume, blood volume, and capillary density, with a decrease in resting heart rate); submaximal exercise changes (increase in anaerobic threshold and stroke volume, with a decrease in lactic acid production, heart rate, and cardiac output); maximal exercise changes (increase in $\dot{V}O_{2max}$, stroke volume, blood flow to active muscles, ability to tolerate higher lactic acid levels, ventilation, and lung diffusion capacity, plus a variable effect on maximal heart rate); and other assorted changes (decrease in total body fat, blood lipids, and recovery heart rate, with an increase in heat acclimatization and the density and strength of bone and connective tissues).
4. The performance gap between the sexes occurs because of important differences between men and women. Women have less hemoglobin, more body fat, less skeletal muscle, smaller lungs and heart, a lower $\dot{V}O_{2max}$, and less strength than their male counterparts at all similar levels of fitness (sedentary to elite status). Most researchers have shown that cardiorespiratory trainability of the elderly does not differ greatly from that of younger adults when groups are compared on a percentage (not absolute) basis. For children and teenagers, researchers have in general concluded that when programs satisfy adult-related criteria for intensity and duration, children demonstrate a similar physiological training effect.
5. The genetic effect is about 10–40% for $\dot{V}O_{2max}$. There is large variability in trainability, and researchers have concluded that the sensitivity of $\dot{V}O_{2max}$ improvement to exercise training depends in part on hereditary factors. Therefore, an exceptionally high performance level will be the result of prior endowment, an adequate training program, and genetic characteristics associated with the status of a high responder to training.
6. Inactivity (through bed rest) affects virtually every physiological system. Early responses involve the fluid, electrolyte, and blood pressure control systems, with significant muscular atrophy and decreases in bone density occurring somewhat later.
7. Detraining (termination of exercise training, but not bed rest) affects the different systems variously, with stroke volume being affected quickly (decreasing to control levels within 1 month), and muscle capillarization dropping only 7% after 84 days of detraining. The respiratory capacity of trained muscles (mitochondrial enzymes) decreases by 50% after 1 week of inactivity. To prevent these detraining effects, it is more important to maintain the intensity of exercise than the frequency of exercise.
8. Factors affecting performance include $\dot{V}O_{2max}$, anaerobic threshold, and exercise oxygen economy. While $\dot{V}O_{2max}$ is most important when evaluating the performance ability of a heterogeneous group, the anaerobic threshold and exercise oxygen economy are most important when comparing athletes of similar ability.

Review Questions

1. *After a person undergoes several months of endurance training, the person's ____ will demonstrate a decrease while at rest (compared to the untrained state).*

   A. Heart rate
   B. Oxygen consumption
   C. Stroke volume
   D. Cardiac output
   E. Ventilation

2. *After a person undergoes several months of endurance training, the person's ____ will demonstrate an increase during submaximal exercise (compared to the untrained state).*

   A. Heart rate
   B. Oxygen consumption
   C. Stroke volume
   D. Cardiac output
   E. Ventilation

3. *After a person undergoes several months of endurance training, the person's ____ will demonstrate no (or slight) change at the point of maximal exertion (compared to the untrained state).*

   A. Heart rate
   B. Oxygen consumption
   C. Stroke volume
   D. Cardiac output
   E. Ventilation

4. *Cardiac output is equal to the stroke volume times the ____.*

   A. Heart rate
   B. Oxygen consumption
   C. Frequency of breathing
   D. Arteriovenous oxygen difference
   E. Ventilation

5. *Beyond a threshold of ____% $\dot{V}O_{2max}$, the stroke volume increases very little with increase in workload.*

A. 25 B. 50 C. 70 D. 80 E. 90

6. *When changing position from lying down to standing, there is a ____ in the stroke volume.*

A. Increase B. Decrease

7. *The ____ reflects the amount of oxygen extracted by the tissues of the body.*

A. Heart rate
B. Stroke volume
C. Frequency of breathing
D. Arteriovenous oxygen difference
E. Ventilation

8. *The resting arteriovenous oxygen difference is ____ ml/100 ml blood.*

A. 5 B. 8 C. 10 D. 15 E. 20

9. *For every liter of oxygen the body consumes during exercise, approximately ____ kilocalories of energy are produced.*

A. 5 B. 8 C. 10 D. 15 E. 20

10. *Oxygen consumed equals the ____ times the arteriovenous oxygen difference.*

A. Heart rate B. Oxygen consumption
C. Stroke volume D. Cardiac output
E. Ventilation

11. *Blood pressures are higher during ____ at the same absolute workload.*

A. Cycling with legs B. Cycling with arms

12. *The mean arterial pressure = ____ (systolic − diastolic pressure) + diastolic pressure*

A. 20% B. 33% C. 45% D. 50% E. 67%

13. *The ____ = TV × f.*

A. Heart rate B. Oxygen consumption
C. Stroke volume D. Cardiac output
E. Ventilation

14. *At rest, the minute ventilation is usually about ____ liters of air per minute.*

A. 2 B. 4 C. 6 D. 12 E. 20

15. *____ = ERC + RV.*

A. IRV B. FRC C. FVC D. TLC E. RMR

16. *Which one of the following increases in a curvilinear fashion from rest to maximal exertion when plotted against the workload?*

A. Heart rate B. Oxygen consumption
C. Stroke volume D. Cardiac output
E. Ventilation

17. *R = ____ /$\dot{V}O_2$.*

A. $\dot{V}CO_2$ B. RV C. IRV D. Q E. HR

18. *When the R value reaches a threshold of ____, this indicates that carbohydrate is the only fuel being used by the working muscles.*

A. 0.8 B. 0.9 C. 1.0 D. 1.25 E. 2.0

19. *With regular aerobic training, many significant changes take place in the muscle cells. Which one of the following is* **not** *included?*

A. Increase in myoglobin content
B. Increase in concentration of mitochondrial enzymes
C. Increase in number of slow-twitch fibers
D. Increased capacity to oxidize fat
E. Increase in number and size of mitochondria

20. *With regular aerobic training, stroke volume at rest will ____.*

A. Increase B. Decrease

21. *At a given submaximal workload, trained individuals will have a ____ respiratory exchange ratio than the untrained.*

A. Higher B. Lower

22. *At a given submaximal workload, trained individuals will have a ____ stroke volume than the untrained.*

A. Higher B. Lower

23. *The major limiting factor to endurance performance is ____.*

A. Maximal heart rate
B. Breathing frequency
C. Respiratory exchange ratio
D. Cardiac output
E. Ventilation

24. *The single biggest difference between endurance-trained and untrained individuals is the size of the ____.*

A. Stroke volume B. Lungs
C. Leg muscles D. Blood compartment
E. Fat compartment

25. ***Which one of the following does* not *occur in response to regular endurance exercise?***

A. Greater ability to exercise in the heat
B. Increase in bone density
C. Decrease in HDL cholesterol
D. Decrease in body fat

26. ***Several changes occur to skeletal muscles in response to strength training. Which one of the following is* not *included?***

A. Increase in size of muscle cells, especially the fast-twitch
B. Large increase in muscle cell numbers
C. Decrease in normal inhibitory nervous impulses from the brain
D. Increase in lean body mass
E. Increase in the thickness of the left ventricle wall

27. ***During detraining of athletes, which one of the following parameters is least affected?***

A. Muscle capillarization **B.** Mitochondrial enzymes
C. $\dot{V}O_{2max}$ **D.** Stroke volume
E. Plasma volume

28. ***Among people varying widely in activity patterns, ____ is the most important variable predicting ability to perform endurance exercise.***

A. $\dot{V}O_{2max}$ **B.** Anaerobic threshold
C. Exercise oxygen economy

29. ***If the arteriovenous oxygen difference is 150 ml oxygen per 1000 ml blood, and the cardiac output is 20,000 ml/min, what is the oxygen consumption?***

A. 3 L/min **B.** 2000 ml/min
C. 10 METs **D.** 45 ml · kg^{-1} · min^{-1}
E. 2750 ml/min

Answers

1. A	**16.** E
2. C	**17.** A
3. A	**18.** C
4. A	**19.** C
5. B	**20.** A
6. B	**21.** B
7. D	**22.** A
8. A	**23.** D
9. A	**24.** A
10. D	**25.** C
11. B	**26.** B
12. B	**27.** A
13. E	**28.** A
14. C	**29.** A
15. B	

REFERENCES

1. Huston TP, Puffer JC, Rodney WM. The athletic heart syndrome. *N Engl J Med* 313:24–31, 1985.
2. Shephard RJ, Åstrand P-O. *Endurance in Sport: The Encyclopaedia of Sports Medicine* (Vol. II) (2nd ed.). Oxford: Blackwell Science, 2000.
3. Bouchard C, Shephard RJ, Stephens T. *Physical Activity, Fitness, and Health: International Proceedings and Consensus Statement.* Champaign, IL: Human Kinetics, 1994.
4. Kraemer WJ. *Strength Training for Sports: Olympic Handbook of Sports Medicine.* Oxford: Blackwell Science, 2001.
5. Baechle TR, Earle RW. *Essentials of Strength Training and Conditioning* (2nd ed.). Champaign, IL: Human Kinetics, 2000.
6. Wilmore JH, Costill DL. *Physiology of Sports and Exercise.* Champaign, IL: Human Kinetics, 2004.
7. Brooks GA, Fahey TD, Baldwin KM. *Exercise Physiology: Human Bioenergetics and Its Applications* (4th ed.). St Louis: McGraw-Hill, 2004.
8. American College of Sports Medicine. *ACSM's Resource Manual for Guidelines for Exercise Testing and Prescription* (4th ed.). Philadelphia: Lippincott Williams & Wilkins, 2005.
9. McArdle WD, Katch FI, Katch VL. *Exercise Physiology: Energy, Nutrition, and Human Performance* (5th ed.). Philadelphia: Lippincott Williams & Wilkins, 2001.
10. Di Carlo LJ, Sparling PB, Millard-Stafford ML, Rupp JC. Peak heart rates during maximal running and swimming: Implications for exercise prescription. *Int J Sports Med* 12:309–312, 1991.
11. Gladden B. Muscle as a consumer of lactate. *Med Sci Sports Exerc* 32:764–771, 2000.
12. McLellan TM, Cheung KSY. A comparative evaluation of the individual anaerobic threshold and the critical power. *Med Sci Sports Exerc* 24:543–550, 1992.
13. Davis JA. Anaerobic threshold: Review of the concept and directions for future research. *Med Sci Sports Exerc* 17:6–18, 1985.
14. Londeree BR. Effect of training on lactate/ventilatory thresholds: A meta-analysis. *Med Sci Sports Exerc* 29:837–843, 1997.
15. Loat CER, Rhodes EC. Relationship between the lactate and ventilatory thresholds during prolonged exercise. *Sports Med* 15:104–115, 1993.
16. Smith TP, McNaughton LR, Marshall KJ. Effects of 4-wk training using $\dot{V}_{max}/T_{max}$ on $\dot{V}O_{2max}$ and performance in athletes. *Med Sci Sports Exerc* 31:892–896, 1999.
17. Hickson RC. Time course of the adaptive responses of aerobic power and heart rate to training. *Med Sci Sports Exerc* 13:17–20, 1981.

18. Wagner PD. Central and peripheral aspects of oxygen transport and adaptations with exercise. *Sports Med* 11:133–142, 1991.
19. Blomqvist CG, Saltin B. Cardiovascular adaptations to physical training. *Annu Rev Physiol* 45:169–189, 1983.
20. Hepple RT. Skeletal muscle: Microcirculatory adaptation to metabolic demand. *Med Sci Sports Exerc* 32:117–123, 2000.
21. Bergh U, Ekblom B, Åstrand PO. Maximal oxygen uptake "classical" versus "contemporary" viewpoints. *Med Sci Sports Exerc* 32:85–88, 2000.
22. Saltin B, Strange S. Maximal oxygen uptake: "Old" and "new" arguments for a cardiovascular limitation. *Med Sci Sports Exerc* 24:30–37, 1992.
23. Richardson RS, Harms CA, Grassi B, Hepple RT. Skeletal muscle: Master or slave of the cardiovascular system? *Med Sci Sports Exerc* 32:89–93, 1999.
24. Richardson RS. What governs skeletal muscle $\dot{V}O_{2max}$? New evidence. *Med Sci Sports Exerc* 32:100–107, 2000.
25. Spina RJ, Chi MMY, Hopkins MG, Nemeth PM, Lowry OH, Holloszy JO. Mitochondrial enzymes increase in muscle in response to 7–10 days of cycle exercise. *J Appl Physiol* 80:2250–2254, 1996.
26. Jansson E, Kaijser L. Substrate utilization and enzymes in skeletal muscle of extremely endurance-trained men. *J Appl Physiol* 62:999–1005, 1987.
27. Ama PFM, Simoneau JA, Boulay MR, et al. Skeletal muscle characteristics in sedentary Black and Caucasian males. *J Appl Physiol* 61:1758–1761, 1986.
28. Pette D. Activity-induced fast to slow transitions in mammalian muscle. *Med Sci Sports Exerc* 16:517–528, 1984.
29. Howard H, Hoppeler H, Cloassen H, et al. Influences of endurance training on the ultrastructural composition of the different muscle fiber types in humans. *Pflugers Arch* 403:369–376, 1985.
30. Cohen JL, Segal KR. Left ventricular hypertrophy in athletes: An exercise-echocardiographic study. *Med Sci Sports Exerc* 17:695–700, 1985.
31. Convertino VA. Blood volume: Its adaptation to endurance training. *Med Sci Sports Exerc* 23:1338–1348, 1991.
32. Hopper MK, Coggan AR, Coyle EF. Exercise stroke volume relative to plasma-volume expansion. *J Appl Physiol* 64:404–408, 1988.
33. Sawka MN, Convertino VA, Eichner ER, Schnieder SM, Young AJ. Blood volume: Importance and adaptation to exercise training, environmental stresses, and trauma/sickness. *Med Sci Sports Exerc* 32:332–348, 2000.
34. Costill DL, Fink WJ, Flynn M, Kirwan J. Muscle fiber composition and enzyme activities in elite female distance runners. *Int J Sports Med* 8 (suppl):103–106, 1987.
35. Martin DE, May DF. Pulmonary function characteristics in elite women distance runners. *Int J Sports Med* 8 (suppl):84–90, 1987.
36. Nieman DC, Tan SA, Lee JW, Berk LS. Complement and immunoglobulin levels in athletes and sedentary controls. *Int J Sports Med* 10:124–128, 1989.
37. Pate RR, Sparling PB, Wilson GE, Cureton KJ, Miller BJ. Cardiorespiratory and metabolic responses to submaximal and maximal exercise in elite women distance runners. *Int J Sports Med* 8 (suppl):91–95, 1987.
38. National Center for Health Statistics, Drury EF (ed.). *Assessing Physical Fitness and Physical Activity in Population-Based Surveys*. DHHS Pub. No. (PHS) 89–1253. Public Health Service. Washington, DC: U.S. Government Printing Office, 1989.
39. Rusko HK. Development of aerobic power in relation to age and training in cross-country skiers. *Med Sci Sports Exerc* 24:1040–1047, 1992.
40. Vogel JA, Patton JF, Mello RP, Daniels WL. An analysis of aerobic capacity in a large United States population. *J Appl Physiol* 60:494–500, 1986.
41. Harms CA. Effect of skeletal muscle demand on cardiovascular function. *Med Sci Sports Exerc* 32:94–99, 2000.
42. Martin WH, Montgomery J, Snell PG, et al. Cardiovascular adaptations to intense swim training in sedentary middle-aged men and women. *Circulation* 75:323–330, 1987.
43. Lutz GJ, Lieber RL. Skeletal muscle myosin II structure and function. *Exerc Sport Sci Rev* 27:63–77, 1999.
44. Abernethy PJ, Jürimäe J, Logan PA, Taylor AW, Thayer RE. Acute and chronic response of skeletal muscle to resistance exercise. *Sports Med* 17:22–38, 1994.
45. Kelley G. Mechanical overload and skeletal muscle fiber hyperplasia: A meta-analysis. *J Appl Physiol* 81:1584–1588, 1996.
46. Hortobágyi T, Devita P, Money J, Barrier J. Effects of standard and eccentric overload strength training in young women. *Med Sci Sports Exerc* 33:1206–1212, 2001.
47. Blazevich AJ, Gill ND, Bronks R, Newton RU. Training-specified muscle architecture adaptation after 5-wk training in athletes. *Med Sci Sports Exerc* 35:2013–2022, 2003.
48. McCall GE, Byrnes WC, Dickinson A, Pattany PM, Fleck SJ. Muscle fiber hypertrophy, hyperplasia, and capillary density in college men after resistance training. *J Appl Physiol* 81:2004–2012, 1996.
49. Taylor NAS, Wilkinson JG. Exercise-induced skeletal muscle growth: Hypertrophy or hyperplasia? *Sport Med* 3:190–200, 1986.
50. Kraemer WJ, Deschenes MR, Fleck SJ. Physiological adaptations to resistance exercise: Implications for athletic conditioning. *Sports Med* 6:246–256, 1988.
51. Akima H, Takahashi H, Kuno SY, Masuda K, Masuda T, Shimojo H, Anno I, Itai Y, Katsuta S. Early phase adaptations of muscle use and strength to isokinetic training. *Med Sci Sports Exerc* 31:588–594, 1999.
52. Bishop D, Jenkins DG, Mackinnon LT, McEniery M, Carey MF. The effects of strength training on endurance performance and muscle characteristics. *Med Sci Sports Exerc* 31:886–891, 1999.
53. Marcinik EJ, Potts J, Schlabach G, Will S, Dawson P, Hurley BF. Effects of strength training on lactate threshold and endurance performance. *Med Sci Sports Exerc* 23:739–743. 1991.
54. Charkoudian N, Joyner MJ. Physiologic considerations for exercise performance in women. *Clin Chest Med* 25:247–255, 2004.
55. Suetta C, Kanstrup IL, Fogh-Andersen N. Hematological status in elite long-distance runners: Influence of body composition. *Clin Physiol* 16:563–574, 1996.
56. Graves JE, Pollock ML, Sparling PB. Body compositions of elite female distance runners. *Int J Sports Med* 8(suppl):96–102, 1987.
57. Sparling PB, O'Donnell EM, Snow TK. The gender difference in distance running performance has plateaued: An analysis of world rankings from 1980 to 1996. *Med Sci Sports Exerc* 30:1725–1729, 1998.
58. Bam J, Noakes TD, Juritz J, Dennis SC. Could women outrun men in ultramarathon races? *Med Sci Sports Exerc* 29:244–247, 1997.
59. Birch K. Female athlete triad. *BMJ* 330:244–246, 2005.

60. Adams Hillard PJ, Deitch HR. Menstrual disorders in the college-age female. *Pediatr Clin North Am* 52:179–197, 2005.
61. American College of Sports Medicine, Position Stand. Exercise and physical activity for older adults. *Med Sci Sports Exerc* 30:992–1008, 1998.
62. Wilson TM, Tanaka H. Meta-analysis of the age-associated decline in maximal aerobic capacity in men: Relation to training status. *Am J Physiol Circ Physiol* 278:H829–H834, 2000.
63. Jackson AS, Wier LT, Ayers GW, Beard EF, Stuteville JE, Blair SN. Changes in aerobic power of women, ages 20–64 yr. *Med Sci Sports Exerc* 28:884–891, 1996.
64. Rowland T, Goff D, Popowski B, DeLuca P, Ferrone L. Cardiac responses to exercise in child distance runners. *Int J Sports Med* 19:385–390, 1998.
65. Sallis JF, Patrick K. Physical activity guidelines for adolescents: Consensus statement. *Pediatric Exerc Sci* 6:302–314, 1994.
66. Baquet G, van Proagh E, Berthoin S. Endurance training and aerobic fitness in young people. *Sports Med* 33:1127–1143, 2003.
67. Committee on Sports Medicine. Strength training, weight and power lifting, and bodybuilding by children and adolescents. *Pediatrics* 86:801–803, 1990.
68. Faigenbaum AD. Strength training for children and adolescents. *Clin Sports Med* 19:593–619, 2000.
69. Falk B, Tenenbaum G. The effectiveness of resistance training in children. A meta-analysis. *Sports Med* 22:176–186, 1996.
70. Guy JA, Micheli LJ. Strength training for children and adolescents. *J Am Acad Orthop Surg* 9:29–36, 2001.
71. Rankinen T, Perusse L, Rauramaa R, Rivera MA, Wolfarth B, Bouchard C. The human gene map for performance and health-related fitness phenotypes: The 2003 update. *Med Sci Sports Exerc* 36:1451–1469, 2004.
72. Pérusse L, Gagnon J, Province MA, Rao DC, Wilmore JH, Leon AS, Bouchard C, Skinner JS. Familial aggregation of submaximal aerobic performance in the HERITAGE family study. *Med Sci Sports Exerc* 33:597–604, 2001.
73. Bouchard C, Lesage R, Lortie G, et al. Aerobic performance in brothers, dizygotic and monozygotic twins. *Med Sci Sports Exerc* 18:639–646, 1986.
74. Bouchard C, An P, Rankinen T. Individual differences in response to regular physical activity. *Med Sci Sports Exerc* 33(6 suppl):S446–S451, 2001.
75. Wilmore JH, Stanforth PR, Gagnon J, Rice T, Mandel S, Leon AS, Rao DC, Skinner JS, Bouchard C. Heart rate and blood pressure changes with endurance training: The HERITAGE family study. *Med Sci Sports Exerc* 33:107–116, 2001.
76. An P, Rice T, Gagnon J, Leon AS, Skinner JS, Bouchard C, Rao DC, Wilmore JH. Familial aggregation of stroke volume and cardiac output during submaximal exercise: The HERITAGE family study. *Int J Sports Med* 21:566–572, 2000.
77. Bouchard C, Dionne FT, Simoneau J-A, Boulay MR. Genetics of aerobic and anaerobic performances. *Exerc Sport Sci Rev* 20:27–58, 1992.
78. Tipton CM, Hargens A. Physiological adaptations and countermeasures associated with long-duration spaceflights. *Med Sci Sports Exerc* 28:974–976, 1996.
79. Convertino VA. Cardiovascular consequences of bed rest: Effect on maximal oxygen uptake. *Med Sci Sports Exerc* 29:191–196, 1997.
80. Watenpaugh DE, Ballard RE, Schneider SM, Lee SM, Ertl AC, William JM, Boda WL, Hutchinson KJ, Hargens AR. Supine lower body negative pressure exercise during bed rest maintains upright exercise capacity. *J Appl Physiol* 89:218–227, 2000.
81. Coyle EF, Hemmert MK, Coggan AR. Effects of detraining on cardiovascular responses to exercise: Role of blood volume. *J Appl Physiol* 60:95–99, 1986.
82. Coyle EF, Martin WH, Sinacore DR, et al. Time course of loss of adaptations after stopping prolonged intense endurance training. *J Appl Physiol* 57:1857–1864, 1984.
83. Coyle EF, Martin WH, Bloomfield SA, et al. Effects of detraining on responses to submaximal exercise. *J Appl Physiol* 59:853–859, 1985.
84. Costill DL. Metabolic characteristics of skeletal muscle during detraining from competitive swimming. *Med Sci Sports Exerc* 17:339–343, 1985.
85. Houmard JA, Hortobagyi T, Johns RA, et al. Effect of short-term training cessation on performance measures in distance runners. *Int J Sports Med* 13:572–576, 1992.
86. Madsen K, Pedersen PK, Djurhuus MS, Klitgaard NA. Effects of detraining on endurance capacity and metabolic changes during prolonged exhaustive exercise. *J Appl Physiol* 75:1444–1451, 1993.
87. Mujika I, Padilla S. Cardiorespiratory and metabolic characteristics of detraining in humans. *Med Sci Sports Exerc* 33:413–421, 2001.
88. McConell GK, Costill DL, Widrick JJ, Hickey MS, Tanaka H, Gastin PB. Reduced training volume and intensity maintain aerobic capacity but not performance in distance runners. *Int J Sports Med* 14:33–37, 1993.
89. Hortobagyi T, Houmard JA, Stevenson JR, Fraser DD, Johns RA, Israel RG. The effects of detraining on power athletes. *Med Sci Sports Exerc* 25:929–935, 1993.
90. Colliander EB, Tesch PA. Effects of detraining following short term resistance training on eccentric and concentric muscle strength. *Acta Physiol Scand* 144:23–29, 1992.
91. Graves JE, Pollock ML, Leggett SH, Braith RW, Carpenter DM, Bishop LE. Effect of reduced training frequency on muscular strength. *Int J Sports Med* 9:316–319, 1988.
92. Hickson RC, Rosenkoetter MA. Reduced training frequencies and maintenance of increased aerobic power. *Med Sci Sports Exerc* 13:13–16, 1981.
93. Hickson RC, Foster C, Pollock ML, Galassi TM, Rich S. Reduced training intensities and loss of aerobic power, endurance, and cardiac growth. *J Appl Physiol* 58:492–499, 1985.
94. Sjodin B, Svedenhag J. Applied physiology of marathon running. *Sports Med* 2:83–99, 1985.
95. Sleivert GC, Rowlands DS. Physical and physiological factors associated with success in the triathlon. *Sports Med* 22:8–18, 1996.
96. Van Ingen Schenau GJ, De Koning JJ, Bakker FC, de Groot G. Performance-influencing factors in homogenous groups of top athletes: A cross-sectional study. *Med Sci Sports Exerc* 28:1305–1310, 1996.
97. Roecker K, Schotte O, Niess AM, Horstmann T, Dickhuth HH. Predicting competition performance in long-distance running by means of a treadmill test. *Med Sci Sports Exerc* 30:1552–1557, 1998.
98. Saunders PU, Pyne DB, Telford RD, Hawley JA. Reliability and variability of running economy in elite distance runners. *Med Sci Sports Exerc.* 36:1972–1976, 2004.
99. Pereira MA, Freedson PS. Intraindividual variation of running economy in highly trained and moderately trained males. *Int J Sports Med* 18:118–124, 1997.
100. Schabort EJ, Killian SC, Gibson ASC, Hawley JA, Noakes TD. Prediction of triathlon race time from laboratory testing in national triathletes. *Med Sci Sports Exerc* 32:844–849, 2000.

101. Marti B, Abelin T, Minder CE. Relationship of training and life-style to 16-km running time of 4000 joggers: The '84 Berne "Grand-Prix" study. *Int J Sports Med* 9:85–91, 1988.

102. Pate RR, Macera CA, Bailey SP, Bartoli WP, Powell KE. Physiological, anthropometric, and training correlates of running economy. *Med Sci Sports Exerc* 24:1128–1133, 1992.

103. Coyle EF, Feltner ME, Kautz SA, Hamilton MT, Montain SJ, Baylor AM, Abraham LD, Petrek GW. Physiological and biomechanical factors associated with elite endurance cycling performance. *Med Sci Sports Exerc* 23:93–107, 1991.

104. Morgan DW, Bransford DR, Costill DL, Daniels JT, Howley ET, Krahenbuhl GS. Variation in the aerobic demand of running among trained and untrained subjects. *Med Sci Sports Exerc* 27:404–409, 1995.

105. Barbeau P, Serresse O, Boulay MR. Using maximal and submaximal aerobic variables to monitor elite cyclists during a season. *Med Sci Sports Exerc* 25:1062–1069, 1993.

106. Coyle EF, Sidossis LS, Horowitz JF, Beltz JD. Cycling efficiency is related to the percentage of type I muscle fibers. *Med Sci Sports Exerc* 24:782–788, 1992.

107. Pate RR, Branch JD. Training for endurance sport. *Med Sci Sports Exerc* 24 (suppl):S340–S343, 1992.

108. Robinson DM, Robinson SM, Hume PA, Hopkins WG. Training intensity of elite male distance runners. *Med Sci Sports Exerc* 23:1078–1082, 1991.

109. Anderson O. The perfect pace. *Runner's World,* May 1992, 43–50.

PHYSICAL FITNESS ACTIVITY 7.1

Labeling Figures That Depict Acute and Chronic Responses to Exercise

The figure below illustrates eight different resting dynamic lung volumes, and acute and chronic changes associated with exercise. As explained in this chapter, the *acute responses to exercise* are the sudden, temporary changes in body function caused by exercise that disappear shortly after the exercise period is finished. The *chronic adaptations to exercise* are the persistent changes in the structure and function of your body following regular exercise training, which apparently enable the body to respond more easily to subsequent exercise bouts.

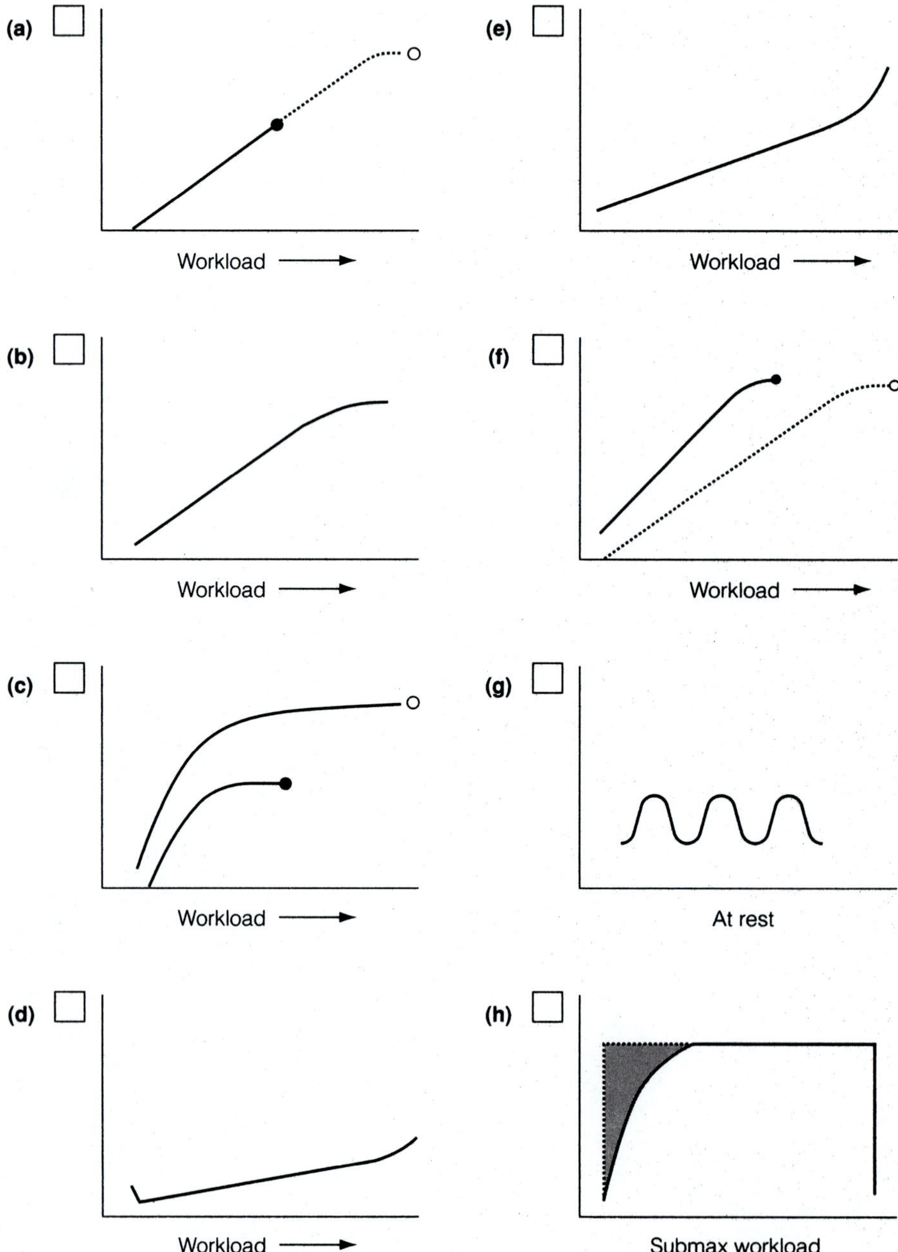

Your assignment is to label each illustration with one of the following listings. In some of the illustrations, the solid line represents the response of an untrained person; the dashed line represents the response of a trained person.

Match these answers with the appropriate illustration (a through h).

1. Respiratory exchange ratio

2. $\dot{V}O_{2max}$

3. Minute ventilation

4. Heart rate differences of trained and untrained people

5. Tidal volume

6. Stroke volume differences of trained and untrained people

7. Oxygen deficit

8. Cardiac-output differences of trained and untrained people

chapter 8

Exercise Prescription

Significant health benefits can be obtained by including a moderate amount of physical activity (e.g., 30 minutes of brisk walking or raking leaves, 15 minutes of running, or 45 minutes of playing volleyball) on most, if not all, days of the week. Through a modest increase in daily activity, most Americans can improve their health and quality of life. Additional health benefits can be gained through greater amounts of physical activity. People who can maintain a regular regimen of activity that is of longer duration or of more vigorous intensity are likely to derive greater benefit.

—Physical Activity and Health: A Report of the Surgeon General, 1996

According to the American College of Sports Medicine (ACSM), exercise prescription is the process of designing a regimen of physical activity in a systematic and individualized manner.[1,2] The art of exercise prescription is the successful integration of the science of exercise physiology with behavior change principles that results in long-term compliance to a physical activity regimen.[1,2] Each exercise prescription has five essential components:

- Frequency
- Duration
- Intensity
- Mode
- Progression

These five components should be used when developing an exercise prescription for individuals of all ages and all fitness and health levels. This chapter places emphasis on exercise prescription principles for apparently healthy individuals, with attention given to a comprehensive fitness approach (both cardiorespiratory and musculoskeletal) (see Box 8.1 for a glossary of terms used in exercise prescription). In other chapters of this book, guidelines for adapting the basic exercise prescription for children and adolescents (Chapter 7), the elderly (Chapter 15), obese individuals (Chapter 13), cardiac patients (Chapter 10), diabetics (Chapter 12), cancer patients (Chapter 11), asthmatics (Chapter 16), arthritis patients (Chapter 15), and pregnant women (Chapter 16) are outlined. ACSM has published a textbook, *Exercise Management for Persons with Chronic Diseases and Disabilities,* that provides additional physical activity guidelines for a wide variety of patients, including those with pulmonary disease, anemia, acquired immune deficiency syndrome (AIDS), chronic fatigue syndrome, stroke, spinal cord injury, epilepsy, cerebral palsy, mental retardation, visual impairment, and other diseases and disabilities.[3]

The major objective of exercise prescription is to facilitate positive changes in a client's personal physical activity habits.[1–10] This chapter reviews basic theories of health-behavior change. Chapter 1 summarized the strategies for increasing physical activity at both the population and individual levels, and the reader is invited to review that chapter once again.

According to the U.S. Surgeon General's report on physical activity and health, despite common knowledge that physical activity is healthful, more than 60% of American adults are not regularly active, and 25% of adults are not active at all (see Chapter 1).[11] Although a significant proportion of people have enthusiastically embarked on vigorous exercise programs at one time or another, most do not sustain that participation. These statistics have led to recent changes in recommendations for physical activity among various governmental and professional groups.

The first position statement from the ACSM on exercise prescription was published in 1978[12] (see Table 8.1). These guidelines recommended an exercise training frequency of 3–5 days per week, an intensity of 60–90% of maximal heart rate (50–85% of maximal oxygen uptake or heart rate reserve), a duration of 15–60 minutes per session, and an exercise mode

Box 8.1

Glossary of Terms Used in Exercise Prescription

activity pyramid: A graphic summary of guidelines underlying both the lifestyle and formal exercise approaches to physical fitness.

aerobic fitness: The ability to continue or persist in strenuous tasks involving large muscle groups for extended periods of time. Heart and lung fitness based on performing such activities as running, cycling, swimming, and sports, 3–5 days per week, at 50–85% $\dot{V}O_{2max}$, for 20–60 minutes each session.

cool-down: The transition period after the aerobic session where one slowly decreases the heart rate by keeping the feet and legs moving for 5–15 minutes through mild aerobic activity.

cross-training: A system of training in which one participates in several different types of aerobic activities to build fitness.

F.I.T. guidelines: Frequency, intensity, and time guidelines for building aerobic fitness.

flexibility exercises: A system of exercises that improve the range of motion around the body's joints.

formal exercise program: An approach to building physical fitness based on specific guidelines for aerobic and muscular fitness. A specific time and place is designated to exercise.

frequency of exercise: The number of exercise sessions per week recommended for building aerobic fitness in the exercise program. To build both aerobic fitness and keep body fat at healthy levels, one needs to exercise at least 3–5 days each week. The lifestyle approach recommends at least 30 minutes of physical activity on most days of the week.

health screening: A process in which individuals at high risk for exercise-induced heart problems are first identified and then referred to appropriate medical care.

high-intensity weight lifting: Development of muscular strength when the weight is heavy and the repetitions to maximum are low, about 4–6.

high or vigorous intensity exercise: Exercise utilizing 75% or higher of the maximum heart rate reserve or $\dot{V}O_{2max}$. This level of effort is for athletes desiring a high level of fitness.

intensity of exercise: The intensity of effort needed to build aerobic fitness: between 50 and 85% of the maximum heart rate reserve. If the fitness level is low, intensity of effort can start at 40%, with a gradual progression toward a higher intensity.

lifestyle approach to physical activity: This approach emphasizes that everyone should attempt to accumulate 30 minutes or more of moderate-intensity physical activity over the course of most, if not all, days of the week.

light intensity exercise: Exercise utilizing 40–59% of the maximum heart rate reserve or $\dot{V}O_{2max}$. This intensity range is reserved for those starting an exercise program after years of inactivity.

low-intensity weight lifting: The development of muscular endurance when the weight is somewhat light and the repetitions to fatigue are high, about 15–20.

maximum heart rate: The maximum attainable heart rate at the point of exhaustion from all-out exertion. The maximum heart rate can be estimated by using the formula 220 minus your age.

maximum heart rate reserve: The difference between the maximum heart rate and the resting heart rate.

moderate-intensity weight lifting: Development of both muscular strength and endurance when the weight is moderate and the repetitions are 8–15.

moderate intensity exercise: Exercise utilizing 60–74% of the maximum heart rate reserve or $\dot{V}O_{2max}$. This is the normal training range for most people.

muscular fitness: Muscular strength, muscular endurance, and flexibility, gained by lifting weights, doing calisthenics, engaging in physical labor, and stretching two to three times per week.

overload principle: To develop muscular strength and endurance, push the muscles to fatigue, lifting weights that are heavier than one is accustomed to.

overtraining: Pushing exercise training beyond one's ability to recover, leading to incapacitating fatigue, injury, and a loss of desire to exercise.

Physical Activity Readiness Questionnaire (PAR-Q): A simple health screening questionnaire that helps determine who should first see a medical doctor prior to starting a moderate exercise program.

principle of specificity: The development of muscular fitness is specific to the muscle groups that are exercised and the intensity of training.

progressive resistance principle: The resistance or pounds of weight against which muscles work should be increased periodically as gains in strength and endurance are made until one reaches the desired level.

repetition: One weight training or calisthenic movement.

(continued)

Box 8.1

Glossary of Terms Used in Exercise Prescription *(continued)*

repetitions maximum: The maximum number of repetitions that one can lift a certain weight.

resting heart rate: The heart rate of a person who is resting quietly. The resting heart rate is best measured in the morning just after a person wakes up.

RPE scale: The rating of perceived exertion scale. A number scale between 6 and 20 that rates a person's subjective assessment of how hard he or she is working at a given moment while exercising.

set: A certain number of weight training or calisthenic repetitions.

static stretching: Exercises that slowly apply a stretch to a muscle group, with this position held for 10–30 seconds.

time: Refers to the duration in minutes of the aerobic exercise session.

total fitness: A comprehensive approach to physical fitness that develops aerobic fitness, muscular fitness (muscular strength, endurance, and flexibility), and body composition.

training heart rate: The exercise heart rate, estimated with this formula: Training heart rate = [(maximum HR − resting HR) × 0.50–0.85] + resting HR.

training heart rate zone: The heart rate range between 50 and 85% of maximum heart rate range for all age groups.

warm-up: The 5–20 minute transition period that precedes the aerobic exercise session. The primary purpose of the warm-up is to prepare the body for vigorous exercise by performing mild-to-moderate aerobic activity.

that used large muscle groups, such as running, walking, swimming, bicycling, rowing, cross-country skiing, and rope skipping. These recommendations addressed only cardiorespiratory fitness and body composition and did not provide guidelines for musculoskeletal fitness or link physical activity patterns to health promotion and disease prevention.

In 1990 (confirmed again in 1998), the ACSM revised the 1978 exercise prescription guidelines by adding the development of musculoskeletal fitness as a major objective[13] (see Table 8.1). The ACSM advised that people engage in resistance training at least 2–3 days a week (minimum of one set of 8–12 repetitions of 8–10 different exercises). The 1990 recommendations also noted that "it is now clear that lower levels of physical activity than recommended by this position statement may reduce the risk for certain chronic degenerative diseases and yet may not be of sufficient quantity or quality to improve maximal oxygen uptake."[2] Recommendations on frequency, intensity, and exercise mode remained similar, but the duration was increased slightly to 20–60 minutes per session.

Epidemiological research since the mid-1970s has shown that health-related benefits are linked to physical activity and fitness in a dose–response manner[5,8,10,11] (see Chapters 10 through 15). The greatest difference in death rates for coronary heart disease and certain forms of cancer has been observed between the least physically active or most unfit and the next higher category.[10] In other words, the most significant public health benefits are experienced when the most sedentary individuals become moderately active. Many of the epidemiological studies used physical activity indices that counted all activities conducted throughout the day. Exercise training studies have also indicated that middle-aged and older persons, obese patients, and individuals with low aerobic fitness can improve both disease risk factors and cardiorespiratory fitness at exercise intensity levels below the 50% threshold urged by the ACSM.[11] A few early controlled studies compared single-session bouts of exercise to multiple bouts spread throughout the day, and reported similar improvements in fitness and risk factors.[14,15]

In response to these research findings, the Centers for Disease Control and Prevention and ACSM (CDC–ACSM) released their most recent physical activity guidelines in 1993 (published in 1995), recommending that all adults perform 30 or more minutes of moderate-intensity physical activity on most, and preferably all, days, either in a single session or accumulated throughout the day in multiple bouts (each lasting 8–10 minutes)[16] (see Figure 8.1, Table 8.1). This recommendation differed from the 1978 and 1990 ACSM statements on three points:

1. The minimum starting exercise intensity was lowered to 40% for patients or individuals with very low fitness.
2. The frequency of exercise sessions was increased from 3–5 days per week to 5–7 days per week.
3. An option was included for allowing people to accumulate the minimum of 30 minutes per day in multiple sessions lasting at least 8–10 minutes.

In 1998, the ACSM revised its position stand on the recommended quantity and quality of exercise, stating that the minimal training intensity threshold is 40–50% of heart rate reserve, especially for the unfit (see Table 8.1).

TABLE 8.1 Exercise Prescription Recommendations

	Intensity (% $\dot{V}O_2R$)	Duration (minutes)	Frequency (days/week)	Purpose
ACSM, 1978[12]	50–85%	15–60	3–5	Develop, maintain fitness, body composition
ACSM, 1990[13]	50–85%	20–60	3–5	Develop, maintain fitness, body composition*
CDC–ACSM, 1995[16]	Moderate/hard	30 or more in bouts of at least 8–10 min	Near daily	Health promotion†
AHA, 1996[18]	40–75%	30–60	3–6	Health promotion and cardiovascular disease prevention*
NIH, 1996[22]	Moderate/hard	30 or more	Near daily	Cardiovascular disease prevention for adults and children†
Surgeon General, 1996[11]	Moderate/hard	30 or more	Near daily	Health promotion, disease prevention†
ACSM, 1998[2]	40/50–85%	20–60	3–5	Develop, maintain cardiorespiratory fitness, body composition, muscular strength and endurance, and flexibility
IOM, 2002	Moderate	≥60	Daily	Weight management and health benefits
USDA, 2005	Moderate/vigorous	≥30 ≥60 60–90	Near daily Near daily Near daily	Reduce disease risk Prevent unhealthy weight gain Sustain weight loss for previously obese people

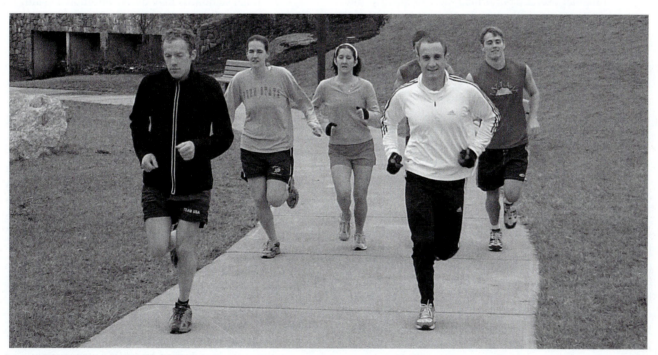

*Also includes recommendations for developing and maintaining muscular strength and endurance (at least one set of 8–12 repetitions of 8–10 exercises that condition the major muscle groups at least 2 days a week).
†Also recommends regular participation in physical activities that develop and maintain muscular strength.

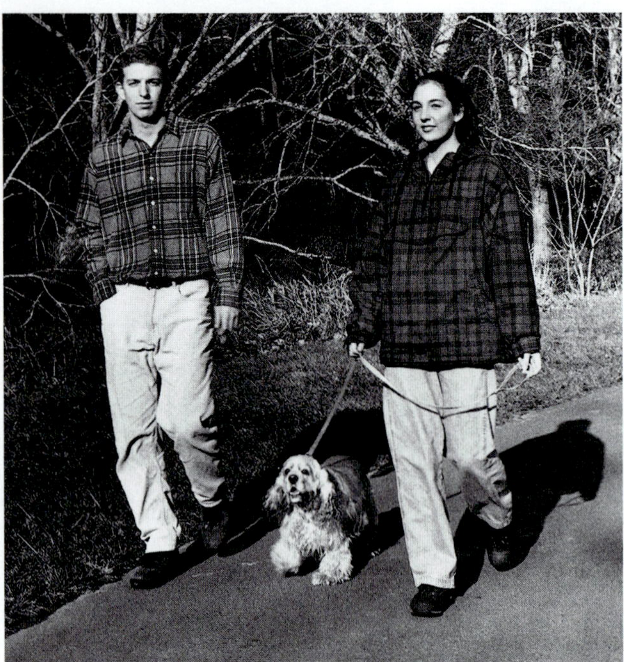

Figure 8.1 The ACSM has urged that for public health benefits, every American adult should accumulate 30 minutes or more of moderate-intensity physical activity over the course of most days of the week.[3]

> The ACSM recognizes the potential health benefits of regular exercise performed more frequently and for a longer duration but at a lower intensity than recommended in the previous editions of this position stand, i.e. 40–49% of maximum $\dot{V}O_2$ reserve and heart rate reserve or 55–65% of maximum heart rate. . . . Thus, the ACSM now views exercise/physical activity for health and fitness in the context of an exercise dose continuum. That is, there is a dose response to exercise by which benefits are derived through varying quantities of physical activity ranging from approximately 700–2,000 plus kilocalories of effort per week.[2]

Other professional and governmental groups have responded by issuing similar reports. In 1992, the American Heart Association (AHA) published a statement identifying physical inactivity as a fourth major risk factor for coronary heart disease (along with smoking, high blood pressure, and high blood cholesterol).[17] The AHA published a second report in 1996 confirming the role of physical inactivity as a risk factor for heart disease and urging that people follow exercise guidelines similar to those released by the CDC–ACSM[18] (see Table 8.1). The AHA also advised that people pay attention to joint flexibility and muscle strength, especially as they age. A consensus statement from the 1993 International Consensus Conference on Physical Activity Guidelines for Adolescents emphasized that youths should be physically active every day, as part of their general lifestyle activities and that they should engage in three or more 20-minute sessions of moderate-to-vigorous exercise each week[19] (see Chapter 7). In 1996, the American Cancer Society listed physical inactivity as a major risk factor for certain forms of cancer (see Chapter 11).[20] That same year, the U.S. Preventive Services Task Force recommended that health-care providers counsel patients regarding the importance of incorporating physical activities into their daily routines to prevent coronary heart disease, hypertension, obesity, and diabetes.[21] The National Institutes of Health Consensus Development Panel on Physical Activity and Cardiovascular Health released a statement in 1995 (published in 1996; see Table 8.1) that encouraged all Americans to

> engage in regular physical activity at a level appropriate to their capacity, needs, and interest. Children and adults alike should set a goal of accumulating at least 30 minutes of moderate-intensity physical activity on most, and preferably all, days of the week. . . . Intermittent or shorter bouts of activity (at least 10 minutes), including occupational, nonoccupational, or tasks of daily living, also have similar cardiovascular and health benefits if performed at a level of moderate intensity (such as brisk walking, cycling, swimming, home repair, and yard work) with an accumulated duration of at least 30 minutes per day. People who currently meet the recommended minimal standards may derive additional health and fitness benefits from becoming more physically active or including more vigorous activity. . . . Developing muscular strength and joint flexibility is also important for an overall activity program to improve one's ability to perform tasks and to reduce the potential for injury.[22]

The surgeon general's report on physical activity and health was released in 1996[11] (see Chapter 1). This landmark report concluded that both the traditional, structured approach to exercise described by the ACSM in 1990 and the lifestyle approach recommended by the CDC–ACSM in 1993 and by the NIH in 1995 can be beneficial and that individual interests and opportunities should determine which is used. Five major recommendations were given[11] (see Table 8.1):

1. All people over the age of 2 years should accumulate at least 30 minutes of endurance-type physical activity, of at least moderate intensity, on most—preferably all—days of the week.
2. Additional health and functional benefits of physical activity can be achieved by adding more time in moderate-intensity activity or by substituting more vigorous activity.
3. Persons with symptomatic cardiovascular disease, diabetes, or other chronic health problems who would like to increase their physical activity should

be evaluated by a physician and provided an exercise program appropriate for their clinical status.

4. Previously inactive men over age 40, women over age 50, and people at high risk for cardiovascular disease should first consult a physician before embarking on a program of vigorous physical activity to which they are unaccustomed.
5. Strength-developing activities (resistance training) should be performed at least twice per week. At least 8–10 strength-developing exercises that use the major muscle groups of the legs, trunk, arms, and shoulders should be performed at each session, with one or two sets of 8–12 repetitions of each exercise.

In 2002, the Institute of Medicine (IOM) recommended at least 60 minutes of moderately intense physical activity each day to prevent weight gain and achieve the full health benefits of activity.[9] This was reiterated by the 2005 *Dietary Guidelines for Americans,* which made the following recommendations:[7]

- *To reduce the risk of chronic disease in adulthood:* Engage in at least 30 minutes of moderate-intensity physical activity, above usual activity, at work or home on most days of the week. For most people, greater health benefits can be obtained by engaging in physical activity of more vigorous intensity or longer duration.
- *To help manage body weight and prevent gradual, unhealthy body weight gain in adulthood:* Engage in approximately 60 minutes of moderate- to vigorous-intensity activity on most days of the week while not exceeding caloric intake requirements.
- *To sustain weight loss in adulthood:* Participate in at least 60 to 90 minutes of daily moderate-intensity physical activity while not exceeding caloric intake requirements.
- *Children and adolescents:* Youth should engage in 60 minutes of physical activity on most, preferably all, days of the week.

Although these recommendations may cause some outcry, notice that the amount of physical activity varies according to an individual's personal goals, with the greatest duration reserved for adults trying to sustain weight loss.

This chapter describes in detail the traditional, structured exercise prescription guidelines published by the ACSM in 1990/1998.[2,13] However, as urged in the 1996 surgeon general's report, individual interests, goals, and opportunities should determine whether the structured or the lifestyle approach is used.[11] Even when the lifestyle approach is used, education on the five components of the structured exercise prescription (frequency, duration, intensity, mode, progression) should be given to the individual desiring to increase physical activity patterns. (See Physical Fitness Activities 8.1 and 8.2 for the two approaches in exercise prescription.)

PHYSICAL ACTIVITY PYRAMID

The ACSM views the CDC–ACSM lifestyle approach[16] and the ACSM formal approach[2] to exercise prescription as components of the same continuum of physical activity recommendations that meet the needs of almost all individuals to improve health status.[1] In other words, accumulating 30 minutes or more of moderate-intensity physical activity on most days of the week is the minimum amount of physical activity that improves the quality of life and decreases disease risk. Additional health and substantially greater fitness benefits can be achieved by adding more time in moderate-intensity activity or by substituting more vigorous activity. Few Americans are willing to adhere to a formal exercise program and find the informal lifestyle approach to physical activity more attractive.

The lifestyle approach seeks to increase opportunities for physical activity throughout the daily routine, while the formal exercise program builds aerobic and muscular fitness to high levels through an exercise system based on specific frequency, intensity, and time guidelines. The activity pyramid shows how the lifestyle and formal exercise approaches to physical fitness can complement each other (see Figure 8.2). The activity pyramid is similar to the food guide pyramid (see Chapter 9) and puts all the recommendations into a simple and easy-to-understand package.

Notice several key features about the activity pyramid (developed by the author for this textbook):

- The lifestyle approach to fitness is at the base of the activity pyramid meaning that everyone should try to accumulate at least 30 minutes of physical activity nearly every day. This is a good start and brings basic health and fitness benefits. But higher levels of aerobic and muscular fitness can be achieved by working up the activity pyramid.
- The formal exercise program is summarized on levels 2 and 3 of the activity pyramid. Aerobic fitness is increased by brisk walking, swimming, cycling, running, or engaging in active sports for 20–60 minutes, 3–5 days per week.
- Muscular fitness is gained by lifting weights, doing calisthenics, engaging in hard physical labor (e.g., chopping wood), and stretching. Perform a minimum of 8–10 separate exercises that train the major muscle groups. Perform one set of 8–12 repetitions of each of these exercises to the point of fatigue, and do this at least 2–3 days per week. For flexibility, stretch at least 2–3 days a week and involve at least four repetitions of several stretches

Reduce inactivity

Reduce time sitting watching TV, playing video games, viewing the Internet, etc.

Exercise for Muscular Fitness, 2–3 times/week

Build muscular strength and endurance through weight lifting, calisthenics, and work

Build joint flexibility through a regular routine of stretching exercises

Exercise for Aerobic Fitness, 20–60 minutes, 3–5 days per week

Participate in fitness aerobic activities like brisk walking, swimming, cycling, or running, or in active sports like basketball, soccer, or racquetball

Lifestyle Physical Activity

Accumulate at least 30 minutes nearly every day

Travel by own leg power; work with your own hands; take active work breaks

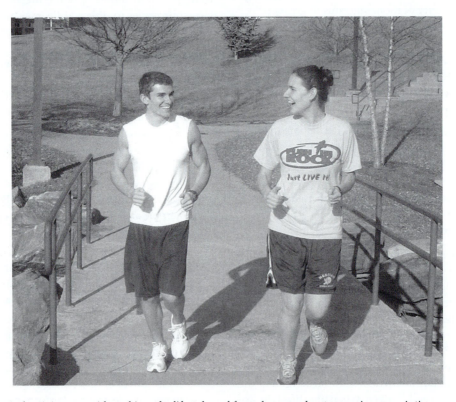

Figure 8.2 The physical activity pyramid combines the lifestyle and formal approaches to exercise prescription.

that are held 10–30 seconds at a position of mild discomfort.

- Sitting time should be reduced because Americans spend far too much time watching TV, playing video games, viewing the Internet, driving cars, and watching other people play sports.

THE INDIVIDUALIZED APPROACH

People vary widely in their health and fitness status, motivation, goals, occupation, age, needs, desires, and education.[1] Thus, to give an *exercise prescription* that best meets a person's needs in a safe and effective manner requires a clear understanding of that person.[1]

Part 2 of this book highlighted the need for obtaining medical, health, and physical fitness information for each participant to be given an exercise prescription. This cannot be emphasized enough. An exercise prescription should not be written before this information is available. In addition, it is a good idea to sit down with the person and discuss interests, felt needs, future goals, reasons for starting an exercise program, and feelings about the results of the physical fitness tests (see Figure 8.3). Once these preliminary requirements have been met, then the participant can be educated about the principles of exercise and given adequate leadership and direction through the use of an exercise prescription.

The focus since the late 1970s has been to use a comprehensive physical fitness approach. During the boom years of the aerobic movement in the 1970s and 1980s, cardiorespiratory conditioning was often the only type of exercise for many, leaving out exercises for flexibility and muscular strength and endurance. This was the reverse of what happened during the 1950s and 1960s, when muscular strength was preeminent, to the detriment of exercises for the heart and lungs. The comprehensive approach that has emerged gives attention to both cardiorespiratory and musculoskeletal fitness. On the other hand, cardiorespiratory training is still the foundation of any exercise prescription because most of the health benefits related to physical activity are associated with dynamic, whole-body, continuous, sustained activity.[11]

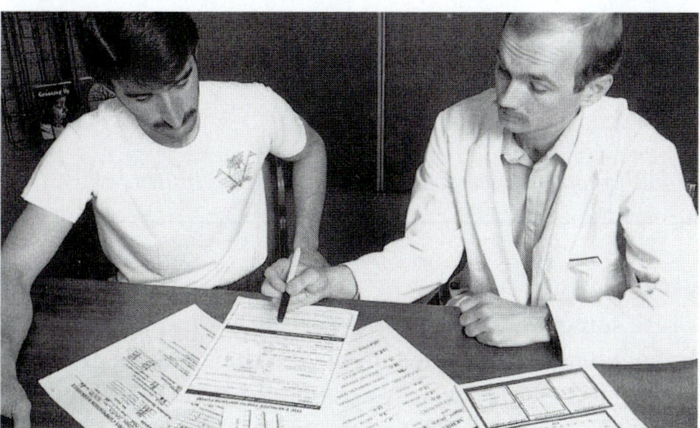

Figure 8.3 A clear understanding of the individual to be given the exercise prescription can be gained by reviewing medical, health, and physical fitness test information.

This chapter will describe a comprehensive approach to physical fitness, emphasizing a five-step approach (i.e., warm-up, aerobic session, warm-down, flexibility exercises, muscular strength and endurance exercises). Each step, in the order given, is considered important for the development of "total fitness."

Before discussing this conditioning format, an important point needs to be made. In order to realize the full benefits of regular exercise and physical activity, the development of physical fitness must be seen as one of several components contributing to wellness and health. Other components include adequate rest, a proper diet, management of stress, wholesome social and family influences, sufficient sunshine, pure air and water, sanitation, and a nurturing sense of spirituality. All these factors work together to promote health, happiness, and "good feelings."

CARDIORESPIRATORY ENDURANCE/BODY COMPOSITION

The cornerstone of a comprehensive physical fitness program is aerobic exercise. As defined in Chapter 2, cardiorespiratory endurance or aerobic fitness is the ability to continue or persist in strenuous tasks involving large muscle groups for extended periods of time. In other words, aerobic fitness is the ability of the heart, blood vessels, blood, and lungs to supply oxygen to the working muscles during such activities as brisk walking, running, swimming, cycling, and other moderate-to-vigorous activities.

The aerobic or cardiorespiratory stage of a comprehensive physical fitness program consists of three segments: the warm-up, aerobic exercise (that conforms to frequency, intensity, and time guidelines), and the cool-down. (See Box 8.2 for a worksheet that organizes the process of aerobic exercise prescription, and see Physical Fitness Activity 8.2.)

Warm-Up

A *warm-up* is defined as a group of exercises performed immediately before an activity, which provides the body with a period of adjustment from rest to exercise.[23] The warm-up can take two forms:[23,24]

1. *Passive.* Use of a warming agent to increase body temperature (e.g., hot baths, infrared light, ultrasound, or sauna)
2. *Active.* Consisting of body movements to moderately increase the heart rate and body temperature; may

Box 8.2

Worksheet: An Exercise Program to Build Aerobic Fitness

Step 1. Warm-Up

Slowly elevate the pulse and body temperature to an aerobic training level by first engaging in 5–20 minutes of easy-to-moderate aerobic activity.

Step 2. Aerobic Exercise

A. F.I.T. Guidelines

Based on current fitness level, follow the F.I.T. guidelines given in the table.

F.I.T. Guidelines	Low Fitness	Average Fitness	High Fitness
Frequency (sessions/week)	3	3–4	5 or more
Intensity (% HR reserve)	40–59	60–74	75–85
Time (minutes/session)	10–19	20–29	30–60

B. Intensity

Calculate personal training heart rate using this formula:

Training heart rate = [(maximum HR − resting HR) × intensity %] + resting HR

________ = [(________ − ________) × ________] + ________

C. Aerobic Exercise Mode

Select 2–3 exercise modes based on personal goals.

Primary mode ________

Secondary mode ________

Backup mode ________

D. Build Exercise into Daily Schedule

Note exercise time on specific days.

Sun ________
Mon ________
Tues ________
Wed ________
Thurs ________
Fri ________
Sat ________

Step 3. Cool-down

Slowly decrease the heart rate and body temperature by engaging in mild-to-moderate aerobic activity for 5–15 minutes.

include light calisthenics, jogging, stationary cycling, or exercises that provide a rehearsal for the actual performance activity (e.g., throwing a ball, swinging a bat, ballet or gymnastic movements)

The extent of the warm-up depends on individual needs, clothing, air temperature, and the intensity of the exercise to follow, but in general, the warm-up should be intense enough to increase the body's core temperature and cause some sweating.[23] However, the warm-up should not be so intense as to cause fatigue or reduce muscle glycogen stores.[24] Generally, warm-ups should take 5–20 minutes, depending on the sport and the environmental conditions.

There has been some debate as to whether *flexibility exercises* (i.e., exercises that are used to increase joint range of motion) should be included within the warm-up routine.[23–27] Some fitness leaders have advocated flexibility exercises prior to light aerobic warm-up activities,[25] while others urge that

Box 8.3

Beneficial Effects of Warm-Up before Strenuous Exercise

1. Increases breakdown of oxyhemoglobin, allowing greater delivery of oxygen to the working muscle.
2. Increases the release of oxygen from myoglobin.
3. Decreases the activation energy for vital cellular metabolic chemical reactions.
4. Decreases muscle viscosity, improving mechanical efficiency and power.
5. Increases speed of nervous impulses and augments sensitivity of nerve receptors.
6. Increases blood flow to the muscles.
7. Decreases number of injuries to muscles, tendons, ligaments, and other connective tissues.
8. Improves the cardiovascular response to sudden, strenuous exercise (especially heart muscle blood flow).
9. Leads to earlier sweating, which reduces risk of high body temperature during exercise.

these exercises be conducted only after the body temperature has been elevated.[23] For instance, the textbook *Science of Flexibility* asserts that "flexibility exercises should always be preceded by a set of mild warm-up exercises, because the increase in the tissue temperature produced by the warm-up exercise will make the stretching both safer and more productive."[23] The ACSM has "recommended that an active warm-up precede vigorous stretching exercises."[1]

Holding *static flexibility* positions before the muscle becomes warm can be potentially injurious.[23] A good plan for athletes is to exercise moderately for 5–10 minutes, then stretch, compete, cool down, and then stretch again. International-class gymnasts have long prepared for performances by running lightly (or engaging in other slow aerobic exercise) to raise body temperature, inducing a light perspiration, and then engaging in flexibility exercises.[28]

The physiological benefits of the warm-up are listed in Box 8.3.[23–36] In general, a thorough warm-up (meaning an elevation in body temperature) before hard aerobic exercise will enhance the activity of enzymes in the working muscles, reduce the viscosity of muscle, improve the mechanical efficiency and power of the moving muscles, facilitate the transmission speed of nervous impulses augmenting coordination, increase muscle blood flow and thus improve delivery of necessary fuel substrates, increase the level of free fatty acids in the blood, help prevent injuries to the muscles and various supporting connective tissues, and allow the heart muscle to adequately prepare itself for aerobic exercise.

For these reasons, researchers advise that the warm-up consist of the specific exercise that will be engaged in during the aerobic session, but at moderate intensity, allowing for a gradual increase in body temperature.[23] This not only warms the body, but also provides a slight rehearsal of the event that is to take place. Flexibility exercises should not be undertaken until the body is warm. Muscle, tendon, and ligament elasticity depends on blood saturation. Cold connective tissues, which have a low blood saturation, can be more susceptible to damage and do not stretch as readily.

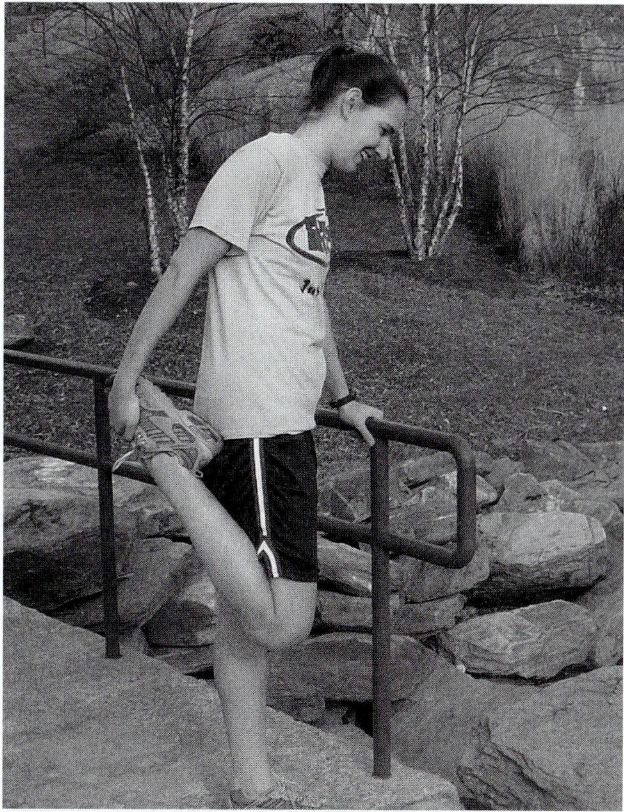

Figure 8.4 Flexibility exercises are best conducted when the body is warm from aerobic activity.

For athletes, the best plan is to stretch just after the warm-up and just after the warm-down. Recreational exercisers can concentrate on flexibility exercises after the aerobic session is over. Stretching at this time has the special advantage of allowing one to stretch warm muscles that have been contracting forcibly during aerobic exercise. It makes sense that muscles that have been continually contracting and shortening should be lengthened after the session is over. This is safer, helps ease the aftereffects of the aerobic exercise, and allows greater stretching because the muscle is warm.

For example, a jogger would start the exercise session by walking for a minute or so, then jogging easily for 2–4 more minutes, and then finally building up speed to elevate the pulse to the training-level intensity. After a warm-down with jogging/walking for several minutes (reversing the warm-up), static flexibility exercises can be performed for at least 5 minutes, emphasizing the posterior leg, lower back, and upper-front chest areas (muscles that are shortened during running) (see Figure 8.4). The same would be true for swimmers or cyclers, except that

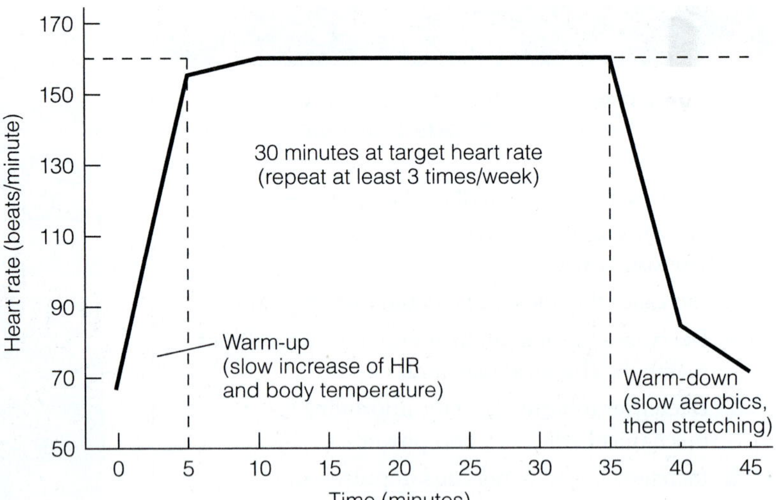

Figure 8.5 The aerobic exercise session: Exercise heart rates and time for an average college student. The aerobic session has three phases (warm-up, exercising at the target heart rate, and warm-down).

flexibility exercises would be directed more toward shoulder and thigh areas, respectively.

The Aerobic Session

To be most effective, an exercise prescription must give specific written instructions for frequency, intensity, and time of exercise (see Figure 8.5). These are known as the F.I.T. criteria of cardiorespiratory endurance training. Box 8.2 outlines the basic guidelines for aerobic exercise prescription, and Figure 8.5 puts this in graphic form. Improvement in $\dot{V}O_{2max}$ is directly related to the F.I.T. criteria followed in training. Depending on the quantity and quality of training, improvement in $\dot{V}O_{2max}$ ranges from 5 to 30%.[1,2] Greater improvement may be found for those with a very low initial level of fitness due to obesity or cardiac disease. Many articles have been written on exercise prescription.[2,6–8,12,16–19] A discussion of the major criteria follows.

Frequency

Frequency of exercise refers to the number of exercise sessions per week in the exercise program. In order to improve cardiorespiratory endurance and keep body fat at optimal levels, most reviewers have concluded that it is necessary to exercise at least three times weekly with no more than 2 days between workouts.[1,2,6] Some studies have shown some cardiorespiratory improvements with an exercise frequency of less than 3 days per week, but such improvements are at most minimal to modest and result in little or no body fat loss.

When a person is initiating an aerobic exercise program, conditioning every other day is recommended. This is especially true for running programs with those who are unfit and have been previously sedentary. For such people, the musculoskeletal system is unable to adapt quickly to hard daily exercise, and it will lead to muscle soreness, fatigue, and injury. If those starting a running program want to exercise more frequently than 3 days per week, jogging days should be mixed with days of walking, bicycling, or swimming, which are easier on the musculoskeletal system.

The ACSM recommends that patients with a low functional capacity (<3 METs) may benefit from multiple short exercise sessions (of about 3–5 minutes each) spread throughout each day.[1] As fitness improves to 3–5 METs, one to two short sessions each day are appropriate, before moving to longer sessions of 20–30 minutes, 3–5 days a week.

In the lifestyle approach advocated by the CDC–ACSM, individuals are urged to accumulate at least 30 minutes of moderate-intensity physical activity on most, preferably all, days of the week.[16] This recommendation emphasizes the benefits of moderate-intensity physical activity that can be accumulated in multiple short bouts. According to the CDC–ACSM, 30 minutes of activity can be accumulated by frequently walking up the stairs instead of taking the elevator, walking instead of driving short distances, doing calisthenics, or pedaling a stationary cycle while watching television.[16] Gardening, housework, raking leaves, dancing, and playing actively with children can also contribute to the 30-minute-per-day total, urges the CDC–ACSM, if performed at an intensity corresponding to brisk walking. Research has demonstrated that people who walk or cycle to work gain substantial health and fitness benefits.[37–39] Unfortunately, less than 1 in 12 Americans walks or cycles to work.[39] On average, inactive people take 2,000 to 4,000 steps per day, moderately active about 5,000 to 7,000, and active people 10,000 steps or more each day.[40] Individuals can wear pedometers to increase their awareness of steps taken on a daily basis. Box 8.4 provides a list of suggestions to increase lifestyle physical activity.

Several experimental studies have addressed the effects of continuous versus intermittent activity on fitness.[14,15,41–48] In general, multiple short bouts compared to one long bout of physical activity are more attractive to most people, enhance health and lower disease risk factors, and improve aerobic fitness if the intensity is moderate to

Box 8.4

Ways to Improve Lifestyle Physical Activity

If you do not like setting aside 20–60 minutes in the midst of your busy schedule for exercise, or dressing in trendy exercise clothes and shoes, or counting your heart rate to keep within the training zone, or running in circles on a track, then the lifestyle approach is for you. Since 1993, most fitness and health organizations including the Office of the Surgeon General have urged that everyone should attempt to accumulate 30 minutes or more of moderate-intensity physical activity over the course of most, if not all, days of the week. This is the minimum amount of physical activity that improves quality of life while decreasing the risk of most chronic diseases. Additional health and fitness benefits can be achieved by adding more time in moderate-intensity activity or by substituting more vigorous activity.

An active lifestyle does not require a regimented, vigorous exercise program. Instead, you can make small changes to increase daily physical activity throughout the entire day. Many people have the perception that they must engage in vigorous exercise for 20–60 continuous minutes to reap health benefits. This is not true. What is important is moving your legs and arms at every opportunity and accumulating activity minutes that total at least 30 nearly every day. In other words, physical activity can accumulate just like loose change. Mix aerobic activities like climbing stairs or brisk walking with calisthenics or vigorous gardening to build both aerobic and muscular fitness. Develop an exercise mentality to counter the technology that can keep you sitting for hours. Consider this list of suggestions:

- Walk, cycle, jog, or skate to work, school, or the store
- Park the car farther away from your destination
- Get on or off the bus several blocks away
- Take the stairs instead of the elevator or escalator
- Walk the dog
- Play sports with the kids
- Take fitness breaks instead of coffee breaks
- Perform gardening, landscaping, or home repair activities
- Avoid labor-saving devices as much as practical
- Take a walk after supper instead of watching TV
- Wear a pedometer and aim for > 7000 steps a day (one mile = 2000 to 2500 steps).

Source: Adapted from U.S. Department of Health and Human Services. *Promoting Physical Activity: A Guide for Community Action.* Champaign, IL: Human Kinetics, 1999.

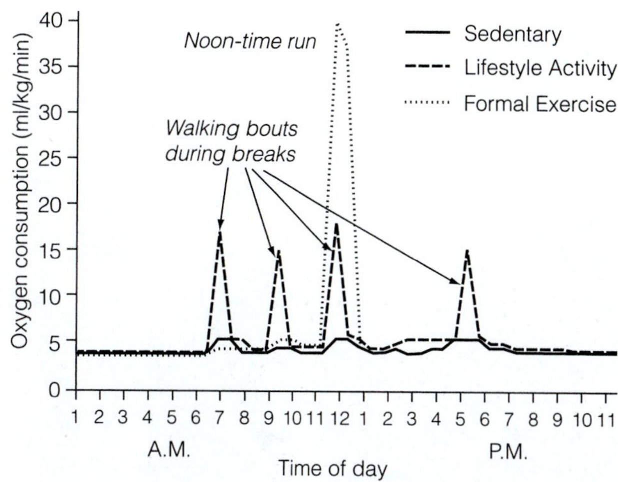

Figure 8.6 Patterns of physical activity in groups following different approaches: lifestyle activity and formal exercise compared to sedentary.

high. Figure 8.6 compares daily patterns of energy expenditure in different groups of individuals.

Athletic endeavor requires a high frequency and intensity of training, as discussed in Chapter 7.[49] Many athletes put in double workouts each day for many years to improve aerobic power, anaerobic threshold, and economy of movement. (See the section on systems of training, later on in this chapter.)

Intensity

As described previously in Chapter 4, the *maximum heart rate* (HR_{max}) represents the maximum attainable heart rate at the point of exhaustion from all-out exertion. During a graded treadmill test, the ECG heart rate recorder measures the maximum heart rate when the person reaches total exhaustion. If the oxygen uptake is measured at this same point, the $\dot{V}O_{2max}$ can be determined ($ml \cdot kg^{-1} \cdot min^{-1}$) (see Figure 8.7).

For healthy adults to develop and maintain cardiorespiratory fitness and proper body composition, the ACSM and others have emphasized that the *intensity of exercise* needs to be between 50 and 85% of *maximum heart rate reserve,* which is approximately the same as 50–85% of maximum oxygen uptake reserve.[1,2] Maximum heart rate reserve (HRR) and maximum $\dot{V}O_2$ reserve ($\dot{V}O_2R$) are calculated from the difference between resting and maximum heart rate and resting and maximum $\dot{V}O_2$, respectively. To estimate training intensity, a percentage of this value is added to the resting heart rate and/or resting $\dot{V}O_2$ and is expressed as a percentage of HRR or $\dot{V}O_2R$.[2] As emphasized earlier in this chapter, when improved health and lowered disease risk are the goals, intensity of exercise can drop to 40%, with duration and frequency becoming the more important standards.[1] These recommendations are based on substantial evidence that low-to-moderate levels of physical activity can reduce risk of heart disease and other chronic conditions, even though they do not produce significant changes in $\dot{V}O_{2max}$,

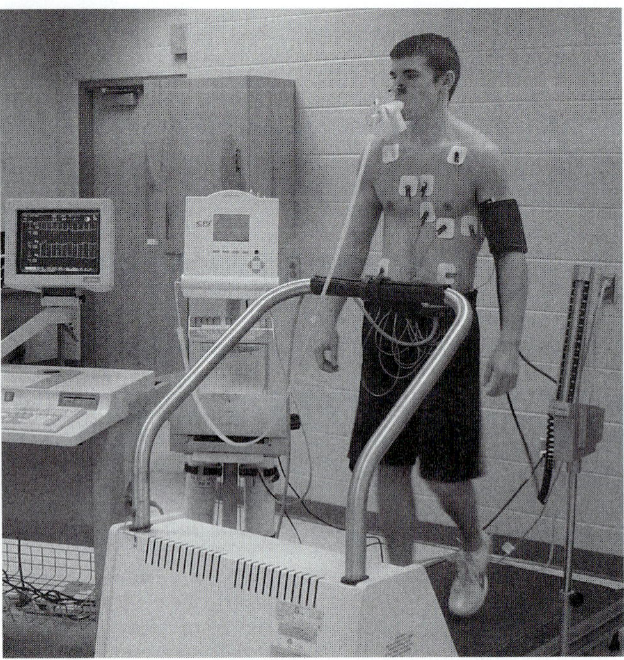

Figure 8.7 Although not required, the process of exercise prescription is enhanced when maximal heart rate and $\dot{V}O_{2max}$ are measured during graded exercise testing.

and that long-term adherence to exercise regimens goes down when intensity rises above moderate levels.[11,16,41–48] However, as noted in the NIH[22] and surgeon general[11] reports, the greatest fitness and health benefits are experienced by individuals who are capable of sustained, high-intensity exercise on a regular basis.

For athletes, the greatest improvements in aerobic power occur when intensity is high (90–100% $\dot{V}O_2R$).[49] When exercise duration exceeds 30–45 minutes, training intensity can be reduced to 70–80% $\dot{V}O_2R$ and training effects will be similar to those from training at higher intensities for shorter durations. Athletes need to balance this information with the consistent finding that high-intensity exercise increases the risk of injury.

Calculating Exercise Intensity Exercise intensity can be assessed using the results of the graded exercise test. Based on the length of time the participant stays on the treadmill, $\dot{V}O_{2max}$ can be estimated (see Chapter 4). This $\dot{V}O_{2max}$ can be expressed in METs (3.5 ml · kg^{-1} · min^{-1} = 1 MET). If the subject desires to exercise at 70% of $\dot{V}O_{2max}$, then the MET value is simply multiplied by 70%. For example, if a participant has a $\dot{V}O_{2max}$ of 10 METs, then 70% times 10 METs is 7 METs. Consult Appendix D for a full compendium of the MET values of physical activities.[50]

However, using a set MET level for exercise can have some disadvantages. Various environmental factors such as wind, hills, sand, snow, heat, cold, humidity, altitude, pollution, and bulky or restrictive clothing, can increase or decrease the amount of actual work being accomplished during a given activity.[1] Also, as the person improves in fitness, different MET levels will be needed to ensure an adequate training stimulus.

For these reasons, either the training heart rate or the rating of perceived exertion (RPE) is often used instead as an indicator of exercise intensity. The heart rate and the RPE are indicators of exercise intensity that adjust for environmental factors and improvement in fitness.

There are several methods of determining the *training heart rate.* The first method used by researchers is to plot the slope of the line between a person's exercise heart rates and the exercise workload in METs or $\dot{V}O_2$ (see Chapter 4).[1] From this relationship, the exercise heart rate pertaining to a given percent of $\dot{V}O_{2max}$ can be obtained.

A second method for determining the exercise heart rate for training is to calculate a given percentage of the maximum heart rate (MHR).[1] However, this method is not the same as using the heart rate reserve and will result in an underestimation of the training heart rate unless an upward adjustment is made.[1] The ACSM recommends that 65–90% of maximum heart rate gives training heart rates similar to 50–85% of HRR or $\dot{V}O_2R$.[2]

The relationship between percent HR_{max}, percent $\dot{V}O_2R$, and percent HRR is summarized in Table 8.2. For light-to-moderate exercise, the estimated difference between % $\dot{V}O_2R$ (% HRR) and % HR_{max} is 17–30%.[1,2] This difference narrows at higher exercise intensities.

The third method for determining training heart rate was developed in Scandinavia.[51,52] The *Karvonen formula* attempts to calculate the training heart rate using a percentage of the HRR, which is the difference between the maximum and resting heart rates (see Figure 8.8).

$$\text{Training heart rate} = [(\text{MHR} - \text{RHR}) \times 40\text{–}85\%] + \text{RHR}$$

[MHR = maximum heart rate; RHR = resting heart rate.] The intensity range of 40–85% of heart rate reserve is approximately equal to 40–85% of $\dot{V}O_{2max}$. See Box 8.2 for recommended intensity ranges based on initial aerobic fitness levels.

A sizeable error exists in the relationship between percent HRR and percent $\dot{V}O_{2max}$ at low exercise intensity, especially for relatively unfit subjects.[53,54] In 1998, the ACSM began relating HRR to $\dot{V}O_{2max}R$ rather than a percentage of $\dot{V}O_{2max}$.[2] Using $\dot{V}O_{2max}R$ improves the accuracy of the relationship, particularly at the lower end of the intensity scale. It is incorrect, according to the ACSM, to relate HRR to a level of $\dot{V}O_2$ that starts from zero rather than a resting level.[2] $\dot{V}O_2R$ is calculated by subtracting 1 MET (3.5 ml · kg^{-1} · min^{-1}) from the subject's $\dot{V}O_{2max}$. The % $\dot{V}O_2R$ is a percentage of the difference between resting $\dot{V}O_2$ and $\dot{V}O_{2max}$ and is calculated by subtracting 1 MET from the measured oxygen uptake, dividing by the subject's $\dot{V}O_2R$ and multiplying by 100%. For example, an individual with a $\dot{V}O_{2max}$ of 35 mL · kg^{-1} · min^{-1} who is exercising at 24 mL · kg^{-1} · min^{-1} would

TABLE 8.2 Classification of Physical Activity Intensity

		Relative Intensity		
		Endurance-Type Activity		Strength-Type Exercise
Intensity	% $\dot{V}O_2R$*, % HRR	% HR_{max}†	RPE‡	% 1-RM§
Very light	<20	<50	<10	<30
Light	20–39	60–63	10–11	30–49
Moderate	40–59	64–76	12–13	50–69
Hard (vigorous)	60–84	77–93	14–16	70–84
Very hard	≥ 85	≥ 94	17–19	>85
Maximal	100	100	20	100

*% $\dot{V}O_2R$ = percent of oxygen uptake reserve; % HRR = percent of heart rate reserve.
†% HR_{max} = percent of maximal heart rate.
‡ Borg rating of perceived exertion 6–20 scale.
§% 1-RM = percent of 1 repitition maximum, the greatest weight that can be lifted once in good form.

Sources: Adapted from Howley ET. Type of activity: Resistance, aerobic and leisure versus occupational physical activity. *Med Sci Sports Exerc* 33 (6 suppl): S364–S369, 2001; ACSM. The recommended quantity and quality of exercise for developing and maintaining cardiorespiratory and muscular fitness, and flexibility in healthy adults. *Med Sci Sports Exerc* 30:975–991, 1998.

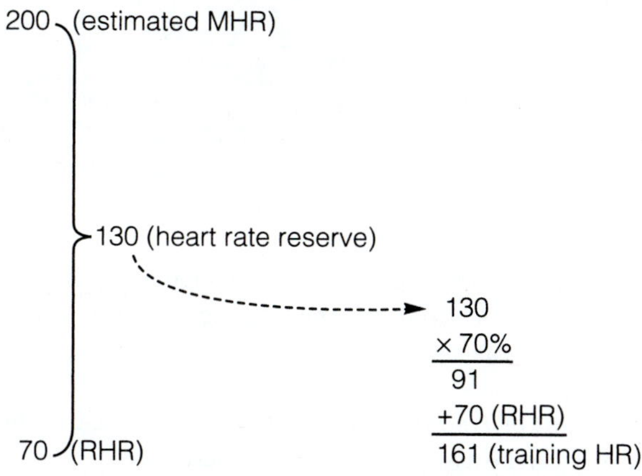

Figure 8.8 Use of the Karvonen formula for a 20-year-old man (average shape, RHR = 70 bpm). The Karvonen formula calculates the training heart rate using a percentage of the *heart rate reserve,* the difference between the maximum and resting heart rates.

be at 65% $\dot{V}O_2R$ ((24 – 3.5)/(35 – 3.5) · 100%). The % $\dot{V}O_2R$ corresponds to the heart rate response when it is expressed as a percentage of the HRR.[2,9]

There are two methods of determining maximum heart rate. The most accurate way is to directly measure the maximum heart rate with an ECG recorder during graded exercise testing. The other way is to estimate MHR by using the simple formula:[1]

$$\text{MHR} = 220 - \text{age}$$

The problem with using this formula is that it is based on population averages, with a standard deviation of ∓ 12 bpm. In other words, there is large variability. For example a 20-year-old would be estimated to have a MHR of 200 bpm, but two thirds of individuals of this age could actually have MHRs varying between 188 and 212 bpm. If estimations are used, the accuracy of the Karvonen formula is lessened. When the training heart rate is based on an estimated maximum heart rate, it should not be used as a precise measure and should be readjusted if the exercise participant complains that perceived exertion (using the Borg scale) is "very hard" or higher. Various attempts have been made to improve the accuracy of estimating MHR. One research group from Ball State University tested 2,010 men and women and found the following equations work better:[55]

Men

$$\text{MHR} = 203.9 - (0.812 \times \text{age}) + (0.276 \times \text{RHR}) - (0.084 \times \text{kg}) - (4.5 \times \text{smoking code})$$

Women

$$\text{MHR} = 204.8 - (0.718 \times \text{age}) + (0.162 \times \text{RHR}) - (0.105 \times \text{kg}) - (6.2 \times \text{smoking code})$$

(MHR = maximum heart rate; RHR = resting heart rate; kg = body weight in kilograms; smoking code: 1 = smoker, 0 = nonsmoker.) These equations account for the fact that people with higher RHRs tend also to have higher MHRs, while smokers and heavyweight people tend to have lower MHRs. Also the "220 – age" equation has been found to underestimate MHR for many older people. For obese people (body fat >30%), this equation has been shown to estimate MHR quite accurately: MHR = 200 – (0.5 × age).[56]

To determine the resting heart rate, it is best to take one's pulse while in a sitting position, upon waking in the morning. This should be done three mornings in a row, and

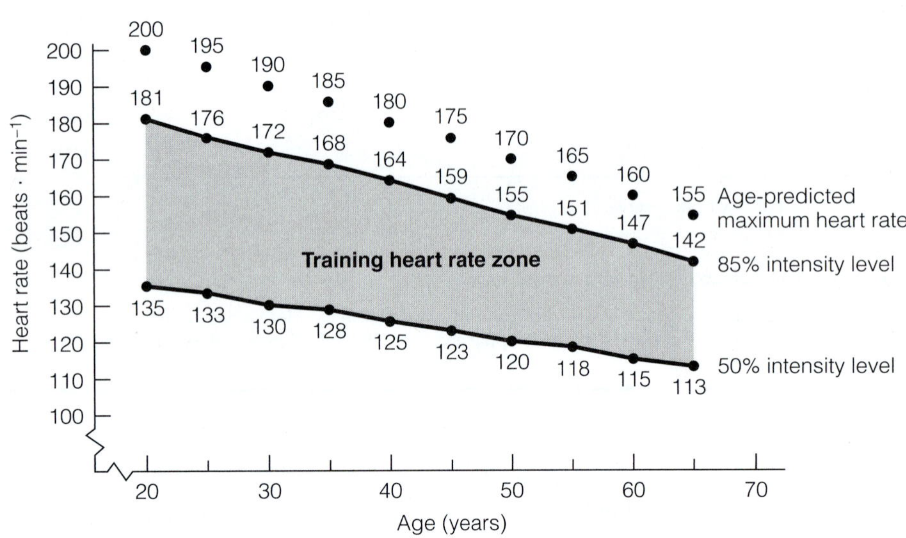

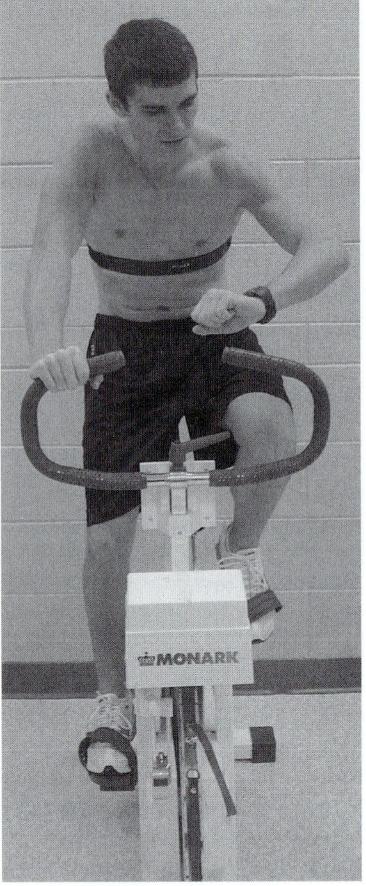

Figure 8.9 Training heart rate zone using the Karvonen formula. Maximal heart rates and the training heart rate zone for people of varying ages using the Karvonen formula. The resting heart rate is assumed to be 70 bpm.

then the values are averaged. After waking, one should allow the heart to calm down, which might mean sitting quietly for a few minutes or emptying the bladder.

Resting heart rates taken prior to graded exercise testing are often elevated because of pretest apprehension. In such situations, it is best to estimate the resting heart rate based on the health and fitness history of the person. (See Appendix A, Table 21, for resting heart rate norms.) Some people are in the habit of taking their RHRs on a periodic, regular basis, and if they are validated with careful questioning, these reported values can be used.

Based on the results of the graded exercise test or exercise history, and the exercise goals of the person, the intensity percentile used in the Karvonen formula can be varied, as summarized in Box 8.2.

To summarize, the exercise training heart rate for a 20-year-old male of average cardiorespiratory fitness and a resting heart rate of 70 bpm would be calculated as follows (see Figure 8.8):

$$(\text{MHR} - \text{RHR}) \times \text{intensity percentage} + \text{RHR} = \text{training heart rate}$$

$$(200 - 70) \times 70\% + 70 = 161 \text{ bpm}$$

So this 20-year-old person of average fitness status would need to exercise at an intensity of 161 bpm, for 20–30 minutes, 3–5 days a week, to develop and maintain a healthy level of cardiorespiratory fitness and proper body composition. Figure 8.9 summarizes the training heart rate zone for people of various ages.

Assessment of Training Heart Rate Training heart rate or intensity can be assessed by four methods:

1. The metabolic method (the use of METs or Calories per minute) (Appendix D).
2. Measurement of the pulse for 10 seconds.
3. The use of the Borg rating of perceived exertion scale.[1]
4. The use of the "talk test."

To measure training heart rate during exercise, the participant should stop every 5 minutes or so during the initial days of the exercise program and count the pulse. It should be located quickly, within 1–2 seconds.

The pulse is best counted using the carotid pulse; when properly done, this method is safe and accurate.[24,25] When palpating the carotid pulse, two fingers of one hand should be placed lightly on one side of the neck adjacent to the larynx or voice box area (see Figure 8.10).

Beginners should compare resting heart rates taken by both carotid and radial palpations (the latter taken on the thumb side of the bottom of the wrist). If the carotid pulse rate is consistently lower than the radial count, it is advis-

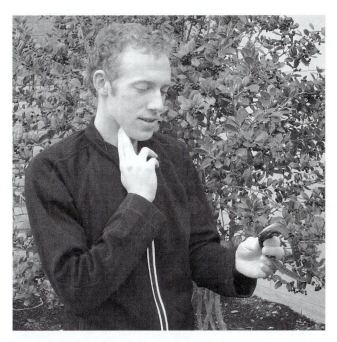

Figure 8.10 To measure the training heart rate during exercise, the participant should stop periodically and count the pulse, using the carotid artery.

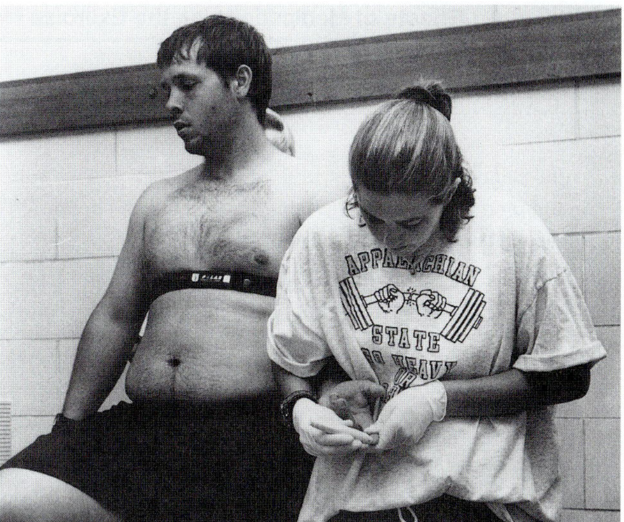

Figure 8.11 Heart rates can be accurately monitored using chest-strap transmitters that wirelessly signal the heart rate to a monitor on the wrist.

TABLE 8.3 10-Second Pulse Count Values for Various Ages, Based on the Karvonen Formula for Average Fitness Status and RHR of 70 BPM

Age Range	10-Second Pulse Count
20–24	27
25–29	26
30–34	25–26
35–39	25
40–44	25
45–49	24–25
50–54	24
55–59	23–24
60–64	23
65–69	22–23

able to use the radial count because some people's heart rates slow down when their carotid pulse is palpated, especially when excessive pressure is applied. However, during exercise, the radial pulse is more difficult to locate because it is smaller and lies among the tendons of the hand and finger flexors. So if possible, it is best to learn to take the carotid pulse properly (as lightly as possible).[24,25]

To estimate the pulse during an exercise bout, count for 10 seconds and then multiply by six. Table 8.3 gives 10-second pulse count values for various age groups. These training heart rate values have been estimated using the Karvonen formula, assuming average fitness status and resting heart rates of 70 bpm.

Various heart rate monitors have been developed to aid the exerciser in counting the pulse. The best ones use chest-strap transmitters that wirelessly signal the heart rate to a monitor on the wrist. These types of heart rate monitors have been found to agree within one or two heartbeats per minute with ECG recordings. (See Figure 8.11).

Although monitoring exercise heart rates with the 10-second carotid pulse count or heart rate monitors has been popular and generally satisfactory, errors do occur, arising from mistakes in counting, difficulty in finding the palpation site, taking too long (and thereby measuring an altered rate), or slippage of the chest-strap transmitter. Various medications can also affect the exercise heart rate (see Table 8.4). Heart rate monitors are also expensive (about \$50–\$500). In addition, some participants do not like to worry about taking their heart rates or feel that it is unnecessary.

To counter these problems, Gunnar Borg, a professor of psychology in Sweden, developed the rating of perceived exertion (RPE) scale in the 1960s.[57] Two types of RPE scales are most commonly used (see Table 8.5). The RPE scale is very easy to use. After some basic instructions on what the numbers mean and the importance of being honest, the people exercising are asked, "How hard do you feel the exercise to be?" Exercisers then give a number from the RPE scale to indicate how the exercise feels to them at that moment. In the original RPE scale, the numbers ranged from 6 to 20 and corresponded roughly to a heart rate range of 60–200 bpm.

Borg's original RPE scale was convenient for indirectly tracking heart rate and oxygen consumption, which increase linearly with increased workload. This scale did not account for variables such as lactic acid and excessive ventilation, which rise in a nonlinear fashion. Consequently, a category scale with ratio properties was developed.[58] The ratio scale uses verbal expressions, which are simple to understand and more accurately describe sensations such as aches and pain. Both scales have been used to rate effort signals from the entire body during exercise.[58–65]

TABLE 8.4 Effects of Medications on the Exercise Heart Rate and Blood Pressure

Medication	Exercise Heart Rate	Exercise Blood Pressure
Beta blockers	↓	↓
Nitrates	↑ or ↔	↓ or ↔
Calcium channel blockers		
Amlodipine Felodopine, isradipine, nicardipine, nifedipine	↑ or ↔	↓
Diltiazem, verapamil	↓	↓
Digitalis	↓ or ↔	↔
Diuretics	↔	↓ or ↔
Vasodilators		
Nonadrenergic	↑ or ↔	↓
ACE inhibitors	↔	↓
Alpha-adrenergic blockers	↔	↓
Antiarrhythmic agents		
Quinidine, disopyramide, procainamide, phenytoin	↑ or ↔	↔
Bronchodilators		
Anticholinergic agents	↑ or ↔	↔
Anthine derivatives	↑ or ↔	↔
Sympathomimetic agents	↑ or ↔	↔ ↓ ↑
Cromolyn sodium, steroida/anti-inflamatories	↔	↔
Antilepemic agents		
Clofibrate, nicotinic acid, probucol, others	↔	↔
Psychotropic medications		
Antidepressants, major tranquilizers	↑ or ↔	↓ or ↔
Lithium	↔	↔
Antihistamines	↔	↔
Cold medications	↑ or ↔	↔ ↓ ↑
Thyroid medications	↑	↑
Insulin, oral hypoglycemic agents	↔	↔
Anticoagulants	↔	↔
Antigout medications	↔	↔
Antiplatelet medications	↔	↔

Source: American College of Sports Medicine. *ACSM's Guidelines for Exercise Testing and Prescription.* Baltimore: Williams & Wilkins, 1995, 2000.

There is widespread consensus that perception of effort during aerobic exercise is determined by a combination of sensory inputs from local factors (sensations of strain or discomfort in the exercising muscles and joints) and central factors (sensations related to rapid heart beat and breathing rates). The RPE scale is often used during graded exercise testing to indicate perceived exertion (see Figure 8.12). Several new RPE scales have been developed for children and adults that use a numerical range of 0 to 10 with mode-specific illustrations.[65] The "OMNI" RPE scales have been developed for walking/running, cycling, stair climbing, weight lifting, and other activity modes.[65]

Available evidence suggests that RPE independently or in combination with pulse rate can be effectively used for prescribing exercise intensity.[58–65] Indeed, an RPE of "somewhat hard or strong" may be more effective for some people than heart rate in estimating the percentage of $\dot{V}O_{2max}$ necessary to elicit a training effect.

Trained and untrained men and women have been found to perceive the exercise intensity at the lactate threshold (intensity at which lactate begins to accumulate in the blood) as "somewhat hard or strong" (13 to 14 on the original RPE Borg scale, 4 on the category-ratio, 10-point scale).[59] In other words, despite gender or state of cardiorespiratory fitness, the "somewhat hard" level correlates with exercising at the lactate threshold, a point that is recommended as the ideal exercise intensity.

When exercising at the "somewhat hard" level, one can think, talk intermittently with a partner, look around and enjoy the scenery, and engage in prolonged endurance activity. When exercising at a "very hard" level, the pulse is too high, and it is difficult to talk or exercise for prolonged periods of time. When exercising below "somewhat hard," the exercise stimulus is not adequate to develop cardiorespiratory endurance. The "talk test" or the ability to talk during exercise without difficulty is a simple but valid method for determining whether the exercise intensity is within accepted ranges and below or at the ventilatory threshold.[60] The level of training intensity that can be tolerated depends on several factors, such as age, experience, fitness status, health, and

TABLE 8.5 Perceived Exertion Category Scales

15-Category RPE Scale		Category-Ratio RPE Scale	
Light Intensity			
6	No exertion at all	0	Nothing at all
7	Extremely light	0.5	Very, very weak (just noticeable)
8			
9	Very light	1	Very weak
10		2	Weak (light)
11	Light	3	Moderate
Moderate Intensity			
12		4	Somewhat strong
13	Somewhat hard	5	Strong (heavy)
14		6	
Vigorous Intensity			
15	Hard (heavy)	7	Very strong
16		8	
17	Very hard	9	
18		10	Very, very strong (almost max)
19	Extremely hard		
20	Maximal exertion	•	Maximal

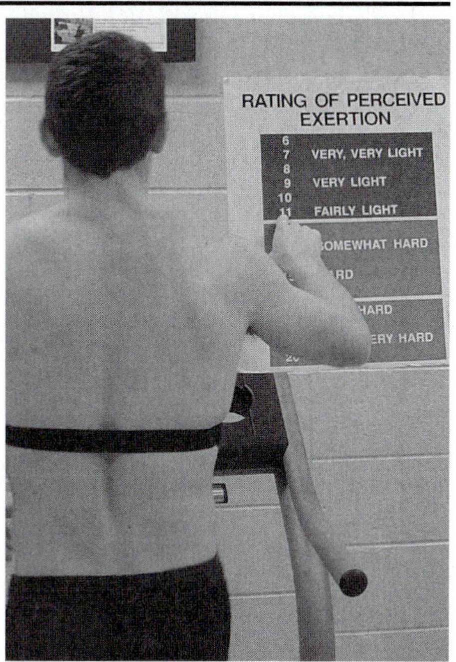

Sources: Noble BJ, Borg GAV, Jacobs I, Ceci R, Kaiser P. A category-ratio perceived exertion scale: Relationship to blood and muscle lactates and heart rate. *Med Sci Sports Exerc* 15:523–528, 1983; Borg G. *An Introduction to Borg's RPE-Scale.* Ithaca, NY: Movement Publications, 1985.

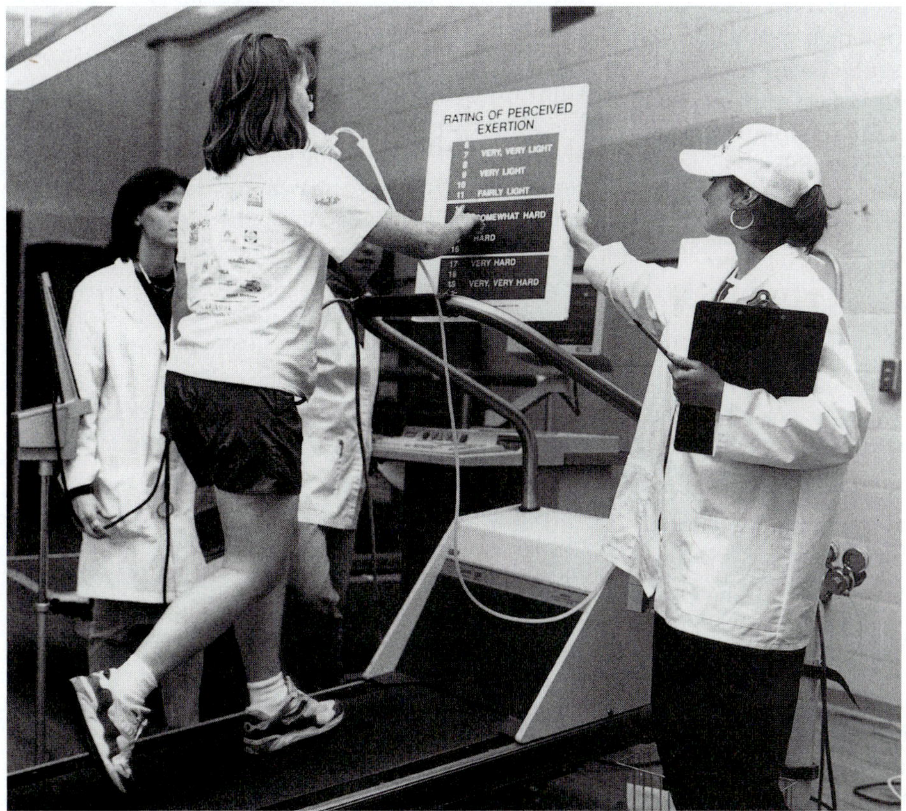

Figure 8.12 The RPE scale is commonly used during graded exercise testing to indicate progress toward maximal exertion.

motivation.[1] Long-distance runners are capable of running 26.2-mile marathons at 80% $\dot{V}O_{2max}$, while most beginners cannot tolerate this level for more than 5–15 minutes. For this reason, beginners should choose a lower intensity level, near 40–60% of heart rate reserve. The intensity percentage can gradually be increased during the ensuing weeks of training.

In summary, the RPE has several advantages:[57–59,61–65]

- It is simple to use, takes only a few seconds, and costs little.
- It has a good correlation to blood lactate and oxygen consumption measures.
- For people on certain types of medications, it is better than the heart rate in determining the proper exercise training zone.
- It teaches people to "listen" to their bodies during exercise.

There are some problems, however, with the RPE method:[57–59,61–65]

- The RPE scale may not give an accurate indication of exercise intensity in children and elderly subjects, and the obese.
- People who were depressed, neurotic, or anxious tend to give high RPE numbers, while extroverts tend to give low numbers. Thus, psychological factors and mood state can affect RPE responses.
- The RPE is less reliable at low versus high workloads.
- Feelings in the legs and the chest both influence the RPE, but depending on the intensity and mode of activity, the most potent sensation determines what RPE number is given. Thus, different exercise modes (running versus cycling, for example) may give different RPE responses despite similar percent $\dot{V}O_{2max}$ levels.
- In the heat, people tend to give RPE numbers that are too high for the effort.
- In the lab, RPE indications tend to differ from those at the same level of effort outside in pleasant surroundings.
- During long exercise bouts (for example, greater than 1 hour), the RPE tends to increase despite no change in the percent $\dot{V}O_{2max}$.

Because of weaknesses and strengths in both the heart rate and the RPE methods, most authorities recommend that exercisers learn to use both. As explained by Borg,

> The aches and the strain we feel may be very important indicators of the real degree of strain, taking all physiological and psychological factors together. We should not rigidly keep to a certain heart rate, e.g., 130 or 150 beats/minute. On one occasion this might be a suitable intensity level. Another day when he or she has a slight infection, has been working hard for many days and been subjected to a very heavy physical and emotional stress, to exercise at 150 beats/minute may feel very hard and stressful. The extra strain he/she then feels in comparison to the usual feeling is most probably an important symptom and a good reason to take it a bit easier.[62]

Time

Time of exercise refers to the duration of time in minutes that the proper intensity level should be maintained to develop $\dot{V}O_{2max}$. Beginners should start with 10–20 minutes of aerobic activity, those in average shape should go for 20–30 minutes, and highly fit people can exercise for 30–60 minutes.[1,2]

In 1998, the ACSM advised that

> duration is dependent on the intensity of the activity; thus lower-intensity activity should be conducted over a longer period of time (30 minutes or more), and, conversely, individuals training at higher levels of intensity should train at least 20 minutes or longer. Because of the importance of total fitness and that it is more readily attained with exercise sessions of longer duration and because of the potential hazards and adherence problems associated with high-intensity activity, moderate-intensity activity of longer duration is recommended for adults not training for athletic competition.[2]

For health benefits, the ACSM recommends accumulating 30 minutes or more of moderate-intensity physical activity during most days.[16] As discussed earlier, this is based on growing evidence that even when fitness is the goal, splitting up the exercise session to several different times of the day is just about as beneficial as doing it all at once.[11,14–16,41–48] Two studies from Finland have shown, for example, that intermittent stair climbing spread throughout the day improves fitness as well as more formal training regimens.[66,67]

An important factor in cardiorespiratory endurance improvement is expending 200–400 Calories (or 4 Calories/kg of body weight) a day in exercise at an intensity of 40–60% HRR or higher several times a week.[1,2] While this is a minimum threshold for health and fitness gains, for the athlete, training long and frequently is critical in order to perform successfully at competitive levels (Chapter 7).

It appears that body fitness and health respond fruitfully to 4–5 days per week of aerobic exercise, with sessions lasting 20–30 minutes. Most of the psychological, cardiorespiratory, and heart disease benefits from physical activity appear to be positively affected within this exercise range.

The proper balance between exercise risks and benefits is hotly debated and is discussed in Chapter 16. Athletes, in their attempts to enhance performance as much as possible, are continuously challenging the delicate balance between training and overtraining. Chapter 16 discusses two terms in more detail:[68]

1. *Overreaching*. An accumulation of training or nontraining stress, resulting in a short-term decrement in performance capacity, with or without related physiological and psychological signs and symptoms of overtraining, in which restoration of performance capacity may take from several days to several weeks.
2. *Overtraining*. An accumulation of training or nontraining stress, resulting in long-term decrement in performance capacity, with or without related physiological and psychological signs and symptoms of overtraining, in which restoration of performance capacity may take several weeks or months.

Mode of Exercise

If frequency, intensity, and duration of training are similar, and a minimum of 150–400 Calories are expended during the session, the training result appears to be independent of the *mode* of aerobic activity.[1,2] Activities should thus be selected on the basis of individual functional capacity, interests, time availability, equipment and facilities, and personal goals and objectives. Exercisers can use any activity that uses large-muscle groups, can be maintained continuously, and is rhythmical and cardiorespiratory in nature. Common examples include running/jogging, walking/hiking, swimming, skating, bicycling, rowing, cross-country skiing, rope skipping, and various endurance sports (see Figures 8.13 and 8.14).

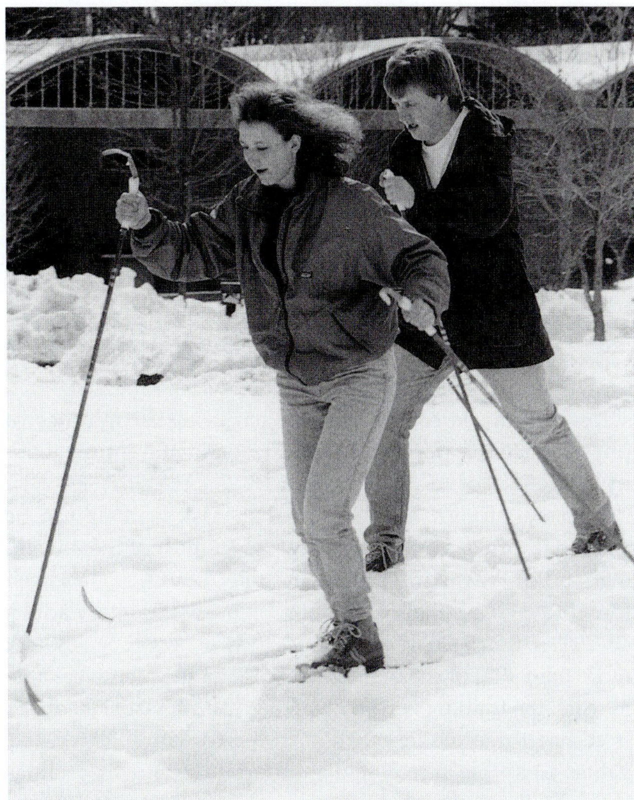

Figure 8.13 Cross-country skiing involves both upper- and lower-body muscles and provides an excellent total body conditioning effect, in addition to a high $\dot{V}O_{2max}$.

One of the trends since the late 1980s has been an emphasis on *cross-training* participation in a variety of aerobic activities, rather than intense concentration on one sport. Cross-training has several benefits, including decreased risk of overuse injury, reduced boredom, increased compliance, and increased overall fitness.[69]

Rating the Cardiorespiratory Exercises As emphasized in Chapter 2, "total fitness" is equated with the development of each of the major exercise components (cardiorespiratory and muscular fitness) through a well-rounded exercise program. Some individuals weight train to develop muscular strength and endurance but pay little attention to aerobic exercise for their cardiorespiratory system. Some runners rank high in heart and lung fitness, but low in upper-body strength. Some modes of exercise even do it all; for instance, rowing, cross-country skiing, swimming, and aerobic dance train both the upper- and lower-body musculature while giving the heart and lung system a good workout (see Figure 8.13). Table 8.6 rates various activities according to their overall potential for developing total fitness.

The 1996 surgeon general's report on physical activity and health emphasized a lifestyle approach to physical activity, urging that people accumulate at least 30 minutes of physical activity on a near-daily basis.[11] According to this report, "People can select activities that they enjoy and that fit into their daily lives. Because amount of activity is a function of duration, intensity, and frequency, the same amount of activity can be obtained in longer sessions of moderately intense activities (such as brisk walking) as in shorter sessions of more strenuous activities (such as running)." Figure 8.15 summarizes different ways that people can engage in physical activity, burning a minimum of 150 Calories per day, or 1,000 Calories per week, as recommended in the surgeon general's report.[11]

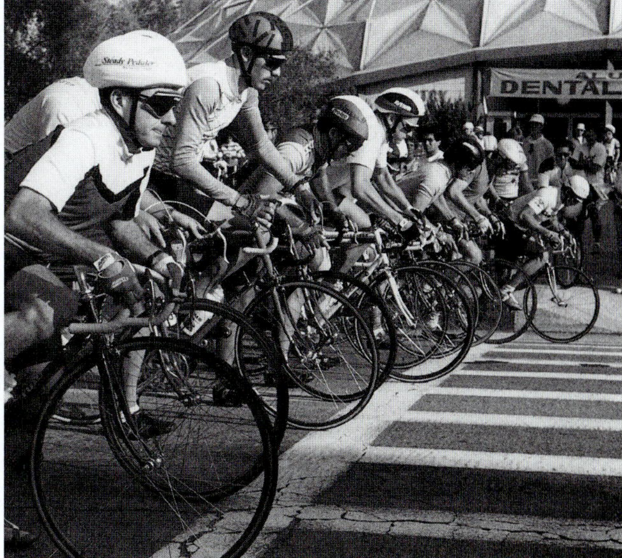

Figure 8.14 Outdoor bicycling causes less trauma to the joints and muscles than running, but high speeds are required for a training effect. Safety is thus a concern unless bicycle paths are available and helmets are worn.

TABLE 8.6 Potential of Various Activities for Development of Total Fitness

The table shows how well each activity builds cardiovascular health, burns fat, and builds muscle strength (1 = not at all, 2 = a little, 3 = moderately, 4 = strongly, and 5 = very strongly). For muslce strength, the activity is rated high if both upper- and lower-body muscles are strengthened.

Activity	Calories per Hour (150-lb person)	Builds Cardiovascular Health and Burns Fat	Builds Muscle Strength
Aerobic dance (vigorous)	474	4	4
Basketball (competitive)	545	4	2
Canoeing or rowing (fast pace)	815	5	4
Cross-country skiing machine	645	5	4
Cycling (fast pace)	680	5	3
Cycling (leisurely pace)	375	3	2
Cycling (stationary, moderate)	475	4	3
Dancing	305	3	2
Gardening	340	3	3
Golf (walking and carrying bag)	375	3	3
Handball (casual)	475	4	3
Lawn mowing (power mower)	305	3	3
Racquetball or squash (casual)	475	4	3
Raking leaves	270	3	3
Rope jumping (moderate to hard)	680	5	3
Running (brisk pace, 8 mph)	920	5	2
Running (moderate pace, 6 mph)	680	5	2
Shoveling dirt or digging	580	4	4
Skating (in-line or ice)	475	4	3
Skiing (cross-country, brisk speed)	610	5	4
Skiing (downhill)	340	3	3
Soccer (casual)	475	4	3
Splitting wood	410	4	4
Stair climbing	610	5	3
Swimming (laps, vigorous)	680	5	4
Swimming (moderate)	545	4	3
Tennis (competitive)	475	4	3
Volleyball (competitive)	270	3	3
Walking (brisk pace, 4 mph)	270	3	2
Walking (slow pace, 2 mph)	170	2	2
Weight training	205	2	5
Yoga	170	1	2

Brisk Walking As emphasized in the surgeon general's report,[11] moderate-intensity activities of longer duration are more acceptable to the masses, increasing the likelihood of a permanent change in lifestyle. Also, the musculoskeletal risk is less, and studies show that health benefits are still realized, especially when total energy expenditure averages at least 1,000 Calories per week.[70–77]

Walking is a popular activity mode, with nearly 40% of adults reporting that they walk for exercise.[71] From a public health viewpoint, brisk walking is probably the best overall exercise for the majority of American adults.[70–72] Walking has been found to have a higher compliance rate than other physical activities because it can easily be incorporated into a busy time schedule, does not require any special skills, equipment, or facility, is companionable, and is much less apt to cause injuries. The accumulation of 10,000 steps per day is comparable to achieving 30 minutes of physical activity per day, which meets the minimum activity guidelines of ACSM and the CDC.[71]

Several studies have shown that brisk walking can be used to improve aerobic capacity.[70–77] In most of these walking studies, a walking pace equal to 60% $\dot{V}O_{2max}$ has been found to increase the $\dot{V}O_{2max}$ of previously sedentary adults 10–20% within 5–20 weeks. In one study of people ages 30–69, more than 90% of the women and 67% of the men were able to reach the training zone by walking.[72] With visual feedback from heart rate monitors, all participants with high $\dot{V}O_{2max}$ values were able to maintain appropriate training heart rates if the walking pace was appropriately adjusted.[72] The researchers concluded that fast walking offers an adequate aerobic training stimulus for nearly all adults. The $\dot{V}O_{2max}$ of competitive race walkers averages 63 $ml \cdot kg^{-1} \cdot min^{-1}$, which

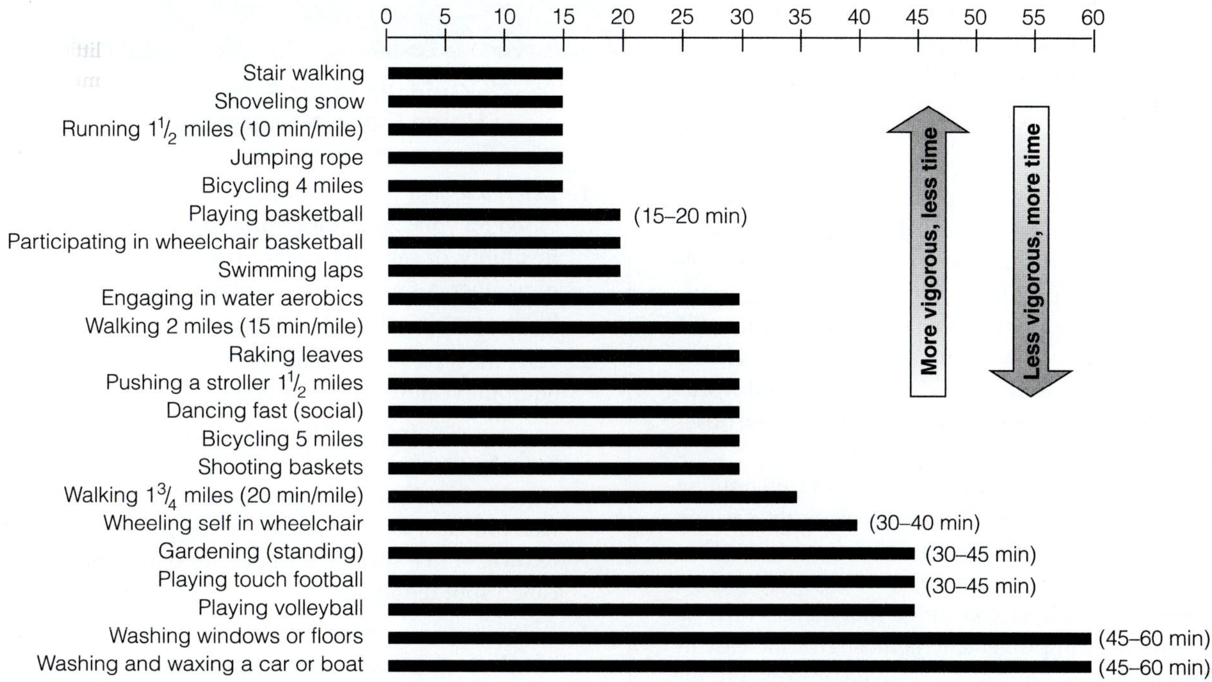

Figure 8.15 Achieving the recommended amount of physical activity can be accomplished by engaging in a variety of moderate- or vigorous-intensity activities. The less vigorous the activity, the more time needed to burn the recommended number of Calories. The more vigorous the activity, the less time needed to burn the same number of Calories. Source: U.S. Department of Health and Human Services. *Physical Activity and Health: A Report of the Surgeon General.* Atlanta, GA: U.S. Department of Health and Human Services, Centers for Disease Control and Prevention, National Center for Chronic Disease Prevention and Health Promotion, 1996.

is an excellent cardiorespiratory fitness level.[24] In one study, most exercise walkers were found to self-select a walking pace that ranged from 40 to 65% of $\dot{V}O_{2max}$, demonstrating that most walkers fall within ACSM guidelines.[77]

While walking burns fewer calories than running, its energy cost can be increased by carrying weights or using walking poles. Many studies have verified that hand/wrist weights increase the energy expenditure of walking significantly more than ankle weights.[78–82] The use of 3-pound hand/wrist weights increases the oxygen cost of walking by 1 MET, with an associated 7–13 bpm increase in exercise heart rate.[78,79] The hand/wrist weights also tend to improve upper-body muscular endurance.

Aerobic Dance Aerobic dance traces its origins to Jacki Sorenson, the wife of a naval pilot, who began conducting exercise classes at a U.S. Navy base in Puerto Rico in 1969.[83] The original aerobic-dance programs consisted of an eclectic combination of dance forms, including ballet, modern jazz, disco, and folk, as well as calisthenic-type exercises.

More recent innovations include water aerobics (done in a swimming pool), nonimpact or low-impact aerobics (one foot on the ground at all times), specific dance aerobics, step aerobics, and "assisted" aerobics with weights on the wrists and/or ankles.

Several studies have shown that when aerobic dancers follow the F.I.T. criteria, aerobic dancing is similar to other aerobic activities in improving the cardiorespiratory system.[83–91] Aerobic dancing also builds the muscular endurance of upper-body muscles, enhancing musculoskeletal fitness.

One cause of concern for the aerobic-dance movement has been the alarming number of reported injuries.[83] This is discussed in greater detail in Chapter 16. *Low-impact aerobics* help reduce the number of injuries.[90] At least one foot touches the floor throughout the aerobic portion. Movements are not ballistic, but focus on large upper-body movements, combined with leg kicks and high-powered steps and lunges. However, to achieve appropriate intensity, low-impact aerobics must be performed at a high rate. Ankle and wrist weights or steps are often used to increase the intensity of exercise.

Aerobic dance in the water uses many of the same upper-body movements practiced on the aerobic dance floor, but without the associated stress on the legs and feet.[91] These aquatic exercise programs are especially beneficial for the obese, elderly, and those with physical disabilities such as arthritis.

Racquet Sports Many people do not like the structure and monotony of the continuous aerobic exercises such as running, swimming, and cycling and have found *racquet sports* such as racquetball, squash, and tennis to be more attractive. The competitive and social aspects of these sports make them enjoyable for many and help promote long-lasting compliance.

When played at appropriate intensity levels, racquet sports provide an adequate cardiorespiratory stimulus.[92–97]

Racquetball participants of intermediate ability expend an average of 600 Calories per hour, playing at 50% $\dot{V}O_{2max}$.[94] Tennis players of intermediate ability average 60% of their heart rate reserve during singles matches, but only 33% playing doubles.[92,95]

Other Modes of Activity Some people find vigorous work activities more satisfying. Appendix D shows that various occupational activities (e.g., wood chopping, heavy shoveling and gardening, using a hand mower for mowing grass, or sawing hardwood) can lead to an energy expenditure of close to 300 Calories in 30 minutes (the recommended amount). In addition, the upper body is given a good workout along with the heart and lungs (and a direct, purposeful task is accomplished).

Some have wondered whether *circuit weight training programs,* which involve 8–12 repetitions with various weight machines at 7–14 stations while moving quickly from one station to the next, develop cardiorespiratory endurance. Most studies have concluded that there is little or no cardiorespiratory improvement (at most a 6% increase in $\dot{V}O_{2max}$) with such regimens.[24,98–101] Nonetheless, circuit weight lifting tends to elevate the heart rate substantially, with average heart rates of 150 (80% of maximum heart rate) reported.[100] However, actual oxygen uptake is relatively low—about 40% of $\dot{V}O_{2max}$. The heavy muscle exertion increases the heart rate through sympathetic nervous system stimulation, but because the involved muscle mass is small, the blood flow and oxygen uptake are low. Caloric expenditure is also modest, averaging 8 Calories for every 1,000 pounds lifted in the weight room.[102]

Such weight-lifting circuits, however, should not be confused with circuit training systems such as the *parcourse,* which emphasize running between stations, each of which calls for various calisthenics or weight-lifting maneuvers. Outdoor circuit training systems of this sort have been shown to burn 400 Calories in 30 minutes and contribute to high improvement in cardiorespiratory endurance.[103]

A training technique called *cardioresistance exercise* intersperses standard sets of resistance exercise with 2½ minutes of cycling, rowing, or treadmill running.[104] A room is set up with resistance training stations in the middle surrounded by aerobic exercise equipment. Participants perform aerobic exercise for 2½ minutes, then a set of resistance exercise, and then repeat this cycle 10–15 times.

For some, the convenience of indoor aerobic-exercise equipment is important, and there is a wide variety of such equipment available today. However, expensive indoor equipment is not needed for a good aerobic workout. Such forms of indoor home exercise as rope skipping, stationary running, or aerobic step dancing have all been shown to be beneficial to the cardiorespiratory system.[105–107]

There are certainly good reasons for preferring home to outdoor exercise—including unpleasant weather, environmental pollution, darkness, and safety concerns. Home exercise equipment can help make exercising convenient. The concern is that such devices will quickly lose their appeal because of lack of motivation and boredom. And one needs to be careful of fraudulent claims regarding exercise equipment (see Box 8.5).[108]

Popular equipment includes stationary bicycles, rowing machines, motorized treadmills, stair climbers, and simulated cross-country skiing machines, each of which has been studied extensively and shown to elicit excellent training responses.[109–114] Rowing and cross-country skiing equip-

Box 8.5

Guidelines for Selecting Home Exercise Equipment

1. *Determine your personal goals.* Select equipment based on your goals for improving strength, flexibility, or cardiovascular fitness. And remember, a single piece of equipment will not likely improve all three areas.
2. *Test equipment prior to purchasing.* Visit a fitness equipment store and sample the equipment.
3. *Be aware of outrageous claims.* A workout that is "easy" or "effortless" is not likely to provide any true benefit. A workout that seems too good to be true probably is. Also know it is *not* possible to reduce fat in a specific area of your body, often called spot reducing.
4. *Be cautious of "scientific evidence."* Research results may be based on a specific population and not the average person. If possible, obtain these results and review them carefully. Consider the strength of the research design, the type of subjects and measurements used, and whether the results are consistent with a majority of other studies and could be replicated by other research teams.
5. *Read the fine print.* Often the advertiser admits the results are only possible when combined with a proper diet or supplemental exercise.
6. *General knowledge.* Exercising at a specific heart rate will burn a similar number of calories regardless of the piece of equipment used (assuming duration is similar). Claims that one piece of equipment burns more calories than another is likely due to incorporation of larger muscle groups, resulting in an increased heart rate.
7. *Be an informed consumer.* Contact the Federal Trade Commission's Consumer Response Center (*www.ftc.gov*) or the American Council on Exercise (ACE) (*www.acefitness.org*) for information regarding exercise equipment.

Source: Adapted from Jung AP, Nieman DC. An evaluation of home exercise equipment claims: Too good to be true. *ACSM's Health & Fitness Journal* 4(5):14–16,30,31, 2000.

ment are especially valuable because they give the entire body musculature a workout, along with the cardiorespiratory system.[110,111] Several studies have shown that people tend to expend more energy on treadmills, than to other equipment.[113,114]

Rate of Progression

Appropriate progression in an exercise conditioning program depends on a person's fitness status, health status, age, needs or goals, family support, and many other factors (see Boxes 8.6 and 8.7 for two case studies). The ACSM defines three progression stages for the aerobic phase of the exercise prescription for apparently healthy people:[1]

- *Initial conditioning stage.* This stage typically lasts 4 weeks but depends on the adaptation of the participant to the program. The ACSM suggests that exercise intensity be 40–60% $\dot{V}O_{2max}$ to help avoid muscle soreness, injury, discomfort, and discouragement. It is best to be conservative when starting an exercise program and then gradually progress. Participants can start at 15 minutes and slowly work up to 30 minutes of exercise during this stage. The ACSM recommends that individuals who are starting a conditioning program exercise three to four times per week.[1]
- *Improvement conditioning stage.* This stage usually lasts 4–5 months and the rate of progression is more rapid. The exercise intensity is increased to 50–85% of HR reserve and the duration of exercise can be increased every 2–3 weeks until participants are able to exercise nonstop for 20–30 minutes. The degree and frequency of progression during this stage depend largely on the participant's age and ability to adapt to the exercise program.
- *Maintenance conditioning stage.* Once the desired level of fitness is reached, the person enters the maintenance stage of the exercise program. This stage usually begins 5–6 months after the start of training and continues on a regular, long-term basis (lifetime commitment). It is important to select aerobic exercises that are enjoyable and establish long-term goals.

Systems of Cardiorespiratory Training

There are several systems of cardiorespiratory training.[24–26]

- *Continuous training.* This involves continuous exercise such as jogging, swimming, walking, or cycling, at "somewhat hard to hard" intensities without rest intervals. The prescribed exercise intensity is maintained consistently throughout the exercise session.
- *Interval training.* This involves a repeated series of exercise work bouts, interspersed with rest periods. Higher intensities can be used during the exercise to overload the cardiorespiratory system because the exercise is discontinuous. A miler training for competition, for example, could use an interval regimen where one lap (400 meters) is run at slightly faster than the race-pace goal, followed by 1 minute of rest or walking, with the cycle repeated 5–20 times. In time, the "rest" interval of walking can gradually be increased in intensity, until the miler can run at a high intensity for four full laps.

  Interval training is necessary for athletes who wish to compete.[49] A good endurance base (at least 1–2 months of regular aerobic training) and a 10-minute warm-up are prerequisites to interval training. In addition, the first interval training sessions should be moderate, with gradual transitions to higher intensity levels. Interval sessions should not number more than one or two per week. Above all, hard anaerobic workouts should not be conducted on consecutive days.
- *Fartlek training.* This is similar to interval training, but it is a free form of training done out on trails or roads. People who abhor track running can do Fartlek training on roads, golf courses, or trails. The exercise–rest cycle is not systematic or precisely timed and measured but is based on the feelings of the participant.
- *Circuit training.* As noted previously, this training involves 10–20 stations of varying calisthenic and weight-lifting exercises, interspersed with running. The parcourse is a good example.

The Question of Supervision

- *Unsupervised exercise programs.* Low risk individuals can usually exercise safely in an unsupervised conditioning program.[1] Participant safety and compliance can be improved by individualizing the exercise prescription and educating participants on signs of overexertion, effects of heat and humidity, and so on. Some people find it more enjoyable to exercise alone at home; some like the group support of a community exercise class.
- *Supervised exercise programs.* Exercise should be supervised for symptomatic and cardiorespiratory disease patients who are considered to be clinically stable and for others who desire instruction in proper exercise techniques. The ACSM recommends that people with two or more coronary artery disease risk factors, known heart disease, or a functional capacity of less than 8 METs exercise under supervision.[1] These programs should be under the combined guidance of a trained ACSM-certified professional and a physician (see Chapter 3). Direct supervision of each session by a physician is, however, not required.

Box 8.6

Case History of a Typical Middle-Age American Female

Data from Medical/Health Questionnaire

Age: 45 years; *height:* 64 inches; *weight:* 154 pounds; *desired weight:* 130 pounds

Smoking status: quit 5 years ago

Exercise habits: sedentary both at work and during leisure for all of adult life

Family history of disease: father died of coronary heart disease at age 52 years

Personal history of disease: negative

Signs or symptoms suggestive of cardiopulmonary or metabolic disease: negative

Dietary habits: fruit/vegetables, 2 servings/day (low); cereals/grains, 5/day (low and refined)

Personal goals: lose weight, improve appearance and muscle tone, decrease risk of heart disease

Preferred modes of aerobic exercise: brisk walking, stationary bicycling

Data from Physical Fitness Testing Session (Physician's Office and Fitness Center)

Resting heart rate: 79 bpm (poor)

Resting blood pressure: 142/93 mm Hg (mild hypertension) (from two measurements on 2 days)

Serum cholesterol: 247 mg/dl (high risk)

HDL cholesterol: 33 mg/dl (low)

Cholesterol-to-HDL-cholesterol ratio: 7.5 (high risk)

Percent body fat: 35% (obese)

$\dot{V}O_{2max}$: estimated from Bruce treadmill test with EKG—23 ml · kg^{-1} · min^{-1} (low); EKG, negative

Sit-and-reach flexibility test: –2 inches from footline (fair)

Hand-grip dynamometer (sum of right and left hands): 55 kg (below average)

Comments

Using the medical/health questionnaire and laboratory data from recent testing, this client was classified as a "moderate risk," using ACSM criteria. This classification was given because she has two or more major coronary risk factors (family history, hypertension, hypercholesterolemia, sedentary lifestyle). Due to the number of risk factors, especially the family history of coronary heart disease, and the client's desire to engage in moderate-to-vigorous exercise, a medical exam and diagnostic exercise test were recommended. The treadmill-ECG test was negative (no evidence of ischemia or arrhythmias), and physician clearance was given for the client to begin a moderate exercise program, with gradual progression. Additional physical fitness tests were conducted at a fitness center to determine body composition and musculoskeletal fitness.

Recommended Exercise Program

A home-based program, using brisk walking and indoor stationary bicycling, supported with calisthenics for general muscle toning is recommended. During the first month, have the client warm up with range-of-motion calisthenics and walking for 5–10 minutes, followed by 15 minutes of brisk walking or stationary cycling at 50–60% heart rate reserve, 3 days per week. After warming down, the client should engage in static stretching activities for 5–10 minutes, followed by toning calisthenics for 10–15 minutes.

After the first month has passed, gradually increase the duration of brisk walking or cycling to 30–45 minutes per session, and the frequency to 5–6 days per week. The intensity of exercise can also be gradually increased to 70% of heart rate reserve. These increases, along with careful control of dietary habits, will help ensure a steady weight loss of about 1 pound per week. Because the client has 24 pounds of body fat to lose, ideal body weight should be attained after 24–30 weeks of training. This degree of weight loss, combined with improvements in physical fitness, should help to bring both hypertension and hypercholesterolemia under control if improvements in dietary quality are made (i.e., less saturated fat and cholesterol, more fruits, vegetables, and whole grains, less sodium and alcohol). The client has a high risk of coronary heart disease, and it is imperative that the risk factors be brought under control through weight loss and dietary and exercise lifestyle changes. Enlist the services of a dietitian to ensure adherence to an antiatherogenic diet.

Retest every 3 months to help ensure motivation and attainment of goals. Long-term compliance can be enhanced by encouraging family support, setting goals and contracting for their achievement, establishing rewards for attainment of goals, and combating time obstacles.

Box 8.7

Case History of a 30-Year-Old Male

Data from Medical/Health Questionnaire

Age: 30 years; *height:* 70 inches; *weight:* 160 pounds; *desired weight:* 175 pounds

Smoking status: never smoked

Exercise habits: plays golf on the weekends, but no other formal exercise; desk job at work

Family history of disease: negative

Personal history of disease: negative

Signs or symptoms suggestive of cardiopulmonary or metabolic disease: negative

Dietary habits: has a healthy diet and tries to follow food pyramid guidelines

Personal goals: increase muscle weight through weight training program; improve aerobic fitness moderately

Preferred modes of aerobic exercise: indoor equipment, especially rowing machine and stationary bicycle

Data from Physical Fitness Testing Session (Fitness Center)

Resting heart rate: 67 bpm (average)

Resting blood pressure: 123/82 mm Hg (normal) (from two measurements on 2 days)

Serum cholesterol: 195 mg/dl (within desirable range)

HDL cholesterol: 46 mg/dl (average)

Cholesterol-to-HDL-cholesterol ratio: 4.2 (average, but above optimal ratio of 3.5)

Percent body fat: 14% (desirable)

$\dot{V}O_{2max}$: estimated from timed Bruce treadmill test—43 ml $\cdot$ kg^{-1} $\cdot$ min^{-1} (average)

Sit-and-reach flexibility test: +2 inches from footline (average)

Hand-grip dynamometer (sum of right and left hands): 110 kg (average)

1-RM bench-press test: 95% of body weight (average)

Pull-ups: 7 (fair)

Push-ups: 25 (above average)

Timed (1 minute) bent-knee sit-ups: 32 (above average)

Comments

This client has no major risk factors for disease and is therefore classified as "low risk," using ACSM guidelines. According to the ACSM, a medical exam or diagnostic exercise test is not needed prior to initiating a vigorous exercise program for this type of client. Although the client has a normal percentage of body fat, his body weight is somewhat low for his height, and he desires to gain 15 pounds through a weight training program while moderately improving his aerobic fitness. He is especially interested in adding muscle bulk to improve his golf game, which is his weekend passion.

Recommended Exercise Program

The client desires an intensive weight training program at the fitness center, 3 days per week, with a moderate aerobic program 2 days a week. Because the client has never lifted weights seriously, a gradual, progressive resistance program should be established. During the first month, a one-set, 10-repetition maximum (RM) program of 10 different exercises will allow the client to adapt to the weight training program without undue fatigue and soreness (which would interfere with his weekend golf game). Over the next 2–3 months, gradually increase the sets to three, with the RM lowered to 6–8.

On 2 days of the week, after 5 minutes of warm-up, the client can use the rowing machine or bicycle for 20–30 minutes at 60–75% of heart rate reserve. On weight-lifting days, it is recommended that the client warm up for 10 minutes, prior to lifting, by rowing or cycling. This will allow additional aerobic training and will help warm up the muscles and joints to allow safe and effective weight lifting.

Establish 1-RM weight-lifting goals for each of the 10 exercises, and retest every 3 months. Also retest aerobic fitness and body composition every 3 months. To facilitate a healthy gain in body weight, consult with a dietitian to provide nutrient and energy analysis of the diet every 3 months. The dietitian can also give recommendations to improve the energy density of the diet.

Warm-Down (Cool-Down)

The purpose of the *warm-down* (cool-down) is to slowly decrease the pulse rate and to lower the body temperature, both of which have been elevated during the aerobic phase. This is effectively and safely done by keeping the feet and legs moving, such as via walking, light jogging, slow swimming, or bicycling. In other words, the warm-down is the warm-up in reverse.

There are at least three important physiological reasons for it:[24–26,115–117]

1. By moving during recovery for about 5–10 minutes (more or less, depending on fitness status, state of fatigue, and environmental factors), muscle and blood lactic acid levels decrease more rapidly than if the exerciser completely rests. In other words, moving during the warm-down promotes faster recovery from fatigue.
2. Mild activity following heavy aerobic exercise keeps the leg muscle "pumps" going and thus prevents the blood from pooling in the legs. The leg muscles promote venous return by the "milking" action of the contraction and relaxation cycle. Preventing the pooling of the blood reduces the possibility of delayed muscular stiffness and also reduces any tendency toward fainting and dizziness.
3. Following very hard aerobic exercise, there is an increase of catecholamines in the blood. Among high-risk people, this can adversely affect the heart, causing cardiac irregularities. The majority of severe cardiac irregularities that can be dangerous appear to occur following exercise, not during it. Although such exercise-related irregularities of the heart are relatively rare, a careful warm-down is recommended for high-risk individuals.

MUSCULOSKELETAL CONDITIONING

Musculoskeletal conditioning includes flexibility exercises and exercises for muscular strength and endurance.

Flexibility Exercises

Exercises to develop flexibility have long been pursued to enhance performance, fitness, and peace of mind. The ancient Greek athletes used flexibility training to enable them to dance, perform acrobatic stunts, and wrestle with greater ease. Stretching positions have been a part of Near Eastern and Far Eastern traditions for thousands of years, and today are practiced by millions in yoga classes to develop equilibrium of body, mind, and spirit. Stretching has long been a vital component of martial arts (e.g., karate and the modern tae kwon do), gymnastics, and ballet.

In the United States, stretching became recognized as an important part of a total fitness program following the publication of the book *Stretching* by Bob Anderson in 1975.[118] This book has since sold more than two million copies in the United States and has been published in 22 languages for worldwide distribution. In 1998, the ACSM included recommendations on flexibility exercise for the first time in its position stand on exercise "based on growing evidence of its multiple benefits."[2]

The word "flexibility" comes from a Latin term meaning "to bend." In Chapter 2, flexibility was defined as the capacity of the joints to move through a full range of movement. Flexibility is specific to each joint of the body. Some people have flexible shoulder joints, for example, but tight hip joints. As a matter of safety and effectiveness, an active aerobic warm-up should precede vigorous stretching sessions.

The major reason for performing flexibility exercises after the aerobic phase is to more safely and effectively stretch the warm muscle groups and joints that were involved in the aerobic exercise.[23,29,32] Appendix B contains pictures and descriptions of eight common flexibility exercises. See Box 8.8 for an exercise program to build flexibility. The *ACSM Fitness Book* describes 22 flexibility exercises for all of the major joints of the body.[119]

A *flexibility program* is defined as a planned, deliberate, and regular program of exercises that can progressively increase the range of motion of a joint or set of joints over a period of time.[23] In 1998, the ACSM included recommendations for flexibility exercise in their position stand for the first time based on growing evidence that flexibility can improve joint range of motion and function, and enhance muscular performance.[2] The ACSM recommends that a basic stretching program be followed at least 2–3 days a week and ideally 5–7 days a week and involve 2 to 4 repetitions of several static stretches that are held 15–30 seconds at a position of tightness at the end of the range of motion but not to pain.[1,2] The ACSM also recommends that major emphasis be placed on the lower back and thigh areas, and all other major muscle/tendon groups.[2]

There are three basic types of flexibility:

- *Static flexibility.* Ability to hold a stretched position (e.g., touching the floor with the fingers with legs straight or performing a "leg split").
- *Dynamic flexibility.* Ability to engage in slow, rhythmic movements throughout the full range of joint motion (e.g., the ability of a ballet dancer to raise and hold her leg above her head).
- *Ballistic flexibility.* Ability to engage in bobbing, bouncing, rebounding, and rhythmic motions (e.g., touching one's toes by bobbing up and down). This type of movement is generally not recommended due to injury potential except when included as an inherent part of a sporting endeavor (e.g., certain gymnastic and dance movements).

Box 8.8

An Exercise Program to Build Flexibility

Step 1. Warm-up Aerobically

Never stretch unless the muscles and joints are warm from 5–15 minutes of moderate aerobic activity.

Step 2. Follow These Minimum Flexibility Program Guidelines

A. Frequency

Perform stretches 2–3 days per week, or after each aerobic workout.

B. Time

Hold each position short of the pain threshold for 10–30 seconds, and repeat four times (total time, about 15 minutes). Relax totally, letting your muscles slowly go limp as the tension of the stretched muscle slowly subsides. Be sure that you do not stretch to the point of pain to avoid injury and a tightening recoil of the muscle.

C. Stretching positions

Improve flexibility in several body areas with eight specific stretching exercises. Follow the order listed below, using the figures in Appendix B. To conduct each stretching exercise, follow the explanations in Appendix B. Do not be worried if you seem "tighter" than other people when practicing these stretches. Flexibility is an individual matter.

Back/hips/hamstrings/legs/calves

1. Lower back–hamstring rope stretch
2. Calf rope stretch
3. Groin stretch
4. Quad stretch
5. Spinal twist
6. Downward dog

Shoulders/arms/upper body

7. Upper body rope stretch
8. Standing side stretch

Factors That Influence Flexibility

Why are some people more flexible than others? Each joint is surrounded by ligaments, tendons, and muscles, and these connective tissues determine whether the joint is tight or loose.[23] Ligaments are special tissues that tie bones together; tendons link muscles to bones; and all of these plus other tissues make up the structural or framework connective tissues. Unusual strain to the joint can stretch the ligaments, leading to a loose joint that is then highly susceptible to injury. Stretching exercises help to lengthen the muscles and tendons, increasing the joint range of motion in a healthy way. Gymnasts and ballet dancers, for example, are capable of amazing feats of flexibility due to spending much time each day stretching.

As a person ages, flexibility decreases, although this is thought to be due more to inactivity than the aging process itself.[23,120] There are good examples of physically active elderly people who have maintained a high degree of flexibility, and studies show that older persons can benefit from flexibility training. In other words, it is never too late in life to perform stretching exercises. But the usual tendency is for people to grow weak and tight as they age. Gender also plays a role, with males tending to have less flexibility than females.

Physically inactive people tend to be less flexible than those who are active.[23] The connective tissues tend to tighten around the joints when the muscles are not used on a regular basis. Warming the joint (either from hot water or aerobic exercise) produces a significant increase in joint range of motion. Thus a good warm-up should precede stretching routines.[23]

Flexible Benefits

The concept behind stretching is simple: When a muscle is extended slightly beyond its normal length (just short of the pain threshold), it gradually adapts and develops a greater range of motion. That improved range accounts for most of the benefits of stretching.

Many claims have been made for the performance-, fitness-, and health-related benefits of flexibility. These include:[23,121–125]

- More graceful body movements
- Enhanced performance of sport skills
- Relaxation of mental stress and tension
- Muscular relaxation and relief of muscular cramps and soreness
- Improved body fitness, posture, symmetry, and self-image
- Reduced risk of low-back pain and other spinal aches and pains
- Prevention of injury
- Rehabilitation/treatment of pain and injury

There is much debate as to whether improved flexibility is related to injury prevention. When questioned, the majority of sports-medicine specialists support the use of flexibility training in injury prevention but also readily admit that there is little scientific support for it.[126] Some studies provide convincing evidence that flexibility training prevents injuries[23,120,127] while others do not.[128–131] Researchers have also published results showing that greater flexibility predicts more injury.[132,133] Part of the problem is that flexibility is a complex characteristic that is highly specific to the type of sport being investigated.[23,134] Most athletic endeavors involve dynamic flexibility or the ability to use a range of joint movement in the performance of a physical activity at either normal or rapid speed. Flexibility is very specific to the type and speed of movement and to the involved joint.[23] Some sports require unique types of flexibility, including Olympic weight lifting, ballet dancing, gymnastics, swimming, and wrestling. Therefore, flexibility training is adapted by trainers to the special needs of the athlete or individual. When researchers attempt to study the relationship between flexibility and injury prevention, they often use static range-of-motion measures that may not translate to the specific dynamic flexibility demands of the sport.

Four types of stretching techniques have been developed by athletes, dancers, and physical therapists.[23,118,125,135–141] *Ballistic methods,* commonly referred to as "bouncing" stretches, use the momentum of the moving body segment to produce the stretch. *Slow movements,* often used by dancers are a second method, in which muscle stretching occurs as the movement progresses gradually from one body position to another and then smoothly returns to the starting point. However, the two other techniques—static stretching and proprioceptive neuromuscular facilitation—discussed here are considered best for developing flexibility.

Static Stretching

Static stretching involves slowly applying stretch to the muscle and then holding it in a lengthened position for a period of 10–30 seconds.[23,118,125] During this easily held stretch, one relaxes, focusing attention on the muscles being stretched. The feeling of slight tension in the stretching muscle should slowly subside. Then one stretches a bit further, until the mild tension is again felt (never any pain), and one holds this position for 30–60 seconds. The tension should again slowly subside. One should be breathing easily and feel relaxed.

Each major joint and muscle group of the body should be stretched. Appendix B contains pictures of eight common static stretching exercises.

Proprioceptive Neuromuscular Facilitation

Studies have shown that proprioceptive neuromuscular facilitation (PNF) flexibility techniques are more effective than conventional stretching methods for increasing joint range of motion.[23,125] Muscle relaxation using PNF is first induced by a contraction of the muscle to be stretched, followed by a static stretching of the same muscle group. There are two ways to do PNF:

1. *Contract–relax.* An isometric contraction of the muscle group being stretched precedes the slow, static stretching (relaxation) of the same muscle group. Theoretically, the isometric contraction of the muscles to be stretched induces a reflex relaxation.
2. *Contract–relax with agonist contraction.* This is the same as the contract–relax technique, except that at the same time the muscle is stretched, the opposing muscle group is submaximally contracted. This is supposed to facilitate even more relaxation in the stretched muscles.

PNF is usually done with a partner. The following steps are recommended:

1. Stretch the muscle group by moving the joint to the end of its range of motion.
2. Have a partner provide resistance as the same muscle group is statically contracted (for example, in a sit-and-reach stretch, after the person stretching has extended his or her reach forward, the partner will push on his or her back as he or she strives to lean back).
3. Have the partner apply pressure to aid in a slow, static stretch of the muscle group, while the person stretching contracts the opposing muscle group (for example, in the sit-and-reach, the partner pushes down on the person's back while the person tries to relax the hamstrings and contract the quadriceps).

PNF appears to produce the largest gains in flexibility.[23] However, it is associated with more pain and muscle stiffness, requires a partner, and takes more time. For these reasons, the static stretching method is often the most practical one. Risk of injury and pain is low with static stretching, and it requires little time and assistance.

Muscular Strength and Endurance Exercises

As described earlier, muscular fitness includes an emphasis on flexibility and muscular strength and endurance. Aerobic and muscular fitness activities can be included in the daily workout routine, or aerobics can be emphasized on one day and then muscular fitness on the next day. A good "total fitness" workout routine that would take about 1–1.5 hours to complete could be organized as follows:

- *Warm-up.* 5–10 minutes of easy-to-moderate aerobic activity
- *Aerobic exercise.* 20–30 minutes of moderate-to-vigorous aerobic activity
- *Cool-down.* 5–10 minutes of mild-to-moderate aerobic activity
- *Stretching.* 5–15 minutes of static stretching, emphasizing all major muscle groups and joints
- *Weight lifting.* 20–30 minutes of weight lifting, one set of 8–12 repetitions of 8–10 different exercises covering all the major muscle groups

This routine could also be split into 2 days, with the first four stages completed during the first day, and the weight training completed the next (with an appropriate warm-up).

There are a wide variety of training programs available, depending on the goals and preferences of the individual.

TABLE 8.7 Recommendations for Improving Muscular Strength and Endurance for the General Adult Population*

	Number of Sets	Number of Reps†	Sessions/ Week	Number of Exercises	Overall Purpose
ACSM[1,2]	1	3–20	2–3	8–10‡	Basic development and maintenance of the fat-free mass
Surgeon general[11]	1–2	8–12	2	8–10	Basic muscular strength and endurance
Cooper Institute for Aerobics Research[146]					
Minimum	1	8–12	2	10	Strength maintenance
Recommended	2	8–12	2	10	Strength improvement
Optimal	3	8–12	2	10	Noticeable gains in strength

*Recommendations for older people (50–60 years of age and above) and cardiac patients are similar, except that lighter weights and more repetitions (10–15) at a reduced intensity (RPE of 12 to 13) are recommended.[144,147–149]
†In all examples listed, repetitions represent maximal weight lifted to fatigue.
‡Minimum of one exercise per major muscle group (e.g., chest press, shoulder press, triceps extension, biceps curl, pull-down, lower-back extension, abdominal crunch/curl-up, quadriceps extension, leg curls, calf raise).

TABLE 8.8 Progression Models* in Resistance Training for Healthy Adults

	Loading	Volume	Frequency
Strength			
Novice	60–70% 1-RM	1–3 sets, 8–12 reps	2–3x/week
Intermediate	70–80% 1-RM	Multiple sets, 6–12 reps	2–4x/week
Advanced	1RM periodized	Multiple sets, 1–12 reps, periodized	4–6x/week
Endurance			
Novice	50–70% 1-RM	1–3 sets, 10–15 reps	2–3x/week
Intermediate	50–70% 1-RM	Multiple sets, 10–15 reps or more	2–4x/week
Advanced	30–80% 1-RM periodized	Multiple sets, 10–25 reps or more, periodized	4–6x/week
Hypertrophy			
Novice	60–70% 1-RM	1–3 sets, 8–12 reps	2–3x/week
Intermediate	70–80% 1-RM	Multiple sets, 6–12 reps	2–4x/week
Advanced	70–100% 1-RM periodized	Multiple sets, 1–12 reps, periodized	4–6x/week

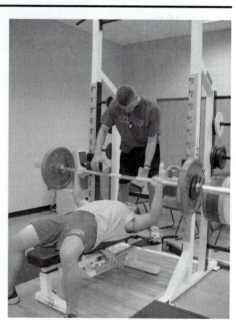

*In order to stimulate further adaptation toward a specific training goal, progression in the type of resistance training protocol used is necessary. The optimal resistance training program includes the use of both concentric and eccentric muscle actions and the performance of both single- and multiple-joint exercises. Specific exercises should be sequenced to optimize the training stimulus (large- before small-muscle group exercises, multiple-joint exercises before single-joint exercises, and higher-intensity before lower-intensity exercises). When training at a specific RM load, a 2–10% increase in load should be applied when the individual can perform the current workload for one to two repetitions over the desired number.

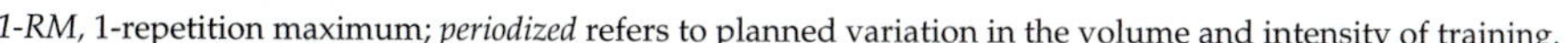

1-RM, 1-repetition maximum; *periodized* refers to planned variation in the volume and intensity of training.

Source: American College of Sports Medicine. Position stand on progression models in resistance training for healthy adults. *Med Sci Sports Exerc* 34:364–380, 2002.

Tables 8.7 and 8.8 and Box 8.9 summarize some of them.[1,2,142–146] The ACSM and the surgeon general's report recommend that at least 2–3 nonconsecutive days per week, people engage in a minimum of one set of 3–20 repetitions to volitional fatigue of 8–10 different exercises that condition all of the major muscle groups (see Box 8.10).[2,11] This strength-training guideline has also been recommended for elderly people and cardiac patients, except that lighter loads and more repetitions are advised.[144,147–149]

The ACSM feels that this is a minimum and basic program that many Americans will have time for.[1,2] Another reason is that most of the strength gains appear to be experienced during the first set.[147–150] This has caused considerable controversy, but the ACSM has been careful to describe these as minimum standards. In 2002, ACSM published a position statement summarizing guidelines for resistance training programs that can be applied to novice, intermediate, and advanced training.[142] These

Box 8.9

Systems of Resistance Training

1. *Single-set system.* Each weight-lifting exercise is performed for one set, 8–12 RM. Although improvement is not as good as with a multiple-set system, this system may be appropriate for those with little time to dedicate to weight training.
2. *Multiple-set system.* A minimum of three sets, 4–6 RM, are performed.
3. *Light-to-heavy system.* As the name implies, the light-to-heavy system entails progressing from light to heavy resistances. A set of 3–5 reps is performed with a relatively light weight. Five pounds are then added to the bar, and another set, 3–5 reps, performed. This is continued until only one repetition can be executed.

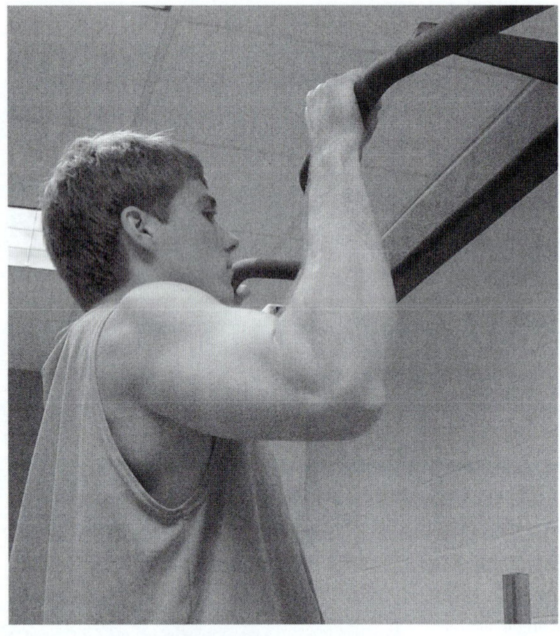

4. *Heavy-to-light system.* This is a reversal of the light-to-heavy system. The research suggests that this produces better strength gains than the light-to-heavy system.
5. *The triangle program.* This consists of the light-to-heavy system followed immediately by the heavy-to-light system. It is used by many power lifters.
6. *Super-set system.* This is used by bodybuilders. Two types are used. In one, multiple sets of two exercises for the same body part but opposing muscle groups (biceps vs. triceps, for example) are performed without any rest in between. The second type of super setting uses one set of several exercises in rapid succession for the same muscle group or body part. Both types of super setting involve many sets of 8–10 reps, with little or no rest between sets or exercises.
7. *Circuit program.* Circuit programs consist of a series of resistance training exercises performed one after the other, with minimal rest (15–30 seconds) between exercises. Approximately 10–15 reps of each exercise are performed per circuit, at a resistance of 40–60% RM. Cardiorespiratory endurance can increase about 5% with such programs.
8. *Split-routine system.* Many bodybuilders use a split-routine system. Bodybuilders like to perform many sets and many types of exercises for each body part, to cause hypertrophy. This is a time-consuming process, and not all parts of the body can be exercised in a single session. A typical split-routine system may entail the training of arms, legs, and abdomen on Monday, Wednesday, and Friday, and chest, shoulders, and back on Tuesday, Thursday, and Sunday.

Source: Fleck SJ, Kraemer WJ. *Designing Resistance Training Programs.* Champaign, IL: Human Kinetics, 1997.

guidelines are summarized in Table 8.8. The Institute for Aerobics Research has chosen to provide three different programs, which differ according to the number of sets.[146] Box 8.9 and Table 8.8 show that athletes go way beyond the recommendations given for the general population, with systems varying according to the sport.[143,145]

Principles of Weight Training

When appropriate weight-training principles are followed, average strength improvement during the first 6 months of training is about 25–30%.[143,145] The effect of exercise training is very specific, however, to the area of the body and training methods utilized and heavily dependent on overloading the muscle groups.[143–160] Although much of the early gain in strength is from neural adaptations, significant hypertrophy of muscle cells can be measured within 2 months.[142–145]

There are three major principles of weight training:[143–160]

1. *Overload principle.* Strength and endurance development is based on what is known as the *overload principle,* which states that the strength, endurance, and size of a muscle will increase only when the muscle performs for a given period of time at its maximal strength and endurance capacity (against workloads that are above those normally encountered). Muscle endurance and strength will improve best when muscle groups are brought to a state of fatigue.

Box 8.10

ACSM Guidelines for Resistance Training in Apparently Healthy Adults

The ACSM recommends the following guidelines for apparently healthy adults engaging in resistance training.

- Perform a minimum of 8–10 separate exercises that train the major muscle groups. A primary goal of the program should be to develop total body strength in a relatively time-efficient manner. Programs lasting longer than 1 hour per session are associated with higher dropout rates.
- Perform one set of 8–12 repetitions of each of these exercises to the point of volitional fatigue. For older and more frail persons (approximately 50–60 years of age and above), 10–15 repetitions may be more appropriate.
- Perform these exercises at least 2–3 days per week. While more frequent training and additional sets or combinations of sets and repetitions elicit larger strength gains, the additional improvement is relatively small.
- Adhere as closely as possible to the specific techniques for performing a given exercise.
- Perform every exercise through a full range of motion.
- Perform both the lifting (concentric phase) and the lowering (eccentric phase) portion of the resistance exercises in a controlled manner.
- Maintain a normal breathing pattern because breath-holding can induce excessive increases in blood pressure.
- If possible, exercise with a training partner who can provide feedback, assistance, and motivation.

Source: American College of Sports Medicine. The recommended quantity and quality of exercise for developing and maintaining cardiorespiratory and muscular fitness, and flexibility in healthy adults. *Med Sci Sports Exerc* 30:975–991, 1998.

2. *Progressive resistance principle.* The resistance (pounds of weight) against which the muscle works should be increased periodically, as gains in strength and endurance are made, until the desired state is reached.
3. *Principle of specificity.* The development of muscular fitness is specific to the muscle group that is exercised, its type of contraction, and the training intensity. In other words, weight-resistance training appears to be motor-skill specific. Thus, weight-training programs should exercise the muscle groups actually used in the sport or activity the person is training for, and they should simulate as closely as possible the movement patterns involved in that activity (see Figure 8.16).

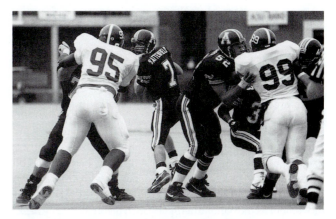

Figure 8.16 Gains in muscle strength and endurance are specific to the type, speed, and intensity of weight-lifting exercises utilized in training. The movement pattern involved in the sports skill should be simulated as closely as possible in the weight room.

Research has also shown that training should be conducted at high speeds because gains in strength and endurance are specific to the speed of training, with maximal gains for activities at velocities equal to or slower, but not faster, than the training velocity.

Systems of Muscular Strength and Endurance Training

Weight lifting centers around five different variables, which can be manipulated according to specific goals.[142,143,145] See Table 8.8.

1. *Repetitions to fatigue.* When repetitions are low (3–5); they build greater strength; when high (15–25), they promote endurance (see Figure 8.17).
2. *Sets.* One set is fine for beginners, but three to five are optimal for strength and muscle size gains.
3. *Rest between sets.* Bodybuilders have a short rest interval (1 minute); 1–2 minutes is typical, and >2 minutes is practiced by Olympic and power lifters.
4. *Order of exercises.* Some lifters exercise the large-muscle groups first, while others start out with

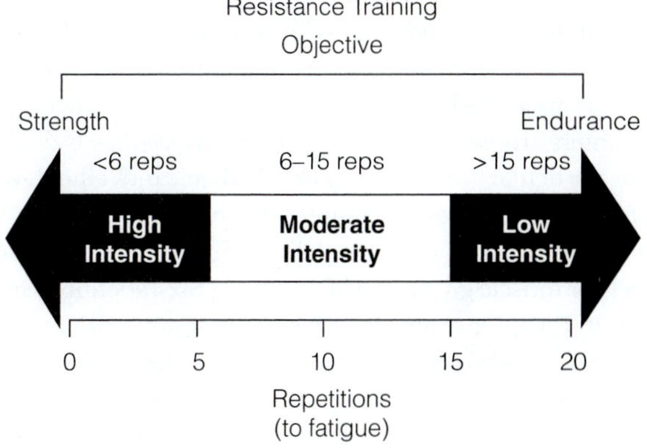

Figure 8.17 When repetitions are low (<6), they build greater strength; when high (>15), they promote endurance.

small-muscle groups. Bodybuilders emphasize working out the front and back of arms and legs.

5. *Type of exercise.* The lift can involve a single joint (e.g., arm curls) or multiple joints (e.g., leg squat). Multiple joint, large-muscle-mass lifts burn more calories.

There are three classifications of muscle contractions: isometric, isotonic (concentric), and isotonic (eccentric).[24–26]

Isometric In *isometrics,* the muscle group contracts against a fixed, immovable resistance. For example, the hands could be placed under a desk while sitting in a chair with arms at a 90-degree angle. The biceps are then contracted, but there is no movement as the hands attempt to push up on the heavy desk.

Maximum gains in strength appear to come from 5–10, 6-second isometric contractions at 100% of maximal strength, repeated at three different points in the full range of motion. Isometric exercises are easy to perform, can be done nearly anywhere, and require little time or expense. It is important to do each exercise at several different angles for each joint because strength gain is specific to the angle at which the isometric exercise is performed.

Isotonic Traditionally, *isotonic training* has involved the use of weights in the form of barbells, dumbbells, and pulleys, or heavy calisthenics such as push-ups, sit-ups, leg squats, etc. Appendix B summarizes the more common calisthenics used to develop muscular endurance and strength.

Isotonic muscular contractions take two forms: *concentric,* muscle contraction with shortening, and *eccentric,* muscular contraction with lengthening. For example, when a heavy weight is lowered, there is eccentric muscle contraction resisting the downward movement of the weight. Running downhill involves eccentric muscle contraction.

A muscle can maximally produce 40% more tension eccentrically than concentrically. However, training with eccentric contractions produces no greater increases in strength than isotonic programs. In fact, at the same relative power level, people performing concentric work will experience greater increases in muscle size and strength than when training with eccentric contractions.[161] However, gains in strength after concentric or eccentric training depend on the muscle action used for training and should be directed toward specific performance goals.[161,162] The major problem with eccentric contraction is its association with muscle soreness (see Figure 8.18; this is discussed in more detail in Chapter 16).

As emphasized earlier, isotonic muscle movement usually centers around sets and repetitions. A *repetition* is defined as one particular weight-lifting or calisthenic movement, with a *set* defined as a certain number of these repetitions. *One-repetition maximum* (1-RM) is defined as the maximal load a muscle or muscle group can lift just once. Six-repetitions maximum (6-RM), for example, is the greatest amount of weight that can be lifted six times. Box 8.9 summarizes the large number of different combinations that are possible.

The isotonic weight-training program should be conducted according to personal goals, with caution given for overtraining.[153] Chronic fatigue can develop from daily training. Some athletes will focus on the upper body one day, and then the lower body the next, allowing 48 hours for exercised muscle groups to recover.

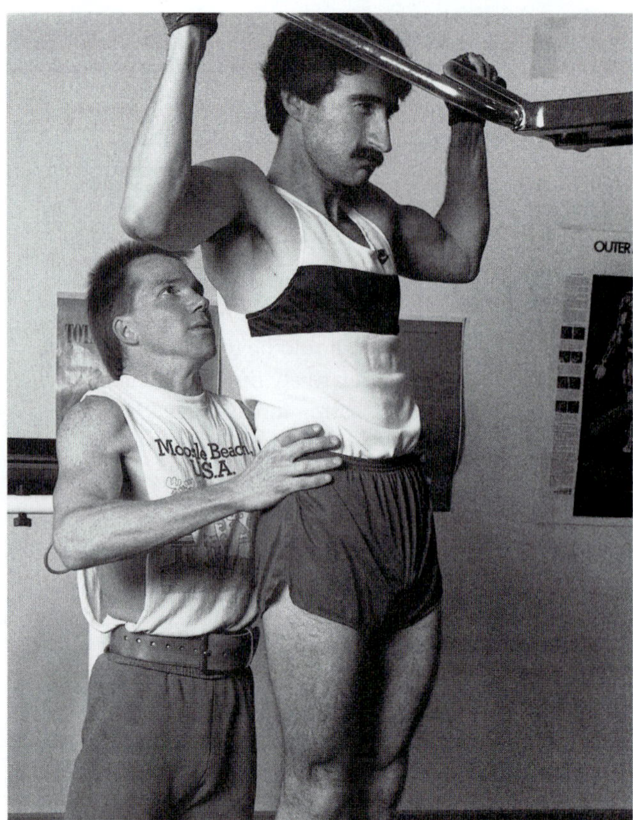

Figure 8.18 *Eccentric muscle contractions* involve the muscle lenghtening as it develops tension. For example, when at the top of a pull-up, if a partner pulls you down, as you attempt to resist the downward action, eccentric muscle contraction will take place. Eccentric muscle contraction is associated with muscle soreness.

Bodybuilding is a unique activity in which competitors work to develop the mass, definition, and symmetry of their muscles, rather than the strength, skill, or endurance required for traditional athletic events.[155,158] In one study of 31 competitive bodybuilders (15 female, 16 male) who were free of steroids, subjects averaged four to six 90-minute weight training workouts each week. Particular muscle groups were generally exercised twice a week, using several different exercises for each muscle group. Each exercise was performed to the point of muscle failure, using a resistance that achieved this effect with 8–15 repetitions. Exercises were repeated for 5–8 sets.[155]

Box 8.11 summarizes some of the more common weight-lifting exercises, with a description of technique, overall benefits, and the muscle groups improved. Consult Appendix C for identification of the muscles involved.

Isokinetic This type of muscular training is relatively new. In joint motion, the muscles controlling the movement have points at which strength is greater and points where it is less. For example, the greatest tension or strength of the elbow

Box 8.11

An Exercise Program to Build Muscular Strength and Endurance

Step 1. Warm-Up Aerobically

Never strength train unless the muscles and joints are warm from 5–15 minutes of moderate aerobic activity.

Step 2. Follow These Minimum Strength Training Program Guidelines

A. Frequency

Strength train at least 2–3 days per week.

B. Set and Reps

Perform a minimum of one set of 8–12 repetitions to the point of volitional fatigue for each exercise.

C. Strength Exercises

Perform a minimum of 8–10 different exercises that condition all the major muscle groups. Try the routine described below. Perform each exercise through a full range of motion. Perform both the lifting and lowering portion of each exercise in a controlled manner. Maintain a normal breathing pattern because breath-holding can induce excessive increases in blood pressure. If possible, exercise with a training partner who can provide feedback, assistance, and motivation.

1. Lat pull down *Part of body benefited.* Side of back (lats) and shoulders *Equipment.* Pulley machine

Description. Kneel below the handle with your hands grasping it, arms straight. Forcefully pull down behind the head. Let the bar rise slowly and under control to the starting position, and repeat.

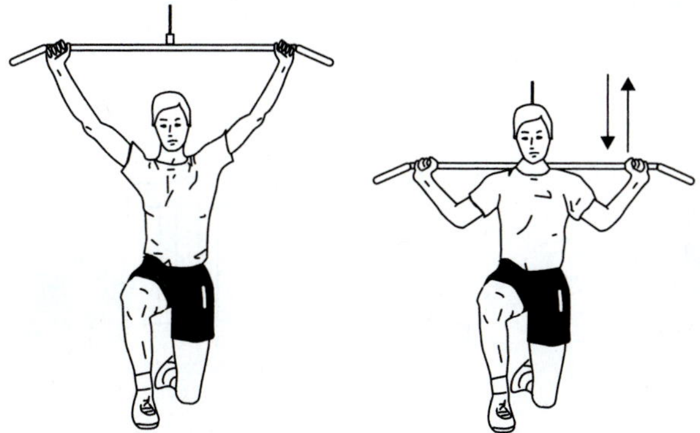

2. Leg press *Part of body benefited.* Front of the thigh and buttocks *Equipment.* Leg press machine

Description. While sitting with the feet on the pedals and hands grasping the handles on the seat, push the foot pedals forward. Keep your buttocks on the seat, and then move the foot pedals backward slowly and under control to the starting position, and repeat.

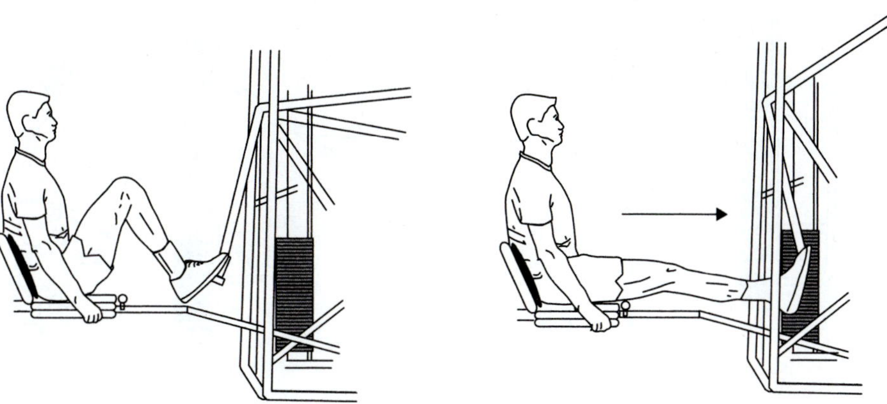

(continued)

Box 8.11

An Exercise Program to Build Muscular Strength and Endurance *(continued)*

3. Bench press — *Part of body benefited.* Front of the chest and back of upper arms (triceps) — *Equipment.* Barbell, bench with rack

Description. Lie down on the bench with your knees bent and feet flat on the floor. Grasp the bar, signal the spotter, and move the bar off the bar shelf. Position the bar over your chest, elbows fully extended. Lower the bar slowly and under control until the bar touches your chest, and then push the bar up to full elbow extension, and repeat.

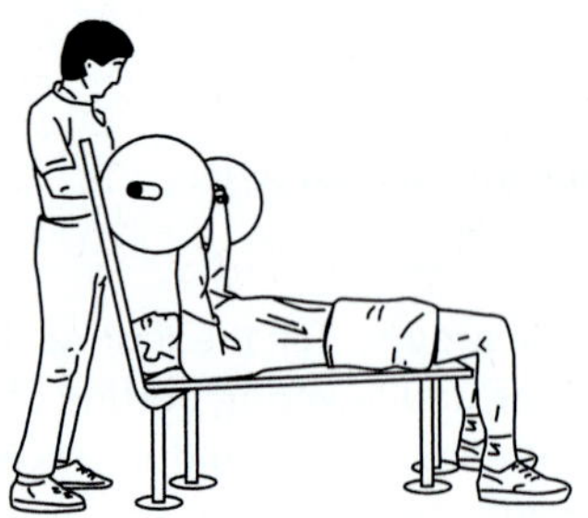
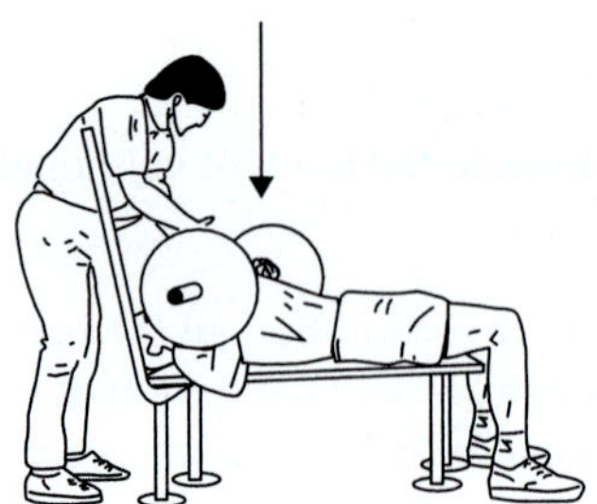
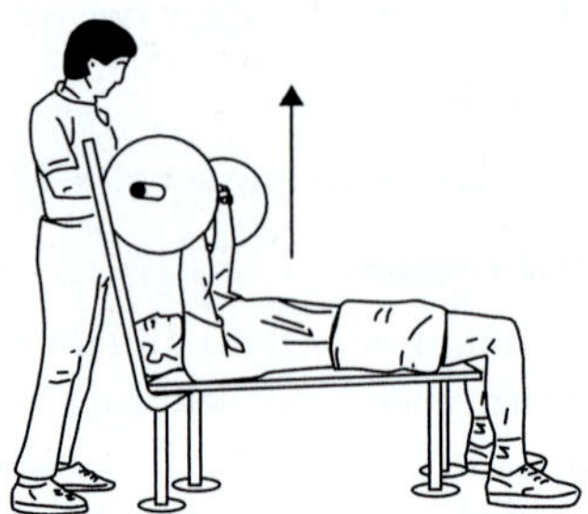

4. Abdominal crunch — *Part of body benefited.* Abdomen — *Equipment.* Padded bench and floor mat

Description. Lie on the mat with your knees hooked over the bench and arms crossed over the chest. Tuck your chin to your chest and curl your upper body toward the thighs until your upper back is off the mat. Lower your shoulders slowly and under control, and repeat.

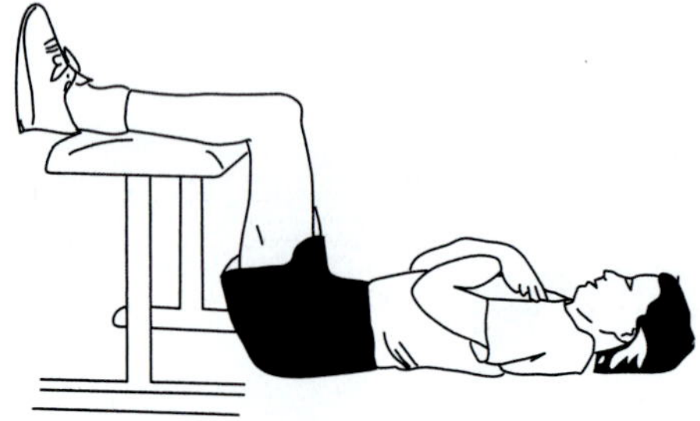
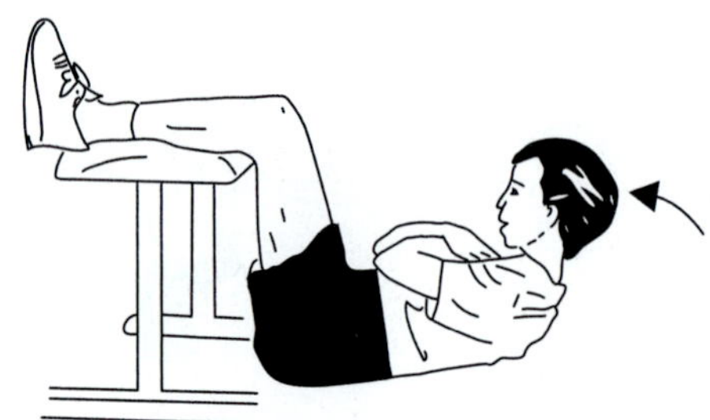

5. Shoulder press — *Part of body benefited.* Shoulders and back of upper arms (triceps) — *Equipment.* Shoulder press machine

Description. Face the machine while seated and push the handles up until the arms are fully extended. Lower the handles slowly and under control to shoulder level, and repeat.

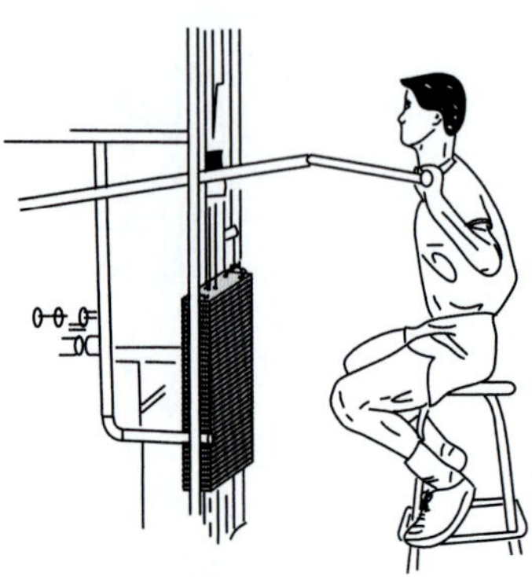
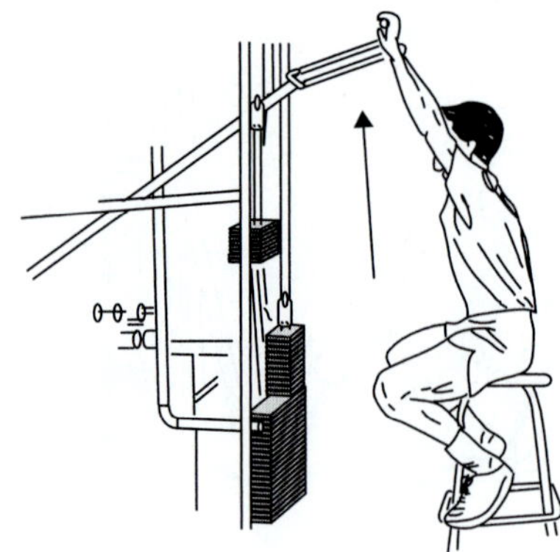

(continued)

Box 8.11

An Exercise Program to Build Muscular Strength and Endurance *(continued)*

6. Seated row — *Part of body benefited.* Upper back, shoulders, front of upper arms (biceps) — *Equipment.* Pulley machine

Description. Sit facing the pulley machine with your feet on the foot supports. With your knees slightly flexed and body erect, pull the handles to your ribs, and then return them slowly and under control, and repeat.

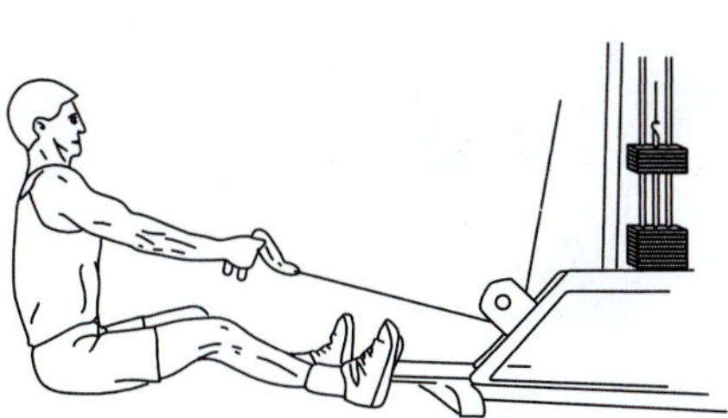

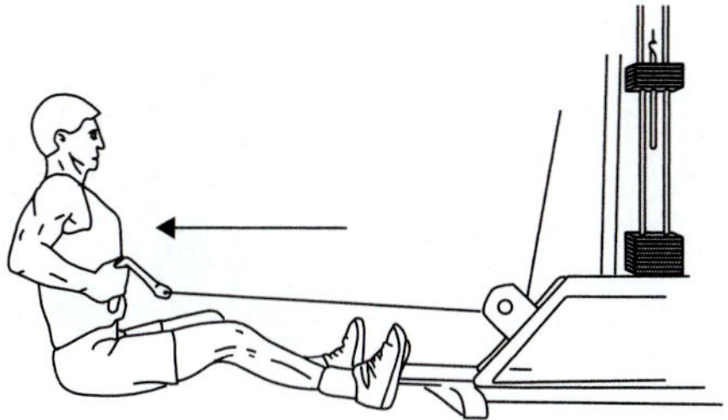

7. Leg extension — *Part of body benefited.* Front of thigh (quadriceps) — *Equipment.* Leg extension machine

Description. Sit on the machine with your ankles locked under the roller pad. With hands grasping the seat handles, extend your legs at the knees until they are straight, and then lower them slowly and under control to the starting position and repeat.

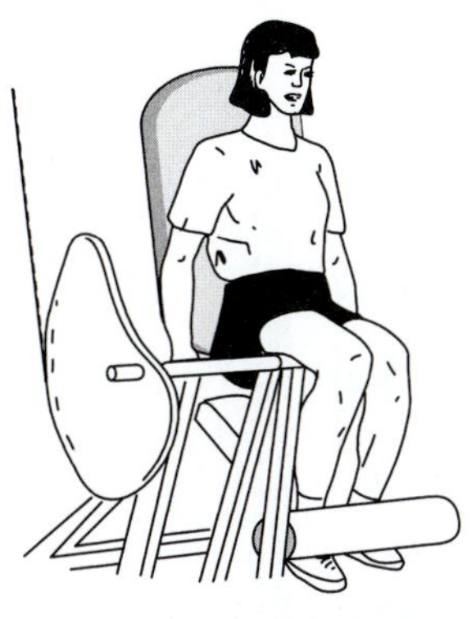

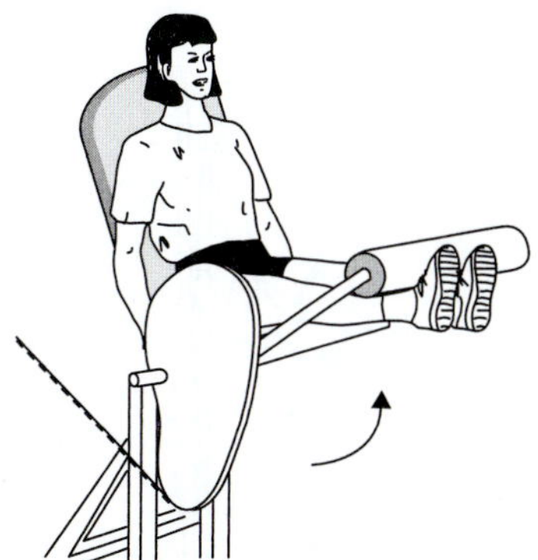

8. Leg curl — *Part of body benefited.* Buttocks and back of legs (hamstrings) — *Equipment.* Leg curl machine

Description. Lie down on the bench with your heels locked under the padded roller, hands grasping the handles. Keep your hips on the bench as you flex your legs at the knees and pull your heels as close to the buttocks as possible. Lower the roller pad slowly and under control to the starting position and repeat.

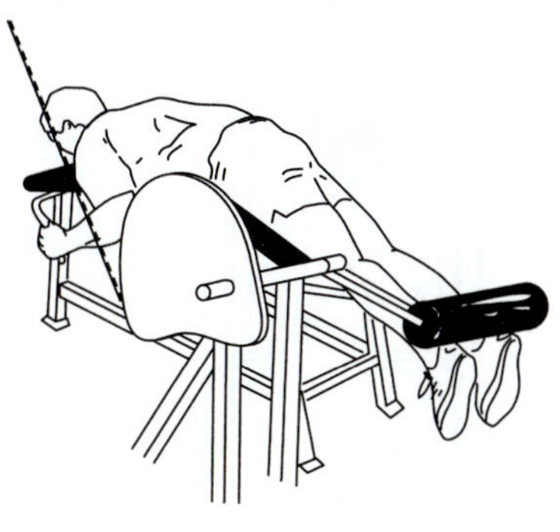

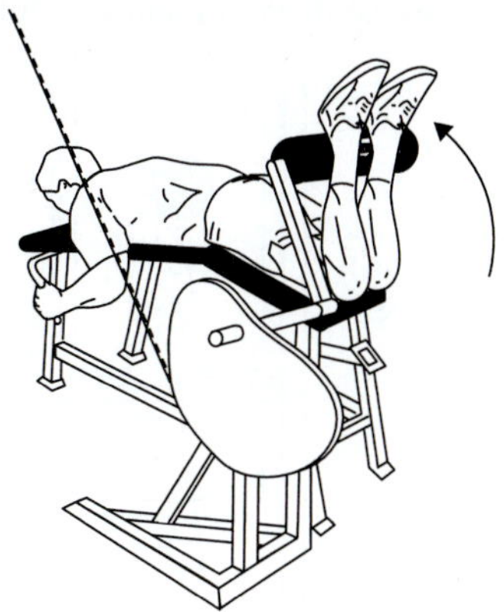

(continued)

Box 8.11

An Exercise Program to Build Muscular Strength and Endurance *(continued)*

9. Biceps curl *Part of body benefited.* Front of upper arm (biceps) *Equipment.* Barbell

Description. With your hands grasping the bar, palms forward, raise the bar in an arc by flexing the arms at the elbows. Keep your upper arms and elbows stationary while maintaining your upright body position. After raising the bar to your shoulders, slowly lower the bar to the starting position and repeat.

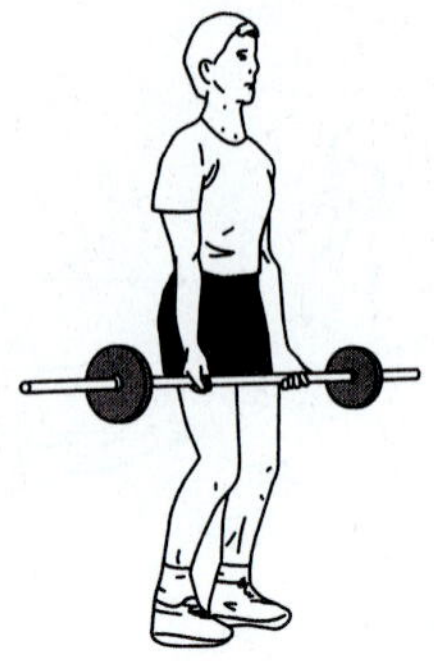

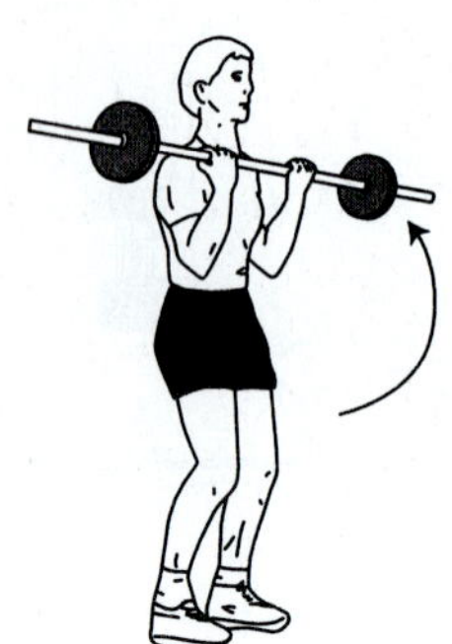

10. Triceps pushdown *Part of body benefited.* Back of upper arm (triceps) *Equipment.* Pulley machine

Description. Grasp the bar with your elbows flexed, palms facing downward. Push the bar down to full elbow extension while keeping your elbows next to your body. Allow the bar to slowly rise up to the starting position and repeat.

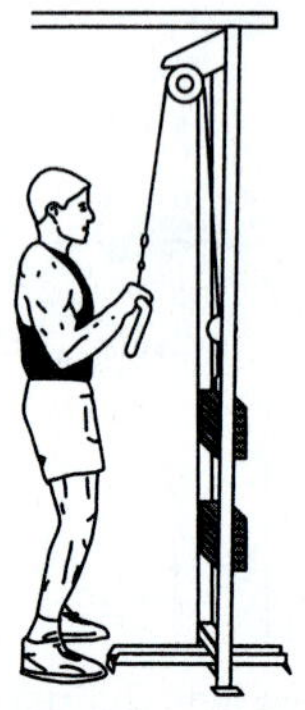

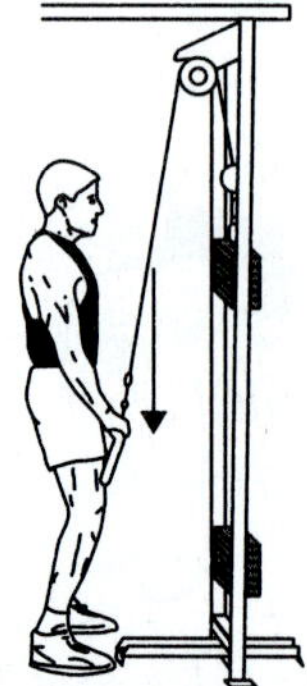

11. Standing heel raise *Part of body benefited.* Back of lower legs (calves) *Equipment.* Barbell, safety rack, and 2-inch platform

Description. Perform this exercise inside of a squat rack with two spotters. Position the bar on your shoulders at the base of your neck. Position the balls of your feet on the raised platform, with your heels down. Push up on your toes as high as possible in a slow, controlled manner while keeping the legs straight. Return under control to the starting position, and repeat.

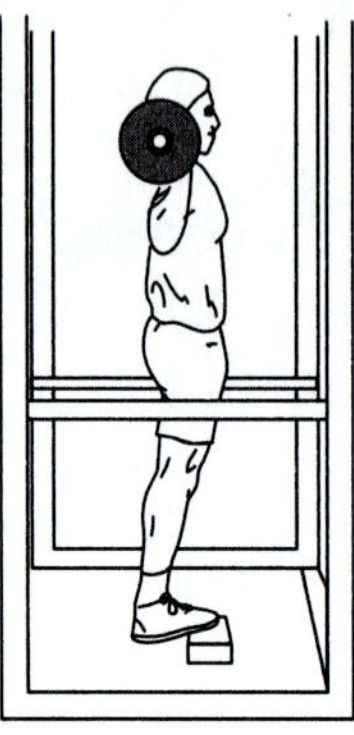

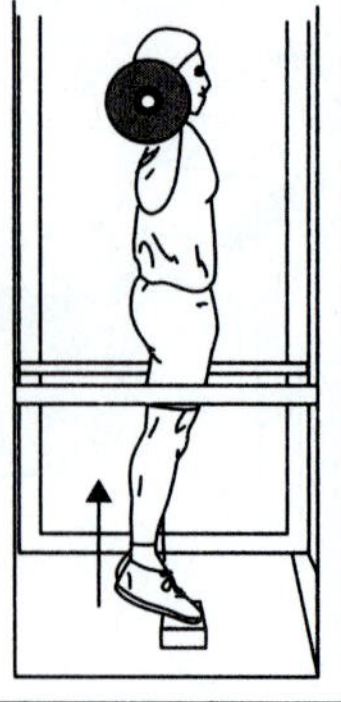

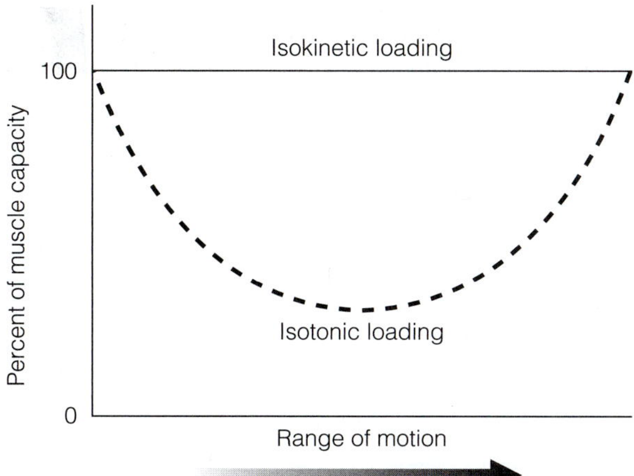

Figure 8.19 Isokinetic versus isotonic exercise. During isotonic muscle contraction, the amount of weight that can be utilized must be adjusted to the weakest point of the lift. Thus the muscle is not operating at 100% capacity during all parts of the lift. With isokinetic exercise, the specialized equipment allows the muscle to contract maximally throughout the entire range of motion.

flexors (biceps, brachialis) is at 120 degrees, with the least tension and strength at 30 degrees. In true isokinetic exercise, the resistance adjusts so that it is exactly matched to the force applied by the muscle throughout the full range of joint motion. This means that the muscle can apply maximal tension during the entire lift. This is accomplished by controlling the speed of the movement (*iso* = same, *kinetic* = motion) with specialized equipment (see Figure 8.19).

Figure 8.20 demonstrates use of an isokinetic device that allows the exercising limb to work at a fixed speed, with a variable resistance that is totally accommodating to the individual throughout the entire range of motion.[154]

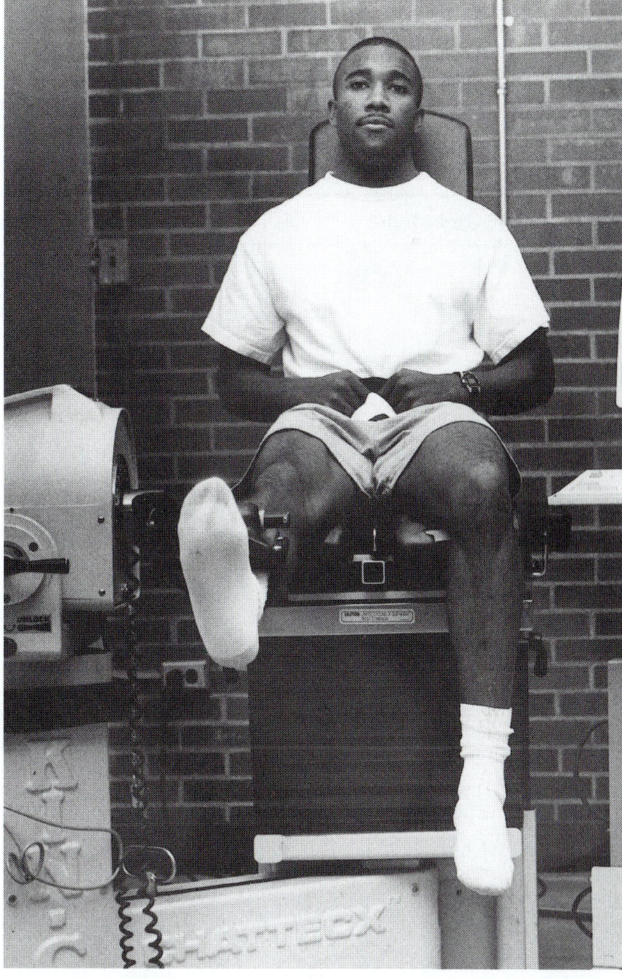

Figure 8.20 The Kincom allows *isokinetic exercise*, keeping all movement at a specific speed while varying the resistance to allow maximal effort throughout the range of motion.

SPORTS MEDICINE INSIGHT

Understanding and Promoting Physical Activity

Only 15% of U.S. adults engage regularly (three times a week for at least 20 minutes each time) in vigorous physical activity during their leisure time.[11] About 25% of adults report no physical activity. Many people have started exercise programs, only to drop out when various barriers present themselves (e.g., time problems, bad weather, family emergencies).[163,164]

Chapter 1 discussed some strategies for promoting physical activity at the population level. Emphasis was placed on four targets of change: (1) the person; (2) organizations; (3) the environment; and (4) public policies. This Sports Medicine Insight discusses models of extensive behavior change in individuals. Lifestyle behaviors do not occur in a vacuum but are affected by many complex factors, including personal beliefs, attitudes, self-esteem, education, ethnicity, income, environment, and culture.

As explained in the surgeon general's report, "as the benefits of moderate, regular physical activity have become more widely recognized, the need has increased for interventions that can promote this healthful behavior."[11] Numerous theories and models have been used to help people improve health behavior and physical activity patterns. These are summarized in Table 8.9.[11]

The transtheoretical model developed by psychologists James O. Prochaska and Carlos C. DiClemente is one of the most effective approaches to health behavior change and to improvement in physical activity habits.[165] This model has been adopted by the Canadian Society of Exercise Physiology in its *Canadian Physical Activity, Fitness & Lifestyle Appraisal* program.[166] Although originally developed for smokers, it has since been applied to other health behavior, including physical activity.

(continued)

SPORTS MEDICINE INSIGHT *(continued)*

Understanding and Promoting Physical Activity

TABLE 8.9 Summary of Theories and Models Used in Physical Activity Research

Theory/Model	Level	Key Concepts
Classic learning theories	Individual	Reinforcement Cues Shaping
Health-belief model	Individual	Perceived susceptibility Perceived severity Perceived benefits Perceived barriers Cues to action Self-efficacy
Transtheoretical model	Individual	Precontemplation Contemplation Preparation Action Maintenance
Relapse prevention	Individual	Skills training Cognitive reframing Lifestyle rebalancing
Social-cognitive theory	Interpersonal	Reciprocal determinism Behavioral capability Self-efficacy Outcome expectations Observational learning Reinforcement

Theory of planned behavior	Interpersonal	Attitude toward the behavior
		  Outcome expectation
		  Value of outcome expectations
		Subjective norm
		  Beliefs of others
		  Motive to comply with others
		Perceived behavioral control

Social support	Interpersonal	Instrumental support Informational support Emotional support Appraisal support

Ecological perspective	Environmental	Multiple levels of influence
		  Intrapersonal
		  Interpersonal
		  Institutional
		  Community
		  Public policy

Source: U.S. Department of Health and Human Services. *Physical Activity and Health: A Report of the Surgeon General.* Atlanta, GA: U.S. Department of Health and Human Services, Centers for Disease Control and Prevention, National Center for Chronic Disease Prevention and Health Promotion, 1996.

(continued)

SPORTS MEDICINE INSIGHT *(continued)*

Understanding and Promoting Physical Activity

In the transtheoretical model, behavior change is described as a five-stage process:

1. *Precontemplation.* Not intending to make changes
2. *Contemplation.* Considering a change
3. *Preparation.* Making small changes or ready to change in the very near future
4. *Action.* Actively engaging in the new behavior
5. *Maintenance.* Sticking with the behavior change

During the first three stages, people experience different processes of knowing and valuing. These include *consciousness raising* (increasing awareness of the problem in order to reduce defensiveness toward any intention to change), *dramatic relief* (expressing a strong emotional reaction to anything associated with the behavioral target), *social liberation* (being aware of enabling conditions in the immediate environment, that support the target behavior), *self-reevaluation* (reappraising personally relevant consequences associated with changing the target behavior), and *environmental reevaluation* (considering how the target behavior affects the social and physical environment).

During the last two stages, people experience certain behavioral processes of change, which include *self-liberation* (choosing and committing to implementation of the target behavior), *counterconditioning* (substituting an alternative behavior to replace a problem behavior that interferes with the desired change), *stimulus control* (removing cues or avoiding situations that trigger the problem behavior), *reinforcement management* (being rewarded by oneself or others for fully changing the target behavior), and *helping relationships* (trusting, accepting, and utilizing the support of caring others in the process of establishing the target behavior).

The amount of confidence people have in their ability to maintain a regular fitness program (self-efficacy) is related to their current stage. People in the early stages have less belief in their ability than those in later stages. Success has a powerful effect on self-efficacy. People often slip, however, and have to recycle through earlier stages.

According to the surgeon general's report, consistent influences on physical activity patterns among adults and young people include:[11]

- Confidence in one's ability to engage in regular physical activity (self-efficacy)
- Enjoyment of physical activity
- Support from others
- Positive beliefs concerning the benefits of physical activity
- Lack of perceived barriers to being physically active

In working with people, long-term interest, enthusiasm, and compliance to an exercise program can be promoted by several strategies, including the following:

- Encourage group participation or exercising with a partner.
- Emphasize variety and enjoyment in the exercise program.
- Minimize musculoskeletal injuries with a moderate exercise intensity and rate of progression.
- Help the client draw up reasonable goals and highlight these in a contract the client signs.
- Recruit the client's spouse or significant other for support.
- Provide progress charts to document achievement of goals.
- Recognize accomplishments through a system of rewards.
- Maximize convenience in terms of time, travel, and disruptions in family relationships.
- Complement fitness activities with nutrition education, stress management, and other health-promotion activities to improve the overall health of the client.

In comparing the different systems, there are several advantages and disadvantages with each.[154] Motivation is generally superior with isotonic exercises because they are self-testing in nature. Also, if heavy calisthenics instead of weight lifting are used for isotonic training, no special equipment is needed (see Appendix B).

Isometrics can also be performed without equipment and can be done anywhere, but gains in strength are joint-angle specific (within 20 degrees), and care must be taken to exercise at several angles. As for isokinetics, studies show that muscular strength and endurance development is somewhat better with such programs, but the specialized, expensive equipment makes this type of training impractical for most people.

It should be noted that Nautilus and similar equipment are not isokinetic in concept (fixed speed, accommodating resistance) but are actually isotonic equipment that attempts imperfectly to vary the resistance using various devices to work around the weak points of each lift.

SUMMARY

A comprehensive approach to exercise prescription should be used to provide all of the elements of physical fitness:

Warm-up. Engage in slow aerobic activity for several minutes, to gradually elevate the pulse and body temperature for hard aerobic activity. This will prepare the body by elevating the pulse, warming the body, and increasing blood flow. Flexibility exercises should not be done before the muscles and joints are warm.

Frequency. Start with 3 days per week and gradually build up to 5 or more days. Less than 3 days per week of aerobic activity does not build adequate fitness or help keep body fat under control. More than 5 days per week brings fewer fitness returns for the time and effort invested.

Intensity. Exercise at 40–85% of maximal capacity, depending on fitness status. The Karvonen formula is helpful for determining the training heart rate. The heart rate should be periodically counted (10-second pulse count) during exercise.

Time. The duration of an aerobic workout should be 20–60 minutes, depending on fitness status, intensity of exercise, and age. Time and intensity are interrelated and can be adjusted, as long as 150 to 400 Calories are expended. Informal exercise for 30–60 minutes a day is advised to complement the formal exercise program.

Mode. If frequency, intensity, and duration of training are similar, and a minimum of 4 Calories/kg are expended during the session, the training result is independent of the mode of exercise. Aerobic activities that are enjoyable should be utilized. A variety of exercises will enhance compliance.

Warm-down. The purpose is to slowly decrease the pulse rate and body temperature, which were elevated during the aerobic phase by engaging in slow aerobics. This will enhance recovery by reducing the muscle and blood lactic acid levels and promoting venous return to the heart.

Flexibility. Engage in flexibility exercises after the aerobic session, to stretch warm muscle groups that have been especially involved in the aerobic activities. Static stretching is advised, with each specific position held for four sets of about 10–30 seconds each.

Conditioning exercises for muscular endurance and strength. Strength, size, and endurance of muscle tissue is enhanced when the muscle performs for a period of time at its maximal strength and endurance capacity, against workloads above those normally encountered. The resistance should be gradually increased until the desired state is achieved. Isometric, isotonic, and isokinetic muscle training systems have been developed.

Review Questions

1. ***The first step of a good warm-up is***

   A. Stretching
   B. Low-intensity aerobic activity
   C. Resistance training
   D. Isometrics

2. ***Depending on the quantity and quality of training, improvement in $\dot{V}O_{2max}$ ranges from 5 to ____%, with greater improvement found for those with a very low initial level of fitness due to obesity or cardiac disease.***

   A. 30 B. 50 C. 100 D. 200 E. 10

3. ***When initiating an aerobic exercise program, conditioning every ____ is recommended.***

   A. Day B. Week
   C. Other day D. Weekend

4. ***If a 30-year-old individual has a maximal heart rate of 185 and a resting heart rate of 65, what is the heart rate reserve?***

   A. 135 B. 120 C. 250 D. 220

5. ***The exercise pulse is best counted using the ____ artery.***

   A. Radial B. Carotid
   C. Aorta D. Femoral

6. ***Exercise prescription has five essential components. Which one of the following is* not *included?***

   A. Periodization B. Progression
   C. Duration D. Frequency
   E. Intensity

7. ***Which mode does* not *improve aerobic fitness to a significant level?***

   A. Weight lifting B. Running
   C. Cross-country skiing D. Bicycling
   E. Swimming

8. ***There are three major principles of weight training. Which one listed below is* not *one of the principles?***

   A. Specificity
   B. Overload principle
   C. Valsalva's maneuver
   D. Progressive resistance principle

9. ***In ____, the muscle group contracts against a fixed, immovable resistance.***

   A. Isometrics B. Isotonic, concentric
   C. Isotonic, eccentric

10. ***A 55-year-old man in very poor cardiorespiratory shape wants to start an exercise program. He is over-***

weight, has high blood pressure and cholesterol, and has never exercised aerobically. He has been cleared by his physician. His resting heart rate is 75. What is his target training rate using the Karvonen formula and ACSM exercise prescription guidelines?

A. 124 B. 120 C. 137 D. 111 E. 161

11. ***What is the recommended rating of perceived exertion (RPE) during exercise training for the average person?***

A. Very hard B. Very, very hard
C. Somewhat hard D. Very light
E. Light

12. ***In 1998, the ACSM recommended that to develop and maintain cardiorespiratory fitness, people should exercise at an intensity of 40/50–85% heart rate reserve for ____ minutes a session, 3–5 days a week.***

A. 10–15 B. 30–75
C. 5–30 D. 20–60
E. 40–80

13. ***What is the estimated maximal heart rate of a 39-year-old man?***

A. 145 B. 165 C. 181 D. 143

14. ***An individual has a $\dot{V}O_{2max}$ of 40 $ml \cdot kg^{-1} \cdot min^{-1}$. He is exercising on a cycle ergometer at 25 $ml \cdot kg^{-1} \cdot min^{-1}$. What intensity is he training at, using percent of $\dot{V}O_2R$?***

A. 59 B. 45 C. 64 D. 39 E. 73

15. ***For light-to-moderate exercise, the estimated difference between %$\dot{V}O_2R$ and %HR_{max} is ____%.***

A. 3–7 B. 5–9 C. 8–12 D. 10–20 E. 17–30

16. ***If frequency, intensity, and duration of training are similar, and a minimum of ____ Calories are expended during the session, the training result appears to be independent of the mode of aerobic activity.***

A. 100–200 B. 150–400
C. 300–500 D. 750–1000
E. 800–1200

17. ***What type of muscle contraction is associated with delayed soreness?***

A. Isometric
B. Eccentric isotonic
C. Concentric isotonic

18. ***During the "down" phase of a push-up, what type of contraction is taking place?***

A. Eccentric, isotonic
B. Concentric, isotonic
C. Isometric

19. ***The ACSM has stated that a minimum muscular strength and endurance program involves 3–20 repetitions of 8–10 different weight lifting exercises conducted at least ____ nonconsecutive days a week.***

A. 4–5 B. 3–6 C. 2–3 D. 5–7 E. 1–2

20. ***If a person holds his or her breath during heavy weight-lifting effort, blood flow to the heart and brain is decreased, which can cause dizziness and blackout. This is called the***

A. Overload principle B. Valsalva maneuver
C. Specificity principle D. Progressive resistance principle

21. ***Three women, each 35 years of age, train at a heart rate of 150 bpm, 30 minutes/session, 5 days a week. One cycles, one runs, and the other uses a rowing machine. Which one will develop the best aerobic fitness?***

A. Woman who cycles
B. Woman who runs
C. Woman who rows
D. All will develop the same level of heart and lung fitness
E. None will improve their fitness because their training program is too easy

22. ***In 1993, the ACSM urged that when improvement in health is of major concern, the intensity can drop to 40%, and people in the general population are urged to accumulate ____ minutes or more of moderate-intensity physical activity over the course of most days of the week.***

A. 10 B. 20 C. 30 D. 45 E. 60

23. ***Which one of the following is* not *regarded as a physiological benefit of warming up before strenuous exercise?***

A. Decreases speed of nervous impulses
B. Increases breakdown of oxyhemoglobin
C. Increases the release of oxygen from muscle myoglobin
D. Decreases muscle viscosity
E. Increases blood flow to muscles

24. ***Less than 1 in ____ Americans walks or cycles to work.***

A. 5 B. 7 C. 20 D. 3 E. 12

25. ***If a participant has a $\dot{V}O_{2max}$ of 10 METs, then a 70% $\dot{V}O_{2max}$ intensity program would be conducted at ____ METs.***

A. 1 B. 7 C. 10 D. 70

26. ***In the heat, people tend to give RPE numbers that are too ____ for the effort.***

A. High B. Low

27. ***____ training is a free form of interval training done on trails or roads.***

A. Continuous B. Circuit
C. Fartlek D. Supervised

28. *The ACSM recommends that a basic stretching program be followed at least 2–3 days a week, and involve 2–4 repetitions of several static stretches that are held ____ seconds.*

A. 1–5 B. 15–30 C. 45–60 D. 60–120

29. *In general, ____ stretching techniques are more effective than conventional stretching methods for increasing joint range of motion.*

A. PNF B. Ballistic
C. Static D. Dynamic

30. *When appropriate weight-training principles are followed, the average strength improvement during the first 6 months of training is about ____ % for most people.*

A. 25–30 B. 50–75
C. 75–100 D. 100–200

31. *Weight lifting centers around five different variables. Which one of the following is* **not** *included?*

A. Repetitions to fatigue B. Order of exercises
C. Type of exercise D. Rest between sets
E. All are included

32. *Which one of the following is* **not** *regarded as an advantage of the RPE method?*

A. Is simple to use, takes only a few seconds, and is low cost
B. Is reliable at both low and high workloads
C. Shows a good correlation with blood lactate and oxygen consumption measures
D. Is preferable for people on certain types of medications
E. Teaches people to listen to their bodies during exercise

33. *In the transtheoretical model, behavior change is described as a five-stage process. Which one of the following is* **not** *included?*

A. Precontemplation B. Contemplation
C. Preparation D. Change
E. Progression

34. *Which one of the following drugs is associated with a decrease in exercise heart rate?*

A. Beta-blockers B. Cold medications
C. Antidepressants D. Thyroid medications
E. Bronchodilators

Answers

1. B	18. A
2. A	19. C
3. C	20. B
4. B	21. D
5. B	22. C
6. A	23. A
7. A	24. E
8. C	25. B
9. A	26. A
10. D	27. C
11. C	28. B
12. D	29. A
13. C	30. A
14. A	31. E
15. E	32. B
16. B	33. E
17. B	34. A

REFERENCES

1. American College of Sports Medicine. *ACSM's Guidelines for Graded Exercise Testing and Prescription* (7th ed.). Philadelphia: Lippincott Williams & Wilkins, 2006.
2. American College of Sports Medicine. The recommended quantity and quality of exercise for developing and maintaining cardiorespiratory and muscular fitness in healthy adults. *Med Sci Sports Exerc* 30:975–991, 1998.
3. American College of Sports Medicine. *ACSM's Exercise Management for Persons with Chronic Diseases and Disabilities.* Champaign, IL: Human Kinetics, 2002.
4. Corbin CB, Pangrazi RP. Physical activity pyramid rebuffs peak experience. *ACSM's Health & Fitness Journal* 2(1):12–17, 1998.
5. Kesaniemi YA, Danforth E, Jensen MD, Kopelman PG, Lefebvre P, Reeder BA. Dose-response issues concerning physical activity and health: An evidence-based symposium. *Med Sci Sports Exerc* 33(6 suppl):S351–S358, 2001.
6. Nieman DC. The exercise test as a component of the total fitness evaluation. *Prim Care* 28:119–135, 2001.
7. U.S. Department of Agriculture. *Dietary Guidelines for Americans.* www.heathierus.gov/dietaryguidelines, 2005.
8. Phillips WT, Pruitt LA, King AC. Lifestyle activity: Current recommendations. *Sports Med* 22:1–7, 1996.
9. Brooks GA, Butte NF, Rand WM, Flatt JP, Caballero B. Chronicle of the Institute of Medicine physical activity recommendation: How a physical activity recommendation came to be among dietary recommendations. *Am J Clin Nutr* 79:921S–930S, 2004.
10. Blair SN, LaMonte MJ, Nichaman MZ. The evolution of physical activity recommendations: How much is enough? *Am J Clin Nutr* 79(suppl):913S–920S, 2004.
11. U.S. Department of Health and Human Services. *Physical Activity and Health: A Report of the Surgeon General.* Atlanta, GA: U.S. Department of Health and Human Services, Centers for Disease Control and Prevention, National Center for Chronic Disease Prevention and Health Promotion, 1996.
12. American College of Sports Medicine. The recommended quantity and quality of exercise for developing and maintaining fitness in healthy adults. *Med Sci Sports Exerc* 10:vii–x, 1978.
13. American College of Sports Medicine. The recommended quantity and quality of exercise for developing and maintain-

ing cardiorespiratory and muscular fitness in healthy adults. *Med Sci Sports Exerc* 22:265–274, 1990.

14. DeBusk RF, Stenestrand U, Sheehan M, et al. Training effects of long versus short bouts of exercise in healthy subjects. *Am J Cardiol* 65:1010–1013, 1990.
15. Ebisu T. Splitting the distance of endurance running: On cardiovascular endurance and blood lipids. *Jap J Phys Educ* 30:37–43, 1985.
16. Pate RR, Pratt M, Blair SN, et al. Physical activity and public health: A recommendation from the Centers for Disease Control and Prevention and the American College of Sports Medicine. *JAMA* 273:402–407, 1995.
17. Fletcher GF, Blair SN, Blumenthal J, et al. Benefits and recommendations for physical activity programs for all Americans. A statement for health professionals by the Committee on Exercise and Cardiac Rehabilitation of the Council on Clinical Cardiology, American Heart Association. *Circulation* 86:340–344, 1992.
18. Fletcher GF, Balady G, Blair SN, et al. Benefits and recommendations for physical activity programs for all Americans. A statement for health professionals by the Committee on Exercise and Cardiac Rehabilitation of the Council on Clinical Cardiology, American Heart Association. *Circulation* 94:857–862, 1996.
19. Sallis JF, Patrick K. Physical activity guidelines for adolescents: Consensus statement. *Pediatric Exerc Sci* 6:302–314, 1994.
20. American Cancer Society. *Cancer Facts & Figures—1996.* Atlanta: American Cancer Society, 1996.
21. U.S. Preventive Services Task Force. *Guide to Clinical Preventive Services* (2nd ed.). Alexandria, VA: International Medical Publishing, 1996.
22. NIH Consensus Development Panel on Physical Activity and Cardiovascular Health. Physical activity and cardiovascular health. *JAMA* 276:241–246, 1996.
23. Alter MJ. *Science of Flexibility* (3rd ed.). Champaign, IL: Human Kinetics, 2004.
24. McArdle WD, Katch FI, Katch VL. *Exercise Physiology: Energy, Nutrition, and Human Performance* (5th ed.). Philadelphia: Lippincott Williams & Wilkins, 2001.
25. Wilmore JH, Costill DL. *Physiology of Sports and Exercise.* Champaign, IL: Human Kinetics, 2004.
26. Brooks GA, Fahey TD, Baldwin KM. *Exercise Physiology: Human Bioenergetics and Its Applications.* St. Louis: McGraw-Hill, 2004.
27. Institute for Aerobics Research. *The Strength Connection.* Dallas: Institute for Aerobics Research, 1990.
28. Maddux GT. *Men's Gymnastics.* Pacific Palisades, CA: Goodyear Publishing Co., Inc., 1970.
29. Shellock FG. Physiological benefits of warm-up. *Phys Sportsmed* 11:134–139, 1983.
30. Kato Y, Ikata T, Takai H, Takata S, Sairyo K, Iwanaga K. Effects of specific warm-up at various intensities on energy metabolism during subsequent exercise. *J Sports Med Phys Fitness* 40:126–130, 2000.
31. Gray SC, DeVito G, Nimmo MA. Effect of active warm-up on metabolism prior to and during intense dynamic exercise. *Med Sci Sports Exerc* 34:2091–2096, 2002.
32. Shellock FG, Prentice WE. Warming-up and stretching for improved physical performance and prevention of sports-related injuries. *Sports Med* 2:267–278, 1985.
33. Strickler T, Malone T, Garrett WE. The effects of passive warming on muscle injury. *Am J Sports Med* 18:141–145, 1990.
34. Houmard JA, Johns RA, Smith LL, Wells JM, Kobe RW, McGoogan SA. The effect of warm-up on responses to intense exercise. *Int J Sports Med* 12:480–483, 1991.
35. Moneta-Chivalbinska J, Hänninen O. Effect of active warming-up on thermoregulatory, circulatory, and metabolic responses to incremental exercise in endurance-trained athletes. *Int J Sports Med* 10:25–29, 1989.
36. Bishop D, Bonetti D, Dawson B. The effect of three different warm-up intensities on kayak ergometer performance. *Med Sci Sports Exerc* 33:1026–1033, 2001.
37. Vuori IM, Oja P, Paronen O. Physically active community to work—testing its potential for exercise promotion. *Med Sci Sports Exerc* 26:844–850, 1994.
38. Hendriksen IJM, Zuiderveld B, Kemper HCG, Bezemer PD. Effect of commuter cycling on physical performance of male and female employees. *Med Sci Sports Exerc* 32:504–510, 2000.
39. Federal Highway Administration, U.S. Department of Transportation. *The National Bicycling and Walking Study: Transportation Choices for a Changing America.* Washington, D.C.: U.S. Government Printing Office, Publication No. FHWA-PD-94-023.
40. Welk GJ, Differding JA, Thompson RW, Blair SN, Dziura J, Hart P. The utility of the Digi-Walker step counter to assess daily physical activity patterns. *Med Sci Sports Exerc* 32(9 suppl):S481–S488, 2000.
41. Thompson DL, Rakow J, Perdue SM. Relationship between accumulated walking and body composition in middle-aged women. *Med Sci Sports Exerc* 36:911–914, 2004.
42. Weyer C, Linkeschowa R, Heise T, Giesen HT, Spraul M. Implications of the traditional and the new ACSM Physical Activity Recommendations on weight reduction in dietary treated obese subjects. *Int J Obesity* 22:1071–1078, 1998.
43. Donnelly JE, Jacobsen DJ, Heelan KS, Seip R, Smith S. The effects of 18 months of intermittent vs. continuous exercise on aerobic capacity, body weight and composition, and metabolic fitness in previously sedentary, moderately obese females. *Int J Obes Relat Metab Disord* 24:566–572, 2000.
44. Hardman AE. Issues of fractionization of exercise (short vs long bouts). *Med Sci Sports Exerc* 33(6 suppl):S421–S427, 2001.
45. Dunn AL, Marcus BH, Kampert JB, Garcia ME, Kohl HW, Blair SN. Comparison of lifestyle and structured interventions to increase physical activity and cardiorespiratory fitness. *JAMA* 281:327–334, 1999.
46. Dunn AL, Garcia ME, Marcus BH, Kampert JB, Kohl HW, Blair SN. Six-month physical activity and fitness changes in Project Active, a randomized trial. *Med Sci Sports Exerc* 30:1076–1083, 1998.
47. Murphy M, Nevill A, Nevill C, Biddle S, Hardman A. Accumulating brisk walking for fitness, cardiovascular risk, and psychological health. *Med Sci Sports Exerc* 9:1468–1474, 2002.
48. Jakicic JM, Winters C, Lang Wei, Wing RR. Effects of intermittent exercise and use of home exercise equipment on adherence, weight loss, and fitness in overweight women. *JAMA* 282:1554–1560, 1999.
49. Pate RR, Branch JD. Training for endurance sport. *Med Sci Sports Exerc* 24(suppl):S340–S343, 1992.
50. Ainsworth BE, Haskell WL, Whitt MC, Irwin ML, Swartz AM, Strath SJ, OBrien WL, Bassett DR, Schmitz KH, Emplaincourt PO, Jacobs DR, Leon AS. Compendium of physical activities: An update of activity codes and MET intensities. *Med Sci Sports Exerc* 32(9 suppl):S498–S516, 2000.
51. Karvonen M, Kentala E, Mustala O. The effects of training on heart rate. A longitudinal study. *Ann Med Exp Biol Fenn* 35:307–315, 1957.

52. Davis JA, Convertino VA. A comparison of heart rate methods for predicting endurance training intensity. *Med Sci Sports Exerc* 7:295–298, 1975.
53. Swain DP, Leutholtz BC. Heart rate reserve is equivalent to %$\dot{V}O_2$reserve, not to % $\dot{V}O_{2max}$. *Med Sci Sports Exerc* 29:410–414, 1997.
54. Swain DP, Leutholtz BC, King ME, Haas LA, Branch JD. Relationship between % heart rate reserve and % $\dot{V}O_2$reserve in treadmill exercise. *Med Sci Sports Exerc* 30:318–321, 1998.
55. Whaley MH, Kaminsky LA, Dwyer GB, Getchell LH, Norton JA. Predictors of over- and underachievement of age-predicted maximal heart rate. *Med Sci Sports Exerc* 24:1173–1179, 1992.
56. Miller WC, Wallace JP, Eggert KE. Predicting max HR and the HR-$\dot{V}O_2$ relationship for exercise prescription in obesity. *Med Sci Sports Exerc* 25:1077–1081, 1993.
57. Borg G. Perceived exertion as indicator of somatic stress. *Scand J Rehabil Med* 2:92–98, 1970.
58. Noble BJ, Borg GAV, Jacobs I, Ceci R, Kaiser P. A category-ratio perceived exertion scale: Relationship to blood and muscle lactates and heart rate. *Med Sci Sports Exerc* 15:523–528, 1983.
59. Robertson RJ, Noble BJ. Perception of physical exertion: Methods, mediators, and applications. *Exerc Sport Sci Rev* 25:407–452, 1997.
60. Persinger R, Foster C, Gibson M, Fater DC, Porcari JP. Consistency of the talk test for exercise prescription. *Med Sci Sports Exerc* 36:1632–1636, 2004.
61. Whaley MH, Woodall T, Kaminsky LA, Emmett JD. Reliability of perceived exertion during graded exercise testing in apparently healthy adults. *J Cardiopulm Rehabil* 17:37–42, 1997.
62. Borg G. *An Introduction to Borg's RPE-Scale.* Ithaca, NY: Movement Publications, 1985.
63. Mahon AD, Stolen KQ, Gay JA. Differentiated perceived exertion during submaximal exercise in children and adults. *Pediatr Exerc Sci* 13:145–153, 2001.
64. Garcin M, Vandewalle H, Monod H. A new rating scale of perceived exertion based on subjective estimation of exhaustion time: A preliminary study. *Int J Sports Med* 20:40–43, 1999.
65. Robertson RJ. *Perceived Exertion for Practitioners: Rating Effort with the OMNI Picture System.* Champaign, IL: Human Kinetics, 2004.
66. Ilmarinen J, Ilmarinen R, Koskela A, Korhonen O, et al. Training effects of stair-climbing during office hours on female employees. *Ergonomics* 22:507–516, 1979.
67. Ilmarinen J, Rutenfranz J, Knauth P, Ahrens M, et al. The effect of an on the job training program, stairclimbing, on the physical working capacity of employees. *Eur J Appl Physiol* 38:25–40, 1978.
68. Kuipers H. Training and overtraining: An introduction. *Med Sci Sports Exerc* 30:1137–1139, 1998.
69. Loy SF, Hoffmann JJ, Holland GJ. Benefits and practical use of cross-training in sports. *Sports Med* 19:1–8, 1996.
70. Porcari JP, Ebbeling CB, Ward A, Freedson PS, Rippe JM. Walking for exercise testing and training. *Sports Med* 8:189–200, 1989.
71. Hultquist CN, Albright C, Thompson DL. Comparison of walking recommendations in previously inactive women. *Med Sci Sports Exerc* 37:676–683, 2005.
72. Porcari J, McCarron R, Kline G, et al. Is fast walking an adequate aerobic training stimulus for 30- to 69-year-old men and women? *Phys Sportsmed* 15(2):119–129, 1987.
73. Davison RCR, Grant S. Is walking sufficient exercise for health? *Sports Med* 16:369–373, 1993.
74. Nieman DC, Custer WF, Butterworth DE, Utter AC, Henson DA. Psychological response to exercise training and/or energy restriction in obese women. *J Psychosom Res* 48:23–29, 2000.
75. Iwane M, Arita M, Tomimoto S, Satani O, Matsumoto M, Miyashita K, Nishio I. Walking 10,000 steps/day or more reduces blood pressure and sympathetic nerve activity in mild essential hypertension. *Hypertens Res* 23(6):573–580, 2000.
76. Lee IM, Rexrode KM, Cook NR, Manson JE, Buring JE. Physical activity and coronary heart disease in women: Is "no pain, no gain" passé? *JAMA* 285:1447–1454, 2001.
77. Spelman CC, Pate RR, Macera CA, Ward DS. Self-selected exercise intensity of habitual walkers. *Med Sci Sports Exerc* 25:1174–1179, 1993.
78. Graves JE, Pollock ML, Montain SJ, et al. The effect of hand-held weights on the physiological responses to walking exercise. *Med Sci Sports Exerc* 19:260–265, 1987.
79. Graves JE, Martin AD, Miltenberger LA, Pollock ML. Physiological responses to walking with hand weights, wrist weights, and ankle weights. *Med Sci Sports Exerc* 20:265–271, 1988.
80. Auble TE, Schwartz L. Physiological effects of exercising with handweights. *Sports Med* 11:244–256, 1991.
81. Porcari JP. Pump up your walk. *ACSM's Health & Fitness Journal* 3(1):25–29, 1999.
82. Claremont AD, Hall SJ. Effects of extremity loading upon energy expenditure and running mechanics. *Med Sci Sports Exerc* 20:167–171, 1988.
83. Garrick JG, Requa RK. Aerobic dance: A review. *Sports Med* 6:169–179, 1988.
84. Grant S, Davidson W, Aitchison T, Wilson J. A comparison of physiological responses and rating of perceived exertion between high-impact and low-impact aerobic dance sessions. *Eur J Appl Physiol* 78:324–332, 1998.
85. Milburn S, Butts NK. A comparison of the training responses to aerobic dance and jogging in college females. *Med Sci Sports Exerc* 15:510–513, 1983.
86. McMurray RG, Hackney AC, Guion WK, Katz VL. Metabolic and hormonal responses to low-impact aerobic dance during pregnancy. *Med Sci Sports Exerc* 28:41–46, 1996.
87. Noreau L, Moffet H, Drolet M, Parent E. Dance-based exercise program in rheumatoid arthritis. Feasibility in individuals with American College of Rheumatology functional class III disease. *Am J Phys Med Rehabil* 76:109–113, 1997.
88. Nelson DJ, Pels AE, Geenen DL, White TP. Cardiac frequency and caloric cost of aerobic dancing in young women. *Res Quart Exerc Sport* 59:229–233, 1988.
89. Williford HN, Blessing DL, Barksdale JM, Smith FH. The effects of aerobic dance training on serum lipids, lipoproteins and cardiopulmonary function. *J Sports Med* 28:151–157, 1988.
90. Tarrant K, McNaughton L. A comparison of the metabolic effects of high and low impact aerobic dance exercise. *Sports Med Training Rehab* 7:255–264, 1997.
91. Sanders ME, Maloney-Hills C. Aquatic exercise for better living on land. *ACSM's Health & Fitness Journal* 2(3):16–23, 1998.
92. Jétte M, Landry F, Tiemann B, Blüumchen G. Ambulatory blood pressure and holter monitoring during tennis play. *Can J Sport Sci* 16:40–44, 1991.
93. Bartoli WP, Slentz CA, Murdoch SD, Pate RR, Davis JM, Durstine JL. Effects of a 12-week racquetball program on maximal oxygen consumption, body composition and blood lipoproteins. *Sports Med Training Rehab* 5:157–164, 1994.

94. Montpetit RR, Beauchamp L, Léger L. Energy requirements of squash and racquetball. *Phys Sportsmed* 15(8):106–112, 1987.

95. Smekal G, Von Duvillard SP, Rihacek C, Pokan R, Hofmann P, Baron R, Tschan H, Bachl N. A physiological profile of tennis match play. *Med Sci Sports Exerc* 33:999–1005, 2001.

96. Locke S, Colquhoun D, Briner M, Ellis L, O'Brien M, Wollstein J, Allen G. Squash racquets. A review of physiology and medicine. *Sports Med* 23:130–138, 1997.

97. Loftin M, Anderson P, Lytton L, Pittman P, Warren B. Heart rate response during handball singles match-play and selected physical fitness components of experienced male handball players. *J Sports Med Phys Fitness* 36:95–99, 1996.

98. Hurley BF. Effects of high-intensity strength training on cardiovascular function. *Med Sci Sports Exerc* 16:483–488, 1984.

99. Gettman LR, Ayres JJ, Pollock ML, Jackson A. The effect of circuit weight training on strength, cardiorespiratory function, and body composition of adult men. *Med Sci Sports Exerc* 10:171–176, 1978.

100. Harris KA, Holly RG. Physiological response to circuit weight training in borderline hypertensive subjects. *Med Sci Sports Exerc* 19:246–252, 1987.

101. Dudley GA, Fleck SJ. Strength and endurance training: Are they mutually exclusive? *Sports Med* 4:79–85, 1987.

102. Kuehl K, Elliot DL, Goldberg L. Predicting caloric expenditure during multi-station resistance exercise. *J Appl Sport Sci Res* 4(5):63–66, 1990.

103. Sleamaker RH. Caloric cost of performing the Perrier Parcourse Fitness Circuit. *Med Sci Sports Exerc* 16:283–286, 1984.

104. Sforzo GA, Micale FG, Bonnani NA, Muir M, Wigglesworth J. A new training technique: Cardioresistance exercise. *ACSM's Health & Fitness Journal* 2(6):11–16, 1998.

105. Berry MJ, Cline CC, Berry CB, Davis M. A comparison between two forms of aerobic dance and treadmill running. *Med Sci Sports Exerc* 24:946–951, 1992.

106. Olson MS, Williford HN, Blessing DL, Greathouse R. The cardiovascular and metabolic effects of bench stepping exercise in females. *Med Sci Sports Exerc* 23:1311–1318, 1991.

107. Quirk JE, Sinning WE. Anaerobic and aerobic responses of males and females to rope skipping. *Med Sci Sports Exerc* 14:26–29, 1982.

108. Jung AP, Nieman DC. An evaluation of home exercise equipment claims: Too good to be true? *ACSM's Health & Fitness Journal* 4(5):14–16, 30,31, 2000.

109. Kuntzleman CT, Wilkerson R. A primer to recommending home aerobic equipment. *ACSM's Health & Fitness Journal* 1(6):24–32, 1997.

110. Hagerman FC, Lawrence RA, Mansfield MC. A comparison of energy expenditure during rowing and cycling ergometry. *Med Sci Sports Exerc* 20:479–488, 1988.

111. Secher NH. Physiological and biomechanical aspects of rowing: Implications for training. *Sports Med* 15:24–42, 1993.

112. Howley ET, Colacino DL, Swensen TC. Factors affecting the oxygen cost of stepping on an electronic stepping ergometer. *Med Sci Sports Exerc* 24:1055–1058, 1992.

113. Zeni AI, Hoffman MD, Clifford PS. Energy expenditure with indoor exercise machines. *JAMA* 275:1424–1427, 1996.

114. Kravitz L, Robergs RA, Heyward VH, Wagner DR, Powers K. Exercise mode and gender comparisons of energy expenditure at self-selected intensities. *Med Sci Sports Exerc* 29:1028–1035, 1997.

115. Carter R, Watenpaugh DE, Wasmund WL, Wasmund SL, Smith ML. Muscle pump and central command during recovery from exercise in humans. *J Appl Physiol* 87:1463–1469, 1999.

116. Ahmaidi S, Granier P, Taoutaou Z, Mercier J, Dubouchaud H, Prefaut C. Effects of active recovery on plasma lactate and anaerobic power following repeated intensive exercise. *Med Sci Sports Exerc* 28:450–456, 1996.

117. Koyama Y, Koike A, Yajima T, Kano H, Marumo F, Hiroe M. Effects of "cool-down" during exercise recovery on cardiopulmonary systems in patients with coronary artery disease. *Jpn Circ J* 64:191–196, 2000.

118. Anderson, B. *Stretching.* Bolinas, CA: Shelter Publications, 1980, 1999 (www.stretching.com).

119. American College of Sports Medicine. *ACSM Fitness Book* (2nd ed.). Champaign, IL: Human Kinetics, 1998.

120. Brown DA, Miller WC. Normative data for strength and flexibility of women throughout life. *Eur J Appl Physiol* 78:77–82, 1998.

121. Malliaropoulos N, Papalexandris S, Papalada A, Papacostas E. The role of stretching in rehabilitation of hamstring injuries: 80 athletes follow-up. *Med Sci Sports Exerc* 36:756–759, 2004.

122. Pope RP, Herbert RD, Kirwan JD, Graham BJ. A randomized trial of preexercise stretching for prevention of lower-limb injury. *Med Sci Sports Exerc* 32:271–277, 2000.

123. Rodenburg JB, Steenbeek D, Schiereck Bar PR. Warm-up, stretching and massage diminish harmful effects of eccentric exercise. *Int J Sport Med* 15:414–419, 1994.

124. Hartigan C, Miller L, Liewehr SC. Rehabilitation of acute and subacute low back and neck pain in the work-injured patient. *Orthop Clin North Am* 27:841–860, 1996.

125. Knudson DV, Magnusson P, McHugh M. Current issues in flexibility fitness. *President's Council on Physical Fitness and Sports, Research Digest* 3(10), June 2000.

126. Thacker SB, Gilchrist J, Stroup DF, Kimsey CD. The impact of stretching on sports injury risk: A systematic review of the literature. *Med Sci Sports Exerc* 36: 371–378, 2004.

127. Krivickas LS, Feinberg JH. Lower extremity injuries in college athletes: Relation between ligamentous laxity and lower extremity muscle tightness. *Arch Phys Med Rehabil* 77:1139–1143, 1996.

128. Jones BH, Knapik JJ. Physical training and exercise-related injuries. Surveillance, research and injury prevention in military populations. *Sports Med* 27:111–125, 1999.

129. Herbert RD, Gabriel M. Effects of stretching before and after exercising on muscle soreness and risk of injury: Systematic review. *BMJ* 325:468–472, 2002.

130. Shrier I. Stretching before exercise does not reduce the risk of local muscle injury: A critical review of the clinical and basic science literature. *Clin J Sport Med* 9:221–227, 1999.

131. Twellaar M, Verstappen FT, Huson A, van Mechelen W. Physical characteristics as risk factors for sports injuries: A four year prospective study. *Int J Sports Med* 18:66–71, 1997.

132. Kirby RL, Simms FC, Symingtom VJ, Garner JB. Flexibility and musculoskeletal symptomatology in female gymnasts and age-matched controls. *Am J Sports Med* 9:160–164, 1981.

133. Bennell KL, Crossley K. Musculoskeletal injuries in track and field: Incidence, distribution and risk factors. *Aust J Sci Med Sport* 28:69–75, 1996.

134. Craib MW, Mitchell VA, Fields KB, Cooper TR, Hopewell R, Morgan DW. The association between flexibility and running economy in sub-elite male distance runners. *Med Sci Sports Exerc* 28:737–743, 1996.

135. Goldberg BA, Scarlat MM, Harryman DT. Management of the stiff shoulder. *J Orthop Sci* 4:462–471, 1999.
136. Etnyre BR, Abraham LD. Antagonist muscle activity during stretching: A paradox re-assessed. *Med Sci Sports Exerc* 20:285–289, 1988.
137. Roberts JM, Wilson K. Effect of stretching duration on active and passive range of motion in the lower extremity. *Br J Sports Med* 33:259–263, 1999.
138. Hutton RS. Neuromuscular basis of stretching exercises. In Komi PV (ed.). *Strength and Power in Sport: The Encyclopaedia of Sports Medicine.* Oxford: Blackwell Scientific Publications, 1992.
139. Moore TM. A workplace stretching program. Physiologic and perception measurements before and after participation. *AAOHN J* 46:563–568, 1998.
140. Godges JJ, MacRae H, Longdon C, Tinberg C, MacRae P. The effects of two stretching procedures on hip range of motion and gait economy. *J Orthop Sports Phys Ther* 10:350–357, 1989.
141. American College of Sports Medicine. Position stand on progression models in resistance training for healthy adults. *Med Sci Sports Exerc* 34:364–380, 2002.
142. Osternig LR, Robertson RN, Troxel RK, Hansen P. Differential responses to proprioceptive neuromuscular facilitation (PNF) stretch techniques. *Med Sci Sports Exerc* 22:106–111, 1990.
143. Baechle TR, Earle RW. *Essentials of Strength Training and Conditioning* (2nd ed.). Champaign, IL: Human Kinetics, 2000.
144. Feigenbaum MS, Pollock ML. Prescription of resistance training for health and disease. *Med Sci Sports Exerc* 31:38–45, 1999.
145. Fleck SJ, Kraemer WJ. *Designing Resistance Training Programs.* Champaign, IL: Human Kinetics Publishers, 2003.
146. Institute for Aerobics Research. *The Strength Connection.* Dallas: Institute for Aerobics Research, 1990.
147. Evans WJ. Exercise training guidelines for the elderly. *Med Sci Sports Exerc* 31:12–17, 1999.
148. American Association of Cardiovascular and Pulmonary Rehabilitation. *Guidelines for Cardiac Rehabilitation Programs* (3rd ed.). Champaign, IL: Human Kinetics, 1998.
149. Hass CJ, Garzarella L, De Hoyos D, Pollock ML. Single versus multiple sets in long-term recreational weightlifters. *Med Sci Sports Exerc* 32:235–242, 2000.
150. Starkey DB, Pollock ML, Ishida Y, Welsch MA, Brechue WF, Graves JE, Feigenbaum MS. Effect of resistance training volume on strength and muscle thickness. *Med Sci Sports Exerc* 28:1311–1320, 1996.
151. Morrissey MC, Harman EA, Johnson MJ. Resistance training modes: Specificity and effectiveness. *Med Sci Sports Exerc* 27:648–660, 1995.
152. Kraemer WJ, Ratamess NA. Fundamentals of resistance training: Progression and exercise prescription. *Med Sci Sports Exerc* 36:674–688, 2004.
153. Fry AC, Kraemer WJ. Resistance exercise overtraining and overreaching: Neuroendocrine responses. *Sports Med* 23:106–129, 1997.
154. Davies GJ. *A Compendium of Isokinetics in Clinical Usage.* Onalaska, WI: S & S Publishers, 1992.
155. Elliot DL, Goldberg L, Kuehl KS, Catlin DH. Characteristics of anabolic- androgenic steroid-free competitive male and female bodybuilders. *Phys Sportsmed* 15(6):169–180, 1987.
156. Braith RW, Graves JE, Pollock ML, Leggett SL, Carpenter DM, Colvin AB. Comparison of 2 vs 3 days/week of variable resistance training during 10- and 18-week programs. *Int J Sports Med* 10:450–454, 1989.
157. Feigenbaum MS, Gentry RK. Prescription of resistance training for clinical populations. *Am J Med Sports* 3:146–158, 2001.
158. Tesch PA. Training for bodybuilding. In Komi PV (ed.). *Strength and Power in Sport: The Encyclopaedia of Sports Medicine.* Oxford: Blackwell Scientific Publications, 2002.
159. Sale DG. Neural adaptation to resistance training. *Med Sci Sports Exerc* 20(suppl):S135–S145, 1988.
160. Rhea MR, Alvar BA, Burkett LN, Ball SD. A meta-analysis to determine the dose response for strength development. *Med Sci Sports Exerc* 35:456–464, 2003.
161. Mayhew TP, Rothstein JM, Finucane SD, Lamb RL. Muscular adaptation to concentric and eccentric exercise at equal power levels. *Med Sci Sports Exerc* 27:868–873, 1995.
162. Higbie EJ, Cureton KJ, Warren GL, Prior BM. Effects of concentric and eccentric training on muscle strength, cross-sectional area, and neural activation. *J Appl Physiol* 81:2173–2181, 1996.
163. U.S. Department of Health and Human Services. *Promoting Physical Activity: A Guide for Community Action.* Champaign, IL: Human Kinetics, 1999.
164. Riebe D, Nigg C. Setting the stage for healthy living. *ACSM's Health & Fitness Journal* 2(3):11–15, 1998.
165. Prochaska JO, Norcross JC, DiClemente CC. *Changing for Good.* New York: William Morrow and Company, Inc., 1994
166. Canadian Society for Exercise Physiology. *The Canadian Physical Activity, Fitness & Lifestyle Appraisal.* Ottawa, Ontario: The Canadian Society for Exercise Physiology, 1996.

PHYSICAL FITNESS ACTIVITY 8.1

The Activity Pyramid: How Do You Rate?

This chapter emphasized a comprehensive approach to physical fitness in which three major components—aerobic fitness, muscular fitness, and body composition—are given balanced attention. In other words, to have total fitness, pay attention to all the muscles of your body, both inside (heart) and out (skeletal), and keep lean by balancing calories burned with those eaten. This comprehensive approach to physical fitness is summarized in the activity pyramid (Figure 8.2).

How comprehensive is your approach to physical fitness? Fill in the blanks below, total your points, and then compare them to the norms to determine how well you adhere to the recommendations of the activity pyramid. Give yourself 5 points for each "yes" answer and 0 points for each "no" answer.

Yes (5 points)	**No** (0 points)	
❑	❑	*Level 1: Lifestyle physical activity.* Do you accumulate at least 30 minutes of physical activity nearly every day?
❑	❑	*Level 2: Exercise for aerobic fitness.* Do you engage in brisk walking, swimming, cycling, running, active sports, or other aerobic activities for 20–60 minutes, 3–5 days per week?
		Level 3: Exercise for muscular fitness.
❑	❑	*A. Muscular strength and endurance exercise.* Do you lift weights, engage in strength calisthenics (push-ups, sit-ups, pull-ups, etc.), or work hard physically (e.g., chopping wood, lifting heavy objects, shoveling dirt) for about 20–30 minutes, two to three times per week?
❑	❑	*B. Flexibility exercise.* Do you engage in a regular stretching routine that affects major muscle groups and joints for about 10–20 minutes, two to three times per week?
❑	❑	*Level 4: Reduce inactivity.* Do you make a conscious effort to reduce sitting time on most days by limiting watching TV, playing video games, viewing the Internet, etc.?

Your total points: ____

Norms	Points	Classification
	25	Excellent
	15 or 20	Good
	10	Fair
	0 or 5	Poor

PHYSICAL FITNESS ACTIVITY 8.2

Your Aerobic Exercise Program

This chapter emphasized that aerobic exercise is the cornerstone of a comprehensive physical fitness program. The aerobic stage of a comprehensive physical fitness program consists of three segments: the warm-up, aerobic exercise (that conforms to frequency, intensity, and time guidelines), and the cool-down. This is summarized in Box 8.2.

Go to Box 8.2 and perform these tasks:

1. ***Fitness level.*** In Chapter 4, you assessed your aerobic fitness level. Circle under step 2 the fitness column that best matches your current aerobic fitness level: low fitness, average, or high.
2. ***Training heart rate.*** Using the intensity range listed for your fitness level, go to step 2B (intensity), and calculate your personal training heart rate. Use the maximum heart rate and resting heart rate that you measured from Chapter 4.
3. ***Aerobic exercise mode.*** Under step 2C (aerobic exercise mode), write down your primary aerobic exercise mode (the one you use most often), a secondary mode, and a backup mode. Consult the section in this chapter on physical activity modes if you are starting an exercise program and want guidelines on making good choices.
4. ***Daily schedule.*** Lack of time is the exercise barrier most frequently listed by people in surveys. Based on your current schedule, go to step 2D (build exercise into daily schedule), and write down the specific times on the specific days you can exercise.

PHYSICAL FITNESS ACTIVITY 8.3

Your Flexibility Exercise Program

In this chapter, several specific guidelines were given for developing flexibility:

Frequency. 2–3 days per week, or after each aerobic workout.

Time. Hold each position short of the pain threshold for 10–30 seconds, and repeat four times (total time, about 15 minutes).

Stretching positions. Improve flexibility in several body areas with specific stretching exercises.

In Box 8.8, instructions for eight flexibility exercises are summarized. With the help of your class instructor, try each of these, and provide your personal comments on how they felt and areas of needed improvement.

Flexibility Exercise	How This Exercise Felt to You: Personal Notes	Improvement in This Area Is Needed (Check "yes" or "no")
1. Lower back–hamstring rope stretch		☐ Yes ☐ No
2. Calf rope stretch		☐ Yes ☐ No
3. Groin stretch		☐ Yes ☐ No
4. Quad stretch		☐ Yes ☐ No
5. Spinal twist		☐ Yes ☐ No
6. Downward dog		☐ Yes ☐ No
7. Upper-body rope stretch		☐ Yes ☐ No
8. Standing side stretch		☐ Yes ☐ No

PHYSICAL FITNESS ACTIVITY 8.4

Your Muscular Strength and Endurance Exercise Program

In this chapter, guidelines for building muscular strength and endurance were described:

Step 1. Warm-Up Aerobically

Never strength train unless the muscles and joints are warm from 5–15 minutes of moderate aerobic activity.

Step 2. Follow These Minimum Strength Training Program Guidelines:

A. Frequency

Strength train at least 2–3 days per week.

B. Set and Reps

Perform a minimum of one set of 8–12 repetitions to the point of volitional fatigue for each exercise.

C. Strength Exercises

Perform a minimum of 8–10 different exercises that condition all of the major muscle groups.

With the help of your class instructor, try the routine described in Box 8.11. Perform each exercise through a full range of motion. Perform both the lifting and lowering portion of each exercise in a controlled manner. Maintain a normal breathing pattern because breath-holding can induce excessive increases in blood pressure. Use a classmate as a spotter. Try each of the strength exercises listed in Box 8.11 and provide your personal comments on how they felt and areas of needed improvement.

Strength Exercise	How This Strength Exercise Felt to You: Personal Notes	Improvement in This Area Is Needed (Check "yes" or "no")
1. Lat pull down		☐ Yes ☐ No
2. Leg press		☐ Yes ☐ No
3. Bench press		☐ Yes ☐ No
4. Abdominal crunch		☐ Yes ☐ No
5. Shoulder press		☐ Yes ☐ No
6. Seated row		☐ Yes ☐ No
7. Leg extension		☐ Yes ☐ No
8. Leg curl		☐ Yes ☐ No
9. Biceps curl		☐ Yes ☐ No
10. Triceps pushdown		☐ Yes ☐ No
11. Standing heel raise		☐ Yes ☐ No

chapter 9

Nutrition and Performance

Aside from the limits imposed by heredity and the physical improvements associated with training, no factor plays a bigger role in exercise performance than does nutrition.

—David Costill[1]

Fitness enthusiasts work out for 30–60 minutes, several times a week. Others are members of athletic teams, training at a high intensity for several days nearly every day. Here are several common questions posed by fitness enthusiasts and athletes:

- What adaptations beyond the prudent diet should be pursued by fitness enthusiasts and athletes?
- Can diet changes improve exercise performance and athletic endeavor?
- What is the optimal diet for athletes?
- Are the nutritional stresses imposed by heavy exertion greater than can be met by the traditional food supply? Are vitamin and mineral supplements needed?
- Do people who lift weights need protein supplements to maximize size and power?
- Are there performance-enhancing aids (called ergogenic aids) that are safe, beneficial, and ethical?

Fitness enthusiasts can obtain all their nutrient requirements by incorporating the recommendations given in *Dietary Guidelines for Americans* (see the section on nutrition basics). The rest of this chapter reviews 10 cardinal sports-nutrition principles that are applicable to the athlete:[2,3]

1. Prudent diet is the cornerstone.
2. Increase total energy intake.
3. Keep the dietary carbohydrate intake high (55–70%) during training.
4. Drink large amounts of fluid during training and the event.
5. Keep a close watch on possible iron deficiency.
6. Vitamin and mineral supplements are not needed.
7. Protein supplements do not benefit the athlete.
8. Rest and emphasize carbohydrates before long endurance events.
9. Use of ergogenic aids is unethical.
10. Fat loading is not recommended for enhanced performance or health.

As time spent in intense exercise (running, swimming, bicycling, weight lifting, etc.) increases above 1 hour a day, several changes in the diet are recommended (above and beyond the dietary recommendations described in the section on nutrition basics). As will be emphasized in this chapter, however, the changes are actually fewer than many athletes expect:

- Increase in energy intake (in other words, more food)
- Increase in the grams per kilogram of body weight coming from carbohydrate
- Increase in fluid intake

Vitamin and mineral supplements are generally not needed by athletes. Contrary to popular opinion, even protein supplements are not needed by strength athletes if they are eating a balanced diet that matches their energy needs. Before reviewing the 10 cardinal sports-nutrition principles, a review will be given of nutrition basics and the recommendations given in *Dietary Guidelines for Americans.*

NUTRITION BASICS

One's diet—the amount and type of food typically eaten—is influenced by many factors, including cultural background and personal food preferences. (See Box 9.1 for a glossary of terms used in nutrition.) On average, Americans tend to eat too much energy in the form of fat, especially the hard saturated fat commonly found in animal products. The Western diet is also too low in starch and fiber, important food components found in plant foods like whole grains, fruits, and vegetables. Such dietary patterns help explain why Americans have high rates of obesity, heart disease, high blood pressure, stroke, diabetes, and certain forms of cancer.[4–7]

Nutrition is the science that looks at how the foods we eat affect the functioning and health of our bodies. Although research into the relationship between diet and health is ongoing, scientists have identified the nutrients necessary for good health and the foods that provide them. In this section, emphasis will be placed on basic nutrition principles and key dietary guidelines for eating smart to maintain lifelong wellness.

Foods contain a variety of compounds that provide energy, build and maintain organs and tissues, and regulate life-sustaining body functions. The energy in food is measured in kilocalories—1 kilocalorie represents the amount of heat needed to raise 1 kilogram of water from 14.5 to 15.5°C. In common usage, the term Calorie is used in place of kilocalorie to represent the amount of energy in food, even though a Calorie is actually a much smaller unit of energy. In this text, the common term Calorie will be used to refer to the energy content of foods. Most American adults consume between 1,600 and 2,500 Calories/day.

Essential Nutrients

For good health, humans need adequate amounts of all the essential nutrients—the nutrients that the body cannot make

Box 9.1

Glossary of Terms Used In Nutrition

antioxidant: An agent that inhibits oxidation and thus prevents rancidity of oils or fats or the deterioration of other materials through oxidative processes (e.g., vitamins A, C, and E).

Calorie (kilocalorie): A unit of heat content or energy. The amount of heat necessary to raise 1 gram of water from 14.5 to 15.5°C. The unit used to measure the energy in food is a kilocalorie (1,000 calories). In this book, Calorie will be used to denote kilocalorie. In many parts of the world, Calorie is being replaced by joule, the international unit equal to 0.239 Calorie.

carbohydrates: An ideal energy source for the body (4 Calories/gram). Compounds made up of carbon, hydrogen, and oxygen and composed of simple sugars (called monosaccharides and disaccharides), as well as long chains of sugars (called starch and glycogen).

carbohydrate loading: The process of eating a very high carbohydrate diet (>70% Calories as carbohydrate) while tapering down exercise prior to a race event. Recommended for endurance athletes competing in cycling, running, swimming, and similar events.

cholesterol: A type of fat found only in animal products. Cholesterol is a soft, waxy substance that helps to form cell membranes and hormones but can also contribute to heart disease.

daily values: Nutrient reference standards for the food label that combine information from the RDA/DRIs and the Dietary Guidelines.

diet: Food and drink in general. A prescribed course of eating and drinking in which the amount and kind of food, as well as the times at which it is to be taken, are regulated for various purposes (e.g., losing weight).

dietary fiber: Plant complex carbohydrates and lignin that are resistant to breakdown by the digestive enzymes in humans. Dietary fiber is either soluble or insoluble in water, and each type has specific effects on health.

Dietary Guidelines for Americans: Guidelines developed and published by the U.S. Department of Agriculture to enhance life quality and prevent disease.

dietary references intakes (DRIs): New nutrient intake standards developed by the Food and Nutrition Board that take into account prevention of nutrient deficiencies and chronic disease.

ergogenic aids: Substances or methods that tend to increase exercise performance capacity.

essential nutrients: Nutrients that the body cannot make on its own and must obtain from foods. There are more than 40 essential nutrients classified into six groups: carbohydrates, fats, proteins, vitamins, minerals, and water.

fat: A chief form of energy (9 Calories/gram). Fats (primarily triglycerides that are made up of three fatty acids and glycerol) are a greasy material found in animal tissues and many plants, and contribute to feelings of fullness at a meal, enhance food's aroma and flavor, cushion the body's vital organs, carry fat-soluble nutrients, and help make up cell membranes.

(continued)

Box 9.1

Glossary of Terms Used In Nutrition *(continued)*

food guide pyramid: A food group plan developed by the U.S. Department of Agriculture to help consumers translate nutrient intake recommendations into a plan for healthy eating.

free radicals: Unstable and reactive oxygen particles that are formed when oxygen is consumed by cells. Free radicals cause oxidative damage on cell membranes and proteins.

hydrogenation: The process of adding hydrogen to unsaturated fatty acids to make the fat stay fresher longer, and makes it more solid and less greasy-tasting.

minerals: Naturally occurring, inorganic chemical elements that represent a very small but important fraction of human body weight (about 5 pounds).

monounsaturated fatty acid: A fatty acid with one point of unsaturation where hydrogens are missing. Olive and canola oils are high in monounsaturated fats.

nutrition: The study of the food and liquid requirements of human beings for normal body function, including energy, growth, muscular activity, reproduction, and lactation.

nutrient-dense foods: Foods high in nutrient value relative to the number of Calories they contain.

phytochemical: Chemical components of plants, many of which have beneficial health effects.

polyunsaturated fatty acid: This fatty acid has two or more points of unsaturation. Most vegetable oils, nuts, and high-fat fish are good sources of polyunsaturated fats.

protein: Large molecules composed of carbon, hydrogen, oxygen, and nitrogen and arranged as strands of amino acids. Protein is three fourths of the dry weight of most cell matter and is involved in structures, hormones, enzymes, muscle contraction, immunological response, and essential life functions.

recommended dietary allowances (RDAs): Nutrient intake standards developed by the Food and Nutrition Board of the National Academy of Sciences.

refined grain products: Processed grain products that have had parts of the grain removed, decreasing fiber and nutrient content.

saturation: Degree of saturation depends on the number of hydrogens in the fatty acid chain. If all of the carbons in the chain are linked to two or more hydrogens, the fatty acid is saturated.

saturated fat: Chemically, this is a type of fat that has no double bonds in the carbon chain and is thus called saturated because it is incapable of absorbing any more hydrogen. Most saturated fats come from animal foods (i.e., meat and dairy products) and tropical oils (e.g., coconut and palm oils). Saturated fats tend to raise blood cholesterol levels and increase the risk of heart disease.

sodium: An essential mineral that plays a role in the regulation of water balance, normal muscle tone, acid–base balance, and the conduction of nerve impulses. The body needs about 500 mg/day of sodium, but up to 2,400 mg/day is compatible with good health.

sugar: A simple type of carbohydrate. Six sugar molecules are important in nutrition: three monosaccharides or single sugars (glucose, fructose, and galactose), and three disaccharides or double sugars (lactose or milk sugar, maltose or malt sugar, and sucrose or table sugar).

***trans*-fatty acids:** During hydrogenation, some fatty acids change their shape as they become saturated. Found in most margarines, shortening, fast foods, and baked products. *Trans*-fatty acids tend to raise blood cholesterol levels.

triglycerides: Triglycerides, or fat, are molecules made up of glycerol and three units of fatty acids.

unsaturated fat: Chemically, this type of fat has a carbon chain with one or more double bonds (e.g., a monounsaturated fatty acid with one double bond in the molecule, and a polyunsaturated fatty acid with two). It is called unsaturated because it is capable of absorbing additional hydrogen. Monounsaturated (e.g., olive oil) and polyunsaturated fats (e.g., plant oils like corn and sunflower oils) tend to decrease blood cholesterol levels when substituted for saturated fat in the diet.

vegetarian diet: A diet plan that excludes meat, poultry, and fish. There are several types of vegetarians, including vegans, who avoid all animal products and only eat plant foods, and lacto-ovo-vegetarians who avoid animal flesh but eat dairy products and eggs.

vitamins: A group of organic substances, present in minute amounts in food, that are essential to normal metabolism; insufficient amounts in the diet may cause deficiency diseases.

whole-grain products: Grain products that contain all the original fiber and grain parts. Whole grain products not only have more fiber, they also contain more nutrients.

on its own and thus must obtain from foods.[3–6] There are more than 40 essential nutrients, classified into six groups: carbohydrates, fats, proteins, vitamins, minerals, and water. Three groups of essential nutrients supply energy:

- Carbohydrates are compounds made up of carbon, hydrogen, and oxygen; they are a main source of energy for the body, providing 4 Calories/gram. Carbohydrates are typically classified into two groups: (1) simple sugars, which are made up of one or two basic sugar units, and (2) complex carbohydrates, or starches, which are made up of long chains of sugar units. Carbohydrates are found in grains, fruits, vegetables, and milk.
- Fats are the most energy-rich of the nutrients, providing 9 Calories/gram. Fats have other functions in addition to providing energy: They enhance the aroma and flavor of foods, contribute to feelings of fullness, and transport certain vitamins. In the body, fats cushion the body's vital organs and help make up cell membranes. Fats are found in animal tissues and in some plants, including grains, nuts, and seeds.
- Proteins are made up of long strands of amino acids, compounds that contain carbon, hydrogen, oxygen, and nitrogen. Proteins form important parts of all the cells and tissues in the body, including skin, muscles, bones, and organs; as enzymes, hormones, and immune cells, proteins help regulate body processes and protect from infection. Proteins can also supply energy; like carbohydrates, they provide 4 Calories/gram. Proteins are found in animal foods, legumes, nuts, and grains.

Alcohol, although not an essential nutrient, also supplies energy at 7 Calories/gram. The recommended breakdown of daily energy intake is 55% of total Calories from carbohydrate, 30% of total Calories from fat, and 15% of total Calories from protein.[6] This breakdown is advocated for Americans of all activity levels, including sedentary people, fitness enthusiasts, and nearly all types of competitive athletes.

The other classes of essential nutrients do not supply energy, but they perform many other critical functions in the body:[4,8]

- Vitamins are organic (carbon-containing) substances that are present in minute amounts in foods. Vitamins are essential to the body because they promote specific chemical reactions in cells, reactions involved in such key processes as digestion, muscular movement, tissue growth, wound healing, and production of energy. Vitamins are classified as either water soluble or fat soluble, depending on whether they dissolve in water or fat; solubility affects how vitamins are transported and stored in your body. The fat-soluble vitamins are vitamins A, D, E, and K; the water-soluble vitamins are vitamin C and the B-complex vitamins. Refer to Table 9.1 for more information about the roles and food sources of specific vitamins.
- Minerals are inorganic (non-carbon-containing) substances that represent a small but important fraction of the weight of the body (about 5 pounds). Minerals are a part of many cells and tissues, including your bones, teeth, and nails. Like vitamins, minerals can also promote chemical reactions and regulate body processes. Major minerals, those present in the body in amounts greater that 5 grams, include calcium, phosphorus, magnesium, sodium, chloride, and potassium. The dozen or so trace minerals, present in the body in amounts less than 5 grams, include iron and zinc (see Table 9.1).
- Water makes up about 60% of the body's weight and has many important functions. Water serves as a solvent and a lubricant, provides a medium for transporting key chemicals, participates in chemical reactions, and aids in the control of body temperature. Water balance is critical for health and exercise performance. Lightly active people need about 8 cups of water or other liquids each day; fluid needs of physically active individuals will be described later in the chapter. Water is found in fruits, vegetables, and other liquids.

Guidelines for Nutrient Intake: Recommended Dietary Allowances (RDAs) and Dietary Reference Intakes (DRIs)

An adequate intake of all essential nutrients is necessary for the proper functioning of the body. What exactly is an adequate intake? For more than 50 years, the Food and Nutrition Board of the National Academy of Sciences has been reviewing nutrition research and defining nutrient requirements for healthy people. Until recently, one set of nutrient intake levels reigned supreme: the recommended dietary allowances (RDAs).[5] When the RDAs were first created in 1941, their primary goal was to prevent diseases caused by vitamin and mineral deficiencies. If a vitamin or mineral is lacking in the diet, characteristic symptoms of deficiency develop based on the particular role that vitamin or mineral plays in the body. For example, an inadequate supply of vitamin C can result in scurvy, a collection of symptoms that includes excessive bleeding, loose teeth, and swollen gums. Fortunately, diseases caused by vitamin and mineral deficiencies are now rare in the United States and other developed nations.

Since the development of the RDAs, scientists have discovered that certain vitamins and minerals are important not just for preventing deficiency diseases but also for preventing chronic diseases such as heart disease, cancer, high blood pressure, diabetes, and osteoporosis. Because the RDAs were not designed to consider these common chronic diseases, the Food and Nutrition Board developed an ambitious plan for revamping the old RDAs. The new standards, known as the dietary reference intakes (DRIs), include intakes for optimal health based on the prevention of both deficiencies and chronic diseases.[9–14] The new focus

TABLE 9.1 RDA, DV, and UL Values for Vitamins and Minerals

Nutrient (other names)	Recommended Dietary Allowance (RDA)	Daily Value (DV)	Good Sources	Upper Level (UL)	Selected Adverse Effects
Vitamins					
Vitamin A (retinol)	Women: 700 μg Men: 900 μg	5,000 IU* (1,500 μg)	Liver, fatty fish, fortified foods (milk, breakfast cereals, etc.)	10,000 IU (3,000 μg)	*Liver toxicity, birth defects.* Inconclusive; bone loss
Carotenoids (alpha-carotene, beta-carotene, beta-cryptoxanthin, lutein, lycopene, zeaxanthin)	None. (NAS advises eating more cartotenoid-rich fruits and vegetables)	None	Orange fruits & vegetables (alpha- and beta-carotene), green leafy vegetables (beta-carotene and lutein), tomatoes (lycopene)	None. Panel said don't take beta-carotene, except to get RDA for vitamin A	Smokers who took high doses of beta-carotene supplements (33,000–50,000 IU a day) had higher risk of lung cancer
Thiamin (vitamin B_1)	Women: 1.1 mg Men: 1.2 mg	1.5 mg	Breads, cereals, pasta, & foods made with "enriched" or whole-grain flour; pork	None	None reported
Riboflavin (vitamin B_2)	Women: 1.1 mg Men: 1.3 mg	1.7 mg	Milk, yogurt, foods made with "enriched" or whole-grain flour	None	None reported
Niacin (vitamin B_3)	Women: 14 mg Men: 16 mg	20 mg	Meat, poultry, seafood, foods made with "enriched" or whole-grain flour	35 mg†	*Flushing (burning, tingling, itching, redness),* liver damage
Vitamin B_6 (pyridoxine)	Ages 19–50: 1.3 mg Women 50+: 1.5 mg Men 50+: 1.7 mg	2 mg	Meat, poultry, seafood, fortified foods (cereals, etc.), liver	100 mg	*Reversible nerve damage (burning, shooting, tingling pains, numbness, etc.)*
Vitamin B_{12} (cobalamin)	2.4 μg	6 μg	Meat, poultry, seafood, dairy foods, fortified foods (cereals, etc.)	None	None reported
Folate (folacin, folic acid)	400 μg	400 μg (0.4 mg)	Orange juice, beans, other fruits & vegetables, fortified cereals, foods made with "enriched" or whole-grain flour	1,000 mg† (1 mg)	*Can mask or precipitate a B_{12}* deficiency, which can cause irreversible nerve damage
Vitamin C (ascorbic acid)	Women: 75 mg Men: 90 mg (Smokers: add 35 mg)	60 mg	Citrus & other fruits, vegetables, fortified foods (cereals, etc.)	2,000 mg	*Diarrhea*
Vitamin D	Ages 19–50: 200 IU‡ Ages 51–70: 400 IU‡ Over 70: 600 IU‡	400 IU	Sunlight, fatty fish, fortified foods (milk, breakfast cereals, etc.)	2,000 IU	*High blood calcium,* which may cause kidney and heart damage
Vitamin E (alpha-tocopherol)	15 mg (33 IU—synthetic) (22 IU—natural)	30 IU (synthetic)	Oils, whole grains, nuts	1,000 mg† (1,100 IU—synthetic) (1,500 IU—natural)	*Hemorrhage* May lower risk of
Vitamin K (phylloquinone)	Women: 90 μg‡ Men: 120 μg‡	80 μg	Green leafy vegetables, oils	None	Interferes with coumadin & other anti-clotting drugs
Calcium	Ages; 19–50: 1,000 mg[3] Over 50: 1,200 mg[3]	1,000 mg	Dairy foods, fortified foods, leafy green vegetables, canned fish (eaten with bones)	2,500 mg	*High blood calcium,* which may cause kidney damage, kidney stones

(continued)

TABLE 9.1 ***(continued)***

Nutrient (other names)	Recommended Dietary Allowance (RDA)	Daily Value (DV)	Good Sources	Upper Level (UL)	Selected Adverse Effects
Chromium	Women: 25 μg[3] Men: 35 μg[3]	120 μg	Whole grains, bran cereals, meat, poultry, seafood	None	Inconclusive: kidney or muscle damage
Copper	900 μg	2 mg (2,000 μg)	Liver, seafood, nuts, seeds, wheat-bran, whole grains, chocolate	10 mg (10,000 μg)	*Liver damage*
Iron	Women 19–50: 18 mg Women 50+: 8 mg Men: 8 mg	18 mg	Red meat, poultry, seafood, foods made with "enriched" or whole-grain flour	45 mg	*Gastrointestinal effects (constipation, nausea, diarrhea)*
Magnesium	Women: 320 mg Men: 420 mg	400 mg	Green leafy vegetables; whole-grain breads, cereals, etc.; nuts	350 mg†	*Diarrhea*
Phosphorus	700 mg	1,000 mg	Dairy foods, meat, poultry, seafood, foods (processed cheese, colas, etc.) made with phosphate additives	Ages 19–70: 4,000 mg Over 70: 3,000 mg	*High blood phosphorus,* which may damage kidneys and bones
Selenium	55 μg	70 μg	Seafood, meat, poultry, grains (depends on levels in soil)	400 μg	Nail or hair loss or brittleness
Zinc	Women: 8 mg Men: 11 mg	15 mg	Red meat, seafood, whole grains, fortified foods (cereals, etc.)	40 mg	*Lower copper levels,* HDL ("good") cholesterol, and immune response

Note: Recommended dietary allowance (RDA). RDAs for adults only.
Daily value (DV). These levels appear on food and supplement labels. Unlike the RDAs, there is only one daily value for everyone over age 4.
Tolerable upper intake level (UL). These levels are upper safe daily limits. ULs for adults only.
Selected adverse effects. What happens if you take too much. *The UL is based on the adverse effect listed in italics.* "Inconclusive" adverse effects are based on inconsistent or sketchy evidence.

Other tolerable upper intake levels.

Boron: 20 mg	Manganese: 11 mg
Choline: 3.5 g	Molybdenum: 2,000 μg (2 mg)
Flouride: 10 mg	Nickel: 1 mg
Iodine: 1,100 μg (1.1 mg)	Vanadium: 1.8 mg

*We get vitamin A both from retinol and carotenoids, but this number assumes that all of the vitamin A comes from retinol.
†From supplements and fortified foods only.
‡Adequate intake (AI). The National Academy of Sciences (NAS) had too little data to set an RDA.

Source: Food and Nutrition Information Center, www.nal.usda.gov/fnic

on chronic diseases has led to increased intake recommendations for some nutrients. For example, the recommended intake for calcium has been raised for both men and women to reflect new research on the link between calcium intake and reduced risk of osteoporosis.

As a general rule, most Americans don't need vitamin and mineral supplements for good health, and pills and capsules are no substitute for healthy dietary habits. As summarized in Table 9.2, intake by adults of most vitamins and minerals is near recommended levels, and when intake seems low, experts caution that this can be related to issues surrounding the difficult task of measuring nutrient intake.[5,15] Supplements of some nutrients, if taken regularly in large amounts, can be harmful. Some nutrients are directly toxic if taken in excess, and large doses of nutrients can also cause problems by interfering with the absorption of other vitamins and minerals. In part because of concerns about people taking high doses of supplements, the DRIs also include standards for upper intake limits, the highest level of daily nutrient intake that is likely to pose no risks of adverse health effects to most individuals (see Table 9.1). (The use of supplements and performance aids by fitness enthusiasts and athletes will be discussed later in the chapter.)

The first group of DRIs was released in 1997, and additional reports were completed by 2004.[9–14] For more information on the DRIs, visit the website of the Food and Nutrition Board. (See Box 9.2 for this and other helpful nutrition-related sites.)

TABLE 9.2 American Adults Aged 20–39 years: Dietary Intake Compared to Recommended Levels (1999–2000)

	Males	Females	Recommended
Energy (Calories)	2,825	2,028	Varies *
Carbohydrate (% total energy)	50.0	52.6	45–65
Fat (% total energy)	32.1	32.3	20–35
Saturated fat (% total energy)	10.8	10.9	<10
Protein (% total energy)	14.9	14.6	10–35
Alcohol (% total energy)	2.6	1.4	Not established
Dietary fiber (g/day)	18.6	13.9	M: 38; F: 25
Cholesterol (mg/day)	350	241	<300
Sodium (mg/day)	4,329	3,161	<2,300
Antioxidants			
Vitamin A (μg/day RAE)	878	961	M: 900; F: 700
Vitamin C (mg/day)	102	85	M: 90; F: 75
Vitamin E (mg/day α-T)	10.4	8.2	15
Vitamin B_6 (mg/day)	2.2	1.6	1.3; 50+ yr, M 1.7, F 1.5
Folate (μg/day DFE)	435	327	400
Calcium (mg/day)	1,025	797	1,000; 50+ yr, 1,200
Iron (mg/day)	17.9	13.7	M: 8; F: 18, 50+ yr, 8
Zinc (mg/day)	14.8	10.1	M: 11; F: 8

*Energy needs vary according to body size and physical activity, with the RDA average set at 2,900 Calories for males, and 2,200 for females. There is evidence that energy intake is underestimated in national surveys. Nonetheless, obesity prevalence is increasing which means that Americans tend to take in more energy than they expend.
RAE = retinol activity equivalents, DFE = dietary folate equivalents

Source: Wright JD, Wang CY, Kennedy-Stephenson J, Ervin RB. Dietary intake of ten key nutrients for public health. United States: 1999–2000. *Advance Data from Vital and Health Statistics,* no., 334. Hyattsville, MD: National Center for Health Statistics. Also: http://www.barc.usda.gov/bhnrc/foodsurvey/home.htm.

Box 9.2

Internet Sources for Sound Nutrition Information

- Tufts University Nutrition Navigator
  http://navigator.tufts.edu

Provides a rating of the accuracy of nutrition content and usability of nutrition websites

- Mayo Health Oasis
  www.mayohealth.org

Provides consumers with good nutrition information in a fun, user-friendly format

- Consumer Information Center
  www.pueblo.gsa.gov

Provides access to hundreds of educational materials

- FDA Center for Food Safety & Applied Nutrition
  vm.cfsan.fda.gov/list.html

Provides government updates on food and nutrition issues and on basic nutrition guidelines

- Meals for You (My Menus)
  www.MealsForYou.com

Provides thousands of recipes with menu plans, shopping lists, and nutritional analysis

- USDA Food and Nutrition Information Center
  www.nal.usda.gov/fnic

Connects readers to the vast nutrition-related resources of the National Agricultural Library

- Healthfinder
  www.healthfinder.gov

Organizes the health and nutrition information from federal and state agencies

- Vegetarian Resource Group
  www.vrg.org

Provides nutrition information and recipes for those interested in the vegetarian diet

- American Dietetic Association
  www.eatright.org

A link for nutrition information for both consumers and dietitians

- International Food Information Council
  www.ific.org

Provides guidelines on nutrition and food safety for consumers and professionals

- Cyberdiet
  www.cyberdiet.com

Gives information on foods, recipes, vitamins and minerals, and food planning

DIETARY GUIDELINES FOR HEALTH AND DISEASE PREVENTION

All individuals, whether sedentary or very active, should consume a prudent diet to enhance quality of life and prevent disease.[16,17] In this text, a prudent diet is defined as one that conforms to the recommendations given in *Dietary Guidelines for Americans,* developed by the U.S. Department of Agriculture (USDA).[7]

The intent of the *2005 Dietary Guidelines* is to summarize and synthesize knowledge regarding individual nutrients and food components into recommendations for a pattern of eating that can be adopted by the public.[7] Key recommendations are grouped under nine interrelated focus areas and are based on available scientific evidence for lowering risk of chronic disease and promoting health. The focus areas are integrated, and taken together they encourage Americans to eat fewer calories, be more active, and make wiser food choices. Here are the nine focus areas (key recommendations will be listed in the focus area sections that follow):

1. Weight Management
2. Physical Activity
3. Food Groups to Encourage
4. Carbohydrates
5. Food Safety
6. Fats
7. Adequate Nutrients within Calorie Needs
8. Sodium and Potassium
9. Alcoholic Beverages

Weight Management; Physical Activity

Key Recommendations[7]

- To maintain body weight in a healthy range, balance calories from foods and beverages with calories expended.
- To prevent gradual weight gain over time, make small decreases in food and beverage calories and increase physical activity.
- Engage in regular physical activity and reduce sedentary activities to promote health, psychological well-being, and a healthy body weight.
  - To reduce the risk of chronic disease in adulthood: Engage in at least 30 minutes of moderate-intensity physical activity, above usual activity, at work or home on most days of the week.
  - For most people, greater health benefits can be obtained by engaging in physical activity of more vigorous intensity or longer duration.
  - To help manage body weight and prevent gradual, unhealthy weight gain in adulthood: Engage in approximately 60 minutes of moderate- to vigorous-intensity activity on most days of the week while not exceeding caloric intake requirements.
  - To sustain weight loss in adulthood: Participate in at least 60 to 90 minutes of daily moderate-intensity physical activity while not exceeding caloric intake requirements. Some people may need to consult with a health-care provider before participating in this level of activity.
- Achieve physical fitness by including cardiovascular conditioning, stretching exercises for flexibility, and resistance exercises or calisthenics for muscle strength and endurance.
- *Children and adolescents.* Engage in at least 60 minutes of physical activity on most, preferably all, days of the week.
- *Pregnant women.* In the absence of medical or obstetric complications, incorporate 30 minutes or more of moderate-intensity physical activity on most, if not all, days of the week. Avoid activities with a high risk of falling or abdominal trauma.
- *Breastfeeding women.* Be aware that neither acute nor regular exercise adversely affects the mother's ability to successfully breastfeed.
- *Older adults.* Participate in regular physical activity to reduce functional declines associated with aging and to achieve the other benefits of physical activity identified for all adults.

During 1971–2000, the prevalence of obesity in the United States doubled from 14.5% to 30.9%,[18] and the prevalence of overweight among children and adolescents also increased substantially. A high prevalence of overweight and obesity is of great public health concern because excess body fat leads to a higher risk for premature death, type 2 diabetes, hypertension, dyslipidemia, cardiovascular disease, stroke, gall bladder disease, respiratory dysfunction, gout, osteoarthritis, and certain kinds of cancers (see Chapter 13).

Ideally, the goal for adults is to achieve and maintain a body weight that optimizes health.[7] However, for obese adults, even modest weight loss (e.g., 10 pounds) has health benefits, and the prevention of further weight gain is very important. For overweight children and adolescents, the goal is to slow the rate of weight gain while achieving normal growth and development. Maintaining a healthy weight throughout childhood may reduce the risk of becoming an overweight or obese adult.

Eating fewer calories while increasing physical activity is the key to controlling body weight. Caloric intake is about 250 Calories/day higher than it was in 1970.[15,19] (See Table 9.2 for a summary of 1999–2000 American diet intake levels, and complete Physical Fitness Activity 9.2 to determine your energy intake.)

Americans tend to be relatively inactive. One in four adult Americans do not participate in any leisure time physical activities, and 4 in 10 students in grades 9 to 12 view television 3 or more hours per day.[7] To reduce the risk of chronic disease, it is recommended that adults engage in at least 30 minutes of moderate-intensity physical activity on most, preferably all, days of the week. For most people, greater health benefits can be obtained by engaging in physical activity of more vigorous intensity or of longer duration.

Regular physical activity is also a key factor in achieving and maintaining a healthy body weight for adults and children. To prevent the gradual accumulation of excess weight in adulthood, approximately 60 minutes of moderate- to vigorous-intensity physical activity on most days of the week may be needed. Though moderate-intensity physical activity can achieve the desired goal, vigorous-intensity physical activity generally provides more benefits than moderate-intensity physical activity. Control of caloric intake is also advisable. However, to sustain weight loss for previously overweight/obese people, about 60 to 90 minutes of moderate-intensity physical activity per day is recommended.

The barrier often given for a failure to be physically active is lack of time. Setting aside 30 to 60 consecutive minutes each day for planned exercise is one way to obtain physical activity, but it is not the only way. Physical activity may include short bouts (e.g., 10-minute bouts) of moderate-intensity activity. The accumulated total is what is important—both for health and for burning calories. Physical activity can be accumulated through three to six 10-minute bouts over the course of a day. Elevating the level of daily physical activity may also provide indirect nutritional benefits. A sedentary lifestyle limits the number of calories that can be consumed without gaining weight. The higher a person's physical activity level, the higher his or her energy requirement and the easier it is to plan a daily food intake pattern that meets recommended nutrient requirements.

Food Groups to Encourage

Key Recommendations[7]

- Consume a sufficient amount of fruits and vegetables while staying within energy needs. Two cups of fruit and 2½ cups of vegetables per day are recommended for a reference 2,000-calorie intake, with higher or lower amounts depending on the calorie level.
- Choose a variety of fruits and vegetables each day. In particular, select from all five vegetable subgroups (dark green, orange, legumes, starchy vegetables, and other vegetables) several times a week.
- Consume 3 or more ounce-equivalents of whole-grain products per day, with the rest of the recommended grains coming from enriched or whole-grain products. In general, at least half the grains should come from whole grains.
- Consume 3 cups per day of fat-free or low-fat milk or equivalent milk products.

The *2005 Dietary Guidelines for Americans* are the basis for federal nutrition policy. The *MyPyramid Food Guidance System* provides food-based guidance to help implement the recommendations of the *Guidelines*.[20] (See Figure 9.1.) *MyPyramid* is based on both the *Guidelines* and the *Dietary Reference Intakes* from the National Academy of Sciences,[6,9–14] while taking into account current consumption patterns of Americans. *MyPyramid* translates the *Guidelines* into a total diet that meets nutrient needs from food sources and aims to moderate or limit dietary components often consumed in excess. An important complementary tool is the *Nutrition Facts* label on food products.

The *MyPyramid Education Framework* provides specific recommendations for making food choices that will improve the quality of an average American diet. These recommendations are interrelated and should be used together. Taken together, they would result in the following changes from a typical diet:

- Increased intake of vitamins, minerals, dietary fiber, and other essential nutrients, especially of those that are often low in typical diets.
- Lowered intake of saturated fats, *trans* fats, and cholesterol, and increased intake of fruits, vegetables, and whole grains to decrease risk for some chronic diseases.
- Calorie intake balanced with energy needs to prevent weight gain and/or promote a healthy weight.

The recommendations in MyPyramid fall under four overarching themes:

- *Variety*—Eat foods from all food groups and subgroups.
- *Proportionality*—Eat more of some foods (fruits, vegetables, whole grains, fat-free or low-fat milk products), and less of others (foods high in saturated or *trans* fats, added sugars, cholesterol, salt, and alcohol).
- *Moderation*—Choose forms of foods that limit intake of saturated or *trans* fats, added sugars, cholesterol, salt, and alcohol.
- *Activity*—Be physically active every day.

Consuming an appropriate number of servings from each food group is important because foods from different groups tend to provide different essential nutrients. Grains and cereals should form the basis of each meal, supplemented with liberal servings of vegetables and fruit, and low-fat servings of meat and dairy products. Box 9.3 summarizes the suggested amounts of food to consume from the basic food groups, subgroups, and oils in *MyPyramid* to meet recommended nutrient intakes at 12 different calorie levels.

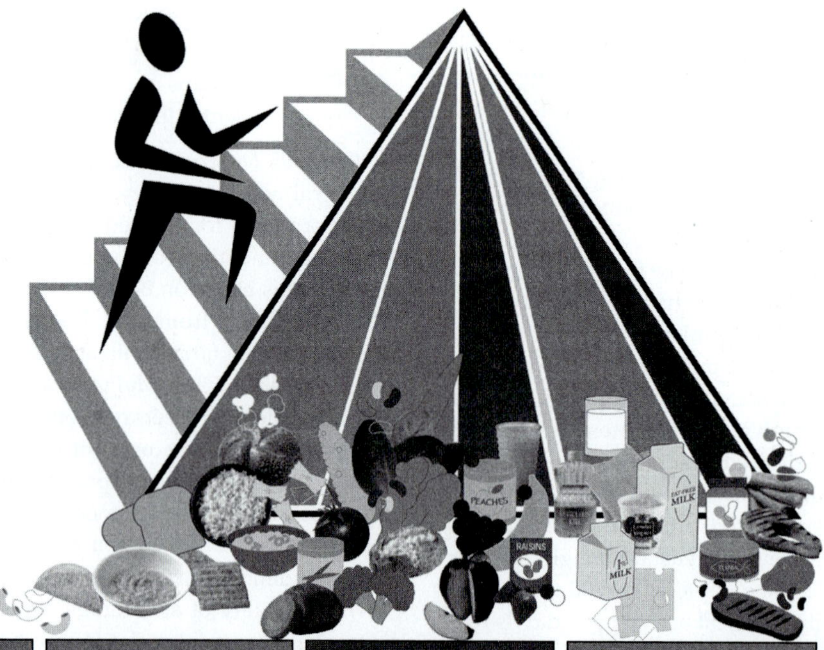

GRAINS Make half your grains whole	VEGETABLES Vary your veggies	FRUITS Focus on fruits	MILK Get your calcium-rich foods	MEAT & BEANS Go lean with protein
Eat at least 3 oz. of whole-grain cereals, breads, crackers, rice, or pasta every day 1 oz. is about 1 slice of bread, about 1 cup of breakfast cereal, or 1/2 cup of cooked rice, cereal, or pasta	Eat more dark-green veggies like broccoli, spinach, and other dark leafy green Eat more orange vegetables like carrots and sweet-potatoes Eat more dry beans and peas like pinto beans, kidney beans, and lentils	Eat a variety of fruit Choose fresh, frozen, canned, or dried fruit Go easy on fruit juices	Go low-fat or fat-free when you choose milk, yogurt, and other milk products If you don't or can't consume milk, choose lactose-free products or other calcium sources such as fortified foods and beverages	Choose low-fat or lean meats and poultry Bake it, broil it, or grill it Vary your protein routine–choose more fish, beans, peas, nuts, and seeds
For a 2,000-calorie diet, you need the amounts below from each food group. To find the amounts that are right for you, go to MyPyramid.com				
Eat 6 oz. every day	Eat 2 1/2 cups every day	Eat 2 cups every day	Get 3 cups every day for kids aged 2 to 8, it's 2	Eat 5 1/2 oz. every day

Find your balance between food and physical activity

- Be sure to stay within your daily calorie needs.
- Be physically active for at least 30 minutes most days of the week.
- About 60 minutes a day of physical activity may be needed to prevent weight gain.
- For sustaining weight loss, at least 60 to 90 minutes a day of physical activity may be required.
- Children and teenagers should be physically active for 60 minutes every day, or most days.

Know the limits on fats, sugars, and salt (sodium)

- Make most of your fat sources from fish, nuts, and vegetable oils.
- Limit solid fats like butter, margarine, shortening, and lard, as well as foods that contain these.
- Check the Nutrition Facts label to keep saturated fats, *trans* fats, and sodium low.
- Choose food and beverages low in added sugars. Added sugars contribute calories with few, if any, nutrients.

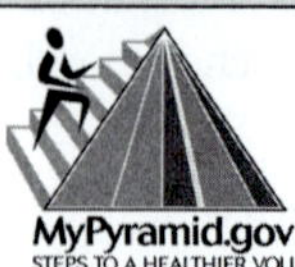

U.S. Department of Agriculture
Center for Nutrition Policy and Promotion
April 2005
CNPP-15
USDA

Figure 9.1

MyPyramid is a personalized approach to healthy eating and physical activity. Source: MyPyramid.gov.

Box 9.3

MyPyramid Food Intake Patterns

Food intake patterns are the suggested amounts of food to consume from the basic food groups, subgroups, and oils to meet recommended nutrient intakes at 12 different calorie levels. Nutrient and energy contributions from each group are calculated according to the nutrient-dense forms of foods in each group (e.g., lean meats and fat-free milk). The table also shows the discretionary calorie allowance that can be accommodated within each calorie level, in addition to the suggested amounts of nutrient-dense forms of foods in each group.

Daily Amount of Food from Each Group

Calorie Level[1]	1,000	1,200	1,400	1,600	1,800	2,000	2,200	2,400	2,600	2,800	3,000	3,200
Fruits[2]	1 cup	1 cup	1.5 cups	1.5 cups	1.5 cups	2 cups	2 cups	2 cups	2 cups	2.5 cups	2.5 cups	2.5 cups
Vegetables[3]	1 cup	1.5 cups	1.5 cups	2 cups	2.5 cups	2.5 cups	3 cups	3 cups	3.5 cups	3.5 cups	4 cups	4 cups
Grains[4]	3 oz-eq	4 oz-eq	5 oz-eq	5 oz-eq	6 oz-eq	6 oz-eq	7 oz-eq	8 oz-eq	9 oz-eq	10 oz-eq	10 oz-eq	10 oz-eq
Meat and Beans[5]	2 oz-eq	3 oz-eq	4 oz-eq	5 oz-eq	5 oz-eq	5.5 oz-eq	6 oz-eq	6.5 oz-eq	6.5 oz-eq	7 oz-eq	7 oz-eq	7 oz-eq
Milk[6]	2 cups	2 cups	2 cups	3 cups	3 cups	3 cups	3 cups	3 cups	3 cups	3 cups	3 cups	3 cups
Oils[7]	3 tsp	4 tsp	4 tsp	5 tsp	5 tsp	6 tsp	6 tsp	7 tsp	8 tsp	8 tsp	10 tsp	11 tsp
Discretionary calorie allowance[8]	165	171	171	132	195	267	290	362	410	426	512	648

[1]**Calorie Levels** are set across a wide range to accommodate the needs of different individuals. The attached table "Estimated Daily Calorie Needs" can be used to help assign individuals to the food intake pattern at a particular calorie level.

[2]**Fruit Group** includes all fresh, frozen, canned, and dried fruits and fruit juices. In general, 1 cup of fruit or 100% fruit juice, or ½ cup of dried fruit can be considered as 1 cup from the fruit group.

[3]**Vegetable Group** includes all fresh, frozen, canned, and dried vegetables and vegetable juices. In general, 1 cup of raw or cooked vegetables or vegetable juice, or 2 cups of raw leafy greens can be considered as 1 cup from the vegetable group.

Vegetable Subgroup Amounts Are per Week

Calorie Level	1,000	1,200	1,400	1,600	1,800	2,000	2,200	2,400	2,600	2,800	3,000	3,200
Dark green veg.	1 c/wk	1.5 c/wk	1.5 c/wk	2 c/wk	3 c/wk	3 c/wk	3 c/wk	3 c/wk	3 c/wk	3 c/wk	3 c/wk	3 c/wk
Orange veg.	.5 c/wk	1 c/wk	1 c/wk	1.5 c/wk	2 c/wk	2 c/wk	2 c/wk	2 c/wk	2.5 c/wk	2.5 c/wk	2.5 c/wk	2.5 c/wk
Legumes	.5 c/wk	1 c/wk	1 c/wk	2.5 c/wk	3 c/wk	3 c/wk	3 c/wk	3 c/wk	3.5 c/wk	3.5 c/wk	3.5 c/wk	3.5 c/wk
Starchy veg.	1.5 c/wk	2.5 c/wk	2.5 c/wk	2.5 c/wk	3 c/wk	3 c/wk	6 c/wk	6 c/wk	7 c/wk	7 c/wk	9 c/wk	9 c/wk
Other veg.	3.5 c/wk	4.5 c/wk	4.5 c/wk	5.5 c/wk	6.5 c/wk	6.5 c/wk	7 c/wk	7 c/wk	8.5 c/wk	8.5 c/wk	10 c/wk	10 c/wk

[4]**Grains Group** includes all foods made from wheat, rice, oats, cornmeal, and barley, such as bread, pasta, oatmeal, breakfast cereals, tortillas, and grits. In general, 1 slice of bread, 1 cup of ready-to-eat cereal, or ½ cup of cooked rice, pasta, or cooked cereal can be considered as 1 ounce equivalent from the grains group. **At least half of all grains consumed should be whole grains.**

[5]**Meat & Beans Group** in general, 1 ounce of lean meat, poultry, or fish, 1 egg, 1 Tbsp. peanut butter, ¼ cup cooked dry beans, or ½ ounce of nuts or seeds can be considered as 1 ounce equivalent from the meat and beans group.

[6]**Milk Group** includes all fluid milk products and foods made from milk that retain their calcium content, such as yogurt and cheese. Foods made from milk that have little to no calcium, such as cream cheese, cream, and butter, are not part of the group. Most milk group choices should be fat-free or low-fat. In general, 1 cup of milk or yogurt, 1½ ounces of natural cheese, or 2 ounces of processed cheese can be considered as 1 cup from the milk group.

[7]**Oils** include fats from many different plants and from fish that are liquid at room temperature, such as canola, corn, olive, soybean, and sunflower oil. Some foods are naturally high in oils, such as nuts, olives, some fish, and avocados. Foods that are mainly oil include mayonnaise, certain salad dressings, and soft margarine.

[8]**Discretionary Calorie Allowance** is the remaining amount of calories in a food intake pattern after accounting for the calories needed for all food groups—using forms of foods that are fat-free or low-fat and with no added sugars.

(continued)

Box 9.3

MyPyramid Food Intake Patterns *(continued)*

Estimated Daily Calorie Needs

To determine which food intake pattern to use for an individual, the following chart gives an estimate of individual calorie needs. The calorie range for each age/sex group is based on physical activity level, from sedentary to active.

	Calorie Range		
Children	**Sedentary**	→	**Active**
2–3 years	1,000	→	1,400
Females			
4–8 years	1,200	→	1,800
9–13	1,600	→	2,200
14–18	1,800	→	2,400
19–30	2,000	→	2,400
31–50	1,800	→	2,200
51+	1,600	→	2,200
Males			
4–8 years	1,400	→	2,000
9–13	1,800	→	2,600
14–18	2,200	→	3,200
19–30	2,400	→	3,000
31–50	2,200	→	3,000
51+	2,000	→	2,800

Source: U.S. Department of Agriculture Center for Nutrition Policy and Promotion, April 2005.

Sedentary means a lifestyle that includes only the light physical activity associated with typical day-to-day life.

Active means a lifestyle that includes physical activity equivalent to walking more than 3 miles per day at 3 to 4 miles per hour, in addition to the light physical activity associated with typical day-to-day life.

Within each group, foods vary in the amount of nutrients and calories they provide. Daily food choices should emphasize nutrient-dense foods, those that are high in nutrients relative to the amount of calories they contain. Within the breads and cereals food group, for example, a slice of whole-wheat bread has more nutrients and fiber, and fewer calories, than a croissant.

Fruits, vegetables, whole grains, and milk products are all important to a healthful diet and can be good sources of key nutrients. When increasing intake of fruits, vegetables, whole grains, and fat-free or low-fat milk and milk products, it is important to decrease one's intake of less-nutrient-dense foods to control calorie intake.

How does the average American diet stack up against the recommendations in the *Guidelines* and *MyPyramid?* As summarized in Figure 9.2, the largest diet changes needed are increases in fruit, low-fat milk, dark green and orange vegetables, legumes, and whole grains.[7,15,21,22] How does your diet compare with the recommendations of *MyPyramid?* Complete Physical Fitness Activity 9.1 at the end of this chapter to evaluate your diet.

The vegetarian diet excludes meat, poultry, and fish.[23,24] Interest in the vegetarian diet continues to grow largely because of health, environmental, and ethical concerns, and is currently followed by over 15 million Americans. Vegetarians avoid animal flesh, but most eat dairy products and eggs, and are called lacto-ovo-vegetarians. Some vegetarians, called vegans, avoid all animal products including eggs and dairy products. All vegetarians emphasize fruits, vegetables, whole grains and cereals, nuts, and seeds in their diets.

Vegetarians enjoy many health benefits including less risk of heart disease, diabetes, certain forms of cancer, obesity, and high blood pressure. Most of these benefits are due to their high intake of fruits and vegetables, which provide fiber and many important vitamins and minerals, and their low intake of saturated fat and cholesterol (found largely in animal products).[23,24]

The lacto-ovo-vegetarian diet provides more than enough protein, vitamins, and minerals for both health and body needs. Instead of using meat for protein, the vegetarian can eat dry beans, eggs, and nuts. In other words, the lacto-ovo-vegetarian can emphasize these foods as meat

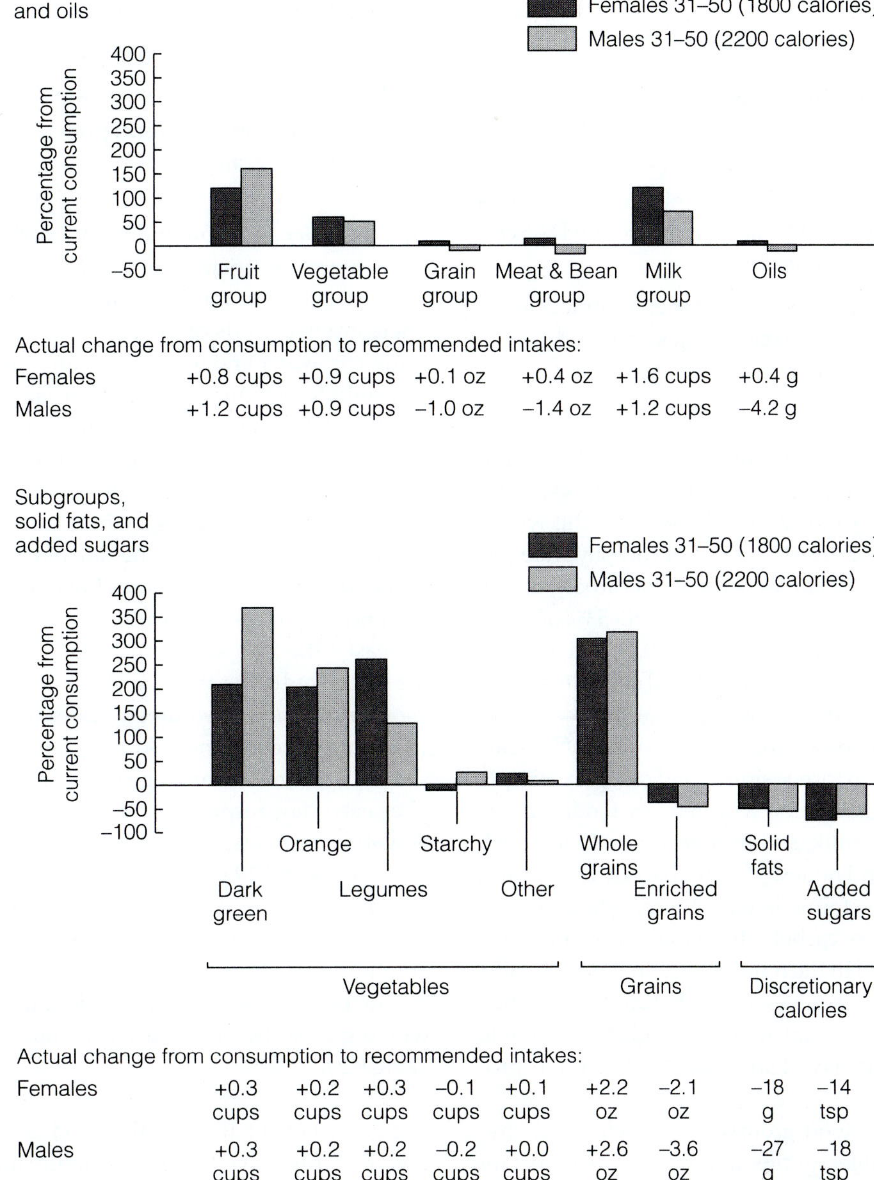

Figure 9.2

Percent increase or decrease from current consumption (zero line) to recommended intakes—a graphical depiction of the degree of change in average daily food consumption by Americans that would be needed to be consistent with the food patterns encouraged by the *Dietary Guidelines* for Americans. The zero line represents average consumption levels from each food group or subgroup by females 31 to 50 years of age and males 31 to 50 years of age. Bars above the zero line represent recommended increases in food group consumption, while bars below the line represent recommended decreases. Source: U.S. Department of Health and Human Services and U.S. Department of Agriculture. *Dietary Guidelines for Americans* (6th ed.). Washington, DC: U.S. Government Printing Office, 2005.

substitutes while using the rest of the Food Guide Pyramid as do nonvegetarians.

The vegan diet can also be nutritious, but more careful planning is needed to ensure intake of several key nutrients including vitamin B_{12}, vitamin D, calcium, iron, and zinc. Vitamin B_{12} is only found in foods of animal origin. Vegans must use a Vitamin B_{12} supplement or look for this nutrient in fortified foods such as breakfast cereals. Vitamin D is made in the skin when exposed to sunlight, and is also added to soy milk and some breakfast cereals. Vegans should seek out foods rich in calcium such as calcium-fortified soy milk or orange juice, nuts and seeds, and dark green vegetables. Iron from meat products is more easily absorbed by the body than iron from plant foods. If a food rich in vitamin C is included with a vegetarian meal, iron absorption is improved. Zinc is found in whole grains, nuts and seeds, and legumes.

Carbohydrates

Key Recommendations[7]

- Choose fiber-rich fruits, vegetables, and whole grains often.
- Choose and prepare foods and beverages with little added sugars or caloric sweeteners, such as amounts suggested by the USDA *MyPyramid* and the DASH Eating Plan (see Chapter 10).
- Reduce the incidence of dental caries by practicing good oral hygiene and consuming sugar- and starch-containing foods and beverages less frequently.

Carbohydrates are part of a healthful diet. The recommended intake of carbohydrates is 45 to 65% of total Calories.[6] For an individual eating 2,000 calories a day, this would be 900–1,300 Calories or 225–325 grams of carbohydrate (divide by 4, the number of Calories per gram of carbohydrate). American male and female adults consume 50–53% of Calories from carbohydrate, respectively (Table 9.2), and much of this carbohydrate is in the form of processed sugar instead of the preferable plant starch.

It is important to choose carbohydrates wisely.[25-27] Carbohydrates come in two forms: simple and complex. Simple carbohydrates are sugars found within many foods such as fruits, vegetables, and milk, and in concentrated form such as processed sugars and honey.[26,27] Complex carbohydrates are plant starches often found in wheat, rice, oats, and corn. Dietary fiber is a type of carbohydrate found only in plants that cannot be digested in the human intestinal tract. Grains and cereals are major sources of both starch and fiber. Whole grain products contain all of the original fiber while refined grain products have had it removed through processing procedures.[25]

Foods in the basic food groups that provide carbohydrates—fruits, vegetables, grains, and milk—are important sources of many nutrients. Choosing plenty of these foods, within the context of a Calorie-controlled diet, can promote health and reduce chronic disease risk. However, the greater the consumption of foods containing large amounts of added sugars, the more difficult it is to consume enough nutrients without gaining weight. Consumption of added sugars provides calories while providing little, if any, of the essential nutrients.

As mapped out by *MyPyramid,* more servings of grain products should be consumed at each meal than any other type of food, followed by fruits and vegetables.[19] Grains (e.g., pasta, rice, wheat, cereals) should form the center of most meals. By choosing more whole-grain products, fruits, and vegetables, intake of total carbohydrate and fiber will increase while intake of total fat, saturated fat, and cholesterol will decrease.[25]

These strategies are recommended by the USDA to incorporate more foods from plant sources into the diet:[7]

- Include grain products, fruits, or vegetables in every meal.
- Choose fruits and vegetables for snacks.
- Choose beans as an alternative to meat.
- Choose whole grains in preference to processed (refined) grains.

Dietary Fiber Although dietary fiber provides no energy, it has many beneficial actions in the body and promotes a low risk of colon cancer, heart disease, and diabetes.[27–29] There are two kinds of dietary fiber: soluble fiber, which is soluble in water and forms a gel, and insoluble fiber, which is insoluble in water. Soluble fiber is found in many fruits and vegetables, and in some grains such as oats. The sticky residue in the bowl after eating oatmeal is the soluble fiber from the oat bran. Insoluble fiber is found in many vegetables and whole grains (e.g., wheat bran).

Soluble fiber controls the rate of blood glucose absorption in the intestine, promotes lower blood cholesterol levels, and improves the health of the colon. Insoluble fiber increases the rate at which food residue moves through the colon, reducing the risk of colon cancer.[27–29]

The recommended dietary fiber intake is 14 grams per 1,000 calories consumed. Although male and female adults should consume an average of 38 and 25 grams of dietary fiber each day, respectively, to encourage good health and bowel movements, current intake is about 14 grams/day for females and 19 grams/day for males (Table 9.2).[7]

Most popular American foods are not high in dietary fiber. Dietary fiber is found solely in plant foods (none in animal-based foods including meats, eggs, and dairy products), and is abundant in legumes, nuts and seeds, whole grains, fresh and dried fruits, and vegetables (see Table 9.3).

The Food Label In 1990, the Food and Drug Administration (FDA) approved a new procedure for nutrition labeling of processed foods and authorized appropriate health claims.[4,5,7] (See Figure 9.3.) Whereas the old food label emphasized vitamin and mineral content, the new food label focuses on the real nutritional shortcomings of Americans: total fat, saturated fat, cholesterol, sodium, dietary fiber, and sugars. The Nutrition Facts food label uses the Daily Values to help consumers plan healthy diets. The Daily Values serve as the nutrient reference values on the food label, combining information from the RDA/DRI and the *Dietary Guidelines for Americans* (see Table 9.1). The Daily Values are based on a 2,000 calorie diet, close to the average American intake. A Daily Value of 20% for total fat means that a serving of this particular food provides 20% of the total fat allowed for the average adult.

An important feature of the FDA's mandate to improve food labels is the regulation of nutrient-content claims and health claims. Nutrient-content claims describe the amount of nutrient in foods such as "cholesterol free," "low fat," "light,"

TABLE 9.3 Selected Sources and Amounts of Dietary Fiber

Food	Amount	Soluble Fiber, g	Total Fiber, g
Legumes (cooked)			
Black beans	1/2 cup	2.1	7.5
Kidney beans	1/2 cup	2.3	5.7
Pinto beans	1/2 cup	2.7	7.4
Vegetables (cooked)			
Green peas	1/2 cup	1.2	4.4
Butternut winter squash	1/2 cup	0.4	3.4
Brussels sprouts	1/2 cup	1.3	2.9
Broccoli	1/2 cup	1.1	2.3
Zucchini	1/2 cup	0.3	2.3
Corn	1/2 cup	0.1	2.2
Spinach	1/2 cup	0.6	2.2
Green beans	1/2 cup	0.8	2.0
Potato	1/2 cup	0.2	0.9
Fruits (raw)			
Apple	1 medium	1.4	3.7
Orange	1 medium	2.1	3.1
Prunes	1/4 cup	1.3	3.0
Banana	1 medium	1.0	2.8
Blueberries	1/2 cup	0.6	2.0
Raisins	1/4 cup	0.5	1.7
Strawberries	1/2 cup	0.6	1.7
Mango slices	1/2 cup	0.9	1.5
Grapefruit	1/2 medium	0.8	1.3
Grapes	1 cup	0.1	0.8
Grains			
Oat bran (dry)	1/3 cup	2.0	4.4
Raisin bran (dry)	1/2 cup	0.5	3.6
Grape-Nuts (dry)	1/3 cup	2.0	3.6
Oatmeal (cooked)	1/2 cup	1.2	2.0
Whole-wheat bread	1 slice	0.4	1.9
Brown rice (cooked)	1/2 cup	0.2	1.8
Nuts and seeds			
Dry roasted almonds	1 oz	0.4	3.9
Dry roasted sunflower seeds	1 oz	1.0	3.1
Dry roasted peanuts	1 oz	0.6	2.3

Note: Within each category, the foods are listed from high to low in total fiber.

Source: The Food Processor, v. 7.0. Salem, OR: ESHA Research.

or "lean." These nutrient-content claims are now based on precise definitions and specific portion sizes to avoid consumer confusion when comparing one food brand with another. For example, "low fat" means 3 grams of fat or less per serving, and "cholesterol free" indicates less than 2 mg of cholesterol per serving. Health claims that link foods with prevention of certain diseases must be scientifically based. The FDA has approved about a dozen health claims, and these include the benefits of fiber for heart disease and cancer, the connection between diets low in saturated fat and cholesterol with heart disease, low-sodium foods and high blood pressure, fruits and vegetables with cancer, and sugar with dental caries.

Anxtioxidants and Phytochemicals Each cell of the body must have oxygen to produce energy. As humans take in oxygen during rest and exercise, some of the oxygen particles change and react with cell membranes and proteins, causing damage. These reactive oxygen particles are highly unstable and are known as free radicals. The oxidative damage caused by free radicals promotes cancer and heart disease, and accelerates aging.

Antioxidants are compounds that protect cells in the body from these reactive oxygen particles. There are many types of antioxidants, including enzymes within the body and certain types of nutrients and chemicals from the diet.

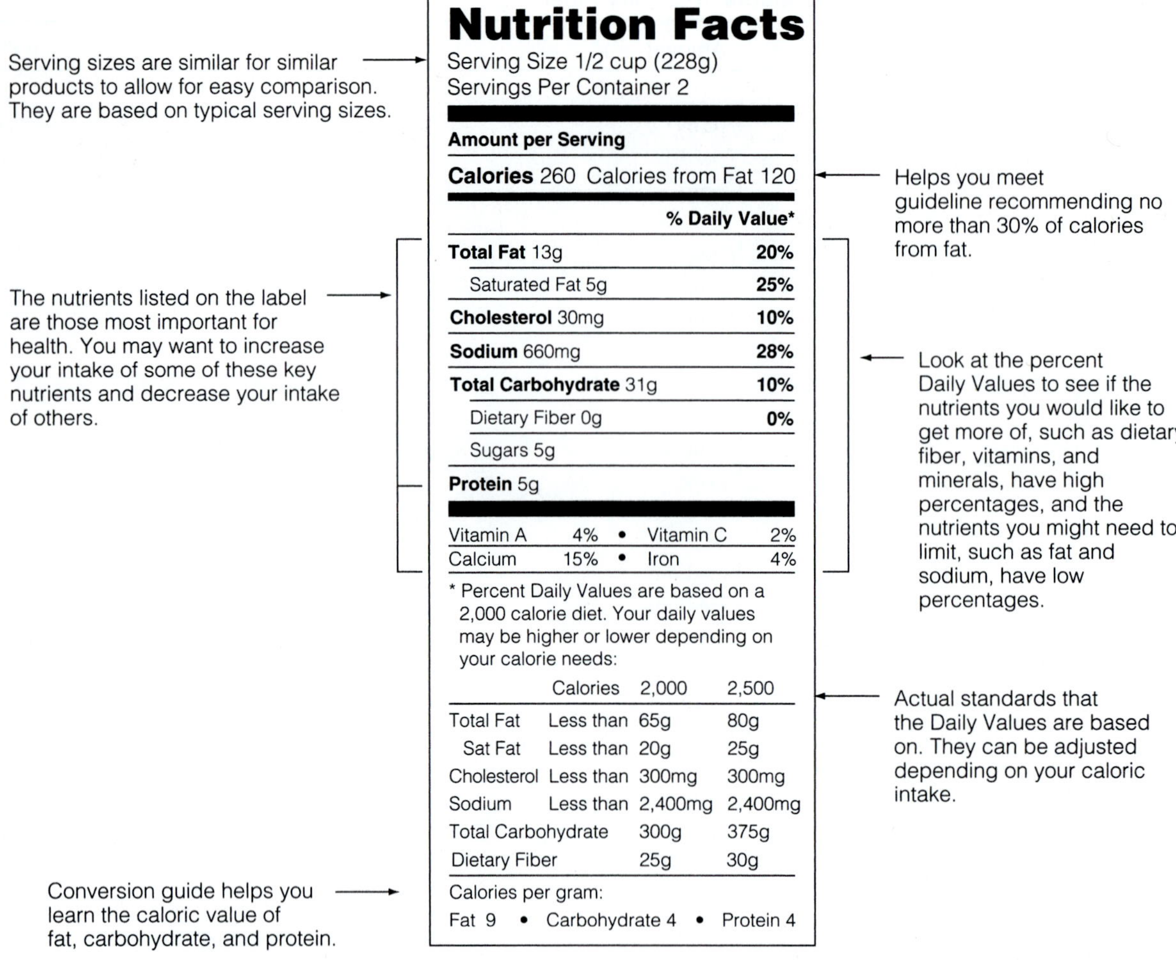

Serving sizes are similar for similar products to allow for easy comparison. They are based on typical serving sizes.
The nutrients listed on the label are those most important for health. You may want to increase your intake of some of these key nutrients and decrease your intake of others.
Conversion guide helps you learn the caloric value of fat, carbohydrate, and protein.
Nutrition Facts
Serving Size 1/2 cup (228g)
Servings Per Container 2
Amount per Serving
Calories 260 Calories from Fat 120
% Daily Value*
Total Fat 13g 20%
Saturated Fat 5g 25%
Cholesterol 30mg 10%
Sodium 660mg 28%
Total Carbohydrate 31g 10%
Dietary Fiber 0g 0%
Sugars 5g
Protein 5g
Vitamin A 4% • Vitamin C 2%
Calcium 15% • Iron 4%
* Percent Daily Values are based on a 2,000 calorie diet. Your daily values may be higher or lower depending on your calorie needs:
Calories 2,000 2,500
Total Fat Less than 65g 80g
Sat Fat Less than 20g 25g
Cholesterol Less than 300mg 300mg
Sodium Less than 2,400mg 2,400mg
Total Carbohydrate 300g 375g
Dietary Fiber 25g 30g
Calories per gram:
Fat 9 • Carbohydrate 4 • Protein 4
Helps you meet guideline recommending no more than 30% of calories from fat.
Look at the percent Daily Values to see if the nutrients you would like to get more of, such as dietary fiber, vitamins, and minerals, have high percentages, and the nutrients you might need to limit, such as fat and sodium, have low percentages.
Actual standards that the Daily Values are based on. They can be adjusted depending on your caloric intake.

Figure 9.3 Guidelines for interpretation of the food label.

Vitamins E and C, and the vitamin A precursor beta-carotene, are strong antioxidants and are found in fruits, vegetables, whole grains, and nuts and seeds.[30–33] Good sources of vitamin E are vegetable oils, nuts and seeds, the wheat germ in whole-grain products, and dark green vegetables. Vitamin C is found in most fruits and vegetables. Beta-carotene is found in orange fruits and vegetables (e.g., carrots, apricots, cantaloupe, squash, sweet potatoes) and dark green vegetables (e.g., spinach, kale, and broccoli).

Phytochemicals are special chemicals within plants that are not vitamins or minerals but have health-protective effects.[30] Some phytochemicals have antioxidant activity, although they work in many other ways, too. Nuts, seeds, whole grains, fruits, and vegetables contain an abundance of phytochemicals that help prevent chronic disease including cancer. The foods and herbs with the highest anticancer activity include garlic, soybeans, cabbage, ginger, carrots, celery, cilantro, parsley, and parsnips. Other foods with cancer-protective activity include onions, citrus fruits, broccoli, brussel sprouts, cabbage, cauliflower, tomatoes, pepper, brown rice, and whole wheat.

Are antioxidant supplements needed to boost defenses against oxygen-free radicals? In general, it is best to follow *MyPyramid* and consume generous amounts of fruits and vegetables each day.[34] Fruits and vegetables are complex foods containing more than 100 beneficial vitamins, minerals, fiber, and other substances, and no pill has captured their protective effects against chronic diseases.

Food Safety

Key Recommendations[7]

- To avoid microbial foodborne illness:
  - Clean hands, food contact surfaces, and fruits and vegetables. Meat and poultry should not be washed or rinsed.
  - Separate raw, cooked, and ready-to-eat foods while shopping, preparing, or storing foods.
  - Cook foods to a safe temperature to kill microorganisms.

- Chill (refrigerate) perishable food promptly and defrost foods properly.
- Avoid raw (unpasteurized) milk or any products made from unpasteurized milk, raw or partially cooked eggs or foods containing raw eggs, raw or undercooked meat and poultry, unpasteurized juices, and raw sprouts.

Avoiding foods that are contaminated with harmful bacteria, viruses, parasites, toxins, and chemical and physical contaminants is vital for healthful eating. The signs and symptoms of foodborne illness range from gastrointestinal symptoms, such as upset stomach, diarrhea, fever, vomiting, abdominal cramps, and dehydration, to more severe systemic illness, such as paralysis and meningitis. The USDA estimates that every year about 76 million people in the United States become ill from pathogens in food; of these, about 5,000 die.[7] Consumers can take simple measures to reduce their risk of foodborne illness, especially in the home.

Foodborne illness is caused by eating food that contains harmful bacteria, toxins, parasites, viruses, or chemical contaminants. According to the USDA, bacteria and viruses, especially *Campylobacter, Salmonella,* and Norwalk-like viruses, are among the most common causes of foodborne illness we know about today.[7] Signs and symptoms after eating just a small portion of an unsafe food may appear within half an hour or may not develop for up to 3 weeks. Pregnant women, young children, older persons, and people with weakened immune systems or certain chronic diseases are at high risk of foodborne illness.

To keep food safe, people who prepare food should clean hands, food contact surfaces, and fruits and vegetables; separate raw, cooked, and ready-to-eat foods; cook foods to a safe internal temperature; chill perishable food promptly; and defrost food properly. For more important information on cooking, cleaning, separating, and chilling, see www.fightbac.org. Seven key steps should be followed to keep food safe:[4,7]

- Wash hands and surfaces often, especially after handling raw meat, poultry, fish, shellfish, or eggs.
- Separate raw, cooked, and ready-to-eat foods while shopping, preparing, or storing.
- Cook foods to a safe temperature. Reheat sauces, soups, marinades, and gravies to a boil, reheat leftovers thoroughly to at least 165°F, and cook whole poultry at 180°F. The danger zone for bacterial growth is 40°F to 140°F.
- Refrigerate perishable foods promptly.
- Serve safely by keeping hot foods hot (140°F or above) and cold foods cold (40°F or below).
- Check and follow label safety instructions.
- When in doubt, throw it out.

Fats

Key Recommendations[7]

- Consume less than 10% of calories from saturated fatty acids and less than 300 mg/day of cholesterol, and keep *trans* fatty acid consumption as low as possible.
- Keep total fat intake between 20 to 35% of calories, with most fats coming from sources of polyunsaturated and monounsaturated fatty acids, such as fish, nuts, and vegetable oils.
- When selecting and preparing meat, poultry, dry beans, and milk or milk products, make choices that are lean, low-fat, or fat-free.
- Limit intake of fats and oils high in saturated and/or *trans* fatty acids, and choose products low in such fats and oils.

The amount and quality of dietary fat has a significant impact on risk of heart disease, cancer, obesity, and other health problems.[6,7,16,35] Diets low in saturated fat and cholesterol decrease risk of heart disease, while high-fat diets promote certain types of cancers and obesity.

Most of the fat in food is triglyceride, a molecule made up of three units known as fatty acids and one unit called glycerol. The fatty acids differ in length and the degree of saturation or the number of hydrogens in the chain.

The saturated fatty acid carries the maximum possible number of hydrogen atoms, with no points of unsaturation (see Figure 9.4). A saturated fat is a triglyceride that contains three saturated fatty acids. Saturated fats are found in all types of dietary fats, but are in greatest concentration in red meat, whole milk, butter, and tropical oils (e.g., palm kernel oil, coconut oil). Saturated fats raise blood cholesterol levels and increase the risk of heart disease.[16]

In the monounsaturated fatty acid, there is one point of unsaturation where hydrogens are missing (Figure 9.4). If there are two or more points of unsaturation, then it is a polyunsaturated fatty acid. Olive and canola oils are particularly high in monounsaturated fats; most other vegetable oils, nuts, and high-fat fish are good sources of polyunsaturated fats. Both kinds of unsaturated fats reduce blood cholesterol when they replace saturated fats in the diet, and thus lower risk of heart disease.[16]

To meet the total fat recommendation of 20 to 35% of calories, most dietary fats should come from sources of polyunsaturated and monounsaturated fatty acids.[7] The upper limit on the grams of fat in the diet depends on total caloric intake. For example, at 2,000 calories per day, the suggested upper limit for total fat is 700 calories (2,000 × 0.35). This is equal to 78 grams of fat (700 ÷ 9, the number of calories each gram of fat provides). For saturated fat, no more than 200 out of 2,000 calories should be ingested, which is 22 grams (200 ÷ 9).

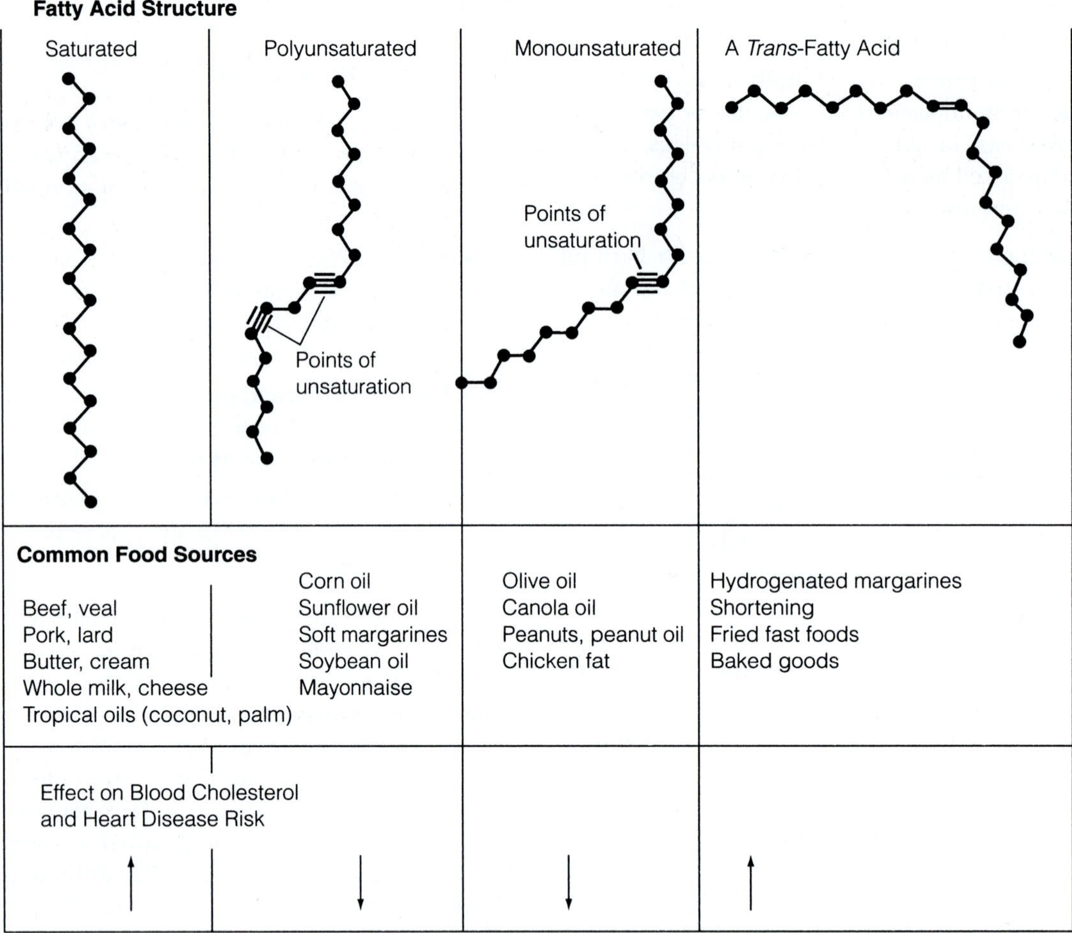

Figure 9.4 Fatty acid structure, common food sources, and influence on blood cholesterol levels and heart disease.

Eicosapentaenoic acid (EPA) and docosahexaenoic acid (DHA) are omega-3 fatty acids that are found in fish and shellfish. Fish that naturally contain more oil (e.g., salmon, trout, herring) are higher in EPA and DHA than are lean fish (e.g., cod, haddock, catfish). Limited evidence suggests an association between consumption of fatty acids in fish and reduced risks of mortality from cardiovascular disease for the general population.[6,7] Other sources of EPA and DHA may provide similar benefits; however, more research is needed.

When manufacturers process foods, they often alter the fatty acids in the food through a process called hydrogenation. Hydrogenation is the process of adding hydrogen to unsaturated fatty acids to make fat stay fresher longer and make it more solid and less greasy-tasting. Some of the unsaturated fatty acids, instead of becoming saturated during the hydrogenation process, end up changing their shapes into *trans*-fatty acids (Figure 9.4).[35] *Trans*-fatty acids raise blood cholesterol levels and are found in most margarines, shortening, fast foods such as french fries, fried chicken and fried fish, chips, and baked goods such as muffins, cakes, doughnuts, crackers, and pies. *Trans*-fat levels must be listed on food labels, and this may prompt companies to provide products without these types of fats.

American adults average about 32% total calories as fat.[15] (See Table 9.2). The most common sources of fat include beef, margarine, salad dressings and mayonnaise, oils, and dairy products. About 11% of total caloric intake is saturated fat, and more than one third of the saturated fat Americans consume comes from cheese, beef, and milk.

Cholesterol is a type of dietary fat found only in animal products. It is a soft, waxy substance that is also made in the body for a variety of purposes, including the formation of cell membranes and certain types of hormones. Dietary cholesterol tends to raise blood cholesterol levels, but not as strongly as saturated fat.[15,22] Cholesterol intake should be below 300 mg/day. Animal products are the source of all dietary cholesterol, egg yolks being one of the richest sources, with each containing about 220 mg of cholesterol. Eggs and beef contribute nearly one half of all the dietary cholesterol Americans ingest.

Limiting Fat Intake For good health, it's best to limit intake of total fat, saturated fat, and cholesterol, and to substitute unsaturated fats for saturated fats. Information about the fat and cholesterol content of packaged foods appears on the food label.[6,7,16]

To limit intake of high-fat foods, especially those containing high amounts of saturated fat, follow these recommendations:

- Replace fat-rich foods with fruits, vegetables, grains, and beans.
- Eat smaller portions of meat and other high-fat foods.
- Choose baked and broiled foods instead of fried foods.
- Select nonfat and low-fat milk and dairy products.
- When eating meat, select lean cuts ("select" or "choice" USDA grade).
- Choose beans, seafood, and poultry as an alternative to beef, pork, and lamb.

What about the new fat replacers? Fat replacers are compounds developed by food manufacturers to taste and feel like fat when eaten; some block the absorption of fat in the intestine.[16] Chemically, fat replacers are not really fat, and have fewer calories. Fat replacers have many different trade and brand names, and are now found in baked goods, chips, salad dressings, sauces, frozen desserts, candy, dairy products, butter, cheese, spreads, and meat products. The American Dietetic Association recommends that when fat replacers are used within a diet that conforms to the Dietary Guidelines for Americans, they are safe and help reduce overall fat intake.[36]

Adequate Nutrients within Calorie Needs

Key Recommendations[7]

- Consume a variety of nutrient-dense foods and beverages within and among the basic food groups while choosing foods that limit the intake of saturated and *trans* fats, cholesterol, added sugars, salt, and alcohol.
- Meet recommended intakes within energy needs by adopting a balanced eating pattern, such as the USDA Food Guide or the DASH Eating Plan.

An important goal is to choose meals and snacks that are high in nutrients but low to moderate in energy content. At the same time, limit saturated and *trans* fats, cholesterol, added sugars, and salt. An additional premise of the *Dietary Guidelines* is that the nutrients consumed should come primarily from foods.[7] Foods contain not only the vitamins and minerals that are often found in supplements, but also hundreds of naturally occurring substances, including carotenoids, flavonoids and isoflavones, and protease inhibitors that may protect against chronic health conditions.

Two examples of eating patterns that exemplify the *Dietary Guidelines* are the DASH Eating Plan and *MyPyramid*. These two similar eating patterns are designed to integrate dietary recommendations into a healthy way to eat and are used in the *Dietary Guidelines* to provide examples of how nutrient-focused recommendations can be expressed in terms of food choices. Both *MyPyramid* and the DASH Eating Plan differ in important ways from common food consumption patterns in the United States. In general, they include:

- *More* dark green vegetables, orange vegetables, legumes, fruits, whole grains, and low-fat milk and milk products
- *Less* refined grains, total fats (especially cholesterol, and saturated and *trans* fats), added sugars, and calories

As defined earlier, sugars are classified as simple carbohydrates whereas starch is defined as a complex carbohydrate. During digestion, the body breaks down all carbohydrates except fibers into sugars. Sugars and starches occur naturally in many foods, including milk, fruits, some vegetables, bread, cereals, and grains. These foods also supply many other important nutrients. On the other hand, so-called added sugars—those added during processing or at the table—supply calories but few nutrients. Foods rich in added sugars include soft drinks and desserts, among others.[26,27]

Carbonated drinks are the single biggest source of added sugars in the American diet (about 8–10 teaspoons per can), supplying one third of all sugar ingested.[26] Carbonated soft drink consumption has been soaring, and now accounts for more than one fourth of Americans' beverage consumption.

Sugar is hidden in many foods. One cup of yogurt, for example, has 7 teaspoons of sugar, 1 cup of canned corn has 3 teaspoons, and 1 tablespoon of ketchup has 1 teaspoon of sugar. Desserts often have more sugar than expected: a glazed donut has 6 teaspoons of sugar, one chocolate eclair or a piece of angel food cake each has 7 teaspoons, 2 ounces of chocolate candy has 8 teaspoons, a piece of iced chocolate cake or berry pie each has 10 teaspoons, and 4 ounces of hard candy has 20 teaspoons. To locate hidden sugars, check the list of ingredients on the food label; sugars are listed by many different names, including brown sugar, corn sweetener, corn syrup, fructose, fruit juice concentrate, glucose or dextrose, high-fructose corn syrup, honey, lactose, maltose, molasses, raw sugar, table sugar or sucrose, and syrup. If one of these appears near the top of the list, the food is probably high in added sugars. The total grams of sugar per serving listed on the Nutrition Facts panel includes both naturally occurring and added sugars.

The average American male and female ingest far too much sugar, about 22 and 16 teaspoons of added sugar on average each day, respectively.[15] (This statistic does not include sugars that occur naturally in foods such as fruit and milk.) The USDA recommends that people learn to choose and prepare foods and beverages with little added sugars or caloric sweeteners. Total discretionary calories (see Box 9.3) should not exceed the allowance for any given calorie level. The discretionary calorie allowance covers all calories from added sugars, alcohol, and the additional fat found in even moderate fat choices from the milk and meat group. For example, the 2,000-calorie pattern includes only about 267 discretionary calories. At 29% of Calories from total fat (including 18 g of solid fat), if no alcohol is consumed, then only 8 teaspoons (32 g) of added sugars can be afforded. This is less than the amount in a typical 12-ounce soft drink. If fat is decreased to 22% of Calories, then 18 teaspoons (72 g) of added sugars is allowed. If fat is increased to 35% of Calories, then no allowance remains for added sugars, even if alcohol is not consumed.

For very physically active people, sugars in sport beverages can be an additional source of energy. However, because maintaining a nutritious diet and a healthy weight is very important, sugars should be used in moderation by most healthy people and sparingly by people with low calorie needs.

Sugar and Health Sugars and starches can both promote tooth decay. The more often foods containing sugars and starches are eaten, and the longer these foods are in the mouth before the teeth are brushed, the greater the risk for tooth decay.

Despite widespread concerns, intake of sugar has not been associated with increased risk of heart disease, cancer, diabetes, or abnormal behavior.[6,7] In a small proportion of people, diets containing large amounts of sugar can increase plasma triglyceride levels, which is bad because this promotes heart disease. However, for most people, sugar consumption does not influence blood cholesterol or fat levels.[37] Some parents feel that sugar affects the behavior of their children, but there is no good scientific support for the belief that sugar causes hyperactivity, impairment in mental function, or abnormal behavior in children.[38]

Sugar Substitutes Sugar substitutes such as sorbitol, saccharin, and aspartame are ingredients in many foods, and have been shown to be safe by many different research teams and professional organizations. Most of the sugar substitutes do not provide significant calories and can be useful if one is trying to lose weight. Foods containing sugar substitutes, however, may not always be lower in calories than similar products that contain sugars.[27] Thus, the food label should be reviewed carefully.

Sodium and Potassium

Key Recommendations[7]

- Consume less than 2,300 mg (approximately 1 tsp of salt) of sodium per day.
- Choose and prepare foods with little salt. At the same time, consume potassium-rich foods, such as fruits and vegetables.
- *Individuals with hypertension, blacks, and middle-aged and older adults:* Aim to consume no more than 1,500 mg of sodium per day, and meet the potassium recommendation (4,700 mg/day) with food.

Sodium is an essential mineral that plays a role in the regulation of water balance, normal muscle tone, acid–base balance, and the conduction of nerve impulses.[4,6,7] The human body needs about 500 mg of sodium per day, but Americans consume much more—about 4000–6000 per day.[15] Sodium intake is a concern for health because for many people, high sodium intake is associated with high blood pressure, a form of cardiovascular disease and a key risk factor for heart attacks and strokes (see Chapter 10).[6,16]

The *Dietary Guidelines* recommend that intake be limited to no more than 2,300 mg of sodium per day, the equivalent of a little more than a teaspoon of table salt.[7] Salt or sodium chloride (NaCl) is 40% sodium. Thus 1 teaspoon of salt (about 5,000 mg) is approximately 2,000 mg of sodium.

Food labels list sodium rather than salt content. When reading a Nutrition Facts on a food product, look for the sodium content. Foods that are low in sodium (less than 140 mg or 5% of the Daily Value [DV]) are low in salt. On average, the natural salt content of food accounts for only about 10% of total intake, while discretionary salt use (i.e., salt added at the table or while cooking) provides another 5 to 10% of total intake. Approximately 75% is derived from salt added by manufacturers. It is important to read the food label and determine the sodium content of food.

The richest sources of sodium are sauces, salad dressings, cheeses, processed meats, soups, and grain-cereal products. Table 9.4 gives sodium values for different types of foods. The USDA recommends several steps to keep sodium intake at healthy levels:[7]

- Learn to read food labels, and limit foods high in sodium. Look for labels that say "low-sodium"—they contain 140 mg or less of sodium per serving.
- Choose more fresh fruits and vegetables, which are very low in sodium.
- Choose fresh or frozen fish, shellfish, poultry, and meat most often. They are lower in salt than most canned and processed forms.
- Reduce the use of salt during cooking, and use herbs, spices, and low-sodium seasonings.
- Avoid using the salt shaker on prepared foods at the table, and go easy on condiments such as soy sauce, ketchup, mustard, pickles, and olives.
- Limit the use of foods with visible salt on them (snack chips, salted nuts, crackers, etc.).

Another dietary measure to lower blood pressure is to consume a diet rich in potassium.[7] A potassium-rich diet also blunts the effects of salt on blood pressure, may reduce the risk of developing kidney stones, and may possibly decrease bone loss with age. The recommended intake of potassium for adolescents and adults is 4,700 mg/day. Recommended intakes for potassium for children 1 to 3 years of age is 3,000 mg/day, 4 to 8 years of age is 3,800 mg/day, and 9 to 13 years of age is 4,500 mg/day. Fruits and vegetables, which are rich in potassium with its bicarbonate precursors, favorably affect acid–base metabolism, which may

TABLE 9.4 Where's the Salt?

Food groups	Sodium, mg
Bread, cereal, rice, and pasta	
Cooked cereal, rice, pasta, unsalted, 1/2 cup	Trace
Ready-to-eat cereal, 1 oz	100–360
Bread, 1 slice	110–175
Vegetable	
Vegetables, fresh or frozen, cooked without salt, 1/2 cup	Less than 70
Vegetables, canned or frozen with sauce, 1/2 cup	140–460
Tomato juice, canned, 3/4 cup	660
Vegetable soup, canned, 1 cup	820
Fruit	
Fruit, fresh, frozen, canned, 1/2 cup	Trace
Milk, yogurt, and cheese	
Milk, 1 cup	120
Yogurt, 8 oz	160
Natural cheeses, 1 1/2 oz	110–450
Processed cheeses, 2 oz	800
Meat, poultry, fish, dry beans, eggs, and nuts	
Fresh meat, poultry, fish, 3 oz	Less than 90
Tuna, canned, water pack, 3 oz	300
Bologna, 2 oz	580
Ham, lean roasted, 3 oz	1,020
Other	
Salad dressing, 1 tbsp	75–220
Ketchup, mustard, steak sauce, 1 tbsp	130–230
Soy sauce, 1 tbsp	1,030
Salt, 1 tsp	2,000
Dill pickle, 1 medium	930
Potato chips, salted, 1 oz	130
Corn chips, salted, 1 oz	235
Peanuts, roasted in oil, salted, 1 oz	120

Source: U.S. Department of Agriculture.

reduce risk of kidney stones and bone loss. Potassium-rich fruits and vegetables include leafy green vegetables, fruit from vines, and root vegetables. Meat, milk, and cereal products also contain potassium, but may not have the same effect on acid–base metabolism.

Alcoholic Beverages

Key Recommendations[7]

- Those who choose to drink alcoholic beverages should do so sensibly and in moderation—defined as the consumption of up to one drink per day for women and up to two drinks per day for men.
- Alcoholic beverages should not be consumed by some individuals, including those who cannot restrict their alcohol intake, women of childbearing age who may become pregnant, pregnant and lactating women, children and adolescents, individuals taking medications that can interact with alcohol, and those with specific medical conditions.
- Alcoholic beverages should be avoided by individuals engaging in activities that require attention, skill, or coordination, such as driving or operating machinery.

About 55% of U.S. adults are current drinkers.[7] The hazards of heavy alcohol consumption are well known and include increased risk of liver cirrhosis, hypertension, cancers of the upper gastrointestinal tract, injury, violence, and death. Alcoholic beverages supply calories but few or no nutrients. Alcohol may have beneficial effects when consumed in moderation. The lowest death rates for coronary heart disease occur at an intake of one to two drinks per day. While it is true that moderate amounts of alcohol lower risk of coronary heart disease, this must be balanced against all the health risks.

TABLE 9.5 Blood Alcohol Content (BAC) and Symptoms

Blood Alcohol Content [g/100 ml of blood or g/(210 L) of breath]*	Symptoms
0.01–0.05	Normal behavior
0.03–0.12	Mild euphoria; increased confidence; slight decrease in attention, judgment, and control
0.09–0.25	Feelings of excitement; emotional instability; loss of critical judgment; impairment of perception, memory, and comprehension; slower reaction time; reduced peripheral vision; impaired balance; drowsiness
0.18–0.30	Confusion, disorientation, dizziness, vision disturbance, slurred speech, lack of coordination while walking, apathy, lethargy
0.25–0.40	Stupor, marked incoordination, inability to stand or walk, vomiting, sleep, inability to control urination
0.35–0.50	Coma, lack of reflexes, low body temperature, reduced heartbeat and breathing
0.45+	Death from inability to breathe

*Ranges overlap due to varying responses from one individual to another.

Source: Intoximeters Inc., at http://intox.com.

Individuals in some situations should avoid alcohol—such as those who plan to drive, operate machinery, or take part in other activities that require attention, skill, or coordination. Some people, including children and adolescents, women of childbearing age who may become pregnant, pregnant and lactating women, individuals who cannot restrict alcohol intake, individuals taking medications that can interact with alcohol, and individuals with specific medical conditions should not drink at all. Even moderate drinking during pregnancy may have behavioral or developmental consequences for the baby. Heavy drinking during pregnancy can produce a range of behavioral and psychosocial problems, malformations, and mental retardation in the baby.[7]

If one chooses to drink alcoholic beverages, they should be consumed in moderate amounts, defined as no more than two drinks a day for men and one drink a day for women. One serving of alcohol, commonly called a drink, delivers 0.5 ounces of pure alcohol and is found in:

12 ounces of regular beer (150 calories)

5 ounces of wine (100 calories)

1.5 ounces of 80-proof distilled spirits (100 calories)

10 ounces of a wine cooler (140 calories)

The amount of alcohol in actual mixed drinks varies widely. While a whiskey sour/highball has about 0.5–0.6 ounces of ethanol, a dry martini has about 1 ounce, and a manhattan 1.15 ounces.

When ingested, alcohol passes from the stomach into the small intestine, where it is rapidly absorbed into the blood and distributed throughout the body.[4,6,7] Peak blood alcohol levels are reached in fasting people within 30 minutes to 2 hours. As a rule of thumb, one standard alcoholic drink consumed within 1 hour will produce a blood alcohol level or content (called BAL or BAC) of 0.02 in a 150-pound male, but this varies depending on body size, gender, food taken along with the alcohol, and tolerance (i.e., less responsive to alcohol because of long-term use). Five beers consumed within 1 hour will cause the BAC to rise on average to 0.10, which violates the drinking and driving laws of most states. The liver enzyme system takes 3 hours on average to clear the body of alcohol from two to three drinks. Table 9.5 summarizes the relationship between BAC and clinical symptoms.

PRINCIPLE 1: PRUDENT DIET IS THE CORNERSTONE

For all Americans, whether physically active or inactive, a "prudent diet" is recommended for general health and prevention of disease.[6,7] In other words, this diet is suitable for fitness enthusiasts (those exercising 3–5 days per week, 20–30 minutes per session) and nearly all athletes, including those in most individual, dual, and team sports, and power events (weight lifting, track and field). For the competitive endurance athlete (who trains more than 90 minutes a day in such sports as running, swimming, and cycling), several adaptations beyond the prudent diet are beneficial, including more energy and carbohydrate, less fat, and more water; for those who are at risk, close attention to iron status is also important.

Dietary Practices of Athletes

A large number of studies have measured the dietary intake and eating behaviors of a wide variety of athletes.[39–81] Table 9.6 summarizes some of the cross-sectional studies that have evaluated dietary intakes by athletes.

Examination of Table 9.6 reveals that there is a wide range of energy intake among athletes. In general, however, athletes tend to be high energy consumers, with the size of the participant and the energy demands of the sport having much to do with the amount of Calories each consumes. Very large athletes training intensively for several hours

TABLE 9.6 Dietary Intakes by Athletes (Reported in Various Studies)

Sport	Daily Calories	Protein Grams/%	Fat Grams/%	Carbohydrate Grams/%
Aerobic				
Males				
Running	2,500–4,000	120/16	107/32	390/52
Cross-country skiing	3,500–5,500	150/13	215/38	600/49
Triathlon	3,600–6,400	130/13	125/28	560/59
Females				
Running	1,700–3,000	80/16	70/32	260/52
Cross-country skiing	2,400–4,000	115/14	145/41	330/42
Swimming	2,030–4,000	100/15	110/38	310/47
Triathlon	1,500–3,500	80/13	85/31	350/56
Aerobic–Anaerobic				
Males				
Soccer	3,000–5,000	140/14	133/30	530/53
Football	2,000–11,000	200/16	215/40	540/44
Basketball	2,000–9,000	180/15	215/41	500/44
Wrestling	1,100–6,700	95/14	100/34	400/52
Females				
Basketball	1,900–3,900	110/14	145/40	380/46
Volleyball	1,100–3,200	100/16	95/34	315/50
Power				
Males				
Track and field	3,500–4,700	175/17	330/36	470/47
Bodybuilding	2,000–5,000	200/23	157/40	320/37
Females				
Track and field	1,500–2,800	95/17	95/38	260/45
Bodybuilding	1,000–4,000	100/20	70/30	250/50
Skill				
Males				
Gymnastics	600–4,300	80/15	90/40	230/45
Ballet dancing	1,740–4,100	122/17	140/42	300/38
Females				
Gymnastics	1,350–1,900	70/15	75/37	225/48
Ballet dancing	900–2,900	70/15	69/34	230/50

Sources: Data taken from references 39–81.

each day (e.g., football players in the early fall) have the highest caloric requirements. Smaller athletes who transport their body mass over long distances on a regular basis (e.g., cross-country skiers and distance runners) also have high caloric requirements. In some studies, energy intake of athletes falls below expected levels, which may be related to underreporting by the athlete during the food-recording process.[43,45,47–51]

Athletes who purposely keep their body weights below natural weight for competition (e.g., wrestlers, gymnasts, bodybuilders, runners, and ballet dancers) tend to have reported caloric intakes that appear to fall way below calculated energy expenditure. Several researchers have reported that athletes in sports that emphasize leanness are exceptionally preoccupied with weight, tend to use unhealthy methods for weight control, tend toward eating disorders, and demonstrate poor nutrition practices.[43,45,52,68–82]

The desire of the highly competitive wrestler to alter body weight without medical supervision has caused much concern among sports-medicine professionals. A high percentage induce dehydration, utilizing sauna baths, fluid restriction, and rubber or plastic suits. Some also resort to laxatives, diuretics, and vomiting. Such practices may endanger health, adversely affect performance, and affect a young person's growth potential[79–82] (see Box 9.4).

As can be seen from Table 9.6, protein in athletes' diets, on average, accounts for about 13–17% of energy intake, but proportions among different athletes can vary from 10 to 36%. Protein intakes tend to be lower among endurance athletes and higher among some groups of power and strength athletes, who can consume more than 20% of their energy as protein.[53,54,57,74] Relative to body weight, protein intakes usually exceed 1.5 g/kg per day, and intakes exceeding 2.0 g/kg per day are common. Although the recommended

Box 9.4

American College of Sports Medicine Recommendations on Weight Loss in Wrestlers*

1. Coaches and wrestlers should be educated about the adverse consequences of prolonged fasting and dehydration on physical performance and health. They
   a. Appear to adversely influence the wrestler's energy reserves and fluid and electrolyte balances, which may affect performance
   b. May alter hormonal status
   c. Diminish protein nutritional status
   d. Can impede normal growth and development
   e. May affect psychological state
   f. Can impair academic performance
   g. May have severe health consequences, such as pulmonary emboli, pancreatitis, and reduced immune function
2. The use of rubber suits, steam rooms, hot boxes, saunas, laxatives, and diuretics for "making weight" should be discouraged.
3. New state or national legislation should be adopted, which would schedule weigh-ins immediately prior to competition.
4. Weigh-ins should be scheduled each day before and after practice, to monitor weight loss and dehydration. Weight lost during practice should be regained through adequate food and fluid intake.
5. The body composition of each wrestler should be assessed prior to the season, using valid techniques. Males 16 years of age and younger with a body fat below 7%, or those over 16 years of age with a body fat below 5%, should be required to have medical clearance before being allowed to compete. Female wrestlers should be required to have a minimal body fat of 12–14%.
6. The need for daily caloric intake obtained from a balanced diet high in carbohydrates (>55% of Calories), low in fat (<30%), with adequate protein (1.0–1.5 grams/kg body weight) should be emphasized and determined on the basis of RDA guidelines and physical activity levels. The minimal caloric intake for wrestlers of high school and college age should range from 1,700 to 2,500 Calories/day, and rigorous training may increase the requirement up to an additional 1,000 Calories/day. Wrestlers should be discouraged by coaches, parents, school officials, and physicians from consuming less than their minimal daily needs.

Source: Data from American College of Sports Medicine. Weight loss in wrestlers. *Med Sci Sports Exerc* 28:ix–xii, 1996.

*In 1998, the NCAA instituted several permanent rule changes across all three divisions intended to make wrestling safer. The minimum wrestling weight for each athlete is based on body composition, body weight, and specific gravity of urine, and most unsafe techniques for making weight have been banned.

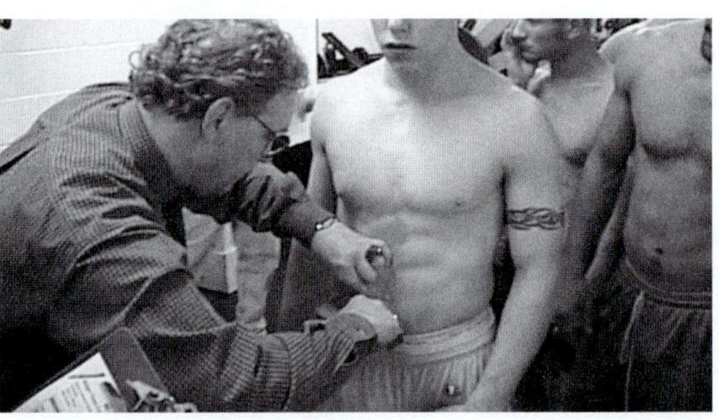

dietary allowance (RDA) is only 0.8 g/kg per day, athletes do not appear to be much different than the nonathletic population, which tends to consume nearly double the RDA.

Table 9.6 also shows that fat accounts for about 36% of athletes' energy intakes. This is above the 32% reported in national diet surveys.[15] Again, the proportions for athletes vary and range from about 20% to more than 50%. Power and strength athletes tend to have higher fat intakes than endurance athletes, and these higher fat intakes are often associated with their higher protein intakes.

Carbohydrate provides about 46% of the energy consumed by athletes, slightly below the percentage for the average American. The range of percentages is wide, and intakes of 22–72% have been reported. Triathletes are unique, in that they tend to have higher carbohydrate intakes than other athletes.[58,63] Several studies have shown that in the days just before, during, and after prolonged endurance events, carbohydrate intake increases dramatically as the athlete attempts to "carbohydrate load."[46,47]

In most studies, the diets of athletes contain vitamins and minerals in excess of the RDA, in part because they eat more food than inactive people.[46,52,55,57,67,78] However, despite the adequacy of minerals and vitamins in their diets, athletes make widespread use of dietary supplements. (This is discussed further in the section on vitamins and minerals in this chapter.) Several large-scale studies have concluded that sports training does not have a negative effect on the nutritional status of athletes (as measured both by diet and biochemical methods) and that the use of supplements is generally unnecessary for the vast majority of athletes.[52,55,61,67,78]

Athletes in sports that emphasize leanness, however, have been found to consume insufficient quantities of vitamins and minerals, largely because of inadequate total food intake. Close to half of all gymnasts, wrestlers, and ballet dancers, for example, have been reported to consume less than two thirds the RDA for various important minerals and vitamins.[68–76]

In general, the quality of the diets of most athletes is somewhat similar to that of the general population, although some endurance athletes are making efforts to increase their carbohydrate intake. Some athletes eat more or less calories, depending on their sport, but usually energy intake increases with the demands of the training program. As a rule of thumb, athletes consume more Calories per kilogram of body weight than the general population. Even though the dietary composition may be similar to those who exercise little, vitamin and mineral intake is usually sufficient for athletes because they are eating more.

PRINCIPLE 2: INCREASE TOTAL ENERGY INTAKE

If an athlete's body weight is normal, energy consumption will need to be higher than that of the average sedentary individual to maintain body weight (see Table 9.7). Many athletes are high energy consumers because of their high working capacities and ability to train at high intensities for long periods of time. Body size is also an important determinant of caloric expenditure, with football players expending much more than gymnasts. In planning additional food consumption, the guidelines of the prudent diet will ensure a proper balance among the energy-providing nutrients.

Athletes Expend Large Amounts of Energy

The amount and intensity of training and body size are the chief determinants of the energy requirements of the athlete[2] (Table 9.6).

As physical activity increases, Calories expended per kilogram of body weight steadily increase. Athletes are capable of amazingly high levels of energy output. A study from Great Britain reported that during a 24-hour cycling time trial in a human performance lab, one athlete cycled 430 miles, expending 20,166 Calories.[83] The athlete lost 1.19 kg of body weight because only 54% of energy needs were met through liquids and food.

Athletes are high energy expenders for two major reasons:[2,84]

1. *High working capacities.* As discussed in Chapter 7, one of the best indicators of fitness is the maximum amount of oxygen one can consume during maximal exercise ($\dot{V}O_{2max}$). Male athletes commonly have maximum oxygen uptakes exceeding 4.5 $L \cdot min^{-1}$ and some can achieve more than 6.0 $L \cdot min^{-1}$. Female athletes, because of their smaller size, have $\dot{V}O_{2max}$ values about 30% lower. For every liter of oxygen consumed, approximately 5 Calories are expended (see Figure 9.5).
2. *Ability to work at high percentage of maximal capacity.* During competition and training, athletes often exercise at levels ranging from 70 to 90% of $\dot{V}O_{2max}$.

During periods of increased exercise or unusually heavy exertion, athletes tend to increase their caloric consumption to match energy expenditure, although periodic rest days improve the overall caloric balance. In some studies, athletes have been reported to be eating far less than the caloric demands of their training program, but this appears to be due to underreporting of caloric intake by the athletes.[2] Measurement of nutrient intake is imprecise and difficult. Athletes must accurately record normal food intake over extended periods, a process that many

TABLE 9.7 The Energy and Quality of Diet Recommended for People Who Exercise Compared to Average American Intake

	Calories*		% of Total Energy Intake		
	Males	Females	Carbohydrate	Fat	Protein
Actual intake of average American	2,800	2,000	51	32	15
Fitness enthusiasts	2,900	2,000	55	30	15
Endurance athletes	2,500–7,500	2,000–4,000	60–70†	15–25	15‡
Team/power athletes	3,000–10,000	2,000–4,000	55	30	15§

*Energy intake can vary widely depending on body size and amount of exercise.
†6–10 grams of carbohydrate per kilogram of body weight per day; the amount required depends upon the athlete's total daily energy expenditure.
‡1.2–1.4 grams of protein per kilogram of body weight per day.
§May be as high as 1.6–1.7 grams of protein per kilogram of body weight per day.

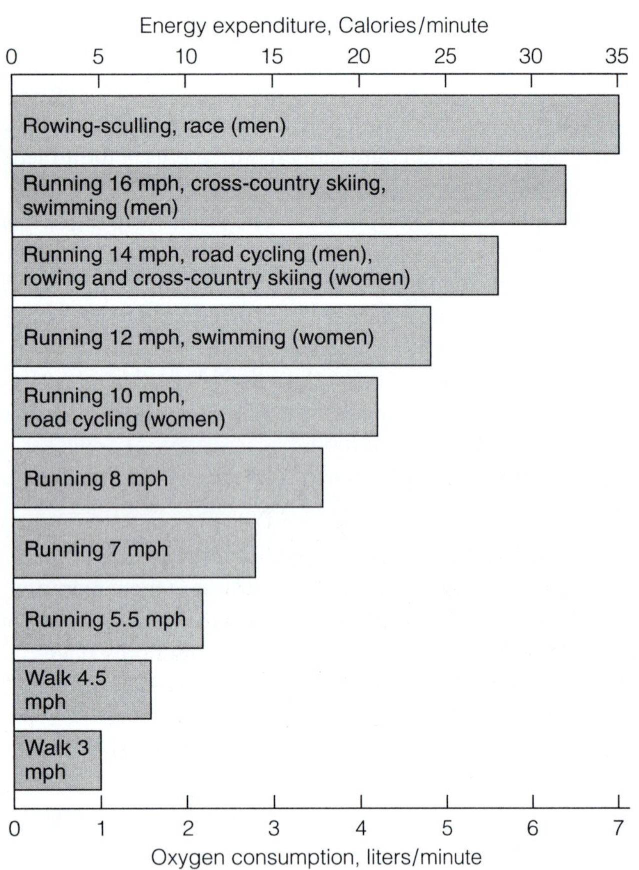

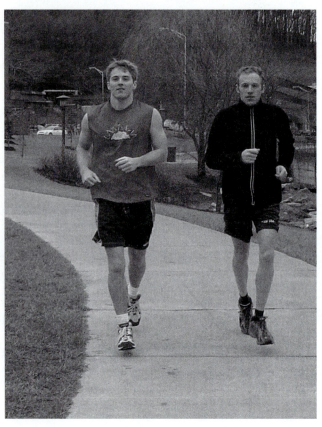

Figure 9.5 Energy-power chart. Some of the best endurance athletes in the world are capable of extremely high energy expenditure rates. Source: Data from Hagerman FC. Energy metabolism and fuel utilization. *Med Sci Sports Exerc* 24: S309–S314, 1992.

subjects find onerous, leading to both dietary changes and underreporting.[5]

Athletes are not only high energy expenders, but they also have a unique pattern of energy utilization, which has important implications for the design of athletic diets. Although endurance athletes tend to expend amounts of energy comparable to those of workers in heavy-labor occupations, they expend a large quantity of their Calories during short time periods—as much as 40% of the daily total in less than 2 hours. This has special nutritional implications for the athlete because of

- High utilization of glycogen (higher carbohydrate needs)
- High sweat rates (higher water needs)
- Musculoskeletal trauma (may affect protein and iron needs)
- Gastrointestinal disturbances (may affect iron balance)

Energy and ATP Production

The energy from food is transferred to the storage molecule called *adenosine triphosphate* (ATP). Muscular contraction for any sport or physical activity is produced by movement within the muscle, powered by energy released from the separation of high-energy phosphate bonds from ATP[85] (see Chapter 7).

Although ATP is the immediate energy source for muscular contraction, the amount of ATP present in a muscle is so small (only about 85 grams) that it must be constantly replenished, or it will be depleted after several seconds of high-intensity exercise. ATP is replenished by two separate systems, the anaerobic system (which produces ATP in the absence of oxygen from the small ATP–creatine phosphate [CP] stores and the lactate system) and the aerobic or oxygen system (see Figures 9.6 and 9.7).

The three sources from which ATP is supplied are

1. *ATP–CP stores.* The body stores a small amount of ATP and CP. The muscles can depend on these stores for up to 10 seconds (e.g., sprinting and weight lifting) before these stores are depleted.
2. *Lactate path.* ATP is produced at a high rate from carbohydrate (glycogen) stores within the muscle (see Chapter 7), during a process called *glycolysis.* Lactic acid is also produced. Because of the lactic acid by-product, which causes muscle fatigue, ATP production from the lactate system can empower intense exercise for only 1–3 minutes (for such

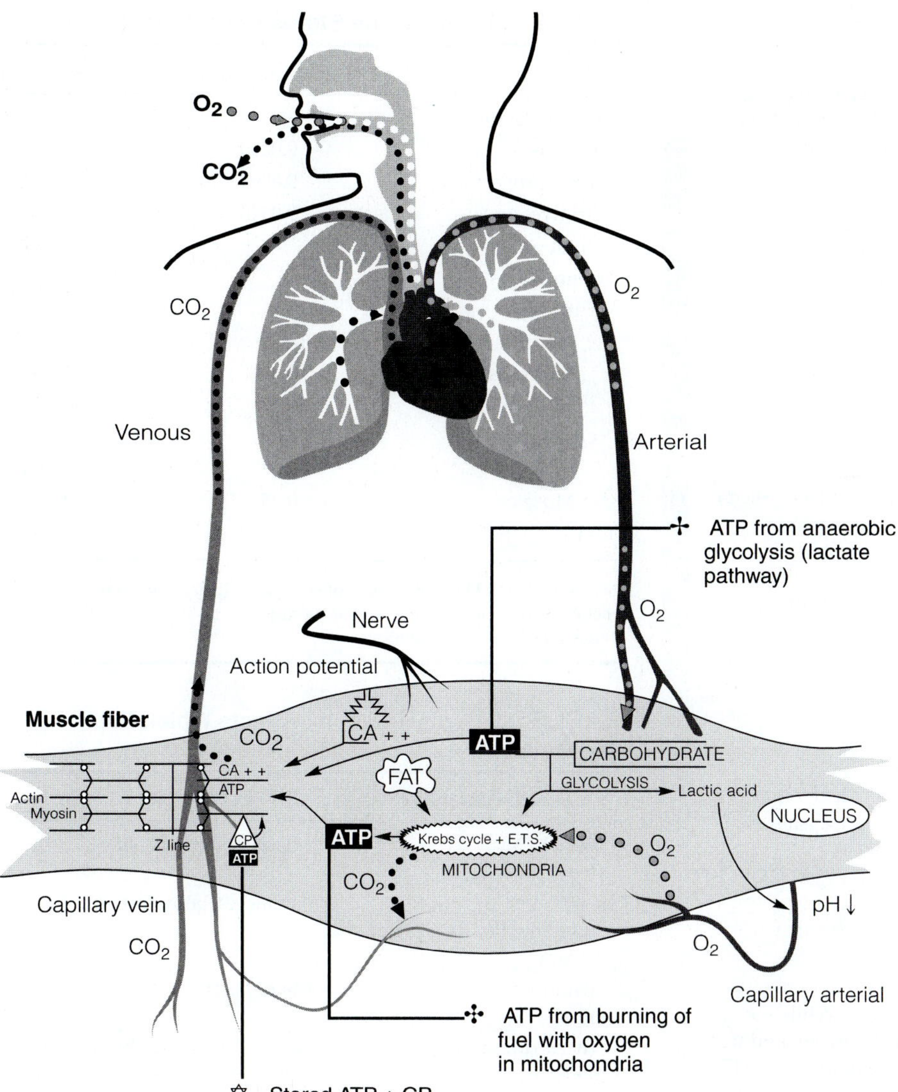

Figure 9.6 ATP is supplied via three pathways: (1) stored ATP and CP, (2) lactate pathway, and (3) mitochondrial oxygen system.

sporting events as 400- to 800-meter runs, 100-meter swimming events, and boxing).

3. *Oxygen system.* This system, which can utilize fatty acids as well as carbohydrates, produces ATP at a slower rate than the other two energy systems. It represents an enormous potential source of energy—the body supply of fats and carbohydrates for exercise are more than enough for 5 continuous days of exercise. Oxygen is required, however, which is why the oxygen utilization capacity of the athlete becomes critically important. The oxygen system is the main provider of ATP in events lasting more than 3 minutes, and in such events as the 26.2-mile marathon, this system becomes by far the main provider of ATP.

The aerobic and anaerobic systems work in tandem. When the exercise rate is pushed beyond the capability of the ventilation–circulation system to provide oxygen in sufficient amounts, the muscle cells rely more and more on the

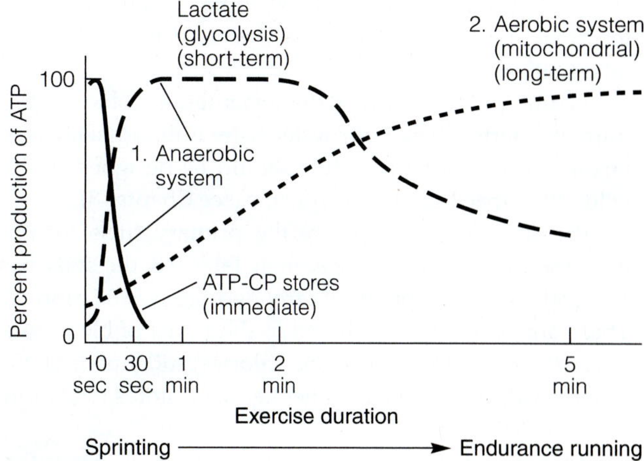

Figure 9.7 Contribution of the two energy systems during exercise of increasing duration. The anaerobic energy system provides ATP to the working myofilaments from ATP–CP stores and the lactate or glycolysis path. The aerobic system supplies ATP from mitochondria, which require oxygen to burn carbohydrates and fats.

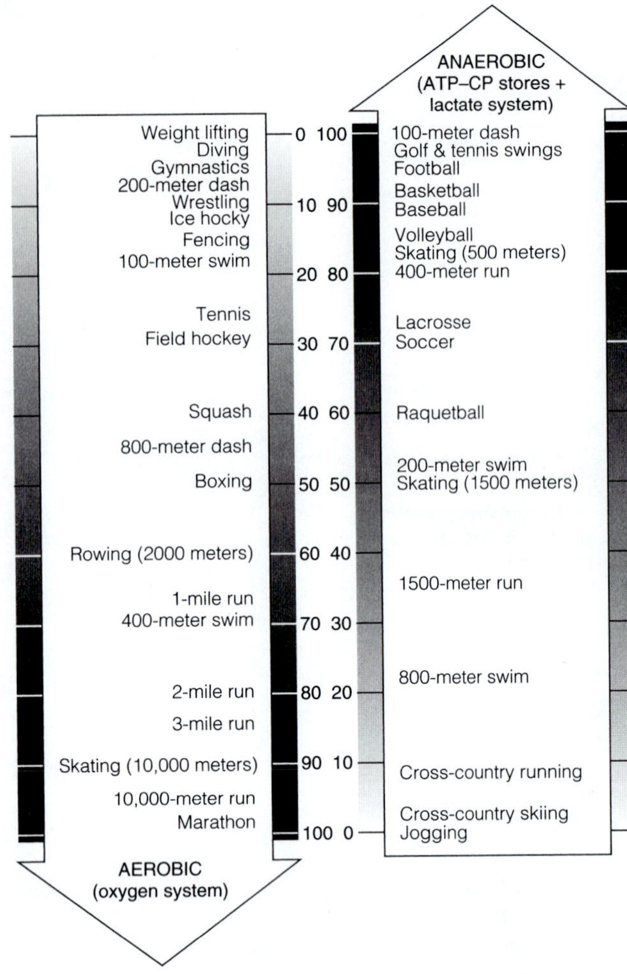

Figure 9.8 The anaerobic–aerobic continuum. While the 100-meter dash is considered a pure anaerobic event, and the marathon a pure aerobic event, most other activities use ATP from both systems. Athletes should train both systems in accordance with the demands of their sport.

lactate system to provide ATP. When this reliance becomes too great, the accumulation of lactic acid may cause debilitating fatigue.

Figure 9.8 summarizes the anaerobic–aerobic continuum. In sports where both systems are utilized (such as in boxing), the training schedule should be designed to develop the capacities of both systems (see Chapter 8).

Fat and carbohydrate are the primary fuels for endurance exercise. As can be seen in Table 9.8, the body has relatively limited supplies of carbohydrate (1,880 Calories). These are generally distributed in the forms of blood glucose (80 Calories), and liver (350 Calories) and muscle (1,450 Calories) glycogen. On the other hand, fat stores total more than 140,000 Calories.[85]

Three factors determine which primary fuel—fat or carbohydrate—will be utilized for ATP production.[85]

1. *Intensity and duration of exercise.* High-intensity, low-duration events (for example, 200-meter sprinting) depend primarily on carbohydrate through the anaerobic system. Carbohydrate is the only fuel that can be used anaerobically.

   As the intensity decreases and duration increases (e.g., hiking), fat becomes the major preferred fuel source. Carbohydrate is still utilized, especially during the beginning portion of the exercise. Table 9.9 summarizes the utilization of metabolic fuels by muscles at different intensities of exercise.[85]

   During prolonged exercise, the usage of carbohydrate is at first high. As the exercise continues, more and more fat is used to supply ATP for the working muscle (see Figures 9.9 and 9.10).[85–87]
2. *Fitness status.* With an improvement in aerobic fitness status, at any given workload there is an increase in the utilization of fat to produce ATP, thereby preserving the limited carbohydrate stores and decreasing the lactate levels[1] (see Figure 9.11).

TABLE 9.8 Substrate Stores of a "Normal Man"

Fuel	Weight (kg)	Energy (Cal)
Circulating Fuels		
Glucose	0.0200	80
Free fatty acids	0.0004	4
Triglycerides	0.0040	40
Total		124
Tissue Stores		
Fat		
Adipose	15.0	140,000
Intramuscular	0.3	2,800
Protein (muscle)	10.0	41,000
Glycogen		
Liver	0.085	350
Muscle	0.350	1,450
Total		185,600

Source: Gollnick PD. Metabolism of substrates: Energy substrate metabolism during exercise and as modified by training. *Federation Proceedings* 44:353–357, 1985.

TABLE 9.9 How Intensity Affects Which Fuel the Muscle Uses

Exercise Intensity	Fuel Used by Muscle
$<$ 30% $\dot{V}O_{2max}$ (easy walking)	Mainly muscle fat stores
40–60% $\dot{V}O_{2max}$ (jogging, brisk walking)	Fat and carbohydrate used evenly
75% $\dot{V}O_{2max}$ (running)	Mainly carbohydrate
$\geq$ 80% $\dot{V}O_{2max}$ (hard running)	Nearly 100% carbohydrate

Source: Data from McCardle WD, Katch FI, Katch VL. *Exercise Physiology: Energy, Nutrition, and Human Performance* (5th ed.), Philadelphia: Lippincott Williams & Wilkens, 2001.

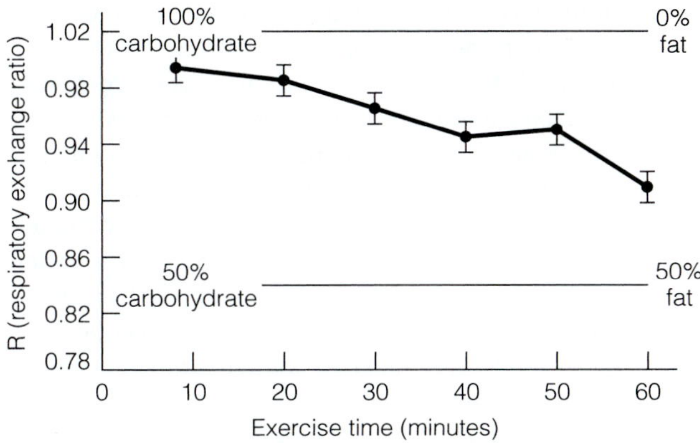

Figure 9.9 Change in use of fuel by muscle mitochondria during a 1-hour run at 70% $\dot{V}O_{2max}$. During a 1-hour run at 70% $\dot{V}O_{2max}$, the muscles gradually use more and more fat to produce ATP. Source: Data from Nieman DC, Carlson KA, Brandstater ME, Naegele RT, Blankenship JW. Running exhaustion in 27-h fasted humans. *J Appl Physiol* 63:2502–2509, 1987.

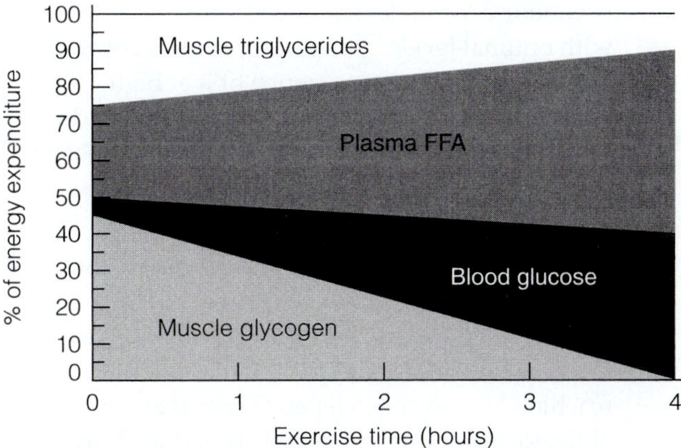

Figure 9.10 Percentage of energy derived from the four major substrates during prolonged exercise at 65–75% of maximal oxygen uptake. Initially, approximately half of the energy is derived each from carbohydrate and fat. As muscle glycogen concentration declines, blood glucose and fats become an increasingly important source of energy for muscle. After 2 hours of exercise, carbohydrate ingestion is needed to maintain blood glucose concentration and carbohydrate oxidation. Source: Coyle EF. Substrate utilization during exercise in active people. *Am J Clin Nutr* 61(suppl):968S–979S, 1995. © American Journal of Clinical Nutrition. American Society for Clinical Nutrition.

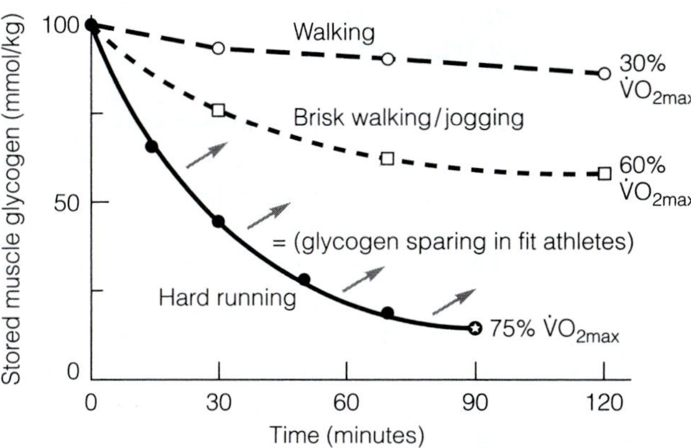

Figure 9.11 Relationship between intensity of exercise and fitness status and use of glycogen during exercise. With increasing intensity of exercise, more and more glycogen is utilized by the muscle. As the arrows depict, with aerobic training, fit athletes tend to use less glycogen during any given workload, sparing the glycogen. Source: Data from Costill DL. Carbohydrates for exercise: Dietary demands for optimal performance. *Int J Sports Med* 9:1–18, 1988.

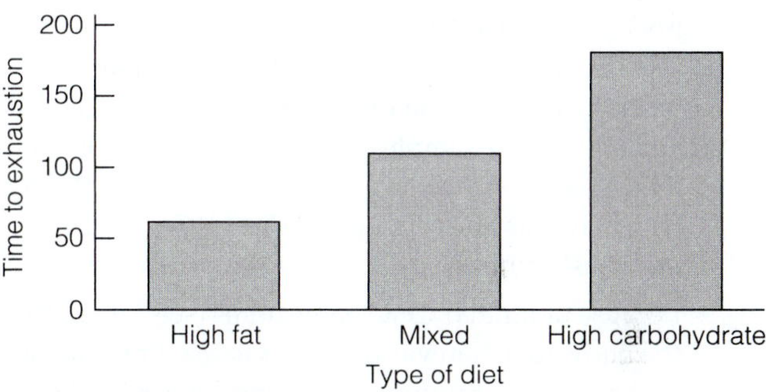

Figure 9.12 Effect of diet on duration of endurance exercise. High-carbohydrate diets allow athletes to perform endurance exercise longer. Source: Data from Bergstrom J, Hermansen L, Hultman E, et al. Diet, muscle glycogen and physical performance. *Acta Physiol Scand* 71:140–150, 1967.

This greater utilization of fat stores (which are relatively unlimited) enables the athlete to perform longer before muscle glycogen stores are depleted.

3. *Previous diet.* During the 1960s, it was discovered that when the pre-event diet was high in carbohydrate, relatively more carbohydrate was stored and available at any given workload for ATP production, and subjects could exercise much longer (Figure 9.12).[1,88] With a high-fat diet, relatively more fat was used, reducing the time of exercise to fatigue. The influence of diet is discussed fully in the following section.

PRINCIPLE 3: KEEP THE DIETARY CARBOHYDRATE INTAKE HIGH (55–70%) DURING TRAINING

A high-carbohydrate diet is probably the most important nutritional principle for both the fitness enthusiast and the endurance athlete. Body carbohydrate stores (glycogen) are critical because they are the primary fuel source for the working muscles. When muscle glycogen levels drop too low, the ability to exercise falls, and one feels more stale and tired and is more prone to injury. Athletes in heavy training may need 6–10 grams of carbohydrate per kilogram of body weight in their diet per day.

The Importance of Carbohydrate during Heavy Training

The story of carbohydrate (CHO) in endurance performance began in 1939, when Scandinavian researchers demonstrated the effect of exercise intensity on the fuel used by the muscle during exercise.[1,89,90] They found that as the intensity of the exercise increased, the relative contribution of CHO as muscular fuel increased.

The development of the biopsy needle in 1962 allowed researchers to extend these findings by measuring the actual amounts of glycogen in the muscle[91] (see Figure 9.13). A series of experiments by other Scandinavian investigators during the late 1960s demonstrated that the ability to exercise at a high intensity was related to the pre-exercise level of muscle glycogen.[1,88,92]

Several basic principles are now clear regarding the relationship between exercise and dietary carbohydrate, and muscle glycogen.[93–122]

- Body glycogen stores play an important role in hard exercise (70–85% of $\dot{V}O_{2max}$) that is either prolonged and continuous (e.g., running, swimming, cycling), or of an extended intermittent, mixed anaerobic–aerobic nature (e.g., soccer, basketball, ice hockey, repeated running intervals). The higher the intensity of exercise, the more dependent the working muscle is on glycogen (see Figure 9.11 and Table 9.9). For example, 2 hours of cycling at 30% of $\dot{V}O_{2max}$ will only reduce muscle glycogen by about 20%, whereas performing at 75% of $\dot{V}O_{2max}$ results in almost complete muscle glycogen depletion.[1]
- Because of limited CHO body stores (see Table 9.8), the body adapts in various ways to maximize its use of these stores. Endurance training leads to higher stored levels of muscle glycogen, nearly double those of untrained people.[85] Endurance training also leads to a greater utilization of fat at any given workload, sparing the glycogen.[96,123] In other words, aerobically fit people consume more fat at any given workload, sparing the glycogen (see Figure 9.11). For example, when fit and unfit people run together at a certain pace (e.g., 8 minutes/mile), the fit will use more fat and less carbohydrate per mile than the unfit. This is advantageous because muscle glycogen is spared, allowing the fit person to exercise longer.
- Exhaustion during prolonged, hard exercise is tied to low muscle glycogen levels. CHO stores are thus the *limiting* factor in exercise bouts lasting longer than 60–90 minutes[1,112–120] (see Figure 9.14). Low glycogen levels are also limiting in various team sports that entail a lot of running. In soccer, for example, players with low glycogen levels have been found to run less and walk more than those with optimal levels.[121] In soccer, players cover an average of 10 kilometers, much of it at high sprinting speeds. Fatigue in shorter events is due to other factors, especially the buildup of metabolic byproducts such as lactic acid and hydrogen ions within the muscle cells.
- When muscle and liver glycogen stores are low, a high work output cannot be maintained. Marathoners use the term "hitting the wall" to describe the fatigue and pain that is associated with reaching low glycogen levels. There is an apparent obligatory requirement of muscle and liver glycogen breakdown for intense exercise. The breakdown of fat cannot sustain metabolic rates during exercise at levels much above 50–65% of $\dot{V}O_{2max}$. In other words, when muscle glycogen levels are low, the exerciser will not be able to exercise at intensities above 50–65% of $\dot{V}O_{2max}$—which for many runners means a painful shuffle or jog.

  For endurance cyclers, low initial glycogen levels have been shown to reduce power output during the end of the race.[122]
- During the first hour of hard exercise, most of the CHO and fat (triglycerides) come from within the muscle, which is a major depot of fuel[116] (see Figures 9.10 and 9.15). As the exercise continues beyond 1 hour, more and more demands are placed upon adipose tissue fat fuel sources and blood glucose as muscle glycogen levels begin to be depleted. The longer the exercise period, the greater the need for glucose from the liver to keep pace with the increasing glucose demands of the glycogen-depleted working muscle.[1,112,114,116] As with muscle glycogen, trained individuals utilize less plasma glucose than the untrained, preserving liver glycogen, minimizing

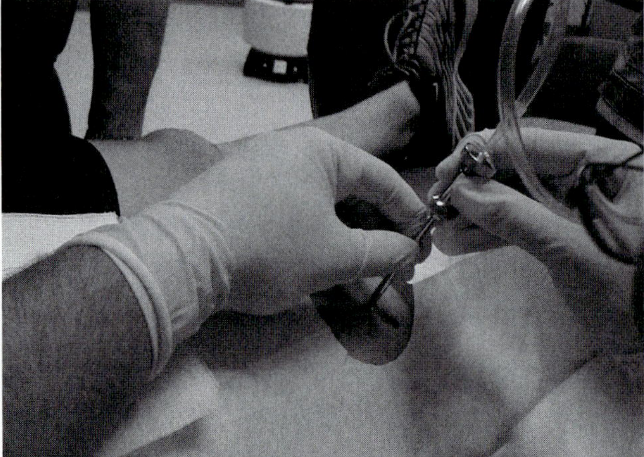

Figure 9.13 The needle biopsy allows researchers to obtain a small sample of muscle tissue to measure the amount of glycogen. A small incision is made in the muscle (after anesthetizing the area), the biopsy needle is inserted, suction pressure is applied, and a small piece of muscle is cut with a sliding knife device in the needle.

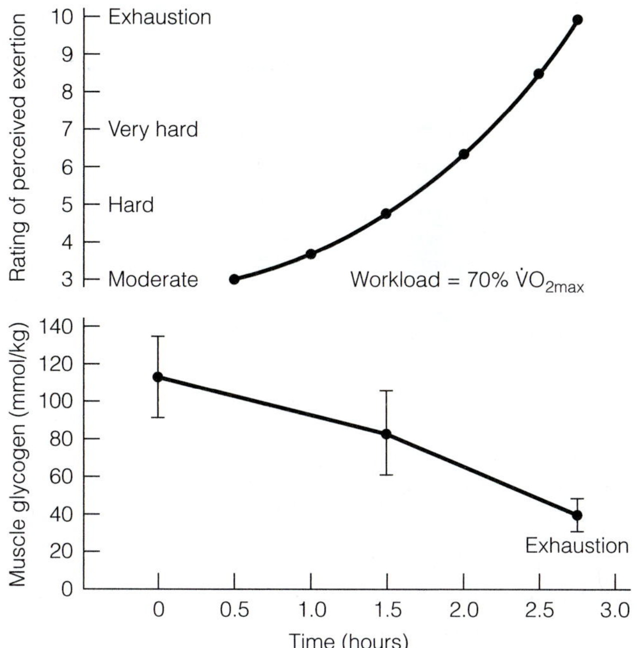

Figure 9.14 Nine experienced marathoners ran for nearly 3 hours on a treadmill at 70% $\dot{V}O_{2max}$. As the muscle glycogen levels fell, the rating of perceived exertion climbed strongly. Exhaustion was associated with low glycogen levels in the muscles of the runners. Source: Data from Nieman DC, Carlson KA, Brandstater ME, Naegele RT, Blankenship JW. Running exhaustion in 27-h fasted humans. *J Appl Physiol* 63:2502–2509, 1987.

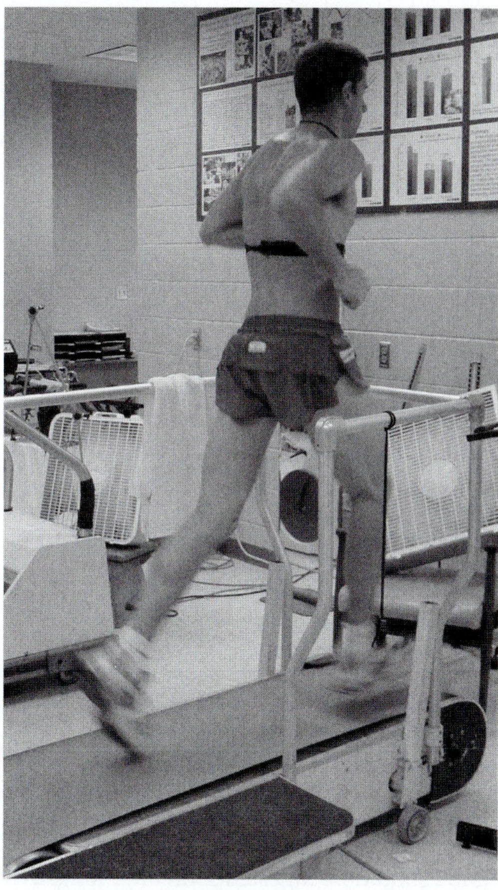

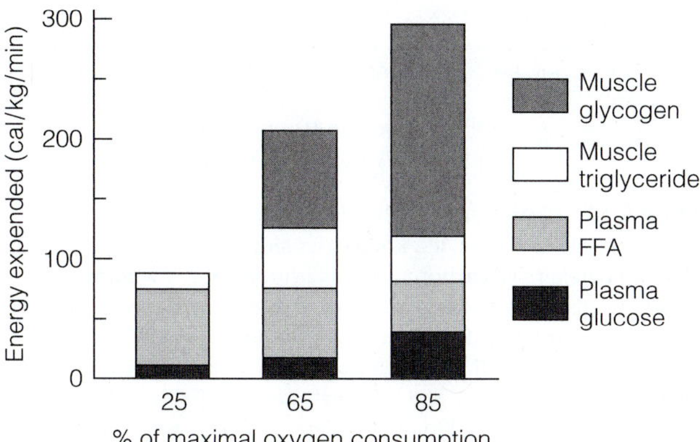

Figure 9.15 Contribution of the four major substrates to energy expenditure after 30 minutes of exercise at 25%, 65%, and 85% of maximal oxygen uptake when fasted. Sources: Coyle EF. Substrate utilization during exercise in active people. *Am J Clin Nutr* 61(suppl):968S–979S, 1995; Coyle EF. *Perspectives in Exercise Science and Sports Medicine, Recent Advances in the Science and Medicine of Sport*, Vol. 10. Reprinted with permission of the author.

the possibility of hypoglycemia, and improving long-term endurance.[114]

- During strenuous training, muscle glycogen stores undergo rapid day-to-day fluctuation.[1,101] Sedentary people on normal mixed diets have glycogen stores of only 70–110 mmol per kilogram wet muscle. Athletes on mixed diets, after 24 hours of rest, have glycogen levels of 130–135 mmol/kg wet muscle, and after 48 hours of rest with a high-carbohydrate diet, they have 140–230 mmol/kg.[1]

  As Figure 9.16 shows, glycogen levels of athletes can be reduced 50% after a 2-hour workout.[124,125] If the carbohydrate content of the diet is low (about 40% of total Calories), little muscle glycogen is restored during the day, and with a 2-hour workout the next day the athlete will be less able to exercise intensely, or exercise will feel harder than normal.[1,113,118,124] This has been demonstrated in rowers, swimmers, and runners, leading most sports-nutrition experts to advise that endurance athletes adopt high-carbohydrate diets[113,115,120,126–128] (see Figure 9.17).
- Endurance athletes compete or train repeatedly on the same day or on consecutive days, and thus the rapid restoration of muscle glycogen is essential. While earlier studies suggested that 48 hours or longer were required to replenish muscle glycogen stores after long endurance exercise, more recent investigations have shown that when 9–16 grams CHO per kilogram body weight are consumed soon after exercise, muscle glycogen stores can be normalized within 1 day, especially in highly trained individuals.[105,129–134] CHO-rich foods or

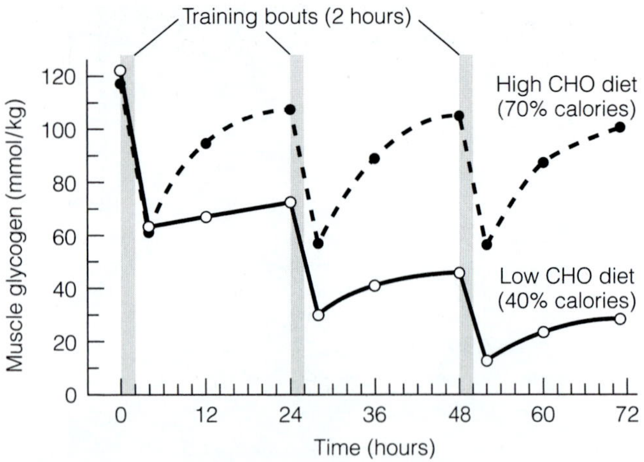

Figure 9.16 The importance of a high-carbohydrate diet during heavy training. Daily, 2-hour workouts deplete muscle glycogen stores by about 50%. A low-carbohydrate diet (40% of Calories) does not adequately restore this depleted glycogen, and there will be a progressive reduction in muscle glycogen as the daily workouts continue. A high-carbohydrate diet (70% of Calories) helps to keep muscle glycogen stores near normal despite heavy training, allowing the athlete to train harder with less effort. Source: Data from Costill DL, Miller JM. Nutrition for endurance sports: Carbohydrate and fluid balance. *Int J Sports Med* 1:2–14, 1980.

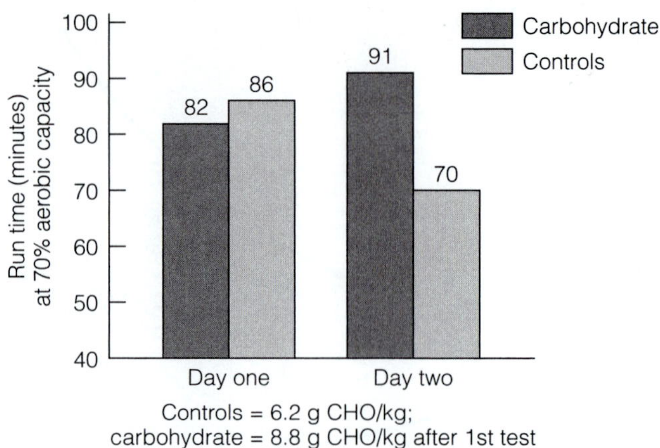

Figure 9.17 Carbohydrate intake and recovery from prolonged exercise. In this study, runners were able to run longer on day 2 when they consumed nearly 9 grams CHO/kg after a hard bout of running the first day. Source: Data from Fallowfield JL, Williams C. Carbohydrate intake and recovery from prolonged exercise. *Int J Sport Nutr* 3:150–164, 1993.

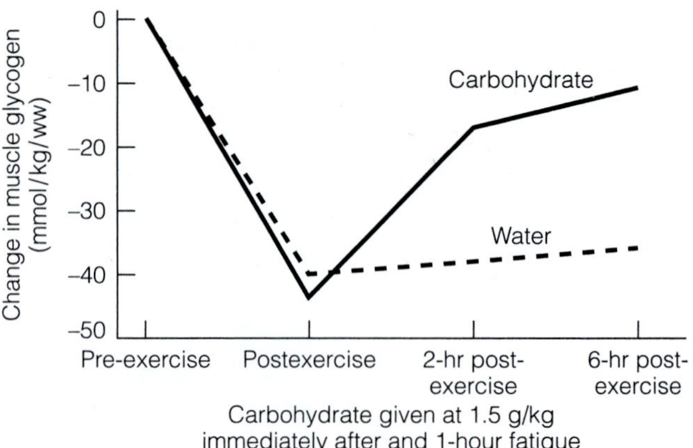

Figure 9.18 Glycogen resynthesis following resistance exercise: 9 sets of 6 reps, leg knee extensions, 70% 1-RM, to fatigue. Postexercise carbohydrate is important for weight trainers to restore muscle glycogen depleted during exercise. Source: Data from Pascoe DD, Costill DL, Fink WJ, Robergs RA, Zachwieja JJ. Glycogen resynthesis in skeletal muscle following resistive exercise. *Med Sci Sports Exerc* 25:349–354, 1993.

fluids should be ingested soon after long-term exercise, until at least 8–10 grams CHO per kilogram of body weight (500–800 grams or 2,000–3,200 CHO Calories, depending on body size) are consumed.[119,129–134] There is some evidence that high-glycemic-index foods promote a greater glycogen storage rate.[106–111,131–135] (see Box 9.5). This is also good advice for weight trainers.[104] In one study, multiple sets of intense leg knee extensions decreased muscle glycogen by about 30%.[130] When subjects took in carbohydrate immediately after the session, most of the muscle glycogen was restored within 6 hours, while there was little change in subjects drinking only water (see Figure 9.18).

Practical Implications for Athletes

In general, glycogen synthesis increases in proportion to the amount of CHO consumed. About 6–10 grams of CHO are needed per kilogram of body weight (about 500–800 total grams) each day for the endurance athlete who is training for more than 60–90 minutes.[1,2] Athletes in heavy training should consume a diet of close to 70% CHO (525 grams per 3,000 Calories), which will restore muscle glycogen within 24 hours, enabling the athlete to continue heavy training. This is especially important after race events and long, intense training bouts.

This is more carbohydrate than most athletes would ordinarily choose, however, and they need to be educated to include this large amount. Athletes commonly underestimate their carbohydrate needs and are thus susceptible to feeling "stale" from glycogen depletion.

Table 9.10 is a sample listing of high-carbohydrate foods, in descending order of amount of the carbohydrate they contain (in grams per cup). Notice that foods high in simple sugars lead the list, followed by dried fruits, cereals, potatoes, rice, legumes, and fruit juices. While high-sugar foods such as honey, jams, and syrups provide high amounts of carbohydrate, too much simple sugar in the diet invites shortages of necessary vitamins and minerals.

Box 9.5

Should Athletes Be Concerned about the Glycemic Index?

Although most athletes know that they should consume liberal amounts of carbohydrate before, during, and after prolonged exercise, few are concerned about the types of carbohydrate foods to select. The glycemic index (GI) has been proposed as an important resource when selecting an ideal carbohydrate food to optimize glycogen storage rates.

The GI categorizes foods containing carbohydrates according to the blood glucose response they elicit. High-GI foods evoke the highest blood glucose response, while low-GI foods produce a relatively low response. The GI was originally developed for diabetics to better control blood glucose levels. The GI is a percentage value, based on the area of the blood glucose response of 50 grams of carbohydrate in a reference food (typically white bread), multiplied by 100:

$$\text{GI} = (\text{blood glucose area of test food}) \div (\text{blood glucose area of reference food}) \times 100$$

The GI approach has been criticized because some foods have been rated as good or bad simply on the basis of their GI. The GI was never intended to be used in isolation. Instead, the user must balance GI information with other measures of diet quality, including dietary fiber; vitamin and mineral content; and the amount of salt, cholesterol, and saturated fat.

Researchers from the University of British Columbia in Vancouver, Canada, have made these recommendations concerning exercise and the GI:[135]

1. Athletes wishing to consume carbohydrates 30–60 minutes before exercise should be encouraged to ingest low-GI foods. This will decrease the likelihood of creating hyperglycemia and hyperinsulinemia at the onset of exercise, while providing exogenous carbohydrate throughout the early stages of exercise. Notice from the following list that low-GI foods include spaghetti, milk, fructose, some fruits and juices, and most legumes.
2. High-GI foods should be consumed during exercise to ensure rapid digestion and absorption, and elevated blood glucose levels. Notice from the following list that high-GI foods include instant rice, glucose, potatoes and other root vegetables, sucrose, bagels, and many types of breakfast cereals. Most sports drinks are a combination of glucose (high GI) and fructose (low GI), so the proportion should be checked carefully, with an emphasis on high-glucose sports drinks.
3. Postexercise meals should consist of high-GI carbohydrates, to enhance glycogen resynthesis.

Foods can be ranked as follows, according to their GI (with white bread used as the standard or a GI of 100):

High (GI > 100)	GI	Moderate (GI = 60–100)	GI	Low (GI < 60)	GI
Carrots	101	Muffin	88	Spaghetti	59
Bagels	103	Oatmeal	87	Apple juice	58
Honey	104	Ice cream	87	Tomato soup	54
Doughnut	108	Rice (white and brown)	80	Apple	52
Waffles	109	Oatmeal cookies	79	Yogurt, low fat	47
Sucrose	117	Corn	78	Dried apricots	44
Corn Chex	118	Banana	76	Kidney beans	42
Cornflakes	119	Orange juice	74	Peach, fresh	40
Baked potatoes	121	Chocolate	70	Whole milk	39
Crispix cereal	124	Lactose	65	Red lentils	36
Rice Chex	127	Orange	62	Fructose	32
Instant rice	128	Grapes	62	Soy beans	25
Glucose	138	All-bran cereal	60	Peanuts	21

Sources: Walton P, Rhodes EC. Glycemic index and optimal performance. *Sports Med* 23:164–172, 1997; Foster-Powell K, Miller JB. International tables of glycemic index. *Am J Clin Nutr* 62:871S–893S, 1995.

TABLE 9.10 High-Carbohydrate Foods—1-Cup Portions

Food	Grams Carbohydrate	Calories per Cup	% Carbohydrate Calories
Honey	272	1040	100
Pancake syrup	238	960	100
Jams/preserves	224	880	100
Molasses	176	720	100
Dates (chopped)	131	489	100
Raisins	115	434	100
Prunes	101	385	100
Grape-Nuts	94	407	92
Whole-wheat flour	85	400	85
Dried apricots (uncooked)	80	310	100
Sweet potato (boiled, mashed)	80	344	93
Sweetened applesauce	51	194	100
Brown rice	50	232	86
Prune juice	45	181	100
Kidney beans	42	230	73
Rolled wheat (cooked)	41	180	91
Macaroni (cooked)	39	190	82
Lentils (cooked)	39	210	74
Grape juice	38	155	98

Source: USDA.

Although high- versus low-glycemic foods promote more rapid glycogen resynthesis, the athlete should choose foods that also promote nutritional health.

Table 9.11 outlines a sample menu for an athlete who is training more than 60–90 minutes a day aerobically. Notice that grain products and fruits predominate in this high-carbohydrate diet. The use of fatty meats and dairy products, nuts, olives, and oils should be limited, to ensure that sufficient carbohydrate is consumed to replete muscle glycogen stores. High-carbohydrate diets are healthy, supply more than 100% of the RDA for all nutrients, help prevent chronic disease, and can therefore be recommended on a daily basis. The process of "carbohydrate loading" before major events is discussed in Principle 8.

PRINCIPLE 4: DRINK LARGE AMOUNTS OF FLUIDS DURING TRAINING AND THE EVENT

The second most important dietary principle for those who exercise is to drink large quantities of fluids. As little as a 2% drop in body weight caused by water loss (primarily from sweat) can reduce exercise capacity. In other words, if an athlete weighs 150 pounds and loses 3 pounds during an exercise bout, performance ability is reduced. A good habit is to measure body weight before and after each exercise session; each pound lost should be replaced with 1 pint (or 2 cups) of fluid.[136,137]

Thirst lags behind actual body needs. So before, during, and after the exercise bout, one should drink plenty of fluids, beyond the demands of thirst. A plan recommended by some sports-medicine experts is to drink 2 cups of water immediately before the exercise bout, 1 cup every 15 minutes during the exercise session, and then 2 more cups after the session. When intense exercise lasts longer than 1 hour, carbohydrates (30–60 grams/hour) and sodium (0.5–0.7 gram/L of water) should be ingested to delay fatigue and promote fluid retention.[136,137]

The Importance of Water for Temperature Regulation during Exercise

As carbohydrate and fat are used by the working muscle to produce energy for movement, about 70–80% is transformed into heat (much like the engine in a car).[138–142] If this were retained by the body, body heat would potentially increase up to 1°C every 5 minutes, resulting in serious heat injury (hyperthermia) within 20–30 minutes.[138,143]

During steady-state exercise at 75% of capacity, average heat loss from the body may range from 900 to 1,500 Calories/hour. An addition of up to 100–150 Calories/hour may be gained from the sun. The body heat is transferred from the warm muscle to the blood and then to the skin, where it is dissipated to the air by evaporation, radiation, or convection.[138,140] On a hot dry day at rest, 55% of heat loss is by radiation and convection, 45% by sweat evaporation. During exercise, sweat evaporation becomes by far the major

TABLE 9.11 Sample Menu—3,500 Calories, High-Carbohydrate (79% Total Calories)

The foods listed here represent a 1-day sample of the type of diet recommended for the average male runner training for long endurance events. This type of diet is also recommended for "carbohydrate loading" during the 3-day period before a long endurance race. This sample diet meets the recommended dietary allowance (RDA) for all nutrients and follows the guidelines of the "prudent diet."

Portion	Food	Calories
Breakfast		
1 cup	Grape-Nuts	404
2 cups	2% lowfat milk	242
1 whole	Banana	105
1/2 cup	Seedless raisins	247
2 cups	Orange juice	224
1 piece	Whole-wheat bread	84
2 tsp	Honey	43
Lunch		
1/2 whole	Fresh tomato	12
1/2 cup	Loose leaf lettuce	5
2 oz	Cooked chicken	108
2 pieces	Whole-wheat bread	168
1 tbs	Low-cal dressing	35
2 cups	Canned pineapple juice	278
Supper		
2 pieces	Whole-wheat bread	168
1 tbs	Peanut butter	96
2 whole	Apple	162
2 cups	Cooked brown rice	464
2 cups	Mixed vegetables	105
1 tsp	Seasonings	5
1 cup	Low-fat yogurt	231
2 whole	Bagels	330

Meal	Calories	Total CHO Grams	% CHO
Breakfast	1,349	290	86
Lunch	606	108	71
Supper	1,561	292	75
Totals	3,516	690	79

Nutrients	Protein	Iron	Zinc	Calcium	Vit C	Vit A	Vit B_1
Day totals	116 g	25 mg	18 mg	1,578 mg	425 mg	15,009 IU	4.2 mg
% RDA	207	250	120	197	708	300	280

avenue of heat loss, accounting for greater than 80%. For every liter of sweat evaporated on the skin, close to 600 Calories are given off, preventing an increase in body temperature of a full 10°C. The body has 2–4 million sweat glands, and, on a hot but dry day, can secrete enough sweat to dissipate all of the heat generated by exercise.[141] For example, if an athlete sweats 1.8 L/hour, 1,000 Calories of heat are removed from the body. Figure 9.19 shows the avenues of heat loss from the exercising human body.

The sweat glands draw fluid from stores between and within the body cells, and then from the plasma volume of the blood in the skin[137,144] (see Figure 9.20). However, the efficiency of sweat evaporation is greatly affected by humidity, especially if it rises above 70% (relative humidity).[136,137,145] If the humidity is so high that the sweat rolls off the skin without evaporation, little heat is given off, and body temperature rises. This can result in heat injury, including heat exhaustion and heat stroke (see Chapter 16). In heat stroke, the brain shuts off the sweat glands to protect blood fluid levels, resulting in dry, hot, and red skin and a deadly rise in body temperature.

Exercise in hot and humid weather can be dangerous. During the 1986 Pittsburgh marathon, for example, the

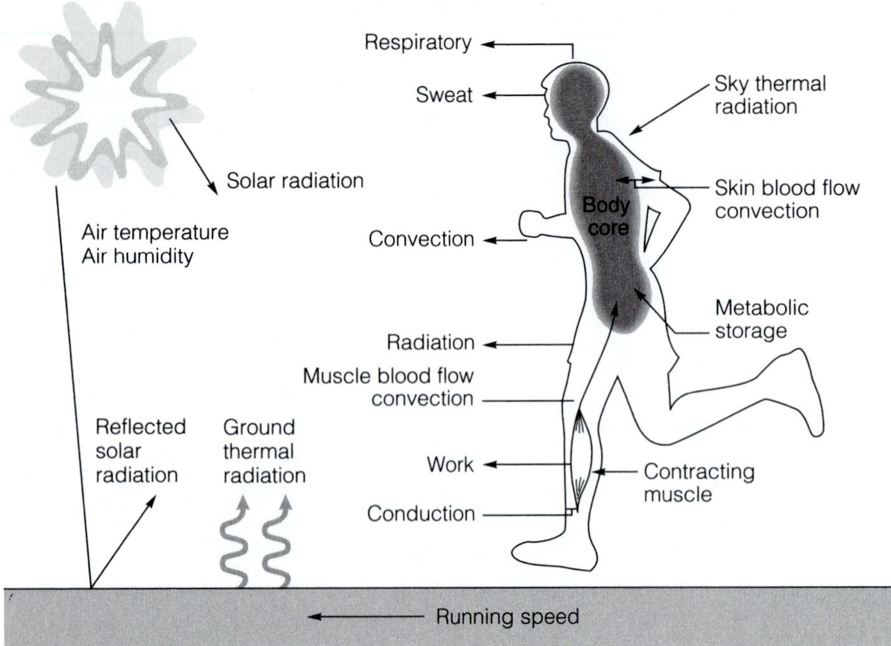

Figure 9.19 As the muscles contract during exercise, heat is produced, causing the core body temperature to rise. A small amount of heat is also gained by the body from the environment. The primary route for this heat to exit is sweat evaporation. Other routes include convection, radiation, conduction, and respiration. Source: Gisolfi CV, Wenger CB. Temperature regulation during exercise: Old concept, new ideas. In Terjung RL (ed.), *Exercise and Sports Sciences Reviews*, Lexington: Collamore Press, 1984.

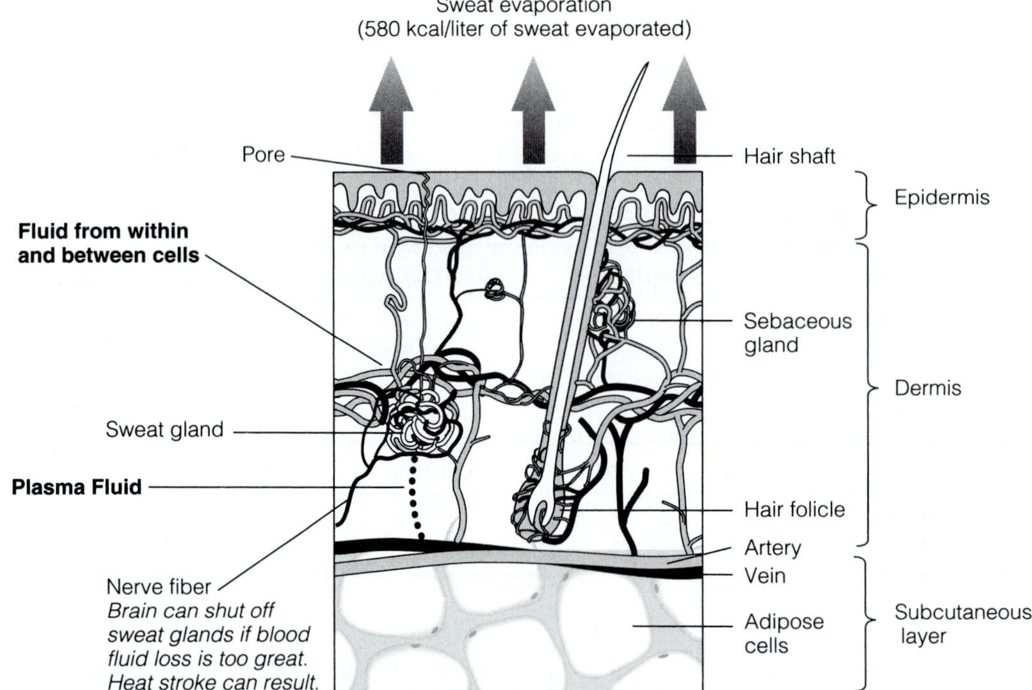

Figure 9.20 Sources of fluid for sweat production. The sweat glands draw fluids from between and within cells and from the blood, to produce sweat during exercise. If blood volume levels fall too low, the brain will shut off sweat gland activity. Continued exercise can then result in heat stroke.

temperature reached 87°F and the humidity 60%; as a result, half of the 2,879 runners were treated for heat injuries.[146] (The American College of Sports Medicine has established guidelines for race directors to follow to avoid this type of disaster; see Chapter 16.)

Figure 9.21 shows the effect of running pace and weather conditions on the sweat rate; rates become extremely high during fast running on hot and humid days.

Sweat losses of 0.5 to 1.5 L/hour are common in endurance sports.[136,137] Under extremely hot conditions,

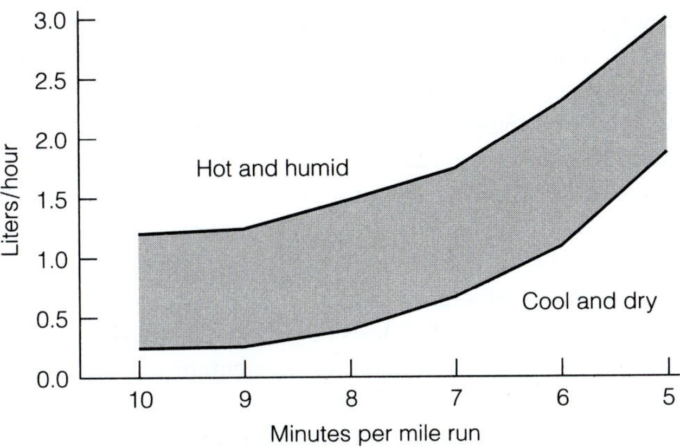

Figure 9.21 Sweat rates in runners. Sweat rates are affected by running pace and weather conditions. The specifics of measuring heat stress, including the relationship of heat and humidity, is described in Chapter 16.
Source: Data from Sawka MN. Physiological consequences of hypohydration: Exercise performance and thermoregulation. *Med Sci Sports Exerc* 24:657–670, 1992.

TABLE 9.12 Adverse Effects of Dehydration*

% Body Wt Loss	Symptoms
1.0	Thirst threshold
2.0	Stronger thirst, vague discomfort, loss of appetite
3.0	Increasing hemoconcentration, dry mouth, reduction in urine
4.0	Decrement of 20–30% in exercise capacity
5.0	Difficulty in concentrating, headache, impatience
6.0	Severe impairment in exercise temperature regulation, increased respiration, extremity numbness and tingling
7.0	Likely collapse if combined with heat and exercise

Physiological Responses to Dehydration

↑ Incidence of gastrointestinal distress	↓ Gastric emptying rate
↑ Plasma osmolality	↓ Splanchnic, renal blood flow
↑ Blood viscosity	↓ Plasma volume
↑ Heart rate	↓ Central blood volume
↑ Core temperature at which sweating begins	↓ Cardiac filling pressure
↑ Core temperature at which skin blood flow increases	↓ Stroke volume and cardiac output
↑ Core temperature at a given exercise intensity	↓ Sweat rate at a given core temperature
	↓ Maximal sweat rate
	↓ Maximal skin blood flow
	↓ Performance

*1% of body weight for a 150-lb person would equal 3 cups of water (1 cup = 0.5 lb).

Sources: Data from Greenleaf JE, Harrison MH. Water and electrolytes. In Layman DK (ed.), *Nutrition and Aerobic Exercise.* Washington, DC: American Chemical Society, 1986; Murray R. Fluid needs in hot and cold environments. *Int J Sport Nutr* 5:S62–S73, 1995.

sweat rates (of fit participants) have been measured at over 2.5 L/hour. During the 1984 Los Angeles Olympic Games, U.S. runner Alberto Salazar lost 12 pounds (8.1% of body weight) during the marathon, despite drinking nearly 2 liters of water during the race. Alberto's sweat rate was 3.7 L/hour, one of the highest ever measured.[147] Sweat rates are influenced by fitness level, temperature and humidity, intensity of exercise, heat acclimation, hydration status, air velocity, and the type of clothing worn.[144] Sweat rates can be calculated using this formula:

(Loss in body weight)
+ (fluids ingested during exercise)
− (urine excreted during exercise) = sweat loss

For example, if an athlete runs intensely for 1 hour and loses 0.5 kilogram of body weight, drinks 500 ml of fluid, and urinates 100 ml, the sweat rate = 1,100 g + 500 − 100 = 1,500 ml/hour.

The average 70-kilogram individual has 42 liters of body water (60% of body weight). The body water is divided into three components:[138]

1. Intracellular fluid (67%)
2. Interstitial (between cells) fluid (27%)
3. Plasma volume (6%)

Loss of body water from sweating beyond 2% of body weight will significantly impair endurance capacity, through elevation of body temperature and decreased cardiac output. When sweat output exceeds water intake, both intracellular and extracellular water levels fall, and plasma volume decreases, resulting in an increase in body temperature, a decrease in the ability of the heart to pump blood, and a decrease in endurance performance. Even a slight amount of dehydration causes physiological consequences. For example, every liter (2.2 lb) of water lost will cause heart rate to be elevated by about eight beats per minute, cardiac output to decline by 1 L/minute, and core temperature to rise by 0.3°C when an individual participates in prolonged exercise in the heat.[137,138,141,148–153]

Table 9.12 outlines the adverse effects of dehydration. Those most vulnerable to dehydration during exercise are obese, unfit, unacclimatized, overclothed people, who are exercising on hot, humid, sunny days. Early warning signals include clumsiness, stumbling, excessive sweat, cessation of sweating, headache, nausea, or dizziness.[136]

People who are accustomed to exercising in the heat go through physiological changes that have been termed the *acclimatization process.*[151–153] Acclimatization (using a gradual progression for safety) can occur within as few as 5–10 days of training in the heat. The acclimatized person has a higher plasma volume (400–700 ml increase) and sweat glands that produce more sweat earlier in the exercise session, with less loss of sodium. During exercise, the acclimatized person's body temperature and heart rate do not rise as strongly as those of unacclimatized people.

Fluid replacement during exercise reduces the adverse effects of dehydration by slowing the rise in core temperature, maintaining plasma volume and cardiac output, improving endurance, and lessening the risk of heat injury.[136,137,154–156]

During prolonged exercise, as the body loses water primarily through sweating, there tends to be a gradual decrease in heartstroke volume, and a corresponding increase in heart rate, making the exercise seem more difficult than normal. Drinking about 1 liter of fluid per hour helps prevent this "cardiovascular drift," making it easier to continue exercising.[150]

Figure 9.22 shows the results of one study in which subjects cycled for 6 hours at 55% of $\dot{V}O_{2max}$ while either avoiding fluids or drinking enough to replace total body water loss (a little over 1 L/hour in an environmental chamber set at 30°C and 50% relative humidity).[154] When fluids were restricted, subjects lost an average of 6.4% of their body weight (10 pounds), experienced high rectal temperatures and heart rates, and found the exercise too difficult to complete, stopping 1.5 hours earlier than subjects who drank enough to maintain body water. These results demonstrate the deleterious effects of dehydration on exercise performance.

How much water should one drink during exercise to avoid dehydration? Figure 9.23 summarizes the water balance needs of sedentary and physically active people. The Institute of Medicine recommends that men ingest 3.7 liters of water each day (3 liters from water and other beverages and 0.7 liters from water in food) and women 2.7 liters each day (2.2 liters from beverages, 0.5 from water in food).[14] In general, most people sweat 0.5–1.5 Liters per hour of exercise and need to replace this by drinking more fluids.[136,137] It is common for athletes to lose 2–4% of body weight during vigorous workouts. Marathoners can lose 6–8% of their body weight in water during the 26.2-mile event, with plasma volume decreasing 13–18%.[157] A 4% drop in body weight for a 150-pound person means a loss of 6 pounds, or about 3 quarts of water. It is not uncommon in a hot environment to lose half a pound per mile after the first hour. That would amount to a cup of water every mile, or every 6–8 minutes.

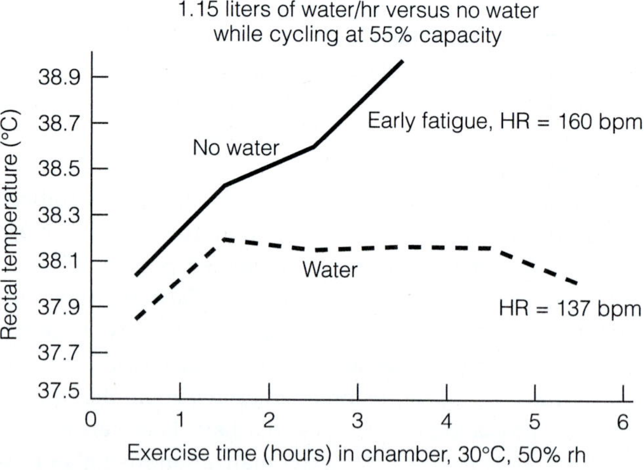

Figure 9.22 Fluid replacement during prolonged exercise: 1.15 liters of water/hr versus no water while cycling at 55% capacity. Drinking about 1.2 liters of water each hour during prolonged exercise in a moderately hot environment prevented dehydration, allowing subjects to exercise for 6 hours. Source: Data from Barr DI, Costill DL, Fink WJ. Fluid replacement during prolonged exercise: Effects of water, saline, or no fluid. *Med Sci Sports Exerc* 23:811–817, 1991.

For most athletes, it is hard to drink this much water, mainly because such intake is beyond the demands of thirst. Exercise tends to blunt thirst, so a systematic plan should be followed for fluid consumption during exercise. In other words, when one is exercising, thirst provides a poor index of body needs, leading to what some researchers call "involuntary dehydration."[136,137] Most athletes are "reluctant" drinkers during exercise and do not drink enough to match body losses. Runners, for example, generally drink only 300–500 ml of fluids per hour of exercise.[136,137] Therefore, fluids need to be "forced down" during exercise.

Box 9.6 summarizes information from the ACSM "Position Stand on Exercise and Fluid Replacement."[136] Notice several key points on fluid consumption:

- Emphasize fluid intake before exercise by drinking adequate fluids during the day before the event, and drink about 500 ml 2 hours before exercise.

Individuals who exercise heavily should make a conscious effort to ingest adequate volumes of fluid throughout the day. Often, the amount of fluid is beyond what is desired. For example, in one study of soccer players in Puerto Rico, players were randomly allocated to a week of voluntary hydration (2.7 L/day of fluid) or a week of hyperhydration (4.6 L/day).[158] Total body water was increased in the athletes forcing down extra fluids and was associated with improved sport performance. The ACSM recommends that fluids be readily available during meal consumption because most people rehydrate during and after meals. To avoid or delay dehydration during exercise, the ACSM recommends that about ½ liter of water be ingested 2 hours before exercise. The 2-hour limit allows the kidneys to adjust total body water stores at optimal pre-exercise levels. Individuals are urged to pay attention to the color, volume, and smell of their urine.[136,137,159] A well-hydrated person excretes a good volume of urine that is light yellow in color (i.e., more like lemonade than the apple-juice-colored urine of a dehydrated person) and without a strong smell.[137]

- Athletes should start drinking early and at regular intervals during exercise to replace nearly all the water lost through sweating.

Avoiding dehydration during exercise is critical. Without adequate fluid replacement during prolonged exercise, rectal temperature and heart rate are elevated above normal levels, impairing performance, and if continued long enough, leading to potentially life-threatening heatstroke.[136,137] Fluid intake must be above the thirst perception and must match

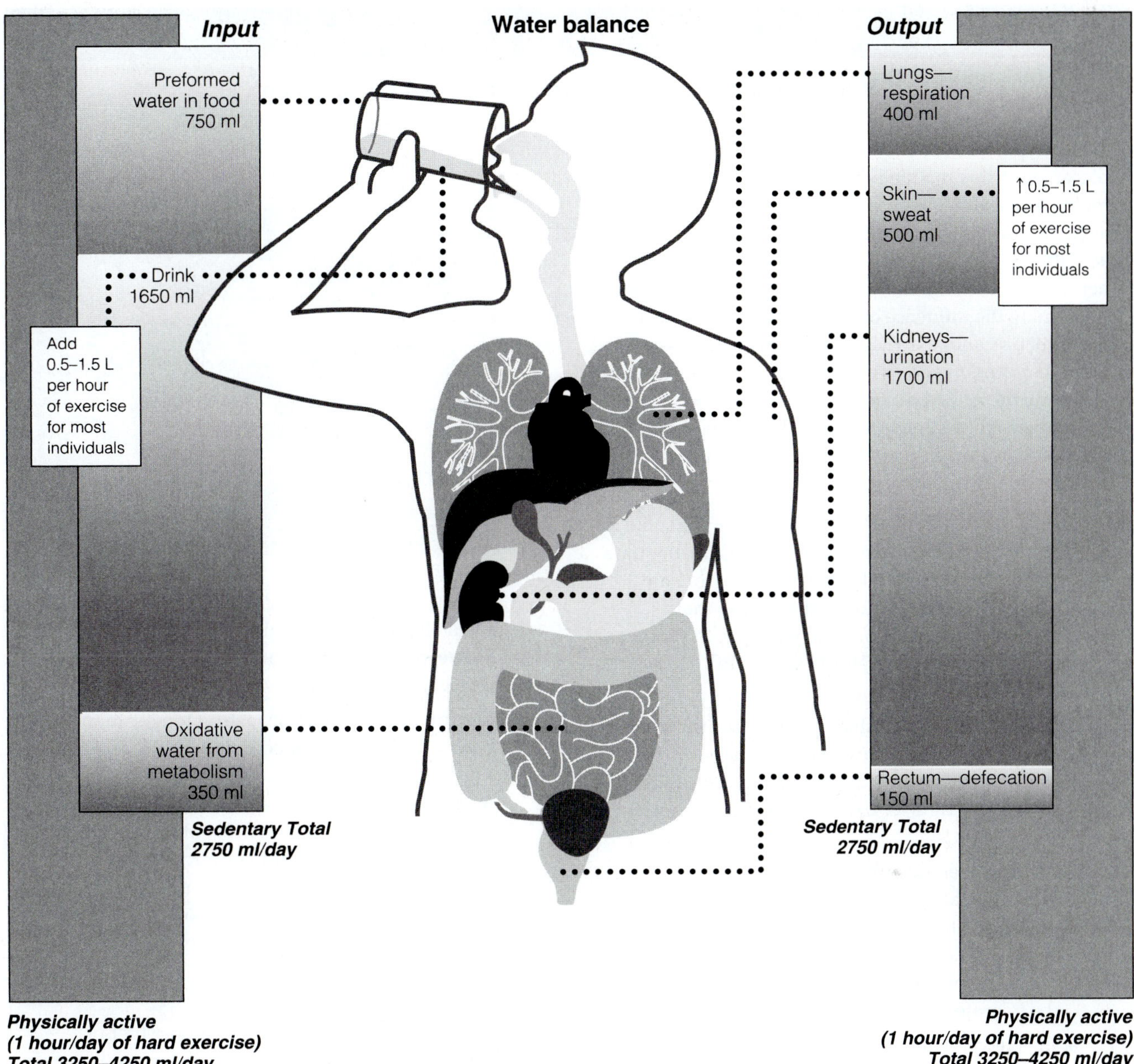

Figure 9.23 Water balance in a sedentary man. Physically active people must increase fluid intake to match sweat rates that are typically between 0.5 and 1.5 L/hour of exertion. Source: Institute of Medicine. *Dietary Reference Intakes for Water, Potassium, Sodium, Chloride, and Sulfate.* Food and Nutrition Board. Washington, DC: The National Academies Press, 2004.

body weight reduction in fluids (1 pint of fluid per pound of weight reduction). For most individuals, matching fluid intake with sweat loss can be accomplished by drinking 0.5–1 cup of water every 10–15 minutes of exercise. For sweat rates above 1.5 L/minute, 1–2 cups of water should be ingested every 10 minutes.[137]

The rate at which the fluid leaves the stomach to be absorbed in the intestine depends on many factors, such as the exercise intensity and the temperature, volume, and composition of the ingested fluid. The most important factor influencing gastric emptying is the fluid volume in the stomach.[136] When gastric volume is maintained at 600 ml or more, most individuals can empty more than 1,000 ml per hour, even when the fluids contain 4–8% carbohydrate concentration. It is advantageous to maintain the largest volume of fluid that can be tolerated in the stomach during exercise (e.g., 400–600 ml).[160] Mild-to-moderate exercise appears to have little or no effect on gastric emptying, whereas heavy exercise at intensities above 80% of maximal capacity may slow gastric emptying.

- Ingested fluids should be cooler than ambient temperature and flavored to enhance palatability and promote fluid replacement.

The ACSM recommends that fluid replacement beverages be sweetened, flavored, and cooled to between 15° and 21°C to stimulate fluid intake.[136,161] Fluids and drinking

Box 9.6

ACSM Position Stand on Exercise and Fluid Replacement

It is the position of the ACSM that adequate fluid replacement helps maintain hydration and, therefore, promotes the health, safety, and optimal physical performance of individuals participating in regular physical activity. This position statement is based on a comprehensive review and interpretation of scientific literature concerning the influence of fluid replacement on exercise performance and the risk of thermal injury associated with dehydration and hyperthermia. Based on available evidence, the ACSM makes the following general recommendations on the amount and composition of fluid that should be ingested in preparation for, during, and after exercise or athletic competition:

1. It is recommended that individuals consume a nutritionally balanced diet and drink adequate fluids during the 24-hour period before an event, especially during the period that includes the meal prior to exercise, to promote proper hydration before exercise or competition.
2. It is recommended that individuals drink about 500 ml (about 17 ounces) of fluid about 2 hours before exercise to promote adequate hydration and allow time for excretion of excess ingested water.
3. During exercise, athletes should start drinking early and at regular intervals in an attempt to consume fluids at a rate sufficient to replace all the water lost through sweating (i.e., body weight loss), or consume the maximal amount that can be tolerated.
4. It is recommended that ingested fluids be cooler than ambient temperature (between 15° and 22°C [59° and 72°F]) and flavored to enhance palatability and promote fluid replacement. Fluids should be readily available and served in containers that allow adequate volumes to be ingested with ease and with minimal interruption of exercise.
5. Addition of proper amounts of carbohydrates and/or electrolytes to a fluid-replacement solution is recommended for exercise events of duration greater than 1 hour because it does not significantly impair water delivery to the body and may enhance performance. During exercise lasting less than 1 hour, there is little evidence of physiological or physical performance differences between consuming a carbohydrate–electrolyte drink and plain water.

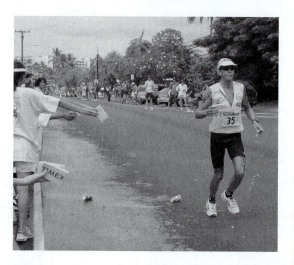

6. During intense exercise lasting longer than 1 hour, it is recommended that carbohydrates be ingested at a rate of 30–60 grams/hour to maintain oxidation of carbohydrates and to delay fatigue. This rate of carbohydrate intake can be achieved without compromising fluid delivery by drinking 600–1,200 ml/hour of solutions containing 4–8% carbohydrates (g/100 ml). The carbohydrates can be sugars (glucose or sucrose) or starch (e.g., maltodextrin).
7. Inclusion of sodium (0.5–0.7 gram per liter of water) in the rehydration solution ingested during exercise lasting longer than 1 hour is recommended because it may be advantageous in enhancing palatability, promoting fluid retention, and possibly preventing hyponatremia in certain individuals who drink excessive quantities of fluid. There is little physiological basis for the presence of sodium in an oral rehydration solution for enhancing intestinal water absorption, as long as sodium is sufficiently available from the previous meal.

Source: Data from American College of Sports Medicine. Position stand on exercise and fluid replacement. *Med Sci Sports Exerc* 28:i–vii, 1996.

containers should be readily available. Overall, several practical recommendations to encourage fluid intake include the following:[137]

- Do whatever it takes to make it easy to drink during physical activity (stash bottles in the bushes along a run course, have a friend on a bike hand you fluid on a long run, crush the top of a paper cup to form a small spout to make drinking easier during exercise, carry money to buy fluid, use a bottle belt to carry fluid, know where to find fluid from water fountains or convenience stores, practice drinking during exercise).
- Start prehydrating the day before a long race or training session.
- Make sure the urine is light-colored before exercising.
- Drink 8–16 fluid ounces (1–2 cups) in the 2 hours before exercise.
- Have plenty of fluid on hand during meals.
- Part of staying well-hydrated during exercise in the heat is to reduce sweat loss. Limit the intensity and duration of warm-up exercises, wear white, lightweight clothing, and get out of the sun when possible.
- During a race, make time to drink.
- Speed gastric emptying by drinking frequently to keep a comfortably full stomach.

Can body temperature be controlled and dehydration prevented by wetting the head and skin during exercise? Although this may be psychologically pleasing, researchers have found that skin wetting does not reduce sweat rates or reduce core body temperature.[137,162] It is far better to drink the water.

Should Electrolytes and Carbohydrates Be Used during Exercise?

A wide variety of sports drinks are available, containing varying levels of electrolyte and carbohydrate (see Table 9.13). There are three reasons for using these drinks:[136,137,163–172]

1. To avoid dehydration
2. To counter the loss of electrolytes
3. To oppose the loss of body carbohydrate stores

Should electrolytes (sodium, potassium, and chloride) be added to the exercise drink? The electrolyte content of sweat is relatively very low. One liter of sweat has 400–1,000 mg of sodium, 500–1,500 mg of chloride, and 120–225 mg of potassium.[172] Although sodium, chloride, potassium, magnesium, calcium, zinc, and some vitamins are excreted with the sweat, most studies have shown that such losses are rarely significant for properly nourished and acclimatized people. Electrolytes are very easily obtained in the diet—1 teaspoon of salt has 2,000 mg of sodium and 3,000 mg of chloride, while 1 cup of orange juice has 500 mg of potassium. In particular, athletes are very unlikely to develop sodium chloride deficiency, even with high sweat rates, because training develops adaptive mechanisms that conserve salt.

There are exceptions to this in extreme endurance events. Low levels of sodium (hyponatremia) have been measured in ultramarathoners and Ironman triathletes.[136,173] If large quantities of plain water are consumed during exercise exceeding 4–6 hours duration, low blood sodium levels (< 135 mEq/L) become a concern. Symptoms include confusion, loss of coordination, extreme muscle weakness, and in severe cases, convulsions and coma. Therefore, athletes engaging in events lasting longer than 4 hours are urged to drink fluids containing electrolytes and to avoid overdrinking of plain water.

The addition of small amounts of sodium to a sports drink enhances palatability, helping people take more fluids during and after exercise. Also fluids with sodium in them lead to less urination than plain water and attenuates the decline in plasma volume during exercise.[136,167,174] Most sports drinks include small amounts of electrolytes for these reasons (see Table 9.13). Sodium does not enhance intestinal fluid absorption, however, or improve endurance performance. The ACSM recommends that 0.5–0.7 gram of sodium be added to each liter of sports drink[136] (see Box 9.6).

Although the results of earlier studies suggested that solutions with more than 2.5% glucose slowed the rate of passage of the fluid through the stomach, recent gastric-emptying studies conducted during 2–4 hours of exercise show that 4–8% CHO solutions, regardless of CHO type,

TABLE 9.13 A Comparison of Leading Sports Drinks (per Cup or 8 Fluid Ounces)

Sports Drink	Type of Carbohydrate	Carbohydrate Concentration (%)	Sodium (mg)	Potassium (mg)	Calories
All Sport	High fructose corn syrup	8	55	55	70
Gatorade	Sucrose / glucose / fructose	6	110	30	50
Powerade	High fructose corn syrup / glucose polymers	8	55	30	70
Orange juice	Fructose / sucrose / glucose	10	6	436	104
Coca-Cola	High fructose corn syrup / sucrose	11	6	0	103

can be emptied from the stomach at rates similar to water.[136,137,164] Overall, the gastrointestinal tract appears capable of delivering up to 1.2 liters of fluid and 72 grams of CHO each hour of exercise, enough to match the needs of most athletes.[165]

Beverages containing simple sugars or glucose polymers (4–6 glucose units) with small amounts of electrolytes minimize disturbances in temperature regulation and cardiovascular function as well as ordinary water, maintain blood glucose levels better than water, and enhance athletic performance more than water. Carbohydrate enhances performance in high-intensity endurance events lasting 1 hour or longer and preserves central nervous system function.[175–178] Sports drinks that contain 4–8% CHO of glucose polymer, glucose, or sucrose in volumes of 200–400 ml consumed every 15–20 minutes are preferable to plain water.[169] A total of 30–60 grams of CHO (120–240 Calories) during each hour of exercise appears to be optimal and is found in 1 liter of most sports drinks.[136] Some research suggests that fructose can cause gastrointestinal distress and may compromise performance, so this type of sugar should be avoided. Fructose is absorbed more slowly than other sugars from the gut and then must be converted into glucose by the liver, limiting the amounts that can be absorbed and metabolized.[171,179] Recent evidence, however, suggests that when fructose is combined with glucose and sucrose, CHO oxidation is higher than when the sports drink only contains glucose.[179]

Figure 9.24 summarizes this information. The importance of CHO in the drink solution lies in its ability to elevate blood glucose levels. Several studies have shown that even when muscle glycogen levels are low, ingestion of CHO solutions during long endurance exercise can counter the drop in blood glucose levels and prolong exercise by as much as 20–30%.[175–178,180,181] The elevated blood glucose levels from the CHO ingestion during exercise can support exercise even at 60–75% $\dot{V}O_{2max}$ levels.

Most athletes prefer to take in sports drinks throughout the event, and this has been shown to be highly effective in improving performance by maintaining blood glucose levels and sparing muscle glycogen levels.[181] Energy bars and gels are also popular sources of CHO. Figure 9.25 shows the results of one study of cyclers in which CHO was consumed every 20 minutes of exercise, prolonging exercise by 1 hour.[182] Runners benefit, too, as shown in Figure 9.26. In this study, runners decreased their 30-kilometer race time by 3 minutes by drinking a 5% CHO solution before and during the event.[180]

In summary, when exercise exceeds 1 hour, the exerciser's fluid, electrolyte, and CHO requirements can be met simultaneously by ingesting 600–1,200 ml per hour of a solution containing 4–8% CHO, and 0.5–0.7 gram/L of sodium[136] (see Box 9.6).

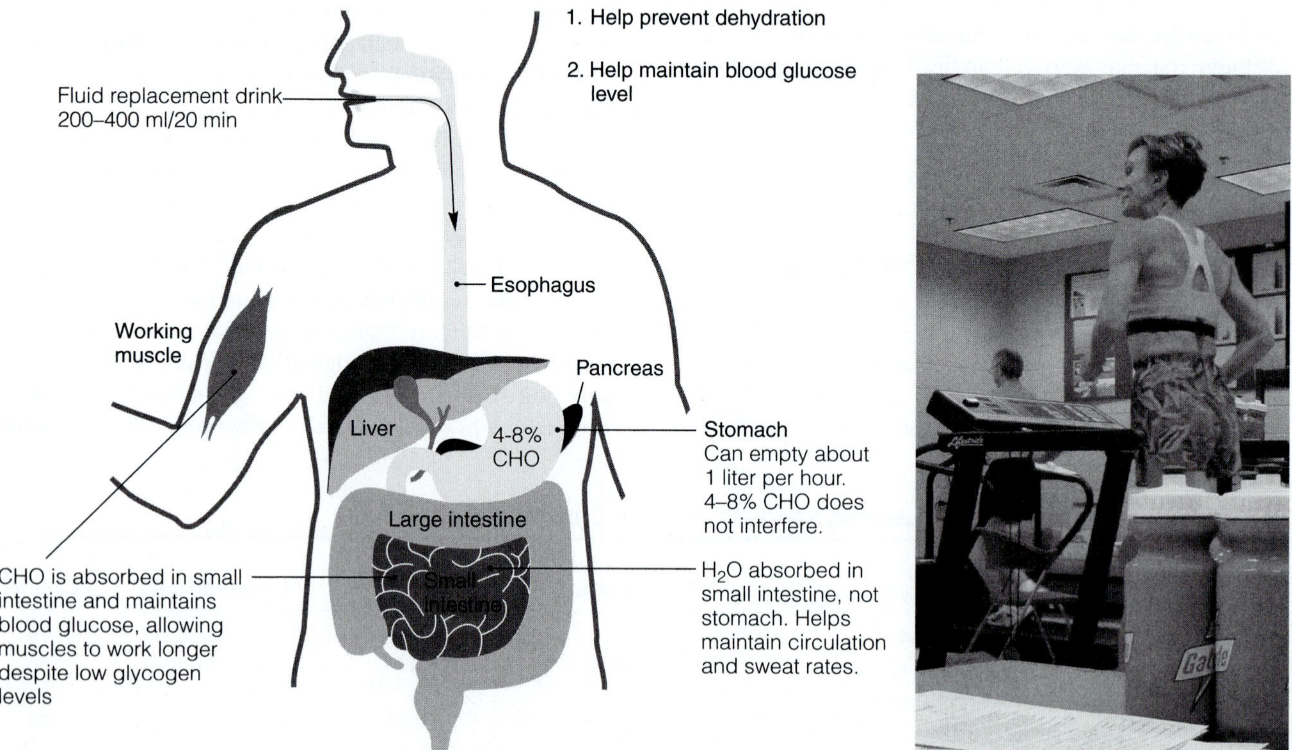

Figure 9.24 Two goals of fluid replacement drinks during exercise. There are two primary goals of fluid replacement during exercise: (1) to prevent dehydration; (2) to help maintain blood glucose levels.

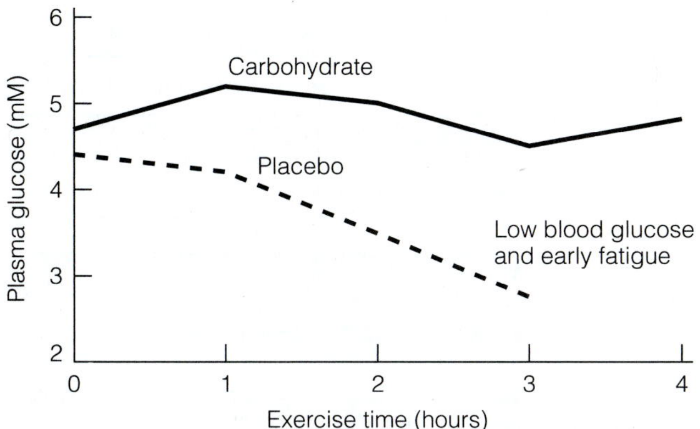

Figure 9.25 Sports drinks improve long-term endurance. Cyclers were able to prolong their exercise time by 1 hour by drinking fluids with sugar every 20 minutes during the event. Source: Data from Coyle EF, Coggan AR, Hemmert MK, Ivy JL. Muscle glycogen utilization during prolonged strenuous exercise when fed carbohydrate. *J Appl Physiol* 61:165–172, 1986.

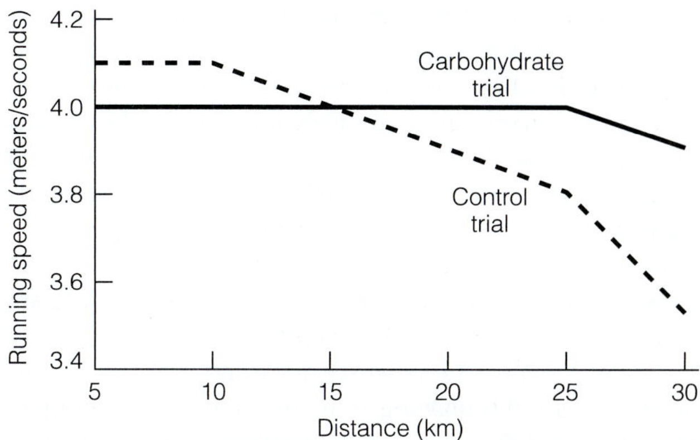

Figure 9.26 Carbohydrate intake improves 30-km race time: 250 ml 5% CHO prior to race, 150 ml/5 km. Total race time: CHO trial = 128 ∓ 19.9; Control = 131.2 ∓ 18.7 min. Runners were able to maintain their race pace longer during a 30-km run by using a sports drink. Source: Data from Tsintzas K, Liu R, Williams C, Campbell I, Gaitanos G. The effect of carbohydrate ingestion on performance during a 30-km race. *Int J Sport Nutr* 3:127–139, 1993.

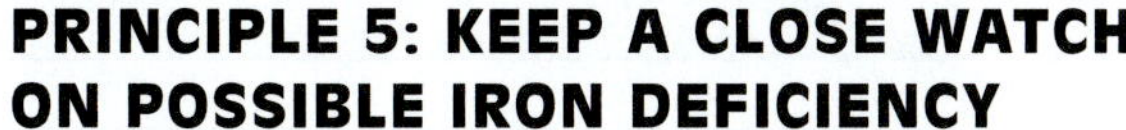

PRINCIPLE 5: KEEP A CLOSE WATCH ON POSSIBLE IRON DEFICIENCY

A number of athletes, especially elite female endurance athletes, test positive for mild iron deficiency, best measured by evaluating serum ferritin levels. On the other hand, very few athletes reach a state of anemia, which is measured when the hemoglobin falls below 12 mg/dl for females and 13 mg/dl for males. In general, fitness enthusiasts do not usually need to be concerned with iron deficiency because moderate amounts of exercise have not been linked to this problem.

The Problem of Iron Deficiency

Endurance athletes, especially females, may be prone to iron deficiency.[183–190]

In the human body, iron is present in all cells and has several vital functions. Too little iron can interfere with these vital functions and lead to morbidity and mortality. Iron has these functions:[183]

- Carrier of oxygen to the tissues from the lungs in the form of hemoglobin
- Facilitator of oxygen use and storage in the muscles as myoglobin
- Transport medium for electrons within the cells in the form of cytochromes
- Integral part of enzyme reactions in various tissues

Iron deficiency is the most common known form of nutritional deficiency. Its prevalence is highest among young children and women of childbearing age (particularly pregnant women).

Iron is the most abundant trace element in the cellular metabolism of all living species and is required for growth. Total body iron averages approximately 3.8 grams in men and 2.3 grams in women, which is equivalent to 50 mg per kilogram of body weight for a 75-kg man and 42 mg per kilogram of body weight for a 55-kg woman.[183] In healthy adults, most iron (>70%) is classified as functional iron, and the remainder is classified as storage or transport iron. More than 80% of functional iron in the body is found in the red-blood-cell mass as hemoglobin, and the rest is found in myoglobin and intracellular respiratory enzymes. Iron is stored in the body in the form of ferritin and hemosiderin in the liver, bone marrow, spleen, and skeletal muscle, and can be used for the formation of hemoglobin and myoglobin when needed. In healthy persons, most iron is stored as ferritin. Small amounts of ferritin circulate in the plasma and correlate with ferritin iron stores. Iron is distributed within the body via transferrin in the plasma. Regulation of iron balance occurs mainly in the gastrointestinal tract through absorption. The normal loss of iron from the body is 1–2 mg/day and is balanced by absorption of dietary iron (which can vary from <1% to >50%, depending on need).

Using serum ferritin levels as a criterion (less than 12 μg/L), between 10% and 80% of female athletes, depending on the study, have been described as having mild iron deficiency. In one review, the prevalence of low serum ferritin concentration averaged 37% in female athletes compared to 23% in untrained female controls.[184]

In nearly all studies, however, it is extremely rare to find that hemoglobin is low (an indication of anemia). Some elite athletes tend to have hemoglobin levels that are somewhat low, but this appears to be due to their expanded plasma volumes and not because of depleted body iron stores.[191,192] Also, iron deficiency has not been a problem for fitness enthusiasts who exercise moderately (20–40 minutes per session, 3–5 sessions per week).[193,194]

Iron deficiency is commonly divided into three stages, which form a continuum, each shading gradually into the other (see Table 9.14 and Figure 9.27).[183,195–197] The first stage is mild iron depletion, which is characterized by decreased or absent iron stores and measured by a drop in plasma ferritin. At this stage, other indices of iron deficiency are normal. Serum ferritin levels below 12 μg/L are associated with very low iron stores.

Stage 2 follows the exhaustion of iron stores and is characterized as a diminishing iron supply to the developing red cell. Iron-deficient *erythropoiesis* (formation of red blood cells) occurs and is measured by increased total iron-binding capacity and reduced serum iron and percent saturation (<16% is abnormal). The red blood cell *protoporphyrin* (a derivative of hemoglobin, which has an atom of iron deleted) increases above normal.[197]

Stage 3 is iron-deficient anemia, characterized by a drop in hemoglobin. Hemoglobin levels below 12 mg/dl for females and 13 mg/dl for males are considered anemic. The range of normal hemoglobin levels is 13–16 mg/dl for men and 12–16 mg/dl for women. During this stage, the bone marrow produces an increasing number of smaller and less brightly colored red blood cells. This is measured when the mean corpuscular volume (MCV) falls below 80 fl.

Anemia is generally acknowledged to be the most common single nutritional deficiency in both developing and developed countries. In the United States, 3–5% of female teenagers and young adults and less than 1% of males are anemic.[197] In one study of 85 female marathon runners, only 2% were anemic.[198] Another study of 111 runners and 65 inactive females found that 3% in each group were anemic (hemoglobin less than 12 mg/dl).[186] These studies show that anemia is extremely rare among athletes (see Figure 9.28).

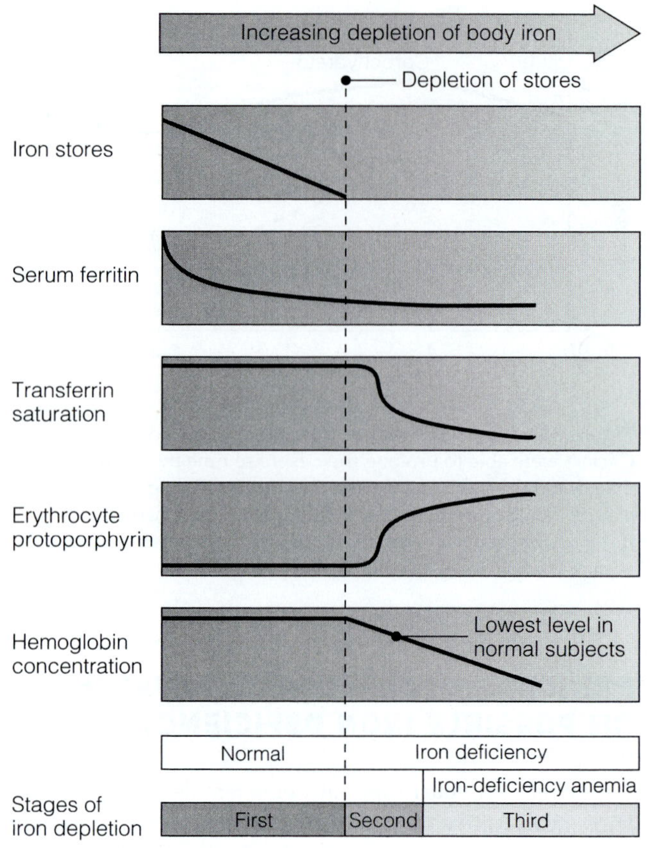

Figure 9.27 Changes in body iron components and laboratory assessments of iron status during the stages of iron depletion. Source: From Life Sciences Research Office, Federation of American Societies for Experimental Biology. *Nutrition Monitoring in the United States: An Update Report on Nutrition Monitoring*. Washington, DC: U.S. Government Printing Office, 1989.

TABLE 9.14 Stages of Iron Deficiency

	Blood Indices* (values indicating deficiency)							
Stage	SF <12 μg/L	FE M <80 μg/dl F <60 μg/dl	TIBC Stage II >390 μg/dl Stage III >410 μg/dl	SAT <16%	HGB M <13 mg/dl F <12 mg/dl	RBC	Iron Stores	Iron Absorption
I. Iron-deficient—mild	D	N	N	N	N	N	0	I
II. Iron-deficient erythropoiesis	D	D	I	D	N	N	0	I
III. Iron-deficient anemia	D	D	I	D	D	D†	0	I

*N = normal; D = decrease; I = increase; 0 = none; SF = serum ferritin; FE = serum iron; TIBC = total iron-binding capacity; SAT = transferrin saturation; HGB = hemoglobin; RBC = red blood cells.

†Red blood cells in iron-deficient anemia become small (microcytic) and less red (hypochromic). The amount of RBC protoporphyrin, a derivative of hemoglobin with one atom of iron deleted, increases (>1.24 μmol/L RBC).

Sources: Herbert V. Recommended dietary intakes (RDI) of iron in humans. *Am J Clin Nutr* 45:679–686, 1987; Expert Scientific Working Group. Summary of a report on assessment of the iron nutritional status of the United States population. *Am J Clin Nutr* 42:1318–1330, 1985.

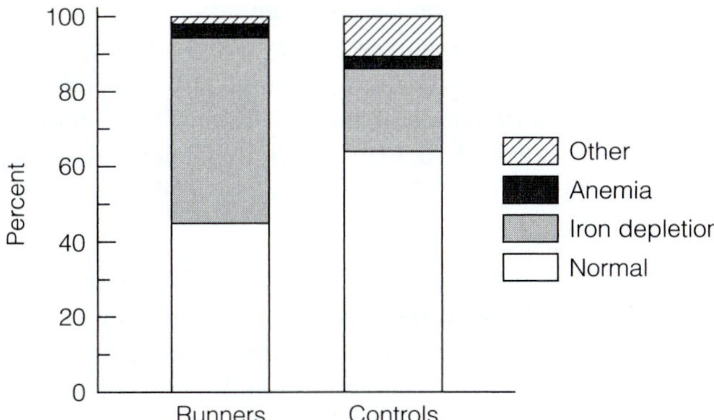

Figure 9.28 Iron status in female runners versus controls. Although female runners tend to have a higher prevalence of iron deficiency compared to inactive controls, anemia is rare. Source: Data from Pate RR, Miller BJ, Davis JM, Slentz CA, Klingshirn LA. Iron status of female runners. *Int J Sport Nutr* 3:222–231, 1993.

Iron is an essential constituent of hemoglobin, myoglobin, and several iron-containing respiratory enzymes, and it plays a vital role in energy production. Relatively small decreases in hemoglobin (1–2 g/dl) have been shown to impair physical performance.[199,200] There is a very close association between the hemoglobin content of the blood and $\dot{V}O_{2max}$.

Although anemia does impair exercise performance, researchers disagree as to whether iron deficiency without anemia is a hindrance. There is a growing consensus, however, that although a significant proportion of athletes has iron deficiency, it has little or no meaningful impact on health or performance.[191,192,201–203] In several studies, for example, when iron-deficient subjects are put on iron therapy, plasma ferritin concentrations rise, but exercise performance is not affected.[204–208] Other studies, however, suggest that iron deficiency without anemia impairs endurance capacity and the ability to favorably adapt to aerobic exercise.[188,209] The high prevalence of iron deficiency among female athletes has led to a large number of investigations seeking to determine the causes.[184,209–217] Three major factors have been researched:

1. *Inadequate dietary iron.* The average Western diet supplies about 7–8 mg of iron per 1,000 Calories (see Table 9.2). Several studies measuring the diets of female athletes have shown that a significant proportion consumes less than the RDA of 18 mg.[184] Also, some female athletes are very conscious of their weight and eat too few Calories or avoid red meat (a rich source of iron), putting themselves at risk for iron deficiency.[184,191] Blood losses due to menstruation and low dietary iron intake are the most important reasons for the high prevalence of iron deficiency among female athletes.[189]
2. *Increased hemolysis.* Several studies suggest that exercise causes an accelerated destruction of red blood cells.[210,211,215] The breakdown of red blood cells inside the capillaries (measured by a decrease in blood haptoglobin), together with kidney excretion of hemoglobin may contribute to the low iron states reported among athletes. Some researchers have attributed this to the mechanical trauma imposed on the capillaries of the feet from running.[211] Other factors may include elevated body temperatures, increased blood flow, acidosis, and the effects of catecholamines. However, only trace amounts of iron can be lost through this route, and it cannot be considered a major factor of iron deficiency.[191]
3. *Increased iron loss in sweat and feces.* Some iron is lost in sweat but the amounts are extremely small and unlikely to cause iron deficiency.[184,212] Running (especially when racing) has been found to induce some gastrointestinal bleeding, which can be measured in the feces.[184,213,214] In the long run, this may occasionally lead to iron deficiency.[213] A thorough examination of the GI tract, especially the colon, is standard practice and may be recommended for some athletes with unexplained anemia.[216]

Practical Implications for Athletes

The so-called sports anemia is for most athletes a false anemia, in that their expanded plasma volumes dilute the blood, lowering hemoglobin concentrations. A very small percentage of athletes develop true anemia when iron losses exceed iron intake and absorption. Also, a significant proportion have iron deficiency without anemia, which probably has little effect on performance but still should be treated to improve body iron stores.

The U.S. Olympic Committee feels that all elite female athletes should have their hemoglobin checked at least once a year.[218] If abnormal, 3–6 months of iron therapy is recommended for menstruating females. If therapy is unsuccessful, a thorough medical evaluation is recommended, including a stool guaiac to check for GI bleeding and lab tests for iron status (serum ferritin, iron-binding capacity, erythrocyte protoporphyrin).[219]

It is very difficult to help a person recover from iron deficiency with diet alone.[195] Oral iron therapy must often be considered, consisting of ferrous sulfate and meat supplements.[184] In addition, ascorbic acid can help enhance absorption.[220] However, for some athletes, effective therapy also involves reducing iron losses by decreasing the amount of exercise to more moderate levels.

Despite the prevalence of iron deficiency among runners, iron supplements should not be given routinely to athletes without medical supervision. In addition to the possibility of inducing deficiencies of other trace minerals, such as copper and zinc, a high iron intake can produce an iron overload in

TABLE 9.15 Iron in 1-Cup Portions of Foods

Food	Iron per Cup of Food (mg)
Pumpkin seeds	20.7
Raisin Bran cereal	16.4
Wheat germ	10.3
Sunflower seeds	9.8
Cashews	8.2
Wheat Chex cereal	7.3
Dried apricots	6.1
Grape-Nuts cereal	4.9
Great Northern beans (cooked)	4.9
Soybeans (cooked)	4.9
Almonds	4.8
Peanut butter	4.6
Red kidney beans (cooked)	4.6
Lentils (cooked)	4.2
Prunes	4.0
Blackeye cowpeas (cooked)	3.6
Lima beans (cooked)	3.5
Raisins	3.0
Fish, bass, broiled	2.9
Turkey	2.5
Ham, extra lean	2.1
Lobster	1.9
Tuna	1.5

Note: Although meats have lower concentrations of iron, their iron (heme iron) is more easily absorbed than iron from plant foods (nonheme iron). Vitamin C, however, greatly improves the availability of iron from plant food.

Source: USDA.

some people.[183] In one study of professional road cyclists, high serum ferritin levels were measured due to routine and excessive iron supplementation.[221] High body iron stores have been linked to health complications such as heart disease. Therefore, athletes should be encouraged to increase iron intake by eating foods high in iron. High-iron foods include fortified breakfast cereals, dried fruit, legumes, molasses, lean meats, and nuts (see Table 9.15).

Animal tissue has an average of 40% heme iron and 60% nonheme iron, while plant products are composed of 100% nonheme iron. Nonheme iron absorption is enhanced by consuming vitamin C during the meal, and absorption from plant sources is also increased if meat is eaten at the same time. Vegetarian athletes, who may be at special risk for iron deficiency, should be sure to include vitamin C foods with each meal.[222]

PRINCIPLE 6: VITAMIN AND MINERAL SUPPLEMENTS ARE NOT NEEDED

Most studies show that the intake of major vitamins and minerals by people who exercise is above recommended levels. People who exercise are at an advantage because they tend to eat more than sedentary people, thereby providing their bodies with more vitamins and minerals beyond the extra demands of their exercise. The American College of Sports Medicine, American Dietetic Association, and Dietitians of Canada have made the following joint statement:

> In general, no vitamin and mineral supplements should be required if an athlete is consuming adequate energy from a variety of foods to maintain body weight. If an athlete is dieting, eliminating foods or food groups, is sick or recovering from injury, or has a specific micronutrient deficiency, a multivitamin/mineral supplement may be appropriate. No single nutrient supplements should be used without a specific medical or nutritional reason (e.g., iron supplements to reverse iron deficiency anemia).[2]

Although a nutritional deficiency can impair physical performance and can cause several other detrimental effects, there is no conclusive evidence of performance enhancement with intakes in excess of the recommended levels.

There is considerable misinformation and exaggeration regarding the relationship between vitamins and minerals, and exercise.[2,184,223–228] Coaches' magazines, popular fitness journals, and training table practices of sports superstars send the message that high levels of vitamins and minerals are needed as an energy boost, to maximize performance, to compensate for less-than-optimal diets, to meet the unusual nutrient demands induced by heavy exercise, and to help alleviate the stress of competition. Advocates of supplementation have exaggerated the needs for all 14 recognized vitamins and have even created some new ones, such as pangamic acid and vitamin B_{15}.

The relationship between vitamins/minerals and exercise can be looked at in two ways:[223]

1. Do vitamin and mineral supplements improve performance?
2. Does exercise impose requirements for vitamins and minerals greater than the amounts obtainable from the diet? (See Figure 9.29.)

Most studies that have examined the vitamin and mineral contents of athletic diets have found that athletes exceed 67% of the RDA for all vitamins and minerals measured, except for iron in some females. Figure 9.30 shows that male and female Los Angeles marathon runners met or exceeded 100% of the RDA for all major nutrients except for vitamin B_6, and iron for women.[78]

Despite what appear to be adequate diets for athletes (mainly because of their high caloric intakes), many athletes feel the need to supplement their diets with vitamins and minerals. Research evidence shows that between 50 and

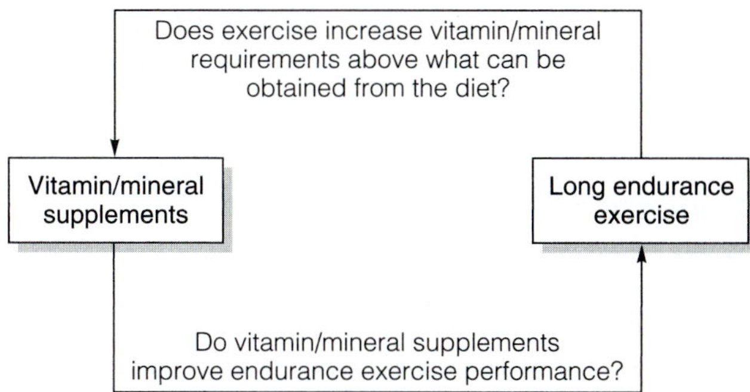

Figure 9.29 Vitamin/mineral–exercise relationship. The relationship between vitamins/minerals and exercise can be looked at in two ways.

90% of elite athletes use vitamin and mineral supplements on a regular basis.[225,229,230] This compares with about 40–47% of the American public, as measured in recent government surveys.[231,232]

The American Medical Association, the American Dietetic Association, the American Institute of Nutrition, the Food and Nutrition Board, and the National Council Against Health Fraud have submitted formal statements to the effect that there are no demonstrated benefits of self-supplementation beyond the recommended dietary allowances except in special cases.[7,232–234] According to the American Dietetic Association, "The best nutritional strategy for promoting optimal health and reducing the risk of chronic disease is to wisely choose a wide variety of foods."[232]

There are several reasons for advising against vitamin and mineral supplementation by athletes. For one thing, research does not support the value of vitamin and mineral supplementation. For another, high intake of supplements may be problematic.

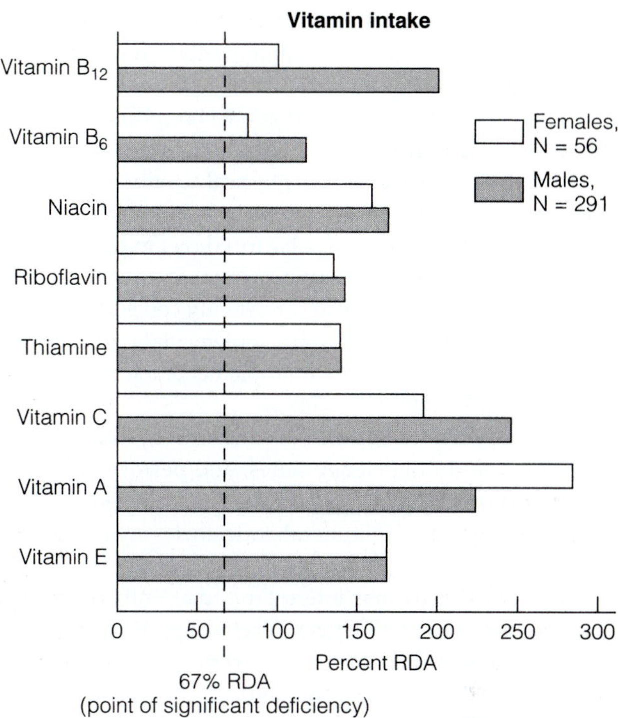

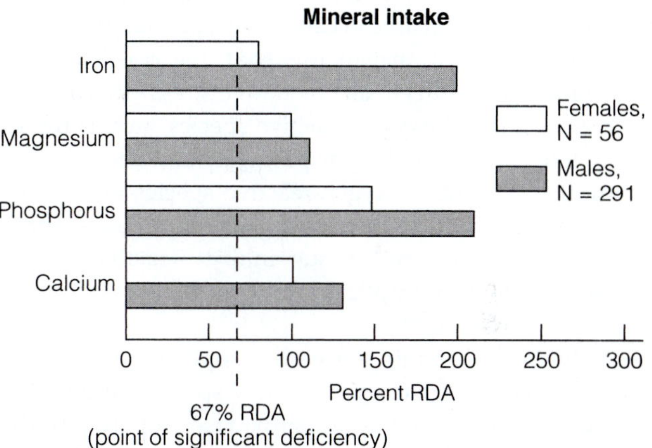

Figure 9.30 In this study of 291 male and 56 female Los Angeles marathon runners, 3-day food records revealed that vitamin (top) and mineral (bottom) intake was adequate except for a slight deficiency of vitamin B_6, and iron for women. Source: Data from Ervin RB, Wright JD, Reed-Billette D. Prevalence of leading types of dietary supplements used in the Third National Health and Nutrition Examination Survey, 1988–94. *Advance Data from Vital and Health Statistics*, 349. Hyattsville, MD: National Center for Health Statistics, 2004.

Lack of Evidence for Benefits

Extensive reviews of the literature have failed to find any convincing support for the role of supplementation in enhancing performance, hastening recovery, or decreasing the rate of injury in healthy, well-nourished adults undergoing athletic training.[62,223–227] After more than 50 years of research, there is no conclusive evidence to suggest that vitamin supplementation improves the performance of adequately nourished people.[184,235–242] For example, in one (double-blind, placebo design) study of 82 athletes from four sports (basketball, gymnastics, rowing, and swimming), 7–8 months of daily supplementation with a high-dose vitamin/mineral tablet failed to affect muscular strength, or aerobic and anaerobic fitness, relative to a control group.[238]

Although heavy endurance exercise is associated with an increased need for many nutrients, including iron, zinc, copper, magnesium, chromium, vitamin B_6, riboflavin, and ascorbic acid, these demands are usually met when the athlete matches energy expenditure through increased consumption of the conventional food supply.[184,223–228,242–248]

In general, when the vitamin and mineral biochemical status of athletes and inactive controls are compared, researchers have concluded that sports training has no negative effect and that supplementation in most instances appears unwarranted.[55,59,247,248]

This approach is supported in a technical support paper from the American Dietetic Association (ADA).[2] The ADA took the position that extended physical activity may increase the need for some vitamins and minerals, but that these could easily be met by consuming a balanced diet in proportion to the extra caloric requirement. Other reviews of the sports-nutrition literature have also consistently concluded that except in special cases (e.g., iron supplementation for anemic athletes), vitamin and mineral supplementation by athletes is unnecessary.[184,185,223–227]

The capacity to exercise is hindered by the development of vitamin-deficiency states, and performance is returned to normal when the deficiency is corrected.[223–227,249] However, vitamin and mineral deficiencies are rare among athletes.[184]

There has been much interest raised recently concerning exercise, generation of oxygen-reactive species or free radicals, and antioxidant nutrients (primarily vitamins E, C, and A, and the mineral selenium).[250–258] During exercise, oxygen consumption can increase 10- to 20-fold compared to rest. Due to various means (which are still being researched, e.g., increases in catecholamines, lactic acid, hyperthermia, and transient hypoxia), the rise in oxygen consumption results in an "oxidative stress" that leads to the generation of oxygen-reactive species such as the superoxide radical, hydrogen peroxide, and the hydroxyl radical.[250,251] These oxygen-reactive species are defined as molecules or ions containing an unpaired electron, which cause cell and tissue injury. Reactive oxygen species have been implicated in certain diseases and in the aging process.[250–253]

The body is equipped with a sophisticated defense system to scavenge oxygen-reactive species. Antioxidant enzymes (e.g., glutathione peroxidase, superoxide dismutase, catalase) provide the first line of defense, with antioxidant nutrients providing a second line of defense.[250] Because strenuous and prolonged exercise promotes production of oxygen-reactive species, considerable concerns have been raised among experts regarding the ability of the body to cope with the increased oxidative stress.[253]

Most studies have shown that chronic physical training augments the physiological antioxidant defenses in several tissues of the body.[250,256,258] The activities of the various antioxidant enzymes are enhanced by physical training, helping to counter the exercise-induced increase in oxygen-reactive species. In general, antioxidant supplementation does not appear necessary and has not been consistently shown to improve performance, minimize exercise-induced oxidative stress, immuno suppression, and muscle cell damage, or maximize recovery.[256,257] However, until more is known, people who exercise regularly and intensely are urged to ingest foods rich in antioxidants (fruits, vegetables, nuts, seeds, and whole grains) to augment the body's defense system against oxygen-reactive species.[257]

Evidence of Possible Problems with High Intake

There are problems associated with very high intakes of vitamins and minerals. Considerable evidence shows that dietary excess of one nutrient may have a detrimental effect on another.[7,232,259–261] High intakes of specific nutrients, especially fat-soluble vitamins such as A, D, E, and K, can be toxic in themselves and indirectly dangerous because they block the action of other nutrients. See Table 9.1 for upper-level (UL) standards set by the National Academy of Sciences. Excessive intake of water-soluble vitamins can also cause problems. Too much niacin can in time lead to liver toxicity, too much vitamin C to red blood cell hemolysis and impaired white blood cell activity, and too much vitamin B_6 to peripheral nervous system toxicity and muscle weakness.

A deficiency of one nutrient can be caused by an excess of another.[232] For instance, zinc supplementation can reduce copper status; excessive vitamin C decreases copper absorption; high levels of folic acid decrease zinc absorption and may mask symptoms of vitamin B_{12} deficiency; excess fructose decreases copper absorption; large amounts of calcium, phytates, and fiber in the diet cause the formation of insoluble iron, zinc, or copper complexes, making these minerals unavailable for absorption; high doses of vitamin E can interfere with vitamin K action; excess manganese decreases iron absorption.

Increasing evidence indicates that antioxidant supplements are not only ineffective in preventing chronic diseases such as cancer and heart disease, they appear to increase overall mortality rates.[261] In other words, too much of a good thing becomes a definite evil. Water and sunshine are both necessary for life, but excesses of either can kill you. Obviously, it is best to eat a varied diet, for it supplies all of the nutrients in the appropriate amounts.

Some coaches and other leaders still feel that giving supplements is beneficial, even if there is no proven physiological benefit, because the athlete thinks the supplement will help and thus performs better (placebo effect). It would be better to help the athlete believe in something that really works, such as a nutritious, varied diet, high in carbohydrate and liquids, providing both physiological and psychological support.

For the athlete who is poorly nourished (often to "make weight"), the best solution is education to provide a better diet. Supplements can reinforce unhealthy eating habits. Dietary imbalances can get worse in this situation. Thus, every effort must be made to convince athletes that their best nutritional resource for optimum performance is proper eating habits. (See Principle 1 on the "prudent diet.") If an athlete is dieting, eliminating foods or food groups, is sick or recovering from injury, or has a specific micronutrient deficiency, a multivitamin/mineral supplement may be appropriate.[2] No single-nutrient supplements should be used without a specific medical or nutritional reason.

PRINCIPLE 7: PROTEIN SUPPLEMENTS DO NOT BENEFIT THE ATHLETE

Many people who exercise, especially weight lifters, feel that consumption of high-protein foods and protein supplements is necessary to build muscle mass. The average sedentary person should consume 0.8 gram of dietary protein per kilogram of body weight. Highly active people may need 50–125% more than this because 5–15% of the energy required for long endurance exercise or weight lifting comes from protein, and extra protein is needed for muscle protein synthesis. So, should athletes use protein supplements—or should they concentrate on high-protein foods in their diets? Most experts feel that the traditional food supply provides all of the protein needed, even for athletes during active muscle-building phases.

Changes in Protein Metabolism during Exercise

Interest in the influence of dietary protein intake on athletic performance has been evident since the days of the ancient Greeks and Romans. Athletes consumed meat-rich diets in the belief that they would achieve the strength of the consumed animal.

The importance of protein for athletics has been debated since the mid-1880s. In 1842, the great German chemist and physiologist Justus von Liebig reported that the primary fuel for muscular contraction was derived from muscle protein, and he suggested that large quantities of meat be eaten to replenish the supply.[262,263] A number of studies during the late 1800s, which measured urinary urea excretion, failed to confirm his results, however, and the concept became established that changes in protein metabolism during exercise are nonexistent or minimal at best.[262]

However, studies using modern technology and improved techniques have concluded that protein is a much more important fuel source during exercise than was previously thought.

Figure 9.31 summarizes protein/amino acid metabolism.[262,263] Amino acids enter the body's free pools from the diet, from body protein, or from carbons contributed from carbohydrate, fat, and ammonia. Amino nitrogen leaves the free pools to form body protein or exit the body in urine, sweat, and feces. Amino carbons can leave the free pools to form body fat or carbohydrate, or they can exit the body as carbon dioxide.

Exercise has a strong effect on protein/amino acid metabolism.[262–277] Four basic changes in protein metabolism take place with exercise (see Figure 9.32).

1. *Depression followed by increase of protein synthesis.* During exercise (endurance exercise or heavy weight lifting) normal protein synthesis is depressed by 17–70%, depending on the intensity and duration of the exercise. This depression leaves amino acids available as fuel for the working muscle. Later, during recovery, muscle protein synthesis increases, augmenting incorporation of amino acids into muscle protein (hypertrophy).[262,263,265,274,276]

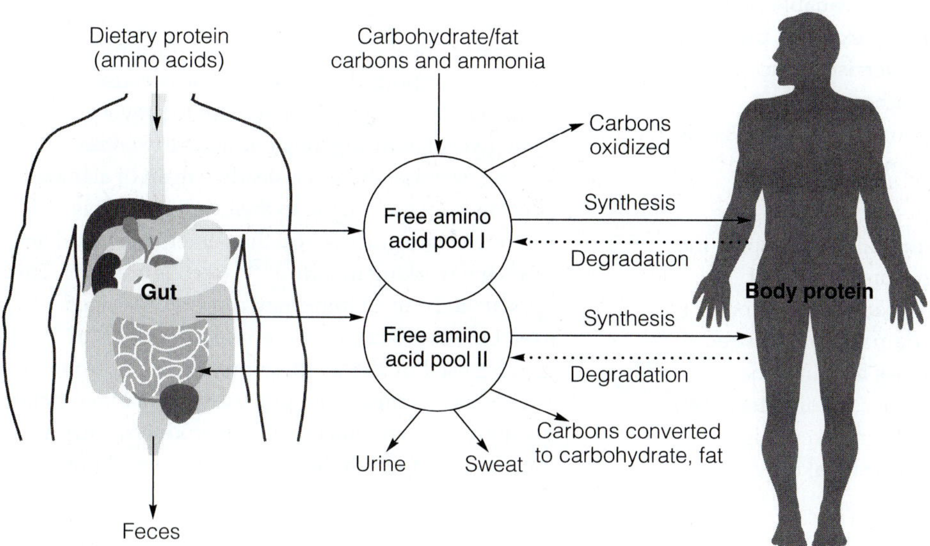

Figure 9.31 Protein/amino acid metabolism. Protein/amino acid metabolism is complex, with amino acids entering and leaving the body's free amino acid pools through several different routes.
Source: Data from Lemon PWR. Protein and amino acid needs of the strength athlete. *Int J Sport Nutr* 1:127–145, 19911 see also *Int J Sport Nutr* 5:S39–S61, 1995.

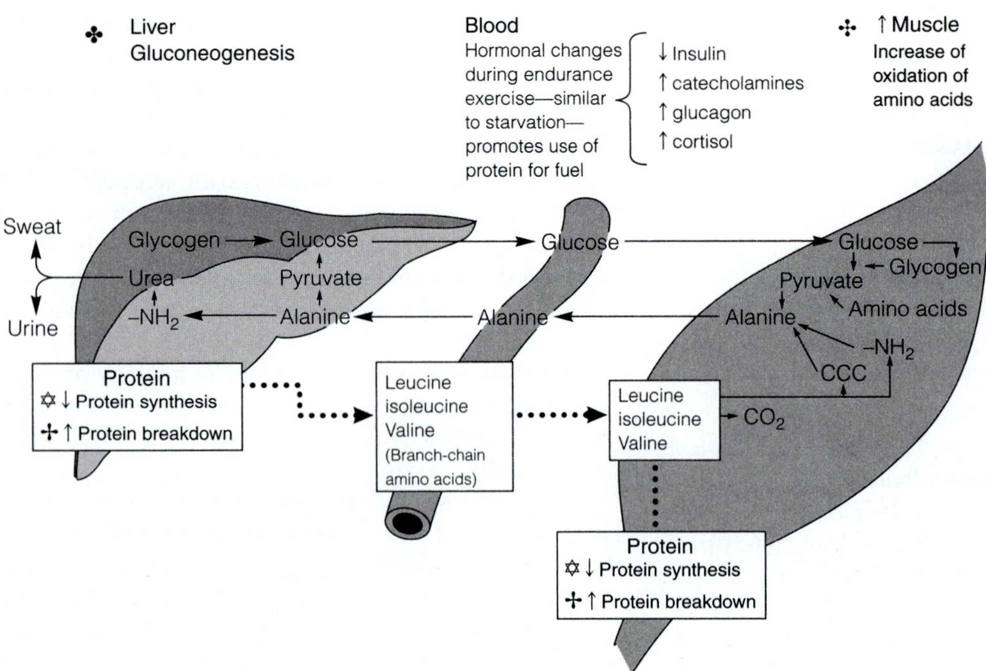

Figure 9.32 Use of protein as fuel during long endurance exercise. This figure summarizes the various pathways by which protein can be used as fuel by the working muscles (see text for an explanation).

The average 70-kg man has 12 kg of protein in his body, nearly half in the actin and myosin myofilaments found in muscle. The body depot of protein is highly labile, with some 200–500 grams (50 grams of nitrogen) of new protein being synthesized every day, and only 10 grams/day of nitrogen excreted. Five tons of protein are thus synthesized in one's lifetime, while total dietary protein intake is only 1 ton, indicating the extensive reutilization of body amino acids. For young adults, muscle accounts for 25–30% of total body protein turnover.

The fact that exercise temporarily interrupts this protein turnover and synthesis is very important, making amino acids immediately available for fuel (Figures 9.31 and 9.32). Following exercise, protein synthesis is accelerated. Thus exercise induces increases in muscle protein synthesis and breakdown (i.e., muscle protein turnover) that is the metabolic basis for cell repair and maintenance in young and old muscle.[276]

2. *Increased muscle breakdown.* Most studies support the concept that exercise leads to a breakdown of muscle protein.[266,268,269] Hard exercise appears to cause significant muscle cell damage that can be measured when muscle enzymes leak into the plasma. Also, long-term resistance training has been shown to increase 3-methylhistidine excretion, which is a marker for myofibrillar breakdown.[262]

With the combination of reduced muscle protein synthesis and increased muscle protein breakdown, more amino acids are available in the body for fuel during exercise and the repair and buildup of muscle cells after exercise.

3. *Increase in amino acid oxidation.* During rest, 10–20% of ATP regeneration comes from protein. Exercise increases the rate of amino acid oxidation.[264,266,275] During cycling exercise, for example, there is a 240% increase in leucine oxidation, with a 21% decrease in leucine synthesis. There is some indication that male endurance athletes may oxidize leucine at a greater rate than female athletes.[262,263]

4. *Increase in gluconeogenesis.* Sixteen of the amino acids that are in the human body can be changed into glucose by the liver. This gluconeogenic process is extremely important during exercise because it can contribute to the supply of glucose to prevent hypoglycemia during long endurance exercise. During exercise, there is a steady stream of alanine passing from the muscle to the liver, where it is converted into glucose and then enters the blood and feeds the working muscle[262,263] (see Figure 9.32). This appears to be most important during prolonged exercise. After 3 hours of exercise, about 60% of glucose used by the working muscle comes from the liver, which is producing glucose from alanine, lactate, glycerol, and other metabolic by-products. Fatty acids are also an important fuel under these conditions.

The increase in liver gluconeogenesis during long endurance exercise and the use of protein for fuel is probably hormonally controlled.[262,263] Exercise causes several changes in blood hormone levels, including a decrease in insulin and increases in catecholamines (epinephrine and norepinephrine), glucagon, and cortisol. These hormonal changes are similar to what happens during starvation (which tends to increase the use of protein for fuel). Endurance exercise and heavy weight lifting cause a transient increase in the use of protein, which is somewhat analogous to the changes caused by starvation.

Practical Implications for Athletes

The practical advice in light of this information is still conjectural. The contribution of protein as an energy source during endurance training is about 3–10% (instead of next to nothing, as previously thought). The actual amount of protein utilized during such exercise depends on the intensity, duration, and fitness status, with long, hard exercise by trained athletes leading to the greatest protein utilization.[262,263]

The current protein RDA is insufficient for both strength and endurance athletes.[262,263] The American Dietetic Association has advised that endurance athletes take in 1.2–1.4 g/kg body weight per day, and strength-trained athletes up to 1.6–1.7 g/kg per day. For some athletes who restrict calories (e.g., wrestlers, gymnasts, female runners), protein needs may be greater because protein will be used to meet energy needs.[262,263] Adequacy of energy intake is paramount when determining absolute protein need (see Table 9.16).

Most endurance athletes are already getting this much protein and do not need to supplement their diets with protein powder or concern themselves with eating high-protein foods. Table 9.11 demonstrates that even on a high-carbohydrate diet with relatively little meat and few dairy products, protein intake is still 116 grams, or 13% of total caloric intake. See Table 9.17 for a list of the protein content of common foods. The sedentary public consumes more than 1 gram of protein per kilogram per day, about 16% of total caloric intake.[17] The general public needs to worry more about exercise supplementation than about protein supplementation!

Several studies have carefully measured the amount of dietary protein needed to keep bodybuilders and weight trainers in positive nitrogen balance.[262,270,271,273] Protein is needed to form increased lean body weight, but more than enough is provided by a normal diet. Most strength and power athletes can enhance muscle development when dietary protein intake ranges between 1.4 and 1.7 g/kg.[262] There is no good evidence that very high protein intakes (>2 g/kg per day) are either necessary or beneficial.[262,263]

There is little scientific evidence that amino acid supplementation enhances the physiological responses to strength training when adequate diets are consumed. Recent evidence indicates, however, that ingestion of small amounts of essential amino acids and carbohydrate following resistance exercise has a small but significant effect on stimulating net muscle protein synthesis.[272,275] Thus ingesting proteins immediately after exercise is an effective strategy to help increase muscle size.

As emphasized by the American Dietetic Association, recommended protein intakes can generally be met through diet alone, without the use of protein or amino acid supplements, if energy intake is adequate to maintain body weight. Athletes should be aware that increasing protein intake beyond the recommended level is unlikely to result in additional increase in lean tissue because there is a limit to the rate at which protein tissue can be accrued.[2] Box 9.7 reviews recommendations for the vegetarian athlete.

TABLE 9.16 Estimated Protein Needs According to Exercise Habits

	Calories* (Body weight in kilograms)		Estimated Protein Needs*		
	Males	Females	g/kg body weight per day	Males, g/day	Females, g/day
Average adult	2,800 (80 kg)	2,000 (65 kg)	0.8	64	52
Fitness enthusiasts	2,900 (75 kg)	2,000 (60 kg)	1.0	75	60
Endurance athletes	3,500 (70 kg)	2,600 (58 kg)	1.2	84	70
Team/power athletes	4,500 (100 kg)	3,500 (80 kg)	1.6	160	128

*All protein requirements fall within 15% of total caloric intake.

TABLE 9.17 Choosing the Best Protein Sources*

	Serving Size	Protein, G	Protein, % of Daily Value†	Calories	Total Fat	Saturated Fat
Animal Foods						
Meat, fish, and seafood						
Chicken breast no skin	3 oz	26.4	53	140	3.1	0.9
Tuna, light, canned in water	3 oz	21.7	43	99	0.7	0.2
Swordfish	3 oz	21.6	43	132	4.4	1.2
Atlantic salmon	3 oz	21.6	43	155	6.9	1.1
Shrimp	3 oz	17.8	36	84	0.9	0.2
Dairy and eggs						
Cottage cheese, nonfat	1/2 cup	15.0	30	80	0.0	0.0
Yogurt, low-fat plain	1 cup	12.9	26	155	3.8	2.5
Milk, nonfat	1 cup	8.4	17	86	0.4	0.3
Cheddar cheese	1 oz	7.1	14	114	9.4	6.0
Egg hard-boiled	1	6.3	13	78	5.3	1.6
Plant Foods						
Legumes, nuts, and seeds						
Tempeh	3 oz	16.1	32	169	6.6	0.9
Peanuts	1/3 cup	12.5	25	276	23.4	3.3
Soy nuts	1/3 cup	10.3	21	126	6.7	0.9
Tofu	1/2 cup	10.0	20	94	5.9	0.9
Lentils	1/2 cup	9.0	18	115	0.4	0.1
Peanut butter, smooth	2 tbsp	8.7	17	191	16.8	3.1
Sunflower seeds	1/4 cup	8.2	16	205	17.9	1.9
Red kidney beans	1/2 cup	7.7	15	112	0.4	0.1
Pinto beans	1/2 cup	7.1	14	117	0.4	0.1
Cashews	1/3 cup	7.0	14	247	20.7	4.1
Grains						
Whole-wheat bread	2 slices	6.8	14	172	2.9	0.6
Rolled oats	1/2 cup	6.4	13	154	2.5	0.4
Millet	1/2 cup	4.2	8	143	1.2	0.2
Barley	1/2 cup	3.7	7	135	1.1	0.2
White rice	1/2 cup	2.8	6	134	0.3	0.1
Brown rice	1/2 cup	2.5	5	108	0.9	0.2

*Fruits and vegetables contain fewer than 3 g of protein per serving.
†The Food and Drug Administration's daily value is based on 50 g of protein in a 2,000-Calorie diet.

Source: USDA.

Box 9.7

Special Issues for Vegetarian Athletes

There have been some concerns that the vegetarian athlete is at risk for protein and mineral deficiencies due to lack of meat products in the diet. At an international conference on vegetarian nutrition in 1997 (Loma Linda University, Loma Linda, CA), these and other health issues were addressed. The following conclusions were drawn:

1. *Performance.* The vegetarian diet per se is not associated with improved aerobic endurance performance; however, other benefits make this dietary regimen worthy of consideration by serious athletes.
2. *Carbohydrate intake.* A plant-based diet facilitates a high intake of carbohydrate, which is essential for prolonged exercise.
3. *Potential for suboptimal intake of iron, zinc, and other minerals.* A well-planned vegetarian diet provides the athlete with adequate levels of all known nutrients, although the potential for suboptimal intake of iron, zinc, and trace elements exists if the diet is too restrictive. However, this concern exists for all athletes, vegetarian or nonvegetarian, who have poor dietary habits.
4. *Protein intake.* Although there has been some concern about protein intake for vegetarian athletes, data indicate that all essential and nonessential amino acids can be supplied by plant food sources alone, as long as a variety of foods is consumed and the caloric intake is adequate to meet energy needs.
5. *Antioxidant nutrients.* Athletes consuming a diet rich in fruits, vegetables, and whole grains receive a high intake of antioxidant nutrients, which help reduce the oxidative stress associated with heavy exertion.
6. *Menstrual irregularity.* There has been some concern that vegetarian female athletes are at increased risk for oligo-amenorrhea, but evidence suggests that low energy intake, not dietary quality, is a major cause.
7. *Health benefits.* While the athlete is most often concerned with performance, long-term health benefits and a reduction in risk of chronic disease have been associated with the vegetarian diet. Studies suggest that a combination of regular physical activity and vegetarian dietary practices provide lower mortality rates than the vegetarian diet or exercise alone.

The vegetarian diet per se is not associated with improved aerobic endurance performance. Although some concerns have been raised about the nutrient status of vegetarian athletes, a varied and well-planned vegetarian diet is compatible with successful athletic endeavor.

Source: Nieman DC. Physical fitness and vegetarian diets: Is there a relation? *Am J Clin Nutr* 70(suppl): 570s–575s, 1999.

PRINCIPLE 8: REST AND EMPHASIZE CARBOHYDRATES BEFORE LONG ENDURANCE EVENTS

The preparation during the last few days and hours before the endurance event can mean the difference between success and failure. In this section, the concept of "carbohydrate loading" (or "glycogen loading") is reviewed. The best scheme for endurance athletes preparing for any exercise event lasting longer than 60–90 minutes is to taper off the exercise gradually during the week before the event, while consuming 8–10 g/kg carbohydrate during the 3 days before the event. If the exercise event lasts less than 60 minutes, carbohydrate loading is unnecessary.

The "pre-event meal" is another important consideration. The meal 3–5 hours before the event should be 500–800 Calories of light, low-fiber starch. There are various pros and cons concerning the use of different sugar solutions.

How to Carbohydrate Load before the Big Event

As discussed earlier, the human body has only limited stores of CHO. Exercise training at 60–80% $\dot{V}O_{2max}$ leads to muscle glycogen depletion after 100–120 minutes.[1] Exercise at 80–95% can lead to muscle glycogen depletion even sooner.

Various researchers have therefore tried to manipulate muscle glycogen stores using a combination of the high-CHO diet and varying levels of exercise and rest to increase glycogen levels above normal, in the belief that exercise time to exhaustion could be prolonged.

The original Scandinavian researchers set up a regimen now known as the "classical" method of "muscle glycogen supercompensation." According to this plan, athletes first depleted their muscles of glycogen by eating a low-carbohydrate diet for 3 consecutive days while engaging in intense, prolonged exercise sessions for at least 2 of these days. Next, athletes would "supercompensate" their muscles with glycogen, by resting for 3 days before competition while eating a very high (90%) carbohydrate diet.

This regimen has been found to create muscle glycogen levels as high as 220 mmol/kg wet muscle (with total body CHO stores of more than 1,000 grams).[1,278] Unfortunately, this program causes several undesirable side effects during the depletion phase, including marked physical and mental fatigue, elevation of fat metabolic by-products in the blood (ketosis), low blood sugar levels (hypoglycemia), muscle cell damage, electrocardiographic abnormalities, depression, and irritability.[1,279] In addition, during the high-carbohydrate phase, the athlete often feels heavy and stiff in the legs.

Because of these side effects, researchers have modified the depletion phase.[1,280,281] Instead of 3 days of a low-carbohydrate diet and hard exercise, the modified scheme utilizes a slow tapering of exercise over a 6-day period, without any intensive exercise the day before competition. During the week, the diet should provide more than 8 g CHO/kg (about 70% CHO).[1,282] (See Table 9.11 for a sample menu.) This modified regimen has been found to create muscle glycogen levels of approximately 200 mmol/kg, nearly the same as the old classical method, without the side effects[1] (see Figure 9.33).

With the muscles "loaded" or "supercompensated" with glycogen, endurance athletes are able to maintain their racing pace for longer periods of time. The overall race time is lower, though the pace per mile does not improve. In other words, athletes can maintain speed longer and thus reduce the total time.[1,282–286] In 30-km time trials, for example, carbohydrate-loaded runners are able to run 4–5 minutes faster than when on low-carbohydrate diets.[283,284]

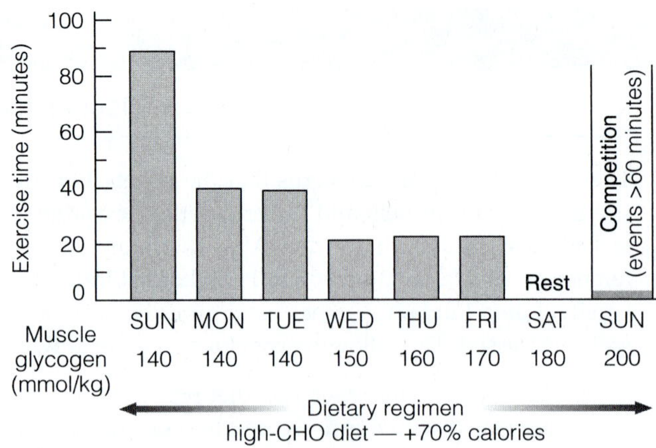

Figure 9.33 Carbohydrate loading with exercise taper. The best scheme for increasing muscle glycogen stores before endurance competition is to consume a high-carbohydrate diet while tapering the exercise to complete rest. Source: Data from Sherman WM, Costill DL, Fink WJ, et al. The effect of exercise diet manipulation on muscle glycogen and its subsequent utilization during performance. *Int J Sports Med* 2:114–118, 1981.

The Pre-Event Meal

The meal before competition can make a difference both physiologically and psychologically. Most sports-nutrition experts advise one or two glasses of water, followed within 20–30 minutes by a light (500–800 Calorie) meal of rapidly digestible, low-fiber starch (e.g., Cream of Wheat hot cereal, white bread, bagels, pasta, refined cereals).[2,3] The food should be consumed 3–5 hours before the event, so that the stomach will be empty at the time of competition to avoid uncomfortable feelings of fullness or cramping. The use of proteins, fats, known gas-forming foods, high-fiber foods, and foods known to act as laxatives is not recommended.[1]

Some athletes feel that drinking sports drinks with sugar 30–60 minutes before hard exertion will enhance performance. Earlier studies examining intakes of glucose or sucrose 30–60 minutes before exercise reported that blood glucose rose sharply, causing an increase in blood insulin concentrations, which then stimulated the muscles to utilize blood glucose. This resulted in rebound low blood sugar levels, and later, accelerated muscle glycogen depletion.[287,288]

More recent studies, however, have not been able to confirm these earlier findings.[289–296] The use of 70- to 80-gram glucose solutions (about 280–320 Calories) 30–60 minutes before endurance performance has not been associated with abnormally low blood glucose levels, increased glycogen depletion, or decreased performance. In fact, some researchers report that a carbohydrate meal 30–60 minutes before exercise increases the amount of glucose available to the working muscle, enhancing endurance performance.[289,290]

In one study of 10 well-trained cyclists, researchers found that the best possible pre-event eating schedule was a 200-gram carbohydrate meal (800 Calories) 4 hours before the event, and a 45-gram carbohydrate snack immediately before high-intensity endurance exercise.[297] Figure 9.34 shows the results of an interesting study comparing a large pre-event carbohydrate meal of 1,300 Calories, to 700 Calories of carbohydrate during the exercise, to both schemes used in combination.[298] Cyclers were able to exercise 44% longer when carbohydrates were used both 3 hours before and during exercise.

Some athletes feel that fasting before long endurance exercise will make them feel lighter and more energetic.[299] In one study, a 1-day fast by male marathon runners resulted in a 45% decrease in endurance performance.[86] Fasting caused significant increases in oxygen uptake, heart rate, rating of perceived exertion, ventilation, and psychological fatigue. In general, the metabolic data appeared to suggest that the responses at the start for the runners who had fasted were like those of the runners who had eaten after 90 minutes of exercise (see Figure 9.35). Most other studies have also shown that fasting causes early fatigue and decreased ability to perform.[299]

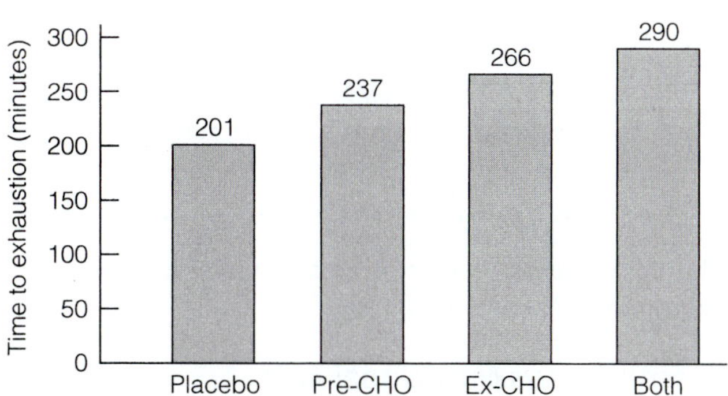

Figure 9.34 Carbohydrate feedings and cycling performance. Three hours prior to exercise, subjects ingested 1,300 Calories as carbohydrate, and during exercise, 700 Calories as carbohydrate. Having carbohydrate in the pre-event meal and during cycling exercise greatly improves endurance time to exhaustion. Source: Data from Wright DA, Sherman WM, Dernbach AR. Carbohydrate feedings before, during, or in combination improve cycling endurance performance. *J Appl Physiol* 71:1082–1088, 1991.

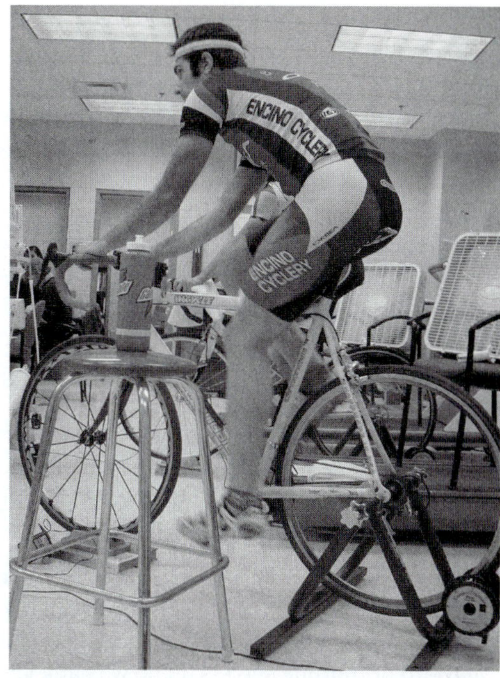

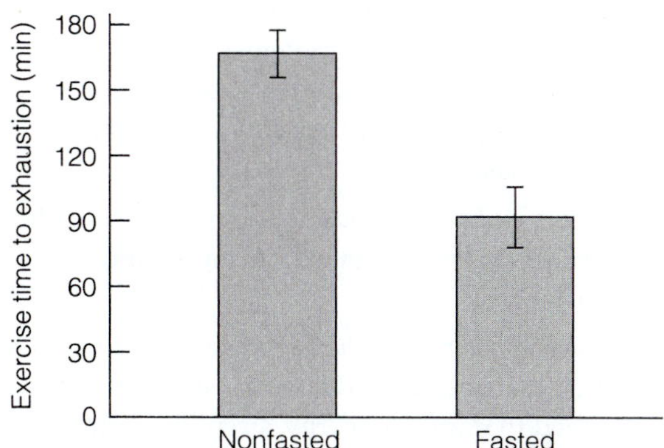

Figure 9.35 The effects of a 1-day fast on running endurance. Fasting for 1 day before long endurance running led to a 45% reduction in exercise time to exhaustion. Source: Data from Nieman DC, Carlson KA, Brandstater ME, Naegle RT, Blankenship JW. Running exhaustion in 27-h fasted humans. *J Appl Physiol* 63:2502–2509, 1987.

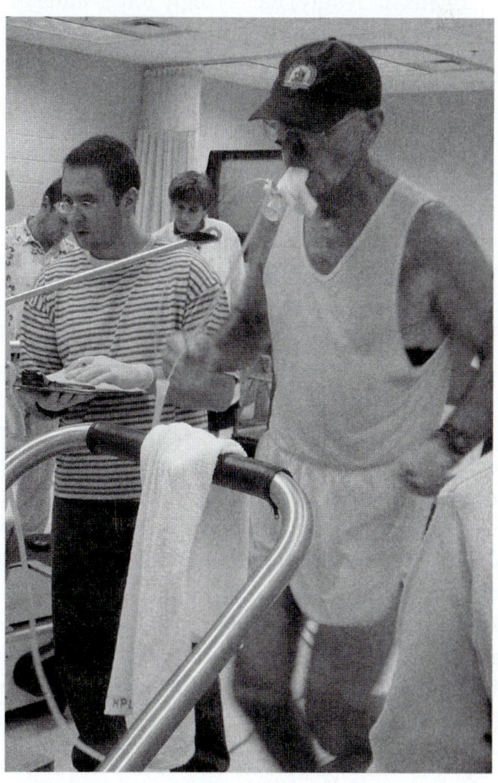

PRINCIPLE 9: USE OF ERGOGENIC AIDS IS UNETHICAL

Ergogenic aids are defined as substances that increase one's ability to exercise harder. Although there are many worthless ergogenic aids (e.g., bee pollen, B_{15} or pangamic acid, alcohol, wheat germ oil, lecithin, kelp, brewer's yeast, phosphates, L-carnitine, and chromium picolinate), others confer impressive benefits (caffeine, sodium bicarbonate, blood doping, steroids, etc.). These may enhance performance, but the ethical issues of equitable competition and fair play claim a higher priority.[300–307]

For thousands of years, warriors and athletes have used a wide variety of substances in the attempt to enhance physical performance.[308] The ancient Greek athletes believed in the value of meat and also consumed special herbs and mushrooms; ancient Muslim warriors used hashish; during World War II, some German soldiers experimented with anabolic–androgen steroid hormones to increase their aggressiveness in combat; American soldiers were given the stimulant amphetamine to improve their endurance and attentiveness; amphetamines became popular among bicycle racers in the 1960s, leading to several deaths; strychnine was used by some of the early prizefighters; and many athletes today use everything from anabolic–androgen steroids to caffeine to doses of blood to improve endurance performance.[308]

Why is the use of drugs and ergogenic aids so pervasive today? This is best answered in a statement made in 1972 by the Medical Commission of the International Olympic Committee.[309]

> The merciless rigor of modern competitive sports, especially at the international level, the glory of victory, and the growing social and economical reward of sporting success (in no way any longer related to reality) increasingly forces athletes to improve their performance by any means available.

As athletic endeavor becomes more competitive and lucrative, many athletes turn to chemical performance enhancement with products such as human growth hormone, anabolic steroids, creatine, beta-hydroxy-geta-methylbutyrate (HMB), amphetamines ("beans" or "greenies"), ephedrine, and androstenedione.[306] Even high school and collegiate athletes are turning to anabolic steroids to gain an advantage. There is increasing usage of and concern over "designer steroids" such as tetrahydrogestrinone (THG) that are chemically modified steroids that are not detected in existing testing protocols.[306] Human growth hormone is widely used despite limited scientific evidence that it improves strength, power, or athletic performance. Amphetamines are the most commonly abused drug in professional baseball.[306] Professional cyclers and other endurance athletes use erythropoietin (EPO). The supplement industry, led by makers of creatine and androstenedione (andro), has become a highly profitable industry. Part of the problem is that regulation of these ergogenic aids is an extremely difficult task. Testing for banned substances requires precise and expensive techniques, and legal resources are necessary to defend test results in court battles that come with suspension of an athlete.

Categories of Ergogenic Aids

The term *ergogenic* means "tending to increase work." Thus ergogenic aids are any substances or methods that tend to increase performance capacity.[300–307] These aids fall into five categories:

1. *Nutritional aids:* carbohydrates, proteins, vitamins, minerals, iron, water, electrolytes, and miscellaneous substances (e.g., bee pollen, B_{15})
2. *Pharmacological aids:* amphetamines, caffeine, anabolic steroids, alcohol, $NaHCO_3$, recombinant erythropoietin (r-EPO)
3. *Physiological aids:* oxygen, blood doping
4. *Psychological aids:* hypnosis, covert rehearsal strategies, stress management
5. *Mechanical aids:* biomechanical aids, physical warm-up

This section reviews some of the more common nutritional and pharmacological aids.

Miscellaneous Nutritional Aids

Athletes are constantly searching for a "performance edge" through the use of dietary supplements, with some taking large amounts of nutrient preparations, far in excess of recommended levels.[310,311] Most studies show that over half of athletes use supplements, with elite athletes using more than college or high school athletes.[311]

A number of nutritional substances are advocated to improve performance. Included are the various vitamins and minerals, and extracts from various foods. (See Principle 6, on vitamin and mineral supplements.)

Nutritional supplements can be organized into eight different classes:[301]

- *Prohormones.* Compounds such as androstenedione, androstenediol, and dehydroepiandrosterone that are purported to increase testosterone, improve recovery, and build muscle mass.
- *Creatine preparations.* Supplements that contain creatine monohydrate and are advertized to improve power performance and build muscle mass.
- *Proteins and amino acids.* Claimed effects include increases in muscle mass, strength, and endurance.
- *Natural and herbal products.* Ginseng, echinacea, saw palmetto, tribulus, and kava kava, which are claimed to improve energy, strength, endurance, and immune function.
- *Diuretics.* Herbal diuretics and stinging nettle, which purportedly prevent water retention, swelling, gout, and high blood pressure.
- *Energy enhancers.* Vitamins, and antioxidants: vanadyl sulfate, taurine, and vitamins, which are postulated to improve recovery, aid in rehydration and glycogen replenishment, and provide added energy.
- *Mental enhancers.* Plant extracts, amino acids, alkaloids (ephedrines and caffeine), minerals, and vitamins that are alleged to modulate mood, boost metabolism, increase adrenaline output, and provide energy and power.
- *Fat burners.* L-carnitine, inositol, and choline that are asserted to increase lean muscle mass and burn fat.

TABLE 9.18 Natural Products and Miscellaneous Nutritional Aids Marketed for Ergogenic Purposes

Product	Claims	Fact
Alcohol	Enhances endurance; alters fatigue; fuel source	Does not enhance endurance; may be ergolytic
Amino acid tablets or capsules	Improves muscle-mass gains, endurance, strength	Most studies show no special benefits
Argentinian bull testes	Potent anabolic agent that increases testosterone	No data to back claims
Arginine/ornithine amino acids	Promotes release of growth hormone and insulin	Studies are inconclusive
Bee pollen	Improves metabolism and endurance performance	Best studies show no effect
Boron	Increases testosterone; strengthens muscles	Best studies show no effect
Branch-chain amino acids	Prevents fatigue during long endurance events	Most studies do not support claim
Carnitine	Fat-loss agent ("cutting"); promotes use of fat for fuel	Insufficient data to back claims
Choline	Increases strength and decreases body fat, delays fatigue	No well-designed studies back claims
Chromium picolinate	Increases insulin activity, increases muscle cell uptake of amino acids, decreases body fat	No good data to support claims
Coenzyme Q10	Enhances aerobic performance	Best studies show no improvement
Creatine	Increases anaerobic power; stimulates muscle growth	Well-designed studies both support claims and show no effect
Dibencozide	Potent anabolic agent; increases oxygen transport	No good support for claims
Gamma oryzanol/ferulic acid	From rice-bran oil; for metabolic activation; anabolic agent	No data to back claims
Ginseng	Weight loss; energy enhancer; improves mental and physical vigor	Limited data to back claims; best studies show no effect
HMB (β-hydroxy-β-methylbutyrate)	Builds muscle size and strength	Limited data are inconclusive
Inosine	Energy enhancer; improves endurance, strength; weight loss	Insufficient data to back claims; may be ergolytic
Lactate supplement	Regular intake promotes lactate clearance during exercise	Studies do not support claim
Ma-huang	Weight loss; energy enhancer; improves strength and endurance	No data to support performance gains
Pangamic acid/vitamin B_{15}	Improves endurance performance	Best studies show no effect
Phosphate salts	Improves endurance performance	Studies are equivocal
Plant sterols	Anabolic agent; increases growth hormone	No support for claims
Pyruvate	Enhances endurance performance, prolonging time to fatigue	No support for claims
Ribose	Enhances high-intensity exercise performance	Best studies show no effect
Smilax compounds	Increases testosterone; improves muscle mass	No support for claims
Sodium citrate	Augments body's buffering capacity, improving anaerobic performance	Best studies show no effect
Tribulus	Enhances blood testosterone, promoting muscle hypertrophy	No support for claims
Tricarboxylic-acid-cycle intermediates	Enhances endurance performance and recovery	Best studies show no effect
Tryptophan	Increases brain serotonin; delays fatigue, resists pain	Best studies show no effect
Vanadyl sulfate	Builds muscle tissue	Best studies show no effect
Yohimbine	Testosterone enhancer	No support for claims

Sources: Based on references 309–337.

Table 9.18 summarizes the ergogenic claims made for a wide variety of natural products and nutritional aids currently available.[309–337] In general, most of the performance claims either are not supported by current research, or research findings have been extrapolated to inappropriate applications. Often, biological functions of some compounds used by the body (e.g., inosine, carnitine, and boron) were amplified as performance claims when used in large-dose supplements.

Bodybuilders and strength athletes are the targets of many companies who push various substances as anabolic agents to "naturally" improve body hormone levels, muscle size, and strength.[338] In one study of 309 male and female bodybuilders, 94% took some type of supplement, and 60% spent $25–$100 each month on supplements.[339] In one review of 250 supplements, only two (HMB and creatine) had published scientific data supporting their use to augment lean mass and strength gains with resistance training.[304] The FDA is cracking down on these companies, and misleading claims and false advertising should diminish. [183] It is hoped that most of these ergogenic products will be tested using appropriate scientific methods (double-blind, placebo controlled) so that truth can be separated from error. The Centers for Disease Control (CDC), in its review of ergogenic aids marketed to bodybuilders, has emphasized that because of false claims, widespread use, and lack of proper labeling guidelines, "unanticipated effects" may occur.[338] The CDC has urged clinicians to report adverse effects of supplement products to appropriate public health authorities.

Despite such evidence, many athletes are convinced that various nutritional substances do lead to improved performance. If these substances have no value, why do athletes continue to use and believe in them? (See Box 9.8 for guidelines in sorting out the hype from the truth.)

The U.S. Food and Drug Administration has concluded that "people are often helped, not by the food or drug being touted, but by a profound belief it will help."[340] In other words, the placebo effect is powerful enough to actually produce a benefit.[341,342] A review of the literature shows that an average of 35% of the members of any group will respond favorably to placebos (with a variation of 0–100%).[341]

The challenge of the health professional working with an athlete is to use this placebo effect to his or her advantage by instilling a "profound belief" in food substances that have proven worth (e.g., carbohydrate, water, and nutritious foods).

The American Dietetic Association (in partnership with the ACSM) has advised health professionals that the 1994

Box 9.8

Tools for Evaluating Research on Dietary Supplements

The following questions represent some of the key points that may be used to sort out the hype from the truth when evaluating research on dietary supplements.

1. Is there a legitimate rationale for the dietary supplement? Theoretically, the dietary supplement should be able to influence physiological processes involved in exercise, or improve body composition.
2. Were appropriate subjects studied? If claims are that the dietary supplement augments a certain type of exercise performance, then subjects who are currently engaging in the specific activity should be selected (e.g., weight lifters vs. bodybuilders, runners vs. swimmers, wrestlers vs. gymnasts).
3. How was exercise performance or changes in body composition evaluated? The exercise or body composition test to evaluate the effect of the dietary supplement should be both valid and reliable.
4. Was a placebo used? The dietary supplement should be provided in the appropriate amount and for an appropriate time period to the experimental group of subjects, but a placebo should be used with a control group of subjects. A dietary supplement may work for some individuals, not because of any bona fide physiological effect, but rather because a psychological placebo effect may modify personal behaviors, which are conducive to modifying exercise performance or body mass.
5. Were the subjects randomly assigned to the treatments? Subjects should be randomly assigned to the dietary supplement or placebo groups. If the study is a crossover design, in which all subjects take both the dietary supplement and the placebo, the order of giving the supplement should be balanced; that is, half of the subjects should take the dietary supplement first, and half take the placebo first. In the second phase of the study, the subjects switch treatments.
6. Was the study double-blind? Neither the subjects nor the investigators interacting with them should know which group receives the dietary supplement or placebo. This is known as a double-blind protocol.
7. Were extraneous factors controlled? Investigators should attempt to control other factors besides the treatment, which may influence exercise performance and body composition. Diet, exercise, and daily physical activities need to be controlled.
8. Were the data analyzed properly? Appropriate statistical techniques should be used to minimize the chance of statistical error.

Well-designed studies published in *peer-reviewed* (reviewed by several other experts) scientific journals serve as the basis for determining the efficacy of dietary supplements. However, a single study does not provide conclusive evidence that a dietary supplement is either effective or ineffective for its stated purpose. The efficacy of dietary supplements must be evaluated by a number of well-designed research studies.

Source: Adapted from Williams M. The gospel truth about dietary supplements. *ACSM's Health & Fitness Journal* 1(1):24–28, 1997.

Dietary Supplement Health and Education Act allows supplement manufacturers to make claims regarding the effect of products on the structure and function of the body, as long as they do not claim to diagnose, mitigate, treat, cure, or prevent a specific disease.[2] In other words, as long as a special supplement label indicates the active ingredients and the entire ingredient list is provided, claims for enhanced performance—be they valid or not—can be made. According to the American Dietetic Association, ergogenic aids can be classified into one of four categories:

- Those that perform as claimed.
- Those that may perform as claimed but for which there is insufficient evidence of efficacy at this time.
- Those that do not perform as claimed.
- Those which are dangerous, banned, or illegal, and consequently should not be used.

Table 9.18 provides a summary of how specific ergogenic aids can be currently classified. Go to www.wada-ama.org for the list of substances and methods prohibited by the International Olympic Committee. The American Dietetic Association and the ACSM have taken the position that "athletes should be counseled regarding the use of ergogenic aids, which should be used with caution and only after careful evaluation of the product for safety, efficacy, potency, and legality."[2]

Use of Caffeine to Improve Performance in Long Endurance Events

Despite the widespread use of caffeinated beverages by Americans, a growing number of studies are providing evidence that this drug is not as benign as once thought.[343–345] Daily caffeine intake has been related to osteoporosis, birth defects, and sleep interference, and this drug exhibits the features of a typical psychoactive substance leading to dependence. Mean caffeine intakes in adults range from 106–170 mg/day (90th percentile intake is 227–382 mg/day).[343] Caffeine is an alkaloid present in more than 60 plant species. Peak plasma levels after ingestion occur within 15–45 minutes, with a plasma half-life ranging from 2.5 to 7.5 hours. The metabolism by the liver, storage, and clearance rate of caffeine may vary greatly between acute and chronic users. Table 9.19

TABLE 9.19 Caffeine Sources

Caffeine Content in Bottled Beverages (mg/12 fl oz)	
Red Bull	116
Full Throttle	100
Java Water	90
Jolt	72
Krank	71
Sun Drop	69
Pepsi One	55
Mountain Dew	55
Mello Yellow	51
Nehi Wild Red	50
Tab	47
Sunkist	41
Pepsi	38
Nestea	39
RC Cola, Diet	36
Coca-Cola	34
Snapple Peach	32
Caffeine Content of Coffee & Teas	
Percolated (7 oz)	140
Drip (7 oz)	115–175
Espresso (1.5–2 oz)	100
Brewed (7 oz)	80–135
Instant (7 oz)	65–100
Decaf, brewed (6 oz)	5
tea, iced (12 oz)	70
tea, black (6 oz)	70
tea, green (6 oz)	35

Caffeine Content of Foods	
Milk Chocolate (1 oz)	1–15
Dark Chocolate (1 oz)	5–35
Bakers Chocolate (1 oz)	26
Coffee Flavored Yogurt (8 oz)	45
Chocolate Flavored Syrup	4
Caffeine Content of Caffeine Pills (mg per tablet)	
Vivarin	200
No-Doz, Maximum Strength	200
Dexatrim	200
Caffedrine	200
Awake, Maximum Strength	200
Stay Awake	200
Caffeine Content of Medications (mg per tablet)	
Anacin	32
Arthriten	65
Cafergot	100
Darvon	32
Dristan	30
Excedrin	65
Midol Max Strength	60
PC - CAP	32
Vanquish	33
Wigraine	100
XS Hangover Reliever	50

Sources: The American Beverage Association, Center for Science and the Public Interest, Erowid, International Food Information, and National Soft Drink Association.

summarizes the caffeine content of various beverages, chocolate, and medications.

There is growing evidence that caffeine ingestion (3–9 mg/kg body weight) prior to exercise increases performance during prolonged endurance exercise and short-term intense exercise lasting about 5 minutes.[346–353] Caffeine taken 1 hour prior to exercise will enhance endurance performance 10–30%, although individual responses can vary widely.[346]

Caffeine tends to elevate catecholamines and free fatty acids in the blood. When exercising muscles are presented with elevated levels of free fatty acids at the beginning of exercise, the muscles will increase their utilization of fat, sparing the muscle glycogen, resulting in improved endurance. Caffeine also appears to have a "neural" effect, decreasing the perception of effort.[347,348]

The ACSM does not recommend the use of caffeine for enhancement of performance. The International Olympic Committee has banned caffeine present in urine at levels greater than 12 μg/ml urine. It takes about 6 cups of brewed coffee (at 100-mg caffeine per cup) during a 2–3 hour period to reach this level. Three tablets of Vivarin® or six tablets of NoDoz® would have the same effect as 6 cups of coffee (see Table 9.19). The ergogenic effects of caffeine are present with urinary caffeine levels that are below the limit of 12 μg/ml, raising serious ethical issues regarding the use of caffeine by athletes.[346,349]

Soda Loading for Anaerobic Exercise

During high-intensity exercise, the requirement for oxygen exceeds the capacity of the aerobic system, increasing glycolysis and therefore lactic acid levels. The buildup of lactic acid finally inhibits the energy-supplying chemical reactions, resulting in fatigue. Exercise of 1- to 4-minute duration is limited by lactic acid buildup.

Several recent studies have shown that sodium bicarbonate (as found in Alka Seltzer) augments the body's buffer reserve, counteracts the buildup of lactic acid, and improves anaerobic exercise performance.[354–358] The use of sodium bicarbonate in doses of 300 mg/kg (taken all at once or spread out over a 1- to 3-hour period and given with water) has been shown to improve 400-meter running times by an average of 1.5 seconds and 800-meter running times by 2.9 seconds.[354,355] In general, such doses improve performance during any exercise bout with a large anaerobic component.[356,357] One review of the literature concluded that anaerobic exercise performance is enhanced 27% when using time to exhaustion as the criterion.[356] For the 800-meter, 2.9 seconds translates to a 19-meter advantage, often the difference between first and last place.

The practical implications are that performance can be enhanced in any event demanding hard exercise over a 1- to 4-minute period because the usual limiting factor, lactic acid, is partially controlled and buffered.

As with all ergogenic aids, however, there are some adverse effects. As many as half of those using soda may suffer from "urgent diarrhea" 1 hour after the soda loading is completed. The effects of repeated ingestion are unknown, and caution is advised.

As with caffeine, this use brings up the ethical issue of equitable competition and fair play. Soda loading should be banned because of the unfair advantage it offers. Bicarbonate rises sharply in the urine after sodium bicarbonate is used and can be measured to detect "soda loaders."

Blood Boosting and Doping for Endurance

Just as Roman gladiators drank the blood of foes to gain strength, modern Olympians have infused the blood of friends, as well as their own, to gain endurance. Increased performance after blood transfusion was first demonstrated in the late 1930s, but the technique did not attract attention until the early 1970s, when it was dubbed "blood doping" by the media. "Blood boosting" is now the preferred term for this practice with "blood doping" used when recombinant human erythropoietin is injected to induce red blood cell formation. Although earlier studies on blood doping reported mixed results, recent studies have shown that this practice has strong ergogenic value.[359–365]

Blood boosting involves removing 900 ml of blood (about 2 units) from a matching donor (homologous) or self (autologous). In autologous blood boosting, the blood is stored at –80° C for 8–12 weeks, and then reinfused into the athlete 1–4 days before the competition (see Figure 9.36). This increases the hemoglobin about 10%, leading to a 4–11% increase in $\dot{V}O_{2max}$.[364]

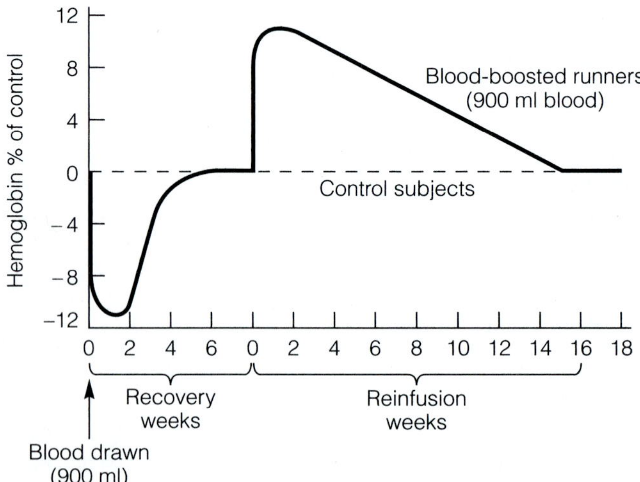

Figure 9.36 Blood-boosting scheme. Blood boosting usually involves removing 900 ml of one's own blood, storing it for 6–8 weeks as the body builds back to its normal amount, and then, shortly before competition, infusing the 900-ml blood to increase blood volume and hemoglobin to higher than normal levels. Source: Gledhill N. The ergogenic effect of blood doping. *Phys Sportsmed* 11:87–90, 1983.

Training with a lower amount of red blood cells and blood triggers a physiological response similar to that which occurs when runners train at high altitudes. In general, a runner's performance will drop by 10–20% immediately after the removal of 900 ml of blood, but it will gradually return to normal over the next 6–8 weeks.

Cardiorespiratory endurance performance is improved following the reinfusion because the oxygen-carrying capacity of the blood is greater, cardiac output is increased, lactate levels are reduced and sweating responses are improved.[359–365] Treadmill time to exhaustion is increased, 10-kilometer (6.2-mile) times drop an average of 69 seconds, 5-mile time performances drop an average of 49 seconds (10 seconds faster per mile), and 3-mile time performances drop an average of 23.7 seconds.[364]

After blood boosting, the hemoglobin level rises about 10% (e.g., to 15–16.5 g/dl). Because the normal range of hemoglobin is 14–18 g/dl, detecting blood boosting has proven to be very difficult. Blood doping was forbidden by the International Olympic Committee after the 1984 Olympics, despite the fact that no methods had been devised for unequivocal detection. The ACSM has taken the position that "any blood doping procedure used in an attempt to improve athletic performance is unethical, unfair, and exposes the athlete to unwarranted and potentially serious health risks."[364]

The Food and Drug Administration approved a new drug, erythropoietin (EPO), during the late 1980s. EPO is a hormone produced by the kidney, to stimulate production of red blood cells by the bone marrow. A synthetic form, recombinant EPO (r-EPO) is used to treat kidney patients who have anemia; r-EPO is considered by athletes to be an easier way to blood dope.[366–370] It causes the percentage of red blood cells (hematocrit) in the blood to increase, enhancing oxygen transport capacity. Administering EPO will slowly increase the number of red blood cells over several weeks, but the increase will be sustained as long as EPO treatment continues.[367]

A typical regimen is to administer 5,000 units of r-EPO three times weekly for 4 weeks. Hematocrit values will typically increase from 40–43% to 50–53%, increasing $\dot{V}O_{2max}$ by 8–10%.[368] Once r-EPO administration is discontinued, red cell mass gradually returns to its original state, but this may take weeks. As a result, an "open window" exists where there is no evidence of r-EPO misuse but where performance is enhanced. Although use of EPO has been prohibited by the International Olympic Committee since 1990, analytical methods to detect its misuse have been only recently developed and still lack strong specificity.[366–369] Blood and urine r-EPO are indistinguishable from endogenous EPO, and elevated EPO levels are only detectable several days after r-EPO administration. Indirect parameters have been introduced (e.g., hematocrit, soluble transferrin receptor, ferritin levels, and other markers of functional iron deficiency), but these also lack strong specificity. Unfortunately, the widespread use of r-EPO by endurance athletes is likely to continue until a valid, low-cost test is produced that can be administered in a random and frequent basis throughout the year to all athletes (a highly unlikely proposition).

Blood boosting and use of EPO may quickly give way to a new method of blood doping with blood substitutes.[370] Blood substitutes based on hemoglobin or hemoglobin-based oxygen carriers (HBOCs) are oxygen-carrying therapeutic agents developed for use in operations and emergencies in place of donated blood. Given the athlete's propensity to experiment with novel ergogenics, it is likely that HBOCs are already in use.

Steroids and Steroid-Like Compounds

Anabolic–androgenic steroids are prescription drugs that have legitimate medical uses, including treatment for anemias, hereditary angioedema, certain gynecological conditions, and protein anabolism.[371–376]

Current estimates indicate that approximately 3 million Americans use anabolic–androgenic steroids.[375] Two thirds of anabolic–androgenic steroid users are noncompetitive recreational bodybuilders or nonathletes who use these drugs for cosmetic purposes. An estimated 10% of steroid users are teens.[375, 377, 378] Steroid use rises to 15–30% among community weight trainers attending gyms and health clubs. Among adolescents, steroid users compared to nonusers are more likely to use other illicit drugs and participate in sports such as football, wrestling, weight lifting, and bodybuilding.[377,378]

The problems of anabolic–androgenic steroids can be considered from three different perspectives: pharmacological—the possibility that these substances may provide a real physiological advantage for the athletes; psychological—the importance of winning and the placebo effect of drugs; and ethical—the concept of violation of fair play.[372–391]

Anabolic steroids are synthetic derivatives of testosterone, a male sex hormone, but have greater anabolic activity (building up the body) relative to androgenic activity (masculinization) than testosterone. *Testosterone* is the principal circulating androgen in humans, concentrated 20 times as much in men as in women, and is a powerful agent to increase muscle mass and reduce body fat.[379,387] For example, in one study, subjects were given weekly muscle injections of testosterone for 12 weeks. The average subject gained 16.5 pounds of lean body mass while losing 7.5 pounds of fat, all without changing normal exercise or diet patterns.[379] The average adult male naturally produces 2.5–11.0 milligrams of testosterone daily. The typical steroid abuser often takes 250–3,200 mg per week through "stacking" or combining several different brands of steroids.[375]

The esterified steroids are usually given intramuscularly, whereas the alkylated steroids are given orally. The effects of steroids depend on the type used, the size and frequency of the doses, the overall length of treatment, and the route of administration. Most users indicate they use injectable formulations of anabolic–androgenic steroids for

4–12 weeks along with steroid accessory drugs such as ephedrine, amphetamines, thyroxine, growth hormone, insulin, diuretics, GHB, androstenedione, creatine, and dihydroepiandrosterone.[375]

A new, alarming trend is the use of "designer" steriods to achieve the "performance-enhancing" effects of steroids.[375,392] These steroid "alternatives" are sought in order to avoid the stiff penalties now in effect against steroid users. A recent example is tetrahydrogestrinone (THG), a chemically modified steroid that when developed could not be detected by existing testing protocols.[306]

Anabolic steroids have been used by athletes for decades, in the belief that they increase body mass, muscle tissue, strength, and aggressiveness. More recently, testosterone has been used because it is more difficult to detect in drug screening programs. Although study results have been mixed, an intensive exercise program, coupled with a high-protein diet and anabolic steroids, will increase muscular strength and size for most people.[373,378] One problem in obtaining research data is that athletes use drug combinations and doses that researchers do not replicate in their studies, often for ethical reasons.

Reasons given by athletes for using steroids include decreasing body fat, increasing muscle mass and strength, improving appearance, increasing red blood cell count, and increasing training tolerance (greater intensity, better recovery).[378] Athletes often take doses 10–1,000 times greater than clinical therapeutic doses.

The side effects are legion[375,378,381–391] (see Box 9.9). Use of these substances can affect the reproductive system, leading to temporary infertility. Among men, such use may result in atrophy of the testicles, decreased production of sperm, and reduced levels of several reproductive hormones. Steroids also produce liver abnormalities, decrease HDL cholesterol and increase LDL cholesterol, and increase the incidence of acne. Among women, androgenic hormones produce masculinizing effects (e.g., clitoris enlargement and increased hair growth).

While most of the effects of anabolic steroid use among adults may be reversible, several studies suggest that they may have more serious biophysical consequences for adolescents, particularly with regard to premature skeletal maturation, spermatogenesis, and an elevated risk of injury. However, the long-term health effects of anabolic steroid use are relatively unstudied.[375,378]

The use of steroids may also expose athletes to a risk of injury to ligaments and tendons, and these injuries may take longer to heal. There is also some evidence of anabolic steroid association with cancer, death, edema, fetal damage, heart disease, prostate enlargement, sterility, swelling of feet or lower legs, and yellowing of the eyes or skin.

It has been known for years that anabolic steroids increase aggressiveness. Athletes using steroids have exhibited increased levels of anger and hostility and overall mood disturbance. Studies also show that in addition to irritability and hostility, steroids increase confusion and forgetfulness, hardly the mental traits coaches desire in their athletes.[386,391]

Box 9.9

Steroid Side Effects

The side effects of steroid ingestion are legion. These include both established effects and less certain effects.

Established Effects

- Low HDL cholesterol
- Elevated blood pressure
- Acne
- Water retention in tissue
- Prostate enlargement
- Yellowing of eyes and skin
- Oily, thickened skin
- Stunted growth (when taken before puberty)
- Fetal damage (when taken during pregnancy)
- Heart muscle hypertrophy
- Heart arrhythmias
- Coronary artery disease
- Sterility, lowered sperm count in men, testicular atrophy
- Mood swings, aggression, mania, depression
- Liver tumors and disease
- Death

Additional effects in women—male-pattern baldness, hairiness, voice deepening, decreased breast size, menstrual irregularities, clitoris hypertrophy

Other Possible Effects

Abdominal pains, hives, chills, diarrhea, fatigue, fever, muscle cramps, headache, nausea, vomiting blood, bone pains, breast development in men, urination problems, gallstones, kidney disease

Sources: See references 374, 375, 381–391.

Prohormones are a class of androgenic steroids that either convert to testosterone directly or mimic testosterone by forming androgen-like derivatives (e.g., nandrolone).[371,376,378,380,393] Their use was popularized by baseball-great Mark McGwire and East German Olympians. As depicted in Figure 9.37, testosterone is formed from cholesterol through two different pathways that include a number of intermediate compounds that have a chemical structure differing slightly from testosterone. These compounds include dehydroepiandrosterone (DHEA); androstenedione, 5-androstenediol, and 4-androstenediol, all now sold as prohormones in the U.S. marketplace. Most sports governing bodies have banned the use of such agents, but they are abundantly available to recreational athletes through retail outlets.

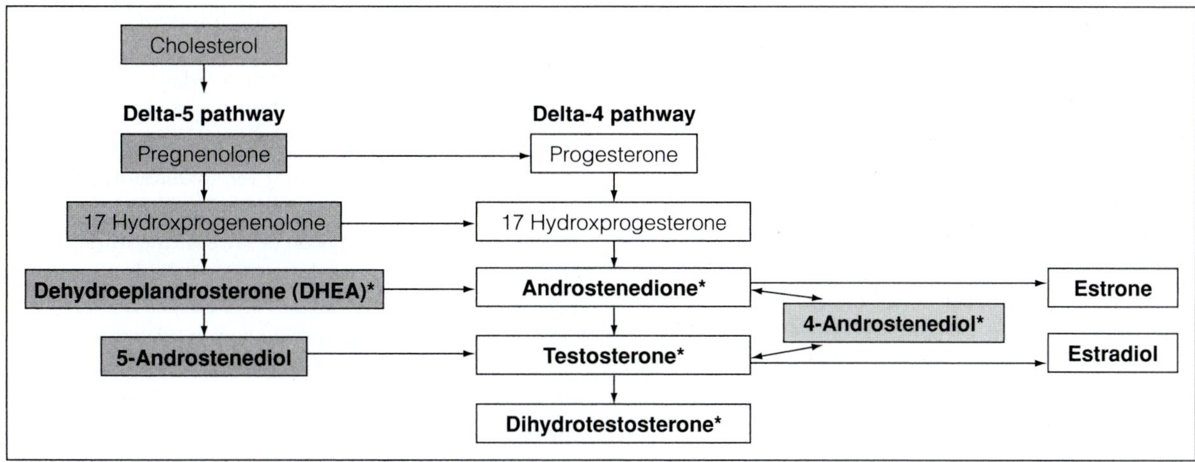

Figure 9.37 Metabolic pathways for androgen biosynthesis. *Currently available on the market.

Most studies indicate that some androgen supplements in sufficient doses do convert to more active components such as testosterone.[376,378,380,393–397] At the same time, however, increases in estrogen subfractions can be measured (as shown in Figure 9.37). The net effect is no increase in protein synthesis, muscle mass, or strength. Thus the athlete using prohormone supplements may test positive for banned anabolic agents while receiving no performance benefit.[393]

Doping with growth hormone has become an increasing problem during the past two decades.[398–400] Growth hormone has a reputation of being effective in building skeletal mass, reducing fat mass, and improving submaximal and maximal aerobic endurance among athletes.[398] Discovery of recombinant growth hormone (rGH) in the possessions of Chinese swimmers bound for the 1998 World Swimming Championships and similar problems at the Tour de France cycling event in 1998 indicate the abuse of growth hormone at the elite athlete level. Use of growth hormone by athletes to enhance performance is banned by the International Olympic Committee and major sporting bodies, but there is currently no approved means of detection.

Growth hormone is crucial in energy metabolism and body anabolism and has multiple benefits when administered to adults with growth hormone deficiencies.[398–400] Insulin like growth factor I (IGF-I) mediates the principal effects of growth hormone. Currently, the effects of rGH or IGF-I in improving athletic performance, muscle strength, and recovery from intensive exercise are unproven. The few controlled studies that have been performed with supraphysiological growth hormone doses to athletes have shown inconsistent performance effects.[398–400]

Creatine Supplementation

Creatine supplementation has become a common ergogenic aid for athletes who engage in repeated bouts of short-term, high-intensity exercise.[401–408] Creatine is found in large quantities in skeletal muscle and binds a significant amount of phosphate, providing an immediate source of energy in muscle cells (ATP). The reason for consuming supplemental creatine is to increase the skeletal muscle creatine content, in the hope that some of the extra creatine binds phosphate, increasing muscle creatine phosphate content. During repeated bouts of high-intensity exercise (for example, five 30-second bouts of sprinting or cycling exercise, separated by 1–4 minutes of rest), the increased availability of creatine phosphate may improve resynthesis and degradation rates, leading to greater anaerobic ATP turnover and high-power exercise performance.

The estimated daily requirement for creatine is about 2 grams. Nonvegetarians typically get about 1 gram of creatine a day from the various meats they ingest, and the body synthesizes another gram in the liver, kidney, and pancreas, using the amino acids arginine and glycine as precursors. Vegetarians have a reduced body creatine pool, suggesting that lack of dietary creatine from avoidance of meat is not adequately compensated by an increase in endogenous creatine production.

Consuming about 20–25 grams of creatine per day for 5–6 days in a row significantly increases muscle creatine in most people, especially those with low levels to begin with, such as vegetarians. Four to five daily doses of 5 grams each are usually consumed by dissolving creatine in about 250 ml of a beverage throughout the day. Each 5-gram dose of creatine is the equivalent of 1.1 kg of fresh, uncooked steak. There do not appear to be any adverse side effects associated with the oral ingestion of supplemental creatine.

A large volume of literature has been published on the ergogenic value of creatine supplementation.[401–408] Despite unprecedented attention given to creatine supplementation by the media and recreational and competitive athletes, research findings have been unclear and confusing. The ACSM submitted a consensus statement on the physiological and health effects of oral creatine supplementation in the year 2000 and concluded the following:[403]

- Creatine supplementation can increase muscle phosphocreatine content, but not in all individuals.
- Exercise performance involving short periods of extremely powerful activity can be enhanced with creatine supplementation (e.g., 5–7 days of 20 grams/day), especially during repeated bouts of activity. Creatine supplementation does not increase maximal isometric strength, the rate of maximal force production, nor aerobic exercise performance.
- Creatine supplementation leads to weight gain within the first few days, likely due to water retention related to creatine uptake in the muscle.
- There is no definitive evidence that creatine supplementation causes gastrointestinal, renal, and/or muscle cramping complications.
- Although creatine supplementation exhibits small but significant physiological and performance changes, the increases in performance are realized during very specific exercise conditions. This suggests that the apparent high expectations for performance enhancement are inordinate.

PRINCIPLE 10: FAT LOADING IS NOT RECOMMENDED FOR ENHANCED PERFORMANCE OR HEALTH

Research has shown that athletes have no guarantee of protection from heart disease unless they continue prudent habits of exercise and diet after their days of competition are over (see Chapter 10). Even during heavy training, a diet high in saturated fats can raise serum cholesterol to high levels. Regular endurance exercise will not fully negate bad nutritional habits. Fitness enthusiasts and endurance athletes are well advised to consider not only performance, but also general health, in making their dietary choices.

Recently, claims for special diets and nutritional supplements that provide more fat and less carbohydrate for endurance performance have been advanced.[409] It is well known that endurance athletes are capable of sparing body carbohydrate stores through increased fat oxidation during exercise.[410] This training-induced effect has led to the premise that a greater availability of fat during exercise, through supplementation or dietary alterations (i.e., "fat loading"), can improve performance by further sparing muscle glycogen.[411]

With endurance training, the muscles become more efficient in using fat for energy, "sparing" the glycogen reserves, allowing the athlete to endure longer before glycogen stores are depleted. One hypothesis is that the increased fat utilization by the endurance athlete at a given work rate increases the intracellular citrate concentration, inhibiting phosphofructokinase (PFK).[411] The inhibition of PFK eventually slows down the rate of glycolysis and glycogenolysis. Because of the ability of the muscle to adapt to aerobic training by increasing fat oxidation, and the well-accepted fact that fatigue is tied to low muscle glycogen levels, it has been speculated that acutely increasing the availability of fatty acids for oxidation through dietary or pharmacological methods might increase the oxidation of fat, sparing muscle glycogen, and therefore improving long-term endurance performance. Before exploring whether this hypothesis is true, the role of fat as a fuel for exercise metabolism is reviewed.

Of the two main fuels stored in the body and used for muscular exercise, fat has several characteristics that would make it a desirable substrate.[412] There is more stored energy (9 Calories/gram) in a gram of fat than in an equal weight of carbohydrate (4 Calories/gram). Typically, about 50,000–60,000 Calories of energy are stored as triglycerides in the body of a normal-weight fit individual.[413] This large amount of energy is stored in a relatively small amount of adipose tissue (about 13–18 pounds), providing an excellent portable depot of fuel as people move from place to place. In contrast, if all of this energy were stored as glycogen, more than 100 pounds of storage weight would be required, due to binding of heavy water molecules.

Triglyceride is also stored in droplets directly within the muscle fibers, in close proximity to the site of oxidation in the muscle mitochondria. Intramuscular triglyceride accounts for 2,000–3,000 Calories of stored energy, making it a larger source of potential energy than muscle glycogen, which can contribute only about 1,500 Calories.[413]

During endurance exercise, lipolysis of triglycerides in both adipose tissue and the muscles is increased after 15–20 minutes by epinephrine stimulation of hormone-sensitive lipase, releasing free fatty acids.[411] Free fatty acids from the blood enter the muscle cell via a carrier-mediated diffusion process. Once inside the muscle cell, the fatty acid is converted to fatty acyl-CoA and then transported across the mitochondrial membrane by an ATP-requiring process via the enzyme complex carnitine palmityl-transferase. In the mitochondria, the acyl-CoA enters the β-oxidation cycle and eventually enters the Krebs cycle, resulting in ATP production.

If the muscle could oxidize fatty acids at a sufficiently high rate during intense exercise, a greater yield of ATP per carbon molecule would occur (1.3-fold) than is possible when relying on carbohydrates. Unfortunately, humans can only slowly convert body fat stores into energy during exercise (less than one third the rate attributed to muscle glycogen).[413] About 75% more oxygen is required to completely oxidize fatty acids than glucose, resulting in a much higher stress to the cardiorespiratory system.[1,411] At rest and during low-intensity exercise, fat is the dominant and preferred substrate.[413] However, as the intensity of exercise increases, an increasing proportion of the energy is supplied by carbohydrates. If high-intensity exercise is continued for several hours, muscle glycogen stores slowly become depleted, forcing the muscle cells to use more fatty acids, increasing the sense of effort and strain to the cardiorespiratory system,

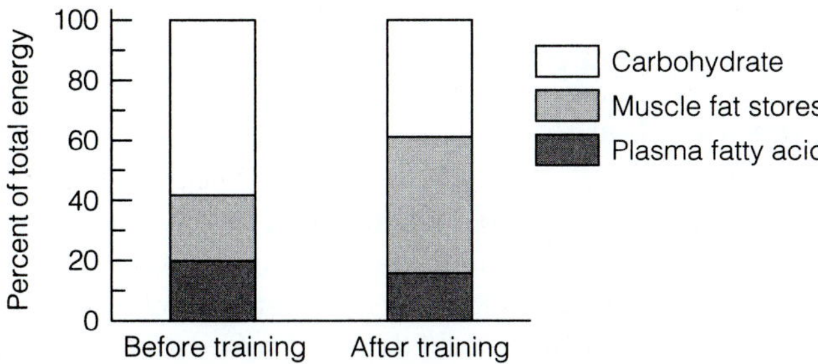

Figure 9.38 Percentage of total energy from carbohydrate and fat during 90–120 minutes cycling at 63% $\dot{V}O_{2max}$ before and after exercise training. Exercise training results in a greater proportion of energy coming from fat, especially fat stored within the muscle. Source: Martin WH, Dalsky GP, Hurly BF, et al. Effect of endurance training on plasma free fatty acid turnover and oxidation during exercise. *Am J Physiol* 265:E708–E714, 1993.

and ultimately causing a reduction in pace.[1] The primary source of free fatty acids during exercise appear to be intramuscular, rather than adipose tissue triglyceride stores, especially in trained individuals (see Figure 9.38).[413]

Dietary and pharmacological methods have been used to increase fatty acid availability and oxidation, in an attempt to spare muscle glycogen and thus enhance long-term endurance performance. Several studies with rats have shown this hypothesis to be true, but the data on humans are at best equivocal.[414]

It is not possible to ingest free fatty acids because they are too acidic and need a protein carrier for intestinal absorption. Thus the only practical way of significantly elevating blood fat levels is by ingesting triglycerides. Normal long-chain dietary triglycerides enter the blood 3–4 hours after ingestion and are bound to chylomicrons. The rate of uptake of triglycerides by muscles during exercise appears to be relatively low. Although medium-chain triglycerides are directly absorbed into the blood and liver and are rapidly broken down to fatty acids and glycerol, only a small amount (about 30 grams) can be ingested without experiencing gastrointestinal discomfort and diarrhea.[415] In general, most studies with medium-chain triglycerides have failed to demonstrate muscle glycogen sparing or enhanced performance.[416]

A technique used in a few research studies to raise plasma levels of free fatty acids is to intravenously infuse a triglyceride emulsion (e.g., Intralipid®), followed by heparin. Thus far, this method has been shown to have minimal, if any, effects on muscle glycogen utilization or performance.[417] Research with normal long-chain dietary triglycerides has centered around the following manipulations:[411]

- High-fat diets for 1–5 days before endurance exercise
- High-fat diets for 2–4 weeks prior to endurance exercise
- High-fat diets immediately before and/or during endurance exercise (after a normal diet)

Nearly all studies have shown that high-fat diets (about 70% of total energy) for several days prior to endurance exercise significantly decrease body carbohydrate stores, reducing endurance time dramatically.[1] Although the relative contribution of fat is increased, performance is impaired because of low muscle glycogen levels. In one study, subjects were fed a high-fat (76% of energy) diet or a high-carbohydrate (76% of energy) diet for 4 days.[418] Subjects then ran to exhaustion on a treadmill at 70% maximal aerobic power. Time to exhaustion following the high-fat diet was decreased by 40%, and all subjects exhibited neurological symptoms of low blood sugar.

A few researchers have studied the effect of 2–4 weeks of a high-fat diet on endurance performance.[419–422] Investigators measured the effect of a 28-day, high-fat diet (with only 20 grams of carbohydrate per day) on the endurance performance of five well-trained cyclists.[422] Muscle glycogen was decreased by nearly half after the high-fat diet, but the cyclists were able to perform at a moderate intensity (60–65% $\dot{V}O_{2max}$) to the same level as before the diet began. However, it should be noted that the results may have been quite different, had the intensity been higher.

Researchers have examined the impact of a fatty meal 1–5 hours before exercise after several days of a normal carbohydrate-rich diet, or the use of fat supplements during exercise.[423–425] Potentially, oil supplements just before or during prolonged endurance exercise could cause the muscles to utilize more free fatty acids for fuel, sparing the muscle glycogen that has been built up by a normal carbohydrate-rich diet. Studies thus far, however, have failed to demonstrate improvement in performance.

Taken together, these studies do not support the use of fat loading to enhance endurance performance.[411,420] It should be noted that few studies have explored the issue of fat loading, and the ones that have been conducted do have various methodological flaws. Nonetheless, physiologically, the use of free fatty acids as a major fuel substrate for high-intensity exercise does not seem probable, and even if long-term, high-fat diets lead to some sort of adaptation that allows long-term, moderate-intensity endurance exercise to be performed without impairment, health considerations would forbid an enthusiastic endorsement.

There are data showing that even in athletes training intensively, changes in dietary composition can substantially alter blood lipoprotein levels.[426–429] High-fat diets have also been associated with increased body fat deposition, increasing the difficulty of maintaining an ideal body weight for competition. Although there has been some concern that extremely high carbohydrate diets may lower HDL cholesterol even within athletes training heavily, it is doubtful that this imposes any real impairment in long-term health because levels still remain above values typical of sedentary subjects.[426,427] Athletes in heavy training should realize, however, that as long as carbohydrate intake is adequate (8–10 g/kg per day), the addition of fat and protein to the diet to meet energy needs does not alter glycogen storage or performance.[430] There is little need for an endurance athlete to be fat-phobic, especially because several studies have shown that total oxidation of fat over the postprandial period is enhanced by long-duration exercise.[431]

SPORTS MEDICINE INSIGHT

Practical Nutrition Scheme for a Marathon

For the highly active endurance athlete, maximizing muscle glycogen stores for the "big event" is vital. This Sports Medicine Insight deals with the necessary preparation and race-day activities for a marathon-type event (more than 2 hours).

1. Train long and hard to help the muscles adapt. During the months of training for the marathon-type event, train at a hard pace for a minimum of 90–120 minutes several times per month, to train the muscles both to store more glycogen and to utilize fat more efficiently (sparing the glycogen stores). Remember, nutrition is not as important as talent and training. The minimum amount of training for a marathon (26.2 miles) is 50 miles per week for 3 months before the event. The best athletes in the world work up to a schedule of 80–120 miles per week, but this takes many months of gradual training progression.
2. During the months of training, emphasize a high-carbohydrate diet with plenty of rest and water. Adequate recovery from hard training means consuming a high-carbohydrate diet (at least 60–70% of total Calories). The carbohydrate should be primarily starch, not sugar, to ensure adequate vitamin and mineral intake. A wide variety of healthful foods should be used to obtain all nutrients without supplementation. A conscious effort must be made to drink more water than desired.
3. During the week before the event, rest and eat primarily carbohydrate-rich foods. The exercise should gradually taper to total rest the day before the event. During the 3 days just before the event, eat a very high carbohydrate diet (close to 70–80% of total Calories).
4. In the 3–4 hours before the event, consume a high-carbohydrate meal. About 20–30 minutes before eating the meal, consume two to four glasses of water to ensure that your body is adequately hydrated to provide digestive juices for the meal. The meal should be consumed 3–4 hours before the event, to allow the stomach time to empty all its contents. If the event is early in the day, get up early. The meal should be light (500–800 Calories) and high in carbohydrate, but low in dietary fiber. Refined hot cereal, fruit juices, bagels, white bread and jam, white rice, or pasta (without any fats added) are good choices. Just before the event (5 minutes before), consuming 150–200 Calories of a diluted CHO solution can help maintain blood glucose levels.
5. During the event, drink about 1 liter/hour of a cold sports drink. (Practice during training with various sports drinks until you find one that suits you.)
6. After the event, consume a high-carbohydrate diet to replenish muscle glycogen stores. Recovery from the marathon-type event is hastened by consuming a high-CHO diet soon after the race.

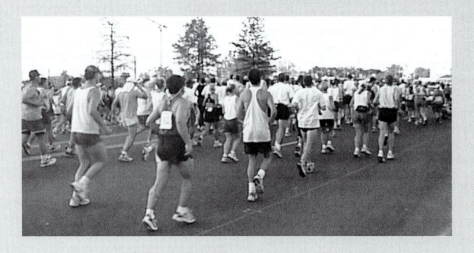

SUMMARY

- Principle 1: Prudent diet is the cornerstone. The same diet that enhances health (the prudent diet) is the one that also maximizes performance for most athletes. For some athletes in heavy training, however (defined as more than 60–90 minutes a day of aerobic or intermittent anaerobic–aerobic activity), several adaptations beyond the prudent diet are beneficial. Heavy training imposes special nutritional stresses because of the high intensity of effort over a relatively short time period, demanding extra energy, carbohydrate, and water.
- Principle 2: Increase total energy intake. Athletes are high energy consumers because of their high working capacities, and high-intensity training levels. Many athletes need more than 50 Calories per kilogram of body weight. Most of this extra energy should come in the form of carbohydrate from grains, dried fruits, breads, and pasta.
- Principle 3: Keep the carbohydrate intake high (55–70%) during training. A high-carbohydrate diet is probably the most important nutritional factor for athletes. Body carbohydrate stores (glycogen) are extremely labile because they are the chief fuel source for the working muscle during high-intensity exercise. When muscle glycogen levels drop too low, exercise performance is impaired, and the athlete feels stale and tired and is more prone to injury. Athletes in heavy training need up to 8–10 g CHO/kg in their diet per day (close to 70% of total Calories as carbohydrate). The high levels of carbohydrate are usually more than athletes want, so they must be trained to eat high-carbohydrate diets.
- Principle 4: Drink large amounts of water during training and the event. Probably the second most important dietary principle for athletes is to drink large quantities of water. As little as a 2% drop in body weight from water loss has been associated with impaired performance. Athletes tend to sweat earlier and more than nonathletes, so they tend to lose more body water with exercise. The thirst desire of an athlete lags behind actual body needs, so athletes should be encouraged to force fluids beyond what is desired. No electrolytes are needed except in ultramarathon events—they are easily obtained with normal meals after the event. Carbohydrate added to the drink taken during exercise can help maintain blood glucose levels.
- Principle 5: Keep a close watch on possible iron deficiency. A number of athletes, especially runners, have stage 1 iron deficiency, best measured by evaluating serum ferritin levels. All elite athletes are urged to have their iron status checked yearly. To help prevent iron deficiency, runners (especially menstruating females) should consume high-iron foods. Under the supervision of a physician, some runners may benefit from moderate iron supplementation.
- Principle 6: Vitamin and mineral supplements are not needed. Most studies show that athletes are above RDA levels for all nutrients (except iron for females). Athletes are at an advantage because their high caloric intakes provide more than adequate quantities of vitamins and minerals. The sedentary are actually at greater risk because of their low caloric intakes. Athletes should not use vitamins or mineral supplements in amounts above the RDA; studies are showing the potential for nutrient imbalances in the body.
- Principle 7: Protein supplements do not benefit the athlete. Although 3–10% of the energy needed in long endurance exercise or weight lifting come from protein, athletes obtain more than enough protein in their normal diets. There is no need for protein supplements.
- Principle 8: Rest and emphasize carbohydrates before long endurance events. The best scheme for preparing for any exercise event lasting longer than 60–90 minutes is to taper the exercise gradually, while consuming more than 70% carbohydrate during the 7 days before the event. (Depletion of muscle glycogen during the initial phase of "glycogen loading" is no longer recommended.) The pre-event meal should be 500–800 Calories, of light, low-fiber starch, 3–5 hours before the event.
- Principle 9: Use of ergogenic aids is unethical. Although there are many worthless ergogenic aids (e.g., bee pollen, B_{15}, alcohol), many provide impressive performance benefits (caffeine, sodium bicarbonate, phosphorus, blood boosting). These enhance performance, but the ethical issue of equitable competition and fair play claim a higher priority.
- Principle 10: Fat loading is not recommended for enhanced performance or health. Research has evaluated the effects of fat in the diet before and during exercise, and performance is not enhanced. Adapting to a high-fat diet for 1 month has been found to aid endurance in some studies, but such adaptation may be harmful to health in the long term. Athletes have no guarantee of protection from heart disease unless they continue prudent habits of exercise and diet after their days of competition are over. Even during heavy training, a diet high in saturated fat can raise serum cholesterol—exercise is not powerful enough to fully negate bad nutritional habits. Athletes can maximize both performance and health through wise dietary choices.

Review Questions

1. *The recommended breakdown of daily energy intake for carbohydrate when considering general health is ____% carbohydrate.*

   A. 15–30 **B.** 30–45 **C.** 45–65 **D.** 65–75 **E.** 75–100

2. *Ten french fries have 158 Calories, with 2.0 grams of protein, 19.8 grams of carbohydrate, and 8.3 grams of fat. What percent of Calories are carbohydrate? ____ What percent of Calories are fat? ____.*

   A. 50 / 47 **B.** 37 / 50 **C.** 40 / 60 **D.** 27 / 70

3. *Which condition would promote a higher use of fat during exercise?*

   A. Athletic versus average fitness status
   B. Short versus long duration
   C. High versus low intensity

4. *If you ran as far as you could for 10 seconds, the primary source of ATP for the working muscles would be the ____.*

   A. ATP–PC stores
   B. Lactate system
   C. Oxygen system

5. *A major limiting factor in ability to perform long endurance exercise is*

   A. Body fat stores **B.** Muscle glycogen levels
   C. Muscle protein stores **D.** Amount of fat in the blood

6. *If you weigh yourself before and after you exercise, and you lose 3 pounds, how much water should you drink to restore what was lost?*

   A. 1 cup **B.** 2 cups
   C. 3 cups **D.** 4 cups
   E. 6 cups

7. *During exercise, the stomach can empty about ____ liters of liquid per hour.*

   A. 0.5 **B.** 1 **C.** 1.5 **D.** 2 **E.** 3

8. *What type of food should be eaten in the greatest quantity each day?*

   A. Vegetables **B.** Fruits
   C. Breads, cereals, rice, pasta **D.** Dairy products
   E. Meats

9. *If you eat 2,000 calories, what is the maximum grams of fat you should include in this diet?*

   A. 50 **B.** 78 **C.** 100 **D.** 400

10. *Which nutrient has been shown to improve performance when supplemented to the diet?*

    A. Vitamin C **B.** Zinc
    C. Magnesium **D.** Vitamin A
    E. None of these

11. *Which ergogenic aid listed below improves 400–800 meter run performance?*

    A. Blood boosting **B.** Wheat germ oil
    C. Ginseng **D.** Sodium bicarbonate
    E. Steroids

12. *Which one of these statements is* **not** *consistent with the 2005 USDA Dietary Guidelines for Americans?*

    A. Eat five servings or more a day of foods high in protein
    B. Choose a diet low in saturated fat and cholesterol and moderate in total fat
    C. Choose and prepare foods with less salt
    D. Aim for a healthy weight
    E. Choose beverages and foods to moderate your intake of sugars

13. *On the energy-power chart (Figure 9.5), which activity ranks highest?*

    A. Running **B.** Road cycling
    C. Rowing **D.** Walking

14. *Which substrate store is in greatest quantity in the average human?*

    A. Protein **B.** Fat
    C. Carbohydrate

15. *When the exercise intensity is <30% $\dot{V}O_{2max}$, the primary fuel by the working muscle is*

    A. Protein **B.** Fat
    C. Carbohydrate

16. *For elite endurance athletes, about ____ grams of carbohydrate are needed per kilogram of body weight each day.*

    A. 1–2 **B.** 3–4 **C.** 4–6 **D.** 6–10

17. *During exercise, the chief avenue of heat loss is*

    A. Radiation **B.** Conduction
    C. Sweat evaporation **D.** Convection

18. *For every liter of sweat evaporated on the skin, close to ____ Calories are given off, preventing an increase in body temperature of a full 10°C.*

    A. 600 **B.** 800 **C.** 1,000 **D.** 2,000 **E.** 3,000

19. *Sweat losses of ____ liters per hour are common in endurance sports.*

A. 1.5 B. 3 C. 5 D. 6 E. 7

20. *Loss of body water from sweating beyond a threshold of ____% of body weight will significantly impair endurance capacity.*

A. 1 B. 2 C. 4 D. 6 E. 8

21. *Sports drinks that contain ____% carbohydrate in volumes of 200–400 ml consumed every 15–20 minutes are preferable to plain water.*

A. 1–2 B. 3–4 C. 4–10 D. 10–20

22. *Anemia is defined as a hemoglobin below a threshold of ____ mg/dl for females.*

A. 5 B. 7 C. 12 D. 15 E. 20

23. *____ is an indicator for stage 1 or mild iron deficiency.*

A. Serum iron
B. Hemoglobin
C. Red blood cell count
D. Transferrin saturation
E. Serum ferritin

24. *Several changes in protein metabolism take place during intensive exercise. Which one of the following is* not *included?*

A. Enhancement of protein synthesis
B. Increased muscle protein breakdown
C. Increase in amino acid oxidation
D. Increase in gluconeogenesis

25. *The average sedentary American needs 0.8 grams of protein per kilogram of body weight. Strength athletes may need up to ____ g/kg/day during intensive training.*

A. 1.0–1.2
B. 1.6–1.7
C. 2.5–3.0
D. 3.3–3.6
E. 4.5–5.0

26. *Which ergogenic aid is claimed (falsely, it now appears) to increase insulin activity and increase muscle cell uptake of amino acids?*

A. Ginseng
B. Inosine
C. Carnitine/choline
D. Tryptophan
E. Chromium picolinate

27. *It takes about ____ cups of strongly brewed coffee to exceed the International Olympic Committee's threshold for urine caffeine.*

A. 2 B. 4 C. 6 D. 8 E. 10

28. *Anabolic steroids are synthetic derivatives of ____.*

A. Testosterone
B. Estrogen
C. Insulin
D. Glucagon
E. Cortisol

29. *Which food listed below does* not *have dietary fiber in it?*

A. Fruit
B. Meat
C. Nuts
D. Whole grains
E. Vegetables

30. *Intake of sugar has been linked to*

A. Heart disease
B. Abnormal behavior
C. Cancer
D. Diabetes
E. None of these

31. *Table salt is ____ % sodium.*

A. 10 B. 25 C. 40 D. 66 E. 90

32. *A standard drink contains ____ ounces of pure alcohol.*

A. 0.5 B. 1 C. 1.5 D. 2.0 E. 0.8

33. *Overall, the gastrointestinal tract appears capable of delivering up to ____ grams of carbohydrate each hour of exercise, enough to match the needs of most athletes.*

A. 25 B. 72 C. 100 D. 200 E. 45

34. *Which food listed has the highest glycemic index?*

A. Peanuts
B. Apple
C. Ice cream
D. Bagels
E. Lentils

35. *During dehydration*

A. Stroke volume and cardiac output decrease
B. Plasma osmolality decreases
C. Heart rate decreases
D. Plasma volume increases
E. Gastric emptying rate increases

36. *Which one of these ergogenic aids has been consistently linked with increased strength?*

A. Boron
B. Amino acid supplements
C. Yohimbine
D. Ma-huang
E. None of these

37. *According to the USDA Dietary Guidelines for Americans, ________ minutes of daily physical activity are recommended to sustain weight loss.*

A. 15–20
B. 30–45
C. 50–75
D. 60–90
E. None of these

38. *Which one of the following is* **not** *a side effect of using steroids on a regular basis?*

A. High sperm counts
B. Acne
C. Low HDL cholesterol
D. Liver disease
E. Yellowing of skin

39. *During the first hour of exercise, most of the carbohydrate and fat metabolized for energy come from the*

A. Liver
B. Blood
C. Brain
D. Colon
E. Muscle

40. *The normal loss of iron from the body each day is ____ mg.*

A. 1–2 B. 3–4 C. 5–6 D. 7–8 E. 9–10

41. *Which factor explains the majority of iron deficiency in athletes?*

A. Foot-strike hemolysis
B. Iron loss in sweat
C. Inadequate dietary iron
D. Gastrointestinal bleeding

42. *What hormone produced by the kidney stimulates production of red blood cells by the bone marrow?*

A. Erythropoietin
B. Insulin
C. Growth hormone
D. Epinephrine
E. Cortisol

43. *IGF-I mediates the principal effects of what hormone?*

A. Erythropoietin
B. Insulin
C. Growth hormone
D. Epinephrine
E. Cortisol

44. *According to the ACSM, creatine supplementation can enhance performance during what specific exercise condition?*

A. Maximal isometric strength
B. Maximal force production
C. Aerobic exercise
D. Short, repeated bouts of powerful activity

45. *Nutrient reference standards for the food label are called*

A. DRI B. DV C. RDA D. UL E. TFA

Answers

1. C	24. A
2. A	25. B
3. A	26. E
4. A	27. C
5. B	28. A
6. E	29. B
7. B	30. E
8. C	31. C
9. B	32. A
10. E	33. B
11. D	34. D
12. A	35. A
13. C	36. E
14. B	37. D
15. B	38. A
16. D	39. E
17. C	40. A
18. A	41. C
19. A	42. A
20. B	43. C
21. C	44. D
22. C	45. B
23. E	

REFERENCES

1. Costill DL. Carbohydrates for exercise: Dietary demands for optimal performance. *Int J Sports Med* 9:1–18, 1988.
2. American College of Sports Medicine, American Dietetic Association, and Dietitians of Canada. Joint position statement. Nutrition and athletic performance. *Med Sci Sports Exerc* 32:2130–2145, 2000; *J Am Diet Assoc* 12:1543–1556, 2000.
3. American Dietetic Association. *Sports Nutrition: A Guide for the Professional Working with Active People.* Chicago: The American Dietetic Association, 2000.
4. Williams MH. *Nutrition for Health, Fitness and Sport.* St. Louis: McGraw-Hill, 2004.
5. Lee RD, Nieman DC. *Nutritional Assessment* (4th ed.). St. Louis: McGraw-Hill, 2006.
6. Institute of Medicine. *Dietary Reference Intakes for Energy, Carbohydrate, Fiber, Fat, Fatty Acids, Cholesterol, Protein, and Amino Acids.* Washington, DC: The National Academies Press, 2002.
7. U.S. Department of Health and Human Services and U.S. Department of Agriculture. *Dietary Guidelines for Americans* 6th ed.). Washington, DC: U.S. Government Printing Office, 2005.
8. CSPI. Vitamins & minerals: How much is too much? *Nutrition Action Healthletter,* June, 2001, pp. 8–11.
9. Institute of Medicine. *Dietary Reference Intakes for Vitamin A, Vitamin K, Arsenic, Boron, Chromium, Copper, Iodine, Iron, Manganese, Molybdenum, Nickel, Silicon, Vanadium and Zinc.* Food and Nutrition Board. Washington, DC: National Academy Press, 2002.
10. Institute of Medicine. *Dietary Reference Intakes for Calcium, Phosphorus, Magnesium, Vitamin D, and Fluoride.* Food and Nutrition Board. Washington, DC: National Academy Press, 1997.

11. Institute of Medicine. *Dietary Reference Intakes for Thiamin, Riboflavin, Niacin, Vitamin B_6, Folate, Vitamin B_{12}, Pantothenic Acid, Biotin, and Choline.* Food and Nutrition Board. Washington, DC: National Academy Press, 1998.
12. Institute of Medicine. *Dietary Reference Intakes for Vitamin C, Vitamin E, Selenium, and Carotenoids.* Food and Nutrition Board. Washington, DC: National Academy Press, 2000.
13. Institute of Medicine. *Dietary Reference Intakes: Use in Dietary Assessment.* Food and Nutrition Board. Washington, DC: National Academy Press, 2000.
14. Institute of Medicine. *Dietary Reference Intakes for Water, Potassium, Sodium, Chloride, and Sulfate.* Food and Nutrition Board. Washington, DC: The National Academies Press, 2004.
15. Wright JD, Wang CY, Kennedy-Stephenson J, Ervin RB. Dietary intake of ten key nutrients for public health, United States: 1999–2000. *Advance Data from Vital and Health Statistics,* no. 334. Hyattsville, MD: National Center for Health Statistics. Also: http://www.barc.usda.gov/bhnrc/foodsurvey/home.htm.
16. Eyre H, Kahn R, Robertson RM. Preventing cancer, cardiovascular disease, and diabetes. A common agenda for the American Cancer Society, the American Diabetes Association, and the American Heart Association. *Diabetes Care* 27:1812–1824, 2004.
17. Byers T, Nestle M, McTiernan A, Doyle C, Currie-Williams A, Gansler T, Thun M. American Cancer Society guidelines on nutrition and physical activity for cancer prevention: Reducing the risk of cancer with healthy food choices and physical activity. *CA Cancer J Clin* 52:92–119, 2002.
18. Flegal KM, Carroll MD, Ogden CL, Johnson CL. Prevalence and trends in obesity among US adults, 1999–2000. *JAMA* 288:1723–1727, 2002.
19. Wright JD, Kennedy-Stephenson J, Wang CY, McDowell MA, Johnson CL. Trends in intake of energy and macronutrients—United States, 1971–2000. *MMWR* 53:80–82, 2004.
20. United States Department of Agriculture. *MyPyramid.* Available at http://www.mypyramid.gov, 2005.
21. Haines PS, Siega-Riz AM, Popkin BM. The Diet Quality Index revised: A measurement instrument for populations. *J Am Diet Assoc* 99:697–704, 1999.
22. Subar AF, Krebs-Smith SM, Cook A, Kahle LL. Dietary sources of nutrients among US adults, 1989 to 1991. *Am J Diet Assoc* 98:537–547, 1998.
23. Messina M, Messina V. *The Dietitian's Guide to Vegetarian Diets. Issues and Applications.* Gaithersburg, MD: Aspen Publishers, Inc., 1996.
24. Sabaté J. *Vegetarian Nutrition.* Boca Raton, FL: CRC Press, 2001.
25. Slavin JL, Jacobs D, Marquart L, Wiemer K. The role of whole grains in disease prevention. *J Am Diet Assoc* 101:780–785, 2002.
26. Guthrie JF, Morton JF. Food sources of added sweeteners in the diets of Americans. *J Am Diet Assoc* 100:43–48, 51, 2000.
27. American Dietetic Association. Position of the American Dietetic Association: Use of nutritive and nonnutritive sweeteners. *J Am Diet Assoc* 98:580–587, 1998.
28. American Dietetic Association. Position of the American Dietetic Association: Health implications of dietary fiber. *J Am Diet Assoc* 97:1157–1159, 1997.
29. Van Horn L. Fiber, lipids, and coronary heart disease. A statement for healthcare professionals from the Nutrition Committee, American Heart Association. *Circulation* 95:2701–2704, 1997.
30. Manach C, Williamson G, Morand C, Scalbert A, Remesy C. Bioavailability and bioefficacy of polyphenols in humans. I. Review of 97 bioavailability studies. *Am J Clin Nutr* 81(1 Suppl):230S–242S, 2005.
31. Moskaug JO, Carlsen H, Myhrstad MC, Blomhoff R. Polyphenols and glutathione synthesis regulation. *Am J Clin Nutr* 81(1 Suppl):277S–283S, 2005.
32. Kris-Etherton PM, Lichtenstein AH, Howard BV, Steinberg D, Witztum JL. Nutrition Committee of the American Heart Association Council on Nutrition, Physical Activity, and Metabolism. Antioxidant vitamin supplements and cardiovascular disease. *Circulation* 110:637–641, 2004.
33. Van Duyn MAS, Pivonka E. Overview of the health benefits of fruit and vegetable consumption for the dietetics professional: Selected literature. *J Am Diet Assoc* 100:1511–1521, 2000.
34. American Dietetic Association. Position of the American Dietetic Association: Food fortification and dietary supplements. *J Am Diet Assoc* 101:115–125, 2001.
35. Wijendran V, Hayes KC. Dietary n-6 and n-3 fatty acid balance and cardiovascular health. *Annu Rev Nutr* 24:597–615, 2004.
36. American Dietetic Association. Position of the American Dietetic Association: Fat replacers. *J Am Diet Assoc* 98:463–467, 1998.
37. Frayn KN, Kingman SM. Dietary sugars and lipid metabolism in humans. *Am J Clin Nutr* 62(suppl):250S–263S, 1995.
38. Wolraich ML, Wilson DB, White W. The effect of sugar on behavior or cognition in children. A meta-analysis. *JAMA* 274:1617–1621, 1995.
39. Rico-Sanz J. Body composition and nutritional assessments in soccer. *Int J Sport Nutr* 8:113–123, 1998.
40. Rico-Sanz J, Frontera WR, Molé PA, Rivera MA, Rivera-Brown A, Meredith CN. Dietary and performance assessment of elite soccer players during a period of intense training. *Int J Sport Nutr* 8:230–240, 1998.
41. Sugiura K, Suzuki I, Kobayashi K. Nutritional intake of elite Japanese track-and-field athletes. *Int J Sport Nutr* 9:202–212, 1999.
42. Krumbach CJ, Ellis DR, Driskell JA. A report of vitamin and mineral supplement use among university athletes in a division I institution. *Int J Sport Nutr* 9:416–425, 1999.
43. Jonnalagadda SS, Benardot D, Dill MN. Assessment of underreporting of energy intake by elite female gymnasts. *Int J Sport Nutr Exerc Metab* 10:315–325, 2000.
44. García-Rovés PM, Terrados N, Fernández S, Patterson AM. Comparison of dietary intake and eating behavior of professional road cyclists during training and competition. *Int J Sport Nutr Exerc Metab* 10:82–98, 2000.
45. Deutz RC, Benardot D, Martin DE, Cody MM. Relationship between energy deficits and body composition in elite female gymnasts and runners. *Med Sci Sports Exerc* 32:659–668, 2000.
46. Peters EM, Goetzsche JM. Dietary practices of South African ultradistance runners. *Int J Sport Nutr* 7:80–103, 1997.
47. Onywera VO, Kiplamai FK, Boit MK, Pitsiladis YP. Food and macronutrient intake of elite Kenyan distance runners. *Int J Sport Nutr Exerc Metab* 14:709–719, 2004.
48. Sjodin AM, Andersson AB, Hogberg JM, Westerterp KR. Energy balance in cross-country skiers: A study using doubly labeled water. *Med Sci Sports Exerc* 26:720–724, 1994.
49. Thompson JL, Manore MM, Skinner JS, Ravussin E, Spraul M. Daily energy expenditure in male endurance athletes with differing energy intakes. *Med Sci Sports Exerc* 27:347–354, 1995.
50. Beidleman BA, Puhl JL, De Souza MJ. Energy balance in female distance runners. *Am J Clin Nutr* 61:303–311, 1995.
51. Horton TJ, Drougas HJ, Sharp TA, Martinez LR, Reed GW, Hill JO. Energy balance in endurance-trained female cyclists and untrained controls. *J Appl Physiol* 76:1937–1945, 1994.

52. Jonnalagadda SS, Benardot D, Nelson M. Energy and nutrient intake of the United States national women's artistic gymnastics team. *Int J Sport Nutr* 8:331–344, 1998.

53. Keith RE, Stone MH, Carson RE, Lefavi RG, Fleck SJ. Nutritional status and lipid profiles of trained steroid-using bodybuilders. *Int J Sport Nutr* 6:247–254, 1996.

54. Nelson Steen S, Mayer K, Brownell KD, Wadden TA. Dietary intake of female collegiate heavyweight rowers. *Int J Sport Nutr* 5:225–231, 1995.

55. Fogelholm GM, Himberg JJ, Alopaeus K, et al. Dietary and biochemical indices of nutritional status in male athletes and controls. *J Am Coll Nutr* 11:181–191, 1992.

56. Butterworth DE, Nieman DC, Butler JV, Herring JL. Feeding patterns of marathon runners. *Int J Sport Nutr* 4:1–7, 1994.

57. Faber M, Spinnler Benadé AJ. Mineral and vitamin intake in field athletes (discus-, hammer-, javelin-throwers and shotputters). *Int J Sport Med* 12:324–327, 1991.

58. Burke LM, Gollan RA, Read RSD. Dietary intakes and food use of groups of elite Australian male athletes. *Int J Sport Nutr* 1:378–394, 1991.

59. Fogelholm GM, Rehunen S, Gref CG, et al. Dietary intake and thiamin, iron, and zinc status in elite nordic skiers during different training periods. *Int J Sport Nutr* 2:351–365, 1992.

60. Van Erp-Baart AMJ, Saris WHM, Binkhorst RA, et al. Nationwide survey on nutritional habits in elite athletes. Part I. Energy, carbohydrate, protein, and fat intake. *Int J Sports Med* 10(suppl 1):S3–S10, 1989.

61. Van Erp-Baart AMJ, Saris WHM, Binkhorst RA, et al. Nationwide survey on nutritional habits in elite athletes. Part II. Mineral and vitamin intake. *Int J Sports Med* 10(suppl 1):S11–S16, 1989.

62. Brotherhood JR. Nutrition and sports performance. *Sports Med* 1:350–389, 1984.

63. Burke LM, Diet GD, Read RSD. Diet patterns of elite Australian male triathletes. *Physician Sportsmed* 15(2):140–155, 1987.

64. Ellsworth NM, Hewitt BF, Haskell WL. Nutrient intake of elite male and female nordic skiers. *Physician Sportsmed* 13(2):78–92, 1985.

65. Hickson JF, Duke MA, Risser WL, et al. Nutritional intake from food sources of high school football athletes. *J Am Diet Assoc* 87:1656–1659, 1988.

66. Nowak RK, Knudsen KS, Schultz LO. Body composition and nutrient intakes of college men and women basketball players. *J Am Diet Assoc* 88:575–578, 1988.

67. Singh A, Evans P, Gallagher KL, Deuster PA. Dietary intakes and biochemical profiles of nutritional status of ultramarathoners. *Med Sci Sports Exerc* 25:328–334, 1993.

68. Sundgot-Borgen J. Risk and trigger factors for the development of eating disorders in female elite athletes. *Med Sci Sports Exerc* 26:414–419, 1994.

69. Petrie HJ, Stover EA, Horswill CA. Nutritional concerns for the child and adolescent competitor. *Nutrition* 20:620–631, 2004.

70. Kirchner EM, Lewis RD, O'Connor PJ. Bone mineral density and dietary intake of female college gymnasts. *Med Sci Sports Exerc* 27:543–549, 1995.

71. O'Connor PJ, Lewis RD, Kirchner EM, Cook DB. Eating disorder symptoms in former female college gymnasts: Relations with body composition. *Am J Clin Nutr* 64:840–843, 1996.

72. Walberg-Rankin J, Edmonds CE, Gwazdauskas FC. Diet and weight changes in female bodybuilders before and after competition. *Int J Sport Nutr* 3:87–102, 1993.

73. Thompson J, Manore MM, Skinner JS. Resting metabolic rate and thermic effect of a meal in low- and adequate-energy intake male endurance athletes. *Int J Sport Nutr* 3:194–206, 1993.

74. Faber M, Benadé AJS, van Eck M. Dietary intake, anthropometric measurements, and blood lipid values in weight training athletes (body builders). *Int J Sports Med* 7:342–346, 1986.

75. Koutedakis Y, Jamurtas A. The dancer as a performing athlete: Physiological considerations. *Sports Med* 34:651–661, 2004.

76. Rosen LW, Hough DO. Pathogenic weight-control behaviors of female college gymnasts. *Physician Sportsmed* 16(9):141–146, 1988.

77. Edwards JE, Lindeman AK, Mikesky AE, Stager JM. Energy balance in highly trained female endurance runners. *Med Sci Sports Exerc* 25:1398–1404, 1993.

78. Nieman DC, Butler JV, Pollett LM, Dietrich SJ, Lutz RD. Nutrient intake of marathon runners. *J Am Diet Assoc* 89:1273–1278, 1989.

79. Horswill CA. Weight loss and weight cycling in amateur wrestlers: Implications for performance and resting metabolic rate. *Int J Sport Nutr* 3:245–260, 1993.

80. Kiningham RB, Gorenflo DW. Weight loss methods of high school wrestlers. *Med Sci Sports Exerc* 33:810–813, 2001.

81. Walberg-Rankin J, Ocel JV, Craft LL. Effect of weight loss and refeeding diet composition on anaerobic performance in wrestlers. *Med Sci Sports Exerc* 28:1292–1299, 1996.

82. American College of Sports Medicine. Weight loss in wrestlers. *Med Sci Sports Exerc* 28:ix–xii, 1996.

83. White JA. Ergogenic demands of a 24-hour cycling event. *Br J Sports Med* 18:165, 1984.

84. Hagerman FC. Energy metabolism and fuel utilization. *Med Sci Sports Exerc* 24:S309–S314, 1992.

85. McArdle WD, Katch FI, Katch VL. *Exercise Physiology: Energy, Nutrition, and Human Performance* (5th ed.). Philadelphia: Lippincott Williams & Wilkins, 2001.

86. Nieman DC, Carlson KA, Brandstater ME, Naegele RT, Blankenship JW. Running exhaustion in 27-h fasted humans. *J Appl Physiol* 63:2502–2509, 1987.

87. Coyle EF, Coggan AR, Hemmert MK, Ivy JL. Muscle glycogen utilization during prolonged strenuous exercise when fed carbohydrate. *J Appl Physiol* 61:165–172, 1986.

88. Bergstrom J, Hermansen L, Hultman E, et al. Diet, muscle glycogen and physical performance. *Acta Physiol Scand* 71:140–150, 1967.

89. Christensen EH, Hansen O. Hypoglykamie, arbeitsfahigkeit and ermudung. *Scand Arch Physiol* 81:172–179, 1939.

90. Christensen EH, Hansen O. Respiratorischer quotient and O_2 aufnahme. *Scand Arch Physiol* 81:180–189, 1939.

91. Fink WJ, Costill DL. Skeletal muscle structure and function. In Maud PJ, Foster C (eds.), *Physiological Assessment of Human Fitness*. Champaign, IL: Human Kinetics, 1995.

92. Bergstrom J, Hultman E. A study of the glycogen metabolism during exercise in man. *Scan J Clin Lab Invest* 19:218–228, 1967.

93. Febbraio MA, Chiu A, Angus DJ, Arkinstall MJ, Hawley JA. Effects of carbohydrate ingestion before and during exercise on glucose kinetics and performance. *J Appl Physiol* 89:2220–2226, 2000.

94. Angus DJ, Hargreaves M, Dancey J, Febbraio MA. Effect of carbohydrate or carbohydrate plus medium-chain triglyceride ingestion on cycling time trial performance. *J Appl Physiol* 88:113–119, 2000.

95. Carrithers JA, Williamson DL, Gallagher PM, Godard MP, Schulze KE, Trappe SW. Effects of postexercise carbohydrate-protein feedings on muscle glycogen restoration. *J Appl Physiol* 88:1976–1982, 2000.

96. Coggan AR, Raguso CA, Gastaldelli A, Sidossis LS, Yeckel CW. Fat metabolism during high-intensity exercise in endurance-trained and untrained men. *Metabolism* 49:122–128, 2000.

97. Rick-Sanz J, Zehnder M, Buchli R, Dambach M, Boutellier U. Muscle glycogen degradation during simulation of a fatiguing soccer match in elite soccer players examined noninvasively by ^{13}C-MRS. *Med Sci Sports Exerc* 31:1587–1593, 1999.

98. Balsom PD, Wood K, Olsson P, Ekblom B. Carbohydrate intake and multiple sprint sports: With special reference to football (soccer). *Int J Sports Med* 20:48–52, 1999.

99. Greiwe JS, Hickner RC, Hansen PA, Racette SB, Chen MM, Holloszy JO. Effects of endurance exercise training on muscle glycogen accumulation in humans. *J Appl Physiol* 87:222–226, 1999.

100. Jacobs KA, Sherman WM. The efficacy of carbohydrate supplementation and chronic high-carbohydrate diets for improving endurance performance. *Int J Sport Nutr* 9:92–115, 1999.

101. Tsintzas K, Williams C. Human muscle glycogen metabolism during exercise. Effect of carbohydrate supplementation. *Sports Med* 25:7–23, 1998.

102. Sugiura K, Kobayashi K. Effect of carbohydrate ingestion on sprint performance following continuous and intermittent exercise. *Med Sci Sports Exerc* 30:1624–1630, 1998.

103. Chryssanthopoulos C, Williams C, Nowitz A, Kotsiopoulou C, Vleck V. The effect of a high carbohydrate meal on endurance running capacity. *Int J Sports Nutr Exerc Metab* 12:157–171, 2002.

104. Roy BD, Tarnopolsky MA. Influence of differing macronutrient intakes on muscle glycogen resynthesis after resistance exercise. *J Apply Physiol* 84:890–896, 1998.

105. Nicholas CW, Green PA, Hawkins RD, Williams C. Carbohydrate intake and recovery of intermittent running capacity. *Int J Sport Nutr* 7:251–260, 1997.

106. Wu CL, Nicholas C, WIlliams C, Took A, Hardy L. The influence of high-carbohydrate meals with different glycemic indices on substrate utilization during subsequent exercise. *Br J Nutr* 90:1049–1056, 2003.

107. Stannard SR, Thompson MW, Miller JCB. The effect of glycemic index on plasma glucose and lactate levels during incremental exercise. *Int J Sport Nutr Exerc Metab* 10:51–61, 2000.

108. Wee SL, Williams C, Gray S, Horabin J. Influence of high and low glycemic index meals on endurance running capacity. *Med Sci Sports Exerc* 31:393–399, 1999.

109. DeMarco HM, Sucher KP, Cisar CJ, Butterfield GE. Pre-exercise carbohydrate meals: Application of glycemic index. *Med Sci Sports Exerc* 31:164–170, 1999.

110. Sparks MJ, Selig SS, Febbraio MA. Pre-exercise carbohydrate ingestion: Effect of the glycemic index on endurance exercise performance. *Med Sci Sports Exerc* 30:844–849, 1998.

111. Kirwan JP, O'Gorman D, Evans WJ. A moderate glycemic meal before endurance exercise can enhance performance. *J Appl Physiol* 84:53–59, 1998.

112. Hargreaves M. Interactions between muscle glycogen and blood glucose during exercise. *Exerc Sport Sci Rev* 25:21–39, 1997.

113. Coyle EF. Substrate utilization during exercise in active people. *Am J Clin Nutr* 61(suppl):968S–979S, 1995.

114. Coggan AR. Plasma glucose metabolism during exercise: Effect of endurance training in humans. *Med Sci Sports Exerc* 29:620–627, 1997.

115. Burke LM, Kiens B, Ivy JL. Carbohydrates and fat for training and recovery. *J Sports Sci* 22:15–30, 2004.

116. Arkinstall MJ, Bruce CR, Clark SA, Rickards CA, Burke LM, Hawley JA. Regulation of fuel metabolism by preexercise muscle glycogen content and exercise intensity. *J Appl Physiol* 97:2275–2283, 2004.

117. O'Brien MJ, Viguie CA, Mazzeo RS, Brooks GA. Carbohydrate dependence during marathon running. *Med Sci Sports Exerc* 25:1009–1017, 1993.

118. Sherman WM, Wimer GS. Insufficient dietary carbohydrate during training: Does it impair athletic performance? *Int J Sport Nutr* 1:28–44, 1991.

119. Ivy JL. Muscle glycogen synthesis before and after exercise. *Sport Med* 11:6–19, 1991.

120. Simonsen JC, Sherman WM, Lamb DR, et al. Dietary carbohydrate, muscle glycogen, and power output during rowing training. *J Appl Physiol* 70:1500–1505, 1991.

121. Kirkendall DT. Effects of nutrition on performance in soccer. *Med Sci Sports Exerc* 26:1370–1374, 1993.

122. Widrick JJ, Costill DL, Fink WJ, et al. Carbohydrate feedings and exercise performance: Effect of initial muscle glycogen concentration. *J Appl Physiol* 74:2998–3005, 1993.

123. Saltin B, Astrand PO. Free fatty acids and exercise. *Am J Clin Nutr* 57 (suppl):752S–758S, 1993.

124. Costill DL, Miller JM. Nutrition for endurance sports: Carbohydrate and fluid balance. *Int J Sports Med* 1:2–14, 1980.

125. Costill DL, Bowers R, Branam G, Sparks K. Muscle glycogen utilization during prolonged exercise on successive days. *J Appl Physiol* 63:2388–2395, 1971.

126. Costill DL, Flynn MG, Kirwan JP, et al. Effects of repeated days of intensified training on muscle glycogen and swimming performance. *Med Sci Sports Exerc* 20:249–254, 1988.

127. Kirwan JP, Costill DL, Mitchell JB, et al. Carbohydrate balance in competitive runners during successive days of intense training. *J Appl Physiol* 65:2601–2606, 1988.

128. Fallowfield JL, Williams C. Carbohydrate intake and recovery from prolonged exercise. *Int J Sport Nutr* 3:150–164, 1993.

129. Sherman WM. Recovery from endurance exercise. *Med Sci Sports Exerc* 24 (suppl):S336–S339, 1992.

130. Pascoe DD, Costill DL, Fink WJ, Robergs RA, Zachwieja JJ. Glycogen resynthesis in skeletal muscle following resistive exercise. *Med Sci Sports Exerc* 25:349–354, 1993.

131. Parkin JA, Carey MF, Martin IK, Stojanovska L, Febbraio MA. Muscle glycogen storage following prolonged exercise: Effect of timing of ingestion of high glycemic index food. *Med Sci Sports Exerc* 29:220–224, 1997.

132. Burke LM, Collier GR, Davis PG, Fricker PA, Sanigorski AJ, Hargreaves M. Muscle glycogen storage after prolonged exercise: Effect of the frequency of carbohydrate feedings. *Am J Clin Nutr* 64:115–119, 1996.

133. Hickner RC, Fisher JS, Hansen PA, Racette SB, Mier CM, Turner MJ, Holloszy JO. Muscle glycogen accumulation after endurance exercise in trained and untrained individuals. *J Appl Physiol* 83:897–903, 1997.

134. Van Den Bergh AJ, Houtman S, Heerschap A, et al. Muscle glycogen recovery after exercise during glucose and fructose intake monitored by ^{13}C-NMR. *J Appl Physiol* 81:1495–1500, 1996.

135. Walton P, Rhodes ED. Glycemic index and optimal performance. *Sports Med* 23:164–172, 1997.

136. American College of Sports Medicine. Position stand on exercise and fluid replacement. *Med Sci Sports Exerc* 28:i–vii, 1996.

137. Coyle EF. Fluid and fuel intake during exercise. *J Sports Sci* 22:39–55, 2004.

138. Sawka MN, Coyle EF. Influence of body water and blood volume on thermoregulation and exercise performance in the heat. *Exerc Sport Sci Rev* 27:167–218, 1999.

139. Sparling PB. Expected environmental conditions for the 1996 Summer Olympic Games in Atlanta. *Clin J Sport Med* 5:220–222, 1995.

140. Kenney WL. Heat flux and storage in hot environments. *Int J Sports Med* 19:S92–S95, 1998.
141. Murray R. Nutrition for the marathon and other endurance sports: Environmental stress and dehydration. *Med Sci Sports Exerc* 24(suppl):S319–S323, 1992.
142. Gleeson M. Temperature regulation during exercise. *Int J Sports Med* 19:S96–S99, 1998.
143. Kenney WL, Johnson JM. Control of skin blood flow during exercise. *Med Sci Sports Exerc* 24:303–312, 1992.
144. Armstrong LE, Maresh CM. Effects of training, environment, and host factors on the sweating response to exercise. *Int J Sports Med* 19:S103–S105, 1998.
145. Gisolfi CV, Wenger CB. Temperature regulation during exercise: Old concepts, new ideas. In Terjung RL (ed.), *Exercise and Sport Sciences Reviews.* Lexington: Collamore Press, 1984.
146. Perlmutter EM. The Pittsburgh Marathon: "Playing weather roulette." *Physician Sportsmed* 14(8):132–138, 1986.
147. Armstrong LE, Hubbard RW, Jones BH, Daniels JT. Preparing Alberto Salazar for the heat of the 1984 Olympic Marathon. *Physician Sportsmed* 14(3)73–81, 1986.
148. Gonzalez-Alonso J, Mora-Rodriguez R, Below PR, Coyle EF. Dehydration reduces cardiac output and increases systemic and cutaneous vascular resistance during exercise. *J Appl Physiol* 79:1487–1496, 1995.
149. Horswill CA. Effective fluid replacement. *Int J Sport Nutr* 8:175–185, 1998.
150. Coyle EF. Cardiovascular drift during prolonged exercise and the effects of dehydration. *Int J Sports Med* 19:S121–S124, 1998.
151. Nielsen B. Heat acclimation—mechanisms of adaptation to exercise in the heat. *Int J Sports Med* 19:S154–S156, 1998.
152. Aoyagi Y, McLellan TM, Shephard RJ. Interactions of physical training and heat acclimation. The thermophysiology of exercising in a hot climate. *Sports Med* 23:173–210, 1997.
153. Pandolf KB. Time course of heat acclimation and its decay. *Int J Sports Med* 19:S157–S160, 1998.
154. Barr SI, Costill DL, Fink WJ. Fluid replacement during prolonged exercise: Effects of water, saline, or no fluid. *Med Sci Sports Exerc* 23:811–817, 1991.
155. Epstein Y, Armstrong LE. Fluid-electrolyte balance during labor and exercise: Concepts and misconceptions. *Int J Sport Nutr* 9:1–12, 1999.
156. Maresh CM, Gabaree-Boulant CL, Armstrong LE, Judelson DA, Hoffman JR, Castellani JW, Kenefick RW, Bergeron MF, Casa DJ. Effect of hydration status on thirst, drinking, and related hormonal responses during low-intensity exercise in the heat. *J Appl Physiol* 97:39–44, 2004.
157. Holtzhausen LM, Noakes TD. The prevalence and significance of post-exercise (postural) hypotension in ultramarathon runners. *Med Sci Sports Exerc* 27:1595–1601, 1995.
158. Rico-Sanz J, Frontera WR, Rivera MA, Rivera-Brown A, Mole PA, Meredith CN. Effects of hyperhydration on total body water, temperature regulation and performance of elite young soccer players in a warm climate. *Int J Sports Med* 17:85–91, 1996.
159. Armstrong LE, Soto JAH, Hacker FT, Casa DJ, Kavouras SA, Maresh CM. Urinary indices during dehydration, exercise, and rehydration. *Int J Sport Nutr* 8:345–355, 1998.
160. Brouns F. Gastric emptying as a regulatory factor in fluid uptake. *Int J Sports Med* 19:S125–S128, 1998.
161. Minehan MR, Riley MD, Burke LM. Effect of flavor and awareness of kilojoule content of drinks on preference and fluid balance in team sports. *Int J Sport Nutr Exerc Metab* 12:81–92, 2002.
162. Bassett DR, Nagle FJ, Mookerjee S, et al. Thermoregulatory responses to skin wetting during prolonged treadmill running. *Med Sci Sports Exerc* 19:28–32, 1987.
163. Burke LM, Hawley JA. Fluid balance in team sports. Guidelines for optimal practices. *Sports Med* 24:38–54, 1997.
164. Jeukendrup AE, Jentjens R. Oxidation of carbohydrate feedings during prolonged exercise: Current thoughts, guidelines and directions for future research. *Sports Med* 29:407–424, 2000.
165. Duchman SM, Ryan AJ, Schedl HP, Summers RW, Bleiler TL, Gisolfi CV. Upper limit for intestinal absorption of a dilute glucose solution in men at rest. *Med Sci Sports Exerc* 29:482–488, 1997.
166. Cunningham JJ. Is potassium needed in sports drinks for fluid replacement during exercise? *Int J Sports Nutr* 7:154–159, 1997.
167. Gisolfi CV, Summers RD, Schedl HP, Bleiler TL. Effect of sodium concentration in a carbohydrate-electrolyte solution on intestinal absorption. *Med Sci Sports Exerc* 10:1414–1420, 1995.
168. Shirreffs SM, Maughan RJ. Rehydration and recovery of fluid balance after exercise. *Exerc Sport Sci Rev* 28:27–32, 2000.
169. Coggan AR, Coyle EF. Carbohydrate ingestion during prolonged exercise: Effects on metabolism and performance. *Exerc Sport Sci Rev* 19:1–40, 1991.
170. Maughan RJ, Merson SJ, Broad NP, Shirreffs SM. Fluid electrolyte intake and loss in elite soccer players during training. *Int J Sport Nutr Exerc Metab* 14:333–346, 2004.
171. Coggan AR, Swanson SC. Nutritional manipulations before and during endurance exercise: Effects on performance. *Med Sci Sports Exerc* 24(suppl):24:S331–S335, 1992.
172. Brouns F, Saris W, Schneider H. Rationale for upper limits of electrolyte replacement during exercise. *Int J Sport Nutr* 2:229–238, 1992.
173. Montain SJ, Sawka MN, Wenger CB. Hyponatremia associated with exercise: Risk factors and pathogenesis. *Exerc Sport Sci Rev* 29:113–117, 2001.
174. Shirreffs SM, Taylor AJ, Leiper JB, Maughan RJ. Post-exercise rehydration in man: Effects of volume consumed and drink sodium content. *Med Sci Sports Exerc* 28:1260–1271, 1996.
175. Jeukendrup A, Brouns F, Wagenmakers AJM, Saris WHM. Carbohydrate-electrolyte feedings improve 1h time trial cycling performance. *Int J Sports Med* 18:125–129, 1997.
176. Tsintzas OK, Williams C, Singh R, Wilson W, Burrin J. Influence of carbohydrate-electrolyte drinks on marathon running performance. *Eur J Appl Physiol* 70:154–160, 1995.
177. Tsintzas OK, Williams C, Boobis L, Greenhaff P. Carbohydrate ingestion and single muscle fiber glycogen metabolism during prolonged running in men. *J Appl Physiol* 81:801–809, 1996.
178. Winnick JJ, Davis JM, Welsh RS, Carmichael MD, Murphy EA, Blackmon JA. Carbohydrate feedings during team sport exercise preserve physical and CNS function. *Med Sci Sports Exerc* 37:306–315, 2005.
179. Jentjens RLPG, Achten J, Jeukendrup AE. High oxidation rates from combined carbohydrates ingested during exercise. *Med Sci Sports Exerc* 36:1551–1558, 2004.
180. Tsintzas K, Liu R, Williams C, Campbell I, Gaitanos G. The effect of carbohydrate ingestion on performance during a 30-km race. *Int J Sport Nutr* 3:127–139, 1993.
181. Yaspelkis BB, Patterson JG, Anderla PA, Ding Z, Ivy JL. Carbohydrate supplementation spares muscle glycogen during variable-intensity exercise. *J Appl Physiol* 75:1477–1485, 1993.

182. Coyle EF, Coggan AR, Hemmert MK, Ivy JL. Muscle glycogen utilization during prolonged strenuous exercise when fed carbohydrate. *J Appl Physiol* 61:165–172, 1986.

183. Centers for Disease Control and Prevention. Recommendations to prevent and control iron deficiency in the United States. *MMWR* 47(No. RR-3):1–29, 1998.

184. Fogelholm M. Indicators of vitamin and mineral status in athletes' blood: A review. *Int J Sport Nutr* 5:267–284, 1995.

185. Shaskey DJ, Green GA. Sports hematology. *Sports Med* 29:27–38, 2000.

186. Pate RR, Miller BJ, Davis JM, Slentz CA, Klingshirn LA. Iron status of female runners. *Int J Sport Nutr* 3:222–231, 1993.

187. Nielsen P, Nachtigall D. Iron supplementation in athletes. Current recommendations. *Sports Med* 26:207–216, 1998.

188. Hinton PS, Giordano C, Brownlie T, Haas JD. Iron supplementation improves endurance after training in iron-depleted, nonanemic women. *J Appl Physiol* 88:1103–1111, 2000.

189. Malczewska J, Raczynski G, Stupnicki R. Iron status in female endurance athletes and in non-athletes. *Int J Sport Nutr Exerc Metab* 10:260–276, 2000.

190. Beard J, Tobin B. Iron status and exercise. *Am J Clin Nutr* 72(2 suppl):594S–597S, 2000.

191. Eichner ER. Anemia and blood boosting. *Sports Science Exchange* 14(2):1–4, 2001.

192. Chatard JC, Mujika I, Guy C, Lacour JR. Anemia and iron deficiency in athletes. Practical recommendations for treatment. *Sports Med* 27:229–240, 1999.

193. Blum SM, Sherman AR, Boileau RA. The effects of fitness-type exercise on iron status in adult women. *Am J Clin Nutr* 43:456–463, 1986.

194. Bourque SP, Pate RR, Branch D. Twelve weeks of endurance exercise training does not affect iron status measures in women. *J Am Diet Assoc* 97:1116–1121, 1997.

195. Herbert V. Recommended Dietary Intakes (RDI) of iron in humans. *Am J Clin Nutr* 45:679–686, 1987.

196. Expert Scientific Working Group. Summary of a report on assessment of the iron nutritional status of the United States population. *Am J Clin Nutr* 42:1318–1330, 1985.

197. Looker AC, Dallman PR, Carroll MD, Gunter EW, Johnson CL. Prevalence of iron deficiency in the United States. *JAMA* 277:973–976, 1997.

198. Matter M, Stittfall T, Graves J, et al. The effect of iron and folate therapy on maximal exercise performance in female marathon runners with iron and folate deficiency. *Clin Sci* 72:415–422, 1987.

199. Perkkio MV. Work performance in iron deficiency of increasing severity. *J Appl Physiol* 58:1477–1480, 1985.

200. Li R, Chen X, Yan H, Deurenberg P, Garby L, Hautvast JGAJ. Functional consequences of iron supplementation in iron-deficient female cotton mill workers in Beijing, China. *Am J Clin Nutr* 59:908–913, 1994.

201. Moore RJ, Friedl KE, Tulley RT, Askew EW. Maintenance of iron status in healthy men during an extended period of stress and physical activity. *Am J Clin Nutr* 58:923–927, 1993.

202. Ashenden MJ, Martin DT, Dobson GP, Mackintosh C, Hahn AG. Serum ferritin and anemia in trained female athletes. *Int J Sport Nutr* 8:223–229, 1998.

203. Zhu YI, Haas JD. Iron depletion without anemia and physical performance in young women. *Am J Clin Nutr* 66:334–341, 1997.

204. Lamanca JJ, Haymes EM. Effects of low ferritin concentration on endurance performance. *Int J Sport Nutr* 2:376–385, 1992.

205. Klingshirn LA, Pate RR, Bourque SP, Davis JM, Sargent RG. Effect of iron supplementation on endurance capacity in iron-depleted female runners. *Med Sci Sports Exerc* 24:819–824, 1992.

206. Powell PD, Tucker A. Iron supplementation and running performance in female cross-country runners. *Int J Sports Med* 12:462–467, 1991.

207. Telford RD, Bunney CJ, Catchpole EA, et al. Plasma ferritin concentration and physical work capacity in athletes. *Int J Sport Nutr* 2:335–342, 1992.

208. Lamanca JJ, Haymes EM. Effects of iron repletion on $\dot{V}O_{2max}$, endurance, and blood lactate in women. *Med Sci Sports Exerc* 25:1386–1392, 1993.

209. Brownlie T, Utermohlen V, Hinton PS, Haas JD. Tissue iron deficiency without anemia impairs adaptation in endurance capacity after aerobic training in previously untrained women. *Am J Clin Nutr* 79:437–443, 2004.

210. O'Toole ML, Hiller WDB, Roalstad MS, Douglas PS. Hemolysis during triathlon races: Its relation to race distance. *Med Sci Sports Exerc* 20:272–275, 1988.

211. Miller BJ, Pate RR, Burgess W. Foot impact force and intravascular hemolysis during distance running. *Int J Sports Med* 9:56–60, 1988.

212. Waller MF, Haymes EM. The effects of heat and exercise on sweat iron loss. *Med Sci Sports Exerc* 28:197–203, 1996.

213. Peters HP, De Vries WR, Vanberge-Henegouwen GP, Akkermans LM. Potential benefits and hazards of physical activity and exercise on the gastrointestinal tract. *Gut* 48:435–439, 2001.

214. McMahon LF. Occult gastrointestinal blood loss in marathon runners. *Ann Intern Med* 100:846–847, 1984.

215. Weight LM, Byrne MJ, Jacobs P. Hemolytic effects of exercise. *Clin Sci* 81:147–152, 1991.

216. Rockey DC, Cello JP. Evaluation of the gastrointestinal tract in patients with iron-deficiency anemia. *N Engl J Med* 329:1691–1695, 1993.

217. Ehn L, Carlmark B, Hoglund S. Iron status in athletes involved in intense physical activity. *Med Sci Sports Exerc* 12:61–64, 1980.

218. International Center for Sport Nutrition, United States Olympic Committee. *Iron and Physical Performance.* Omaha, NE: Author, 1990.

219. Zoller H, Vogel W. Iron supplementation in athletes—first do no harm. *Nutrition* 20:615–619, 2004.

220. Schmid A, Jakob E, Berg A, et al. Effect of physical exercise and vitamin C on absorption of ferric sodium citrate. *Med Sci Sports Exerc* 28:1470–1473, 1996.

221. Zotter H, Robinson N, Zorzoli M, Schattenberg L, Saugy M, Mangin P. Abnormally high serum ferritin levels among professional road cyclists. *Br J Sports Med* 38:704–708, 2004.

222. Nieman DC. Physical fitness and vegetarian diets: Is there a relation? *Am J Clin Nutr* 70(suppl):570S–575S, 1999.

223. Belko AZ. Vitamins and exercise—an update. *Med Sci Sports Exerc* 19:S191–S196, 1987.

224. Clarkson PM, Thompson HS. Antioxidants: What role do they play in physical activity and health? *Am J Clin Nutr* 72(2 suppl):637S–646S, 2000.

225. Herbold NH, Visconti BK, Frates S, Bandini L. Traditional and nontraditional supplements used by collegiate female varsity athletes. *Int J Sport Nutr Exerc Metab* 14:586–593, 2004.

226. Lukaski HC. Magnesium, zinc, and chromium nutriture and physical activity. *Am J Clin Nutr* 72:(2 suppl):585S–593S, 2000.

227. Clarkson PM, Haymes EM. Trace mineral requirements for athletes. *In J Sport Nutr* 4:104–119, 1994.

228. Manore MM. Effect of physical activity on thiamine, riboflavin, and vitamin B_6 requirements. *Am J Clin Nutr* 72(2 suppl):598S–606S, 2000.

229. Froiland K, Koszewski W, Hingst J, Kopecky L. Nutritional supplement use among college athletes and their sources of information. *Int J Sport Nutr Exerc Metab* 14:104–120, 2004.

230. Nieman DC, Gates JR, Butler JV, Pollett LM, Dietrich SJ, and Lutz RD. Supplementation patterns in marathon runners. *J Am Diet Assoc* 89:1615–1619, 1989.

231. Ervin RB, Wright JD, Reed-Billette D. Prevalence of leading types of dietary supplements used in the Third National Health and Nutrition Examination Survey, 1988–94. *Advance Data from Vital and Health Statistics,* 349. Hyattsville, MD: National Center for Health Statistics, 2004.

232. American Dietetic Association. Position of The American Dietetic Association: Food fortification and dietary supplements. *J Am Diet Assoc* 101:115–125, 2001.

233. Council on Scientific Affairs. Vitamin preparations as dietary supplements and as therapeutic agents. *JAMA* 257:1929–1936, 1987.

234. Callaway CW, McNutt K, Rivlin RS. Statement on vitamin and mineral supplements. *Am J Clin Nutr* 46:1075, 1987.

235. Barnett DW, Conlee RK. The effects of a commercial dietary supplement on human performance. *Am J Clin Nutr* 40:586–590, 1984.

236. Keys A. Vitamin supplementation of U.S. Army rations in relation to fatigue and the ability to do muscular work. *J Nutr* 23:259–269, 1942. See also: *Am J Physiol* 144:5, 1945.

237. Singh A, Papanicolaou DA, Lawrence LL, Howell EA, Chrousos GP, Deuster PA. Neuroendocrine responses to running in women after zinc and vitamin E supplementation. *Med Sci Sports Exerc* 31:536–542, 1999.

238. Telford RD, Catchpole EA, Deakin V, Hahn AG, Plank AW. The effect of 7 to 8 months of vitamin/mineral supplementation on athletic performance. *Int J Sport Nutr* 2:135–153, 1992.

239. Singh A, Moses FM, Deuster PA. Chronic multivitamin-mineral supplementation does not enhance performance. *Med Sci Sports Exerc* 24:726–732, 1992.

240. Nielsen AN, Mizuno M, Ratkevicius A, Mohr T, Rohde M, Mortensen SA, Quistorff B. No effect of antioxidant supplementation in triathletes on maximal oxygen uptake, ^{31}P-NMRS detected muscle energy metabolism and muscle fatigue. *Int J Sports Med* 20:154–158, 1999.

241. Finstad EW, Newhouse IJ, Lukaski HC, McAuliffe JE, Stewart CR. The effects of magnesium supplementation on exercise performance. *Med Sci Sports Exerc* 33:493–498, 2001.

242. Rokitzki L, Sagredos AN, Feub F, Buchner M, Keul J. Acute changes in vitamin B_6 status in endurance athletes before and after a marathon. *Int J Sport Nutr* 4:154–165, 1994.

243. Soares MJ, Satvanaravana K, Famii MS, Jacob CM, Ramana YV, Rao SS. The effect of exercise on the riboflavin status of adult men. *Br J Nutr* 69:541–551, 1993.

244. Manore MM, Helleksen JM, Merkel MS, Skinner JS. Longitudinal changes in zinc status in untrained men: Effects of two different 12-week exercise training programs and zinc supplementation. *J Am Diet Assoc* 93:1165–1168, 1993.

245. Webster MJ. Physiological and performance responses to supplementation with thiamin and pantothenic acid derivatives. *Eur J Appl Physiol* 77:486–491, 1998.

246. Virk RS, Dunton NJ, Young JC, Leklem JE. Effect of vitamin B_6 supplementation on fuels, catecholamines, and amino acids during exercise in men. *Med Sci Sports Exerc* 31:400–408, 1999.

247. Lukaski HC, Hoverson BS, Gallagher SK, Bolonchuk WW. Physical training and copper, iron, and zinc status of swimmers. *Am J Clin Nutr* 51:1093–1099, 1990.

248. Fogelholm M. Micronutrient status in females during a 24-week fitness-type exercise program. *Ann Nutr Metab* 36:209–218, 1992.

249. Van der Beck EJ, van Dokkum W. Schrijver J, et al. Thiamin, riboflavin, and vitamins B_6 and C: Impact of combined restricted intake on functional performance in man. *Am J Clin Nutr* 48:1451–1462, 1989.

250. Ji LL. Exercise, oxidative stress, and antioxidants. *Am J Sports Med* 24:S20–S24, 1996.

251. Powers SK, Ji LL, Leeuwenburgh C. Exercise training-induced alterations in skeletal muscle antioxidant capacity: A brief review. *Med Sci Sports Exerc* 31:987–997, 1999.

252. Jenkins RR. Exercise and oxidative stress methodology: A critique. *Am J Clin Nutr* 72(2 suppl):670S–674S, 2000.

253. Evans WJ. Vitamin E, vitamin C, and exercise. *Am J Clin Nutr* 72(2 suppl):647S–652S, 2000.

254. Viitala P, Newhouse IJ. Vitamin E supplementation, exercise and lipid peroxidation in human participants. *Eur J Appl Physiol* 93:108–115, 2004.

255. Nieman DC, Henson DA, McAnulty SR, McAnulty LS, Morrow JD, Ahmed A, Heward CB. Vitamin E and immunity after the Kona Triathlon World Championship. *Med Sci Sports Exerc* 36:1328–1335, 2004.

256. Nieman DC, Henson DA, McAnulty SR, McAnulty L, Swick NS, Utter AC, Vinci DM, Opiela SJ, Morrow JD. Influence of vitamin C supplementation on oxidative and immune changes following an ultramarathon. *J Appl Physiol* 92:1970–1977, 2002.

257. Urso ML, Clarkson PM. Oxidative stress, exercise, and antioxidant supplementation. *Toxicology* 189:41–54, 2003.

258. Tessier F, Margaritis I, Richard MJ, Moynot C, Marconnet P. Selenium and training effects on the glutathione system and aerobic performance. *Med Sci Sports Exerc* 27:390–396, 1995.

259. Wood RJ, Zheng JJ. High dietary calcium intakes reduce zinc absorption and balance in humans. *Am J Clin Nutr* 65:1803–1809, 1997.

260. Yadrick MK, Kenney MA, Winterfeldt EA. Iron, copper, and zinc status: Response to supplementation with zinc or zinc and iron in adult females. *Am J Clin Nutr* 49:145–150, 1989.

261. Bjelakovic G, Nikolova D, Simonetti RG, Gluud C. Antioxidant supplements for prevention of gastrointestinal cancers: A systematic review and meta-analysis. *Lancet* 364(9441):1219–1228, 2004.

262. Lemon PWR. Effects of exercise on dietary protein requirements. *Int J Sport Nutr* 8:426–447, 1998.

263. Lemon PWR. Protein and amino acid needs of the strength athlete. *Int J Sport Nutr* 1:127–145, 1991; see also *Int J Sport Nutr* 5:S39–S61, 1995.

264. LaMont LS, McCullough AJ, Kalhan SC. Comparison of leucine kinetics in endurance-trained and sedentary humans. *J Appl Physiol* 86:320–325, 1999.

265. Gibala MJ. Regulation of skeletal muscle amino acid metabolism during exercise. *Int J Sport Nutr Exerc Metab* 11:87–108, 2001.

266. Poortmans JR, Dellalieux O. Do regular high protein diets have potential health risks on kidney function in athletes? *Int J Sport Nutr Exerc Metab* 10:28–38, 2000.

267. Bowtell JL, Leese GP, Smith K, Watt PW, Nevill A, Rooyackers O, Wagenmakers AJM, Rennie MJ. Modulation of whole body protein metabolism during and after exercise, by variation of dietary protein. *J Appl Physiol* 86:1744–1752, 1998.

268. Roy BD, Fowlers JR, Hill R, Tarnopolsky MA. Macronutrient intake and whole body protein metabolism following resistance exercise. *Med Sci Sports Exerc* 32:1412–1418, 2000.

269. Dohm GL, Tapscott EB, Kasperek GJ. Protein degradation during endurance exercise and recovery. *Med Sci Sports Exerc* 19:S166–S171, 1987.

270. Tarnopolsky MA, Atkinson SA, MacDougall JD, et al. Evaluation of protein requirements for trained strength athletes. *J Appl Physiol* 73:1986–1995, 1992.

271. Lemon PWR, Tarnopolsky MA, MacDougall JD, Atkinson SA. Protein requirements and muscle mass/strength changes during intensive training in novice bodybuilders. *J Appl Physiol* 73:767–775, 1992.

272. Tipton KD, Elliott TA, Cree MG, Wolf SE, Sanford AP, Wolfe RR. Ingestion of casein and whey proteins result in muscle anabolism after resistance exercise. *Med Sci Sports Exerc* 36:2073–2081, 2004.

273. Tarnopolsky MA, MacDougall JD, Atkinson SA. Influence of protein intake and training status on nitrogen balance and lean body mass. *J Appl Physiol* 64:187–193, 1988.

274. Tipton KD, Ferrando AA, Williams BD, Wolfe RR. Muscle protein metabolism in female swimmers after a combination of resistance and endurance exercise. *J Appl Physiol* 81:2034–2038, 1996.

275. Borsheim E, Aarsland A, Wolfe RR. Effect of an amino acid, protein, and carbohydrate mixture on net muscle protein balance after resistance exercise. *Int J Sport Nutr Exerc Metab* 14:255–271, 2004.

276. Sheffield-Moore M, Yeckel CW, Volpi E, Wolf SE, Morio B, Chinkes DL, Paddon-Jones D, Wolfe RR. Postexercise protein metabolism in older and younger men following moderate-intensity aerobic exercise. *Am J Physiol Endocrinol Metab* 287:E513–E522, 2004.

277. Wagenmakers AJM. Muscle amino acid metabolism at rest and during exercise: Role in human physiology and metabolism. *Exerc Sport Sci Rev* 26:287–314, 1998.

278. Acheson KJ, Schutz Y, Bessard T, et al. Glycogen storage capacity and de novo lipogenesis during massive carbohydrate overfeeding in man. *Am J Clin Nutr* 48:240–247, 1988.

279. Goss FL, Karam C. The effects of glycogen supercompensation on the electrocardiographic response during exercise. *Res Quart Exerc Sport* 58:68–71, 1987.

280. Sherman WM, Costill DL, Fink WJ, et al. The effect of exercise diet manipulation on muscle glycogen and its subsequent utilization during performance. *Int J Sports Med* 2:114–118, 1981.

281. Blom PCS, Costill DL, Vollestad NK. Exhaustive running: Inappropriate as a stimulus of muscle glycogen supercompensation. *Med Sci Sports Exerc* 19:398–403, 1987.

282. Hawley JA, Schabort EJ, Noakes TD, Dennis SC. Carbohydrate-loading and exercise performance: An update. *Sports Med* 24:73–81, 1997.

283. Williams C, Brewer J, Walker M. The effect of a high carbohydrate diet on running performance during a 30-km treadmill time trial. *Eur J Appl Physiol* 65:18–24, 1992.

284. Karlsson J, Saltin B. Diet, muscle glycogen, and endurance performance. *J Appl Physiol* 31:203–206, 1971.

285. Rauch LHG, Rodger I, Wilson GR, Belonje JD, Dennis SC, Noakes TD, Hawley JA. The effects of carbohydrate loading on muscle glycogen content and cycling performance. *Int J Sport Nutr* 5:25–36, 1995.

286. Maughan RJ, Greenhaff PL, Leiper JB, Ball D, Lambert CP, Gleeson M. Diet composition and the performance of high-intensity exercise. *J Sports Sci* 15:265–275, 1997.

287. Foster C, Costill DL, Fink WJ. Effects of preexercise feedings on endurance performance. *Med Sci Sports Exerc* 11:1–5, 1979.

288. Keller K, Schwarzkopf R. Preexercise snacks may decrease exercise performance. *Physician Sportsmed* 12:89–91, 1984.

289. Gleeson M, Maugham RJ, Greenhaff PL. Comparison of the effects of pre-exercise feeding of glucose, glycerol, and placebo on endurance and fuel homeostasis in man. *Eur J Appl Physiol* 55:645–653, 1986.

290. Sherman WM, Peden MC, Wright DA. Carbohydrate feedings 1 h before exercise improves cycling performance. *Am J Clin Nutr* 54:866–870, 1991.

291. Hargreaves M, Costill DL, Fink WJ, et al. Effect of pre-exercise carbohydrate feedings on endurance cycling performance. *Med Sci Sports Exerc* 19:33–36, 1987.

292. Burelle Y, Peronnet F, Massicotte D, Brisson GR, Hillaire-Marcel C. Oxidation of ^{13}C-glucose and ^{13}C-fructose ingested as a preexercise meal: Effect of carbohydrate ingestion during exercise. *Int J Sport Nutr* 7:117–127, 1997.

293. Short KR, Sheffield-Moore M, Costill DL. Glycemic and insulinemic responses to multiple preexercise carbohydrate feedings. *Int J Sport Nutr* 7:128–137, 1997.

294. Hendelman DL, Ornstein K, Debold EP, Volpe SL, Freedson PS. Preexercise feeding in untrained adolescent boys does not affect responses to endurance exercise or performance. *Int J Sport Nutr* 7:207–218, 1997.

295. Febbraio MA, Stewart KL. Carbohydrate feeding before prolonged exercise: Effect of glycemic index on muscle glycogenolysis and exercise performance. *J Appl Physiol* 81:1115–1120, 1996.

296. Van Zant RS, Lemon PW. Preexercise sugar feeding does not alter prolonged exercise muscle glycogen or protein catabolism. *Can J Appl Physiol* 22:268–279, 1997.

297. Neufer PD, Costill DL, Flynn MG, et al. Improvements in exercise performance: Effects of carbohydrate feedings and diet. *J Appl Physiol* 62:983–988, 1987.

298. Wright DA, Sherman WM, Dernback AR. Carbohydrate feedings before, during, or in combination improve cycling endurance performance. *J Appl Physiol* 71:1082–1088, 1991.

299. Aragon-Vargas LF. Effects of fasting on endurance exercise. *Sports Med* 16:255–265, 1993.

300. Williams MH. Ergogenic aids: A means to *citius, altius, fortius,* and Olympic gold? *Res Q Exerc Sport* 67(suppl):58–64, 1996.

301. Kamber M, Baume N, Saugy M, Rivier L. Nutritional supplements as a source for positive doping cases? *Int J Sport Nutr Exerc Metab* 11:258–263, 2001.

302. Williams MH. The gospel truth about dietary supplements. *ACSM's Health & Fitness Journal* 1(1):24–29, 1997.

303. Catlin DH, Murray TH. Performance-enhancing drugs, fair competition, and Olympic sport. *JAMA* 276:231–237, 1996.

304. Nissen SL, Sharp RL. Effect of dietary supplements on lean mass and strength gains with resistance exercise: A meta-analysis. *J Appl Physiol* 94:651–659, 2003.

305. Juhn M. Popular sports supplements and ergogenic aids. *Sports Med* 33:921–939, 2003.

306. Tokish JM, Kocher MS, Hawkins RJ. Ergogenic aids: A review of basic science, performance, side effects, and status in sports. *Am J Sports Med* 32:1543–1553, 2004.

307. Bucci LR. Selected herbals and human exercise performance. *Am J Clin Nutr* 72(2 suppl):624S–636S, 2000.

308. Strauss RH. *Drugs and Performance in Sports.* Philadelphia: W.B. Saunders Company, 1987.

309. Percy EC. Ergogenic aids in athletics. *Med Sci Sports Exerc* 10:298–303, 1978.

310. Consumer Reports. Sports-supplement dangers. *Consumer Reports,* June 2001, pp. 40–42.

311. Sobal J, Marquart LF. Vitamin/mineral supplement use among athletes: A review of the literature. *Int J Sport Nutr* 4:320–334, 1994.

312. Brass EP. Supplemental carnitine and exercise. *Am J Clin Nutr* 72(2 suppl):618S–623S, 2000.

313. Bahrke MS, Morgan WR. Evaluation of the ergogenic properties of ginseng: An update. *Sports Med* 29:113–133, 2000.

314. Villani RG, Gannon J, Self M, Rich PA. L-carnitine supplementation combined with aerobic training does not promote weight loss in moderately obese women. *Int J Sport Nutr Exerc Metab* 10:199–207, 2000.

315. Van Someren K, Fulcher K, McCarthy J, Moore J, Horgan G, Langford R. An investigation into the effects of sodium citrate ingestion on high-intensity exercise performance. *Int J Sport Nutr* 8:356–363, 2000.

316. Brouns F, Fogelholm M, van Hall G, Wagenmakers A, Saris WHM. Chronic oral lactate supplementation does not affect lactate disappearance from blood after exercise. *Int J Sport Nutr* 5:117–124, 1995.

317. Antonio J, Uelmen J, Rodriguez R, Earnest C. The effects of *Tribulus Terrestris* on body composition and exercise performance in resistance-trained males. *Int J Sport Nutr Exerc Metab* 10:208–215, 2000.

318. Campbell WW, Joseph LJO, Davey SL, Cyr-Cambell D, Anderson RA, Evans WJ. Effects of resistance training and chromium picolinate on body composition and skeletal muscle in older men. *J Appl Physiol* 86:29–39, 1999.

319. Fawcett JP, Farquhar SJ, Walker RH, Thou T, Lowe G, Goulding A. The effect of oral vanadyl sulfate on body composition and performance in weight-training athletes. *Int J Sport Nutr* 6:382–390, 1996.

320. Weston SB, Zhou S, Weatherby RP, Robson SJ. Does exogenous coenzyme Q10 affect aerobic capacity in endurance athletes? *Int J Sport Nutr* 7:197–206, 1997.

321. Warber JP, Patton JF, Tharion WJ, Zeisel SH, Mello RP, Kemnitz CP, Lieberman HR. The effects of choline supplementation on physical performance. *Int J Sport Nutr Exerc Metab* 10:170–181, 2000.

322. McNaughton L, Dalton B, Tarr J. Inosine supplementation has no effect on aerobic or anaerobic cycling performance. *Int J Sport Nutr* 9:333–344, 1999.

323. Walker LS, Bemben MG, Bemben DA, Knehans AW. Chromium picolinate effects on body composition and muscular performance in wrestlers. *Med Sci Sports Exerc* 30:1730–1737, 1998.

324. Eschbach LC, Webster MJ, Boyd JC, McArthur PD, Evetovich TK. The effect of Siberian Ginseng (*Eleutherococcus Senticosus*) on substrate utilization and performance during prolonged cycling. *Int J Sport Nutr Exerc Metab* 10:444–451, 2000.

325. Svensson M, Malm C, Tonkonogi M, Ekblom B, Sjödin B, Sahlin K. Effect of Q10 supplementation on tissue Q10 levels and adenine nucleotide catabolism during high-intensity exercise. *Int J Sport Nutr* 9:166–180, 1999.

326. Brown AC, MacRae HSH, Turner NS. Tricarboxylic-acid-cycle intermediates and cycle endurance capacity. *Int J Sport Nutr Exerc Metab* 14:720–729, 2004.

327. O'Brien CP, Lyons F. Alcohol and the athlete. *Sports Med* 29:295–300, 2000.

328. Mottram DR. Banned drugs in sport. Does the International Olympic Committee (IOC) list need updating? *Sports Med* 27:1–10, 1999.

329. Sukala WR. Pyruvate: Beyond the marketing hype. *Int J Sport Nutr* 8:241–249, 1998.

330. Stensrund T, Ingjer F, Holm H, Stromme SB. L-tryptophan supplementation does not improve running performance. *Int J Sports Med* 6:481–485, 1992.

331. Wheeler KB, Garleb KA. Gamma oryzanol-plant sterol supplementation: Metabolic, endocrine, and physiologic effects. *Int J Sport Nutr* 1:170–177, 1991.

332. Gallagher PM, Carrithers JA, Godard MP, Schulze KE, Trappe SW. β-hydroxy-β-methylbutyrate ingestion, part I: Effects on strength and fat free mass. *Med Sci Sports Exerc* 32:2109–2115, 2000.

333. Sen CK, Packer L. Thiol homeostasis and supplements in physical exercise. *Am J Clin Nutr* 72(2 suppl):653S–669S, 2000.

334. Ferrando AA, Green NR. The effect of boron supplementation on lean body mass, plasma testosterone levels, and strength in male bodybuilders. *Int J Sport Nutr* 3:140–149, 1993.

335. Davis JM, Welsh RS, Aldersen NA. Effects of carbohydrate and chromium ingestion during intermittent high-intensity exercise to fatigue. *Int J Sport Nutr Exerc Metab* 10:476–485, 2000.

336. Ivy JL. Effect of pyruvate and dihydroxyacetone on metabolism and aerobic endurance capacity. *Med Sci Sports Exerc* 30:837–843, 1998.

337. Kreider RB, Melton C, Greenwood M, Rasmussen C, Lundberg J, Earnest C, Almada A. Effects of oral D-ribose supplementation on anaerobic capacity and selected metabolic markers in health males. *Int J Sport Nutr Exerc Metab* 13:76–86, 2003.

338. Philen RM, Ortiz DI, Auerbach SB, Falk H. Survey of advertising for nutritional supplements in health and bodybuilding magazines. *JAMA* 268:1008–1011, 1992.

339. Brill JB, Keane MW. Supplementation patterns of competitive male and female bodybuilders. *Int J Sport Nutr* 4:398–412, 1994.

340. Larkin T. Bee pollen as a health food. *FDA Consumer,* April, 1984, p. 21.

341. Fennema O. The placebo effect of foods. *Food Technology,* December 1984, pp. 57–67.

342. Turner JA, Deyo RA, Loeser JD, Von Korff M, Fordyce WE. The importance of placebo effects in pain treatment and research. *JAMA* 271:1609–1614, 1994.

343. Knight CA, Knight I, Mitchell DC, Zepp JE. Beverage caffeine intake in US consumers and subpopulations of interest: Estimates from the Share of Intake Panel Survey. *Food Chem Toxicol* 42:1923–1930, 2004.

344. Sinclair CJ, Geiger JD. Caffeine use in sports. A pharmacological review. *J Sports Med Phys Fitness* 40:71–79, 2000.

345. James JE. Critical review of dietary caffeine and blood pressure: A relationship that should be taken more seriously. *Psychosom Med* 66:63–71, 2004.

346. Doherty M, Smith PM. Effects of caffeine ingestion on exercise testing: A meta-analysis. *Int J Sport Nutr Exerc Metab* 14:626–646, 2004.

347. Bell DG, Jacobs I, Ellerington K. Effect of caffeine and ephedrine ingestion on anaerobic exercise performance. *Med Sci Sports Exerc* 33:1399–1403, 2001.

348. Paluska SA. Caffeine and exercise. *Curr Sports Med Rep* 2:213–219, 2003.

349. Magkos F, Kavouras SA. Caffeine and ephedrine: Physiological, metabolic and performance-enhancing effects. *Sports Med* 34:871–889, 2004.

350. Van Baak MA, Saris WHM. The effect of caffeine on endurance performance after nonselective β-adrenergic blockade. *Med Sci Sports Exerc* 32:499–503, 2000.

351. Van Soeren MH, Graham TE. Effect of caffeine on metabolism, exercise endurance, and catecholamine responses after withdrawal. *J Appl Physiol* 85:1493–1501, 1998.

352. Bruce CR, Anderson ME, Fraser SF, Stepto NK, Klein R, Hopkins WG, Hawley JA. Enhancement of 2000-m rowing performance after caffeine ingestion. *Med Sci Sports Exerc* 32:1958–1963, 2000.

353. Kovacs EMR, Stegen JHCH, Brouns F. Effect of caffeinated drinks on substrate metabolism, caffeine excretion, and performance. *J Appl Physiol* 85:709–715, 1998.

354. Wilkes D, Gledhill N, Smyth R. Effect of acute induced metabolic alkalosis on 800-m racing time. *Med Sci Sports Exerc* 15:277–280, 1983.

355. Goldfinch J, Naughton LM, Davies P. Induced metabolic alkalosis and its effects on 400-m racing time. *Eur J Appl Physiol* 57:45–48, 1988.

356. Matson LG, Tran ZV. Effects of sodium bicarbonate ingestion on anaerobic performance: A meta-analytic review. *Int J Sport Nutr* 3:2–28, 1993.

357. Montfoort MCE, Van Dieren L, Hopkins WG, Shearman JP. Effects of ingestion of bicarbonate, citrate, lactate, and chloride on sprint running. *Med Sci Sports Exerc* 36:1239–1243, 2004.

358. McNaughton L, Dalton B, Palmer G. Sodium bicarbonate can be used as an ergogenic aid in high-intensity, competitive cycle ergometry of 1 h duration. *Eur J Appl Physiol* 80:65–69, 1999.

359. Leigh-Smith S. Blood boosting. *Br J Sports Med* 38:99–101, 2004.

360. Shaskey DJ, Green GA. Sports hematology. *Sports Med* 29:27–38, 2000.

361. Ekblom BT. Blood boosting and sport. *Baillieres Best Pract Res Clin Endocrinol Metab* 14:89–98, 2000.

362. Sawka MN, Young AJ. Acute polycythemia and human performance during exercise and exposure to extreme environments. *Ex Sport Sci Rev* 17:265–293, 1989.

363. Jones M, Pedoe DST. Blood doping—a literature review. *Br J Sport Med* 23:84–88, 1989.

364. American College of Sports Medicine: Position stand on the use of blood doping as an ergogenic aid. *Med Sci Sports Exerc* 28:i–vii, 1996.

365. Young AJ, Sawka MN, Muza SR, Boushel R, Lyons T, Rock PB, Freund BJ, Waters R, Cymerman A, Pandolf KB, Valeri CR. Effects of erythrocyte infusion on $\dot{V}O_{2max}$ at high altitude. *J Appl Physiol* 81:252–259, 1996.

366. Abellan R, Ventura R, Pichini S, Remacha AF, Pascual JA, Pacifici R, Di Giovannandrea R, Zuccaro P, Segura J. Evaluation of immunoassays for the measurement of erythropoietin (EPO) as an indirect biomarker of recombinant human EPO misuse in sport. *J Pharm Biomed Anal* 35:1169–1177, 2004.

367. Nissen-Lie G, Birkeland K, Hemmersbach P, Skibeli V. Serum sTfR levels may indicate charge profiling of urinary r-hEPO in doping control. *Med Sci Sports Exerc* 36:588–593, 2004.

368. Birkeland KI, Stray Gundersen J, Hemmersbach P, Hallen J, Haug E, Bahr R. Effect of rhEPO administration on serum levels of sTfR and cycling performance. *Med Sci Sports Exerc* 32:1238–1243, 2000.

369. Lippi G, Guidi G. Laboratory screening for erythropoietin abuse in sports: An emerging challenge. *Clin Chem Lab Med* 38:13–19, 2000.

370. Goebel C, Alma C, Howe C, Kazlauskas R, Trout G. Methodologies for detection of hemoglobin-based oxygen carriers. *J Chromatogr Sci* 43:39–46, 2005.

371. Foster ZJ, Housner JA. Anabolic-androgenic steroids and testosterone precursors: Ergogenic aids and sport. *Curr Sports Med Rep* 3:234–241, 2004.

372. Yesalis CE, Kennedy NJ, Kopstein AN, Bahrke MS. Anabolic–androgenic steroid use in the United States. *JAMA* 270:1217–1221, 1993.

373. American College of Sports Medicine. Position statement on the use of anabolic–androgenic steroids in sports. *Med Sci Sports Exerc* 19:534–539, 1987.

374. Hartgens F, Kuipers H. Effects of androgenic–anabolic steroids in athletes. *Sports Med* 34:513–554, 2004.

375. Evans NA. Current concepts in anabolic–androgenic steroids. *Am J Sports Med* 32:534–542, 2004.

376. Bahrke MS, Yesalis CE. Abuse of anabolic androgenic steroids and related substances in sport and exercise. *Curr Opinion Pharmacol* 4:614–620, 2004.

377. Bahrke MS, Yesalis CE, Kopstein AN, Stephens JA. Risk factors associated with anabolic–androgenic steroid use among adolescents. *Sports Med* 29:397–405, 2000.

378. Ziegenfuss TN, Berardi JM, Lowery LM. Effects of prohormone supplementation in humans: A review. *Can J Appl Physiol* 27:628–646, 2002.

379. Forbes GB, Porta CR, Herr BE, Griggs RC. Sequence of changes in body composition induced by testosterone and reversal of changes after drug is stopped. *JAMA* 267:397–399, 1992.

380. Leder BZ, LeBlanc KM, Longcope C, Lee H, Catlin DH, Finkelstein JS. Effects of oral androstenedione administration on serum testosterone and estradiol levels in postmenopausal women. *J Clin Endocrinol Metab* 87:5449–5454, 2002.

381. Mottram DR, George AJ. Anabolic steroids. *Baillieres Best Pract Res Clin Endocrinol Metab* 14:55–69, 2000.

382. Glazer G. Atherogenic effects of anabolic steroids on serum lipid levels: A literature review. *Arch Intern Med* 151:1925–1933, 1991.

383. Blue JG, Lombardo JA. Steroids and steroid-like compounds. *Clin Sports Med* 18:667–689, 1999.

384. Pope HG, Katz DL. Affective and psychotic symptoms associated with anabolic steroid use. *Am J Psychiatry* 145:487–490, 1988.

385. Su T-P, Pagliaro M, Schmidt PJ, et al. Neuropsychiatric effects of anabolic steroids in male normal volunteers. *JAMA* 269:2760–2764, 1993.

386. Bricout V, Wright F. Update on nandrolone and norsteroids: How endogenous or xenobiotic are these substances? *Eur J Appl Physiol* 92:1–12, 2004.

387. Bhasin S, Storer TW, Berman N, et al. The effects of supraphysiologic doses of testosterone on muscle size and strength in normal men. *N Engl J Med* 335:1–7, 1996.

388. Bronson FH, Matherne CM. Exposure to anabolic-androgenic steroids shortens life span of male mice. *Med Sci Sports Exerc* 29:615–619, 1997.

389. Melchert RB, Welder AA. Cardiovascular effects of androgenic–anabolic steroids. *Med Sci Sports Exerc* 27:1252–1262, 1995.

390. Cohen LI, Hartford CG, Rogers GG. Lipoprotein(a) and cholesterol in bodybuilders using anabolic androgenic steroids. *Med Sci Sports Exerc* 28:176–179, 1996.

391. Bahrke MS, Yesalis CE, Wright JE. Psychological and behavioral effects of endogenous testosterone and anabolic–androgenic steroids. An update. *Sports Med* 22:367–390, 1996.

392. Dodd SL, Powers SK, Vrabas IS, Criswell D, Stetson S, Hussain R. Effects of clenbuterol on contractile and biochemical properties of skeletal muscle. *Med Sci Sports Exerc* 28:669–676, 1996.

393. Earnest CP. Dietary androgen "supplements." Separating substance from hype. *Physician Sportsmed* 29(5):63–79, 2001.

394. Brown GA, Vukovich MD, Reifenrath TA, Uhl NL, Parsons KA, Sharp RL, King DS. Effects of anabolic precursors on serum testosterone concentrations and adaptations to resistance training in young men. *Int J Sport Nutr Exerc Metab* 10:340–359, 2000.

395. Leder BZ, Longcope C, Catlin DH, Ahrens B, Schoenfeld DA, Finkelstein JS. Oral androstenedione administration and serum testosterone concentrations in young men. *JAMA* 283:779–782, 2000.

396. Ballantyne CS, Phillips SM, MacDonald JR, Tarnopolsky MA, MacDougall JD. The acute effects of androstenedione supplementation in healthy young males. *Can J Appl Physiol* 25:68–78, 2000.

397. Broeder CE, Quindry J, Brittingham K, Panton L, Thomson J, Appakondu S, Breuel K, Byrd R, Douglas J, Earnest C, Mitchell C, Olson M, Roy T, Yarlagadda C. The Andro project: Physiological and hormonal influences of androstenedione supplementation in men 35 to 65 years old participating in a high-intensity resistance training program. *Arch Intern Med* 160:3093–3104, 2000.

398. Stacy JJ, Terrell TR, Armsey TD. Ergogenic aids: Human growth hormone. *Curr Sports Med Rep* 3:229–233, 2004.

399. DePalo EF, Gatti R, Lancerin F, Cappellin E, Spinella P. Correlations of growth hormone (GH) and insulin-like growth factor I (IGF-I): Effects of exercise and abuse by athletes. *Clin Chim Acta* 305:1–17, 2001.

400. Healy ML, Gibney J, Russell-Jones DL, Pentecost C, Croos P, Sönksen PH, Umpleby AM. High dose growth hormone exerts an anabolic effect at rest and during exercise in endurance-trained athletes. *J Clin Endocrinol Metab* 88:5221–5226, 2003.

401. Mujika I, Padilla S. Creatine supplementation as an ergogenic aid for sports performance in highly trained athletes: A critical review. *Int J Sports Med* 18:491–496, 1997.

402. Juhn MS. Oral creatine supplementation. Separating fact from hype. *Physician Sportsmed* 27(5):47–61, 1999.

403. ACSM Roundtable. The physiological and health effects of oral creatine supplementation. *Med Sci Sports Exerc* 32:706–717, 2000.

404. Casey A, Greenhaff PL. Does dietary creatine supplementation play a role in skeletal muscle metabolism and performance? *Am J Clin Nutr* 72(2 suppl):607S–617S, 2000.

405. Branch JD. Effect of creatine supplementation on body composition and performance: A meta-analysis. *Int J Sport Nutr Exerc Metab* 13:198–226, 2003.

406. Jacobs I. Dietary creatine monohydrate supplementation. *Can J Appl Physiol* 24:503–514, 1999.

407. Volek JS, Rawson ES. Scientific basis and practical aspects of creatine supplementation for athletes. *Nutrition* 20:609–614, 2004.

408. Greenhaff PL. Creatine and its applications as an ergogenic aid. *Int J Sport Nutr* 5:S100–S110, 1995.

409. Pendergast DR, Horvath PJ, Leddy JJ, Venkatraman JT. The role of dietary fat on performance, metabolism, and health. *Am J Sports Med* 24:S53–S58, 1996.

410. Ranallo RF, Rhodes EC. Lipid metabolism during exercise. *Sports Med* 26:29–42, 1998.

411. Sherman WM, Leenders N. Fat loading: The next magic bullet. *Int J Sport Nutr* 5:S1–S12, 1995.

412. Saltin B, Åstrand P-O. Free fatty acids and exercise. *Am J Clin Nutr* 57(suppl):752S–758S, 1993.

413. Coyle EF. Substrate utilization during exercise in active people. *Am J Clin Nutr* 61(suppl):968S–979S, 1995.

414. LaPachet RAB, Miller WC, Arnall DA. Body fat and exercise endurance in trained rats adapted to a high-fat and/or high-carbohydrate diet. *J Appl Physiol* 80:1173–1179, 1996.

415. Jeukendrup AE, Thielen JJHC, Wagenmakers AJM, Brouns F, Saris WHM. Effect of medium-chain triacylglycerol and carbohydrate ingestion during exercise on substrate utilization and subsequent cycling performance. *Am J Clin Nutr* 67:397–404, 1998.

416. Goedecke JH, Clark VR, Noakes TD, Lambert EV. The effects of medium-chain triacylglycerol and carbohydrate ingestion on ultra-endurance exercise performance. *Int J Sport Nutr Exerc Metab* 14:15–27, 2005.

417. Vukovich MD, Costill DL, Hickey MS, Trappe SW, Cole EJ, Fink WJ. Effect of fat emulsion infusion and fat feeding on muscle glycogen utilization during cycle exercise. *J Appl Physiol* 75:1513–1518, 1993.

418. Johannessen A, Hagen C, Galbo H. Prolactin, growth hormone, thyrotropin, 3,5,3-triiodothyronine, and thyroxine responses to exercise after fat- and carbohydrate-enriched diet. *J Clin Endocrine Metab* 52:56–61, 1981.

419. Helge JW, Wulff B, Kiens B. Impact of a fat-rich diet on endurance in man: Role of the dietary periods. *Med Sci Sports Exerc* 30:456–461, 1998.

420. Hawley JA. Effect of increased fat availability on metabolism and exercise capacity. *Med Sci Sports Exerc* 34:1485–1491, 2002.

421. Lambert EV, Speechly DP, Dennis SC, Noakes TD. Enhanced endurance in trained cyclists during moderate intensity exercise following 2 weeks adaptation to a high fat diet. *Eur J Appl Physiol* 69:287–293, 1994.

422. Phinney SD, Bistrian BR, Evans WJ, Gervina E, Blackburn GL. The human metabolic response to chronic ketosis without caloric restriction: Preservation of submaximal exercise capability with reduced carbohydrate oxidation. *Metabolism* 32:769–776, 1983.

423. Okano G, Sato Y, Murata Y. Effect of elevated blood FFA levels on endurance performance after a single fat meal ingestion. *Med Sci Sports Exerc* 30:763–768, 1998.

424. Costill DL, Coyle EF, Dalsky G, Evans W, Fink W, Hoopes D. Effects of elevated plasma free fatty acids and insulin on muscle glycogen usage during exercise. *J Appl Physiol* 43:695–699, 1977.

425. Satabin P, Portero P, Defer G. Metabolic and hormonal responses to lipid and carbohydrate diets during exercise in man. *Med Sci Sports Exerc* 19:218–223, 1987.

426. Leddy J, Horvath P, Rowland J, Pendergast D. Effect of a high or a low fat diet on cardiovascular risk factors in male and female runners. *Med Sci Sports Exerc* 29:17–25, 1997.

427. Lukaski HC, Bolonchuk WW, Klevay LM, Mahalko JR, Milne DB, Sandstead HH. Influence of type and amount of dietary lipid on plasma lipid concentrations in endurance athletes. *Am J Clin Nutr* 39:35–44, 1984.

428. Thompson PD, Cullinane EM, Eshleman R, Kantor MA, Herbert PN. The effects of high-carbohydrate and high-fat diets on the serum lipid and lipoprotein concentrations of endurance athletes. *Metabolism* 33:1003–1010, 1984.

429. Brown RC, Cox CM. Effects of high fat versus high carbohydrate diets on plasma lipids and lipoproteins in endurance athletes. *Med Sci Sports Exerc* 30:1677–1683, 1998.

430. Burke LM, Collier GR, Beasley SK, Davis PG, Fricker PA, Heeley P, Walder K, Hargreaves M. Effects of coingestion of fat and protein with carbohydrate feedings on muscle glycogen storage. *J Appl Physiol* 78:2187–2192, 1995.

431. Tsetsonis N, Hardman AE, Mastana SS. Acute effects of exercise on postprandial lipemia: A comparative study in trained and untrained middle-aged women. *Am J Clin Nutr* 65:525–533, 1997.

PHYSICAL FITNESS ACTIVITY 9.1

Rating Your Diet with *MyPyramid*

The food pyramid shown early in this chapter is an excellent guide to help you eat healthfully while obtaining all known vitamins and minerals. How close is your diet to the recommendations of *MyPyramid?*

Step 1 Write down *everything* (all fluids and foods) that you ate yesterday. Be exact!

Food or Beverage	**How Much (cups, tablespoons, slices, etc.)?**

Step 2 Refer to Table 9.20, and fill in the blanks. Go to www.mypyramid.gov for more information. *Note:* The worksheet in Table 9.20 is for a 2,800-Calorie diet. Go to www.mypyramid.gov and use the interactive program to determine your Calorie needs. Then use Box 9.3 to determine the amount of food you need for each food group and adjust Table 9.20.

TABLE 9.20 MyPyramid Worksheet

MyPyramid Worksheet—2,800-Calorie Food Intake Pattern

Check how you did today and set a goal to aim for tomorrow

Write in Your Choices for Today	Food Group	Tip	Goal	List Each Food Choice in its Food Group*	Estimate Your Total
	Grains	Make at least half your grains whole grains	**10-ounce equivalents** (1 ounce equivalent is about 1 slice bread, 1 cup dry cereal, or ½ cup rice or pasta)		____ ounce equivalents
	Vegetables	Try to have vegetables from several subgroups each day	**4 cups** Subgroups: Dark Green, Orange, Starchy, Dry Beans and Peas, Other Veggies		____ cups
	Fruits	Make most choices fruit, not juice	**2 ½ cups**		____ cups
	Milk	Choose fat-free or low-fat most often	**3 cups** (1 ½ ounces cheese = 1 cup milk)		____ cups
	Meat and Beans	Choose lean meat and poultry. Vary your choices—more fish, beans, peas, nuts, and seeds	**7-ounce equivalents** (1 ounce equivalent is 1 ounce meat, poultry or fish, 1 T. peanut butter, ½ ounce nuts, ¼ cup dry beans or peas)		____ ounce equivalents
	Physical Activity	Build more physical activity into your daily routine at home or work	At least **30 minutes** of moderate to vigorous activity a day, 10 minutes or more at a time	*Some foods don't fit into any group. These "extras" may be mainly fat or sugar—limit your intake of these.	____ minutes

How did you do today? ☐ Great ☐ So-So ☐ Not so Great

My food goal for tomorrow is: ____________________

My activity goal for tomorrow is: ____________________

PHYSICAL FITNESS ACTIVITY 9.2

Analyzing Your Energy and Nutrient Intake

Directions: Take the food list from Physical Fitness Activity 9.1 (where you listed all foods and their amounts ingested during the previous day) and enter the foods into one of the following Internet diet analysis programs. Follow the simple instructions given at the Internet site. List your intake of Calories and nutrients in the table provided and compare to recommended levels. What areas need special attention?

MyPyramid Tracker

http://www.mypyramidtracker.gov
MyPyramid Tracker is an online dietary and physical activity assessment tool that provides information on your diet quality, physical activity status, related nutrition messages, and links to nutrient and physical activity information. The Food Calories/Energy Balance feature automatically calculates your energy balance by subtracting the energy you expend from physical activity from your food calories/energy intake. Use of this tool helps you better understand your energy balance status and enhances the link between good nutrition and regular physical activity. MyPyramid Tracker translates the principles of the 2005 *Dietary Guidelines for Americans* and other nutrition standards developed by the U.S. Departments of Agriculture and Health and Human Services.

The online dietary assessment provides information on your diet quality, related nutrition messages, and links to nutrient information. After providing a day's worth of dietary information, you will receive an overall evaluation by comparing the amounts of food you ate to current nutritional guidance. To give you a better understanding of your diet over time, you can track what you eat up to a year.

The physical activity assessment evaluates your physical activity status and provides related energy expenditure information and educational messages. After providing a day's worth of physical activity information, you will receive an overall "score" for your physical activities that looks at the types and duration of each physical activity you did and then compares this score to the physical activity recommendation for health. A score over several days or up to a year gives a better picture of your physical activity lifestyle over time.

Nutrition Analysis Tool (NAT)

http://nat.crgq.com
NAT is provided as an Internet public service by the Food Science and Human Nutrition Department at the University of Illinois. The database used by NAT is composed of the USDA Handbook 8 and information from food companies. The tabular report compares intake from a 1-day food record with the RDA for 19 nutrients. NAT provides a strong help function, and users can save food intake data to a CD.

Agricultural Research Service Nutrient Data Laboratory

www.nal.usda.gov/fnic/foodcomp/Data
This Internet page provides access to the USDA Nutrient Database for Standard Reference, Release 17. You can either view the data or download the data files and documentation in several different formats for use later on your computer. A search tool is also provided so you can look up the nutrient content (over 28 nutrients and a complete breakdown of fatty acids and amino acids) of over 6,800 different foods directly from this home page. Users can view the nutrient content for one food at a time but cannot enter a 1-day food record for analysis.

List your nutrient intake in the table provided and then comment on areas where you need to improve.

	Your Intake	Recommended
Energy (Calories)	___	Varies *
Carbohydrate (% total energy)	___	45–65
Fat (% total energy)	___	20–35
Saturated fat (% total energy)	___	<10
Protein (% total energy)	___	10–35
Dietary fiber (g)	___	M: 38; F: 25
Cholesterol (mg)	___	<300
Sodium (mg)	___	<2,300
Vitamin C (mg)	___	M: 90; F: 75
Calcium (mg)	___	1000; 50+ yr, 1200
Iron (mg)	___	M: 8; F: 18, 50+ yr, 8

*Energy needs vary according to body size and physical activity, with the RDA average set at 2,900 Calories for males and 2,200 Calories for females.

Comment on areas of needed improvement (consult the text for ideas):

PHYSICAL FITNESS ACTIVITY 9.3

Case Study: Female Vegetarian Fitness Enthusiast with Anemia

Review the data summarized here, which was gathered from a female vegetarian who had been exercising faithfully each day for more than 10 years. Answer the following questions, based on information presented in this chapter, and then discuss your answers with your instructor.

Demographic Data

Age	47 years
Weight	130 pounds
$\dot{V}O_{2max}$	43.5 ml · kg^{-1} · min^{-1} ("good")
Exercise habits	Daily brisk walking, 30–45 minutes; more than 10 years
Height	66.25 inches
Percent body fat	16% ("lean")

3-Day Food Record Nutrient Intake

Energy intake	2602 Calories/day
Protein	37 g (6%)
Cholesterol	30.1 mg (<300)
Iron	17.9 mg (119% RDA)
Copper	2.3 mg (within RDA range)
Vitamin B_6	2.62 mg (164%)
Vitamin A	1328 μg RE (166%)
Vitamin E	4.82 mg α-TE (60%)
Carbohydrate	560 g (86%)
Fat	23 g (8%)
Dietary fiber	29.4 g (20–35)
Zinc	12.2 mg (102%)
Calcium	499 mg (62%)
Vitamin B_{12}	1.2 μg (60%)
Vitamin C	137 mg (228%)

Food exchanges (servings per day)

Meat	1.4 (from legumes)
Bread	6.6
Vegetable	2.7
Milk	0
Fruit	12

Blood Lipid and Iron Status

Serum cholesterol	178 mg/dl
HDL cholesterol	51 mg/dl (3:4 ratio)
Hematocrit	31.4% (37–47)
Serum iron	32 μg/dl (60–180)
Hemoglobin	10.2 g/dl (12–16)

1. What would you recommend that this vegetarian woman do to improve her iron status?

____

____

2. What changes would you recommend in her diet? (Consider iron, protein, and vegetarian issues.)

____

____

part

IV

Physical Activity and Disease

chapter 10

Heart Disease

Regular physical activity or cardiorespiratory fitness decreases the risk of cardiovascular disease mortality in general and of coronary heart disease in particular. The level of decreased risk of coronary heart disease attributable to regular physical activity is similar to that of other lifestyle factors such as keeping free from cigarette smoking.
—*Physical Activity and Health:* A Report of the Surgeon General, 1996

The circulatory system includes the heart, lungs, arteries, and veins. The normal heart is a strong, muscular pump a little larger than the human fist; within the normal lifetime, it will faithfully beat nearly 3 billion times, pumping 42 million gallons of blood (see Figure 10.1). Unfortunately, many hearts have their work cut short by various diseases related to unhealthy lifestyles.[1,2]

Heart disease is the leading killer of people in the United States and developed countries worldwide (see Figure 10.2).[3] In this chapter, each of the major risk factors for heart disease are reviewed, with special attention given to prevention.

HEART DISEASE

Heart disease, or cardiovascular disease (CVD), comprises diseases of the heart and its blood vessels. CVD is not a single disorder, but a general name for more than 20 different diseases of the heart and its vessels. (See Box 10.1 for a glossary of terms.) The American Heart Association has reminded us that although we have made tremendous progress in fighting CVD, it has been the leading cause of death among Americans in every year but one (1918) since 1900.[1] Every 34 seconds, an American dies of CVD, the underlying cause of just under 1 million deaths annually. Four of every 10 U.S. coffins contain victims of CVD (see Table 10.1).[1] About one third of CVD deaths occur prematurely (before the age of 75 years).

Deaths, however, do not tell the whole story, in that of the 300 million Americans alive today, nearly one in four live with some form of CVD. Also, 64% of U.S. adults has one or more CVD risk factors.[1] In other words, an alarming number of Americans either have CVD or are headed in that direction.

Cancer, according to most surveys, is the disease people fear the most. CVD deserves more respect, however, maintains the National Center for Health Statistics. According to their most recent computations, if all forms of major CVD were eliminated, total life expectancy would rise by nearly 7 years. If all forms of cancer were abolished, the gain would be just 3 years.[1]

Atherosclerosis, the buildup of fatty, plaque material in the inner layer of blood vessels, is the underlying factor in 85% of CVD.[4–7] When atherosclerotic plaque blocks one or more of the heart's coronary blood vessels, the diagnosis is coronary heart disease (CHD), the major form of CVD (see Figure 10.3).

Often, a blood clot forms in the narrowed coronary blood artery, blocking the blood flow to the part of the heart muscle supplied by that artery. This causes a heart attack, or what clinicians call a myocardial infarction (MI). Each year, as many as 1,200,000 Americans have a heart attack, and about 4 in 10 die as a result.[1,2]

Atherosclerosis can also block blood vessels in the brain (leading to a stroke) or legs (defined as peripheral artery disease).[1] Stroke kills over 160,000 Americans each year and is the third largest cause of death. Peripheral artery disease affects up to 20% of older people and leads to

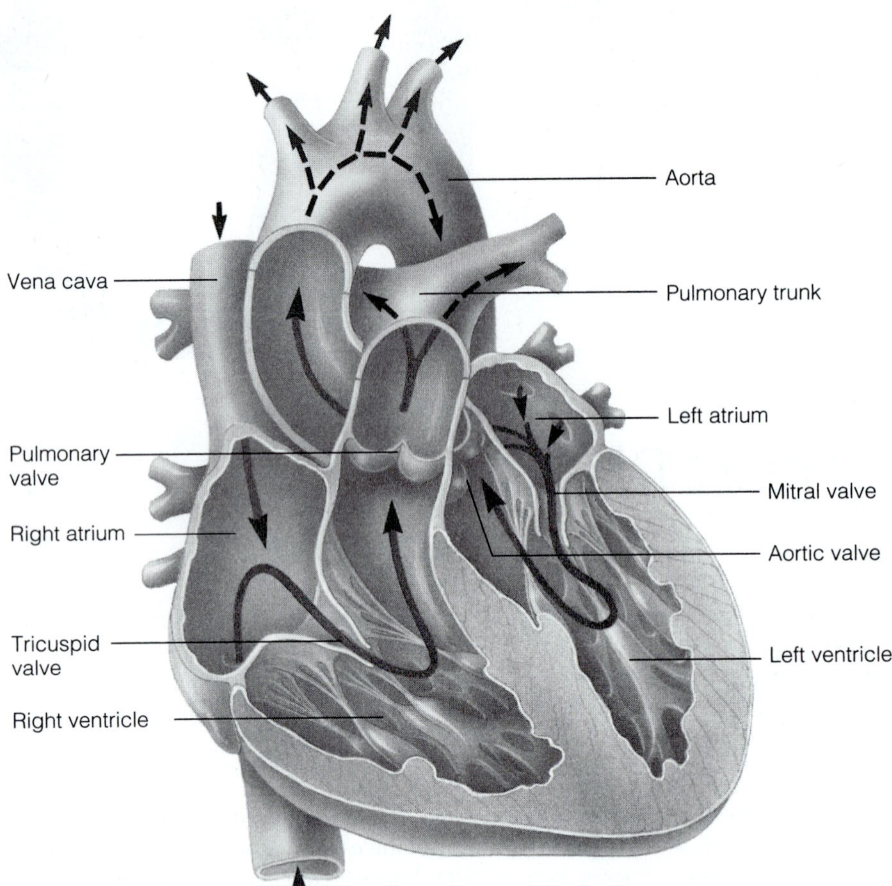

Figure 10.1 Within the normal lifetime, the average heart will beat nearly 3 billion times, pumping 42 million gallons of blood.

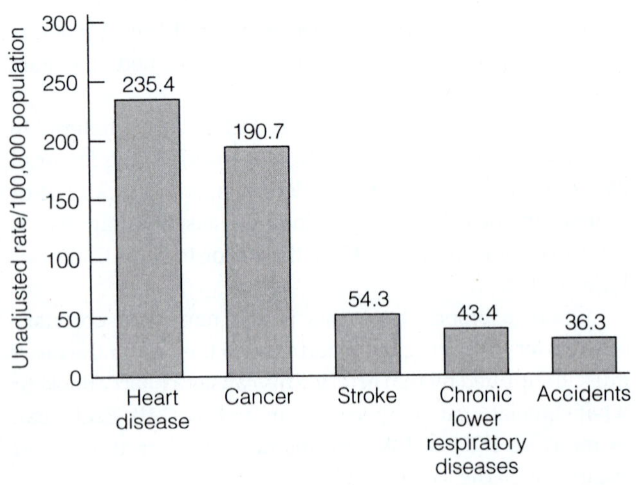

Figure 10.2 Current comparison of death rates. Death rates for the top five leading causes of death in the United States. Source: Data from Hoyert DL, Kung HC, Smith BL. Deaths: Preliminay data for 2003. *National Vital Statistics Reports* 53(15). Hyattsville, MD: National Center for Health Statistics, 2005.

pain in the legs brought on by walking (intermittent claudication). Patients with peripheral artery disease are able to walk only short distances before they must rest to relieve the pain in their legs, brought on by poor circulation due to atherosclerosis. The atherosclerotic plaques range from small yellow streaks to advanced lesions with ulceration, *thrombosis* (formation or existence of a blood clot within the blood vessel system), hemorrhage, and calcification.[4–7]

There are several stages in the development of atherosclerosis[4–7] (see Figure 10.4). First, the arterial wall is injured

Box 10.1

Glossary of Terms Used in Heart Disease

Following is a list of terms related to heart disease.

aneurysm: A ballooning-out of the wall of a vein, an artery, or the heart, due to weakening of the wall by disease, injury, or an abnormality present at birth.

angina pectoris: Medical term for chest pain due to coronary heart disease; a condition in which the heart muscle does not receive enough blood, resulting in pain in the chest.

angiocardiography: An x-ray examination of the blood vessels or chambers of the heart, by tracing the course of a special fluid (called a contrast medium or dye) visible by x-ray, which has been injected into the bloodstream. The x-ray pictures made are called "angiograms."

angioplasty: A procedure sometimes used to dilate (widen) narrowed arteries; a catheter with a deflated balloon on its tip is passed into the narrowed artery segment, the balloon is inflated, and the narrowed segment is widened.

arrhythmia (or dysrhythmia): An abnormal rhythm of the heart.

arteriosclerosis: Commonly called "hardening of the arteries," this includes a variety of conditions that cause artery walls to thicken and lose elasticity.

atherosclerosis: A form of arteriosclerosis, in which the inner layers of artery walls become thick and irregular due to deposits of fat, cholesterol, and other substances; this buildup is sometimes called "plaque"; as the interior walls of arteries become lined with layers of these deposits, the arteries become narrowed, and the flow of blood through them is reduced.

blood clot: A jellylike mass of blood tissue formed by clotting factors in the blood; this clot can then stop the flow of blood from an injury; blood clots can also form inside an artery with walls damaged by atherosclerotic buildup and can cause a heart attack or stroke.

blood pressure: The force or pressure exerted by the heart in pumping blood; the pressure of blood in the arteries.

bradycardia: Slowness of the heartbeat.

capillaries: Microscopically small blood vessels between arteries and veins, which distribute oxygenated blood to the body's tissues.

cardiac arrest: The stopping of the heartbeat, usually because of interference with the electrical signal (often associated with coronary heart disease).

cardiopulmonary resuscitation (CPR): A technique combining chest compression and mouth-to-mouth breathing; used during cardiac arrest to keep oxygenated blood flowing to the heart muscle and brain until advanced cardiac life support can be started or an adequate heartbeat resumes.

cardiovascular: Pertaining to the heart and blood vessels ("cardio" means heart; "vascular" means blood vessels); the circulatory system of the heart and blood vessels is the cardiovascular system.

carotid artery: A major artery in the neck.

catheterization: The process of examining the heart by introducing a thin tube (catheter) into a vein or artery and passing it into the heart.

cerebral embolism: A blood clot formed in one part of the body and then carried by the bloodstream to the brain, where it blocks an artery.

cerebral hemorrhage: Bleeding within the brain, resulting from a ruptured aneurysm or a head injury.

cerebral thrombosis: Formation of a blood clot in an artery that supplies part of the brain.

cerebrovascular accident: Also called "cerebral vascular accident," "apoplexy," or "stroke"; an impeded blood supply to some part of the brain, resulting in injury to brain tissue.

cholesterol: A fat-like substance found in animal tissue and present only in foods from animal sources, such as whole-milk dairy products, meat, fish, poultry, animal fats, and egg yolks.

circulatory system: Pertaining to the heart, blood vessels, and the circulation of the blood.

collateral circulation: A system of smaller arteries closed under normal circumstances, which may open up and start to carry blood to part of the heart when a coronary artery is blocked; can serve as alternative routes of blood supply.

coronary arteries: Two arteries arising from the aorta, which arch down over the top of the heart, and then branch and provide blood to the heart muscle.

coronary artery disease: Conditions that cause narrowing of the coronary arteries, so blood flow to the heart muscle is reduced.

coronary bypass surgery: Surgery to improve blood supply to the heart muscle; most often performed when narrowed coronary arteries reduce the flow of oxygen-containing blood to the heart itself.

(continued)

Box 10.1

Glossary of Terms Used in Heart Disease *(continued)*

coronary heart disease: Disease of the heart caused by atherosclerotic narrowing of the coronary arteries, likely to produce angina pectoris or heart attack; a general term. Used interchangeably with *coronary artery disease.*

coronary occlusion: An obstruction of one of the coronary arteries, thereby hindering blood flow to some part of the heart muscle.

coronary thrombosis: Formation of a clot in one of the arteries that conduct blood to the heart muscle; also called coronary occlusion.

echocardiography: A diagnostic method in which pulses of sound are transmitted into the body, and the echoes returning from the surfaces of the heart and other structures are electronically plotted and recorded to produce a "picture" of the heart's size, shape, and movements.

electrocardiogram (ECG or EKG): A graphic record of electrical impulses produced by the heart.

embolus: A blood clot that forms in a blood vessel in one part of the body and then is carried to another part of the body.

endarterectomy: Surgical removal of plaque deposits or blood clots in an artery.

endothelium: The smooth inner lining of many body structures, including the heart (endocardium) and blood vessels.

heart attack: Death of, or damage to, part of the heart muscle, due to an insufficient blood supply.

ischemia: Decreased blood flow to an organ, usually due to constriction or obstruction of an artery.

ischemic heart disease: Also called "coronary artery disease" and "coronary heart disease"; applied to heart ailments caused by narrowing of the coronary arteries, and therefore characterized by a decreased blood supply to the heart.

lipoprotein: The combination of lipid surrounded by a protein, which makes it soluble in blood.

lumen: The opening within a tube, such as a blood vessel.

myocardial infarction: The injury to or death of an area of the heart muscle ("myocardium"), resulting from a blocked blood supply to that area.

myocardium: The muscular wall of the heart; contracts to pump blood out of the heart and then relaxes as the heart refills with returning blood.

nitroglycerin: A drug that causes dilation of blood vessels and is often used in treating angina pectoris.

plaque: Also called "atheroma"; a deposit of fatty (and other) substances in the inner lining of the artery wall, characteristic of atherosclerosis.

risk factor: An element or condition involving certain hazard or danger; when referring to the heart and blood vessels, a risk factor is associated with an increased chance of developing cardiovascular disease, including stroke.

stroke: Also called "apoplexy," "cerebrovascular accident," or "cerebral vascular accident"; loss of muscle function, vision, sensation, or speech, resulting from brain cell damage, caused by an insufficient supply of blood to part of the brain.

subarachnoid hemorrhage: Bleeding from a blood vessel on the surface of the brain into the space between the brain and the skull.

thrombus: A blood clot that forms inside a blood vessel or cavity of the heart.

transient ischemic attack (TIA): A temporary stroke-like event that lasts for only a short time and is caused by a temporarily blocked blood vessel.

ventricular fibrillation: A condition in which the ventricles contract in a rapid, unsynchronized, uncoordinated fashion, so no blood is pumped from the heart.

Source: American Heart Association. *Heart Disease and Stroke Statistics—2005 Update.* Dallas, TX: American Heart Association, 2005.

TABLE 10.1 Statistics on Cardiovascular Disease

Prevalence	70,100,000	Cardiovascular disease
	65,000,000	Hypertension (adults)
	13,000,000	Coronary heart disease
	5,400,000	Stroke
Cardiovascular disease deaths	927,448	38% of all deaths; 32% occur before age 75
Heart attack deaths	494,382	Number 1 cause of death
	1,200,000	Projected heart attacks of which 41% will die
Stroke deaths	162,672	5,400,000 victims alive today; number 3 cause of death
CAB (coronary artery bypass) surgery	515,000	Coronary bypass operations ($60,853 average cost)
PTCA procedures	1,204,000	Balloon angioplasty ($28,558 average cost)

Source: American Heart Association. *Heart Disease and Stroke Statistics—2005 Update.* Dallas, TX: American Heart Association, 2005.

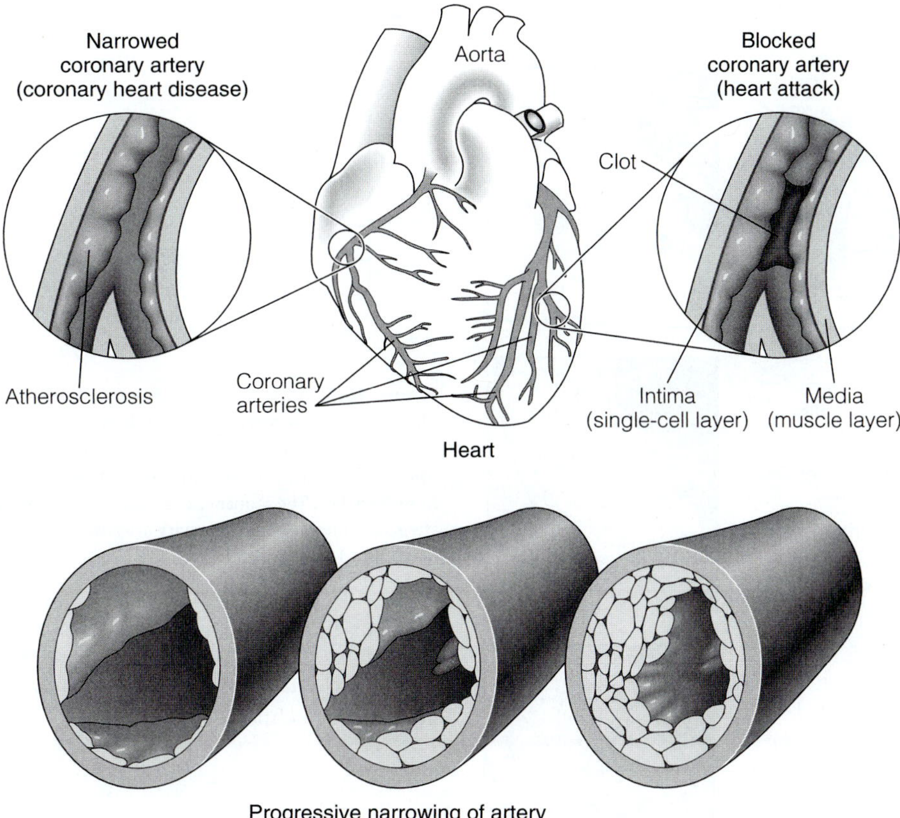

Figure 10.3 Atherosclerosis can form in the coronary arteries, resulting in a progressive narrowing of the lumen (artery passage). If a clot forms, blood flow through the coronary artery can be blocked, resulting in a heart attack.

by a variety of factors, including high blood pressure (*hypertension*), high blood cholesterol levels (*hypercholesterolemia*), oxidized low-density lipoproteins (LDL), cigarette smoking, toxins and viruses, and blood flow turbulence.

These injuries lead to a change or impairment in the normal function of the *endothelium* (the lining cells), and a chronic inflammatory response ensues.[4,6] There is increasing evidence that inflammation and immunologic mechanisms play a major role in the formation of atherosclerosis.[6,7] In response to the injury, monocytes and T cells (both are special types of immune cells) penetrate through the endothelium into the underlying *intima* (inner layer of the arterial wall).[5,6] The monocytes are then converted to *macrophages,* scavenger cells that ingest oxidized LDL and other substances. Key to the entire process is the interaction of LDL particles, especially the oxidized form, with the endothelium and the monocytes.[5] As reviewed in Chapter 9, a high intake of saturated fats and cholesterol, combined with a low fruit and vegetable intake, has been implicated in the formation of oxidized LDL. By accumulating large amounts of cholesterol from oxidized LDL, the macrophages are transformed into foam cells. In addition, oxidized LDL causes further injury to the endothelium, attracting even more monocytes, inducing a vicious cycle that leads to the development of a fatty streak, a precursor to plaque.[5]

The injured and impaired endothelial cells attract platelets and begin to release growth factors that stimulate the migration of smooth-muscle cells from the outer layers of the artery wall into the intima, where they proliferate abnormally. The macrophages and smooth-muscle cells begin to release collagen and other proteins, which form the fibrous component of atherosclerosis. The engorged foam cells then die and release cholesterol debris into the artery wall.[2]

The mature plaque is made up of a complex mixture of foam cells, smooth-muscle cells, cholesterol debris, and fibrous proteins. Over time, the plaque may become hardened or calcified and then develop cracks and ulcers, prompting the formation of blood clots that can suddenly close up the narrowed artery lumen, causing a heart attack.[1,4–7] Later in this chapter, important issues such as the treatment and reversal of atherosclerosis are discussed.

There is increasing evidence that atherosclerosis begins in childhood and progresses from fatty streaks to raised lesions in adolescence and young adulthood (see Figure 10.5).[8–10] In one autopsy study of 1,079 men and 364 women who had died from external causes between the

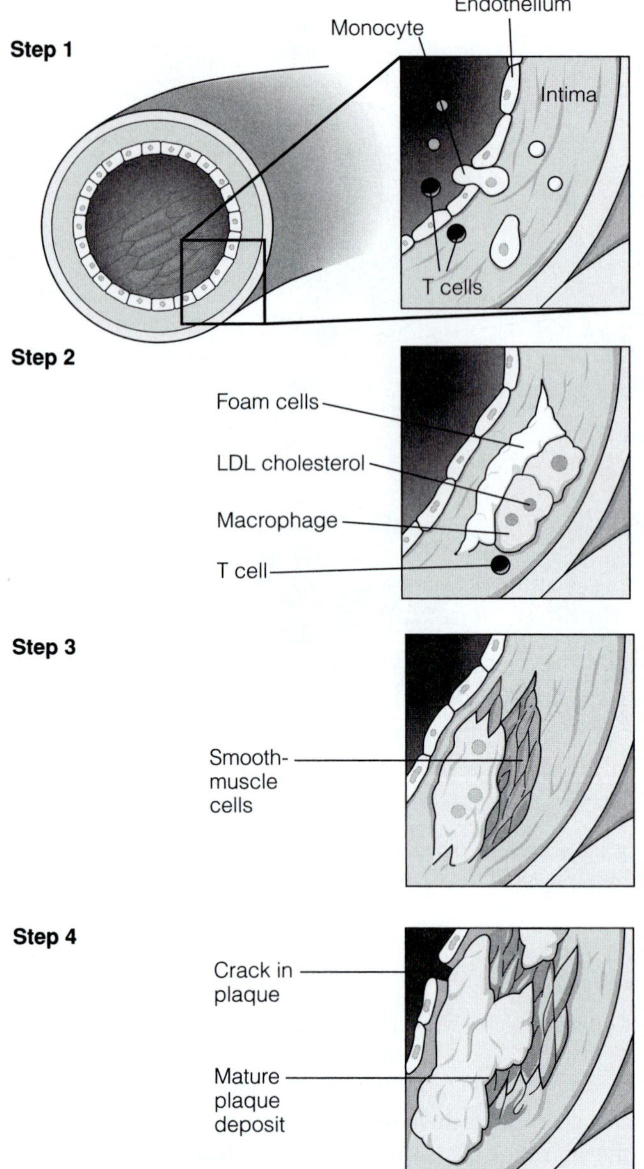

Figure 10.4 How atherosclerosis develops. *Step 1*—Injury to inner lining of intima. Monocytes and T cells penetrate into intima. *Step 2*—Monocytes are converted to macrophages and scavenge oxidized LDL, turning into foam cells. *Step 3*—Smooth-muscle cells migrate into intima and divide. Macrophages and smooth-muscle cells release collagen and other proteins. *Step 4*—The mature plaque is a complex collection of foam cells, proteins, smooth-muscle cells, and cholesterol debris. The plaque can harden, crack, and then cause blood clots to form. Source: *The Johns Hopkins White Papers.* Baltimore, MD: Johns Hopkins Medical Institutions, 1996.

ages of 15 and 34, researchers found dramatic differences in the severity of atherosclerosis, depending on blood LDL cholesterol levels and lifestyle habits such as smoking and fat-rich diets.[9] Men and women who smoked and/or had elevated LDL cholesterol experienced the greatest amount of atherosclerosis. The researchers warned that teenagers

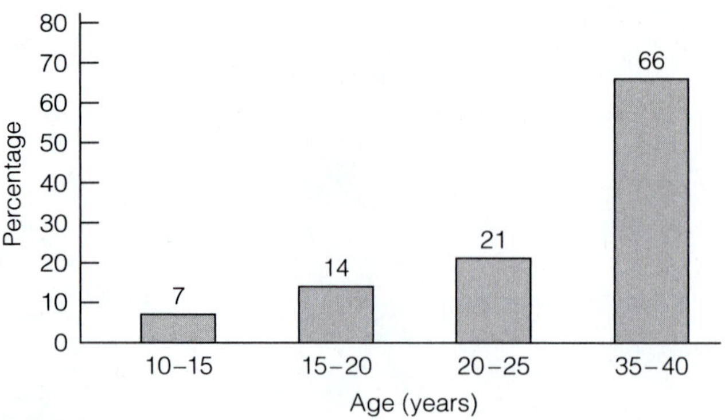

Figure 10.5 Prevalence of atherosclerosis in coronary blood vessels, according to age. Evidence of atherosclerosis is noticeable among children and is almost universal among middle-aged individuals in Western societies. Source: Data from Stary HC. The sequence of cell and matrix changes in atherosclerotic lesions of coronary arteries in the first 40 years of life. *Eur Heart J* 11(suppl):3–19, 1990.

and young adults place themselves at increased risk of early heart attack unless good lifestyle habits are practiced beginning in childhood.

CORONARY HEART DISEASE

Coronary heart disease (CHD) (also referred to as *coronary artery disease* [CAD]) is the major form of heart disease.[1] Nearly one of every five deaths is the result of CHD, making it the single leading cause of death in the United States. About every 26 seconds, an American suffers from a heart attack, and each minute an American dies from one.[1]

The heart muscle, like every other organ of the body, needs its own blood supply. The heart is not nourished by the blood that is being pumped to the lungs and body (Figure 10.1). The heart's blood is supplied through the *coronary arteries* (three major branches) (Figure 10.3). The narrowing, hardening, and blocking of these arteries by atherosclerosis leads to CHD. A blood clot may form in a narrowed coronary artery and block the flow of blood to the part of the heart muscle supplied by that artery. This is referred to as a *myocardial infarction* or *heart attack.*

When part of the heart muscle does not get enough blood (oxygen and nutrients), it begins to die. CHD can cause chest pain, called *angina pectoris,* which can occur during emotional excitement or physical exertion. (The treadmill ECG test for victims of angina pectoris can cause a depression of the ST segment. See Chapter 4.) Over 6 million Americans have angina pectoris.[1]

The first indications of a heart attack may be any of several warning signals, including those listed in Box 10.2. Unfortunately, in half of men and two thirds of women who died suddenly of CHD, there were no previous symptoms of this disease.[1]

Box 10.2

Warning Signals of a Heart Attack

If any of the following signals are experienced, seek help immediately, or go as quickly as possible to an emergency room. Each year 335,000 Americans die from heart attack before reaching the hospital. Studies indicate that half of all heart attack victims wait more than 2 hours before going for help. This is too long. Watch for these signals:

- An uncomfortable pressure, fullness, squeezing, or pain in the center of the chest, which lasts more than a few minutes or goes away and returns
- Pain that spreads to the shoulders, neck, or arms
- Chest discomfort with lightheadedness, fainting, sweating, nausea, or shortness of breath

Source: American Heart Association. *Heart Disease and Stroke Stastics—2005 Update.* Dallas, TX: American Heart Association, 2005.

STROKE

Stroke is a form of cardiovascular disease that affects the blood vessels supplying oxygen and nutrients to the brain[1] (see Figure 10.6).

Most strokes occur because the arteries in the brain become narrow from either a buildup of plaque material or atherosclerosis. Atherosclerosis is the underlying factor for both heart attacks and strokes (sometimes called "brain attacks"). Clots can then totally block the blood flow, causing the stroke. These clots are of two types: A clot that forms in the area of the narrowed brain blood vessel is called a thrombus; a clot that floats in from another area is an embolus. About 9 in 10 strokes are caused by these clots that plug narrowed brain arteries[1,11] (see Figure 10.7).

Other strokes occur when a blood vessel in the brain or on its surface ruptures and bleeds (hemorrhagic stroke). A subarachnoid hemorrhage occurs when a defective blood vessel on the surface of the brain ruptures and bleeds into the space between the brain and the skull (but not into the brain itself). Another type of hemorrhagic stroke (cerebral

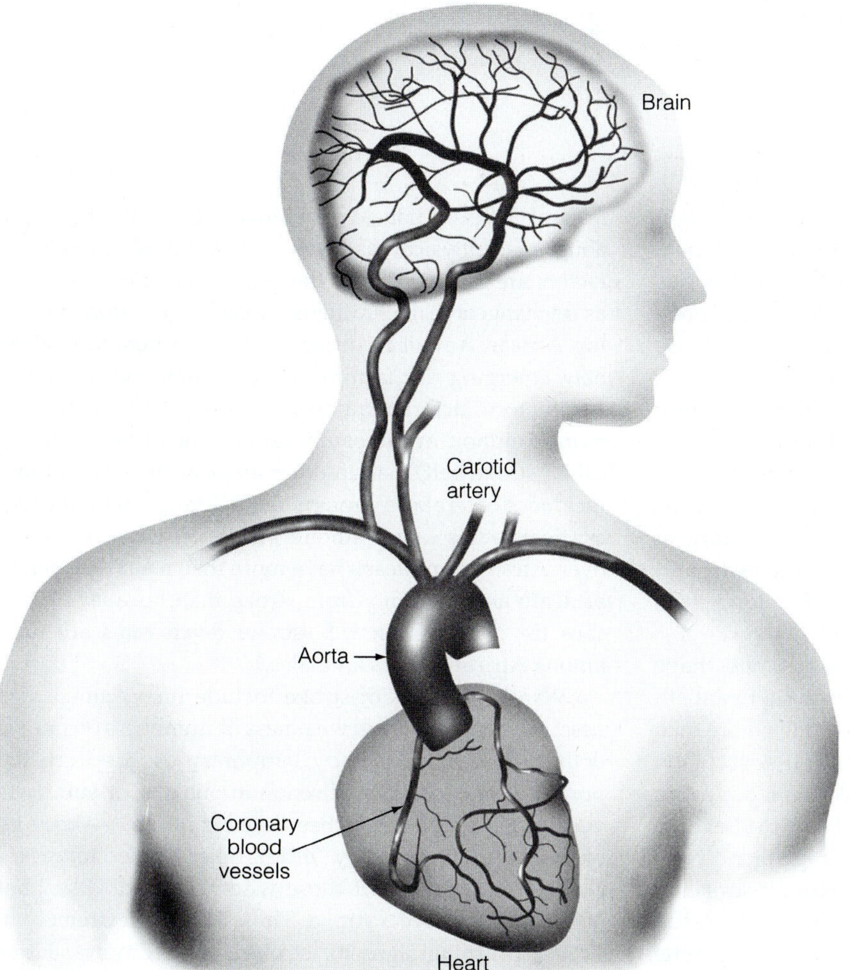

Figure 10.6 Stroke is a form of CVD that affects the arteries of the central nervous system. A stroke (or "brain attack") occurs when a blood vessel carrying oxygen and nutrients to the brain bursts or is clogged by a blood clot or some other particle. Deprived of oxygen, brain nerve cells cannot function and die within minutes.

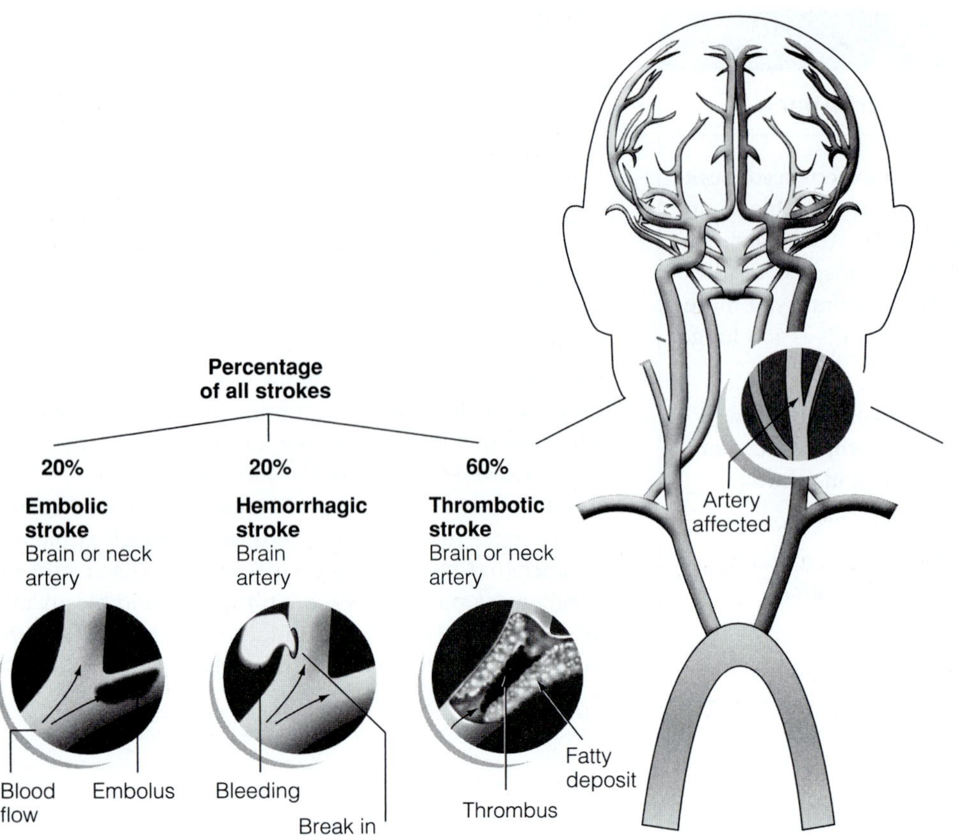

Figure 10.7 The three types of stroke—embolic, hemorrhagic, and thrombotic.

hemorrhage) occurs when a defective artery in the brain bursts, flooding the surrounding tissue with blood.[1] Often, the hemorrhage occurs when a spot in a brain artery has been weakened from atherosclerosis or high blood pressure. Hemorrhagic strokes are less common than those caused by clots but are far more lethal.

About 700,000 Americans suffer a new or recurrent stroke each year.[1] About 1 in 4 people who have a stroke die within a year, increasing to 5 in 10 within 8 years. Each year, stroke kills over 160,000 Americans, accounting for 1 of every 15 U.S. deaths. It is the third largest cause of death, ranking behind diseases of the heart and cancer. Of those who survive, 15–30% suffer long-term disabilities.

The good news about stroke is that death rates have fallen dramatically during the latter part of the twentieth century. Since 1950, stroke death rates have fallen more than 70%.[1,11] (see Figure 10.8). The American Heart Association urges that the best way to prevent a stroke from occurring is to reduce the risk factors for stroke (see Box 10.3). Seventy percent of all strokes occur in people with high blood pressure, making it the most important risk factor for stroke. In fact, stroke risk varies directly with blood pressure. Additional risk factors that can be treated include cigarette smoking, obesity, excessive alcohol intake, high blood cholesterol levels, diabetes mellitus, poor nutrition, drug abuse, and physical inactivity.[1,11] Several other stroke risk factors are categorized by the American Heart Association as unchangeable, including increasing age, being male, being African American, prior stroke, and heredity. Several new, emerging risk factors such as high blood clot and inflammatory factors require more research.[11,12] Strokes are more common in the southeastern United States, the so-called stroke belt, than in other areas of the United States. Incidence of stroke is strongly related to age, with the highest death rates found among people 85 years of age and over. African Americans have more than a 60% greater risk of death and disability from stroke than European Americans do. The highest U.S. stroke death rates are found among African American males.[1,11,12]

Warning signals of stroke include unexplained dizziness; sudden temporary weakness or numbness on one side of the face, arm, leg, or body; temporary loss of speech; temporary dimness or loss of vision in one eye; or sudden severe, unexplained headaches[1] (see Figure 10.9). About 10% of strokes are preceded by "little strokes," called *transient ischemic attacks* (TIA). Of those who have had TIAs, about 36% will later have a stroke. Thus, TIAs are extremely important warning signs for stroke.[1,11] See Physical Fitness Activity 10.3 to assess your stroke risk.

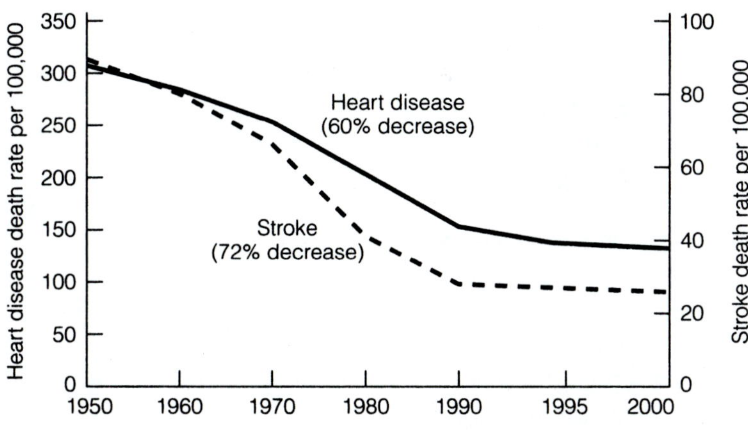

Figure 10.8 Trends in age-adjusted death rates: Heart disease and stroke. Death rates from heart disease and stroke have fallen sharply since 1950. Source: National Center for Health Statistics. *Health, United States, 2005*. Hyattsville, MD: 2005. Available at www.cdc.gov/nchs.

Box 10.3

Risk Factors for Stroke

Nonmodifiable Risk Factors

1. *Age.* Stroke risk doubles in each successive decade after 55 years of age.
2. *Sex.* Stroke is more prevalent in men than in women.
3. *Race/ethnicity.* African Americans and some Hispanic Americans have high stroke death rates compared with European Americans.
4. *Family history.* Paternal/maternal stroke history associated with stroke risk.

Well-Documented Modifiable Risk Factors

1. *Hypertension.* A major risk factor for stroke, with an increased relative risk of 2–4 for individuals aged 50–70 years.
2. *Smoking.* Long recognized as a major risk factor for stroke (increased relative risk of 1.8).
3. *Diabetes.* Increased relative risk of stroke is two- to sixfold in diabetics.
4. *Carotid artery disease.* Neck carotid arteries damaged by atherosclerosis may become blocked with a clot, resulting in a stroke.
5. *Heart disease.* People with heart problems (e.g., coronary heart disease, atrial fibrillation) have a high stroke risk.
6. *Sickle cell disease.* A genetic disorder that increases stroke risk.
7. *Hyperlipidemia.* Abnormalities in blood lipids and lipoproteins increase stroke risk.

Less Well Documented or Potentially Modifiable Risk Factors

1. *Obesity.* Increases stroke risk, especially if it is abdominal obesity.
2. *Physical inactivity.* There is increasing evidence that an inverse association exists between level of physical activity and stroke incidence.
3. *Poor diet and nutrition.* A healthy diet containing at least five daily servings of fruit and vegetables may decrease the risk of stroke.
4. *Alcohol abuse.* Excessive drinking and binge drinking can raise blood pressure and increase stroke risk, especially hemorrhagic stroke.
5. *Hyperhomocysteinemia.* There is increasing evidence that high blood homocysteine levels increase stroke risk.
6. *Drug abuse.* Intravenous drug abuse increases stroke risk from cerebral emboli; cocaine use is closely related to increased stroke risk.
7. *Hypercoagulability.* Several blood factors may increase the likelihood of clot formation, increasing stroke risk.
8. *Inflammatory processes.* Several markers of inflammation (e.g., C-reactive protein, cytokines, activated T cells and macrophages) have been linked to elevated stroke risk.

Source: Goldstein LB, Adams R, Becker K, et al. AHA Scientific Statement. Primary prevention of ischemic stroke. A statement for healthcare professionals from the Stroke Council of the American Heart Association. *Circulation* 103:163–182, 2001.

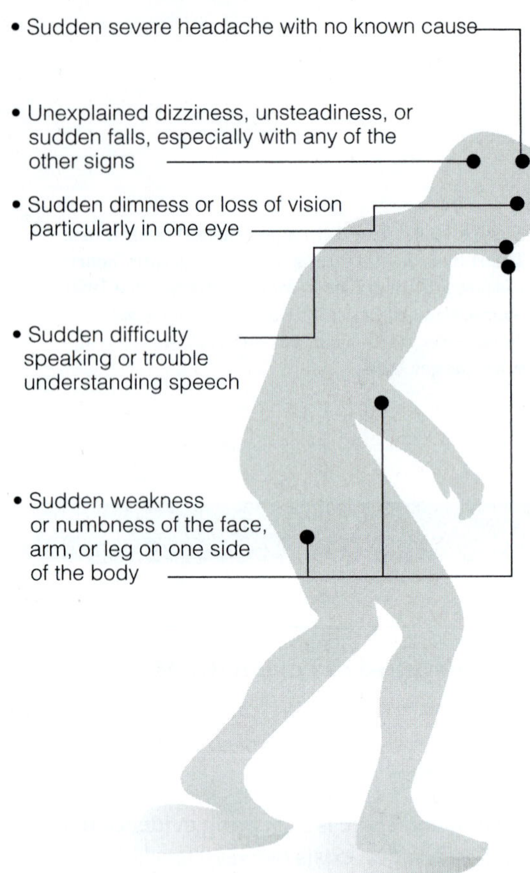
Warning Signs of a Stroke
• Sudden severe headache with no known cause
• Unexplained dizziness, unsteadiness, or sudden falls, especially with any of the other signs
• Sudden dimness or loss of vision particularly in one eye
• Sudden difficulty speaking or trouble understanding speech
• Sudden weakness or numbness of the face, arm, or leg on one side of the body

Signs of a Stroke

If you or someone else has one or more of these warning signs, don't wait. Call 911 immediately, even if the signs go away. Other, less common signs include double vision, drowsiness, nausea, or vomiting.

Figure 10.9 The warning signs of stroke should lead to immediate requests for medical help.

TRENDS IN CARDIOVASCULAR DISEASE

From 1920 to 1950, there was a sharp rise in deaths from heart disease, primarily from acute myocardial infarction among men. The causes are unknown, but during this time, Americans moved off farms into cities, began driving cars, and increased their consumption of saturated fats and cigarettes. In 1953, awareness of the increasing epidemic grew, with the publication of a study of American soldiers killed in action in Korea.[13] Of 300 autopsies on soldiers, whose average age was 22 years, 77.3% of the hearts showed some gross evidence of coronary arteriosclerosis. Of all cases, 12.3% had plaques causing luminal narrowing of more than 50%.

Since the 1950s, the trend has reversed—the sharp rise of the earlier period has been followed by an equally sharp fall in deaths from heart disease.[14–17] Since 1950, CVD death rates dropped by 60%, which is one of the greatest public health successes of the twentieth century (see Figure 10.8).[14] Men and women of all races shared in the encouraging downward mortality trend. Despite the pronounced overall reduction in heart disease mortality in the United States, Americans still experience higher death rates than their counterparts in many industrialized nations.[1]

The death rate attributable to stroke has been declining since the early 1900s.[14] Increasing control of hypertension (through lifestyle adjustments and modification) is probably the major cause of this decline. About 72% of people with high blood pressure report taking action to bring it under control, and 18% have achieved success.[2]

Much has been written regarding the causes of this dramatic turnaround.[1,2,15–18] Although estimates vary, about half of the decline in CVD mortality rates has been related to risk-factor improvements, and the other half to improvements in the treatment of CVD.

Americans appear to be heeding the extensive health information about reducing risk factors for heart disease.[1,14,17,18] Since the early 1970s, Americans have become increasingly health conscious and appreciative of the importance of preventive medicine. Despite these hopeful trends in CVD and CHD, much work remains. The lifetime risk for developing CHD is very high in the United States: One of every two males and one of every three females aged 40 years and under will develop CHD sometime in their life.[1] Figure 10.10 summarizes the *Healthy People 2010* goals for heart disease risk factors.[2]

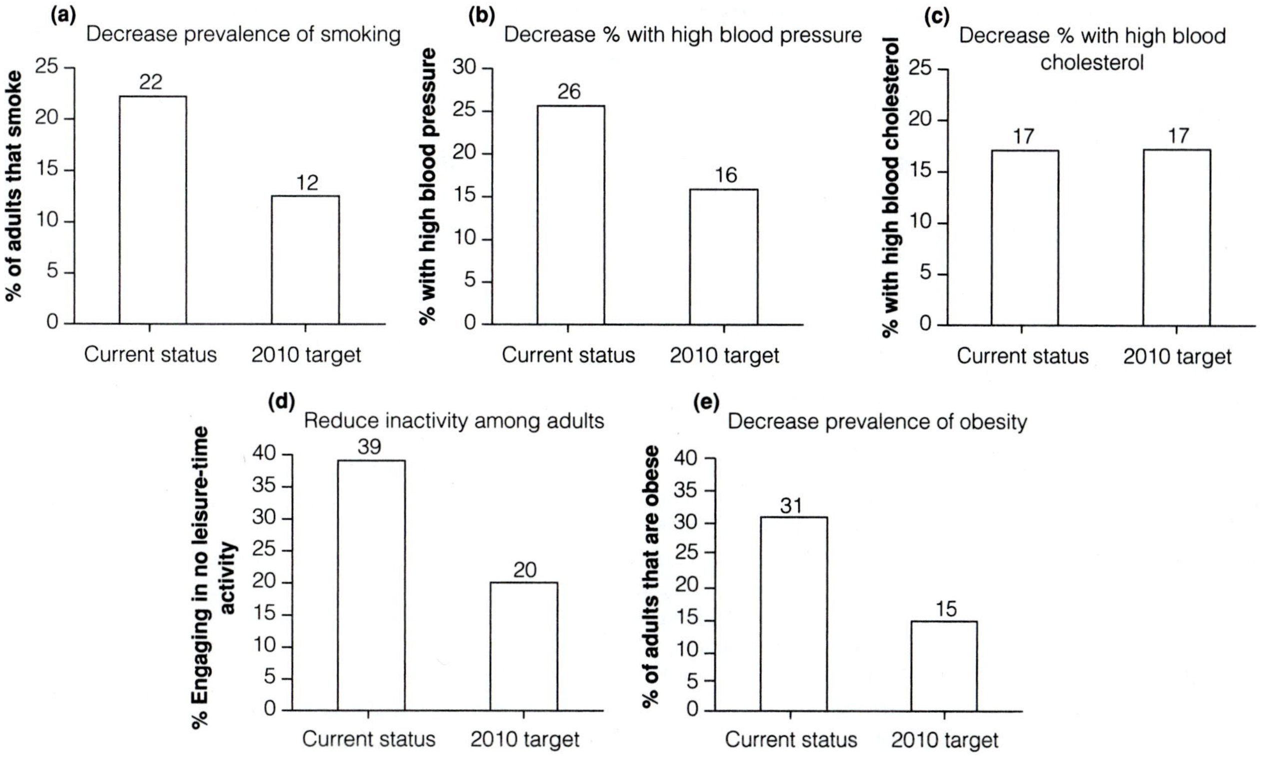

Figure 10.10 *Healthy People 2010* target goals for five major heart disease risk factors. Source: U.S. Dept. of Health and Human Services.

RISK FACTORS FOR HEART DISEASE

Risk factors are defined as personal habits or characteristics that medical research has shown to be associated with an increased risk of heart disease. Up until 1992, the American Heart Association did not include physical inactivity in its list of "major risk factors that can be changed," which included cigarette smoking, high blood pressure, and high blood cholesterol. Inactivity was listed along with obesity, stress, and diabetes as "contributing factors."[1,19] In 1998, obesity and diabetes were upgraded from "contributing" risk factors to "major" risk factors.

Heredity, sex (being a male), and increasing age have been listed for many years as "risk factors that cannot be changed." Table 10.2 outlines the current list of heart disease risk factors observed by the American Heart Association, along with the prevalence of each factor. Notice that among the risk factors listed, inactivity is by far the most prevalent.

Why did the American Heart Association wait so long to include physical inactivity as a major risk factor for heart disease? The primary reason was that good research data to support this relationship had been lacking until recently. Most of the earlier studies showed that physically active compared to inactive people had a lower risk for heart disease, but critics contended that such findings did not control for other important factors. The importance of physical inactivity as a risk factor for CVD is reviewed later in this chapter.

TABLE 10.2 Risk Factors for Heart Disease, According to the American Heart Association

Risk Factors	% U.S. Adults with Risk Factor
Major risk factors that *can* be changed	
1. Cigarette/tobacco smoke	22%
2. High blood pressure	26% (≥140/90 mm Hg)
3. High blood cholesterol	17% (≥240 mg/dl)
4. Physical inactivity	39%
5. Obesity	31% (body mass index ≥30 kg/m^2)
6. Diabetes	6.7%
Major risk factors that *cannot* be changed	
1. Heredity	
2. Being male	
3. Increasing age	13% (over age 65)
Contributing factor	
1. Individual response to stress	

Source: American Heart Association. *Heart Disease and Stroke Statistics—2005 Update.* Dallas, TX: American Heart Association, 2005.

The risk factors listed in Table 10.2 explain the majority of CHD. Most studies show that 90% of CHD patients have prior exposure to at least one of these major risk factors.[20] Table 10.3 summarizes major risk factors, life-habit

TABLE 10.3 National Cholesterol Education Program (Adult Treatment Panel III) Risk Factors*

	Description
Major risk factors (exclusive of LDL cholesterol†)	
Cigarette smoking	
Hypertension	BP ≥ 140/90 mm Hg or on antihypertensive medication
Low HDL cholesterol‡	<40 mg/dl
Family history of premature CHD	CHD in male first-degree relative <55 years; CHD in female first-degree relative <65 years
Age	Men ≥45 years; women ≥55 years
Life-habit risk factors	
Obesity	BMI ≥ 30
Physical inactivity	
Atherogenic diet	A diet high in saturated fat and cholesterol
Emerging risk factors	
Lipoprotein(a)	A distinct lipoprotein complex that promotes atherogenesis and clot formation
Homocysteine	Fasting plasma levels ≥ 16 μmol/L increases the risk for CVD and is related to low folate intake from fruits and vegetables
Prothrombotic factors	Factors that promote clot formation (e.g., fibrinogen, prothrombin, factor V Leiden, protein C deficiency)
Proinflammatory factors	Factors that reflect chronic inflammation such as interleukin-6, C-reactive protein, activated T cells and macrophages, acute-phase reactants
Impaired fasting glucose	Fasting glucose levels of 110–125 mg/dl (above normal plasma levels of <110 mg/dl)
Subclinical atherosclerosis	Atherosclerosis that is below clinical detection levels and does not produce symptoms in patients

*In ATP III, diabetes is regarded as a CHD risk equivalent (risk for major coronary events equal to that in established CHD).

†LDL cholesterol ≥ 160 mg/dl is regarded as high risk. ATP III determines the risk factor count separate from LDL cholesterol, and then recommends therapeutic changes based on the LDL cholesterol.

‡High-density lipoprotein (HDL) cholesterol ≥ 60 mg/dl counts as a "negative" risk factor; its presence removes one risk factor from the total count.

Source: Third Report of the National Cholesterol Education Program (NCEP) Expert Panel on Detection, Evaluation, and Treatment of High Blood Cholesterol in Adults (Adult Treatment Panel III), 2001. www.nhlbi.nih.gov.

risk factors, and emerging risk factors according to the National Cholesterol Education Program.[21] Notice that many of the CHD risk factors considered as "emerging" are also listed as potential risk factors for stroke (Box 10.3).

Other potential risk factors include stature (short people have higher risk), baldness, low social support, high uric acid levels, hyperinsulinemia, emotional distress, a hostile personality, low blood levels of antioxidants, and a host of others.[22–32]

People with a family history of premature CHD are at a risk two to five times that of those with no family CHD history, particularly if first-degree relatives are involved. The role of genetic factors in atherosclerosis is difficult to evaluate precisely, however, because various coronary risk factors tend to cluster within families, as well.[1,33,34]

The danger of heart attack increases with the number of risk factors (see Figure 10.11). Often, people who are stricken with heart disease have several risk factors, each of which is only marginally abnormal.

The Harvard Medical School has summarized what can be expected in regard to lowering heart disease risk when people quit smoking, decrease their blood cholesterol or blood pressure, become active, or maintain ideal weight.[35]

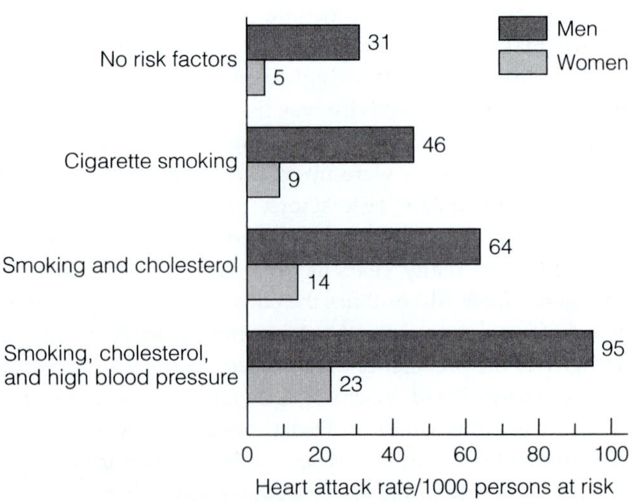

Figure 10.11 Chance of heart attack within 8 years, by risk factors present. This chart shows that a combination of three risk factors can increase the likelihood of heart attack. This chart uses an abnormal blood pressure level of 150 mm Hg (systolic) and a cholesterol level of 260 mg/dl in a 55-year-old male and female. Source: American Heart Association. *Heart Disease and Stroke Statistics—2005 Update.* Dallas, TX: American Heart Association, 2005.

- Quitting cigarette smoking
  50–70% decrease within 5 years
- Decreasing blood cholesterol
  2–3% decrease for each 1% drop in cholesterol
  (among people with an elevated level)
- Decreasing high blood pressure
  2–3% decrease for each 1 mm Hg drop in diastolic pressure
- Becoming physically active
  45% decrease for those who maintain active lifestyle
- Maintenance of ideal body weight
  35–55% decrease for maintaining ideal weight vs. obesity
  (obesity defined as more than 20% above desirable weight)

Figure 10.12 Lifestyle and heart disease risk reduction: Achievable reductions in risk (independent contribution of each risk factor). Improving lifestyle and altering risk factors has a powerful impact on lowering heart disease risk.
Source: Data from Manson JE, Tosteson H, Ridker PM, et al. The primary prevention of myocardial infarction. *N Engl J Med* 326:1406–1413, 1992.

TABLE 10.4 Strategies for Primary Prevention of Heart Disease and Stroke

Risk Factor	Strategies*
High blood pressure ($\geq$140/90 mm Hg)	Weight reduction, promotion of physical activity, reduced salt and alcohol intake
Smoking	Smoking cessation programs, physician counseling, nicotine patches, legislation
High serum cholesterol ($\geq$240 mg/dl)	Reduced saturated fat intake, weight reduction, physical activity (to raise HDL cholesterol)
Obesity (>20% desirable weight)	Low-fat, low-energy diet; promotion of long-term physical activity; behavior change
Physical inactivity and irregular exercise habits	Worksite fitness programs, community fitness facilities, physician counseling
Diabetes and impaired glucose tolerance	Weight reduction, promotion of physical activity, dietary improvement
Estrogens	Consider estrogen replacement therapy in postmenopausal women, especially those with multiple CHD risk factors

*The first goal of prevention is to prevent the development of risk factors. People should be instructed about adopting healthy life habits to prevent CVD, and this education should be family oriented. Ideally, risk-factor prevention begins in childhood.

Source: Data from Bronner LL, Kanter DS, Manson JE. Primary prevention of stroke. *N Engl J Med* 333:1392–1400, 1995.

This is summarized in Figure 10.12. These data show that primary prevention of CVD is an effective strategy that should be integrated throughout American society (see Table 10.4).[19,36] See Physical Fitness Activities 10.1 and 10.2 to assess heart disease risk.[37]

TREATMENT OF HEART DISEASE

When a person's heart muscle does not get as much blood as it needs, due to blockage of the coronary blood vessels (called myocardial ischemia), the person may experience chest pain, called angina pectoris. Angina pectoris can be treated with drugs that affect either the supply of blood to the heart muscle or the heart's demand for oxygen.[1] Nitroglycerin is the drug most often used, as it relaxes the veins and coronary arteries. Other drugs can be used to reduce blood pressure and thus decrease the heart's workload and need for oxygen.

Invasive techniques may also be used, which improve the blood supply to the heart. In 1959, cardiologists first began to insert thin tubes (catheters) into the coronary arteries of patients with angina, to inject a liquid contrast agent to detect atherosclerotic plaques.[1] This procedure is called *coronary angiography.*

For the next two decades, when this procedure detected severe narrowing of the coronary arteries, there was usually only one recourse—coronary artery bypass graft surgery (CABGS). In this surgery, surgeons take a blood vessel from another part of the body (usually from the leg or inside the chest wall) and construct a detour around the blocked part of a coronary artery (see Figure 10.13). One end of the vessel is attached above the blockage, and the other to the coronary artery just beyond the blocked area, restoring blood supply to the heart muscle.[38]

In 1977, a Swiss cardiologist revolutionized cardiology by developing a technique to open coronary arteries with special catheters bearing inflatable balloons on the tips (called percutaneous transluminal coronary angioplasty [PTCA]).[39] In PTCA, the balloon is positioned using a catheter and wire adjacent to the atherosclerotic plaque and then inflated. This squashes and cracks the plaque, widening the narrowed coronary artery (see Figure 10.13).

Although PTCA and CABGS techniques are common and fairly successful in at least alleviating pain symptoms, various problems and limitations have led many researchers to investigate new techniques. One problem with PTCA is that in 25–50% of patients, the coronary artery renarrows, usually within the first 6 months. Also, in about 5% of cases, physicians cannot open the vessel using PTCA. On the other hand, CABGS is expensive, and long-term studies have not been able to determine that the procedure significantly lengthens the life of the patient.[2,38]

Percutaneous Transluminal Coronary Angioplasty (PTCA)
A catheter is inserted into a groin artery and threaded up to the blocked coronary artery. The balloon is then inflated several times, compressing the plaque against the arterial wall.

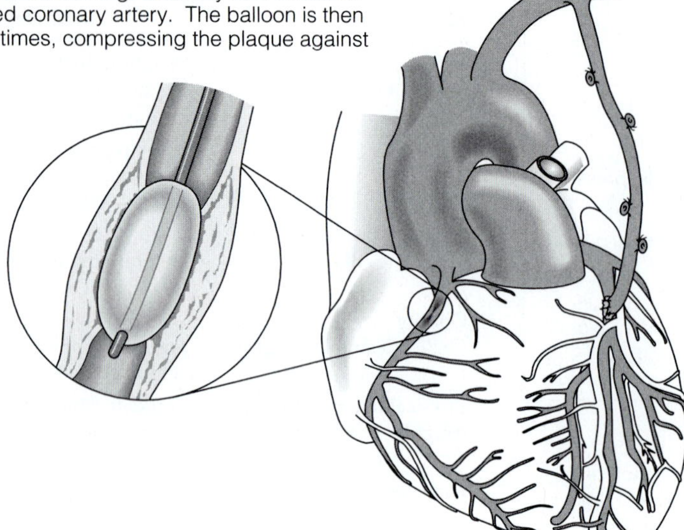

Coronary Artery Bypass Surgery
A segment of a blood vessel from another part of the body (the saphenous vein in the leg or the preferred choice, the internal mammary artery in the chest) is used as a graft. A venous graft is performed by sewing one end of the vein into the aorta and the other end into the blocked artery at a point beyond the blockage. Alternatively, an internal mammary artery is redirected to a place beyond the obstructed coronary artery. Thus, blood is carried around the point of obstruction, effectively "bypassing" the blockage. If necessary, multiple coronary artery blockages can be bypassed in a single operation.

Atherectomy utilizes a mechanical device—either a rotating blade or a drill—to shave plaque off of the artery wall. The tiny pieces of plaque debris are then swept or suctioned into a small compartment in the device and removed when the catheter is withdrawn.

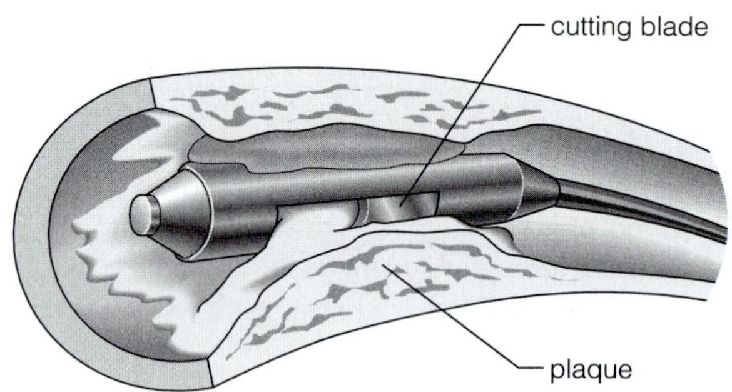

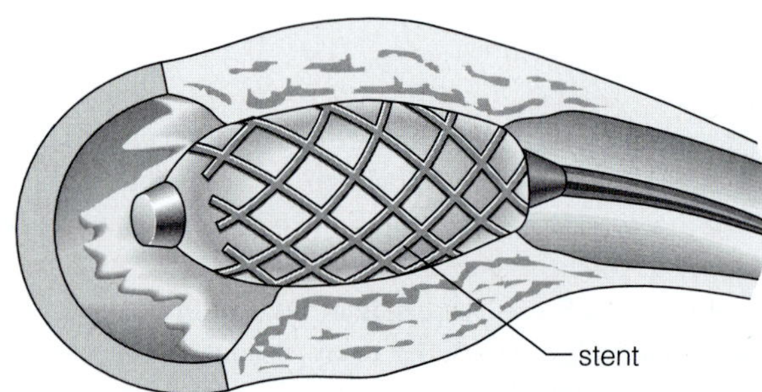

Coronary stents —flexible, stainless steel tubes that are permanently implanted in a coronary artery to keep it propped open—are used in conjunction with balloon angioplasty. The stent is initially collapsed around a deflated balloon and is threaded to the site of the blockage. When the balloon is inflated, the stent expands and locks into position.

Laser ablation does not actually use a laser beam to vaporize plaque. Instead, laser light, emitted from the tip of the catheter, is used to heat a probe that burns plaque away from the artery wall, layer by layer.

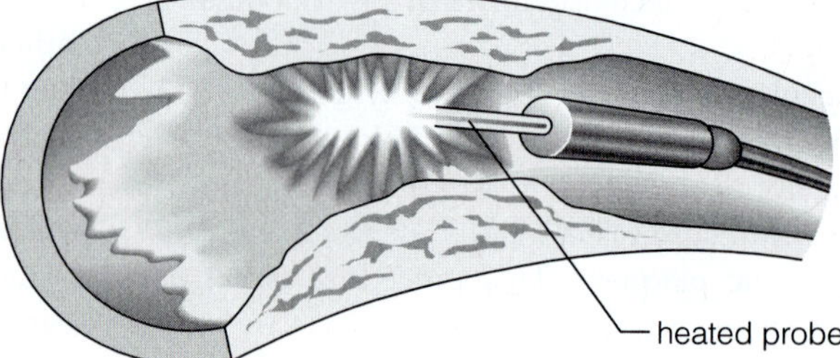

Figure 10.13 Treatment of coronary heart disease. Source: *The Johns Hopkins White Papers.* Baltimore, MD: Johns Hopkins Medical Institutions, 1996.

Three new techniques are laser angioplasty (or ablation), directional coronary atherectomy (DCA), and coronary stent (see Figure 10.13). With *laser angioplasty*, light, heat, and other strategies are used to burn away plaque material. With *DCA*, a special cutting device with a balloon is positioned by the atherosclerotic plaque material. The opening in the cylinder is turned toward the plaque, and the balloon is inflated, to force the plaque into the window of the cylinder. An external motor rotates the cutting blade at approximately 1800 revolutions per minute, grinding up plaque material, which is then sucked into the catheter by a vacuum pressure device. The *coronary stent* is a metallic wire tube that is implanted at the site of a narrowed coronary artery to keep the vessel open. Stents are now used in most of PTCA procedures and reduce the acute risk of major complications and restenosis.[39] Each of these techniques has various strengths and limitations, and research is ongoing to determine the circumstances in which each applies best.

CAN ATHEROSCLEROSIS BE REVERSED WITHOUT SURGERY?

Obviously, preventing atherosclerosis from forming in the first place is the primary goal for all who value their health. If an individual has had a heart attack, however, or is at high risk for one because of poor lifestyle habits, can the accumulation of atherosclerotic plaque be reversed through improvements in diet, exercise, weight loss, smoking cessation, and stress management, and initiation of drug therapy?[40–50] (This is termed "secondary prevention."[49])

Since early in the twentieth century, regression of atherosclerosis has been demonstrated in many different types of animals, including rabbits, roosters, pigs, and monkeys.[40] In the typical animal experiment, atherosclerosis is promoted by diets high in fat and cholesterol, followed by a vegetarian "regression" diet that leads to a reduction in plaque size within 20–40 months.[41] (The earliest human studies were with World War II prisoners who had been subjected to semistarvation diets in prisoner camps and were found at autopsy to have far less atherosclerosis than well-nourished people.)

Since the mid-1970s, controlled trials have convincingly demonstrated that intensive drug and diet therapy to lower LDL cholesterol and raise HDL cholesterol retards the progression of coronary atherosclerosis, promotes regression, and thus decreases the incidence of coronary events.[40–50] In general, secondary prevention stabilizes progression of atherosclerosis in about half of patients and induces regression in about one fourth of patients.[49] In patients with CHD, when blood pressure and blood lipids are brought below recommended levels through vigorous drug and diet therapy, stabilization and regression of atherosclerosis occurs in 75% of cases.[50]

In several trials, the effect of lifestyle interventions without drug therapy was investigated.[44,45,47–50] In patients combining exercise with a low-fat diet, coronary artery disease progresses at a slower pace than for a control group on standard care. The challenge is getting patients to adhere to the improved lifestyle over long time periods.

Obviously, prevention of atherosclerosis in the first place is the best strategy to follow, and this can be accomplished for most people by avoidance of smoking, eating a diet low in saturated fat and cholesterol, maintaining ideal weight, exercising regularly, managing stress, and keeping blood pressure and cholesterol under control. Such a healthy lifestyle prevents 80–90% of coronary heart disease events.[51] The rest of this chapter deals with prevention of heart disease by emphasizing management of the major risk factors.

CIGARETTE SMOKING

Cigarette smoking is the single most preventable cause of premature death in the United States.[52] The Office of the Surgeon General of the United States has been vigilant in warning Americans about the negative consequences of cigarette smoking. On January 11, 1964, the surgeon general released the first report on smoking and health, concluding that "cigarette smoking is causally related to lung cancer." This historic report was widely covered by the media and brought an immediate outcry from the tobacco industry, which continues unabated to the present.

A Leading Cause of Death

The Department of Health and Human Services has ranked tobacco as the leading cause of death in the United States, followed by diet and inactivity, and then alcohol (see Figure 10.14).[53] Nearly one out of every five deaths is the result of cigarette smoking. Approximately 435,000 Americans die each year from diseases caused by smoking, and (as shown in Figure 10.15) smoking kills more through cardiovascular disease than through cancer.[54] Smoking causes an additional 9 million Americans to suffer increased rates of various debilitating and chronic diseases, including bronchitis, emphysema, and arteriosclerosis.[54] Attainment of a tobacco-free society would add 15 years of life to each of the more than 435,000 individuals who would have experienced tobacco-related deaths.

Smoking is a strong and independent risk factor for all forms of CVD, including CHD, stroke, and peripheral artery disease.[55–58] As many as 30% of all CHD deaths in the United States are attributable to cigarette smoking. Smoking also doubles the risk of ischemic stroke.[56] Using data from the multiple risk factor intervention trial (MRFIT), death from CHD has been shown to be about three times greater among heavy

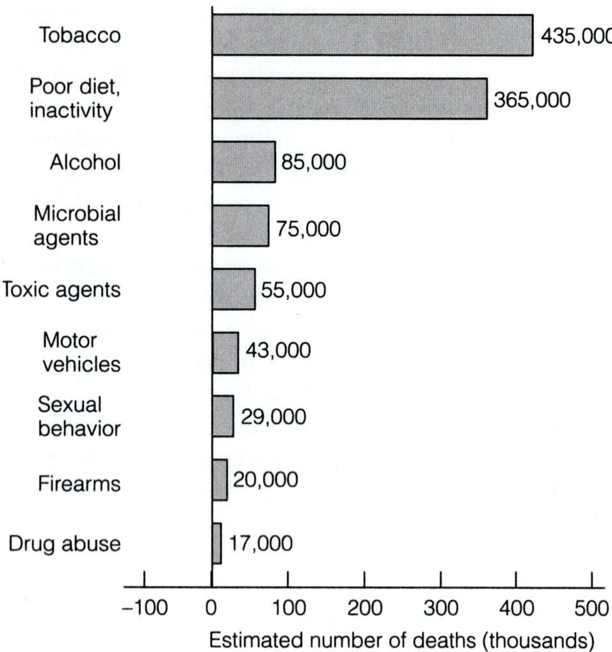

Figure 10.14 Actual causes of death in the United States. The Department of Health and Human Services has ranked tobacco as the leading cause of death in the United States. Source: Data from Mokdad AH, Marks JS, Stroup DF, Gerberding JL. Actual causes of death in the United States, 2000. *JAMA* 291:1238–1245, 2004.

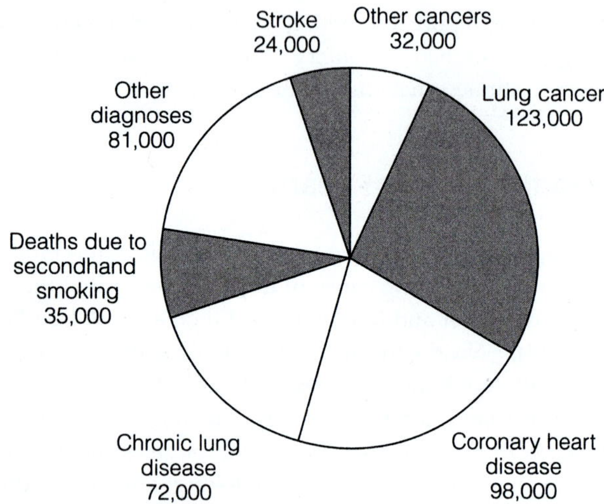

Figure 10.15 Each year approximately 435,000 deaths in the United States are attributed to cigarette smoking. Sources: Data from Mokdad AH, Marks JS, Stroup DF, Gerberding JL. Actual causes of death in the United States, 2000. *JAMA* 291:1238–1245, 2004; CDC. Cigarette smoking-attributable mortality and years of potential life lost—United States. *MMWR* 46(20):444–451, 1997; CDC. Cigarette smoking-attributable morbidity—United States, 2000. *MMWR* 52:842–843, 2003.

smokers (more than 25 cigarettes a day) than among nonsmokers (see Figure 10.16).[55] Data from the MRFIT study have also demonstrated that at every level of serum cholesterol or blood pressure, smoking doubles or triples the death rate from

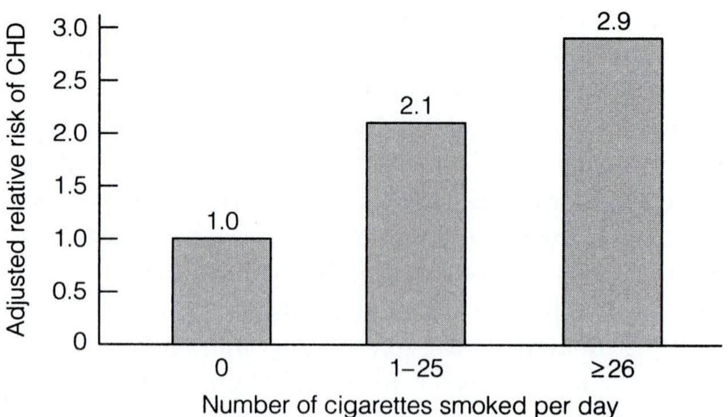

Figure 10.16 Cigarette smoking and coronary heart disease. Risk of coronary heart disease is nearly tripled for heavy smokers. Source: Data from Neaton JD, Wentworth D. Serum cholesterol, blood pressure, cigarette smoking, and death from coronary heart disease. *Arch Intern Med* 152:56–64, 1992.

CHD.[55] These three risk factors work closely together, with the result that smokers with high blood cholesterol and blood pressure levels have CHD death rates approximately 20 times greater than those found among nonsmokers with low blood cholesterol and low blood pressure.

Many underlying mechanisms have been proposed as leading to the hazardous effects of smoking on cardiovascular health. Exposure to tobacco smoke causes abnormalities in endothelial cell function, promotes formation of blood clots, decreases HDL cholesterol levels, and increases the stiffness of both muscular and elastic arteries.[56–58]

Cigarette smoking causes several kinds of cancer (lung, larynx, esophagus, pharynx, mouth, and bladder), and contributes to cancer of the pancreas, kidney, and cervix[2,52] (see Chapter 11). Smoking during pregnancy causes spontaneous abortions, low birth weight, and sudden death syndrome. Other forms of tobacco are not safe alternatives to smoking cigarettes. Use of spit tobacco causes a number of serious oral health problems, including cancer of the mouth and gum, periodontitis, and tooth loss. Cigar use causes cancer of the larynx, mouth, esophagus, and lung.[2] In recent years, reports have shown an increase in the popularity of bidis. Bidis are small brown cigarettes, often flavored, consisting of tobacco hand-rolled in tendu or temburni leaf and secured with a string at one end. Research shows that bidis are a significant health hazard to users, increasing the risk of CHD and cancer of the mouth, pharynx and larynx, lung, esophagus, stomach, and liver.[2]

Recent Trends

As shown in Figure 10.17, the proportion of U.S. adults who smoke has fallen since the 1960s, so that today only 22% still have the habit.[14,59] Unfortunately, smoking prevalence did not decline much during the past decade, and the year 2010 goal of 12% is unlikely to be met.[2] Table 10.5 shows that cigarette smoking is still a major problem among some

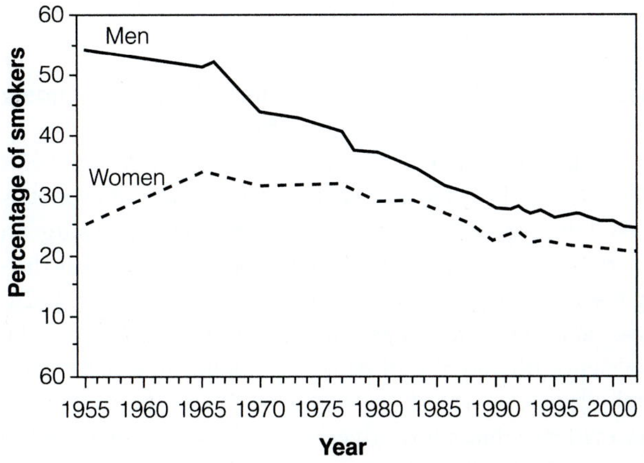

Figure 10.17 Prevalence of smoking among adults since 1955. Source: National Center for Health Statistics. *Health, United States, 2005*. Hyattsville, MD: 2005. www.cdc.gov/nchs.

TABLE 10.5 Percentage of Persons Aged ≥ 18 Years Who Were Current Smokers*, by Selected Characteristics—National Health Interview Survey, United States, 2002

	Men (n = 13,332)		Women (n = 17,374)		Total (n = 30,706)	
Characteristic	%	(95% CI†)	%	(95% CI)	%	(95% CI)
Race/ethnicity§						
White, non-Hispanic	25.5	(±1.1)	21.8	(±1.0)	**23.6**	**(±0.8)**
Black, non-Hispanic	27.1	(±2.4)	18.7	(±1.8)	**22.4**	**(±1.6)**
Hispanic	22.7	(±2.2)	10.8	(±1.3)	**16.7**	**(±1.2)**
American Indian/ Alaska Native¶	40.5	(±13.9)	40.9	(±12.8)	**40.8**	**(±9.8)**
Asian**	19.0	(±4.0)	6.5	(±2.2)	**13.3**	**(±2.4)**
Education††						
0–12 yrs (no diploma)	32.0	(±2.2)	23.8	(±1.8)	**27.6**	**(±1.4)**
<8 yrs	*25.4*	*(±3.2)*	*13.5*	*(±2.2)*	***19.3***	***(±2.0)***
9–11 yrs	*38.1*	*(±3.7)*	*30.9*	*(±2.9)*	***34.1***	***(±2.1)***
12 yrs (no diploma)	*32.3*	*(±6.8)*	*29.7*	*(±6.1)*	***31.0***	***(±4.4)***
GED (diploma)§§	47.4	(±5.6)	37.2	(±5.0)	**42.3**	**(±3.7)**
12 yrs (diploma)	29.8	(±2.0)	22.1	(±1.5)	**25.6**	**(±1.3)**
Associate degree	24.1	(±2.9)	19.6	(±2.2)	**21.5**	**(±1.7)**
Some college (no degree)	24.8	(±2.2)	21.6	(±1.6)	**23.1**	**(±1.4)**
Undergraduate degree	13.6	(±1.7)	10.5	(±1.4)	**12.1**	**(±1.1)**
Graduate degree	7.8	(±1.6)	6.4	(±1.5)	**7.2**	**(±1.1)**
Age group (yr)						
18–24	32.4	(±2.8)	24.6	(±2.5)	**28.5**	**(±2.0)**
25–44	28.7	(±1.4)	22.8	(±1.3)	**25.7**	**(±1.0)**
45–64	24.5	(±1.4)	21.1	(±1.2)	**22.7**	**(±0.9)**
≥65	10.1	(±1.4)	8.6	(±1.1)	**9.3**	**(±0.8)**
Poverty level¶¶						
At or above	24.8	(±1.1)	19.7	(±0.9)	**22.2**	**(±0.7)**
Below	36.9	(±3.3)	30.1	(±2.8)	**32.9**	**(±2.3)**
Unknown	23.0	(±1.8)	16.9	(±1.3)	**19.7**	**(±1.1)**
Total	**25.2**	**(±0.9)**	**20.0**	**(±0.8)**	**22.5**	**(±0.6)**

*Persons who reported smoking ≥ 100 cigarettes during their lifetimes and who reported at the time of interview smoking every day or some days. Excludes 338 respondents whose smoking status was unknown.
†Confidence interval.
§Excludes 343 respondents of unknown, multiple, and other racial/ethnic categories.
¶Wide variances among estimates reflect small sample sizes.
**Does not include native Hawaiians or other Pacific Islanders.
††Persons aged ≥25 years. Excludes 369 persons with unknown years of education.
§§General Educational Development.
¶¶Published 2000 poverty thresholds from the U.S. Bureau of the Census were used in these calculations.
Source: CDC. Cigarette smoking among adults—United States, 2002. *MMWR* 53(20):427–431, 2004.

segments of American society, particularly those with low income and education, and various minority groups.

Cigarette smoking almost always begins in the adolescent years. Among U.S. adults who have ever smoked daily, 82% tried their first cigarette before age 18 years.[2] Approximately 6,000 young persons try a cigarette each day, with half becoming daily smokers.[2] In other words, more than 1 million young persons start to smoke each year, adding about $10 billion during their lifetimes to the cost of health care in the United States. The prevalence of tobacco use among adolescents rose during the 1990s but has since declined to a current 22%, just 6% above the 2010 goal of 16%[60] (see Figure 10.18). Factors the might have contributed to the decline in cigarette use among teenagers include (1) a 90% increase in the retail price of cigarettes from December 1997 to May 2003, (2) increases in school-based efforts to prevent tobacco use, and (3) increases in the proportion of young persons who have been exposed to smoking-prevention campaigns.[60] Cigarette smoking among adolescents has also been linked to other problems, including marijuana use, binge drinking, and fighting.[61]

The mean number of cigarettes smoked daily per smoker is 20, or one pack a day. Per capita consumption of cigarettes peaked during the 1960s, around the time of the first surgeon general's report, and has since fallen sharply, particularly during the 1980s and 1990s (see Figure 10.19).[52,59,62] Social influences and legislation have had a strong impact on the prevalence of smoking in America. Public attitudes toward smoking have changed, in large part due to the contemporary evidence that many adverse health effects are related to passive smoking (breathing someone else's cigarette smoke).

The National Cancer Institute has concluded that "there is no longer any doubt that exposure to environmental tobacco smoke (ETS) is a cause of death and disease among nonsmokers."[63] A panel of science advisors also told the Environmental Protection Agency (EPA) in October of 1992 that there was enough evidence to classify secondhand to-

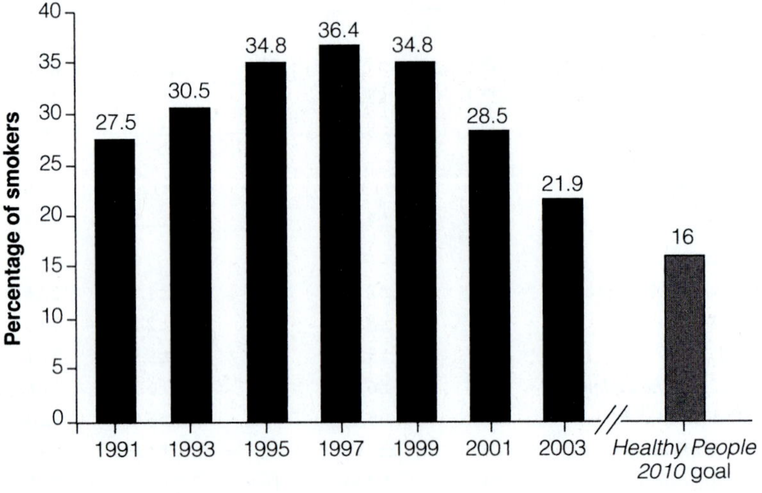

Figure 10.18 Prevalence of smoking among high school students. High school students who reported current cigarette smoking (one or more cigarettes during previous 30 days. Source: National Center for Health Statistics. *Health, United States, 2005.* Hyattsville, MD: 2005, www.cdc.gov/nchs.

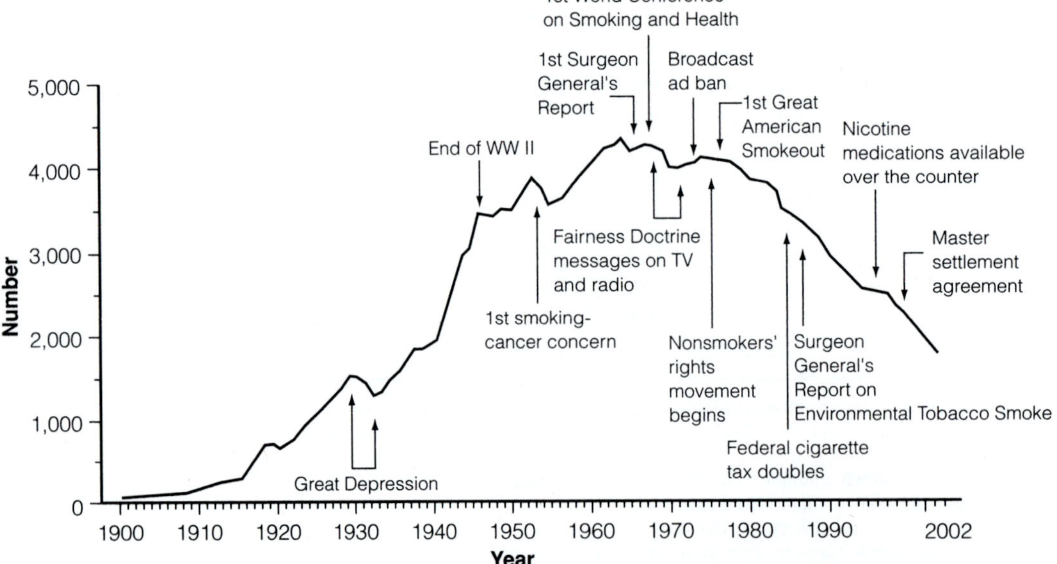

Figure 10.19 Trends in per capita cigarette consumption. Annual adult per capita cigarette consumption and major smoking and health events—United States, 1900–1998. Source: *MMWR* 49(39): 881–884, 2000.

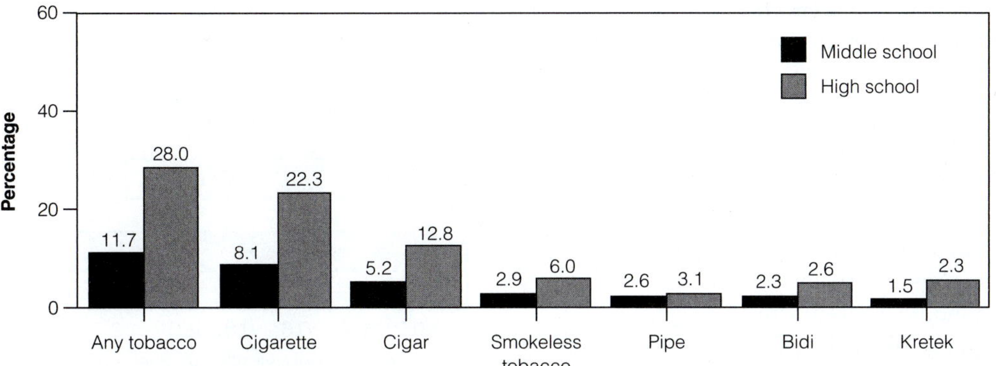

Figure 10.20 Tobacco use among students. Sources: CDC. Cigarette use among high school students—United States, 1991–2003. *MMWR* 53(23):499–502, 2004; CDC. Tobacco use, access, and exposure to tobacco in media among middle and high school students—United States, 2004. *MMWR* 54(12):297–301, 2005.

bacco smoke as a cause of cancer for humans and of serious respiratory problems for infants and young children. In January of 1993, after 2 years of revisions and intense debate, the EPA put its stamp of approval on this historic report.[64]

The report estimated that 3,000 lung cancer deaths each year can be attributed to ETS, and that parental smoking causes as many as 300,000 lung infections, including bronchitis and pneumonia, among children each year. Of equal importance, the EPA estimates that ETS is causally related to additional episodes and increased severity of preexisting asthma among children and exacerbates symptoms of approximately 20% of the estimated 2–5 million asthmatic children annually. There is increasing evidence that ETS increases the risk for CHD.[65,66] The National Institute for Occupational Safety and Health (NIOSH) recommends eliminating smoking in all workplaces.[67] The only alternative, according to NIOSH, is restricting smoking to completely separated smoking lounges, with independent ventilation systems exhausting secondhand smoke outside.

Smokeless Tobacco

Two types of *smokeless tobacco*—snuff and chewing tobacco—are in current use.[68] *Snuff* is a cured, finely ground tobacco that either can be taken nasally or, more commonly today, placed in small quantities between cheek and gum. *Chewing tobacco* comes in several forms, including loose-leaf, plug, and twist, all of which can be chewed directly and then spit out.

Consumption of moist snuff, now the most popular (and dangerous) form of smokeless tobacco, tripled from the 1970s to the 1990s.[69] An estimated 5% of U.S. male adults are users of smokeless tobacco, with prevalence highest among those 18–24 years of age.[2] About 6% of high school students use smokeless tobacco (see Figure 10.20).[2,60,69]

The resurgence in popularity of smokeless tobacco can be linked to advertising campaigns by tobacco companies to promote users as "macho." Adolescent and young adult males are the target of marketing strategies by tobacco companies that link such use with athletic performance and virility. Use of oral snuff is widespread among professional baseball players (about 4 out of 10), encouraging this behavior among adolescent and young adult males.[70]

Snuff and chewing tobacco are associated with a variety of serious adverse effects, especially oral cancer.[68] Holding tobacco in the mouth brings multiple carcinogenic chemicals into contact with the lining of the mouth. This can lead to the formation of white patches called leukoplakia (present in 46% of professional baseball players using smokeless tobacco), some of which then make the final transformation to cancer. Smokeless tobacco may also affect reproduction, longevity, the cardiovascular system, and oral health (bad breath, abrasion of teeth, gum recession, periodontal bone loss, and tooth loss), and it is highly addictive.[68]

Smoking Cessation

The nicotine from tobacco is highly addictive, making smoking cessation one of the most difficult of all health behaviors to change.[71] In 2000, clinical practice guidelines for treating tobacco use and dependence were published by the Public Health Service, U.S. Department of Health and Human Services.[72] These guidelines contain strategies and recommendations designed to assist clinicians, smoking cessation specialists, and allied health personnel in delivering and supporting effective treatments for tobacco use and dependence. In the same year, the surgeon general released guidelines on reducing tobacco use.[73] Key recommendations from these two reports include the following:

- Tobacco dependence is a chronic condition that often requires repeated intervention. However, effective treatments exist that can produce long-term or even permanent abstinence.
- Approaches with the largest span of impact (economic, regulatory, and comprehensive) are likely to have the greatest long-term population impact.
- Educational strategies, conducted in conjunction with community- and media-based activities, can postpone or prevent smoking onset in 20–40% of adolescents.
- It is essential that clinicians and health-care delivery systems (including administrators, insurers, and purchasers) institutionalize the consistent identification, documentation, and treatment of every tobacco user seen in a health-care setting.

- Brief tobacco dependence treatment is effective, and every patient who uses tobacco should be offered at least brief treatment.
- Pharmacologic treatment of nicotine addiction, combined with behavioral support, will enable 20–25% of users to remain abstinent at 1 year posttreatment.
- Numerous effective pharmacotherapies for smoking cessation now exist. Except in the presence of contraindications, these should be used with all patients attempting to quit smoking. Five first-line pharmacotherapies reliably increase long-term abstinence rates: bupropion hydrochloride, nicotine gum, nicotine inhaler, nicotine nasal spray, and nicotine patch. Two second-line pharmacotherapies are efficacious if first-line methods are not effective: Clonidine and Nortriptyline.
- An optimal level of excise taxation on tobacco products will reduce the prevalence of smoking, the consumption of tobacco, and the long-term health consequences of tobacco use.

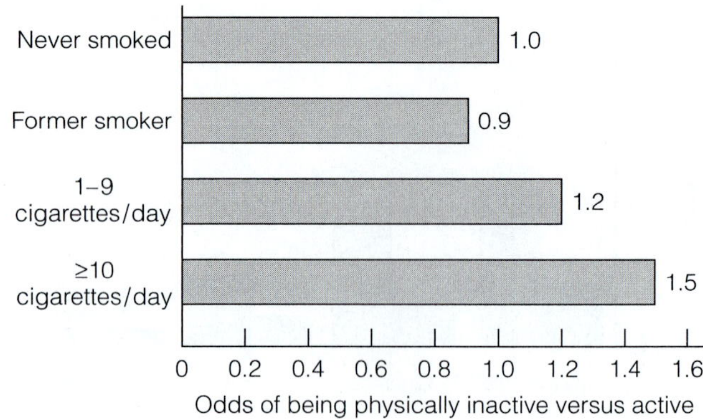

Figure 10.21 Odds of being a physically inactive person by smoking habit: Study of 30,000 Americans, by the Centers for Disease Control and Prevention. The odds of being physically inactive rise with the increasing use of cigarettes. Source: Data from Simoes EJ, Byers T, Coates RJ, Serdula MK, Mokdad AH, Heath GW. The association between leisure-time physical activity and dietary fat in American adults. *Am J Public Health* 85:240–244, 1995.

Exercise and Tobacco

Smoking and sports do not mix, and today it is quite rare to find an elite athlete who smokes. When Michael Jordan, who does not smoke, won his first National Basketball Association title, *Sports Illustrated* put him on the cover with a cigar in his mouth, prompting many readers to scold the magazine for portraying their icon in such a misleading fashion.

The prevalence of smoking among people who exercise is much lower than that of the general population. Studies show a reduced likelihood of incidence of smoking among adolescents involved in vigorous physical activity and interscholastic sports than among those exercising little.[74] Other studies have shown that youths who smoke exercise less than those who abstain, and they are prone to other high-risk behaviors, such as drinking, drug use, carrying weapons, failure to wear seat belts, and engaging in physical fights.[75]

Many studies have confirmed that smokers are less fit and tend to exercise less than nonsmokers.[76–81] Among military personnel, the amount of physical activity has been found to vary inversely with the number of cigarettes smoked.[79,80] Among the 3,300 offspring in the Framingham study, increasing levels of physical activity were associated with fewer cigarettes smoked per day.[81] As depicted in Figure 10.21, the odds of being physically inactive are highest in those smoking more than 10 cigarettes per day.[76]

Smokers may be less likely than nonsmokers to make regular exercise a part of their lives because exercise is more difficult for them. Smoking is associated with a decrease in the ability to perform vigorous exercise because of decreased lung function, increased blood levels of carboxyhemoglobin, a blunted heart rate response to exercise, and decreased maximal oxygen consumption.[79,80,82–94]

At rest, and to a smaller extent during exercise, nicotine from smoking cigarettes increases the heart rate and blood pressure, decreases the heart's blood output, and increases the oxygen demands of the heart muscle.[83,84] Nicotine also increases lactate levels in the blood during exercise, which can make people feel fatigued or feel like quitting exercise when it rises high enough.[86,90] When smokers abstain from cigarettes for one week, exercise performance improves.[94]

The resistance to airflow after smoking is increased in the lung passageways, making it harder to deliver air and oxygen to the lungs during hard exercise.[82,83,85,88,89,92] In some people, cigarette smoke can trigger asthma symptoms, making it nearly impossible to exercise until symptoms subside.[88]

In one study of 1,000 young recruits in the Air Force, the distance each was able to run in 12 minutes was directly related to the amount of cigarettes smoked, with those smoking more than 30 cigarettes a day in the worst shape.[93] In Switzerland, nearly 7,000 19-year-old military conscripts were studied, and performance in the 12-minute run was found to be inversely related to both the number of cigarettes smoked and the number of years with the habit[80] (see Figure 10.22).

A 7-year study of 1,400 Norwegians showed that physical fitness and lung function declined at a significantly faster rate in those who smoked, compared to nonsmokers.[82] In other words, smokers are less fit to begin with, because of their smoking, and then they lose more fitness and lung function as time passes.

Can the initiation of an exercise program be used to improve success in smoking cessation? Ken Cooper of the Cooper Institute for Aerobics Research in Dallas, Texas, has

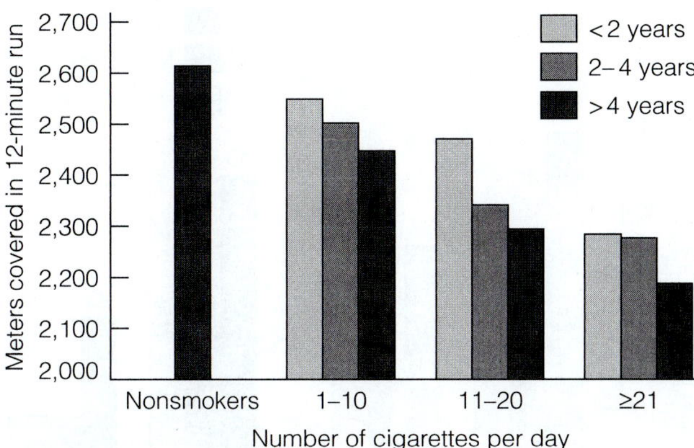

Figure 10.22 Performance in 12-minute run, according to smoking status of 6,592 Swiss 19-year-old military conscripts. The number of meters covered in the 12-minute run was lowest in military conscripts smoking more than a pack a day for more than 4 years. Source: Data from Marti B, Abelin T, Minder CE, Vader JP. Smoking, alcohol consumption, and endurance capacity: An analysis of 6,500 19-year-old conscripts and 4,100 joggers. *Prev Med* 17:79–92, 1988.

written that "smokers who get involved in aerobic exercise become more aware of how smoking has decreased their ability to process oxygen. In short, they find they become winded more easily than their fellow exercisers. This helps create a desire to quit smoking."[95]

Proof of this assertion has been hard to come by, however. A cross-sectional study by the Centers for Disease Control and Prevention reported that 81% of men and 75% of women runners who had smoked cigarettes quit after beginning recreational running.[96] Another study of 347 marathon runners, 38% of whom were former smokers, showed that about two thirds of them claimed that running had helped them quit.[97] Two prospective studies, however, have failed to confirm this finding.[98,99] The Aerobics Research Center was unable to show that individuals voluntarily increasing their physical fitness level were more likely than nonexercisers to reduce smoking.[98] Similarly, a 1-year, randomized, controlled, exercise training study of 160 women and 197 men failed to demonstrate any effect of exercise on smoking cessation.[99]

However, a randomized, controlled trial of 281 female smokers showed that vigorous exercise facilitates short- and long-term smoking cessation, improves aerobic fitness, and delays weight gain.[100] In another study of 2,086 smokers living in New England, those who were successful in quitting smoking were more likely than nonquitters to report efforts to increase exercise.[101]

There is not yet conclusive evidence that exercise helps people stop smoking, but most smoking cessation programs include exercise as a vital component. Several studies indicate that 5 to 20 minutes of moderate-to-vigorous exercise is linked to a short-term reduction in desire to smoke and tobacco withdrawal symptoms.[102] Thus brief exercise bouts are useful in quelling strong urges to smoke and can be injected into stop-smoking regimens as one method to achieve success.

Although nearly all smokers admit that their habit increases the risk of early death from cancer and heart disease, many are still unwilling to quit, frequently citing their fear of weight gain.[103–108] The use of smoking as a weight-control strategy, risky though it may be, appears to be a powerful motivation for continued smoking among a large percentage of smokers.

Cigarettes have long been associated with slenderness. As early as 1925, Lucky Strike launched its "Reach for a Lucky Instead of a Sweet" campaign, using testimonials from famous women such as Amelia Earhart and Jean Harlow.[103,107] This campaign continues. Advertisements targeted at women still emphasize ultraslimness, sophistication, beauty, luxury, and popularity with men.

Unfortunately, there is an element of truth to these advertisements—smoking does promote weight loss. Studies have established that the average smoker weighs about 7 pounds less than a comparable nonsmoker.[105] People who start smoking lose weight, while those who quit gain, with women adding on an average of 8 pounds and men 6 pounds. A 10-year study of 9,000 Americans by the Centers for Disease Control and Prevention confirmed that major weight gain (more than 28.6 pounds) can be expected for 10% of men and 13% of women who quit smoking[104] (see Figure 10.23). The relative risk of major weight gain in those who quit smoking (as compared with those who continued to smoke) was 8:1 in men and 5:8 in women. Two thirds of all smokers who quit gained weight, with the odds increasing for those who smoked more than 15 cigarettes per day. The researchers concluded that major weight gain is strongly related to smoking cessation, but that the average weight gain is rather small and unlikely to negate the health benefits of smoking cessation.

Not only do smokers tend to weigh less than nonsmokers, some studies even suggest they have less body fat, despite eating the same amount and exercising less.[109] It appears that smoking elevates the metabolic rate by 6–10%, and that when people quit, the rate falls back to its original level.[110–113] Then if appetite and food intake are increased, as is commonly reported by those who quit, weight gain is inevitable.

As reviewed by the surgeon general,[107] most studies show that food intake, especially of sweet foods, increases after quitting, resulting in 200–250 extra Calories a day. About one third of the weight gain has been ascribed to the fall in metabolic rate, one third to an increase in caloric consumption, and the other third to unmeasured factors.[111]

For several reasons, then, regular exercise is especially recommended for people quitting smoking.[107] First of all, smokers typically have poor levels of fitness, and initiation of regular exercise can improve their fitness and help improve their general health status. Second, because weight gain is common, burning extra Calories through exercise may help to bring the body into better caloric balance. For

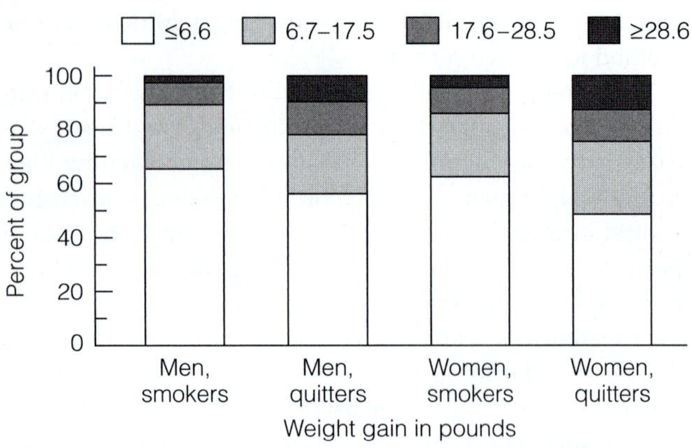

Figure 10.23 Weight gain over a 10-year period by smoking status: Mean adjusted weight gain for quitters was 6.2 pounds for men, 8.4 pounds for women. In this 10-year study of 9,000 Americans, major weight gain (more than 28.6 pounds) occurred in 9.8% of the men and 13.4% of the women who quit smoking. Source: Data from Williamson DF, Madans J, Anda RF, et al. Smoking cessation and severity of weight gain in a national cohort. *N Engl J Med* 324:739–745, 1991.

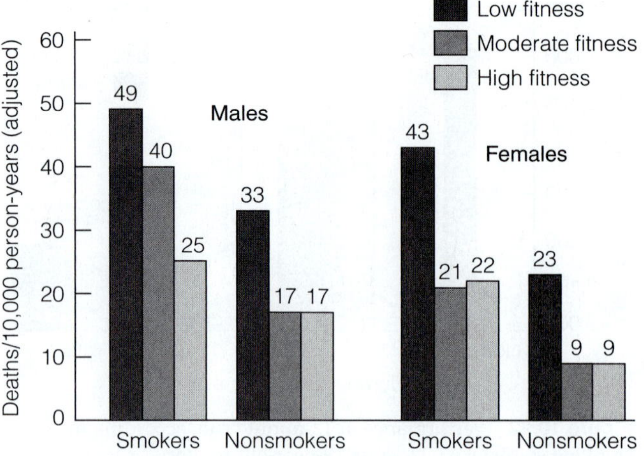

Figure 10.24 Death rates according to fitness status and smoking status. Fit smokers have lower death rates than unfit nonsmokers. Source: Data from Blair SN, Kampert JB, Kohl HW, et al. Influences of cardiorespiratory fitness and other precursors on cardiovascular disease and all-cause mortality in men and women. *JAMA* 276:205–210, 1996.

example, data from the Nurses' Health Study showed that weight gain after smoking cessation was cut in half when subjects simultaneously increased their level of physical activity.[114] Regular exercise can decrease the levels of various risk factors and can reduce the risk for heart disease and some cancers, helping to counter some of the negative disease consequences of smoking.[107] There is also some evidence that exercise enhances long-term maintenance of smoking cessation.[115]

Finally, many individuals use smoking as a method of coping with stress and find the habit to be relaxing. Within 2 hours after quitting, typical feelings of nicotine withdrawal include irritability, frustration, anger, difficulty in concentrating, restlessness, depression, impatience, disrupted sleep, and impaired ability to work.[107] These feelings peak within the first 24 hours, then gradually decline, usually subsiding completely within 1 month.

As emphasized in Chapter 14, exercise is an excellent substitute for smoking in improving psychological mood state and alleviating anxiety and depression, thereby helping the quitter cope with some of the immediate negative mood states.[116] As reported by Ken Cooper, "I have received hundreds of letters from cigarette smokers telling me how they could never break the habit until they started exercising."[95]

For smokers who cannot or will not quit, exercise is still encouraged, to reduce risk of heart disease and early death. Data from the Cooper Institute for Aerobics Research have shown that smokers who maintain a high level of physical fitness have lower death rates from all causes than do low-fitness nonsmokers.[117] The lowest death rates, however, are found among men and women who avoid smoking while maintaining moderate-to-high physical fitness levels (see Figure 10.24).

HYPERTENSION

As described in Chapter 4, *blood pressure* is the force of the blood pushing against the walls of the arteries. The heart beats about 60–75 times each minute, and the blood pressure is at its greatest when the heart contracts, pumping blood into the arteries. This is called *systolic blood pressure.* When the heart is resting briefly between beats, the blood pressure falls, termed *diastolic blood pressure.* According to the National High Blood Pressure Education Program, *hypertension* is defined to be present when diastolic measurements on at least two separate occasions average 90 mm Hg or higher, and/or systolic measurements are 140 mm Hg or higher[118] (see Table 4.1).

In the United States and most other Western societies, the large majority of residents experience a progressive age-related rise in blood pressure (see Figure 4.2). As a result, the incidence and prevalence of hypertension rise steadily with each additional decade of life. Two million new hypertensives are added each year to the pool of patients in the United States, so that by old age, about two thirds of Americans have this disease[119] (see Figure 10.25). In the United States, normotensive individuals at age 55 years have a 90% lifetime risk for developing hypertension.[118]

It is important to stress that in unacculturated societies, age-related increases in blood pressure are uncommon. Thus, it does not appear that hypertension is the inevitable consequence of old age. In societies where salt and alcohol intakes are high, potassium intake is low, and physical inactivity and obesity are the norm, incidence of hypertension is high.[119–121]

Current estimates indicate that approximately 65 million, or 26%, of all adults in the United States have high blood pressure, while another 31% have prehypertension.[4,119,122] The year 2010 target for hypertension preva-

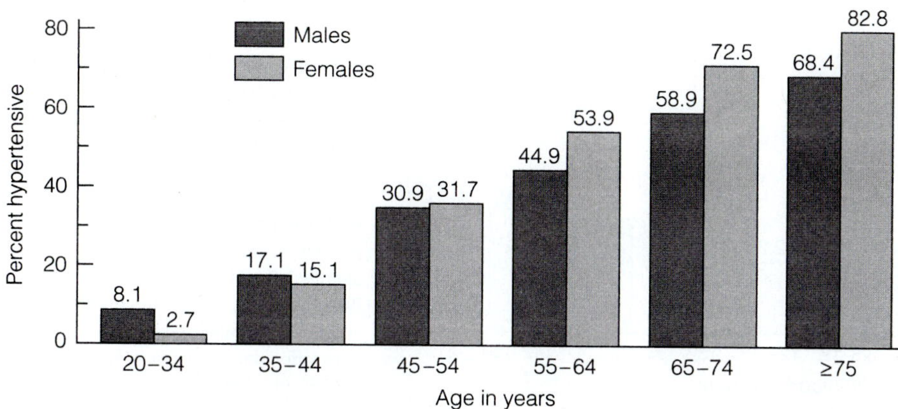

Figure 10.25 Hypertension prevalence by age and sex. Source: National Center for Health Statistics. *Health, United States, 2005.* Hyattsville, MD: 2005. www.cdc.gov/nchs.

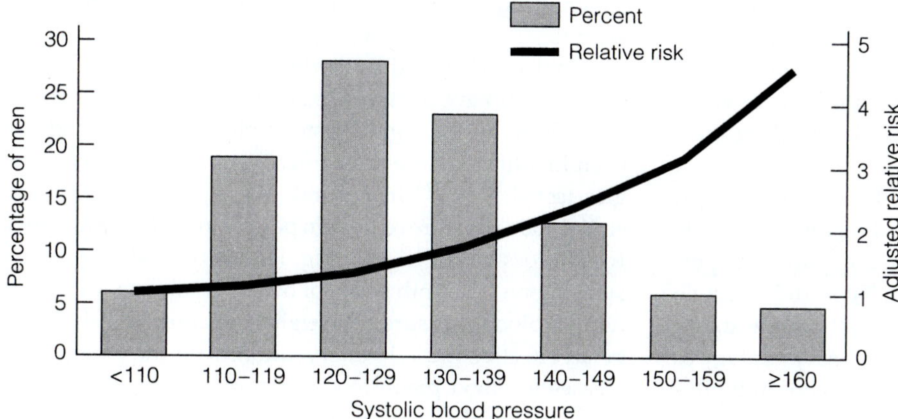

Figure 10.26 Systolic blood pressure and cardiovascular mortality: 12.5-year study of 347,978 men (MRFIT)—prevalence and risk. Data from the MRFIT study have shown that risk of cardiovascular mortality rises sharply with increase in systolic blood pressure. Source: Data from Stamler J, Stamler R, Neaton JD. Blood pressure, systolic and diastolic, and cardiovascular risks: US population data. *Arch Intern Med* 153:598–615, 1993.

lence is 16%. (See Figure 10.10). Only 34% of adults with high blood pressure have it under control, yet 70% are taking some kind of action to control their blood pressure.[2,118]

Blood pressure has increased over the past decade among children and adolescents, and is in part due to an increased prevalence of overweight.[123]

Health Problems

High blood pressure usually does not give early warning signs; for this reason, it is known as the "silent killer." High blood pressure kills more than 37,000 Americans each year and contributes to the deaths of more than 700,000, reports the National Center for Health Statistics.[124] High blood pressure increases the risk for coronary heart disease and other forms of heart disease, stroke, and kidney failure.[124–127]

According to the National Heart, Lung, and Blood Institute, when blood pressure is not detected and treated, it can cause[124]

- The heart to get larger, which may lead to heart failure
- Small blisters (aneurysms) to form in the brain's blood vessels, which may cause a stroke[126]
- Blood vessels in the kidneys to narrow, which may cause kidney failure
- Arteries throughout the body to harden faster, especially those in the heart, brain, and kidneys, which can cause a heart attack, stroke, or kidney failure[125,127]

High blood pressure also affects the brain. People with elevated blood pressure in middle age are more likely to suffer 25 years later from loss of cognitive abilities—memory, problem solving, concentration, and judgment.[128] This loss further translates into a diminished capacity to function independently in old age.

Using data from the large-scale MRFIT study, researchers have documented that cardiovascular and stroke mortality increases progressively with incremental increases in blood pressure from the optimal level of less than 120/80 mm Hg[119,120] (see Figures 10.26 and 10.27). The risk of CVD beginning at 155/75 mm/Hg doubles with each increment of 20/10 mm/Hg.[118]

Treatment of Hypertension

The goal of treatment for individuals with high blood pressure is the reduction of cardiovascular and kidney disease.[118] Studies clearly show that several classes of drugs (see Table 10.6) are highly effective in both treating high

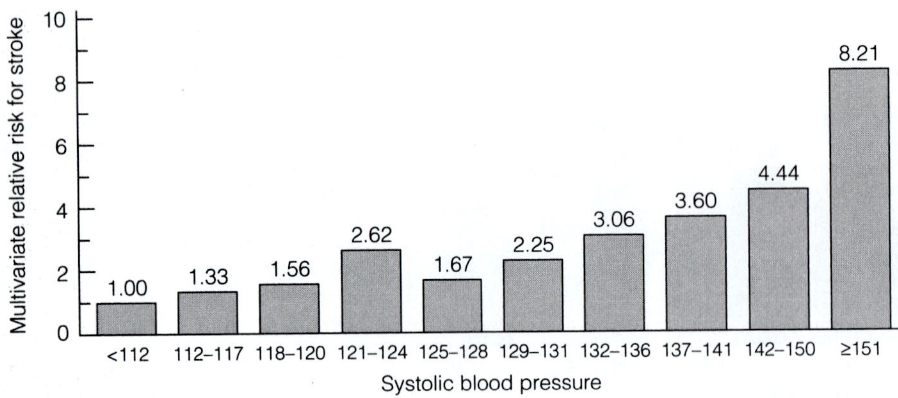

Figure 10.27 Systolic blood pressure and stroke mortality: 12.5-year study of 347,978 men (MRFIT). Data from the MRFIT study have shown that risk of stroke mortality rises sharply with increase in systolic blood pressure. Source: Data from Stamler J, Stamler R, Neaton JD. Blood pressure, systolic and diastolic, and cardiovascular risks: US population data. *Arch Intern Med* 153:598–615, 1993.

blood pressure and preventing medical complications.[118,119,129–131] Adoption of healthy lifestyles is even more critical for the prevention and treatment of high blood pressure.[118,119,132–134] Figure 10.28 shows the relative value of lifestyle treatment alone versus lifestyle and drug therapy combined.[136,137]

The National High Blood Pressure Education Program of the National Heart, Lung, and Blood Institute supports lifestyle modifications as an indispensable part of hypertension management.[118] As outlined in Table 10.7, lifestyle modification should be encouraged for all Americans to prevent high blood pressure and as the primary strategy of treatment for individuals with prehypertension. Individuals with stage 1 and 2 hypertension should combine lifestyle modifications with appropriate drug therapy that is adjusted for individuals with or without compelling indications such as heart failure, post-heart attack, high CHD risk, diabetes, chronic kidney disease, and recurrent stroke prevention. Thiazide-type diuretics should be used in drug treatment for most patients with uncomplicated hypertension, either alone or combined with drugs from other classes. Most patients with hypertension will require lifestyle modifications and two or more antihypertensive medications to achieve goal blood pressure (defined as <140/90 mm Hg, or <130/80 mm Hg for patients with diabetes or chronic kidney disease).

Lifestyle Modifications to Lower Blood Pressure

Box 10.4 outlines the lifestyle modifications for preventing and treating hypertension, as recommended by the Joint National Committee on Detection, Evaluation, and Treatment of High Blood Pressure.[118]

Weight Control

Studies have identified a strong relationship between body weight and blood pressure.[118,119,134–143] (See discussion in Chapter 13.) Being overweight results in a two- to sixfold increase in the risk of developing hypertension, with the risk climbing in a stepwise manner with increasing body weight.

Clinical trials with hypertensive and even normotensive subjects have documented that loss of excess weight reduces both systolic and diastolic blood pressure and has been identified as the most effective of the lifestyle strategies tested.[119,140,143] In general, average systolic and diastolic blood pressure reduction per kilogram (2.2 pounds) of weight loss is 1.6/1.1 mm Hg. Figure 10.29 shows the results of one 18-month study of over 500 subjects with high-normal blood pressure.[138] Weight reduction was shown to be an effective lifestyle intervention, with the greatest decreases in blood pressure correlating with those who lost the most weight. Although the goal for subjects randomized to the weight-loss group was to achieve a weight loss of at least 10 pounds through diet and exercise modifications, only 45% of the men and 26% of the women were able to meet this. As discussed in Chapter 13, weight loss is a difficult task for most people, and requires unusual discipline and motivation.

Reduced Sodium Chloride Intake

Most people in Western societies consume a diet that contains between 2,500 and 5,000 mg of sodium (about 6–12 g of salt or sodium chloride) per person per day. As discussed in Chapter 9, average daily sodium intake from food alone exceeds 4,000 mg for each U.S. man and 3,000 mg for each woman. These values do not include sodium from salt added to foods at the table. This is far in excess of the physiological need for salt and appears to be substantially more than that eaten by our ancestors or people living in isolated societies. When high salt intake is prolonged throughout the lifetime of a population, the majority will eventually experience a rise in blood pressure.[119]

Sodium is essential for a wide variety of functions in the body. Although needs vary from person to person, a minimum of 500 mg sodium per day is considered necessary to maintain physiological balance for adults, although up to 2,000–3,000 mg per day is considered safe and adequate. As reviewed in Chapter 9, 1 teaspoon of salt (5 g) has 2,000 mg

TABLE 10.6 Oral Antihypertensive Drugs*

Class	Drug (Trade Name)
Thiazide diuretics	chlorothiazide (Diuril) chlorthalidone (generic) hydrochlorothiazide (Microzide, HydroDIURIL[†]) polythiazide (Renese) indapamide (Lozol[†]) metolazone (Mykrox) metolazone (Zaroxolyn)
Loop diuretics	bumetanide (Bumex[†]) furosemide (Lasix[†]) torsemide (Demadex[†])
Potassium-sparing diuretics	amiloride (Midamor[†]) Triamterene (Dyrenium)
Aldosterone receptor blockers	eplerenone (Inspra) spironolactone (Aldactone[†])
Beta-blockers	atenolol (Tenormin[†]) betaxolol (Kerlone[†]) bisoprolol (Zebeta[†]) metoprolol (Lopressor[†]) metoprolol extended release (Toprol XL) nadolol (Corgard[†]) propranolol (Inderal[†]) propranolol long-acting (Inderal LA[†]) timolol (Blocadren[†])
Beta-blockers with intrinsic sympathomimetic activity	acebutolol (Sectra[†]) penbutolol (Levatol) pindolol (generic)
Combined alpha- and beta-blockers	carvedilol (Coreg) labetalol (Normodyne, Trandate[†])
ACE inhibitors	benazepril (Lotensin[†]) captopril (Capoten[†]) enalapril (Vasotec[†]) fosinopril (Monopril) lisinopril (Prinivil, Zestril[†]) moexipril (Univasc) perindopril (Aceon) quinapril (Accupril) ramipril (Altace) trandolapril (Mavik)
Angiotensin II antagonists	candesartan (Atacand) eprosartan (Tevetan) irbesartan (Avapro) losartan (Cozaar) olmesartan (Benicar) telmisartan (Micardis) valsartan (Diovan)
Calcium channel blockers—non-Dihydropyridines	diltiazem extended release (Cardizem CD, Dilacor XR, Tiazac[†]) diltiazem extended release (Cardizem LA) verapamil immediate release (Calan, Isoptin[†]) verapamil long acting (Calan SR, Isoptin SR[†]) verapamil—Coer (Covera HS, Verelan PM)
Calcium channel blockers—Dihydropyridines	amiodipine (Norvasc) felodipine (Plendil) isradipine (Dynacirc CR) nicardipine sustained release (Cardene SR) nifedipine long-acting (Adalat CC, Procardia XL) nisoldipine (Sular)
Alpha$_1$-blockers	doxazosin (Cardura) prazosin (Minipress[†]) terazosin (Hytrin)
Central alpha$_2$-agonists and other centrally acting drugs	clonidine (Catapres[†]) clonidine patch (Catapres-TTS) methyldopa (Aldomet[†]) reserpine (generic) guanfacine (generic)
Direct vasodilators	hydralazine (Apresoline[†]) minoxidil (Loniten[†])

*These dosages may vary from those listed in the "Physicians' Desk Reference."
[†]Are now or will soon become available in generic preparations.

Source: National High Blood Pressure Education Program. *The Seventh Report of the Joint National Committee on Detection, Evaluation, and Treatment of High Blood Pressure.* National Heart, Lung, and Blood Institute, National Institutes of Health, NIH Publication No. 03-5233. Bethesda, MD: National Institutes of Health, 2003.

TABLE 10.7 Classification and Management of Blood Pressure for Adults*

				Initial Drug Therapy	
BP Classification	**SBP* mm Hg**	**DBP* mm Hg**	**Lifestyle Modification**	**Without Compelling Indication**	**With Compelling Indications (See Table 10.8)**
Normal	<120	and <80	Encourage		
Prehypertension	120–139	or 80–89	Yes	No antihypertensive drug indicated.	Drug(s) for compelling indications.[‡]
Stage 1 Hypertension	140–159	or 90–99	Yes	Thiazide-type diuretics for most. May consider ACEI, ARB, BB, CCB, or combination.	Drug(s) for the compelling indications.[‡] Other antihypertensive drugs (diuretics, ACEI, ARB, BB, CCB) as needed.
Stage 2 Hypertension	≥160	or ≥100	Yes	Two-drug combination for most[†] (usually thiazide-type diuretic and ACEI or ARB or BB or CCB).	

DBP, diastolic blood pressure; SBP, systolic blood pressure.

Drug abbreviations: ACEI, angiotensin converting enzyme inhibitor; ARB, angiotensin receptor blocker; BB, beta-blocker; CCB, calcium channel blocker.

*Treatment determined by highest BP category.

†Initial combined therapy should be used cautiously in those at risk for orthostatic hypotension.

‡Treat patients with chronic kidney disease or diabetes to BP goal of <130/80 mm Hg.

Source: National High Blood Pressure Education Program. *The Seventh Report of the Joint National Committee on Detection, Evaluation, and Treatment of High Blood Pressure.* National Heart, Lung, and Blood Institute, National Institutes of Health, NIH Publication No. 03-5233. Bethesda, MD: National Institutes of Health, 2003.

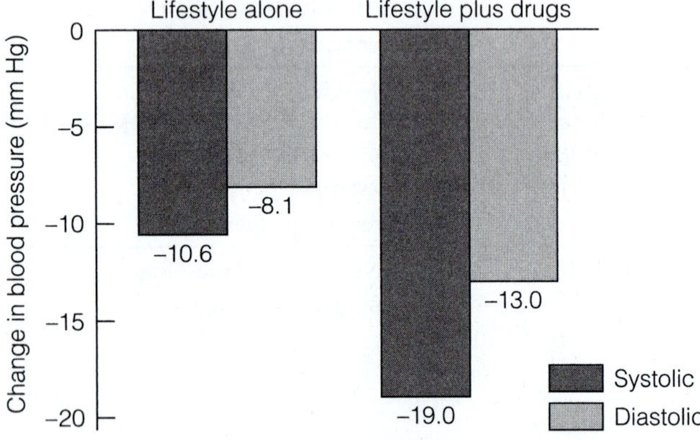

Figure 10.28 Treatment of mild hypertension in 900 people across 1 year: Lifestyle (weight loss, decrease in sodium, and exercise) and drug therapy. Lifestyle modifications have proven to be an effective first-step treatment for persons with mild hypertension. Source: Data from Treatment of Mild Hypertension Research Group. The Treatment of Mild Hypertension Study: A randomized, placebo-controlled trial of a nutritional-hygienic regimen along with various drug monotherapies. *Arch Intern Med* 151:1413–1423, 1991.

of sodium. The Joint National Committee on Detection, Evaluation, and Treatment of High Blood Pressure recommends less than 2,400 mg a day to prevent hypertension.[118]

In the INTERSALT study, a large international epidemiological study of 10,000 people living in 32 countries, a 1-teaspoon difference in salt consumption was associated with a 2.2 mm Hg difference in systolic blood pressure.[144,145] The same study showed that consuming 1 teaspoon less salt a day was associated with a 9 mm Hg attenuation in the rise of systolic blood pressure between the ages of 25 and 55 years.[144,145] In another study of 47,000 individuals, 1 teaspoon of salt was associated with differences in systolic blood pressure that ranged from 5 mm Hg at ages 15–19, to 10 mm Hg at ages 60–69, with the difference even larger for those with higher blood pressures.[146] In general, the risk of hypertension is lower when salt intake is lower.[147]

In clinical trials with hypertensive patients, lowering salt consumption by 1/2 teaspoon a day reduces systolic blood pressure by about 5 mm Hg and diastolic blood pressure by 2.5 mm Hg.[118] Adaptation to long-term salt reduction is possible with appropriate counseling. Although the taste for salt is innate, this can be altered, resulting in a decreased intake of 30–50%.

Approximately 75% of dietary sodium is added to food during its processing and manufacturing. Only 10% of dietary salt comes from foods' natural content. Therefore, a high dietary salt intake is associated with diets in which a large portion of the daily Calories consists of processed foods (see www.nhlbi.nih.gov). Sauces, dressings, processed meats, cheese, soup, and some breakfast cereals are especially high in sodium. Nutrition experts recommend these steps for keeping sodium intake below recommended levels:[124]

Box 10.4

Lifestyle Modifications to Manage Hypertension*†

Modification	Recommendation	Approximate SBP Reduction (Range)
Weight reduction	Maintain normal body weight (body mass index 18.5–24.9 kg/m^2).	5–20 mm Hg/10 kg weight loss
Adopt DASH eating plan	Consume a diet rich in fruits, vegetables, and lowfat dairy products with a reduced content of saturated and total fat.	8–14 mm Hg
Dietary sodium reduction	Reduce dietary sodium intake to no more than 100 mmol per day (2.4 g sodium or 6 g sodium chloride).	2–8 mm Hg
Physical activity	Engage in regular aerobic physical activity such as brisk walking (at least 30 min per day, most days of the week).	4–9 mm Hg
Moderation of alcohol consumption	Limit consumption to no more than 2 drinks (1 oz or 30 mL ethanol; e.g., 24 oz beer, 10 oz wine, or 3 oz 80-proof whiskey) per day in most men and to no more than 1 drink per day in women and lighter weight persons.	2–4 mm Hg

DASH, Dietary Approaches to Stop Hypertension.

*For overall cardiovascular risk reduction, stop smoking.

†The effects of implementing these modifications are dose and time dependent, and could be greater for some individuals.

Source: National High Blood Pressure Education Program. *The Seventh Report of the Joint National Committee on Detection, Evaluation, and Treatment of High Blood Pressure.* National Heart, Lung, and Blood Institute, National Institutes of Health, NIH Publication No. 03-5233. Bethesda, MD: National Institutes of Health, 2003.

- Learn to read food labels, and avoid foods high in sodium.
- Choose more fresh fruits and vegetables.
- Reduce use of salt during cooking, and use herbs, spices, and low-sodium seasonings.
- Avoid using the salt shaker on prepared foods at the table.
- Limit the use of foods with visible salt on them (snack chips, salted nuts, crackers, etc.).

Potassium helps reduce blood pressure by increasing the amount of sodium excreted in the urine and by promoting other favorable physiological changes.[119,148] The potassium recommendation is 4,700 mg a day. The *sodium-to-potassium ratio* (Na:K) is a useful indicator of hypertension risk. In the INTERSALT study, changing the Na:K from 3 to 1 equated to a 3.4 mm Hg drop in systolic blood pressure.[144] The average Na:K ratio in the United States is 1.2–1.3, but 0.50 is recommended (which means consuming more potassium than sodium from the diet). This can be achieved by eating diets that have a high proportion of fruits, vegetables, and legumes.

Although some studies have indicated that low calcium and magnesium intake may be associated with an increased prevalence of hypertension, the data are inconsistent, and there appears to be no justification for using supplements beyond what is obtained in a varied and balanced diet.[118,119,147]

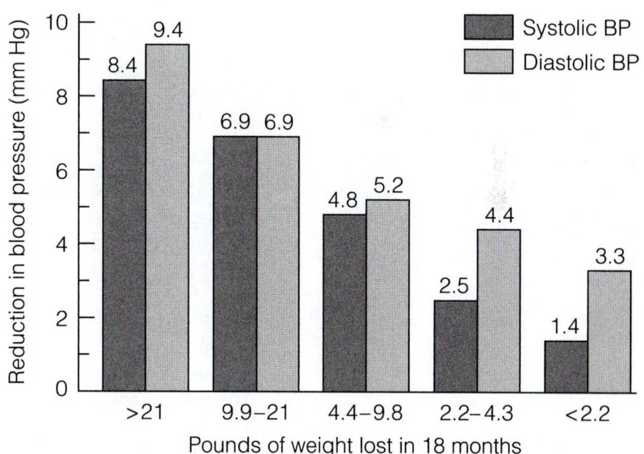

Figure 10.29 Weight loss and effect on blood pressure: 18-month study of more than 500 subjects with high-normal blood pressures. Among subjects with high-normal blood pressure (diastolic blood pressure between 80 and 89 mm Hg), those losing the most weight experienced the greatest reduction in blood pressure. Source: Data from Stevens VJ, Corrigan SA, Obarzanek E, et al. Weight loss intervention in phase I of the trials of hypertension prevention. *Arch Intern Med* 153:849–858, 1993.

In 1997, the National Heart, Lung, and Blood Institute of the National Institutes of Health released an eating plan that was found in clinical studies with hypertensives to lower systolic blood pressure by 11 mm Hg and diastolic blood pressure by 6 mm Hg.[149,150] Blood pressure reductions can be measured within 2 weeks of starting the meal

Box 10.5

Following the DASH Diet

The DASH eating plan given here is based on 2,000 Calories a day. The number of daily servings in a food group may vary from those listed depending on your caloric needs.

Use this chart to help you plan your menus or take it with you when you go to the store.

Food Group	Daily Servings (except as noted)	Serving Sizes	Examples and Notes	Significance of Each Food Group to the DASH Eating Plan
Grains and grain products	7–8	1 slice bread 1 cup dry cereal* 1/2 cup cooked rice, pasta, or cereal	Whole-wheat bread, English muffin, pita bread, bagel, cereals, grits, oatmeal, crackers, unsalted pretzels and popcorn	Major sources of energy and fiber
Vegetables	4–5	1 cup raw leafy vegetable 1/2 cup cooked vegetable 6 oz vegetable juice	Tomatoes, potatoes, carrots, green peas, squash, broccoli, turnip greens, collards, kale, spinach, artichokes, green beans, lima beans, sweet potatoes	Rich sources of potassium, magnesium, and fiber
Fruits	4–5	6 oz fruit juice 1 medium fruit 1/4 cup dried fruit 1 1/2 cup fresh, frozen, or canned fruit	Apricots, bananas, dates, grapes, oranges, orange juice, grapefruit, grapefruit juice, mangoes, melons, peaches, pineapples, prunes, raisins, strawberries, tangerines	Important sources of potassium, magnesium, and fiber
Low-fat or fat-free dairy foods	2–3	8 oz milk 1 cup yogurt 1 1/2 oz cheese	Fat-free (skim) or low-fat (1%) milk, fat-free or low-fat buttermilk, fat-free or low-fat regular or frozen yogurt, low-fat and fat-free cheese	Major sources of calcium and protein
Meats, poultry, and fish	2 or less	3 oz cooked meats, poultry, or fish	Select only lean; trim away visible fats; broil, roast, or boil, instead of frying; remove skin from poultry	Rich sources of protein and magnesium
Nuts, seeds, and dry beans	4–5 per week	1/3 cup or 1 1/2 oz nuts 2 tbsp or 1/2 oz seeds 1/2 cup cooked dry beans	Almonds, filberts, mixed nuts, peanuts, walnuts, sunflower seeds, kidney beans, lentils, and peas	Rich sources of energy, magnesium, potassium, protein, and fiber
Fats and oils†	2–3	1 tsp soft margarine 1 tbsp low-fat mayonnaise 2 tbsp light salad dressing 1 tsp vegetable oil	Soft margarine, low-fat mayonnaise, light salad dressing, vegetable oil (such as olive, corn, canola, or safflower)	Besides fats added to foods, remember to choose foods that contain less fats
Sweets	5 per week	1 tbsp sugar 1 tbsp jelly or jam 1/2 oz jelly beans 8 oz lemonade	Maple syrup, sugar, jelly, jam, fruit-flavored gelatin, jelly beans, hard candy, fruit punch, sorbet, ices	Sweets should be low in fat

*Serving sizes vary between 1/2–1 1/4 cups. Check the product's nutrition label.

†Fat content changes serving counts for fats and oils; for example, 1 tbsp of regular salad dressing equals 1 serving; 1 tbsp of a low-fat dressing equals 1/2 serving; 1 tbsp of a fat-free dressing equals 0 servings.

Source: www.nhlbi.nih.gov.

plan and are experienced by men, women, whites, and minorities alike. This meal plan, called Dietary Approaches to Stop Hypertension (DASH), is summarized in Box 10.5. The DASH eating plan is rich in whole grains, fruits, vegetables, and low-fat dairy foods, resulting in a nutrient intake that is high in potassium, calcium, magnesium, and fiber, and low in saturated fat, cholesterol, and sodium.

Moderation of Alcohol Intake

Studies have identified a positive association between an alcohol intake of 40 grams of ethanol per day (3 drinks or more) and increased blood pressure.[118,119] The prevalence of high blood pressure is four times greater for heavy drinkers than for those who abstain. Also, when hyperten-

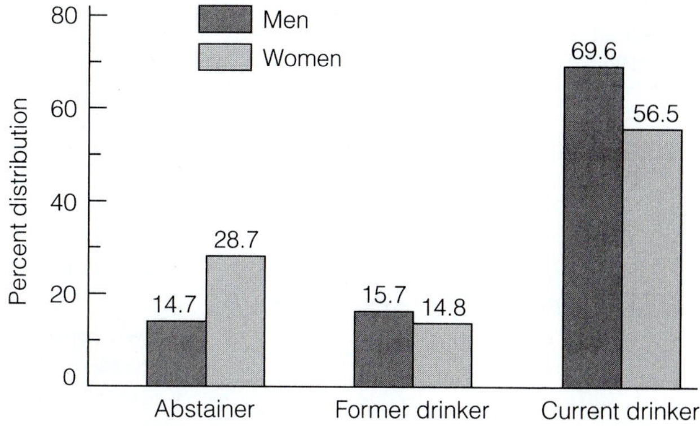

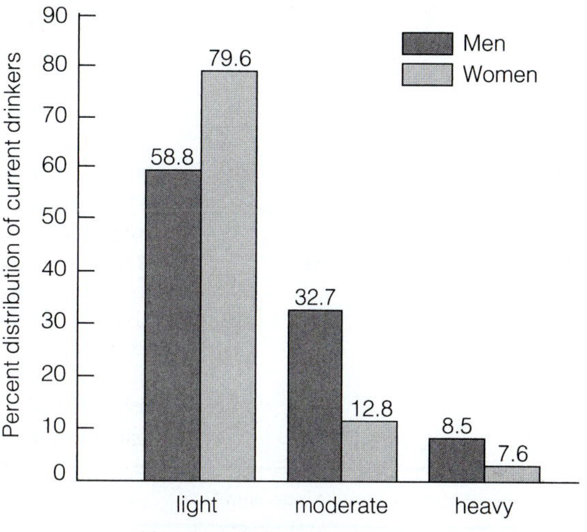

*Drinks/week

	Males	Females
Light	≤3	≤3
Moderate	4–14	4–7
Heavy	>14	>7

Figure 10.30 Alcohol drinking status and consumption.
Source: National Center for Health Statistics. *Health, United States, 2005*. Hyattsville, MD: 2005. www.cdc.gov/nchs.

sive men who are heavy drinkers discontinue their alcohol intake, their blood pressure falls. For these reasons, male hypertensive patients who drink alcohol-containing beverages should be counseled to limit their daily intake to 1 ounce of ethanol a day and for females 0.5 ounces a day.[118] As reviewed in Chapter 9, a standard drink contains 0.5 ounces or 15 grams of ethanol (as found in one 12-oz can of beer, one 5-oz glass of wine, 2 oz of 100-proof spirits or 1.5 oz of 80-proof distilled spirits).

Alcoholism has been defined as[151]

> a primary, chronic disease with genetic, psychosocial, and environmental factors influencing its development and manifestations. The disease is often progressive and fatal. It is characterized by impaired control over drinking, preoccupation with the drug alcohol, use of alcohol despite adverse consequences, and distortions in thinking, most notably denial. Each of these symptoms may be continuous or periodic.

Several questionnaires have been developed to help people determine whether they have alcoholic tendencies.[152] (See Physical Fitness Activity 10.4 at the end of this chapter.) Approximately 50–60% of the risk for developing alcoholism is genetic.[153]

The National Institute on Alcohol Abuse and Alcoholism reports that 14 million (7.4%) in the United States are either alcoholics or alcohol abusers.[153] As summarized in Figure 10.30, 70% of men and 57% of women are current drinkers.[14] Of current drinkers, 8.5% of men and 7.6% of women drink heavily. Alcohol consumption on a per capita basis has been gradually declining since peaking during the late 1970s.[153]

Alcohol affects almost every organ system in the body, either directly or indirectly.[153] The liver (the primary site of alcohol metabolism) is most susceptible. Alcohol alters immune regulation in the liver, causing much of the damage in this organ. The effects of alcohol on the liver include inflammation (alcoholic hepatitis) and cirrhosis (progressive liver scarring). In the gastrointestinal tract, regular alcohol use can precipitate inflammation of the esophagus and pancreas, exacerbate existing peptic ulcers, and cause some cancers (e.g., breast cancer in women, head and neck cancers, and digestive tract cancers). When alcohol accounts for a high percentage of caloric intake, it can lead to significant nutritional deficiencies. Alcohol affects immune, endocrine, and reproductive functions and is a well-documented cause of neurological problems, including dementia, blackouts, seizures, hallucinations, and peripheral neuropathy.

Alcohol is the third leading cause of death in the United States, causing over 100,000 deaths yearly from injuries, certain types of cancer, and liver disease, and it is related to a large percentage of the violence in this country. Nearly half of the trauma beds in the United States are occupied by patients who were injured while under the influence of alcohol.[154] Each year, alcohol-related motor-vehicle crashes result in more than 16,000 deaths, one third of them involving people under the age of 25 years.[153,155]

As a rule of thumb, one standard drink consumed within 1 hour will produce a blood alcohol level (BAL; also BAC, for blood alcohol concentration) of 0.02 in a 150-pound male. Five beers consumed within 1 hour will cause the BAL to rise to 0.10, which violates the drinking and driving laws of most states. (See Table 10.8 for a summary of the relationship between blood alcohol content and clinical symptoms.) About 40% of all Americans will be involved in an alcohol-related crash during their lifetime.[155]

In contrast to these negative effects, alcohol use has been consistently related to lowered risk of coronary heart

TABLE 10.8 Summary of the Relationship between Blood Alcohol Concentration (BAC) and Clinical Symptoms

BAC (g/100 ml of blood or g/210 L of breath)	Stage	Clinical Symptoms
0.01–0.05	Subclinical	Behavior nearly normal by ordinary observation
0.03–0.12	Euphoria	Mild euphoria, sociability, talkativeness Increased self-confidence; decreased inhibitions Diminution of attention, judgment, and control Beginning of sensorimotor impairment Loss of efficiency in finer performance tests
0.09–0.25	Excitement	Emotional instability; loss of critical judgment Impairment of perception, memory, and comprehension Decreased sensory response; increased reaction time Reduced visual acuity, peripheral vision, and glare recovery Sensorimotor incoordination, impaired balance Drowsiness
0.18–0.30	Confusion	Disorientation, mental confusion; dizziness Exaggerated emotional stages Disturbances of vision and of perception of color, form, motion, and dimensions Increased pain threshold Increased muscular incoordination; staggering gait; slurred speech Apathy, lethargy
0.25–0.40	Stupor	General inertia; approaching loss of motor functions Markedly decreased response to stimuli Marked muscular incoordination; inability to stand or walk Vomiting; incontinence Impaired consciousness; sleep or stupor
0.35–0.50	Coma	Complete unconsciousness Depressed or abolished reflexes Subnormal body temperature Incontinence Impairment of circulation and respiration Possible death
0.45+	Death	Death from respiratory arrest

Source: Intoximeters Inc.: http://www.intox.com/.

disease for both men and women, usually on the order of 20–50%.[156–163]

There are more than 60 prospective studies that suggest an inverse relationship between moderate alcoholic beverage consumption and coronary heart disease.[153,156] A consistent coronary protective effect occurs with consumption of one to two alcoholic drinks per day. Although intake of more than two alcoholic drinks per day is also linked to reduced coronary heart disease, mortality from all causes is increased, negating any heart disease protective effect.[153,156] Thus the cardioprotective effects of moderate alcohol consumption must be balanced against disease risks and the entire picture of costs and social consequences. This is summarized in Figure 10.31. According to the National Institute on Alcohol Abuse and Alcoholism, "Among teenagers and young adults in particular, the risks of alcohol use outweigh any benefits that may accrue later in life, since alcohol abuse and dependence and alcohol-related violent behavior and injuries are all too common in young people and not easily predicted. To determine the likely net outcome of alcohol consumption, the probable risks and benefits for each drinker must be weighed."[153]

Researchers from Harvard reported that alcohol consumption reduces risk of coronary heart disease for both men and women, but have written, "Our society is so lacking in effective social controls on alcohol abuse and pays such a heavy price for its inadequate response that . . . the thought of a public policy promoting alcohol consumption runs strongly against the grain, however much it might capture at least some hearts."[160] In other words, there are too many problems associated with drinking in our society to recommend this approach for heart disease reduction. The cure would be far worse than the disease.

The epidemiological evidence suggests that all alcoholic beverages are similarly protective, and that there is no special effect of red wine over beer or spirits.[158,160,161] The cardioprotective effect of alcohol appears to be due to its effect in raising HDL cholesterol 10–15% and reducing clot formation.[153,156] Alcoholics, however, have an increased risk of death from heart disease due to ultrastructural changes in the heart tissue resulting from chronic exposure to ethanol.[153] This can lead to sudden death from abnormal heart arrhythmias. Long-term heavy alcohol consumption also increases risk for stroke, especially hemorrhagic stroke.[153]

Physical Activity

As explained in Chapter 4, when a person engages in aerobic exercise, the systolic blood pressure and heart rate will increase, while the diastolic blood pressure changes little. Immediately following the exercise bout, the systolic blood pressure will fall below pre-exercise values for about 22 hours, with the greatest effects seen in those with the highest baseline blood pressure (see Figure 10.32).[164–166] There are many potential mechanisms for this "postexercise hypotensive effect," including relaxation and vasodilation of blood vessels in the legs and visceral organ areas.[164] The blood vessels may relax after each exercise session because of body warming effects, local production of certain chemicals (e.g., lactic acid and nitric oxide), decreases in nerve activity, and changes in certain hormones and their receptors.[164–167] Over time, as the exercise is repeated, there is growing evidence that a long-lasting reduction in resting blood pressure can be measured, which may in part be due to the acute drop in blood pressure that occurs after each bout.[165]

Interestingly, if the blood pressure surges too steeply (i.e., well above 200 mm Hg) during a standardized exercise test, risk of future hypertension or heart disease is elevated, even in subjects with normal resting blood pressures[168,169] (see Figure 10.33). The American College of Sports Medicine (ACSM) has urged that more research is needed, however, and that current studies do not justify the use of exercise testing to predict future hypertension.[170]

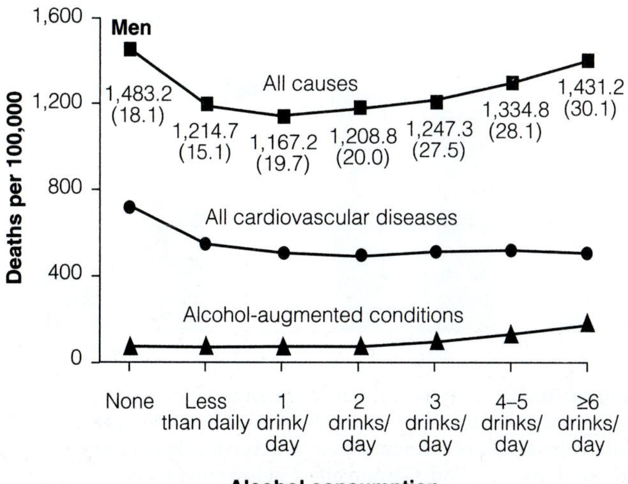

Figure 10.31 Rates of death from all causes, all cardiovascular diseases, and alcohol-augmented conditions according to alcohol consumption. Source: Data from National Institute on Alcohol Abuse and Alcoholism. *Tenth Special Report to the U.S. Congress on Alcohol and Health.* U.S. Department of Health and Human Services, 2000. www.niaaa.nih.gov/.

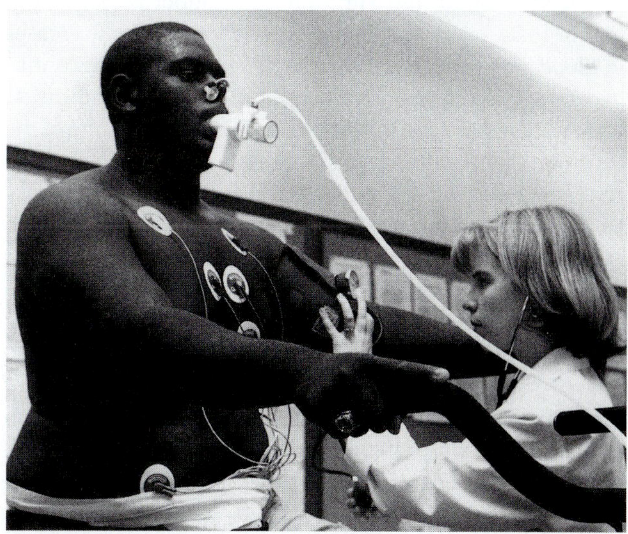

Figure 10.33 People with normal resting blood pressures who experience elevated blood pressure responses during graded exercise testing are at increased risk of developing future resting hypertension.

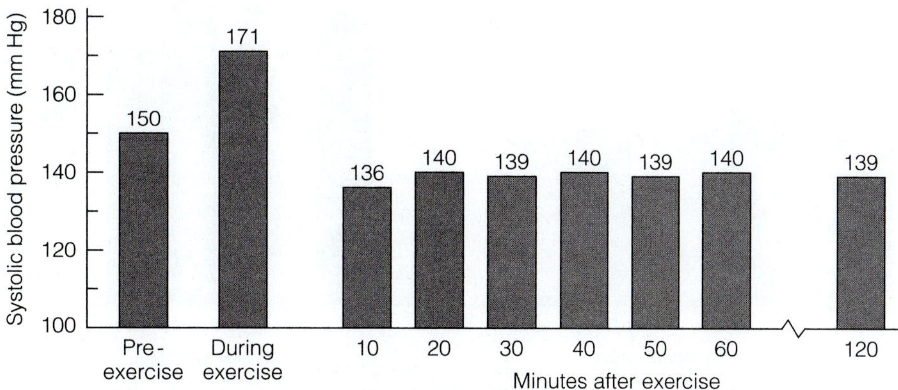

Figure 10.32 The systolic blood pressure response to 45 minutes of exercise: Treadmill walking, 70% of heart rate reserve, in 18 men with high blood pressure. In this study of men with high blood pressure, 45 minutes of brisk treadmill walking lowered the blood pressure below resting levels for at least 2 hours. The decrease was related to a widening and relaxation of the blood vessels. Source: Data from Rueckert PA, Slane PR, Lillis DL, Hanson, P. Hemodynamic patterns and duration of post-dynamic exercise hypotension in hypertensive humans. *Med Sci Sports Exerc* 28:24–32, 1996.

Exercise has a strong effect in treating high blood pressure. The ACSM and other reviewers have concluded that people with mild hypertension can expect systolic and diastolic blood pressures to fall an average of 5 to 7 mm Hg in response to regular aerobic exercise.[170–174] This benefit is independent of changes in body weight or diet (which can result in greater reductions). Even for people with normal resting blood pressures, exercise training can be expected to lower the systolic and diastolic blood pressures by an average of 4 mm Hg and 3 mm Hg, respectively.[171]

Figure 10.34 shows the results of one study of African American men with severe hypertension.[173] Subjects exercised for several months, engaging in stationary cycling, three times a week, 20 to 60 minutes a session at 60–80% of maximum heart rate. As a safety precaution, prior to initiating exercise training, diastolic blood pressures were reduced at least 10 mm Hg with medication. As shown in Figure 10.34, exercise subjects experienced strong decreases in blood pressure after 16 weeks. Exercise training continued for an additional 16 weeks, and doses of medication were reduced in 71% of the exercise subjects, but none of the controls. The results suggest that severe hypertension can be managed effectively with a combination of drug therapy and regular, moderately intense exercise. Most important, medications necessary to control blood pressure without exercise can be curtailed substantially as patients continue exercising.

Most studies show that exercise training acts quickly to improve blood pressure among hypertensives, with most of the effect taking place within the first few weeks. Further reductions in blood pressure may occur if the exercise training is maintained for more than 3 months. Figure 10.35 summarizes results from a study in which hypertensives exercised aerobically three times a week for 10 weeks, while taking a diuretic, a beta-blocker, or a placebo.[174] Exercise alone without drugs resulted in an impressive 8 mm Hg drop in the diastolic blood pressure within the first month, with drug therapy adding a little extra benefit. Interestingly, most of the improvement in blood pressure occurred during the first week, with some additional progress measured as the training continued.

The aerobic exercise program does not have to be too demanding to improve resting blood pressure. The important exercise criterion is frequency—near-daily moderate-intensity activity for 30 minutes and longer helps the body experience the beneficial blood-pressure-lowering effects of regular exercise.[170]

The ACSM recommends weight training as a supplement to aerobic training for hypertensives.[170] Weight training has a modest effect in lowering blood pressure and is an excellent way to increase muscular strength and overall

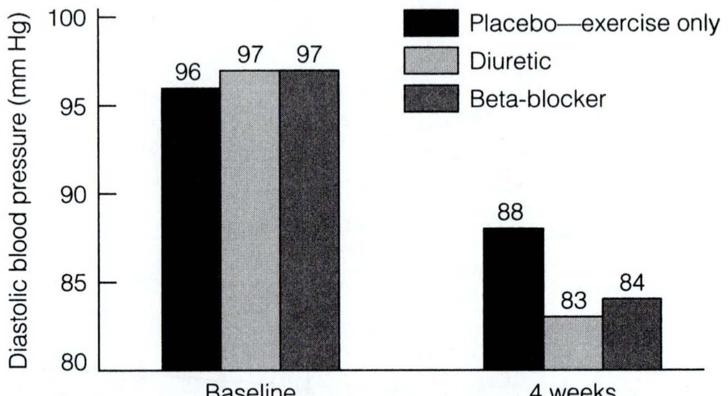

Figure 10.35 Exercise versus drug therapy for hypertension: All subjects exercised three times per week and were randomly assigned to a placebo or a drug group. Exercise training had a strong effect in lowering blood pressure, with drug therapy having only a small additional effect. Source: Data from Kelemen MH, Effron MB, Valenti SA, Stewart KJ. Exercise training combined with antihypertensive drug therapy: Effects on lipids, blood pressure, and left ventricular mass. *JAMA* 263:2766–2771, 1990.

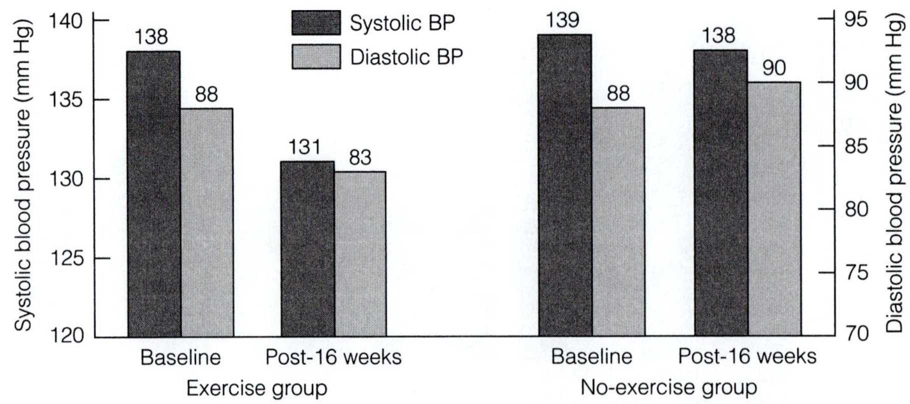

Figure 10.34 Effects of exercise in African American men with severe hypertension: 16 weeks of cycling, three sessions per week, 20–60 minutes per session, at 60–80% maximum heart rate. Moderate exercise training was effective in reducing blood pressure in African Americans with severe hypertension. All subjects were on medication. Source: Data from Kokkinos PF, Narayan P, Colleran JA, et al. Effects of regular exercise on blood pressure and left ventricular hypertrophy in African-American men with severe hypertension. *N Engl J Med* 333:1462–1467, 1995.

physical fitness.[170,175] Experts recommend, however, that hypertensives avoid maximal lifts and instead emphasize weight lifts that they can repeat for 10–15 repetitions.[170]

Can regular exercise training prevent hypertension from developing? Several major epidemiological studies support this idea.[176–178] In general, sedentary and unfit normotensive individuals have a 20–50% increased risk of developing hypertension during follow-up when compared with their more active and fit peers[170] (see Figure 10.36). In a 6- to 10-year study of 15,000 Harvard male alumni, for example, those who did not engage in vigorous sports and activity were at 35% greater risk of hypertension than those who did, and this relationship held at all ages, 35–74 years.[176] In a 4-year study in Dallas, unfit individuals were found to be 52% more likely to develop hypertension than were those who were fit.[177]

Studies on both adults and children have consistently shown that physical activity and fitness are linked to a more favorable blood pressure level, compared to an inactive lifestyle.[170,179–181] In one study of 8,283 male recreational runners, those running more than 50 miles a week, compared to less than 10 miles a week, showed a 50% reduction in prevalence of hypertension and a 50% reduction in the use of medications to lower blood pressure.[179] A study of nearly 5,000 Dutch women showed that blood pressure was lowest in those spending the most time exercising in various sports.[180]

People with high blood pressure have been shown to be less fit (about 30%) than those with normal blood pressures.[182] Thus, regular aerobic exercise is critical for hypertensive patients to improve physical fitness and life quality, and to lower risk of heart disease. Data from the Cooper Institute for Aerobics Research have shown that death rates are lower in highly fit people, even when their blood pressures are high, as compared to people with low aerobic fitness and normal blood pressures.[117]

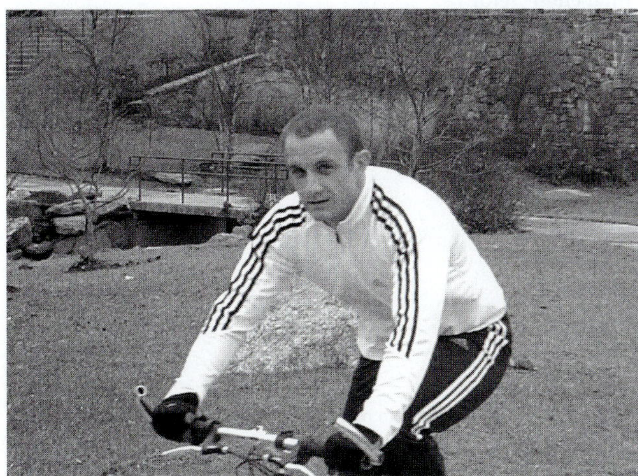

Figure 10.36 Regular exercise is associated with a lower risk of developing high blood pressure.

HIGH BLOOD CHOLESTEROL

As reviewed earlier in this chapter, high blood cholesterol is a major risk factor for heart disease.[21,183–186] Figure 10.37 shows that risk of CHD rises sharply with increase in blood cholesterol levels.[55]

The body makes its own cholesterol and also absorbs cholesterol from certain kinds of foods, specifically all animal products (i.e., meats, dairy products, and eggs). Cholesterol is essential for the formation of bile acids (used in fat digestion) and some hormones, and it is a component of cell membranes and of brain and nerve tissues.[185]

Thus, some cholesterol is necessary to keep the body functioning normally. However, when blood cholesterol levels are too high, some of the excess (especially the oxidized form of LDL cholesterol) is deposited in the artery walls, increasing the risk of heart disease.[4–10, 183] In contrast, according to many studies, when blood cholesterol levels are lowered through lifestyle changes and medication, risk of coronary heart disease decreases.[40–46] For every 1% reduction in blood cholesterol, the occurrence of coronary heart disease is reduced 2–3%.[35,37]

Prevalence of High Blood Cholesterol

Experts urge that everyone know their cholesterol level and have it checked at least once every 5 years (or every year if heart disease risk is high).[21,187] Americans are more "cholesterol conscious" than ever before with 67% having had their blood cholesterol checked in the previous 5 years.[2] Figure 10.38 summarizes the blood cholesterol levels of Americans. Notice the strong increase in serum cholesterol levels with age.[14,188,189]

According to the National Cholesterol Education Program, blood cholesterol levels can be categorized as

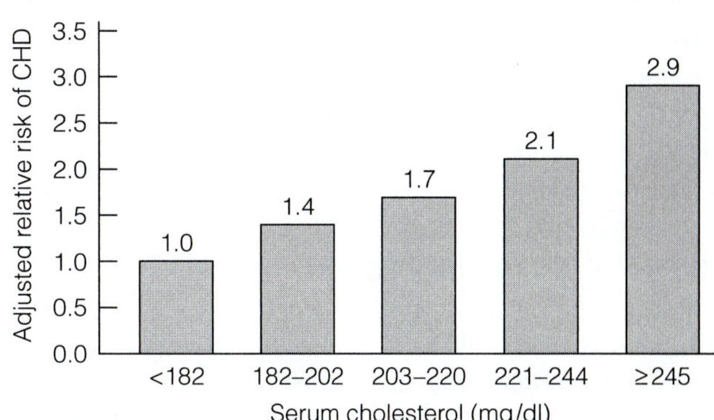

Figure 10.37 Serum cholesterol and coronary heart disease: MRFIT of 316,099 white men, with 12-year follow-up, including 6,327 CHD deaths. In this 12-year study (MRFIT) of more than 300,000 men, risk of coronary heart disease climbed sharply with increase in serum cholesterol. Source: Data from Neaton JD, Wentworth D. Serum cholesterol, blood pressure, cigarette smoking, and death from coronary heart disease. *Arch Intern Med* 152:56–64, 1992.

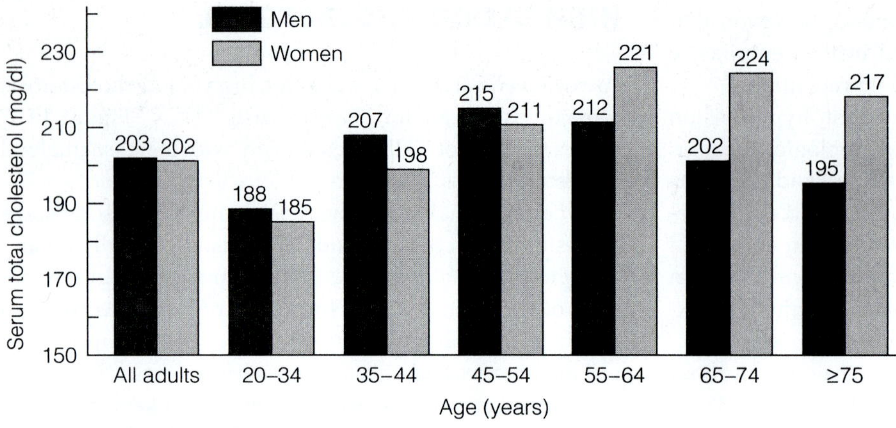

Figure 10.38 Mean serum total cholesterol levels among U.S. adults. Source: National Center for Health Statistics. *Health, United States, 2005.* Hyattsville, MD: 2005. www.cdc.gov/nchs.

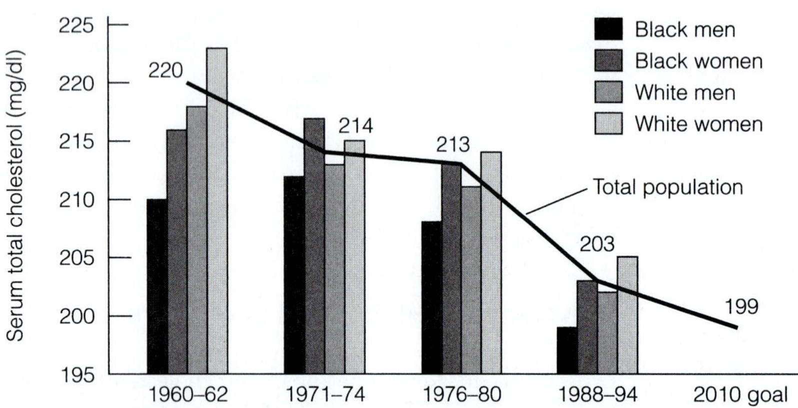

Figure 10.39 Declining serum total cholesterol levels among U.S. adults. Source: National Center for Health Statistics. *Health, United States, 2005.* Hyattsville, MD: 2005. www.cdc.gov/nchs.

summarized in Table 10.9.[21] Despite an impressive drop from the 1960s, 17% of Americans still have high blood cholesterol levels, and 30% have borderline-high levels[14] (see Figures 10.39 and 10.40). The American average for serum cholesterol is 203 mg/dl, and if present trends continue, the *Healthy People 2010* goal of 199 mg/dl will probably be achieved.[2,14] Some populations around the world with very low risk of heart disease have blood cholesterol levels below 160 mg/dl, a level now regarded by some experts as within the "optimal" zone.[184] In the Framingham Heart Study, for example, a study initiated during the 1950s, heart disease has been extremely rare among those with blood cholesterol levels within the optimal zone.[190]

Description of Lipoproteins

To transport the cholesterol and triglycerides, the body utilizes various protein packets, called lipoproteins. There are three major lipoproteins in the fasting blood: *high-density lipoprotein* (HDL), *low-density lipoprotein* (LDL), and *very-low density lipoprotein* (VLDL). Each lipoprotein is composed of several subtypes. Figure 10.41 outlines the protein and lipid composition of each lipoprotein. HDL is the smallest and densest lipoprotein, being nearly half protein. LDL carries the most cholesterol (60–70% of all the serum cholesterol). VLDL is mostly triglyceride.[185,191,192]

TABLE 10.9 Classification of LDL, Total, and HDL Cholesterol, and Triglycerides*

	Primary Target of Therapy
LDL cholesterol	
<100	Optimal
100–129	Near optimal/above optimal
130–159	Borderline high
160–189	High
≥ 190	Very high
Total cholesterol	
<200	Desirable
200–239	Borderline high
≥ 240	High
HDL cholesterol	
<40	Low
≥ 60	High
Triglycerides	
<150	Normal
150–199	Borderline high
200–499	High
≥ 500	Very high

*Numerical values are given in milligrams per deciliter. Obtain complete lipoprotein profile after 9- to 12-hour fast.

Source: Third Report of the National Cholesterol Education Program (NCEP) Expert Panel on Detection, Evaluation, and Treatment of High Blood Cholesterol in Adults (Adult Treatment Panel III), 2001. www.nhlbi.nih.gov.

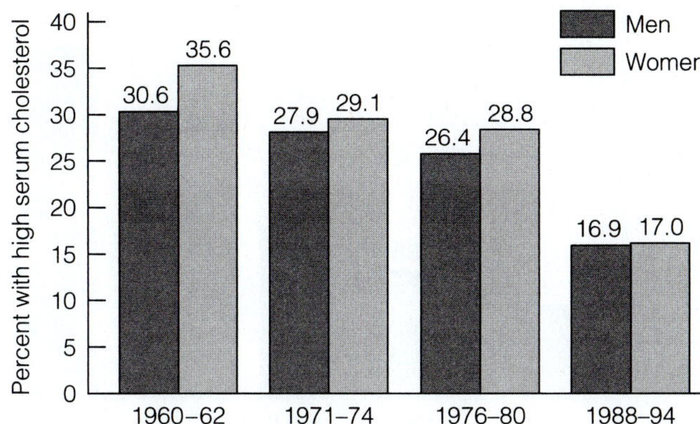

Figure 10.40 Percentage of population with high serum cholesterol (≥240 mg/dl). Source: National Center for Health Statistics. *Health, United States, 2005.* Hyattsville, MD: 2005. www.cdc.gov/nchs.

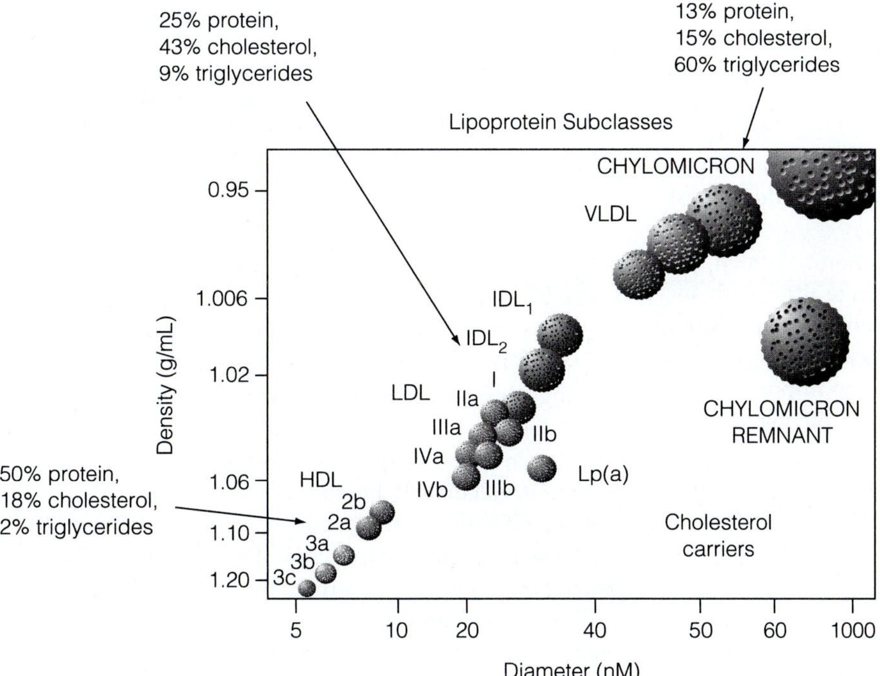

Figure 10.41 There are 3 major types of lipoproteins in fasting blood, and each has several subtypes.

The protein part of the lipoprotein is called *apoprotein.* Apoproteins are important in activating or inhibiting certain enzymes involved in the metabolism of fats. They are identified by letters. HDL, for example, has several different apoproteins, the important ones being Apo A-I and Apo A-II. LDL is high in Apo B.

The HDL particle appears to act as a type of shuttle as it takes up cholesterol from the blood and body cells and transfers it to the liver, where it is used to form bile acids.[159,186,193–195] The bile acids are involved in the digestion process, with some of them passing out with the stool, thus providing the body with a major route for excretion of cholesterol. HDLs have for this reason been called the "garbage trucks" of the blood system, collecting cholesterol and dumping it into the liver.

LDL, on the other hand, is formed after VLDL gives up its triglycerides to body cells. LDLs are high in cholesterol and take their cholesterol to various body cells, where it is deposited for cell functions. When LDL cholesterol is too high and becomes oxidized, it contributes to the buildup of atherosclerosis (see Figure 10.42).[21,191]

LDL cholesterol (LDL-C) levels are classified by the National Cholesterol Education Program (NCEP) of the National Heart, Lung, and Blood Institute, National Institutes of Health (see Table 10.9).[21]

LDL-C levels should be as low as possible, with optimal levels falling below 100 mg/dl. In individuals with a very high risk of CVD, an LDL-C goal of <70 mg/dl is a therapeutic option.[191]

HDL cholesterol (HDL-C) concentration is emerging as an important measure of heart disease risk, and the National Institutes for Health have urged that HDL-C determinations accompany measurements of total cholesterol when healthy individuals are being assessed for coronary heart disease risk.[21,193] Various studies have shown that a 1% rise in HDL-C reduces coronary heart disease risk 2–3%,

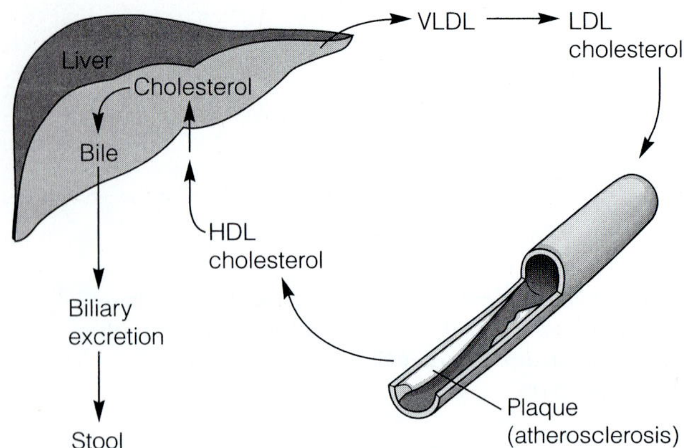

Figure 10.42 Functions of lipoproteins. LDL and HDL have opposing functions. HDL takes cholesterol to the liver, where it is changed to bile and eventually excreted in the stool. This is the body's major method of reducing its cholesterol stores.

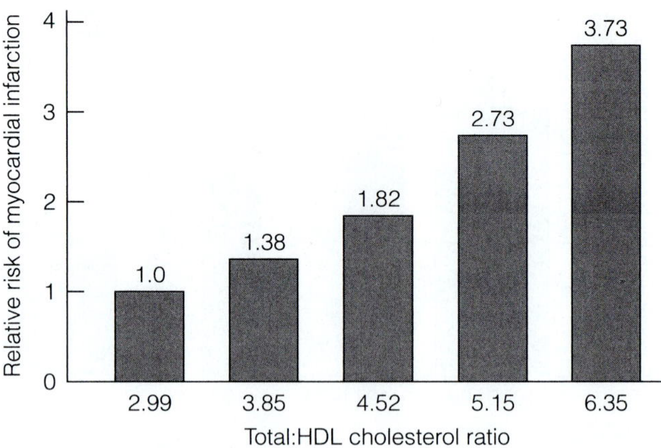

Figure 10.43 Total:HDL cholesterol ratio and myocardial infarction: Physicians' health study, Harvard Medical School; 246 case–control pairs. In this case–control study of heart attack victims, risk climbed sharply with rise in the total: HDL cholesterol ratio. Source: Data from Stampfer MJ, Sacks FM, Salvini S, Willett WC, Hennekens CH. A prospective study of cholesterol, apolipoproteins, and the risk of myocardial infarction. *N Engl J Med* 325:373–381, 1991.

and that people with the highest HDL-C have heart disease death rates 2–3 times lower than those with the lowest HDL-C levels.[194,196,197]

Mean HDL-C levels are higher among women (56 mg/dl) than men (46 mg/dl) and change little with increase in age. HDL-C is also higher among blacks than whites.[188] The National Cholesterol Education Program regards HDL-C levels below 40 mg/dl as an important risk factor, with optimal values rising above 60 mg/dl (see Table 10.9).[21]

Because of the importance of HDL-C, various ratios have been used to improve prediction of heart disease risk. HDL-C can be expressed as a percentage of the total cholesterol, or more commonly, as[195,198,199]

$$\frac{\text{total cholesterol}}{\text{HDL-C}}$$

This ratio has been extremely useful in estimating heart disease risk, as shown in Figure 10.43. In this study of 246 men who had suffered a heart attack versus 246 controls, risk of heart attack climbed sharply with increase in the ratio.[199] A ratio below 3.0 is optimal, while 5.0 and above is considered high risk. For every unit the ratio falls (e.g., 5.0 to 4.0), risk of coronary heart disease decreases 53%.[199] The average American adult male has a 4.6 ratio, the average female, 4.0.[195] The elderly, the obese, and smokers have higher ratios, while females, alcohol users, blacks, and active people have lower ratios.[195]

The status of serum triglyceride levels as a risk factor for heart disease is less clear. Table 10.9 summarizes NCEP guidelines for classifying serum triglycerides.[21] In studies, a high triglyceride level has been found to predict heart disease, but when adjusted for other risk factors, its usefulness as an independent predictor is lost.[193,200,201] However, in cases of people with low HDL-C levels, diabetes, obesity (especially central), and hypertension, and of young adults with multiple risk factors, risk of heart disease increases as the triglyceride level increases.[193] Figure 10.44 shows the average serum triglyceride levels for American males and females.[188] Optimal triglyceride values are less than 110 mg/dl, and the levels for athletes are usually below 80 mg/dl.[192] Triglycerides can be lowered by losing weight, exercising aerobically, and reducing alcohol intake. High-sugar diets may increase triglyceride levels for some people.

Most medical laboratories do not measure the LDL-C, but rather calculate it, based on measurements of total cholesterol, HDL-C, and triglycerides. As shown in Figure 10.41, all three lipoproteins carry cholesterol. Thus, the total cholesterol equals the cholesterol in the LDL, HDL, and VLDL. In the indirect procedure, an estimate of the VLDL-C is made by multiplying triglycerides by 20%. The equation is as follows:[202]

$$\text{LDL-C} = \text{total cholesterol} - [\text{HDL-C} + (0.20 \times \text{triglycerides})]$$

For example, if the total cholesterol is 200 mg/dl, HDL-C is 50 mg/dl, and triglycerides are 100 mg/dl:

$$\text{LDL-C} = 200 - [50 + (0.20 \times 100)] = 130 \text{ mg/dl}$$

Treatment of Hypercholesterolemia

In 2001, the National Cholesterol Education Program (NCEP) released their third report on the detection, evaluation, and treatment of high blood cholesterol (Adult Treatment Panel III, [ATP III]).[21,191] These are clinical guidelines for physicians, with support provided by other health professionals. The NCEP recommends the following nine-step approach for cholesterol testing and management:

- *Step 1.* Determine the complete lipoprotein profile after 9 to 12 hours of fasting. Use Table 10.9 for classification.

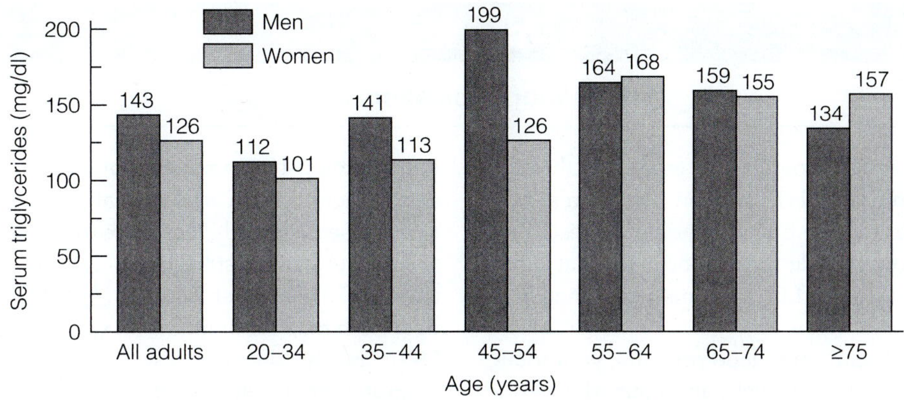

Figure 10.44 Mean serum triglyceride levels among U.S. adults. Source: Johnson CL, Rifkind BM, Sempos CT, et al. Declining serum total cholesterol levels among US adults. The National Health and Nutrition Examination Surveys. *JAMA* 269:3002–3008, 1993.

- *Step 2.* Review medical history to determine the presence of coronary heart disease, diabetes, peripheral artery disease, carotid artery disease, or abdominal aortic aneurysm.
- *Step 3.* Determine the presence of major risk factors (other than LDL-C). (Use NCEP major risk factors from Table 10.3.)
- *Step 4.* If two or more risk factors are present without diabetes or heart disease, assess the 10-year CHD risk using the Framingham risk test outlined in Box 10.6.
- *Step 5.* Determine the risk category summarized in Box 10.6 (low-to-moderate, moderately high, high, or very high). From the risk category, establish the LDL-C goal of therapy, determine the need for therapeutic lifestyle changes (TLC), and the level for drug consideration (summarized in Box 10.6). For example, an individual with two or more NCEP major coronary risk factors and a 10-year heart-attack risk under 10% (moderately high risk group) should start lifestyle changes if the LDL-C level is 130 mg/dl or higher and should consider drug therapy if the LDL-C is 160 mg/dl or higher and lifestyle changes do not bring the LDL-C under 130 mg/dl after 3 months.
- *Step 6.* Initiate TLC if the LDL-C is above the goal. TLC features are summarized in Box 10.7. Notice that the NCEP recommends strong changes in the diet combined with weight reduction and increased physical activity. LDL-C should be remeasured several times to evaluate progress and the need for intensifying TLC efforts during a 4–6 month period.
- *Step 7.* Consider adding drug therapy after 3 months if LDL-C exceeds target levels, using the guidelines given in Box 10.6. See Table 10.10 for a summary of drugs that affect lipoprotein metabolism.
- *Step 8.* Identify if the metabolic syndrome is present. If present, treat, after 3 months of TLC. The metabolic syndrome is summarized in Table 10.11 and is identified by several risk factors including abdominal obesity, high triglycerides, low HDL-C, high blood pressure, and impaired fasting glucose. The underlying causes of the metabolic syndrome are obesity and physical inactivity.
- *Step 9.* Treat elevated triglycerides (see Table 10.9 for a classification). Elevated triglycerides are best treated with increased physical activity and weight reduction. If triglycerides are above 200 mg/dl after the LDL goal is reached, consider adding drug therapy.

Diet and Other Lifestyle Measures

Several organizations have published dietary recommendations for both the prevention and the treatment of hypercholesterolemia.[21,185,203] The AHA guidelines are summarized in Box 10.8. In general, the guidelines urge Americans to consume less saturated animal fat and cholesterol and include more carbohydrates and fiber while moderating sodium, energy, and alcohol intake (see Physical Fitness Activity 10.5).[203] These guidelines are based on extensive literature.[203–216]

Table 10.12 outlines a 3-day menu that meets the AHA diet guidelines and meets all vitamin and mineral intake recommendations. Notice the wide variety of fruits and vegetables that provide "antioxidant" vitamins, now thought to be crucial in reducing oxidized LDL.

To have a favorable total cholesterol:HDL-C ratio, the total cholesterol and LDL-C must be lowered and the HDL-C elevated through an application of both dietary and lifestyle factors. Aerobic exercise, weight reduction, smoking cessation, and moderate alcohol consumption, each favorable, affects HDL-C, while dietary changes and weight reduction lower LDL-C.[204] As is emphasized in the next section, aerobic exercise has little independent effect on LDL-C and on total cholesterol.

Box 10.6

Find Your Cholesterol Plan

The following two-step program will guide you through the National Cholesterol Education Program's new treatment guidelines. The first step helps you establish your overall coronary risk; the second uses that information to determine your LDL treatment goals and how to reach them.

You'll need to know your blood pressure, your total-, LDL-, and HDL-cholesterol levels, and your triglyceride and fasting-glucose levels. If you're not sure of those numbers, ask your doctor and, if necessary, schedule an exam to get them. (Everyone should have a complete lipid profile every 5 years, starting at age 20.)

Step 1: Take the Heart-Attack Risk Test

This test will identify your chance of having a heart attack or dying of coronary disease in the next 10 years. (People with previously diagnosed coronary disease, diabetes, aortic aneurysm, or symptomatic carotid or peripheral artery disease already face more than a 20% risk; they can skip the test and go straight to step 2.) The test uses data from the Framingham Heart Study, the world's longest-running study of cardiovascular risk factors. The test is limited to established, major factors that are easily measured.

Circle the point value for each of the risk factors shown in the tables.

① Age

Years	Women	Men
20–34	−7	−9
35–39	−3	−4
40–44	0	0
45–49	3	3
50–54	6	6
55–59	8	8
60–64	10	10
65–69	12	11
70–74	14	12
75–79	16	13

② Total Cholesterol

	Age 20–39		Age 40–49		Age 50–59		Age 60–69		Age 70–79	
mg/dl	Women	Men	Women	Men	Women	Men	Women	Men	Women	Men
<160	0	0	0	0	0	0	0	0	0	0
160–199	4	4	3	3	2	2	1	1	1	0
200–239	8	7	6	5	4	3	2	1	1	0
240–279	11	9	8	6	5	4	3	2	2	1
280+	13	11	10	8	7	5	4	3	2	1

③ HDL Cholesterol

mg/dl	Women and Men
60+	−1
50–59	0
40–49	1
<40	2

④ Systolic Blood Pressure (the Higher Number)

	Untreated		Treated	
mm/Hg	Women	Men	Women	Men
<120	0	0	0	0
120–129	1	0	3	1
130–139	2	1	4	2
140–159	3	1	5	2
>159	4	2	6	3

⑤ Smoking

Age 20–39		Age 40–49		Age 50–59		Age 60–69		Age 70–79	
Women	Men	Women	Men	Women	Men	Women	Men	Women	Men
9	8	7	5	4	3	2	1	1	1

Total your points: __________

Now find your total-point score in the men's or women's column at right, and then locate your 10-year risk in the far-right column.

Women's Score	Men's Score	Your 10-Year Risk
Less than 20	Less than 12	Less than 10%
20–22	12–15	10–20%
Greater than 22	Greater than 15	Greater than 20%

(continued)

Box 10.6

Find Your Cholesterol Plan *(continued)*

Step 2: Find your LDL Treatment Plan

Consult the table below to learn how your overall coronary risk affects whether you need to lower your LDL-cholesterol level and, if you do, by how much. First, locate your coronary risk in the left-hand column. (That's based on the 10-year heart-attack risk that you just calculated as well as your coronary risk factors and any heart-threatening diseases you may have.) Then look across that row to see whether you should make lifestyle changes and take cholesterol-lowering medication, based on your current LDL level.

Coronary-Risk Group	Start Lifestyle Changes if Your LDL Level is . . .* (See Box 10.7)	Add Drugs if Your LDL Level is . . . (See Table 10.10)
Very high		
1. 10-year heart-attack risk of 20% or more or 2. History of coronary heart disease, diabetes, peripheral artery disease, carotid artery disease, or aortic aneurysm	≥100 mg/dl (Aim for an LDL under 100.) Get retested after 3 months	≥130 (Drugs are optional if your LDL is between 100 and 130.)
High		
1. 10-year heart-attack risk of 10–20% and 2. Two or more major coronary risk factors†	≥130 (Aim for an LDL under 130.) Get retested after 3 months	≥130 and lifestyle changes don't achieve your LDL goal in 3 months
Moderately high		
1. 10-year heart-attack risk under 10% and 2. Two or more major coronary risk factors†	Same as for high risk	160 or higher, and lifestyle changes don't achieve your LDL goal in 3 months‡
Low to moderate		
1. One or no major coronary risk factors†,§	≥160 (Aim for an LDL under 160.) Get retested after 3 months	≥190 and lifestyle changes don't achieve your LDL goal in 3 months. (Drugs are optional if your LDL is between 160 and 189.)

*People who have the metabolic syndrome should make lifestyle changes, even if their LDL level alone doesn't warrant it. You have the metabolic syndrome if you have three or more of these risk factors: HDL under 40 in men, 50 in women; systolic blood pressure of 130 or more or diastolic pressure of 85 or more; fasting glucose level of 110–125; triglyceride level of 150 or more; and waist circumference over 40 inches in men, 35 inches in women (see Table 10.11). People with the syndrome should limit their carbohydrate intake, get up to 30–35% of their Calories from total fat (more than usually recommended), and make the other lifestyle changes, including restriction of saturated fat.

†The major coronary risk factors are cigarette smoking; coronary disease in a father or brother before age 55 or a mother or sister before age 65; systolic blood pressure of 140 or more, a diastolic pressure of 90 or more, or being on drugs for hypertension; and an HDL level under 40. If your HDL is 60 or more, subtract one risk factor. (High LDL is a major factor, of course, but it's already figured into the table.)

‡While the goal is to get LDL under 130, the use of drugs in these people usually isn't worthwhile, even if lifestyle steps fail to achieve that goal.

§People in this group usually have less than 10% 10-year risk. Those who have a higher risk should ask their doctor whether they need more aggressive treatment than shown here.

Source: Third Report of the National Cholesterol Education Program (NCEP) Expert Panel on Detection, Evaluation, and Treatment of High Blood Cholesterol in Adults (Adult Treatment Panel III), 2001. www.nhlbi.nih.gov.

In summary, to lower LDL-C, the most important lifestyle modifications in order of importance are:[203–218]

- Reduction of dietary saturated fats (especially meat and dairy fats) and *trans*-fatty acids (mainly from hydrogenated fats)
- Reduction in body weight (or maintenance of normal body weight)
- Reduction in dietary cholesterol intake (found in all animal foods)

Box 10.7

Therapeutic Lifestyle Changes in LDL-Lowering Therapy

The ATP III recommends a multifaceted lifestyle approach to reduce risk for CHD. This approach is designated *therapeutic lifestyle changes* (TLC). Its essential features are

- Reduced intakes of saturated fats (<7% of total Calories) and cholesterol (<200 mg/day) (see the table to the right for overall composition of the TLC diet)
- Therapeutic options for enhancing LDL lowering such as plant stanols/sterols (2 grams/day) and increased viscous (soluble) fiber (10–25 grams/day)
- Weight reduction
- Increased physical activity

Source: Third Report of the National Cholesterol Education Program (NCEP) Expert Panel on Detection, Evaluation, and Treatment of High Blood Cholesterol in Adults (Adult Treatment Panel III), 2001. http://www.nhlbi.nih.gov.

Nutrient Composition of the TLC Diet

Nutrient	Recommended Intake
Saturated fat*	Less than 7% of total Calories
Polyunsaturated fat	Up to 10% of total Calories
Monounsaturated fat	Up to 20% of total Calories
Total fat	25–35% of total Calories
Carbohydrate†	50–60% of total Calories
Fiber	20–30 grams/day
Protein	Approximately 15% of total Calories
Cholesterol	Less than 200 mg/day
Total Calories (energy)‡	Balance energy intake and expenditure to maintain desirable body weight and prevent weight gain

**Trans*-fatty acids are another LDL-raising fat that should be kept at a low intake.

†Carbohydrate should be derived predominantly from foods rich in complex carbohydrates including grains, especially whole grains, fruits, and vegetables.

‡Daily energy expenditure should include at least moderate physical activity (contributing approximately 200 Calories/day).

A Model of Steps in Therapeutic Lifestyle Changes (TLC)

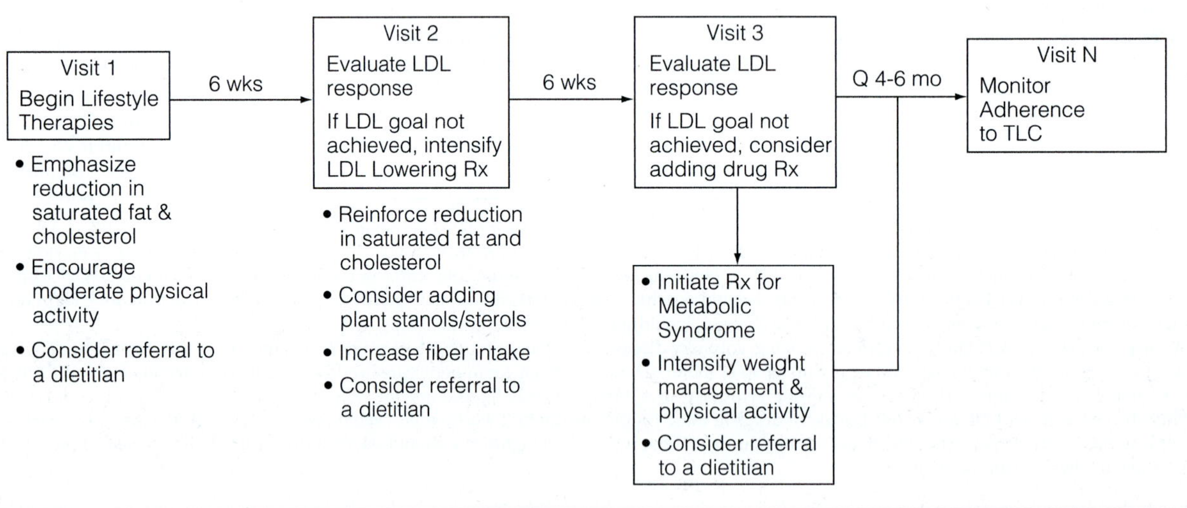

- Increase in dietary polyunsaturated, omega-3, and monounsaturated fatty acids (found in plant foods, fish, and olives)
- Increase in whole grain carbohydrates and dietary water-soluble fibers (especially fruits and vegetables, beans, and oat products)

To increase HDL-C, the most important lifestyle modifications in order of importance are:[203–218]

- Aerobic exercise, at least 90 minutes per week
- Weight reduction and leanness
- Smoking cessation
- Moderate alcohol consumption

Diets using nonhydrogenated unsaturated fats as the predominant form of dietary fat, whole grains as the main form of carbohydrates, an abundance of fruits and vegetables, and

TABLE 10.10 Drugs Affecting Lipoprotein Metabolism

Drug Class	Agents and Daily Doses	Lipid/Lipoprotein Effects	Side Effects	Contraindications
HMG CoA reductase inhibitors (statins)	Lovastatin (20–80 mg), pravastatin (20–40 mg), simvastatin (20–80 mg), fluvastatin (20–80 mg), atorvastatin (10–80 mg), cerivastatin (0.4–0.8 mg)	LDL-C ↓ 18–55% HDL-C ↑ 5–15% TG ↓ 7–30%	Myopathy Increased liver enzymes	Absolute: • Active or chronic liver disease Relative: • Concomitant use of certain drugs*
Bile acid sequestrants	Cholestyramine (4–16 g), colestipol (5–20 g); colesevelam (2.6–3.8 g)	LDL-C ↓ 15–30% HDL-C ↑ 3–5% TG No change or increase	Gastrointestinal distress Constipation Decreased absorption of other drugs	Absolute: • Dysbeta-lipoproteinemia • TG > 400 mg/dl Relative: • TG > 200 mg/dl
Nicotinic acid	Immediate release (crystalline) nicotinic acid (1.5–3 g), extended release nicotinic acid (Niaspan) (1–2 g), sustained release nicotinic acid (1–2 g)	LDL-C ↓ 5–25% HDL-C ↑ 15–35% TG ↓ 20–50%	Flushing Hyperglycemia Hyperuricemia (or gout) Upper GI distress Hepatotoxicity	Absolute: • Chronic liver disease • Severe gout Relative: • Diabetes • Hyperuricemia • Peptic ulcer disease
Fibric acids	Gemfibrozil (600 mg BID),† fenofibrate (200 mg), clofibrate (1000 mg BID)	LDL-C ↓ 5–20% (may be increased in patients with high TG) HDL-C ↑ 10–20% TG ↓ 20–50%	Dyspepsia Gallstones Myopathy	Absolute: • Severe renal disease • Severe hepatic disease

*Cyclosporine, macrolide antibiotics, various antifungal agents, and cytochrome P-450 Inhibitors (fibrates and niacin should be used with appropriate caution).

†BID = two times per day.

Source: Third Report of the National Cholesterol Education Program (NCEP) Expert Panel on Detection, Evaluation, and Treatment of High Blood Cholesterol in Adults (Adult Treatment Panel III), 2001. www.nhlbi.nih.gov.

TABLE 10.11 Clinical Identification of the Metabolic Syndrome*

Risk Factor	Defining Level
Abdominal obesity†	Waist circumference‡
Men	>102 cm (>40 in)
Women	>88 cm (>35 in)
Triglycerides	≥150 mg/dl
HDL cholesterol	
Men	<40 mg/dl
Women	<50 mg/dl
Blood pressure	≥130/≥85 mm Hg
Fasting glucose	≥110 mg/dl

*Patient is determined to have the metabolic syndrome if at least three of the risk factors are present.

†Overweight and obesity are associated with insulin resistance and the metabolic syndrome. However, the presence of abdominal obesity is more highly correlated with the metabolic risk factors than is an elevated body mass index (BMI). Therefore, the simple measure of waist circumference is recommended to identify the body weight component of the metabolic syndrome.

‡Some male patients can develop multiple metabolic risk factors when the waist circumference is only marginally increased, e.g., 94–102 cm (37–39 in). Such patients may have a strong genetic contribution to insulin resistance. They should benefit from changes in life habits, similarly to men with categorical increases in waist circumference.

Treatment of the metabolic syndrome

- Treat underlying causes (overweight/obesity and physical inactivity):
  - –Intensify weight management
  - –Increase physical activity
- Treat lipid and nonlipid risk factors if they persist despite these lifestyle therapies:
  - –Treat hypertension
  - –Use aspirin for CHD patients to reduce prothrombotic state
  - –Treat elevated triglycerides and/or low HDL

Source: Third Report of the National Cholesterol Education Program (NCEP) Expert Panel on Detection, Evaluation, and Treatment of High Blood Cholesterol in Adults (Adult Treatment Panel III), 2001. www.nhlbi.nih.gov.

Box 10.8

American Heart Association Guidelines for Reducing the Risk of Cardiovascular Disease by Dietary and Other Lifestyle Practices

These guidelines are designed to assist individuals in achieving and maintaining:

1. A healthy eating pattern including foods from all major food groups
   - **A.** Consume a variety of fruits and vegetables; choose five or more servings per day.
   - **B.** Consume a variety of grain products, including whole grains; choose six or more servings per day.
2. A healthy body weight
   - **A.** Match intake of total energy (calories) to overall energy needs.
   - **B.** Achieve a level of physical activity that matches (for weight maintenance) or exceeds (for weight loss) energy intake. Walk or do other activities for at least 30 minutes on most days.
3. A desirable blood cholesterol and lipoprotein profile
   - **A.** Limit intake of foods with high content of cholesterol-raising fatty acids.
     - Keep saturated fat intake at less than 10% of energy (<7% for those with high LDL-C). Include fat-free and low-fat milk products, fish, legumes (beans), skinless poultry, and lean meats. Choose fats with 2 grams or less saturated fat per serving, such as liquid and tub margarines, canola oil, and olive oil. Limit intake of full-fat milk products, fatty meats, and tropical oils.
     - Limit intake of *trans*-fatty acids, the major contributor of which is hydrogenated fat.
   - **B.** Limit the intake of foods high in cholesterol.
     - Limit dietary cholesterol intake to less than 300 mg/day on average (<200 mg/day for individuals with elevated LDL-C, diabetes, and/or cardiovascular disease.
   - **C.** Substitute grains and unsaturated fatty acids from fish, vegetables, legumes, and nuts.
4. A desirable blood pressure
   - **A.** Limit salt (sodium chloride) intake to 6 grams/day (100 mmol or 2,400 mg of sodium).
   - **B.** Maintain a healthy body weight.
   - **C.** Limit alcohol intake among those who drink (no more than two drinks per day for men, and one drink per day for women).
   - **D.** Maintain a dietary pattern that emphasizes fruits, vegetables, and low-fat dairy products and is reduced in fat.

Issues That Merit Further Research

- *Antioxidants.* High intake of dietary antioxidants from plant foods is recommended; insufficient evidence to support antioxidant supplements.
- *B vitamins and homocysteine lowering.* The normal metabolism of homocysteine requires an adequate supply of folate, vitamin B_6, vitamin B_{12}, and riboflavin. High plasma homocysteine levels have been related to increased coronary risk in most but not all studies.
- *Soy protein and isoflavones.* The consumption of soy protein in place of animal protein tends to lower blood levels of total cholesterol, LDL-C, and triglycerides without affecting HDL-C (but may require the presence of soy isoflavones, which have been removed in some commercial soy products).
- *ω-3 fatty acid supplements.* Consumption of one fatty fish meal per day (or alternatively, a fish oil supplement) could result in an ω-3 fatty acid intake of about 900 mg/day, an amount shown to beneficially affect mortality rates in patients with coronary heart disease.
- *Stanol/sterol ester-containing foods.* Foods containing stanol/sterol ester (plant sterols) have been shown to decrease blood cholesterol levels. Plant sterols (currently isolated from soybean and tall oils, esterified, and then incorporated into food products) decrease total cholesterol and LDL-C by decreasing intestinal absorption of dietary cholesterol.
- *Fat substitutes.* Fat substitutes mimic one or more of the roles of fat in a food and tend to reduce fat and energy intake.

Source: American Heart Association. AHA Scientific Statement. AHA dietary guidelines. Revision 2000: A statement for healthcare professionals from the Nutrition Committee of the American Heart Association. *Circulation* 102:2284–2299, 2000.

TABLE 10.12 Three-Day Menu Outline for a Healthy Heart

All vitamins and minerals exceed recommended intake levels.

Nutrient Information

Calories	2,000 per day		Cholesterol	140 milligrams	
Protein	86 grams	(17% of Calories)	Saturated fat	13 grams	(6% of Calories)
Fat	55 grams	(25% of Calories)	Dietary fiber	30 grams	
Carbohydrate	290 grams	(58% of Calories)	Caffeine	170 milligrams	
Sodium	2,800 milligrams				

Day 1 Breakfast

½	Grapefruit: raw, white, all areas
4	Pancakes: plain, and buttermilk, made with eggs and milk, 4-inch diameter
2 tsp	Margarine: soft, unspecified oils with salt
1 cup	Applesauce: canned, unsweetened, without ascorbic acid
¼ tsp	Cinnamon, ground
½ cup	Milk, cow's, low-fat, 1% fat
8 fl. oz	Coffee, brewed, prepared with tap water

Day 1 Lunch

2 oz	Fish/shellfish; tuna, canned drained solids, light meat, canned in water
2 slices	Bread: whole wheat
1 piece	Lettuce: iceberg, raw, leaf
2 tsp	Salad dressing: mayonnaise, soybean oil, with salt
1	Carrot, raw
1	Apple, raw, with skin
1 cup	Soup: tomato rice, with water
6	Crackers: saltines
¾ cup	Grape juice: canned/bottled, unsweetened

Day 1 Dinner

3 oz	Beef: composite of trimmed retailed cuts, all grades, separated lean, cooked, 0-in fat
1	Potato: baked, flesh only, without salt
1 cup	Broccoli: frozen, chopped, boiled, drained, without salt
1 ear	Corn: sweet, yellow, boiled, drained, without salt
3 tsp	Margarine: soft, unspecified oils, with salt
2	Peaches, raw
1 cup	Milk: cow's, low-fat, 1% fat

Day 2 Breakfast

1 cup	Yogurt: fruit flavored, low-fat
1	English muffin, plain
1	Orange, raw, all varieties
2 tsp	Margarine: soft, unspecified oils, with salt added
8 fl. oz	Coffee: brewed, prepared with tap water

Day 2 Lunch

¾ cup	Sauce: spaghetti, canned
1 cup	Spaghetti: enriched, cooked with no salt
1½ cup	Lettuce: iceberg, raw
½	Tomato: red, ripe, raw
¼ cup	Carrots: raw, shredded
¼ cup	Cucumber: not pared, raw, sliced
2 tbs	Salad dressing: Italian, diet, with salt
1 tbs	Seeds: sunflower seed kernels, dried
1 slice	Bread: French or Vienna, enriched
1 tsp	Margarine: soft, unspecified oils, with salt added
⅛ tsp	Garlic powder
1 serving	Grapes: European type (adherent skin)
1 cup	Tea: brewed

Day 2 Dinner

3 oz	Chicken: breast, meat only, roasted
¾ cup	Rice: brown, long, cooked, without salt
1 cup	Carrots: boiled, drained, without salt
1	Roll/bun: brown and serve, enriched
2 tsp	Margarine: soft, unspecified oils, with salt
1 cup	Milk: cow's, low-fat, 1% fat
1 cup	Strawberries: raw
1 slice	Cake: angel food, baked from mix, enriched, made with water and flavorings

Day 3 Breakfast

2	Cereal: shredded wheat, large biscuits
2 tsp	Sugar: brown, pressed down
2 slices	Bread: whole wheat, toasted
1	Banana
4 tsp	Nuts: peanut butter, with salt
1 cup	Milk: cow's, low-fat, 1% fat
8 fl. oz	Coffee: brewed, prepared with tap water

Day 3 Lunch

2 oz	Turkey: light, no skin, roasted
1 oz	Cheese: natural, mozzarella, part skim
2 slices	Bread: whole wheat
2 tsp	Salad dressing: mayonnaise, soybean oil, with salt
½ cup	Broccoli: raw, chopped
½ cup	Cauliflower: raw, 1-inch pieces
2 tbs	Salad dressing: Thousand Island, low-calorie, with salt
1	Pear, raw
3	Cookies: oatmeal with raisins
1½ cup	Carbonated beverages low-calorie, cola, with aspartame

Day 3 Dinner

3 oz	Pork: cured, ham, whole, separated lean only, roasted
1	Sweet potato: baked, flesh only
1 cup	Beans: snap, green, boiled with salt
2 tsp	Margarine: soft, unspecified oils, with salt added
1 cup	Apple juice: canned/bottled, unsweetened, without added ascorbic acid
1 cup	Melon: cantaloupe, raw, cubed
½ cup	Ice milk: vanilla, soft serve

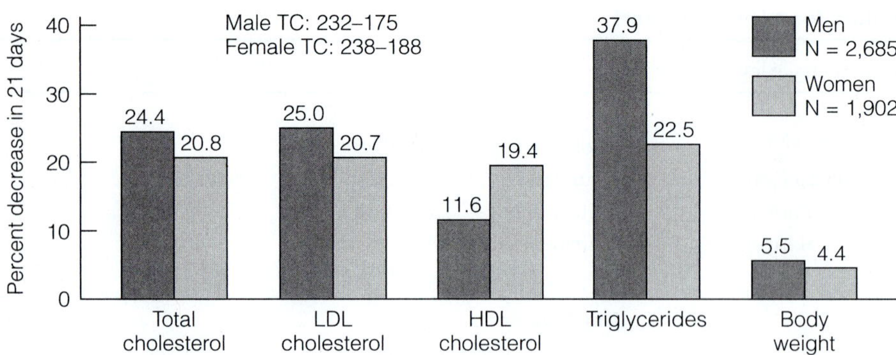

Figure 10.45 Effects of lifestyle modification on serum lipids: Pritikin Program—21 days, <10% fat, high-fiber, carb diet, 1–2 h exercise per day. Source: Data from Barnard RJ. Effects of lifestyle modification on serum lipids. *Arch Intern Med* 151:1389–1394, 1991.

adequate omega-3 fatty acids from fish offer significant protection against CHD. Such diets together with regular physical activity, avoidance of smoking, and maintenance of a healthy body weight prevents the majority of CVD in Western populations.[205]

Improvements in lifestyle can have strong, relatively quick effects on total cholesterol, HDL-C, and LDL-C, depending on the initial levels and the degree of change.[215,216] The Pritikin Program is a 21-day residential program in which high-risk individuals are put on an extremely low-fat (<10% Calories), high-fiber, high-carbohydrate, primarily vegetarian diet, with 1–2 hours of daily moderate exercise.[215]

As shown in Figure 10.45, major improvements are seen in total cholesterol, LDL-C, and triglycerides, with most of the changes occurring within the first 2 weeks. Notice that HDL-C fell 12–19%, which is common during periods where large improvements are being made in the diet. Over time, as the body weight is stabilized and exercise continues, the HDL-C tends to increase a bit. Although the Pritikin diet is extreme for most people and probably can't be followed for extended periods, it does show what is possible when used therapeutically for several weeks.

Role of Exercise

In the 1970s, several published studies showed that low levels of HDL-C were related to coronary heart disease.[192] About the same time, the first reports that exercise may be related to improved HDL-C levels were published.[192,217] In an early Stanford University study of male and female long-distance runners and sedentary controls, HDL-C was found to be substantially higher in the runners[217,218] (see Figure 10.46). Total blood cholesterol, LDL-C, and triglycerides were reported to be much lower among the runners. Because of the cross-sectional nature of the research design, however, group disparities in blood fats and lipoproteins could have been due to factors other than exercise, including diet, body fat, and genetic background.[219–221]

In two more recent and larger studies of male and female runners, a dose–response relationship between miles run per week and HDL-C has been reported[179,222] (see Figure 10.47). In both of these studies, runners training the

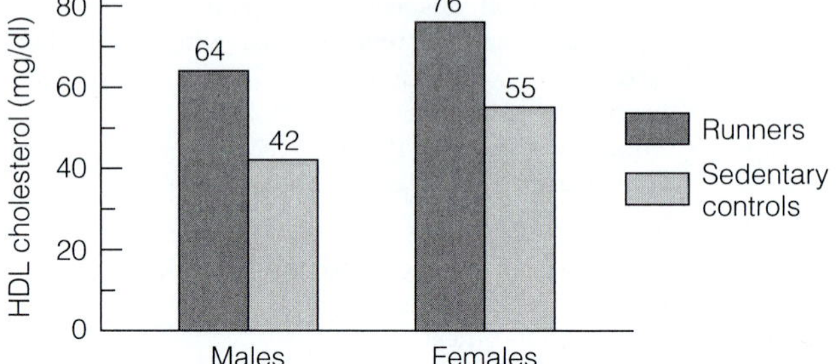

Figure 10.46 High-density lipoprotein cholesterol in male and female runners and sedentary controls. Source: Data from Wood PD, Haskell WL, Stern MP, Lewis S, Perry C. Serum lipoproteins distributions in male and female runners. *Ann NY Acad Sci* 301:748–763, 1977.

most had the highest HDL-C, and no evidence of a plateau or ceiling effect was seen. In other words, moderate amounts of running were better than little or none, while even more running was related to even higher HDL-C levels.[223] For the male, but not the female, runners, LDL-C and triglyceride levels dropped sharply with increase in running distance. However, once again, whether the improved blood lipoprotein profile among the more serious runners was due to genetics, or to a superior diet and body composition, could not be fully determined.

Weight loss, in and of itself, has a powerful effect on blood fats and lipoproteins. With weight loss, the total cholesterol, LDL-C, and triglycerides decrease greatly, while HDL-C increases (but only when weight loss has been maintained and stabilized)[224–226] (see Chapter 13). Some researchers have estimated that the total cholesterol drops about 1 mg/dl for every pound lost (decreases are greatest for those with the highest blood cholesterol levels).[227] In other words, if a subject changes weight from 180 to 160 pounds, blood cholesterol could be expected, on average, to decrease 20 mg/dl (e.g., from 205 to 185 mg/dl).

As discussed in the previous section, improvements in dietary habits also have a favorable effect on blood lipids and lipoproteins.[225–227] Going from the typical American diet to the one recommended by the American Heart Association can decrease the total cholesterol by 5–15% (depending on the initial level). Going to more extreme diets, such as the 21-day Pritikin Program diet (<10% total fat),

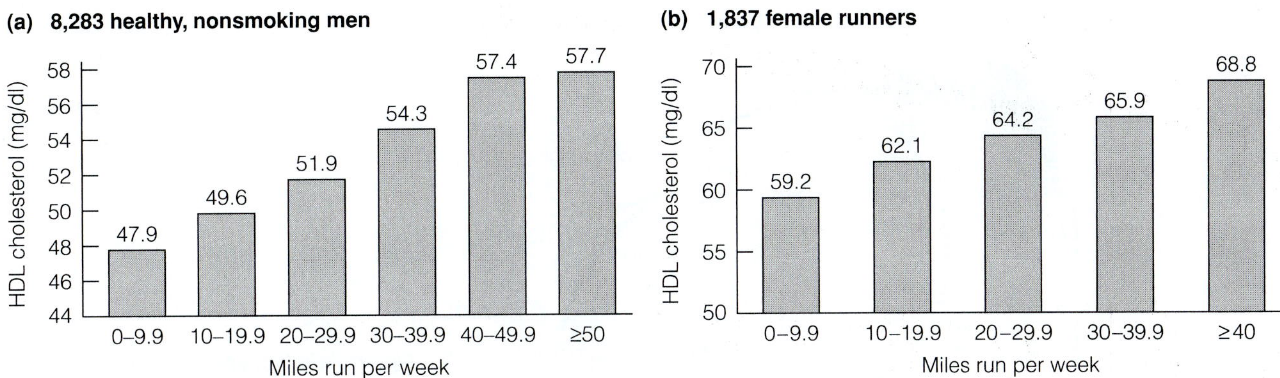

Figure 10.47 Miles run per week and HDL cholesterol. For both men and women, HDL cholesterol levels rise with increase in miles run. Sources: Data from Williams PT. Relationship of distance run per week to coronary heart disease risk factors in 8283 male runners. The National Runners' Health Study. *Arch Intern Med* 157:191–198, 1997; Williams PT. High-density lipoprotein cholesterol and other risk factors for coronary heart disease in female runners. *N Engl J Med* 334:1298–1303, 1996.

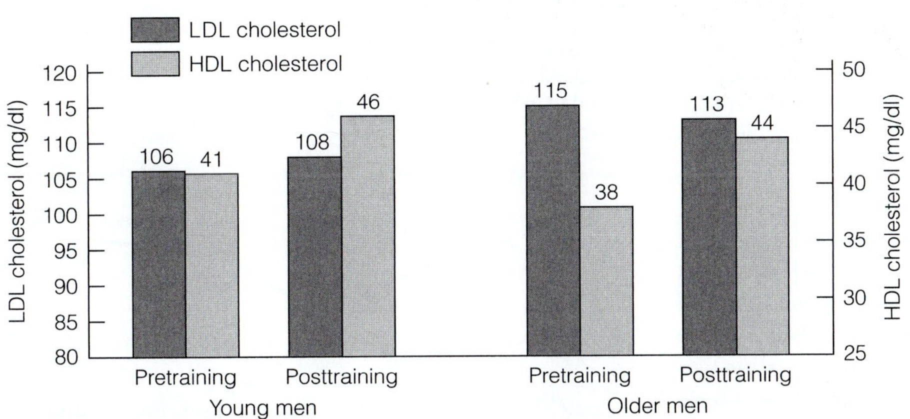

Figure 10.48 Exercise and lipoproteins in young and older men, without change in weight or diet; 6 months exercise, 5 days/week, 45 minutes/session, high intensity. Source: Data from Schwartz RS, Cain KC, Shuman WP, et al. Effect of intensive endurance training on lipoprotein profiles in young and older men. *Metabolism* 41:649–654, 1992.

can have very strong effects on the total cholesterol and LDL-C (20–25% decreases), and triglycerides (20–40% decreases)[215] (Figure 10.45).

These studies show that weight loss and dietary changes can have dramatic effects on the blood lipids and lipoproteins. Often, when people begin exercise programs, improvements in dietary habits and body composition occur. Studies using randomized, controlled designs have carefully demonstrated that changes in blood cholesterol and fats with exercise training are very much affected by parallel changes in body weight and diet.[224–229]

A growing consensus among investigators is that when changes in body weight and dietary habits are controlled for, exercise training alone can be expected to increase HDL-C and to decrease triglyceride levels, with little or no effect on LDL-C.[217–237] Figure 10.48 summarizes the results of one study where changes in body weight and diet in both young and old men were minimized and controlled.[229] After 6 months of training intensely 5 days a week, 45 minutes per session, aerobic fitness in the young and older subjects improved 18% and 22%, respectively. No significant changes in LDL-C were found (because diet and body weight were kept near prestudy levels), while HDL-C improved 14–15%.

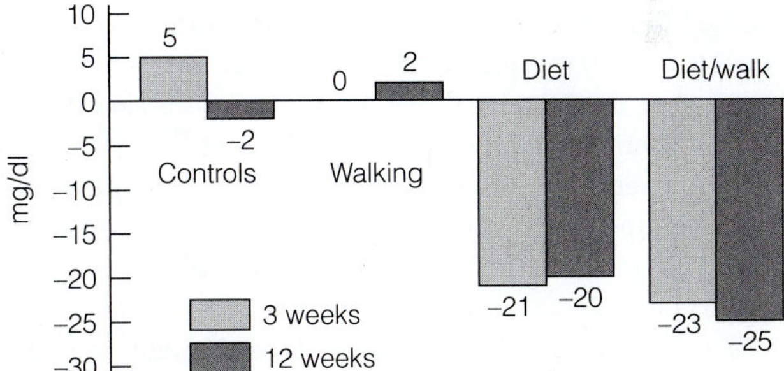

Figure 10.49 Cholesterol changes in response to diet and exercise (12 weeks) in 90 overweight women, randomized to one of four groups. Source: Data from Nieman DC, Brock DW, Butterworth D, Utter AC, Nieman CN. Reducing diet and/or exercise training decreases the lipid and lipoprotein risk factors of moderately obese women. *J Am College Nutr* 21:344–350, 2002.

Triglycerides were low in the young subjects before starting the study, so exercise training had no further effect. For the older subjects, triglycerides fell strongly.

Figure 10.49 shows the results of a 12-week study of 90 overweight women, randomized to one of four groups: controls, walking (five 45-minute sessions per week, 60–75%

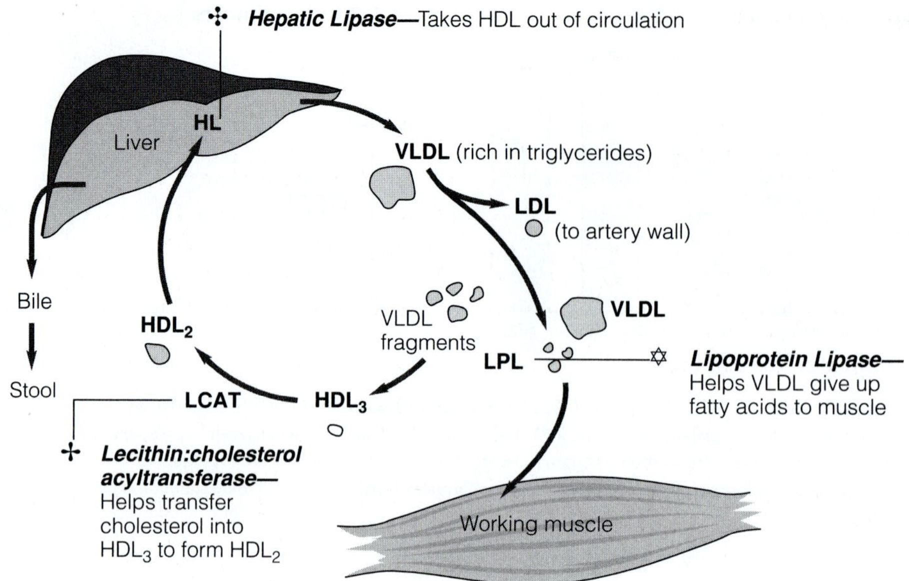

Figure 10.50 Formation and elimination of HDL. HDL is formed within the blood by the action of two key enzymes (lipoprotein lipase [LPL] and lecithin: cholesterol acyltransferase [LCAT]) and then taken out of circulation by hepatic lipase (HL). Active people tend to have higher LPL and LCAT and lower HL enzyme activity levels.

maximum heart rate), diet (1,200–1,300 Calories per day), and diet and walking.[237] Subjects in the two diet groups lost an average of 17 pounds in 12 weeks, while the control and walking groups stayed within 2 pounds of their starting weight. Notice that serum cholesterol did not change in the control or walking groups but decreased 20–25% in the two diet groups. Most of the improvement in serum cholesterol occurred within the first 3 weeks.

How much exercise is necessary to improve the lipid profile? Most researchers agree that an exercise program equal to a moderate jog or brisk walk for at least 30 minutes per session, three to five times per week, is necessary before improvements in HDL-C can be measured.[217,231,232,238] In terms of energy expenditure, about 1,000 Calories per week of moderate-to-high intensity, aerobic-type exercise is required to produce favorable changes in blood fats and lipoproteins.

At this basic, minimum exercise level, changes in HDL-C and triglyceride levels are sometimes small and variable, depending on the individual. Exercise programs with high duration (e.g., 45 minutes or longer), intensity, and frequency (i.e., near daily) produce the strongest effects on HDL-C and triglycerides. Total cholesterol and LDL-C, however, appear to be little affected by exercise training, even when it is intensive, unless body weight is decreased or dietary saturated fats are lowered at the same time.

Many studies testing the effect of moderate amounts of walking on HDL-C in women have failed to show significant changes.[221,230,231,237] However, when researchers increase the overall exercise volume and intensity, HDL-C does improve.[222,231,234] In other words, women require greater volumes of exercise than men to improve their HDL-C because of their initially higher levels.[239]

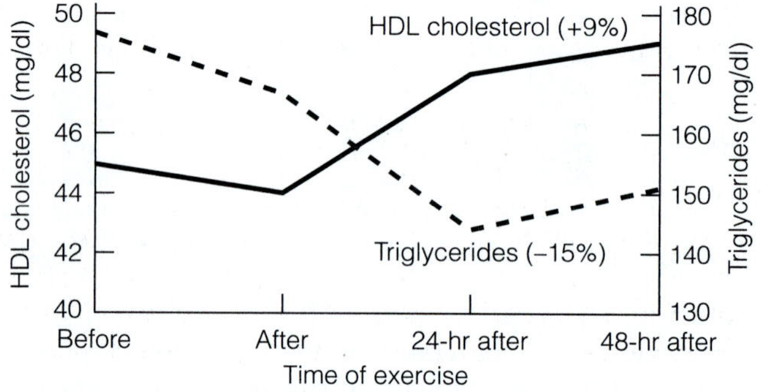

Figure 10.51 Changes in HDL cholesterol and trigylceride levels after exercise in 39 middle-aged men with high cholesterol, who cycled 30–60 minutes, burning 350 Calories. Source: Data from Crouse SF, O'Brien BC, Rohack JJ, et al. Changes in serum lipids and apolipoproteins after exercise in men with high cholesterol: Influence of intensity. *J Appl Physiol* 79:279–286, 1995.

Although there is increasing evidence that regular aerobic exercise increases HDL-C and lowers blood triglyceride levels, the exact mechanism explaining these positive changes is still being determined. At present, most researchers have concentrated their efforts on the interplay of important enzymes that regulate the breakdown and formation of HDL-C and triglycerides.[239–244] Regular exercise alters the activity of the regulatory enzymes in a favorable manner. The end result is that aerobically fit, compared to unfit, individuals appear to clear triglycerides from the blood more quickly, produce more HDL-C, and keep HDL-C in circulation longer (see Figure 10.50).

Studies have shown that single bouts of aerobic exercise, especially when prolonged and intense, result in immediate and significant increases in HDL-C[245–251] (Figure 10.51). This

TABLE 10.13 The Influence of Endurance Exercise on Blood Lipids and Lipoproteins

Component	Acute (Short-term) Change	Chronic (Long-term) Change
Total cholesterol	No change	No change
Low-density lipoprotein	No change	No change, slight decrease
High-density lipoprotein	No change, increase	Increase
Triglycerides	Decrease	Decrease

acute increase in HDL-C has been linked to the breakdown of triglycerides during exercise.[249] Certain enzymes (especially lipoprotein lipase in the walls of the capillaries) break down the triglycerides during exercise, allowing the muscles to take in fat for fuel and energy production.

As the exercise program is maintained on a regular basis, the acute changes in HDL-C and triglycerides, which persist for at least 24–48 hours, result in a chronic improvement. In other words, the favorable lipid profiles of trained individuals may actually be related to short-term changes that occur during or immediately after a single bout of exercise, which over time add up to higher HDL-C and lower triglyceride levels. (See Table 10.13 for a summary.)

The largest acute increase in HDL-C occurs following unusually heavy exertion.[246,250,251] For example, after a marathon race, HDL-C can increase 15–25%.[250,251] Triglycerides drop sharply at the same time, as the muscles use fats for fuel. In one report of 29 triathletes who finished the 1994 Hawaii Ironman World Championship, blood triglyceride levels dropped an average of 39%.[246]

EXERCISE AND CORONARY HEART DISEASE PREVENTION

Up until 1992, the American Heart Association did not include physical inactivity in their list of "major risk factors that can be changed," which included cigarette smoking, high blood pressure, and high blood cholesterol[252,253] (see Table 10.2). Previously, inactivity was listed along with obesity, stress, and diabetes as "contributing factors." Until recently, good research data to support the relationship between CHD and inactivity had been lacking. Most of the earlier studies showed that physically active, compared to inactive, people had a lower risk for CHD, but critics contended that other important factors (e.g., diet, family history) were not controlled for.

For example, in one of the earliest (1953) published studies, London bus drivers who sat and drove were found to be at higher risk for CHD than the conductors who moved through the double-decker buses collecting tickets.[254] However, critics claimed that the drivers may have been at higher risk for CHD to begin with, and self-selected themselves to an easier, sit-down type of job.

Ralph Paffenbarger of Stanford University has done more than any other researcher to silence the criticism and to advance the cause of exercise as a valuable preventive measure. In 1970, Paffenbarger published data showing that San Francisco longshoremen who engaged in little physical labor on the job were at 60% greater risk for CHD death than colleagues engaging in physically demanding work.[255]

In 1978, the first of several reports on college alumni were released, demonstrating that active alumni were at lower CHD risk than their inactive counterparts.[256] In these studies, Paffenbarger carefully controlled for other CHD risk factors, showing that the sedentary lifestyle in and of itself was related to CHD.[255–259]

Physical activity habits are difficult to measure and are largely based on information provided by the subjects. Cardiorespiratory fitness, however, is an objective measure and can be assessed rather easily. Steven Blair of the Cooper Institute for Aerobics Research has been a leader in evaluating the relationship between fitness and coronary heart and cardiovascular diseases.[117,260] He has used maximal treadmill testing to measure cardiorespiratory fitness in a large group of men and women since 1970. Blair has found that a low level of fitness is a strong risk factor for CVD, in both men and women[260] (see Figure 10.52).

Although more research is needed with women, several studies suggest that physical inactivity affects CHD risk to the same degree in both men and women. In one study of older women in the Seattle area, CHD risk was decreased 50% with moderate amounts of exercise.[261] A large study of 73,743 postmenopausal women showed that both walking and vigorous exercise were linked with substantial reductions in incidence of cardiovascular events.[262] As depicted in Figure 10.53, results from a 7 year study of more than 40,000 Iowa women showed that increasing frequency of both moderate and vigorous physical activity was associated with a reduced risk of death from cardiovascular disease.[263]

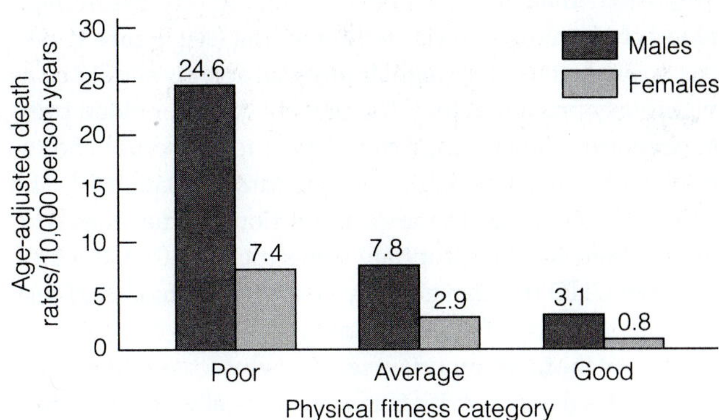

Figure 10.52 Physical fitness and cardiovascular mortality: 8-year study of 10,224 men and 3,120 women. Source: Data from Blair SN, Kohl HW, Paffenbarger RS, Clark DG, Cooper KH, Gibbons LW. Physical fitness and all-cause mortality: A prospective study of healthy men and women. *JAMA* 262:2395–2401, 1989.

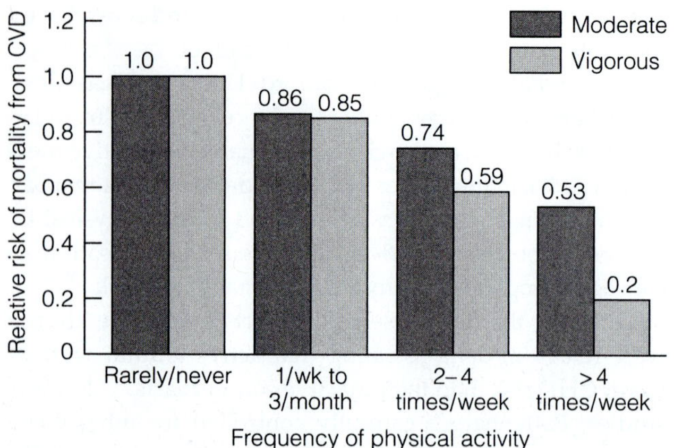

Figure 10.53 Physical activity and CVD mortality in postmenopausal women. Source: Data from Kushi LH, Fee RM, Folsom AR, Mink PJ, Anderson KE, Sellers TA. Physical activity and mortality in postmenopausal women. *JAMA* 277:1287–1292, 1997.

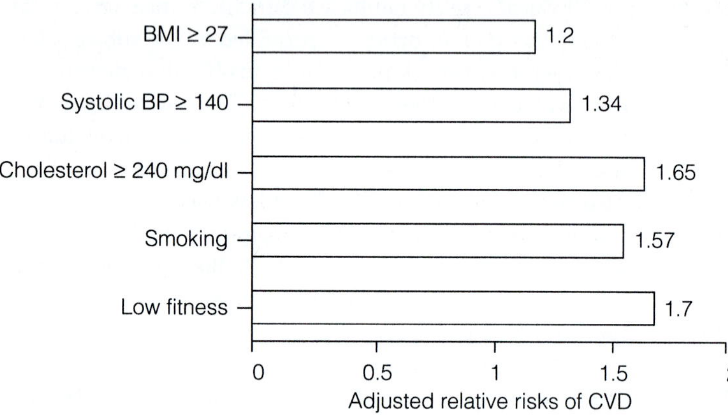

Figure 10.54 Adjusted relative risks for cardiovascular disease in 25,341 male patients tested at the Cooper Clinic in Dallas. Source: Data from Farrell SW, Kampert JB, Kohl HW, Barlow CE, Macera CA, Paffenbarger RS, Gibbons LW, Blair SN. Influences of cardiorespiratory fitness levels and other predictors on cardiovascular disease mortality in men. *Med Sci Sports Exerc* 30:899–905, 1998.

In 1987, a landmark review article was published by researchers from the Centers for Disease Control and Prevention (CDC).[264] Forty-three studies were reviewed, and not one reported a greater risk for CHD among active participants. Two thirds of the studies supported the finding that physically active versus inactive people have less CHD, and the studies following the best research design were the ones most likely to support this relationship.

In general, the risk for CHD among physically inactive people is twice that of people who are relatively active.[254–284] This risk is similar to that reported for high blood pressure, high blood cholesterol, and cigarette smoking (see Figure 10.54). According to the CDC, regular physical activity should be as vigorously promoted for CHD prevention as for blood pressure control, dietary improvements to lower serum cholesterol and control weight, and smoking cessation.[264] The CDC feels that given the large proportion of Americans who do not exercise at appropriate levels (nearly 60%), the incidence of CHD that can actually be attributed to lack of regular physical activity is significant.

One of the most important reasons why active people have less CHD is that other risk factors are typically under control, as well[285–288] (see Figure 10.55). For example, relatively few active people smoke cigarettes, are obese or diabetic, have high blood cholesterol, or experience high blood pressure. Active people have lower blood triglycerides, more HDL-C,

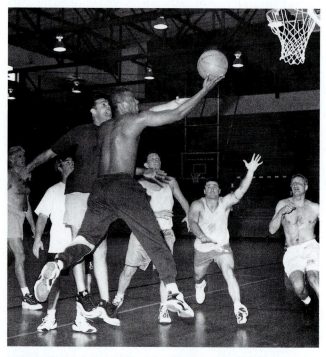

Figure 10.55 Regular physical activity is associated with a lower prevalence for most of the major risk factors of coronary heart disease.

and generally report less anxiety and depression. Although there is some controversy as to whether exercise or self-selection is responsible for these reduced risk factors, most experts feel that exercise does have a direct effect in bringing many CHD risk factors under control.[287]

There are other important reasons why regular exercise is identified with lower CHD risk. Coronary arteries of endurance-trained individuals can expand more, are less stiff in older age, and are wider than those of unfit subjects.[289,290] Even if some plaque material is present, the coronary arteries of fit people are wide enough to diminish the risk of total closure leading to a heart attack. Although the issue is not yet settled, there is some evidence that exercise may decrease the potential for clot formation.[291–293] In other words, with larger, more compliant coronary arteries, and a diminished likelihood of forming clots, the active individual is at lower risk for a heart attack. The heart muscle itself becomes bigger and stronger with regular exercise. Although still under study, there is some indication that the fit heart develops extra blood vessels, enhancing blood and oxygen delivery.[294]

Exercise must be regular in order for CHD risk to be lowered. In college alumni studies, Paffenbarger noted that current physical activity habits were much more important when considering CHD risk than were those from early adulthood.[259] Former college athletes who dropped their sports-playing habits had higher death rates thereafter than their teammates who continued to exercise moderately vigorously into middle or later age.[257] In contrast, college students who had avoided athletics in college but subsequently took up a more active lifestyle experienced the same low risk of mortality as alumni who had been moderately vigorous all along.

More recent results from the college alumni studies also support this concept. Risk of premature death from CHD was increased if physical activity was reduced below favorable levels, and risk was lowered if physical activity was increased.[295] Adopting a regular exercise program was found to be as beneficial in lowering CHD risk as quitting smoking and avoiding obesity and hypertension.

These results are similar to those of Blair, who showed that individuals maintaining or improving fitness over a 5-year span were less likely to die from CVD than those who stayed unfit.[296] Men in the Aerobics Center Longitudinal Study who improved their fitness during the 5-year study had a 64% reduction in risk of death, greater than for any of the other risk factors.

There has been some debate as to the volume and intensity of exercise essential for lowering CHD risk. Some studies have indicated that regular and vigorous exercise is necessary, while others suggest that exercise of moderate duration and intensity is sufficient to reduce CHD risk.[297] There is increasing consensus that while moderate exercise is a sufficient threshold for lowering CHD risk, additional benefit is gained when people are willing to exercise more vigorously for longer periods of time.[297,298] However, the relationship does not appear to be linear. The greatest benefit in lowering CHD risk occurs when sedentary people adopt moderate physical activity habits, with some additional protection gained as the duration and intensity of exercise are raised to a higher level (see Figure 10.56).

Blair has emphasized that as little as 2 miles of brisk walking on most days of the week would result in the moderate level of fitness shown to be protective in the Aerobics Center Longitudinal Study.[260] Other studies suggest a level of activity just a bit higher, the equivalent of 2–3 miles of brisk walking each day of the week.[259,277,281,283]

An expert panel convened by the National Institutes of Health concluded that activity that reduces CVD risk factors does not require a structured or vigorous exercise program.[298] The majority of benefits of physical activity can be gained by performing moderate-intensity activities. The NIH recommends that all children and adults set a long-term goal to accumulate at least 30 minutes or more of

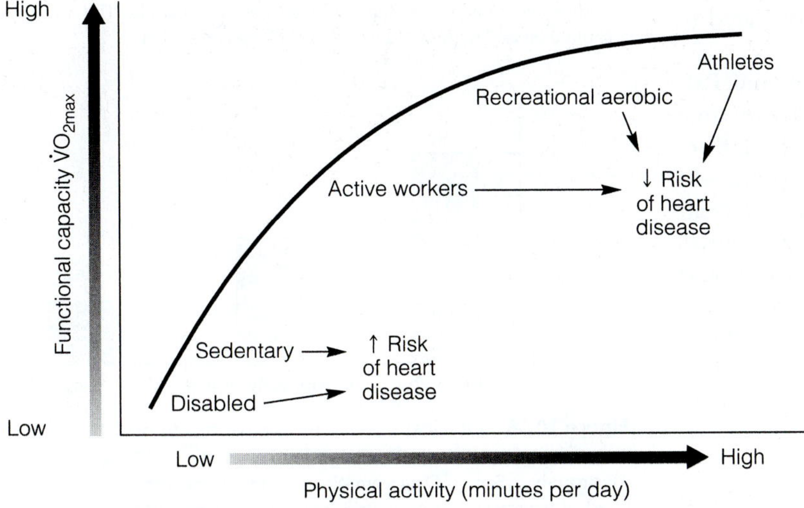

Figure 10.56 The spectrum of physical activity and cardiovascular fitness. Very high $\dot{V}O_{2max}$ values are not necessary to reduce risk of CHD. However, at least moderate physical activity is important and is usually associated with higher than average $\dot{V}O_{2max}$ values.

moderate-intensity physical activity on most, or preferably all, days of the week.

Some researchers, however, urge that people should not be misled to believe that a casual approach to fitness is sufficient. In one study from Finland, 1,453 middle-aged men who were initially free of CHD for 5 years were followed, classified according to the frequency and intensity of their leisure-time physical activity.[281] Men who engaged in moderate-to-strenuous activity for at least 2.2 hours per week had a risk of heart attack that was less than half that of the least active men. Only moderate-to-strenuous aerobic activities such as brisk walking, jogging, bicycling, or cross-country skiing were shown to confer protection. Nonconditioning activities such as slow walking, fishing, easy yard work or gardening, hunting, or picking berries did not lower CHD risk.

EXERCISE AND STROKE PREVENTION

Physical inactivity is still not recognized by the American Heart Association as a primary risk factor for stroke.[1] Instead, physical inactivity is classified as a "less well-documented or potentially modifiable risk factor."[11]

A growing number of research studies have established a link between physical activity and decrease in stroke, although the link has not been as firmly established as the link to CHD.[36] Recent studies using the best research designs have reported a strong protective effect of regular exercise for both men and women.[299] Although some earlier studies did not report a protective effect, no study has found that regular exercise *increases* the risk for stroke.

It makes sense that if regular physical activity *lowers* CHD risk (a relationship that is well established), stroke risk should also be lowered, given the common underlying cause (atherosclerosis). The first research study providing evidence that physical activity may be related to a decreased risk of stroke was published by Paffenbarger in 1967.[300] Among 50,000 college alumni, those men who were not varsity athletes during their college years had nearly a twofold increased risk of death from stroke, compared to that of the varsity athletes.

In an extended follow-up of 17,000 college alumni, Paffenbarger rated the men according to their leisure-time physical activity. Men in the lowest category of physical activity (those expending less than 500 Calories per week) died from stroke at a rate that was 1.7 times higher than that for those who were most active (more than 2,000 Calories per week).[257] Another study of Dutch stroke patients and controls also established that men and women exercising the most during their leisure time exhibited the lowest risk of stroke (73%), when compared to those who were sedentary.[301] However, even those reporting regular light activity during their leisure time (walking or cycling each week) experienced a 51% decreased risk of stroke.

Studies published since 1990 have provided the best evidence that physically active men and women suffer less from strokes.[302–309] In one study of 105 stroke patients and 161 controls, an increasing protection from stroke was experienced as the duration of exercise in earlier years increased.[302] Risk of stroke fell 56% in those who had engaged in regular and vigorous exercise from ages 15 to 25, with some additional protection afforded those who exercised throughout adulthood.

In a 22-year study of 7,530 men of Japanese ancestry living in Hawaii, physical inactivity was found to be a strong risk factor for stroke caused by clots among nonsmoking middle-aged men (relative risk of 2.8) and for hemorrhagic stroke in older men ages 55–68 (relative risk of 3.7)[303] (see Figure 10.57).

Although the evidence is far from conclusive, data from several studies suggest that while moderate physical activity is sufficient to lower the risk for stroke, further benefit is gained with increasing amounts and intensity of exercise.[304,307,308] For example, in one 9.5-year study of 7,735 British middle-aged men, those who were moderately active experienced a 40% decrease in stroke risk, while those who were vigorously active had an even greater decrease (70%)[304] (see Figure 10.58). In a study of 72,488 nurses, risk of stroke was lowest in the most physically active women.[307] Brisk walking but not casual walking was linked to a lower risk of stroke in these women.

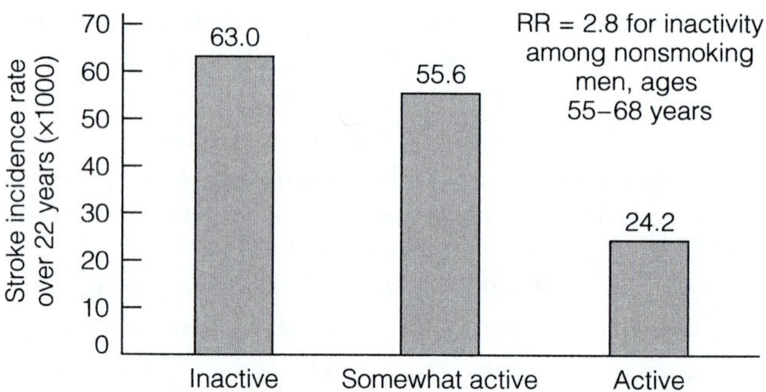

Figure 10.57 Stroke risk and physical activity, in Japanese men living in Hawaii. Incidence rates for stroke among 7,530 Japanese men living in Hawaii were much higher in those who were physically inactive versus active. Source: Data from Abbott RD, Rodriguez BL, Burchfiel CM, Curb JD. Physical activity in older middle-aged men and reduced risk of stroke: The Honolulu Heart Program. *Am J Epidemiol* 139:881–893, 1994.

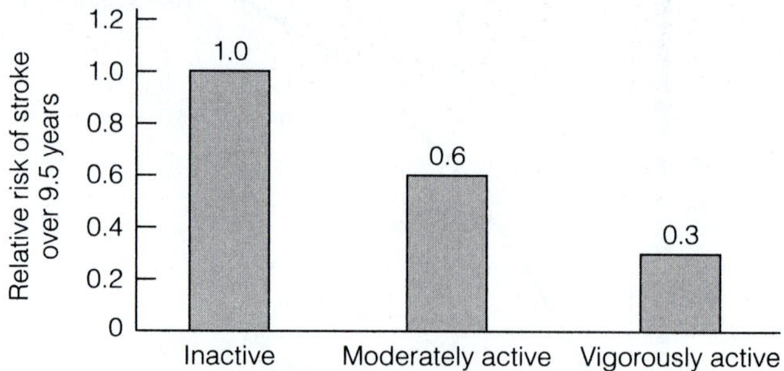

Figure 10.58 Physical activity and stroke risk in British men. Risk of stroke was lowest in British men exercising vigorously. Source: Data from Wannamethee G, Shaper AG. Physical activity and stroke in British middle aged men. *BMJ* 304:597–601, 1992.

SPORTS MEDICINE INSIGHT

Cardiac Rehabilitation

As discussed earlier in this chapter, each year, about 1.5 million Americans have a heart attack.[1] Although one third die soon after, the majority live to face an uncertain future. People who survive the acute stage of a heart attack have a chance of illness and death two to nine times higher than the general population. During the first year after having a heart attack, 27% of men and 44% of women will die. More than 12 million Americans alive today have a history of heart attack, angina pectoris (chest pain), or both.

Cardiovascular operations and procedures to treat heart disease are part of a growing industry. Total vascular and cardiac surgeries now number over 4.4 million per year, including diagnostic cardiac catheterizations, coronary artery bypass graft surgery, percutaneous transluminal coronary angioplasty, open-heart surgery, heart transplants, and pacemaker insertions.[1]

Cardiac rehabilitation programs were first developed in the 1950s in response to the growing epidemic of heart disease.[310–312] Participants include people who have CHD, those who have had a heart attack, and surgery patients. Many programs admit people who have multiple CHD risk factors but have not yet been diagnosed with CVD. The goal is to prepare cardiac patients to return to productive, active, and satisfying lives, with a reduced risk of recurring health problems (see Box 10.9).

In cardiac rehabilitation programs, the emphasis is usually on lifestyle change, optimization of drug therapy, vocational counseling, and group and family therapy. Regarding lifestyle change, exercise is considered the cornerstone, but weight control, smoking cessation, and dietary therapy are also essential.[310,311] During the early days of cardiac rehabilitation, it was common practice to have the heart attack patient stay in bed a minimum of 2–3 weeks. As research began to demonstrate the importance of early and progressive physical activity, a four-phase plan was developed, which is now standard in most programs (see Figure 10.59).

Patients with no complications are expected to progress from phase I through phase III within 1 year after an acute cardiac event. Phase IV is designed for lifelong exercise participation. Phase I involves easy walking and bed exercises during the first 5–14 days while the patient is in the coronary care unit of the hospital. Phase II is an outpatient program lasting 1–3 months, with the patient exercising aerobically in the hospital or clinic under careful supervision. Phase III lasts 6–12 months and is a supervised aerobic exercise program in a community setting.

Exercise programs for cardiac patients should be highly individualized and should involve an initial slow, gradual progression of the exercise duration and intensity. Aerobic activities should be emphasized, with a minimum

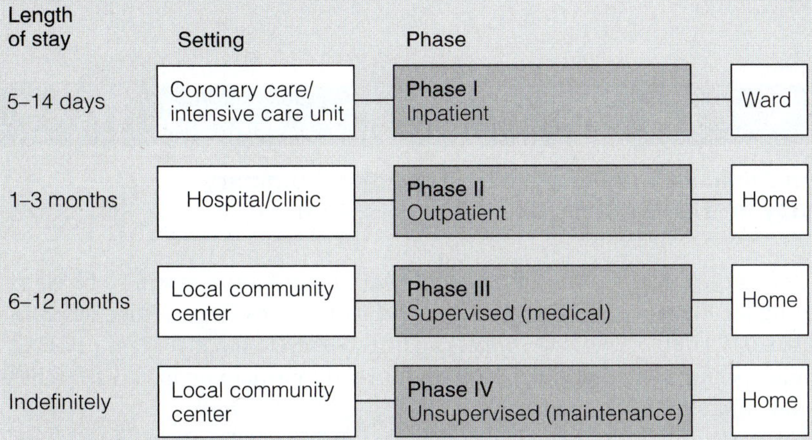

Length of stay
Setting
Phase
5–14 days
Coronary care/ intensive care unit
Phase I Inpatient
Ward
1–3 months
Hospital/clinic
Phase II Outpatient
Home
6–12 months
Local community center
Phase III Supervised (medical)
Home
Indefinitely
Local community center
Phase IV Unsupervised (maintenance)
Home

Figure 10.59 Modern cardiac rehabilitation program summary. There are four phases to the modern cardiac rehabilitation program. Participants include people who have CHD, people who have had a myocardial infarction (MI), those with coronary artery disease who have not had an MI, and surgery patients. Patients with no complications are expected to progress from phase I through phase III within 1 year after an acute cardiac event. Phase IV is designed for lifelong participation. Cardiac rehabilitation programs are found at many different sites, including hospitals, YMCAs, universities, community centers, and medical clinics.
Source: Adapted from Wilson PK. Cardiac rehabilitation: Then and now. *Phys Sportsmed* 16(9):75–84, 1988.

(continued)

SPORTS MEDICINE INSIGHT *(continued)*

Cardiac Rehabilitation

frequency of 3 days per week, 20–40 minutes each session, at a moderate, comfortable intensity. Some resistance exercise, but at a low intensity, is recommended to help build up weakened muscles.[313]

Unfortunately, only 15% of eligible cardiac patients (>2 million) actually participate in cardiac rehabilitation programs.[310] For a variety of reasons, these programs are not feasible or desirable for the vast majority of patients. One problem is that phases II and III involve medical supervision at a designated site (hospital, clinic, or fitness center). This presents time and transportation obstacles for many patients. Home-based programs are an attractive alternative and provide a convenient setting that can also involve the support of family members.

Several pertinent questions have been raised regarding cardiac rehabilitation programs. Do they increase the aerobic fitness of cardiac patients? Do they lengthen life and lower the risk of new cardiac events? Are they safe?

Many studies have clearly shown that cardiac patients who exercise regularly improve their aerobic fitness.[310,312] $\dot{V}O_{2max}$ increases by an average of 20%, according to most studies, and anginal symptoms often disappear or take longer to develop during a certain exercise load.

Researchers have been unable to provide a clear picture as to whether exercise by cardiac patients leads to longer life or fewer subsequent heart attacks.[314,315] Two review articles have shown that when all studies are gathered together, total and CVD mortality are reduced 20–25% for patients in cardiac rehabilitation programs, compared to those not participating.[310,312,314,315] However, the programs involved more than just exercise training, so it is difficult to quantify the role of exercise alone.

Comprehensive cardiac rehabilitation programs that include exercise, diet, and other health behavior changes do help patients keep their CHD risk factors under tighter control.[310] Perhaps more important, studies show that patients in cardiac rehabilitation programs report an improved quality of life.

Cardiac rehabilitation programs are safe.[310,312,316] The estimated incidence of heart attack in supervised cardiac rehabilitation programs is only 1/50,000 to 1/120,000 patient-hours, and of death, 1 per 784,000 patient-hours.[310] Over 80% of patients who have been reported to suffer a cardiac arrest have been successfully resuscitated with prompt defibrillation.

Box 10.9

Cardiac Rehabilitation Clinical Care Guidelines: Executive Summary from the Agency for Health Care Policy and Research

Cardiovascular disease is the leading cause of morbidity and mortality in the United States, accounting for more than 50% of all deaths. Coronary heart disease (CHD), with its clinical manifestations of stable angina pectoris, unstable angina, acute myocardial infarction, and sudden cardiac death, affects 13.5 million Americans. The almost 1 million survivors of myocardial infarction and the 7 million patients with stable angina pectoris are candidates for cardiac rehabilitation, as are the 309,000 patients who undergo coronary artery bypass graft (CABG) surgery and the 362,000 patients who undergo percutaneous transluminal coronary angioplasty (PTCA) and other transcatheter procedures each year. An estimated 4.7 million patients with heart failure may also be eligible. Although beneficial outcomes from cardiac rehabilitation services can be expected in most of these patients, few such patients currently participate in cardiac rehabilitation programs.

The U.S. Public Health Service definition of *cardiac rehabilitation*, used by the panel, states that "cardiac rehabilitation services are comprehensive, long-term programs involving medical evaluation, prescribed exercise, cardiac risk factor modification, education, and counseling. These programs are designed to limit the physiologic and psychological effects of cardiac illness, reduce the risk for sudden death or reinfarction, control cardiac symptoms,

(continued)

Box 10.9

Cardiac Rehabilitation Clinical Care Guidelines: Executive Summary from the Agency for Health Care Policy and Research *(continued)*

stabilize or reverse the atherosclerotic process, and enhance the psychosocial and vocational status of selected patients." This set of guidelines provides recommendations for cardiac rehabilitation services for patients with CHD and with heart failure, including those awaiting or following cardiac transplantation.

These guidelines are designed for use by health practitioners who provide care to patients with cardiovascular disease. These include physicians (primary care, cardiologists, and cardiovascular surgeons), nurses, exercise physiologists, dietitians, behavioral medicine specialists, psychologists, and physical and occupational therapists. The information can guide clinical decision making regarding referral and follow-up of patients for cardiac rehabilitation services, as well as administrative decisions regarding the availability of and access to cardiac rehabilitation services.

These guidelines detail the outcomes that result from cardiac rehabilitation services. The interventions examined involve two parallel applications: (1) exercise training and (2) education, counseling, and behavioral interventions. The panel emphasizes the added effectiveness of multifactorial cardiac rehabilitation services integrated in a comprehensive approach.

Outcomes of Cardiac Rehabilitation Services

The results of cardiac rehabilitation services, based on reports in the scientific literature, are summarized in these guidelines. The most substantial benefits include

- Improvement in exercise tolerance
- Improvement in symptoms
- Improvement in blood lipid levels
- Reduction in cigarette smoking
- Improvement in psychosocial well-being and reduction of stress
- Reduction in mortality

Improvement in Exercise Tolerance

Cardiac rehabilitation exercise training improves objective measures of exercise tolerance in both men and women, including elderly patients, with CHD and with heart failure. This functional improvement occurs without significant cardiovascular complications or other adverse outcomes. Appropriately prescribed and conducted exercise training should be an integral component of cardiac rehabilitation services and particularly benefits patients with decreased exercise tolerance. Maintenance of exercise training is required to sustain improvement in exercise tolerance.

Improvement in Symptoms

Cardiac rehabilitation exercise training decreases symptoms of angina pectoris in patients with CHD and decreases symptoms of heart failure in patients with left ventricular systolic dysfunction. Following exercise rehabilitation, improvement in clinical measures of myocardial ischemia, as identified by electrocardiographic (ECG) and nuclear cardiology techniques, provides objective support for the reported symptomatic improvement. Exercise training of patients with left ventricular systolic dysfunction provides added symptomatic improvement to that achieved by appropriate medication management.

Improvement in Blood Lipid Levels

Multifactorial cardiac rehabilitation in patients with CHD, including exercise training and education, results in improved lipid and lipoprotein levels. Exercise training as a sole intervention has not effected consistent improvement in lipid profiles. Optimal lipid management requires specifically directed dietary and, when medically indicated, pharmacological management as a component of multifactorial cardiac rehabilitation.

Reduction in Cigarette Smoking

Multifactorial cardiac rehabilitation, with well-designed educational and behavioral components, reduces cigarette smoking. Between 16% and 26% of patients can be expected to stop smoking. These smoking cessation rates enhance the spontaneously high smoking cessation rates in most populations following a coronary event. Scientific evidence, consensus reports, and scientific reviews in the nonrehabilitation setting, including the surgeon general's messages since 1965, lend strong support that education, counseling, and behavioral interventions are beneficial for smoking cessation.

Improvement in Psychosocial Well-Being and Stress Reduction

Exercise training enhances measures of psychological and social functioning, particularly as a component of multifactorial cardiac rehabilitation. Improvement in psychological status and functioning, including measures of

(continued)

Box 10.9

Cardiac Rehabilitation Clinical Care Guidelines: Executive Summary from the Agency for Health Care Policy and Research *(continued)*

emotional stress and reduction of the Type-A behavior pattern, is consistent with the improvement in psychosocial outcomes that occurs in nonrehabilitation settings.

Reduction in Mortality

A survival benefit for patients who participate in cardiac rehabilitation exercise training is suggested from the scientific data, but this cannot be attributed solely to exercise training because many studies involved multifactorial interventions. Meta-analysis of the randomized controlled trials of exercise rehabilitation in patients following myocardial infarction establishes a reduction in mortality approximating 25% at 3-year follow-up. This reduction in mortality approaches that resulting from pharmacological management of patients following myocardial infarction with beta-blocking drugs or patients with left ventricular systolic dysfunction with angiotensin-converting enzyme (ACE) inhibitor therapy. The reduction in cardiovascular mortality was 26% in multifactorial randomized trials of cardiac rehabilitation and 15% in trials that involved only an exercise intervention. The panel concludes that multifactorial cardiac rehabilitation services can reduce mortality in patients following myocardial infarction.

Safety

The safety of cardiac rehabilitation exercise training is inferred from aggregate analysis of clinical experience. None of the more than three dozen randomized controlled trials of cardiac rehabilitation exercise training in patients with CHD, involving over 4,500 patients, described an increase in morbidity or mortality in rehabilitation, compared with control patient groups. A survey of 142 cardiac rehabilitation programs in the United States, involving patients participating in exercise rehabilitation from 1980 to 1984, reported, based on aggregate data, a low rate of nonfatal myocardial infarction of 1 per 294,000 patient-hours; the cardiac mortality rate was 1 per 784,000 patient-hours. A total of 21 episodes of cardiac arrest occurred, with successful resuscitation of 17 patients. Thus, the safety of exercise rehabilitation is established by the very low rates of occurrence of myocardial infarction and cardiovascular complications during exercise training.

Source: Agency for Health Care Policy and Research. Full text can be downloaded from http://www.ahrg.gov/.

SUMMARY

1. Death from heart disease (also called cardiovascular disease [CVD]) is the leading killer among people in developed countries worldwide.
2. Atherosclerosis is the underlying factor in 85% of CVD deaths. Coronary heart disease (CHD) is the major form of heart disease and is caused by atherosclerosis and clotting in the coronary arteries.
3. An estimated 65 million Americans have hypertension (systolic BP $\geq$ 140 mm Hg and/or diastolic BP $\geq$ 90 mm Hg), making it the most prevalent form of CVD.
4. Nearly 1 million Americans die each year from CVD, representing 38% of all deaths. Nearly half a million die from heart attacks each year.
5. Since the 1950s, CHD deaths have dropped by 60% and stroke deaths by 72%. Half of the decline in CHD is related to changes in lifestyle.
6. Risk factors for heart disease include being male, family history, cigarette smoking, hypertension, inactivity, high serum cholesterol, low HDL-C, history of stroke or peripheral vascular disease, and severe obesity. The danger of heart attack increases with the number of risk factors.
7. Cigarette smoking is the most important of the known modifiable risk factors for CHD.
8. The relationship between exercise and smoking is complex. Many studies have shown that smoking before exercise adversely affects performance. Very few active people smoke. More studies are needed to determine the role of physical activity in reducing the desire for cigarette smoking. Weight gain is a likely outcome of smoking cessation and is related to the effect of smoking on energy expenditure.
9. The 2003 Joint National Committee on Detection, Evaluation, and Treatment of High Blood Pressure has organized a treatment scheme emphasizing nondrug approaches (especially weight reduction, salt restriction, exercise, and moderation of alcohol consumption) and various drugs to treat hypertension.
10. Heavy drinking has been consistently associated with increased risk of death from heart disease. Ethanol use alters lipoprotein metabolism and blood lipid profiles, increasing HDL-C and VLDL-C. There is good evidence that moderate drinking has a protective effect against coronary heart disease, but recommendations to increase alcohol

consumption are ill-advised because of other overriding health concerns.

11. Following a bout of aerobic exercise, blood pressures fall for 22 hours. Studies have shown that both physical fitness and habitual aerobic activity are associated with a decreased risk of hypertension. Exercise training is associated with lower blood pressures among hypertensive people.
12. Seventeen percent of Americans have blood cholesterol levels above 240 mg/dl. Death rates for CHD climb steadily when serum cholesterol levels rise.
13. There are three major lipoproteins in the fasting blood: HDL, LDL, and VLDL. LDL and HDL have opposing functions. HDL takes cholesterol to the liver, where it is changed to bile and eventually excreted in the stool. LDL takes cholesterol to the artery wall. The level of HDL-C and the ratio of total cholesterol to HDL-C are important measures of heart disease risk.
14. The National Cholesterol Education Program (NCEP) guidelines for classification and treatment of hypercholesterolemia were reviewed. The AHA dietary recommendations are based on reduction of dietary saturated fat and cholesterol, with increased intake of complex carbohydrate foods.
15. Lifestyle factors that increase HDL-C include aerobic exercise, weight control, smoking cessation, and moderate alcohol consumption. Lifestyle factors that decrease LDL-C center around low intake of saturated fat and cholesterol with weight reduction.
16. A consistent finding is that with weight loss, the total cholesterol, LDL-C, and triglyceride levels decrease, while HDL-C levels increase. The independent effect of aerobic exercise during weight loss, however, is limited to improving the magnitude of change in the triglycerides and HDL-C, but not total cholesterol and LDL-C.
17. HDL is formed within the blood by the action of two key enzymes, LPL and LCAT, and then taken out of circulation by hepatic lipase. Active people tend to have higher LPL and LCAT and lower HL enzyme activity levels.
18. Epidemiological studies have left little doubt as to the existence of a strong inverse relationship between physical exercise and risk of CHD. These observations suggest that in CHD prevention programs, regular physical activity should be promoted as vigorously as control of blood pressure, dietary modification to lower serum cholesterol, and smoking cessation.
19. The favorable effect of physical activity in decreasing CVD is probably due to several factors. One of the major factors is that regular physical activity is associated with a reduction of the major risk factors of heart disease.
20. Cardiac rehabilitation has been organized to help restore coronary artery bypass surgery patients and other heart disease patients to productive life. The emphasis in cardiac rehabilitation is usually on lifestyle changes, as well as optimization of drug therapy. Exercise is considered the cornerstone of cardiac rehabilitation, but weight control; cessation of cigarette smoking; group therapy and family counseling; vocational counseling; a low-calorie, low-fat diet; systematic follow-up examinations; and careful drug therapy are also important. There are four phases to the modern cardiac rehabilitation program.

Review Questions

1. *Which subgroup listed has the highest smoking prevalence?*

   A. People with a college education
   B. American Indian/Alaskan Native
   C. Blacks
   D. The elderly
   E. Asians

2. *The third leading "actual cause" of death in the United States is*

   A. Alcohol
   B. Poor diet, inactivity
   C. Tobacco
   D. Sexual behavior
   E. Drug abuse

3. *Smoking kills over 430,000 Americans each year. What is the number 2 ranked killer of smokers?*

   A. Lung cancer **B.** Chronic lung disease
   C. Coronary heart disease **D.** Stroke

4. *The* **Healthy People 2010** *goal for smoking prevalence among adults is ____%.*

   A. 25 **B.** 33 **C.** 5 **D.** 18 **E.** 12

5. *Chest pain that radiates to the neck and arms because of CHD is called*

   A. Cerebrovascular accident (CVA)
   B. Myocardial infarction
   C. Angina pectoris
   D. Thrombus
   E. Endarterectomy

6. *Which one of these risk factors is considered by the American Heart Association to be a contributing (but not major) factor that can be changed?*

   A. Stress **B.** Cigarette smoking
   C. Physical inactivity **D.** High blood pressure
   E. High blood cholesterol

7. *NCEP ATP III lists five major risk factors (exclusive of LDL cholesterol). Which one of the following is* **not** *included?*

   A. Cigarette smoking
   B. Low HDL cholesterol of 45 mg/dl and below
   C. Family history of premature CHD
   D. Age, with men ≥ 45 yr, and women ≥ 55 yr
   E. Hypertension

8. *Which type of stroke is least common but still a potent cause of disability and death?*

   A. Cerebral aneurism **B.** Cerebral thrombosis
   C. Endothelial **D.** Cerebral hemorrhage
   E. Intima

9. *Which one of these risk factors is* **not** *used by the American Heart Association (AHA)?*

   A. Obesity **B.** High blood pressure
   C. High homocysteine **D.** Stress
   E. High total serum cholesterol

10. *Several factors are included in the "metabolic syndrome." Which of the listed factors is* **not** *included?*

    A. Abdominal obesity
    B. Raised blood pressure
    C. Insulin resistance
    D. Large LDL particles and high HDL cholesterol
    E. Prothrombotic state

11. *____ is defined as the formation of a clot in one of the arteries that conduct blood to the heart muscle.*

    A. Coronary thrombosis **B.** Cerebrovascular accident
    C. Cerebral embolism **D.** Congestive heart failure
    E. Bradycardia

12. *Excessive alcohol intake tends to increase the risk of what type of stroke?*

    A. Cerebral hemorrhage **B.** Cerebral thrombosis
    C. Cerebral embolism **D.** TIA
    E. CHD

13. *What percentage of American adults have hypertension or prehypertension?*
    A. 57% **B.** 26% **C.** 39% **D.** 65%

14. *When the systolic blood pressure is greater than a threshold of ____ mm Hg, this is an indication of high blood pressure (when based on two or more readings).*

    A. 160 **B.** 170 **C.** 80 **D.** 140 **E.** 90

15. *The average woman who quits smoking gains ____ pounds.*

    A. 8 **B.** 15 **C.** 3 **D.** 20 **E.** 1

16. *A heart attack is also called a*

    A. Stroke **B.** Myocardial infarction
    C. Angina pectoris **D.** Cerebral thrombus

17. *Sudden temporary weakness or numbness on one side of the face is a sign of a*

    A. Heart attack **B.** Myocardial infarction
    C. Stroke **D.** Angina pectoris

18. *All Americans are urged to consume no more than ____ grams of sodium a day to prevent hypertension.*

    A. 1 **B.** 1.5 **C.** 2.4 **D.** 3.5 **E.** 4

19. *More than a threshold of ____ alcoholic drinks a day can lead to high blood pressure.*

    A. 1 **B.** 2 **C.** 3 **D.** 5

20. *____ is the smallest and most dense lipoprotein-carrying cholesterol.*

    A. LDL **B.** HDL **C.** VLDL

21. *A total cholesterol:HDL-C ratio below a threshold of ____ is considered optimal.*

    A. 1 **B.** 2 **C.** 3 **D.** 5 **E.** 10

22. *If the blood cholesterol level falls 25%, CHD risk falls ____ according to most studies.*

    A. 10–20% **B.** 25–30%
    C. 35–45% **D.** 50–75%

23. *Aerobic exercise, weight reduction, and ____ help to increase the HDL-C.*

    A. Smoking cessation **B.** Low-fat diet
    C. Low-cholesterol diet **D.** High-fiber diet

24. *In a 150-pound person, five alcoholic drinks in 1–2 hours will raise the blood alcohol level to ____.*

    A. 0.5 **B.** 0.1 **C.** 1.0 **D.** 0.2 **E.** 3.0

25. *The single most important lifestyle-change measure to reduce high blood pressure is*

   A. Cigarette smoking cessation
   B. Reduction of body weight
   C. Control of high blood cholesterol levels
   D. Sodium restriction
   E. Alcohol restriction

26. *The approximate systolic blood pressure reduction with adoption of the DASH eating plan is*

   A. 2–4 mm Hg **B.** 8–14 mm Hg
   C. 4–9 mm Hg **D.** 2–8 mm Hg

27. *An optimal LDL-C level (according to the NCEP) is less than a threshold of ____ mg/dl.*

   A. 100 **B.** 130 **C.** 160 **D.** 200

28. *Which factor listed has the overall best effect in both increasing the HDL-C and lowering the LDL-C?*

   A. Weight reduction and leanness
   B. Smoking cessation
   C. Decrease in dietary saturated fat intake
   D. Aerobic exercise
   E. Decrease in dietary cholesterol intake

29. *If body weight and quality of diet are kept constant, aerobic exercise alone can be expected to cause*

   A. An increase in HDL-C
   B. A decrease in LDL-C
   C. A decrease in total cholesterol
   D. A decrease in triglycerides
   E. Both A and D

30. *Which factor listed is most important in decreasing LDL-C and total serum cholesterol?*

   A. Control of stress
   B. Decrease in coffee consumption
   C. Decrease in dietary cholesterol intake
   D. Decrease in dietary saturated fat intake
   E. Increase in water-soluble fiber intake

31. *Triglycerides divided by ____ equals the VLDL-C.*

   A. 10 **B.** 5 **C.** 2 **D.** 14 **E.** 22

32. *The HDL-C level is considered "too low" by the National Cholesterol Education Program (NCEP) when under a threshold of ____ mg/dl.*

   A. 25 **B.** 40 **C.** 45 **D.** 65 **E.** 55

33. *If a person has a total cholesterol level of 280 mg/dl, HDL-C of 55 mg/dl, and triglycerides of 120 mg/dl, what is the LDL-C level?*

   A. 256 **B.** 190 **C.** 201 **D.** 178 **E.** 226

34. *The National Cholesterol Education Program has established that total serum cholesterol levels of ____ mg/dl indicate "borderline-high" levels.*

   A. 180–200
   B. 200–239
   C. 220–279
   D. 240–299
   E. 130–160

35. *Which lipoprotein has the highest percent of weight as cholesterol?*

   A. LDL **B.** HDL
   C. VLDL **D.** TC
   E. TC:HDL-C

36. *There are several major nonpharmacologic therapies recommended for hypertension control. Which one of the following is* **not** *included?*

   A. Restriction of alcohol
   B. Increased intake of vitamin C
   C. Restriction of sodium
   D. Weight reduction
   E. Exercise

37. *In the United States, normotensives at age 55 years have a ____ lifetime risk for developing hypertension.*

   A. 30% **B.** 4%
   C. 50% **D.** 75%
   E. 90%

38. *Another name for "stroke" is*

   A. Coronary thrombosis
   B. Cerebrovascular accident
   C. Cerebral embolism
   D. Congestive heart failure
   E. Arteriosclerosis

39. *The* **Healthy People 2010** *goal for the mean serum cholesterol level among adults is no more than ____ mg/dl.*

   A. 160 **B.** 184 **C.** 199 **D.** 222 **E.** 240

40. *Which one of the following is* **not** *a "well-documented modifiable" risk factor for stroke (according to the AHA)?*

   A. Diabetes **B.** Sickle cell disease
   C. Smoking **D.** Carotid artery disease
   E. High white blood cell count

41. *Which of the statements regarding alcohol consumption is true?*

A. It is inversely related to coronary heart disease.
B. It decreases risk for various cancers.
C. It decreases risk for hypertension.
D. One drink raises the blood alcohol level to 0.10.
E. It decreases the HDL-C level.

42. *Which one of the following is* **not** *considered effective in lowering LDL-C and total cholesterol?*

A. Reduce dietary cholesterol intake
B. Increase soluble fiber intake
C. Reduce saturated fat intake
D. Increase polyunsaturated fat intake
E. Increase aerobic exercise

43. *Regular aerobic exercise in individuals with high blood pressure lowers systolic blood pressure by an average of ____ mm Hg.*

A. 15–20 B. 5–7 C. 20–30 D. 1–2 E. 3–6

44. *Which one of the following lifestyle factors has* **not** *been linked to lower triglyceride levels?*

A. Aerobic exercise
B. Loss of body weight
C. Reduced sodium intake
D. Reduced alcohol intake

45. *Single bouts of prolonged endurance exercise cause an acute ____ in HDL-C.*

A. Increase B. Decrease
C. No change

46. *As a general rule of thumb, the risk for CHD among physically inactive people is ____ that of people who are relatively active.*

A. Twice B. Triple
C. Half D. One third

47. *Which one of the following is* **not** *regarded as a mechanism for the reduced risk of CHD among active people?*

A. Coronary arteries expand more and are less stiff in older age.
B. Coronary arteries are larger.
C. Other risk factors are under better control.
D. Clot formation aptitude is increased.
E. Heart muscle is bigger and stronger.

48. *Triglyceride levels under ____ mg/dl are considered normal by the NCEP.*

A. 100 B. 150 C. 400 D. 1,000 E. 80

49. *There are several emerging risk factors for heart disease according to the NCEP. Which one of the following is* **not** *included?*

A. Obesity
B. Prothrombotic factors
C. Impaired fasting glucose
D. Homocysteine
E. Lipoprotein(a)

50. *Which drug listed is used to reduce LDL cholesterol?*

A. Beta-blocker B. Calcium channel blocker
C. Bile acid sequestrant D. ACE inhibitor
E. Diuretic

51. *The metabolic syndrome is identified using several factors, including*

A. Triglycerides ≥ 150 mg/dl
B. Blood pressure ≥ 125/83 mm Hg
C. Fasting glucose ≥ 100 mg/dl
D. Waist circumference in men of > 35 inches
E. HDL cholesterol in men of < 50 mg/dl

52. *Lifestyle changes are recommended for people in all coronary risk groups depending on their LDL cholesterol level. NCEP ATP III recommends a multifaceted lifestyle approach to reduce risk for CHD. Which one of the following is* **not** *included?*

A. Reduced intakes of saturated fats, <7% of total Calories
B. Weight reduction
C. Stress management
D. Reduced intakes of cholesterol, <200 mg/day
E. Therapeutic options such as plant stanols/sterols (2 grams/day) and viscous (soluble) fiber (10–25 grams/day).

53. *In 2000, the American Heart Association revised its dietary and lifestyle guidelines for reducing the risk of cardiovascular disease. Which one of the following is listed in the section, "Issues That Merit Further Research?"*

A. Limit intake of *trans*-fatty acids.
B. Keep saturated fat intake at less than 10% of energy.
C. Walk or do other activities for at least 30 minutes on most days.
D. Consume one fatty fish meal per day.
E. Limit salt intake to 6 grams/day.

Answers

1. B	**6.** A	**11.** A	**16.** B	**21.** C	**26.** B	**31.** B	**36.** B	**41.** A	**46.** A	**51.** A
2. A	**7.** B	**12.** A	**17.** C	**22.** D	**27.** A	**32.** B	**37.** E	**42.** E	**47.** D	**52.** C
3. C	**8.** D	**13.** A	**18.** C	**23.** A	**28.** A	**33.** C	**38.** B	**43.** B	**48.** B	**53.** D
4. E	**9.** C	**14.** D	**19.** C	**24.** B	**29.** E	**34.** B	**39.** C	**44.** C	**49.** A	
5. C	**10.** D	**15.** A	**20.** B	**25.** B	**30.** D	**35.** A	**40.** E	**45.** A	**50.** C	

REFERENCES

1. American Heart Association. *Heart Disease and Stroke Statistics—2005 Update.* Dallas, TX: American Heart Association, 2005.
2. U.S. Department of Health and Human Services. *Healthy People 2010.* Washington DC: January, 2000. http://www.health.gov/healthypeople/.
3. Hoyert DL, Kung HC, Smith BL. Deaths: Preliminary data for 2003. *National Vital Statistics Reports* 53(15). Hyattsville, MD: National Center for Health Statistics, 2005.
4. McGill HC, McMahan CA, Herderick EE, Malcom GT, Tracy RE, Strong JP. Origin of atherosclerosis in childhood and adolescence. *Am J Clin Nutr* 72(5 suppl):1307S–1315S, 2000.
5. Van Oostrom AJ, van Wijk J, Cabezas MC. Lipemia, inflammation and atherosclerosis: Novel opportunities in the understanding and treatment of atherosclerosis. *Drugs* 64(Suppl 2):19–41,2004.
6. Kullo IJ, Ballantyne CM. Conditional risk factors for atherosclerosis. *Mayo Clin Proc* 80:219–230, 2005.
7. Zhu J, Nieto FJ, Horne BD, Anderson JL, Muhlestein JB, Epstein SE. Prospective study of pathogen burden and risk of myocardial infarction or death. *Circulation* 103:45–50, 2001.
8. Stary HC. The sequence of cell and matrix changes in atherosclerotic lesions of coronary arteries in the first 40 years of life. *Eur Heart J* 11(suppl):3–19, 1990.
9. McGill HC, McMahan CA, Malcom GT, Oalmann MC, Strong JP. Effects of serum lipoproteins and smoking on atherosclerosis in young men and women. The PDAY Research Group. Pathobiological determinants of atherosclerosis in youth. *Arterioscler Thromb Vasc Biol* 17:95–106, 1997.
10. Kavey REW, Daniels SR, Lauer RM, Atkins DL, Hayman LL, Taubert K. American Heart Association guidelines for primary prevention of atherosclerotic cardiovascular disease beginning in childhood. *Circulation* 107:1562–1566, 2003.
11. Goldstein LB, Adams R, Becker K, et al. AHA Scientific Statement. Primary prevention of ischemic stroke. A statement for healthcare professionals from the Stroke Council of the American Heart Association. *Circulation* 103:163–182, 2001.
12. Gorelick PB, Sacco RL, Smith DB, et al. Prevention of first stroke. A review of guidelines and a multidisciplinary consensus statement from the National Stroke Association. *JAMA* 281:1112–1120, 1999.
13. Enos WF, Holmes RH, Beyer J. Coronary disease among United States soldiers killed in action in Korea. *JAMA* 152:1090–1093, 1953.
14. National Center for Health Statistics. *Health, United States, 2005.* Hyattsville, MD: 2005. www.cdc.gov/nchs.
15. Hunink MGM, Goldman L, Tosteson ANA, et al. The recent decline in mortality from coronary heart disease, 1980–1990. The effect of secular trends in risk factors and treatment. *JAMA* 277:535–542, 1997.
16. Cooper R, Cutler J, Desvigne-Nickens P, et al. Trends and disparities in coronary heart disease, stroke, and other cardiovascular diseases in the United States. *Circulation* 102:3137–3147, 2000.
17. National Center for Chronic Disease Prevention and Health Promotion, CDC. Decline in deaths from heart disease and stroke—United States, 1900–1999. *MMWR* 48(30):649–656, 1999.
18. Capewell S, Beaglehole R, Seddon M, McMurray J. Explanation for the decline in coronary heart disease mortality rates in Auckland, New Zealand, between 1982 and 1993. *Circulation* 102:1511–1516, 2000.
19. Grundy SM, Balady GJ, Criqui MH, et al. Guide to primary prevention of cardiovascular diseases. A statement for healthcare professionals from the task force on risk reduction. *Circulation* 95:2329–2331, 1997.
20. Greenland P, Knoll MD, Stamler J, Neaton JD, Dyer AR, Garside DB, Wilson PW. Major risk factors as antecedents of fatal and nonfatal coronary heart disease events. *JAMA* 290:891–897, 2003.
21. *Third Report of the National Cholesterol Education Program (NCEP) Expert Panel on Detection, Evaluation, and Treatment of High Blood Cholesterol in Adults* (Adult Treatment Panel III), 2001. http://www.nhlbi.nih.gov/.
22. Smith SC, Greenland P, Grundy SM. Prevention Conference V. Beyond secondary prevention: Identifying the high-risk patient for primary prevention. Executive summary. *Circulation* 101:111–116, 2000.
23. Langlois M, Duprez D, Delanghe J, De Buyzere M, Clement DL. Serum vitamin C concentration is low in peripheral arterial disease and is associated with inflammation and severity of atherosclerosis. *Circulation* 103:1863–1870, 2001.
24. Anderson JL, Muhlestein JB, Horne BD, Carlquist JF, Bair TL, Madsen TE, Pearson RR. Plasma homocysteine predicts mortality independently of traditional risk factors and C-reactive protein in patients with angiographically defined coronary artery disease. *Circulation* 102:1227–1233, 2000.
25. Stec JJ, Silbershatz H, Tofler GH, Matheney TH, Sutherland P, Lipinska I, Massaro JM, Wilson PFW, Muller JE, D'Agostino RB. Association of fibrinogen with cardiovascular risk factors and cardiovascular disease in the Framingham offspring population. *Circulation* 102:1634–1640, 2000.
26. Hebert PR, Rich-Edwards JW, Manson JE, et al. Height and incidence of cardiovascular disease in male physicians. *Circulation* 88:1437–1443, 1993.
27. Fang J, Alderman MH. Serum uric acid and cardiovascular mortality. The NHANES I epidemiologic follow-up study, 1971–1992. National Health and Nutrition Examination Survey. *JAMA* 283:2404–2410, 2000.

28. Lotufo PA, Chae CU, Ajani UA, Hennekens CH, Manson JE. Male pattern baldness and coronary heart disease: The Physicians' Health Study. *Arch Intern Med* 160:165–171, 2000.

29. Danesh J, Collins R, Peto R. Lipoprotein(a) and coronary heart disease. Meta-analysis of prospective studies. *Circulation* 102:1082–1089, 2000.

30. Volpato S, Guralnik JM, Ferrucci L, Balfour J, Chaves P, Fried LP, Harris TB. Cardiovascular disease, interleukin-6, and risk of mortality in older women. The Women's Health and Aging Study. *Circulation* 103:947–952, 2001.

31. Myers GL, Rifai N, Tracy RP, et al. CDC/AHA workshop on markers of inflammation and cardiovascular disease. Application to clinical and public health practice. Report from the Laboratory Science Discussion Group. *Circulation* 110:e545–e549, 2004.

32. Deary IJ, Fowkes FGR, Donnan PT, Housley E. Hostile personality and risks of peripheral arterial disease in the general population. *Psychosomatic Med* 56:197–202, 1994.

33. Sorensen TIA, Nielsen GG, Andersen PK, Teasdale TW. Genetic and environmental influences on premature death in adult adoptees. *N Engl J Med* 318:727–732, 1988.

34. Marenberg ME, Risch N, Berkman LF, Floderus B, De Faire U. Genetic susceptibility to death from coronary heart disease in a study of twins. *N Engl J Med* 330:1041–1046, 1994.

35. Manson JE, Tosteson H, Ridker PM, et al. The primary prevention of myocardial infarction. *N Engl J Med* 326:1406–1413, 1992.

36. Bronner LL, Kanter DS, Manson JE. Primary prevention of stroke. *N Engl J Med* 333:1392–1400, 1995.

37. Grundy SM, Pasternak R, Greenland P, Smith S, Fuster V. Assessment of cardiovascular risk by use of multiple-risk-factor assessment equations. A statement of healthcare professionals from the American Heart Association and the American College of Cardiology. *Circulation* 100:1481–1492, 1999.

38. American College of Cardiology and American Heart Association. ACC/AHA 2004 guideline update for coronary artery bypass graft surgery. www.americanheart.org.

39. American College of Cardiology and American Heart Association. ACC/AHA guidelines for percutaneous coronary intervention (revision of the 1993 PTCA guidelines)—Executive summary. *Circulation* 103:3019–3041, 2001.

40. Loscalzo J. Regression of coronary atherosclerosis. *N Engl J Med* 323:1337–1339, 1990.

41. Brown BG, Zhao XQ, Sacco DE, Albers JJ. Lipid lowering and plaque regression: New insights into prevention of plaque disruption and clinical events in coronary disease. *Circulation* 87:1781–1789, 1993.

42. Nissen SE, Tuzcu EM, Schoenhagen P, Brown BG, Ganz P, Vogel RA, Crowe T, Howard G, Cooper CJ, Brodie B, Grines CL, DeMaria AN; REVERSAL Investigators. Effect of intensive compared with moderate lipid-lowering therapy on progression of coronary atherosclerosis: A randomized controlled trial. *JAMA* 291:1071–1080, 2004.

43. Sever PS, Dahlof B, Poulter NR, Wedel H, Beevers G, Caulfield M, Collins R, Kjeldsen SE, Kristinsson A, McInnes GT, Mehlsen J, Nieminen M, O'Brien E, Ostergren J; ASCOT Investigators. Prevention of coronary and stroke events with atorvastatin in hypertensive patients who have average or lower-than-average cholesterol concentrations, in the Anglo-Scandinavian Cardiac Outcomes Trial—Lipid Lowering Arm (ASCOT_LLA): A multicenter randomized controlled trial. *Drugs* 64(suppl 2):43–60, 2004.

44. Ornish D, Scherwitz LW, Billings JH, Brown SE, Gould KL, Merritt TA, Sparler S, Armstrong WT, Ports TA, Kirkeeide RL, Hogeboom C, Brand RJ. Intensive lifestyle changes for reversal of coronary heart disease. *JAMA* 280:2001–2007, 1998.

45. Ornish D, Brown SE, Scherwitz LW, et al. Can lifestyle changes reverse coronary artery heart disease? *Lancet* 336:129–133, 1990.

46. Watts GF, Lewis B, Brunt JNH, et al. Effects on coronary artery disease of lipid-lowering diet, or diet plus cholestyramine, in the St Thomas' Atherosclerosis Regression Study (STARS). *Lancet* 339:563–569, 1992.

47. Hambrecht R, Niebauer J, Marburger C, et al. Various intensities of leisure time physical activity in patients with coronary artery disease: Effects on cardiorespiratory fitness and progression of coronary atherosclerotic lesions. *J Am Coll Cardiol* 22:468–477, 1993.

48. Schuler G, Hambrecht R, Schlierf G, et al. Regular physical exercise and low-fat diet: Effects on progression of coronary artery disease. *Circulation* 86:1–11, 1992.

49. Merz CN, Rozanski A, Forrester JS. The secondary prevention of coronary artery disease. *Am J Med* 102:572–581, 1997.

50. Feeman WE, Niebauer J. Prediction of angiographic stabilization/regression of coronary atherosclerosis by a risk factor graph. *J Cardiovasc Risk* 7:415–423, 2000.

51. Stampfer MJ, Hu FB, Manson JE, Rimm EB, Willett WC. Primary prevention of coronary heart disease in women through diet and lifestyle. *N Engl J Med* 343:16–22, 2000.

52. U.S. Department of Health and Human Services. *The Health Consequences of Smoking: A Report of the Surgeon General.* U.S. Department of Health and Human Services, Centers for Disease Control and Prevention, National Center for Chronic Disease Prevention and Health Promotion, Office on Smoking and Health, 2004.

53. Mokdad AH, Marks JS, Stroup DF, Gerberding JL. Actual causes of death in the United States, 2000. *JAMA* 291:1238–1245, 2004.

54. CDC. Cigarette smoking-attributable mortality and years of potential life lost—United States. *MMWR* 46(20):444–451, 1997. See also: CDC. Cigarette smoking-attributable morbidity—United States, 2000. *MMWR* 52:842–843, 2003.

55. Neaton JD, Wentworth D. Serum cholesterol, blood pressure, cigarette smoking, and death from coronary heart disease. *Arch Intern Med* 152:56–64, 1992.

56. Ockene IS, Miller NH. Cigarette smoking, cardiovascular disease, and stroke. A statement for healthcare professionals from the American Heart Association. *Circulation* 96:3243–3247, 1997.

57. Howard G, Wagenknecht LE, Burke GL, Diez-Rioux A, Evans GW, McGovern P, Nieto J, Tell GS. Cigarette smoking and progression of atherosclerosis. The Atherosclerosis Risk in Communities (ARIC) study. *JAMA* 279:119–124, 1998.

58. Kaufmann PA, Gnecchi-Riscone T, Di Terlizzi M, Schafers KP, Luscher TF, Camici PG. Coronary heart disease in smokers. Vitamin C restores coronary microcirculatory function. *Circulation* 102:1233–1239, 2000.

59. CDC. Cigarette smoking among adults—United States, 2002. *MMWR* 53(20):427–431, 2004.

60. CDC. Cigarette use among high school students—United States, 1991–2003. *MMWR* 53(23):499–502, 2004. See also: CDC. Tobacco use, access, and exposure to tobacco in media among middle and high school students—United States, 2004. *MMWR* 54(12):297–301, 2005.

61. Escobedo LG, Reddy M, DuRant RH. Relationship between cigarette smoking and health risk and problem behaviors among US adolescents. *Arch Pediatr Adolesc Med* 151:66–71, 1997.

62. U.S. Department of Health and Human Services. *Strategies to Control Tobacco Use in the United States: A Blueprint for Public Health Action in the 1990's.* USDHHS, Public Health Service, National Institutes of Health, National Cancer Institute. NIH Publication No. 92–3316, 1991.

63. U.S. Department of Health and Human Services. *Major Local Tobacco Control Ordinances in the United States.* USDHHS, Public Health Service, National Institutes of Health, National Cancer Institute. NIH Publication No. 93–3532, 1993.

64. U.S. Environmental Protection Agency. *Respiratory Health Effects of Passive Smoking: Lung Cancer and Other Disorders.* U.S. Environmental Protection Agency, Office of Research and Development. Washington, DC: U.S. EPA, 1992.

65. Steenland K, Thun M, Lally C, Heath C. Environmental tobacco smoke and coronary heart disease in the American Cancer Society CPS-II cohort. *Circulation* 94:622–628, 1996.

66. National Cancer Institute. *Health Effects of Exposure to Environmental Tobacco Smoke: The Report of the California Environmental Protection Agency. Smoking and Tobacco Control Monograph no. 10.* Bethesda, MD. U.S. Department of Health and Human Services, National Institutes of Health, National Cancer Institute, NIH Pub. No. 99–4645, 1999.

67. National Institute for Occupational Safety and Health. *Current Intelligence Bulletin 54: Environmental Tobacco Smoke in the Workplace: Lung Cancer and Other Health Effects.* U.S. Department of Health and Human Services, Centers for Disease Control, National Institute for Occupational Safety and Health, June 1991. DHHS Publication No. (NIOSH) 91–108.

68. U.S. Department of Health and Human Services. *Smokeless Tobacco and Health: An International Perspective.* USDHHS, Public Health Service, National Institutes of Health, National Cancer Institute. NIH Publication No. 93–3461,1992.

69. CDC. Use of smokeless tobacco among adults—United States, 1991. *MMWR* 42(14):263–266, 1993. See also: *MMWR* 45(20):413–418, 1996; *MMWR* 49(SS-10):1–50, 2000.

70. Ernster VL, Grady DG, Greene JC, et al. Smokeless tobacco use and health effects among baseball players. *JAMA* 264:218–224, 1990.

71. Report of the Surgeon General. *The Health Consequences of Smoking: Nicotine Addiction.* Washington, DC: U.S. Department of Health and Human Services, Publication No. CDC 88–8406, 1988.

72. Fiore MC, Bailey WC, Cohen SJ, et al. *Treating tobacco use and dependence.* Clinical practice guidelines. Summary. Rockville, MD: U.S. Department of Health and Human Services. Public Health Service. June 2000. (Reprinted, *Respiratory Care* 45(10):1196–1262, 2000).

73. U.S. Department of Health and Human Services. *Reducing Tobacco Use: A Report of the Surgeon General—Executive Summary.* Atlanta, GA: U.S. Department of Health and Human Services, Centers for Disease Control and Prevention, National Center for Chronic Disease Prevention and Health Promotion, Office on Smoking and Health, 2000.

74. Audrain-McGovern J, Rodriguez D, Moss HB. Smoking progression and physical activity. *Cancer Epidemiol Biomarkers Prev* 12:1121–1129, 2003.

75. Williard JC, Schoenborn CA. Relationship between cigarette smoking and other unhealthy behaviors among our nation's youth: United States, 1992. *Advance Data from Vital and Health Statistics,* no 263. Hyattsville, MD: National Center for Health Statistics, 1995.

76. Simoes EJ, Byers T, Coates RJ, Serdula MK, Mokdad AH, Heath GW. The association between leisure-time physical activity and dietary fat in American adults. *Am J Public Health* 85:240–244, 1995.

77. Bernaards CM, Twisk JWR, Van Mechelen W, Snel J, Kemper HCG. A longitudinal study on smoking in relationship to fitness and heart rate response. *Med Sci Sports Exerc* 35:793–800, 2003.

78. Lazarus NB, Kaplan GA, Cohen RD, Leu D-J. Smoking and body mass in the natural history of physical activity: Prospective evidence from the Alameda County Study, 1965–1974. *Am J Prev Med* 5:127–135, 1989.

79. Huerta M, Grotto I, Shemla S, Ashkenazi I, Shpilberg O, Kark JD. Cycle ergometry estimation of physical fitness among Israeli soldiers. *Mil Med* 169:217–220, 2004.

80. Marti B, Abelin T, Minder CE, Vader JP. Smoking, alcohol consumption, and endurance capacity: An analysis of 6,500 19-year-old conscripts and 4,100 joggers. *Prev Med* 17:79–92, 1988.

81. Dannenberg AL, Keller JB, Wilson WF, Castelli WP. Leisure time physical activity in the Framingham offspring study. *Am J Epidemiol* 129:76–88, 1989.

82. Erikssen SL, Thaulow E. Smoking habits and long-term decline in physical fitness and lung function in men. *Br Med J* 311:715–718, 1995.

83. Huie MJ. The effects of smoking on exercise performance. *Sports Med* 22:355–359, 1996.

84. Symons JD, Stebbins CL. Hemodynamic and regional blood flow responses to nicotine at rest and during exercise. *Med Sci Sports Exerc* 28:457–467, 1996.

85. Gold DR, Wang X, Wypij D, Speizer FE, Ware JH, Dockery DW. Effects of cigarette smoking on lung function in adolescent boys and girls. *N Engl J Med* 335:931–937, 1996.

86. Colberg SR, Casazza GA, Horning MA, Brooks GA. Metabolite and hormonal response in smokers during rest and sustained exercise. *Med Sci Sports Exerc* 27:1527–1534, 1995.

87. McDonough P, Moffatt RJ. Smoking-induced elevations in blood carboxyhemoglobin levels. Effect on maximal oxygen uptake. *Sports Med* 27:275–283, 1999.

88. Agudo A, Bardagi S, Romero PV, Gonzalez CA. Exercise-induced airways narrowing and exposure to environmental tobacco smoke in schoolchildren. *Am J Epidemiol* 140:409–417, 1994.

89. Frette C, Barrett-Connor E, Clausen JL. Effect of active and passive smoking on ventilatory function in elderly men and women. *Am J Epidemiol* 143:757–765, 1996.

90. Huie MJ, Casazza GA, Horning MA, Brooks GA. Smoking increases conversion of lactate to glucose during submaximal exercise. *J Appl Physiol* 80:1554–1559, 1996.

91. Kobayashi Y, Takeuchi T, Hosoi T, Loeppky JA. Effects of habitual smoking on cardiorespiratory responses to sub-maximal exercise. *J Physiol Anthropol Appl Human Sci* 23:163–169, 2004.

92. Higgins MW, Enright PL, Kronmal RA, et al. Smoking and lung function in elderly men and women: The cardiovascular health study. *JAMA* 269:2741–2748, 1993.

93. Cooper KH, Gey GO, Bottenberg RA. Effects of cigarette smoking on endurance performance. *JAMA* 203(3):123–126, 1968.

94. Hashizume K, Yamaji K, Kusaka Y, Kawahara K. Effects of abstinence from cigarette smoking on the cardiorespiratory capacity. *Med Sci Sports Exerc* 32:386–391, 2000.

95. Cooper KH. *Aerobics.* New York: Bantam Books, 1968. *The New Aerobics.* New York: Bantam Books, 1970.

96. Koplan JP, Powell KE, et al. An epidemiologic study of the benefits and risks of running. *JAMA* 248:3118–3121, 1982.

97. Nieman DC, Butler JV, Pollett LM, Dietrich SJ, Lutz RD. Nutrient intake of marathon runners. *J Am Diet Assoc* 89:1273–1278, 1989.
98. Blair SN, Goodyear NN, Wynne KL, Saunders RP. Comparison of dietary and smoking habit changes in physical fitness improvers and nonimprovers. *Prev Med* 13:411–420, 1984.
99. King AC, Haskell WL, Taylor CB, Kraemer HC, DeBusk RF. Group- versus home-based exercise training in healthy older men and women. *JAMA* 266:1535–1542, 1991.
100. Marcus BH, Albrecht AE, King TK, Parisi AF, Pinto BM, Roberts M, Niaura RS, Abrams DB. The efficacy of exercise as an aid for smoking cessation in women: A randomized controlled trial. *Arch Intern Med* 159:1229–1234, 1999.
101. Derby CA, Lasater TM, Vass K, Gonzalez S, Carleton RA. Characteristics of smokers who attempt to quit and of those who recently succeeded. *Am J Prev Med* 10:327–334, 1994.
102. Daniel J, Cropley M, Ussher M, West R. Acute effects of a short bout of moderate versus light intensity exercise versus inactivity on tobacco withdrawal symptoms in sedentary smokers. *Psychopharmacology (Berl)* 174:320–326, 2004.
103. Gritz ER, Klesges RC, Meyers AW. The smoking and body weight relationship: Implications for intervention and postcessation weight control. *Ann Beh Med* 11(4):144–153, 1989.
104. Williamson DF, Madans J, Anda RF, et al. Smoking cessation and severity of weight gain in a national cohort. *N Engl J Med* 324:739–745, 1991.
105. Klesges RC, Meyers AW, Winders SE, French SN. Determining the reasons for weight gain following smoking cessation: Current findings, methodological issues, and future directions for research. *Ann Beh Med* 11(4):134–143, 1989.
106. O'Hara P, Connett JE, Lee WW, Nides M, Murray R, Wise R. Early and late weight gain following smoking cessation in the Lung Health Study. *Am J Epidemiol* 148:821–830, 1998.
107. U.S. Department of Health and Human Services. *The Health Benefits of Smoking Cessation.* U.S. Department of Health and Human Services, Public Health Service, Centers for Disease Control, Center for Chronic Disease Prevention and Health Promotion, Office on Smoking and Health. DHHS Publication No. (CDC) 90–8416. Washington, DC: Superintendent of Documents, 1990.
108. Filozof C, Fernandez-Pinilla MC, Fernandez-Cruz A. Smoking cessation and weight gain. *Obes Rev* 5:95–103, 2004.
109. Klesges RC, Eck LH, Isbell TR, Fulliton W, Hanson CL. Smoking status: Effects on the dietary intake, physical activity, and body fat of adult men. *Am J Clin Nutr* 51:784–789, 1990.
110. Perkins KA, Epstein LH, Stiller RL, et al. Metabolic effects of nicotine after consumption of a meal in smokers and nonsmokers. *Am J Clin Nutr* 52:228–233, 1990.
111. Moffatt RJ, Owens SG. Cessation from cigarette smoking: Changes in body weight, body composition, resting metabolism, and energy consumption. *Metabolism* 40:465–470, 1991.
112. Collins LC, Cornelius MF, Vogel RL, Walker JF, Stamford BA. Effect of caffeine and/or cigarette smoking on resting energy expenditure. *Int J Obes Relat Metab Disord* 18:551–556, 1994.
113. Hofstetter A, Schutz Y, Jequier E, Wahren J. Increased 24–hour energy expenditure in cigarette smokers. *N Eng J Med* 314:79–82, 1986.
114. Kawachi I, Troisi RJ, Rotnitzky AG, Coakley EH, Colditz GA. Can physical activity minimize weight gain in women after smoking cessation? *Am J Public Health* 86:999–1004, 1996.
115. Marcus B, Albrecht AE, Niaura RS, et al. Exercise enhances the maintenance of smoking cessation in women. *Addict Behav* 20:87–92, 1995.
116. Brown DR, Croft JB, Anda RF, Barrett DH, Escobedo LG. Evaluation of smoking on the physical activity and depressive symptoms relationship. *Med Sci Sports Exerc* 28:233–240, 1996.
117. Blair SN, Kampert JB, Kohl HW, et al. Influences of cardiorespiratory fitness and other precursors on cardiovascular disease and all-cause mortality in men and women. *JAMA* 276:205–210, 1996.
118. National High Blood Pressure Education Program. *The Seventh Report of the Joint National Committee on Detection, Evaluation, and Treatment of High Blood Pressure.* National Heart, Lung, and Blood Institute, National Institutes of Health, NIH Publication No. 03-5233. Bethesda, MD: National Institutes of Health, 2003.
119. National High Blood Pressure Education Program. Working Group Report on Primary Prevention of Hypertension. National Heart, Lung, and Blood Institute. Hyattsville, MD: National Institutes of Health, 1992.
120. Stamler J, Stamler R, Neaton JD. Blood pressure, systolic and diastolic, and cardiovascular risks: US population data. *Arch Intern Med* 153:598–615, 1993.
121. Cooper R, Rotimi C, Ataman S, et al. The prevalence of hypertension in seven populations of West African Origin. *Am J Public Health* 87:160–168, 1997.
122. Wang Y, Wang QJ. The prevalence of prehypertension and hypertension among US adults according to the new Joint National Committee guidelines. *Arch Intern Med* 164:2126–2134, 2004.
123. Muntner P, He J, Cutler JA, Wildman RP, Whelton PK. Trends in blood pressure among children and adolescents. *JAMA* 291:2107–2113, 2004.
124. National Heart, Lung, and Blood Institute. *High Blood Pressure: Treat It for Life.* Washington, DC: U.S. Government Printing Office, 1994.
125. Kannel WB. Blood pressure as a cardiovascular risk factor: Prevention and treatment. *JAMA* 275:1571–1576, 1996.
126. Psaty BM, Furberg CD, Kuller LH, Cushman M, Savage PJ, Levine D, O'Leary DH, Bryan N, Anderson M, Lumley T. Association between blood pressure level and the risk of myocardial infarction, stroke, and total mortality. The Cardiovascular Health Study. *Arch Intern Med* 161:1183–11922, 2001.
127. Agmon Y, Khandheria BK, Meissner I, Schwartz GL, Petterson TM, O'Fallon WM, Gentile F, Whisnant JP, Wiebers DO, Seward JB. Independent association of high blood pressure and aortic atherosclerosis: A population-based study. *Circulation* 102:2087–2093, 2000.
128. Launer LJ, Masaki K, Petrovitch H, Foley D, Havlik RJ. The association between midlife blood pressure levels and late-life cognitive function. The Honolulu-Asia Aging Study. *JAMA* 274:1846–1851, 1995.
129. Taylor AA. Combination drug treatment of hypertension: Have we come full circle? *Curr Cardiol Rep* 6:421–426, 2004.
130. Gress TW, Nieto FJ, Shahar E, Wofford MR, Brancati FL. Hypertension and antihypertensive therapy as risk factors for type 2 diabetes mellitus. Atherosclerosis Risk in Communities Study. *N Engl J Med* 342:905–912, 2000.
131. Pontremoli R, Leoncini G, Parodi A. Use of nifedipine in the treatment of hypertension. *Expert Rev Cardiovasc Ther* 3:43–50, 2005.
132. Weir MR, Maibach EW, Bakris GL, Black HR, Chawla P, Messerli FH, Neutel JM, Weber MA. Implications of a health lifestyle and medication analysis for improving hypertension control. *Arch Intern Med* 160:481–490, 2000.
133. Wofford MR, Hall JE. Pathophysiology and treatment of obesity hypertension. *Curr Pharm Des* 10:3621–3637, 2004.

134. Nowson CA, Worsley A, Margerison C, Jorna MK, Godfrey SJ, Booth A. Blood pressure change with weight loss is affected by diet type in men. *Am J Clin Nutr* 81:983–989, 2005.

135. Appel LJ, Champagne CM, Harsha DW, Cooper LS, Obarzanek E, Elmer PJ, Stevens VJ, Vollmer WM, Lin PH, Svetky LP, Stedman SW, Young DR; Writing Group of the PREMIER Collaborative Research Group. Effects of comprehensive lifestyle modification on blood pressure control: Main results of the PREMIER clinical trial. *JAMA* 289:2083–2093, 2003.

136. Neaton JD, Grimm RH, Prineas RJ, et al. Treatment of mild hypertension study: Final results. *JAMA* 270:713–724, 1993.

137. Treatment of Mild Hypertension Research Group. The Treatment of Mild Hypertension Study: A randomized, placebo-controlled trial of a nutritional-hygienic regimen along with various drug monotherapies. *Arch Intern Med* 151:1413–1423, 1991.

138. Stevens VJ, Corrigan SA, Obarzanek E, et al. Weight loss intervention in phase I of the trials of hypertension prevention. *Arch Intern Med* 153:849–858, 1993.

139. Davis BR, Blaufox MD, Oberman A, et al. Reduction in long-term antihypertensive medication requirements: Effects of weight reduction by dietary intervention in overweight persons with mild hypertension. *Arch Intern Med* 153:1773–1782, 1993.

140. The Trials of Hypertension Prevention Collaborative Research Group. The effects of nonpharmacologic interventions on blood pressure of persons with high normal levels. *JAMA* 267:1213–1220, 1992.

141. Wilsgaard T, Schirmer H, Arnesen E. Impact of body weight on blood pressure with a focus on sex differences: The Tromso Study, 1986–1995. *Arch Intern Med* 160:2847–2853, 2000.

142. Curhan GC, Chertow GM, Willett WC, et al. Birth weight and adult hypertension and obesity in women. *Circulation* 94:1310–1315, 1996.

143. The Trials of Hypertension Prevention Collaborative Research Group. Effects of weight loss and sodium reduction intervention on blood pressure and hypertension incidence in overweight people with high-normal blood pressure. *Arch Intern Med* 157:657–667, 1997.

144. Stamler J. The INTERSALT Study: Background, methods, findings, and implications. *Am J Clin Nutr* 65(suppl):626S–642S, 1997.

145. Stamler J, Rose G, Stamler R, Elliott P, Dyer A, Marmot M. INTERSALT study findings: Public health and medical care implications. *Hypertension* 14:570–577, 1989.

146. Law MR, Frost CD, Wald NJ. By how much does dietary salt reduction lower blood pressure? Analysis of observational data among populations. *Br J Med* 302:811–815, 1991.

147. He FJ, MacGregor GA. Effect of longer-term modest salt reduction on blood pressure. *Cochrane Database Syst Rev* 3:CD004937, 2004.

148. Tobian L. Dietary sodium chloride and potassium have effects on the pathophysiology of hypertension in humans and animals. *Am J Clin Nutr* 65(suppl):606S–611S, 1997.

149. Karanja NM, Obarzanek E, Lin PH, McCullough ML, Phillips KM, Swain JF, Champagne CM, Hoben KP. Descriptive characteristics of the dietary patterns used in the Dietary Approaches to Stop Hypertension trial. *J Am Diet Assoc* 99(suppl):S19–S27, 1999.

150. Sacks FM, Svetkey LP, Vollmer WM, Appel LJ, Bray GA, Harsha D, Obarzanek E, Conlin PR, Miller ER, Simons-Morton DG, Karanja N, Lin PH. DASH-Sodium Collaborative Research Group. Effects on blood pressure of reduced dietary sodium and the Dietary Approaches to Stop Hypertension (DASH) diet. *N Engl J Med* 344:3–10, 2001.

151. Morse RM, Flavin DK. The definition of alcoholism. *JAMA* 268:1012–1014, 1992.

152. Kitchens JM. Does this patient have an alcohol problem? *JAMA* 272:1782–1787, 1994.

153. National Institute on Alcohol Abuse and Alcoholism. *Tenth Special Report to the U.S. Congress on Alcohol and Health.* U.S. Department of Health and Human Services, 2000. www.niaaa.nih.gov/.

154. Gentilello LM, Donovan DM, Dunn CW, Rivara FP. Alcohol interventions in trauma centers. Current practice and future directions. *JAMA* 274:1043–1048, 1995.

155. Liu S, Siegel PZ, Brewer RD, Mokdad AH, Sleet DA, Serdula M. Prevalence of alcohol-impaired driving. Results from a national self-reported survey of health behaviors. *JAMA* 277:122–125, 1997.

156. Goldberg IJ, Mosca L, Piano MR, Fisher EA. Wine and your heart. A science advisory for healthcare professionals from the Nutrition Committee, Council on Epidemiology and Prevention, and Council on Cardiovascular Nursing of the American Heart Association. *Circulation* 103:472–475, 2001.

157. Gronbaek M, Becker U, Johansen D, Gottschau A, Schnohr P, Hein HO, Jensen G, Sorensen TIA. Type of alcohol consumed and mortality from all causes, coronary heart disease, and cancer. *Ann Int Med* 133:411–419, 2000.

158. Mukamal KJ, Conigrave KM, Mittleman MA, Camargo CA, Stampfer MJ, Willett WC, Rimm EB. Roles of drinking pattern and type of alcohol consumed in coronary heart disease in men. *N Engl J Med* 348:109–118, 2003.

159. Berger K, Ajani UA, Kase CS, Gaziano JM, Buring JE, Glynn RJ, Hennekens CH. Light-to-moderate alcohol consumption and risk of stroke among U.S. male physicians. *N Engl J Med* 341:1557–1564, 1999.

160. Stampfer MJ, Rimm EB, Walsh DC. Commentary: Alcohol, the heart, and public policy. *Am J Public Health* 83:801–804, 1993.

161. Wannamethee SG, Shaper AG. Type of alcoholic drink and risk of major coronary heart disease events and all-cause mortality. *Am J Public Health* 89:685–690, 1999.

162. Camargo CA, Hennekens CH, Gaziano JM, Glynn RJ, Manson JE, Stampfer MJ. Prospective study of moderate alcohol consumption and mortality in US male physicians. *Arch Intern Med* 157:79–85, 1997.

163. Fuchs CS, Stampfer MJ, Colditz GA, et al. Alcohol consumption and mortality among women. *N Engl J Med* 332:1245–1250, 1995.

164. Halliwill JR. Mechanisms and clinical implications of post-exercise hypotension in humans. *Exerc Sports Sci Rev* 29:65–70, 2001.

165. MacDonald JR, Hogben CD, Tarnopolsky MA, MacDougall JD. Post exercise hypotension is sustained during subsequent bouts of mild exercise and simulated activities of daily living. *J Hum Hypertens* 15:567–571, 2001.

166. Rueckert PA, Slane PR, Lillis DL, Hanson P. Hemodynamic patterns and duration of post-dynamic exercise hypotension in hypertensive humans. *Med Sci Sports Exerc* 28:24–32, 1996.

167. Krieger EM, Da Silva GJ, Negrao CE. Effects of exercise training on baroreflex control of the cardiovascular system. *Ann N Y Acad Sci* 940:338–347, 2001.

168. Sharabi Y, Ben-Cnaan R, Hanin A, Martonovitch G, Grossman E. The significance of hypertensive response to exercise as a predictor of hypertension and cardiovascular disease. *J Hum Hypertens* 15:353–356, 2001.

169. Mundal R, Kjeldsen SE, Sandvik L, Erikssen G, Thaulow E, Erikssen J. Exercise pressure predicts mortality from myocardial infarction. *Hypertension* 27:324–329, 1996.

170. ACSM Position Stand. Exercise and hypertension. *Med Sci Sports Exerc* 36:1–21, 2004.

171. Kelley G, Tran ZV. Aerobic exercise and normotensive adults: A meta-analysis. *Med Sci Sports Exerc* 27:1371–1377, 1995.

172. Fagard RH. Exercise characteristics and the blood pressure response to dynamic physical training. *Med Sci Sports Exerc* 33(No. 6, suppl):S484–S492, 2001.

173. Kokkinos PF, Narayan P, Colleran JA, et al. Effects of regular exercise on blood pressure and left ventricular hypertrophy in African-American men with severe hypertension. *N Engl J Med* 333:1462–1467, 1995.

174. Kelemen MH, Effron MB, Valenti SA, Stewart KJ. Exercise training combined with antihypertensive drug therapy: Effects on lipids, blood pressure, and left ventricular mass. *JAMA* 263:2766–2771, 1990.

175. Kelley G. Dynamic resistance exercise and resting blood pressure in adults: A meta-analysis. *J Appl Physiol* 82:1559–1565, 1997.

176. Paffenbarger RS, Wing AL, Hyde RT, Jung DL. Physical activity and incidence of hypertension in college alumni. *Am J Epidemiol* 117:245–256, 1983.

177. Blair SN, Goodyear NN, Gibbons LW, et al. Physical fitness and incidence of hypertension in healthy normotensive men and women. *JAMA* 252:487–490, 1984.

178. Paffenbarger RS, Jung DL, Leung RW, Hyde RT. Physical activity and hypertension: An epidemiological view. *Ann Med* 23:319–327, 1991.

179. Williams PT. Relationship of distance run per week to coronary heart disease risk factors in 8283 male runners. The National Runners' Health Study. *Arch Intern Med* 157:191–198, 1997.

180. Pols MA, Peeters PHM, Twisk JWR, Kemper HCG, Grobbee DE. Physical activity and cardiovascular disease risk profile in women. *Am J Epidemiol* 146:322–328, 1997.

181. Dwyer T, Gibbons LE. The Australian schools health and fitness survey. Physical fitness related to blood pressure but not lipoproteins. *Circulation* 89:1539–1544, 1994.

182. Lim PO, MacFadyen RJ, Clarkson PBM, MacDonald TM. Impaired exercise tolerance in hypertensive patients. *Ann Intern Med* 124:41–55, 1996.

183. Grundy SM. Cholesterol and coronary heart disease. The 21st century. *Arch Intern Med* 157:1177–1184, 1997.

184. Verschuren WMM, Jacobs DR, Bloemberg BPM, et al. Serum total cholesterol and long-term coronary heart disease mortality in different cultures. Twenty-five year follow-up of the seven countries study. *JAMA* 274:131–136, 1995.

185. National Research Council. *Diet and Health: Implications for Reducing Chronic Disease Risk.* Washington, DC: National Academy Press, 1989.

186. Stamler J, Daviglus ML, Garside DB, Dyer AR, Greenland P, Neaton JD. Relationship of baseline serum cholesterol levels in 3 large cohorts of younger men to long-term coronary, cardiovascular, and all-cause mortality and to longevity. *JAMA* 284:311–318, 2000.

187. Task Force on Risk Reduction, American Heart Association. Cholesterol screening in asymptomatic adults: No cause to change. *Circulation* 93:1067–1068, 1996.

188. Johnson CL, Rifkind BM, Sempos CT, et al. Declining serum total cholesterol levels among US adults. The National Health and Nutrition Examination Surveys. *JAMA* 269:3002–3008, 1993.

189. Sempos CT, Cleeman JI, Carroll MD, et al. Prevalence of high blood cholesterol among US adults. *JAMA* 269:3009–3014, 1993.

190. Castelli WP, Garrison RJ, Wilson PWF, et al. Incidence of coronary heart disease and lipoprotein cholesterol levels: The Framingham Study. *JAMA* 256:2835–2838, 1986.

191. Grundy SM, Cleeman JI, Merz CNB, et al. Implications of recent clinical trials for the National Cholesterol Education Program Adult Treatment Panel III Guidelines. *Circulation* 110:227–239, 2004.

192. Haskell WL. The influence of exercise on the concentrations of triglyceride and cholesterol in human plasma. *Exerc Sport Sci Rev* 12:205–244, 1984.

193. NIH Consensus Development Panel on Triglyceride, High-Density Lipoprotein, and Coronary Heart Disease. Triglyceride, high-density lipoprotein, and coronary heart disease. *JAMA* 269:505–510, 1993.

194. Kwiterovich PO. The antiatherogenic role of high-density lipoprotein cholesterol. *Am J Cardiol* 82(9A):13Q–21Q, 1998.

195. Linn S, Fulwood R, Carroll M, et al. Serum total cholesterol:HDL cholesterol ratios in US white and black adults by selected demographic and socioeconomic variables (NHANES II). *Am J Public Health* 81:1038–1043, 1991.

196. Whitney EJ, Krasuski RA, Personius BE, Michalek JE, Maranian AM, Kolasa MW, Monick E, Brown BG, Gotto AM Jr. A randomized trial of a strategy for increasing high-density lipoprotein cholesterol levels: Effects on progression of coronary heart disease and clinical events. *Ann Intern Med* 142:95–104, 2005.

197. Jacobs DR, Mebane IL, Bangdiwala SI, et al. High density lipoprotein cholesterol as a predictor of cardiovascular disease mortality in men and women: The follow-up study of the Lipid Research Clinics Prevalence Study. *Am J Epidemiol* 131:32–47, 1990.

198. Grover SA, Coupal L, Hu XP. Identifying adults at increased risk of coronary disease. How well do the current cholesterol guidelines work? *JAMA* 274:801–806, 1995.

199. Stampfer MJ, Sacks FM, Salvini S, Willett WC, Hennekens CH. A prospective study of cholesterol, apolipoproteins, and the risk of myocardial infarction. *N Engl J Med* 325:373–381, 1991.

200. LaRosa JC. Triglycerides and coronary risk in women and the elderly. *Arch Intern Med* 157:961–968, 1997.

201. Criqui MH, Heiss G, Cohn R, et al. Plasma triglyceride level and mortality from coronary heart disease. *N Engl J Med* 328:1220–1225, 1993.

202. DeLong DM, Delong ER, Wood PD, et al. A comparison of methods for the estimation of plasma low- and very low-density lipoprotein cholesterol. *JAMA* 256:2372–2377, 1986.

203. American Heart Association. AHA Scientific Statement. AHA dietary guidelines. Revision 2000: A statement for healthcare professionals from the Nutrition Committee of the American Heart Association. *Circulation* 102:2284–2299, 2000.

204. Yu-Poth S, Zhao G, Etherton T, Naglak M, Jonnalagadda S, Kris-Etherton PM. Effects of the National Cholesterol Education Program's Step I and Step II dietary intervention programs on cardiovascular disease risk factors: A meta-analysis. *Am J Clin Nutr* 69:632–646, 1999.

205. Hu FB, Willett WC. Optimal diets for prevention of coronary heart disease. *JAMA* 288:2569–2578, 2002.

206. Jensen MK, Koh-Banerjee P, Hu FB, Franz M, Sampson L, Grønbaek M, Rimm EB. Intakes of whole grains, bran, and germ and the risk of coronary heart disease in men. *Am J Clin Nutr* 80:1492–1499, 2004.

207. Joshipura KJ, Hu FB, Manson JE, Stampfer MJ, Rimm EB, Speizer FE, Colditz G, Ascherio A, Rosner B, Spiegelman D, Willett WC. The effect of fruit and vegetable intake on risk for coronary heart disease. *Ann Intern Med* 134:1106–1114, 2001.

208. Kris-Etherton P, Eckel RH, Howard BV, St. Jeor S, Bazzarre TL. AHA Science Advisory. Lyon Diet Heart Study. Benefits of a Mediterranean-Style, National Cholesterol Education Program/American Heart Association Step I dietary pattern on cardiovascular disease. *Circulation* 103:1823–1825, 2001.

209. Hegsted DM, Ausman LM, Johnson JA, Dallal GE. Dietary fat and serum lipids: An evaluation of the experimental data. *Am J Clin Nutr* 57:875–883, 1993.

210. Esposito K, Marfella R, Ciotola M, Di Palo C, Giugliano F, Giugliano G, D'Armiento M, D'Andrea F, Giugliano D. Effect of a Mediterranean-style diet on endothelial dysfunction and markers of vascular inflammation in the metabolic syndrome: A randomized trial. *JAMA* 292:1440–1446, 2004.

211. Erdman JW. AHA Science Advisory. Soy protein and cardiovascular disease. A statement for healthcare professionals from the Nutrition Committee of the AHA. *Circulation* 102:2555–2559, 2000.

212. Howell WH, McNamara DJ, Tosca MA, Smith BT, Gaines JA. Plasma lipid and lipoprotein responses to dietary fat and cholesterol: A meta-analysis. *Am J Clin Nutr* 65:1747–1764, 1997.

213. Van Horn L. Fiber, lipids, and coronary heart disease. A Statement for Healthcare Professionals From the Nutrition Committee, American Heart Association. *Circulation* 95:2701–2704, 1997.

214. Lichtenstein AH. *Trans* fatty acids, plasma lipid levels, and risk of developing cardiovascular disease. A statement for healthcare professionals from the Nutrition Committee, American Heart Association. *Circulation* 95:2588–2590, 1997.

215. Barnard RJ. Effects of life-style modification on serum lipids. *Arch Intern Med* 151:1389–1394, 1991.

216. Walford RL, Harris SB, Gunion MW. The calorically restricted low-fat nutrient-dense diet in biosphere 2 significantly lowers blood glucose, total leukocyte count, cholesterol, and blood pressure in humans. *Proc Natl Acad Sci* 89:11533–11537, 1992.

217. Wood PD. Physical activity, diet, and health: Independent and interactive effects. *Med Sci Sports Exerc* 26:838–843, 1994.

218. Wood PD, Haskell WL, Stern MP, Lewis S, Perry C. Serum lipoproteins distributions in male and female runners. *Ann NY Acad Sci* 301:748–763, 1977.

219. Carroll S, Cooke CB, Butterly RJ. Metabolic clustering, physical activity and fitness in nonsmoking, middle-aged men. *Med Sci Sports Exerc* 32:2079–2086, 2000.

220. Whaley MH, Kampert JB, Kohl HW, Blair SN. Physical fitness and clustering of risk factors associated with the metabolic syndrome. *Med Sci Sports Exerc* 31:287–293, 1999.

221. Nieman DC, Warren BJ, O'Donnell KA, Dotson RG, Butterworth DE, Henson DA. Physical activity and serum lipids and lipoproteins in elderly women. *J Am Geriatr Assoc* 41:1339–1344, 1993.

222. Williams PT. High-density lipoprotein cholesterol and other risk factors for coronary heart disease in female runners. *N Engl J Med* 334:1298–1303, 1996.

223. Kokkinos PF, Holland JC, Narayan P, Colleran JA, Dotson CO, Papademetriou V. Miles run per week and high-density lipoprotein cholesterol levels in healthy, middle-aged men: A dose-response relationship. *Arch Intern Med* 155:415–420, 1995.

224. Katzel LI, Bleecker ER, Colman EG, Rogus EM, Sorkin JD, Goldberg AP. Effects of weight loss vs aerobic exercise training on risk factors for coronary disease in healthy, obese, middle-aged and older men. *JAMA* 274:1915–1921, 1995.

225. Patalay M, Lofgren IE, Freake HC, Koo SI, Fernandez ML. The lowering of plasma lipids following a weight reduction program is related to increased expression of the LDL receptor and lipoprotein lipase. *J Nutr* 135:735–739, 2005.

226. Andersen RE, Wadden TA, Bartlett SJ, Vogt RA, Weinstock RS. Relation of weight loss to changes in serum lipids and lipoproteins in obese women. *Am J Clin Nutr* 62:350–357, 1995.

227. Nieman DC, Haig JL, Fairchild KS, De Guia ED, Dizon GP, Register UD. Reducing diet and exercise training effects on serum lipids and lipoproteins in mildly obese women. *Am J Clin Nutr* 52:640–645, 1990.

228. Schwartz RS. The independent effects of dietary weight loss and aerobic training on high density lipoproteins and apolipoprotein A-1 concentrations in obese men. *Metabolism* 36:165–171, 1987.

229. Schwartz RS, Cain KC, Shuman WP, et al. Effect of intensive endurance training on lipoprotein profiles in young and older men. *Metabolism* 41:649–654, 1992.

230. Hinkleman L, Nieman DC. The effects of moderate exercise training on body composition and serum lipids and lipoproteins in mildly obese women. *J Sports Med Phys Fit* 33:49–58, 1993.

231. Kelley GA, Kelly KS, Tran ZV. Aerobic exercise and lipids and lipoproteins in women: A meta-analysis of randomized controlled trials. *J Womens Health (Larchmt)* 13:1148–1164, 2004.

232. Tran ZV, Weltman A. Differential effects of exercise on serum lipid and lipoprotein levels seen with changes in body weight. *JAMA* 254:919–924, 1985.

233. Wood PD, Stefanick MI, Williams PT, Haskell WL. The effects on plasma lipoproteins of a prudent weight-reducing diet, with or without exercise, in overweight men and women. *N Engl J Med* 325:461–466, 1991.

234. Varady KA, Ebine N, Vanstone CA, Parsons WE, Jones PJ. Plant sterols and endurance training combine to favorably alter plasma lipid profiles in previously sedentary hypercholesterolemic adults after 8 wk. *Am J Clin Nutr* 80:1159–1166, 2004.

235. King AC, Haskell WL, Young DR, Oka RK, Stefanick ML. Long-term effects of varying intensities and formats of physical activity on participation rates, fitness, and lipoproteins in men and women aged 50 to 65 years. *Circulation* 91:2596–2604, 1995.

236. Leon AS, Sanchez OA. Response of blood lipids to exercise training alone or combined with dietary intervention. *Med Sci Sports Exerc* 33(suppl):S502–S515, 2001.

237. Nieman DC, Brock DW, Butterworth D, Utter AC, Nieman CN. Reducing diet and/or exercise training decreases the lipid and lipoprotein risk factors of moderately obese women. *J Am College Nutr* 21:344–350, 2002.

238. Kraus WE, Houmard JA, Duscha BD, Knetzger KJ, Wharton MB, McCartney JS, Bales CW, Henes S, Samsa GP, Otvos JD, Kulkarni KR, Slentz CA. Effects of the amount and intensity of exercise on plasma lipoproteins. *N Engl J Med* 347:1483–1492, 2002.

239. Wilmore JH. Dose-response: Variation with age, sex, and health status. *Med Sci Sports Exerc* 33(suppl):S622–S634, 2001.

240. Tsetsonis NV, Hardman AE, Mastana SS. Acute effects of exercise on postprandial lipemia: A comparative study in trained and untrained middle-aged women. *Am J Clin Nutr* 65:525–533, 1997.

241. Ziogas GG, Thomas TR, Harris WS. Exercise training, postprandial hypertriglyceridemia, and LDL subfraction distribution. *Med Sci Sports Exerc* 29:986–991, 1997.

242. Ferguson MA, Alderson NL, Trost SG, Essig DA, Burke JR, Durstine JL. Effects of four different single exercise sessions on lipids, lipoproteins, and lipoprotein lipase. *J Appl Physiol* 85:1169–1174, 1998.

243. Thompson PD, Crouse SF, Goodpaster B, Kelley D, Moyna N, Pescatello L. The acute versus the chronic response to exercise. *Med Sci Sports Exerc* 33(suppl):S438–S445, 2001.

244. Seip RL, Semenkovich CF. Skeletal muscle lipoprotein lipase: Molecular regulation and physiological effects in relation to exercise. *Exerc Sport Sci Rev* 26:191–218, 1998.

245. Crouse SF, O'Brien BC, Rohack JJ, et al. Changes in serum lipids and apolipoproteins after exercise in men with high cholesterol: Influence of intensity. *J Appl Physiol* 79:279–286, 1995.

246. Ginsburg GS, Agil A, O'Toole M, Rimm E, Douglas PS, Rifai N. Effects of a single bout of ultraendurance exercise on lipid levels and susceptibility of lipids to peroxidation in triathletes. *JAMA* 276:221–225, 1996.

247. Gordon PM, Fowler S, Warty V, Danduran M, Visich P, Keteyian S. Effects of acute exercise on high density lipoprotein cholesterol and high density lipoprotein subfractions in moderately trained females. *Br J Sports Med* 32:63–67, 1998.

248. Lee R, Nieman DC, Raval R, Blankenship J, Lee J. The effects of acute moderate exercise on serum lipids and lipoproteins in mildly obese women. *Int J Sports Med* 12:537–542, 1991.

249. Borsheim E, Knardahl S, Hostmark AT. Short-term effects of exercise on plasma very low density lipoproteins (VLDL) and fatty acids. *Med Sci Sports Exerc* 31:522–530, 1999.

250. Skinner ER, Watt C, Maughan RJ. The acute effect of marathon running on plasma lipoproteins in female subjects. *Eur J Appl Physiol* 56:451–456, 1987.

251. Goodyear LJ, van Houten DR, Fronsoe MS, et al. Immediate and delayed effects of marathon running on lipids and lipoproteins in women. *Med Sci Sports Exerc* 22:588–592, 1990.

252. American Heart Association. Statement on exercise: Benefits and recommendations for physical activity programs for all Americans. *Circulation* 86:340–343, 1992.

253. Fletcher GF, Balady G, Blair SN, et al. Statement on exercise. Benefits and recommendations for physical activity programs for all Americans. *Circulation* 94:857–862, 1996.

254. Morris JN, Heady JA, Raffle PAB, Parks JW. Coronary heart disease and physical activity of work. *Lancet* 2:1053–1057, 1953.

255. Paffenbarger RS, Laughlin ME, Gima AS, et al. Work activity of longshoremen as related to death from coronary heart disease and stroke. *N Engl J Med* 282:1109–1114, 1970.

256. Paffenbarger RS, Wing AL, Hyde RT. Physical activity as an index of heart attack risk in college alumni. *Am J Epidemiol* 108:161–175, 1978.

257. Paffenbarger RS, Hyde RT, Wing AL, Steinmetz CH. A natural history of athleticism and cardiovascular health. *JAMA* 252:491–495, 1984.

258. Paffenbarger RS, Hyde RT, Wing AL, Lee I-M, Jung DL, Kampert JB. The association of changes in physical-activity level and other lifestyle characteristics with mortality among men. *N Engl J Med* 328:538–545, 1993.

259. Paffenbarger RS, Kampert JB, Lee IM. Physical activity and health of college men: Longitudinal observations. *Int J Sports Med* 18(suppl 3):S200–S203, 1997.

260. Blair SN, Kohl HW, Paffenbarger RS, Clark DG, Cooper KH, Gibbons LW. Physical fitness and all-cause mortality: A prospective study of healthy men and women. *JAMA* 262:2395–2401, 1989.

261. Lemaitre RN, Heckbert SR, Psaty BM, Siscovick DS. Leisure-time physical activity and the risk of nonfatal myocardial infarction in postmenopausal women. *Arch Intern Med* 155:2302–2308, 1995.

262. Manson JE, Greenland P, LaCroix AZ, Stefanick ML, Mouton CP, Oberman A, Perri MG, Sheps DS, Pettinger MB, Siscovick DS. Walking compared with vigorous exercise for the prevention of cardiovascular events in women. *N Engl J Med* 347:716–725, 2002.

263. Kushi LH, Fee RM, Folsom AR, Mink PJ, Anderson KE, Sellers TA. Physical activity and mortality in postmenopausal women. *JAMA* 277:1287–1292, 1997.

264. Powell KE, Thompson PD, Caspersen CJ, Kendrick JS. Physical activity and the incidence of coronary heart disease. *Ann Rev Public Health* 8:253–287, 1987.

265. Berlin JA, Colditz GA. A meta-analysis of physical activity in the prevention of coronary heart disease. *Am J Epidemiol* 132:612–628, 1990.

266. Wei M, Kampert JB, Barlow CE, Nichaman MZ, Gibbons LW, Paffenbarger RS, Blair SN. Relationship between low cardiorespiratory fitness and mortality in normal-weight, overweight, and obese men. *JAMA* 282:1547–1453, 1999.

267. Lee IM, Rexrode KM, Cook NR, Manson JE, Buring JE. Physical activity and coronary heart disease in women: Is "no pain, no gain" passé? *JAMA* 285:1447–1454, 2001.

268. Laukkanen JA, Lakka TA, Rauramaa R, Kuhanen R, Venaiainen JM, Salonen R, Salonen JT. Cardiovascular fitness as a predictor of mortality in men. *Arch Intern Med* 161:825–831, 2001.

269. Hu FB, Stampfer MJ, Solomon C, Liu S, Colditz GA, Speizer FE, Willett WC, Manson JE. Physical activity and risk for cardiovascular events in diabetic women. *Ann Intern Med* 134:96–105, 2001.

270. Manson JE, Hu FB, Rich-Edwards JW, Colditz GA, Stampfer MJ, Willett WC, Speizer FE, Hennekens CH. A prospective study of walking as compared with vigorous exercise in the prevention of coronary heart disease in women. *N Engl J Med* 341:650–658, 1999.

271. Blair SN, Cheng Y, Holder JS. Is physical activity or physical fitness more important in defining health benefits. *Med Sci Sports Exerc* 33(suppl):S379–S399, 2001.

272. Tanasescu M, Leitzmann MF, Rimm EG, Willett WC, Stampfer MJ, Hu FB. Exercise type and intensity in relation to coronary heart disease in men. *JAMA* 288:1994–2000, 2002.

273. Kohl HW. Physical activity and cardiovascular disease: Evidence for a dose response. *Med Sci Sports Exerc* 33(suppl):S472–S483, 2001.

274. Morris JN, Clayton DG, Everitt MG, Semmence AM, Burgess EH. Exercise in leisure time: Coronary attack and death rates. *Br Heart J* 63:325–334, 1990.

275. Sesso HD, Paffenbarger RS, Lee IM. Physical activity and coronary heart disease in men. The Harvard Alumni Health Study. *Circulation* 102:975–980, 2000.

276. Lee IM, Sesso HD, Paffenbarger RS. Physical activity and coronary heart disease risk in men. Does the duration of exercise episodes predict risk? *Circulation* 102:981–986, 2000.

277. Richardson CR, Kriska AM, Lantz PM, Hayward RA. Physical activity and mortality across cardiovascular disease risk groups. *Med Sci Sports Exerc* 36:1923–1929, 2004.

278. Folsom AR, Arnett DK, Hutchinson RG, Liao F, Clegg LX, Cooper LS. Physical activity and incidence of coronary heart disease in middle-aged women and men. *Med Sci Sports Exerc* 29:901–909, 1997.

279. Goldberg RJ, Burchfiel CM, Benfante R, Chiu D, Reed DM, Yano K. Lifestyle and biologic factors associated with atherosclerotic disease in middle-aged men. 20-year findings from the Honolulu Heart Program. *Arch Intern Med* 155:686–694, 1995.

280. Leon AS, Myers MJ, Connett J. Leisure time physical activity and the 16-year risks of mortality from coronary heart disease

and all-causes in the Multiple Risk Factor Intervention Trial (MRFIT). *Int J Sports Med* 18(suppl 3):S208–S215, 1997.

281. Lakka TA, Venalainen JM, Rauramaa R, Salonen R, Tuomilehto J, Salonen JT. Relation of leisure-time physical activity and cardiorespiratory fitness to the risk of acute myocardial infarction in men. *N Engl J Med* 330:1549–1554, 1994.

282. Kaplan GA, Strawbridge WJ, Cohen RD, Hungerford LR. Natural history of leisure-time physical activity and its correlates: Associations with mortality from all causes and cardiovascular disease over 28 years. *Am J Epidemiol* 144:793–797, 1996.

283. Haapanen N, Miilunpalo S, Vuori I, Oja P, Pasanen M. Characteristics of leisure time physical activity associated with decrease risk of premature all-cause and cardiovascular disease mortality in middle-aged men. *Am J Epidemiol* 143:870–880, 1996.

284. Farrell SW, Kampert JB, Kohl HW, Barlow CE, Macera CA, Paffenbarger RS, Gibbons LW, Blair SN. Influences of cardiorespiratory fitness levels and other predictors on cardiovascular disease mortality in men. *Med Sci Sports Exerc* 30:899–905, 1998.

285. O'Donovan G, Owen A, Bird SR, Kearney EM, Nevill AM, Jones DW, Woolf-May K. Changes in cardiorespiratory fitness and coronary heart disease risk factors following 24 wk of moderate- or high-intensity exercise of equal energy cost. *J Appl Physiol* 98:1619–1625, 2005.

286. Thompson PD, Buchner D, Pina IL, et al. Exercise and physical activity in the prevention and treatment of atherosclerotic cardiovascular disease. *Circulation* 107:3109–3116, 2003.

287. Williams PT. Health effects resulting from exercise versus those from body fat loss. *Med Sci Sports Exerc* 33(suppl): S611–S621, 2001.

288. LaMonte MJ, Eisenman PA, Adams TD, Shultz BB, Ainsworth BE, Yanowitz FG. Cardiorespiratory fitness and coronary heart disease risk factors. The LDS Hospital Fitness Institute Cohort. *Circulation* 102:1623–1628, 2000.

289. Haskell WL, Sims C, Myll J, Bortz WM, Goar FG, Alderman EL. Coronary artery size and dilating capacity in ultradistance runners. *Circulation* 87:1076–1082, 1993.

290. Tanaka H, Dinenno FA, Monahan KD, Clevenger CM, DeSouza CA, Seals DR. Aging, habitual exercise, and dynamic arterial compliance. *Circulation* 102:1270–1275, 2000.

291. Koenig W, Ernst E. Exercise and thrombosis. *Coron Artery Dis* 11:123–127, 2000.

292. Koenig W, Sund M, Doring A, Ernst E. Leisure-time physical activity but not work-related physical activity is associated with decreased plasma viscosity. *Circulation* 95:335–341, 1997.

293. Rauramaa R, Li G, Vaisanen SB. Dose-response and coagulation and hemostatic factors. *Med Sci Sports Exerc* 33(suppl):S516–S520, 2001.

294. Laughlin MH, Oltman CL, Bowles DK. Exercise training-induced adaptations in the coronary circulation. *Med Sci Sports Exerc* 30:352–360, 1998.

295. Paffenbarger RS, Kampert JB, Lee I-M, Hyde RT, Leung RW, Wing AL. Changes in physical activity and other lifeway patterns influencing longevity. *Med Sci Sports Exerc* 26: 857–865, 1994.

296. Blair SN, Kohl HW, Barlow CE, Paffenbarger RS, Gibbons LW, Macera CA. Changes in physical fitness and all-cause mortality: A prospective study of healthy and unhealthy men. *JAMA* 273:1093–1098, 1995.

297. U.S. Department of Health and Human Services. *Physical Activity and Health: A Report of the Surgeon General.* Atlanta, GA: U.S. Department of Health and Human Services, Centers for Disease Control and Prevention, National Center for Chronic Disease Prevention and Health Promotion, 1996.

298. NIH Consensus Development Panel on Physical Activity and Cardiovascular Health. Physical activity and cardiovascular health. *JAMA* 276:241–246, 1996.

299. Wendel-Vos GC, Schuit AJ, Feskens EJ, Boshuizen HC, Verschuren WM, Saris WH, Kromhout D. Physical activity and stroke. A meta-analysis of observational data. *Int J Epidemiol* 33:787–798, 2004.

300. Paffenbarger RS, Williams JL. Chronic disease in former college students XII: Early precursors of fatal stroke. *Am J Public Health* 57:1290–1299, 1967.

301. Herman B, Schmitz B, Leyten ACM, et al. Multivariate logistic analysis of risk factors for stroke in Tilburg, the Netherlands. *Am J Epidemiol* 118:514–525, 1983.

302. Shinton R, Sagar G. Lifelong exercise and stroke. *BMJ* 307:231–234, 1993.

303. Abbott RD, Rodriquez BL, Burchfiel CM, Curb JD. Physical activity in older middle-aged men and reduced risk of stroke: The Honolulu Heart Program. *Am J Epidemiol* 139:881–893, 1994.

304. Wannamethee G, Shaper AG. Physical activity and stroke in British middle aged men. *BMJ* 304:597–601, 1992.

305. Oguma Y, Shinoda-Tagawa T. Physical activity decreases cardiovascular disease risk in women: Review and meta-analysis. *Am J Prev Med* 26:407–418, 2004.

306. Gillum RF, Mussolino ME, Ingram DD. Physical activity and stroke incidence in women and men. The NHANES I Epidemiologic Follow-up Study. *Am J Epidemiol* 143:860–869, 1996.

307. Hu FB, Stampfer MJ, Colditz GA, Ascherio A, Rexrode KM, Willett WC, Manson JE. Physical activity and risk of stroke in women. *JAMA* 283:2961–2967, 2000.

308. Lee IM, Paffenbarger RS. Physical activity and stroke incidence: The Harvard Alumni Health Study. *Stroke* 29:2049–2054, 1998.

309. Ellekjaer H, Holmen J, Ellekjaer E, Vatten L. Physical activity and stroke mortality in women. Ten-year follow-up of the Nord-Trondelag health survey, 1984–1986. *Stroke* 31:14–18, 2000.

310. Leon AS, Franklin BA, Costa F, Balady GJ, Berra KA, Stewart KJ, Thompson PD, Williams MA, Lauer MS. Cardiac rehabilitation and secondary prevention of coronary heart disease. *Circulation* 111:369–376, 2005.

311. Leon AS. Exercise following myocardial infarction. Current recommendations. *Sports Med* 29:301–311, 2000.

312. Haskell WL. The efficacy and safety of exercise programs in cardiac rehabilitation. *Med Sci Sports Exerc* 26:815–823, 1994.

313. Perk J, Veress G. Cardiac rehabilitation: Applying exercise physiology in clinical practice. *Eur J Appl Physiol* 83:457–462, 2000.

314. O'Conner GT, Buring JE, Yusaf S, et al. An overview of randomized trials of rehabilitation with exercise after myocardial infarction. *Circulation* 80:234, 1989.

315. Jolliffe JA, Rees K, Taylor RS, Thompson D, Oldridge N, Ebrahim S. Exercise-based rehabilitation for coronary heart disease (Cochrane Review). *Cochrane Database Syst Rev* 1:CD001800, 2001.

316. Van Camp SP, Peterson RA. Cardiovascular complications of outpatient cardiac rehabilitation programs. *JAMA* 256:1160–1163, 1986.

PHYSICAL FITNESS ACTIVITY 10.1

Heart Disease Risk

Playing the Odds—What Is Your Heart Disease Risk Score?

Heart disease continues to be the cause of the greatest number of deaths among adult Americans. Using this simple worksheet, you can calculate your heart disease risk score. Following each risk factor, circle the number that applies to you. Total your score, and compare it with the norms. You will need your systolic blood pressure (the higher pressure when the heart beats) and blood cholesterol measurements to take this test. If you have not been measured, we highly recommend you see your doctor or local public health department very soon.

Risk Factor 1—Heredity

Do you have a father or brother who had heart disease before age 55, or a mother or sister with heart disease before age 65?

No	0
Yes but just 1 individual in family	3
Yes, with more than 1 individual	4

Risk Factor 2—Age/gender

Are you a male 45 years of age or older, or a female 55 years of age or older?

No	0
Yes	4

Risk Factor 3—Cigarette smoking

Never have smoked or quit more than 15 years ago	0
Ex-smoker (quit less than 15 years ago)	1
Smoke 1–20 cigarettes/day	2
Smoke 21–40 cigarettes/day	3
Smoke 41 or more cigarettes/day	4

Risk Factor 4—High blood pressure

Your systolic blood pressure is

≤ 120 mm Hg	0
121–129 mm Hg	1
130–139 mm Hg	2
140–149 mm Hg	3
≥ 150 mm Hg	4

Risk Factor 5—High blood cholesterol

Your serum cholesterol is

< 200 mg/dl	0
200–219 mg/dl	1
220–239 mg/dl	2
240–259 mg/dl	3
≥ 260 mg/dl	4

Risk Factor 6—Inactivity

How often do you usually engage in physical exercise that moderately or strongly increases your breathing and heart rate, and makes you sweat, for at least a total of 30 minutes a day, such as in brisk walking, cycling, swimming, jogging, or manual labor?

5 or more times per week	0
3 or 4 times per week	1
2 times per week	2
1 time per week	3
None	4

Risk Factor 7—Obesity

How would you rate your body weight?

Close to ideal	0
About 10–20 pounds overweight	1
About 21–50 pounds overweight	2
About 51–100 pounds overweight	3
More than 100 pounds overweight	4

Risk Factor 8—Stress

How would you describe the stress you experience?

Low or moderate levels of stress	0
High stress but am able to cope with it	1
High stress and often feel unable to cope	2
Very high stress but trying to cope with it	3
Very high stress and unable to cope with it	4

Risk Factor 9—Diabetes

Have you been diagnosed with diabetes by a doctor?

No	0
Yes	4

Your Heart Disease Risk Score

Classification	Total Points
Very low risk	Less than 5
Low risk	6–10
Moderately high risk	11–15
High risk	16–20
Very high risk	More than 20

Sources: Based on information from the Framingham Heart Study (*Circulation* 83:356–362, 1991) and the MRFIT research project (*Arch Intern Med* 152:56–64, 1992).

PHYSICAL FITNESS ACTIVITY 10.2

Coronary Heart Disease Risk

Estimating 10-Year Risk for Men and Women

Coronary heart disease is the leading cause of death in the United States despite an impressive decline in rates during the past several decades. Risk assessment for determining the 10-year risk for developing CHD is carried out using Framingham risk scoring (separate tables for men and women). The risk factors included in the Framingham calculation of 10-year risk are age, total cholesterol, HDL cholesterol, systolic blood pressure, treatment for hypertension, and cigarette smoking. The first step is to calculate the number of points for each risk factor. Total cholesterol and HDL cholesterol should be the average of at least two measurements. The average of several blood pressure measurements is needed for an accurate measure. The designation "smoker" means any cigarette smoking in the past month. The total risk score sums the points for each risk factor. The 10-year risk for CHD is estimated from total points. This estimation of 10-year CHD risk can also be calculated on the Internet at www.nhlbi.nih.gov.

Estimate of 10-year Risk for Men

Age	Points
20–34	−9
35–39	−4
40–44	0
45–49	3
50–54	6
55–59	8
60–64	10
65–69	11
70–74	12
75–79	13

Point Total	10-Year Risk (%)
<0	<1
0	1
1	1
2	1
3	1
4	1
5	2
6	2
7	3
8	4
9	5
10	6
11	8
12	10
13	12
14	16
15	20
16	25
≥17	≥30

Total Cholesterol	Points at Age 20–39	Points at Age 40–49	Points at Age 50–59	Points at Age 60–69	Points at Age 70–79
<160	0	0	0	0	0
160–199	4	3	2	1	0
200–239	7	5	3	1	0
240–279	9	6	4	2	1
≥280	11	8	5	3	1

	Points at Age 20–39	Points at Age 40–49	Points at Age 50–59	Points at Age 60–69	Points at Age 70–79
Nonsmoker	0	0	0	0	0
Smoker	8	5	3	1	1

HDL	Points
≥60	−1
50–59	0
40–49	1
<40	2

Systollic BP	If Untreated	If Treated
<120	0	0
120–129	0	1
130–139	1	2
140–159	1	2
≥160	2	3

Source: Third Report of the National Cholesterol Education Program (NCEP) Expert Panel on Detection, Evaluation, and Treatment of High Blood Cholesterol in Adults (Adult Treatment Panel III), 2001.

Estimate of 10-year Risk for Women

Age	Points
20–34	−7
35–39	−3
40–44	0
45–49	3
50–54	6
55–59	8
60–64	10
65–69	12
70–74	14
75–79	16

Total Cholesterol	Points at Age 20–39	Points at Age 40–49	Points at Age 50–59	Points at Age 60–69	Points at Age 70–79
<160	0	0	0	0	0
160–199	4	3	2	1	1
200–239	8	6	4	2	1
240–279	11	8	5	3	2
≥280	13	10	7	4	2

	Points at Age 20–39	Points at Age 40–49	Points at Age 50–59	Points at Age 60–69	Points at Age 70–79
Nonsmoker	0	0	0	0	0
Smoker	9	7	4	2	1

HDL	Points
≥60	−1
50–59	0
40–49	1
<40	2

Systollic BP	If Untreated	If Treated
<120	0	0
120–129	1	3
130–139	2	4
140–159	3	5
≥160	4	6

Point Total	10-Year Risk (%)
<9	<1
9	1
10	1
11	1
12	1
13	2
14	2
15	3
16	4
17	5
18	6
19	8
20	11
21	14
22	17
23	22
24	27
≥25	≥30

 **PHYSICAL FITNESS ACTIVITY 10.3**

Stroke Risk

Stroke has been the third leading cause of death in the United States since 1938. Using this simple worksheet, you can calculate your 10-year risk of stroke. Circle the points associated with your personal risk factor information. To estimate stroke risk, you must know your systolic blood pressure and medical history.

Stroke

Women

Step 1.

Find the points for your age.

Age	Women
54–56	0
57–59	1
60–62	2
63–65	3
66–68	4
69–71	5
72–74	6
75–77	7
78–80	8
81–83	9
84–86	10

Step 2.

Find the points for your other risk factors.

SBP	Points
95–104	0
105–114	1
115–124	2
125–134	3
135–144	4
145–154	5
155–164	6
165–174	7
175–184	8
185–194	9
195–204	10

HYP RX

No = 0

If yes, add these points, depending on your SBP level:

SBP	Points
95–104	6
105–124	5
125–134	4
135–154	3
155–164	2
165–184	1

Risk factor	Points
Diabetes	No = 0 Yes = 3
Cigarette smoker	No = 0 Yes = 3
CVD	No = 0 Yes = 2
AF	No = 0 Yes = 6
LVH	No = 0 Yes = 4

Men

Step 1.

Find the points for your age.

Age	Men
54–56	0
57–59	1
60–62	2
63–65	3
66–68	4
69–71	5
72–74	6
75–77	7
78–80	8
81–83	9
84–86	10

Step 2.

Find the points for your other risk factors.

SBP	Points
95–105	0
106–116	1
117–126	2
127–137	3
138–148	4
149–159	5
160–170	6
171–181	7
182–191	8
192–202	9
203–213	10

Risk factor	No	Yes
HYP RX	No = 0	Yes = 2
Diabetes	No = 0	Yes = 2
Cigarette smoker	No = 0	Yes = 3
CVD	No = 0	Yes = 3
AF	No = 0	Yes = 4
LVH	No = 0	Yes = 6

Step 3.

Total the points for all your risk factors.

Age	+____
SBP	+____
HYP RX	+____
Diabetes	+____
Cigarette Smoker	+____
CVD	+____
AF	+____
LVH	+____
Total points	____

Compare Your Risk

Compare your stroke risk to that of an average person your age.

Age	Men	Women
55–59	3%	6%
60–64	5%	8%
65–69	7%	11%
70–74	11%	14%
75–79	16%	18%
80–84	24%	22%

What's Your Risk

Here's your risk of having a stroke within the next 10 years.

Points	Men	Women
1	3%	1%
2	3%	1%
3	4%	2%
4	4%	2%
5	5%	2%
6	5%	3%
7	6%	4%
8	7%	4%
9	8%	5%
10	10%	6%
11	11%	8%
12	13%	9%
13	15%	11%
14	17%	13%
15	20%	16%
16	22%	19%
17	26%	23%
18	29%	27%
19	33%	32%
20	37%	37%
21	42%	43%
22	47%	50%
23	52%	57%
24	57%	64%
25	63%	71%
26	68%	78%
27	74%	84%
28	79%	
29	84%	
30	88%	

Notes:

AF—Has a doctor ever told you that you have atrial fibrillation (irregular heart beats in the upper chambers of your heart)?

CVD—Have you ever had any of these five conditions?

1. Heart attack
2. Angina (chest pain during physical activity)
3. Unstable angina or coronary insufficiency (the symptoms of a heart attack, but with no increase in the enzymes that signal heart muscle damage)
4. Intermittent claudication (severe leg pain, usually upon exertion, that results from an inadequate blood supply)
5. Congestive heart failure (symptoms like breathlessness and severely swollen ankles caused by the heart's failure to pump enough blood and oxygen)

HYP RX—Do you take medication to lower your blood pressure?

LVH—Has an electrocardiogram ever shown that you have left ventricular hypertrophy (an enlarged heart muscle)?

SBP—Your systolic blood pressure (the higher of your two blood pressure numbers)

Source: Data from the Framingham Heart Study. *Circulation* 97:1837, 1998.

PHYSICAL FITNESS ACTIVITY 10.4

Testing for Alcoholism: The Alcohol Use Disorders Identification Test (AUDIT) from the World Health Organization

	Points					
Questions	**0**	**1**	**2**	**3**	**4**	**Your Tally**
1. How often do you have a drink containing alcohol?	Never	Monthly or less	2–3 times per month	2–3 times per week	4 or more times per week	____
2. How many drinks do you have on a typical day when you are drinking?	None	1–2	3–4	5–6	7–9*	____
3. How often do you have more than 3 drinks (women) or 5 drinks (men) on one occasion?	Never	Less than monthly	Monthly	Weekly	Daily or almost daily	____
4. How often during the past year have you found that you were unable to stop drinking once you had started?	Never	Less than monthly	Monthly	Weekly	Daily or almost daily	____
5. How often during the past year have you failed to do what was normally expected from you because of drinking?	Never	Less than monthly	Monthly	Weekly	Daily or almost daily	____
6. How often during the past year have you needed a first drink in the morning to get yourself going after a heavy drinking session?	Never	Less than monthly	Monthly	Weekly	Daily or almost daily	____
7. How often during the past year have you had a feeling of guilt or remorse after drinking?	Never	Less than monthly	Monthly	Weekly	Daily or almost daily	____
8. How often during the past year have you been unable to remember what happened the night before because you had been drinking?	Never	Less than monthly	Monthly	Weekly	Daily or almost daily	____
9. Have you or someone else ever been injured as a result of your drinking?	Never	Yes, but not in past year (2 points)		Yes, during the past year (4 points)		____
10. Has a relative, doctor, or other health worker been concerned about your drinking or suggested you cut down?	Never	Yes, but not in past year (2 points)		Yes, during the past year (4 points)		____

Scoring: A score of 8 points or more indicates a possible drinking problem and the need for a thorough assessment. Total = ____

*Score 5 points if your response is 10 or more drinks on a typical day.

Source: U.S. Preventive Services Task Force. *Guide to Clinical Preventive Services* (2nd ed.). Baltimore: Williams & Wilkins, 1996.

PHYSICAL FITNESS ACTIVITY 10.5

How "Heart Healthy" Is Your Diet?

As discussed in this chapter, all Americans have been advised by the National Cholesterol Education Program to adopt heart-healthy diets. The following questionnaire "MEDFICTS" has been developed by the National Heart, Lung, and Blood Institute to help Americans see how well they are adhering to these dietary recommendations.

MEDFICTS: Dietary Assessment Questionnaire

In each food category for both group 1 and group 2 foods, check one box from the "Weekly Consumption" column (number of servings eaten per week) and then check one box from the "Serving Size" column. If you check Rarely/never, do not check a serving size box. See end of questionnaire for scoring.

Food Category	Weekly Consumption			Serving Size			Score
Meats ■ • Recommended amount per day: ≤6 oz (equal in size to 2 decks of playing cards). • Base your estimate on the food you consume most often. • Beef and lamb sections are trimmed to ⅛ inch fat.	Rarely/ never	3 or less	4 or more	Small <6 oz/day 1 pt	Average 6 oz/day 2 pts	Large >6 oz/day 3 pts	
1. 10 gm or more total fat in 3-oz cooked portion							
Beef. Ground beef, ribs, steak (T-bone, flank, Porterhouse, tenderloin), chuck blade roast, brisket, meatloaf (w/ground beef), corned beef **Processed meats.** ¼-lb burger or lg. sandwich, bacon, lunch meat, sausage/knockwurst, hot dogs, ham (bone-end), ground turkey **Other meats, Poultry, Seafood.** Pork chops (center loin), pork roast (Blade, Boston, sirloin), pork spareribs, ground pork, lamb chops, lamb (ribs), organ meats,* chicken w/skin, eel, mackerel, pompano	☐	☐ 3 pts	☐ 7 pts	× ☐ 1 pt	☐ 2 pts	☐ 3 pts	___
2. Less than 10 g total fat in 3-oz cooked portion							
Lean beef. Round steak (eye of round, top round), sirloin,† tip & bottom round,† chuck arm pot roast,† top loin† **Low-fat processed meats.** Low-fat lunch meat, Canadian bacon, "lean" fast-food sandwich, boneless ham **Other meats, Poultry, Seafood.** Chicken, turkey (w/o skin)§ most seafood,* lamb leg shank, pork tenderloin, sirloin top loin, veal cutlets, sirloin, shoulder, ground veal, venison, veal chops and ribs,† lamb (whole leg, loin, fore-shank, sirloin)†	☐	☐	☐	× ☐	☐	☐‡ 6 pts	___

				Check the number of eggs eaten each time			
Eggs ■ Weekly consumption is the number of times you eat eggs each week				≤1	2	≥3	
1. Whole eggs, yolks	☐	☐ 3 pts	☐ 7 pts	× ☐ 1 pt	☐ 2 pts	☐ 3 pts	___
2. Egg whites, egg substitutes (1/2 c)	☐	☐	☐	× ☐	☐	☐	___
Dairy ■							
Milk. Average serving 1 cup 1. Whole milk, 2% milk, 2% buttermilk, yogurt (whole milk)	☐	☐ 3 pts	☐ 7 pts	× ☐ 1 pt	☐ 2 pts	☐ 3 pts	___ ___
2. Skim milk, 1% milk, skim buttermilk, yogurt (nonfat, 1% lowfat)	☐	☐	☐	× ☐	☐	☐	___
Cheese. Average serving 1 oz 1. Cream cheese, cheddar, Monterey Jack, colby, swiss, American processed, blue cheese, regular cottage cheese (1/2 c), and ricotta (1/4 c)	☐	☐ 3 pts	☐ 7 pts	× ☐ 1 pt	☐ 2 pts	☐ 3 pts	___
2. Low-fat & fat-free cheeses, skim milk mozzarella, string cheese, low-fat, skim milk & fat-free cottage cheese (1/2 c) and ricotta (1/4 c)	☐	☐	☐	× ☐	☐	☐	___
Frozen Desserts ■ Average serving 1/2 c 1. Ice cream, milk shakes	☐	1 ☐ 3 pts	☐ 7 pts	× ☐ 1 pt	☐ 2 pts	☐ 3 pts	___
2. Ice milk, frozen yogurt	☐	☐	☐	☐	☐	☐	___
Frying Foods ■ Average servings: see below. This section refers to method of preparation for vegetables and meat.							
1. French fries, fried vegetables (1/2 c), fried chicken, fish, meat (3 oz)	☐	☐ 3 pts	☐ 7 pts	× ☐ 1 pt	☐ 2 pts	☐ 3 pts	___
2. Vegetables, not deep fried (1/2 c), meat, poultry, or fish-prepared by baking, broiling, grilling, poaching, roasting, stewing: (3 oz)	☐	☐	☐	× ☐	☐	☐	___
Baked Goods ■ 1 Average serving							
1. Doughnuts, biscuits, butter rolls, muffins, croissants, sweet rolls, danish, cakes, pies, coffee cakes, cookies	☐	☐ 3 pts	☐ 7 pts	× ☐ 1 pt	☐ 2 pts	☐ 3 pts	___
2. Fruits bars, Low-fat cookies/cakes/pastries, angel food cake, homemade baked goods with vegetable oils, breads, bagels	☐	☐	☐	× ☐	☐	☐	___
Convenience Foods ■							
1. Canned, packaged, or frozen dinners: e.g., pizza (1 slice), macaroni & cheese (1 c), pot pie (1), cream soups (1 c), potato, rice & pasta dishes with cream/cheese sauces (1/2 c)	☐	☐ 3 pts	☐ 7 pts	× ☐ 1 pt	☐ 2 pts	☐ 3 pts	___
2. Diet/reduced-calorie or reduced-fat dinners (1), potato, rice & pasta dishes without cream/cheese sauces (1/2 c)	☐	☐	☐	× ☐	☐	☐	___
Table Fats ■ Average serving: 1 tbsp							
1. Butter, stick margarine, regular salad dressing, mayonnaise, sour cream (2 tbsp)	☐	☐ 3 pts	☐ 7 pts	× ☐ 1 pt	☐ 2 pts	☐ 3 pts	___
2. Diet and tub margarine, low-fat & fat-free salad dressings, low-fat & fat-free mayonnaise	☐	☐	☐	× ☐	☐	☐	___

Snacks ■							
1. Chips (potato, corn, taco), cheese puffs, snack mix, nuts (1 oz), regular crackers (½ oz), candy (milk chocolate, caramel, coconut) (about 1 ½ oz), regular popcorn (3 c)	☐	☐ 3 pts	☐ 7 pts	× ☐ 1 pt	☐ 2 pts	☐ 3 pts	___
2. Pretzels, fat-free chips (1 oz), low-fat crackers (½ oz), fruit, fruit rolls licorice, hard candy (1 med piece), bread sticks (1-2 pc), air-popped or low-fat popcorn (3 c)	☐	☐	☐	× ☐	☐	☐	___

*Organ meats, shrimp, abalone, and squid are low in fat but high in cholesterol.
†Only lean cuts with all visible fat trimmed. If not trimmed of all visible fat, score as if in group 1.
‡Score 6 pts if this box is checked.
§All parts not listed in group 1 have < 10 g total fat.

Total from page 1 ___
Total from page 2 ___
Final Score ___

To score: For each food category, multiply points in weekly consumption box by points in serving size box and record total in score column. If group 2 foods checked, no points are scored (except for group 2 meats, large serving = 6 pts).

Example:

☐	☐ 3 pts	☑ 7 pts	× ☐ 1 pt	☐ 2 pts	☑ 3 pts	21

Add scores on page 1 and page 2 to get final score.

Key:
≥70 Need to make some dietary changes
40–70 Very good
<40 Excellent

Source: Kris-Etherton P. Eissenstat B, Jaax S, Srinath U, Scott L, Rader J, Pearson T. Validation for MEDFICTS, a dietary assessment instrument for evaluating adherence to total and saturated fat recommendations of the National Cholesterol Education Program Step 1 and Step 2 diets. *J Am Diet Assoc* 101:81–86, 2001.

chapter 11

Cancer

For the majority of Americans who do not use tobacco, improving diet, increasing physical activity, and maintaining a healthy weight are the most important approaches to reducing the risk of developing cancer.

—American Cancer Society, 2005

There are many types of cancers, but they can all be characterized by uncontrolled growth and spread of abnormal cells.[1,2] If the spread is not controlled, it can result in death, as vital passageways are blocked and the body's oxygen and nutrient supplies are diverted to support the rapidly growing cancer (see Figure 11.1).

Cancer is a general term used to indicate any of the more than 100 types of malignant tumors or neoplasms.[1,2] A *neoplasm* is defined as an abnormal tissue that grows by cellular proliferation more rapidly than normal and continues to grow after the stimuli that initiated the new growth cease. Neoplasms show a lack of structural organization and coordination with the surrounding normal tissue, and they usually form a distinct mass of tissue, which may be either benign (noncancerous tumor) or malignant (cancer). A *malignant cancer* is one that invades surrounding tissues and is usually capable of producing *metastases* (the spread of cancer cells from one part of the body to another). Often, the malignant cancer may recur after attempted removal and is likely to cause death unless adequately treated through radiation, chemotherapy, and surgery.

Two classifications of tumors are carcinoma and sarcoma. A *carcinoma* is any of the various malignant neoplasms derived from epithelial tissue (the lining or covering cells of tissues). Carcinomas occur more frequently in the skin and large intestine, the lung and prostate gland in men, and the lung and breast in women. A *sarcoma* is a connective-tissue neoplasm and is usually highly malignant. See Box 11.1 for a description of cancer staging, or the process of describing the extent and spread of cancer.

Humans are made up of approximately 60 trillion cells. Each cell contains *DNA,* the blueprint for making enzymes that drive unique chemical reactions. Researchers have estimated that the DNA in each cell receives a "hit" once every 10 seconds from damaging molecules.[3] Most of the DNA injury comes from a class of chemicals known as *oxidants,* byproducts of the normal process by which cells turn food into energy. Although much of the damage is repaired, over a lifetime, unrepaired damage accumulates. Both aging and cancer can be attributed in large part to the accumulation of damage to DNA. Alteration of the DNA affects more than the cell in which it occurs; when the affected cell divides, the defective blueprint is passed on to all the descendants of that cell.

Normally, the cells that make up the body reproduce and divide in an orderly manner, so that old cells are replaced and cell injuries repaired. Certain environmental (e.g., oxidants and other chemicals, radiation, and viruses) and internal (e.g., hormones, immune conditions, and inherited mutations) factors contribute to the process by which some cells undergo abnormal changes and begin the process toward becoming cancer cells.[1] These abnormal cells may grow into tumors, some of which are cancerous, but others benign. The formation of cancer (*carcinogenesis*) is a long process (often longer than 10 years) and goes through three stages: initiation, promotion, and progression (see Box 11.1). The end result is a loss of control over cellular proliferation.

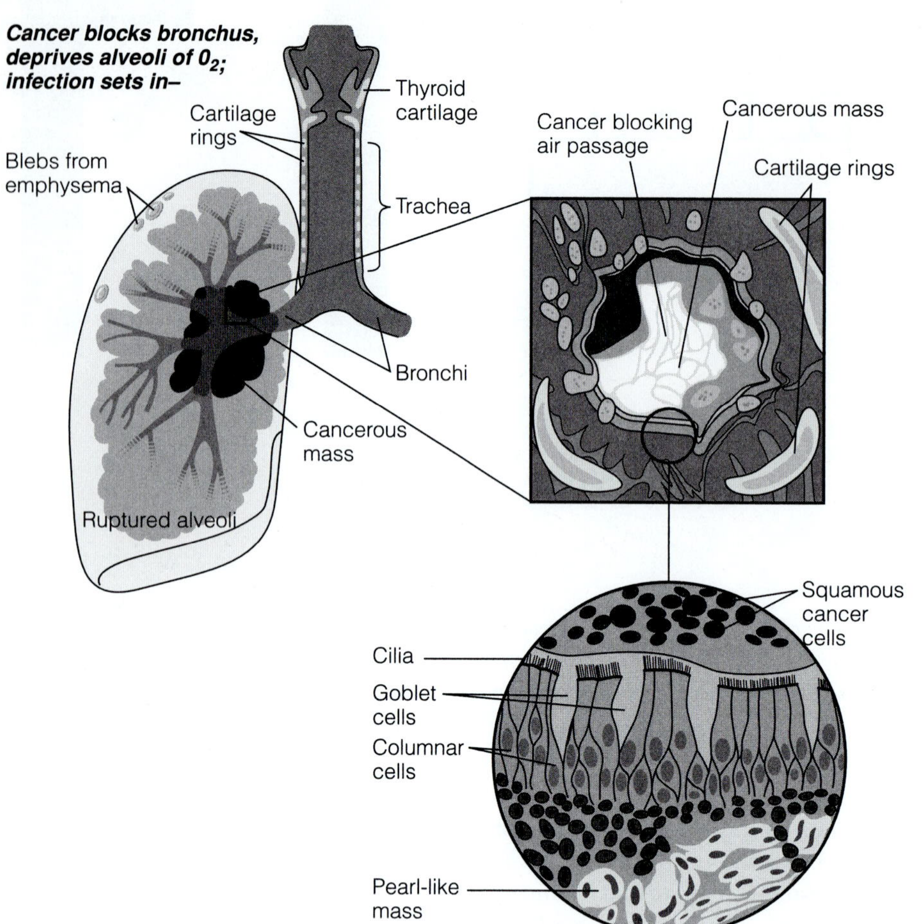

Figure 11.1 Lung cancer. Squamous cancer cells completely line the bronchial wall. Numerous hard, pearl-like masses, made of keratin, have been deposited in the cancerous tissue. With the cancer unchecked and uncontained, the conquest is all but complete. Cancer, blocking the bronchus, also deprives the alveoli of oxygen and makes them ripe for infection by bacteria, which flourish in defenseless tissue.

CANCER STATISTICS

Although heart disease has been the leading cause of death in the United States since the 1950s, cancer will probably replace heart disease as the top killer soon after the year 2010.[4–7] (see Table 11.1 and Figure 11.2). Since the 1950s, death rates for heart disease have fallen steeply (60%). Meanwhile, the war against cancer has been largely unsuccessful.[5] Between 1950 and 1990, age-adjusted death rates for cancer rose 7.7%, due primarily to the sharp increase in lung cancer.[1,6,7] As depicted in Figure 11.3, death rates for many other major cancer sites have leveled off or declined since the 1930s.

Box 11.1

Cancer Growth and Staging

How Does Cancer Begin?

This box provides a simplified explanation of the stages that occur before cancer becomes evident.

The first stage, called initiation, occurs when a normal cell is exposed to a carcinogen, such as chemicals, viruses, radiation, or specific dietary factors. Essentially, anything that causes damage to the cell membrane or the DNA material within the cell can be classified as a carcinogen. DNA repair mechanisms can usually restore the cell to its normal state. If the cell is unable to repair itself, however, it mutates. A mutated, or initiated cell, passes on its mutation when it replicates, thus advancing from the initiation to the promotion stage.

At the promotion stage, the cell may experience spontaneous remission back to the initiation stage, or it may be exposed to growth inhibitors or antipromoters, such as antioxidants and phytochemicals, that will allow regression back to the initiation stage. However, the mutated cell may eventually lose its integrity and develop into a premalignant lesion such as dysplasia, carcinoma in situ, or polyps.

(continued)

Box 11.1

Cancer Growth and Staging *(continued)*

As the cell continues to lose control over its function and structural integrity, progression to the clinical stage of cancer occurs with disruption of normal body functions. The entire process, from exposure to a carcinogen to development of cancer typically takes years.

Cancer Staging

Staging is the process of describing the extent of the disease or the spread of cancer from the site of origin. (See, for example, Stages of Prostate Cancer.)

- **TNM system**

  T = primary tumor

  N = absence or presence of regional lymph node involvement

  M = absence or presence of distant metastases
- Once TNM is determined, then a stage of I, II, III, or IV is assigned:

  I = early stage

  IV = advanced stage
- **Summary staging**

  In situ (cancer cells present only in layers of cells where developed)

  Local

  Regional

  Distant

Stages of Prostate Cancer

The older ABCD system of staging prostate tumors has largely been replaced by the TNM (tumor, nodes, metastases) system, which clinical-stage gauges the severity of cancer on an escalating scale.

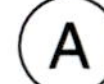

Stage T1
Tumor is microscopic and confined to prostate but is undetectable by a digital rectal exam (DRE) or by ultrasound. Usually discovered by PSA tests or biopsies.

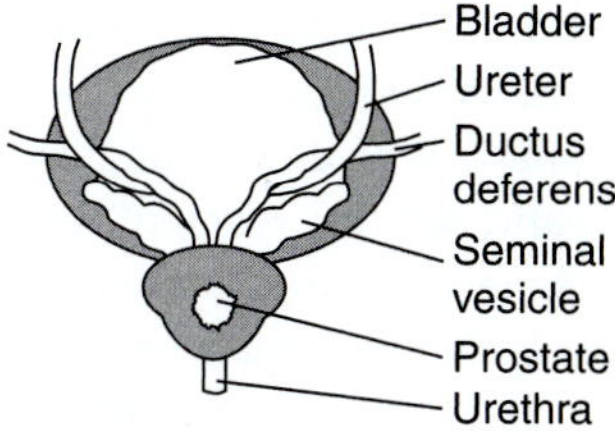

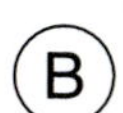

Stage T2
Tumor is confined to prostate and can be detected by DRE or ultrasound.

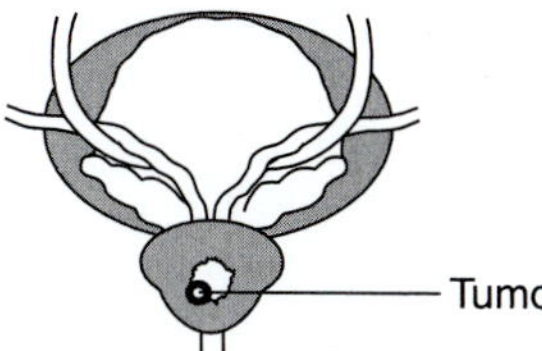

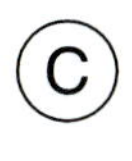

Stage T3 or T4
In stage T3, the cancer has spread to tissue adjacent to the prostate or to the seminal vesicles. Stage T4 tumors have spread to organs near the prostate, such as the bladder.

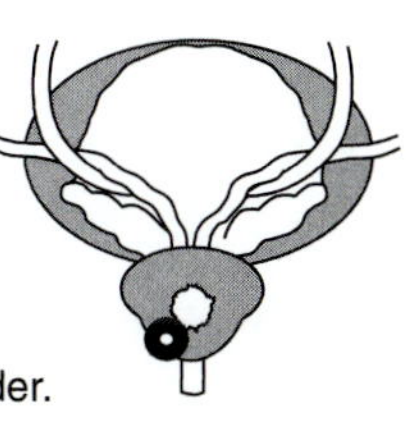

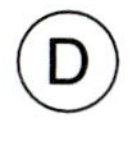

Stage N+ or M+
Cancer has spread to pelvic lymph nodes (N+) or to lymph nodes, organs, or bones distant from the prostate (M+).

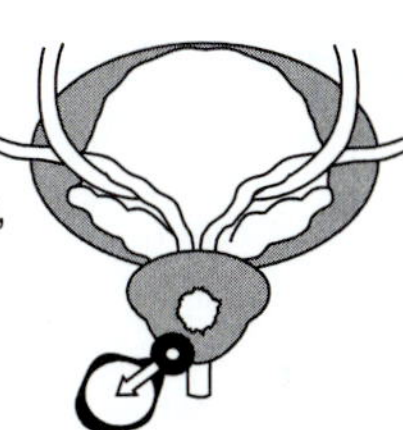

Sources: American Cancer Society. *Cancer Facts & Figures, 2005.* Atlanta: American Cancer Society, 2005, and the IFIC Foundation, Washington, DC: 2005.

TABLE 11.1 Ten Leading Causes of Death, United States, 2003

Rank	Cause of Death	Age-Adjusted Death Rate per 100,000 Population	Percent of Total Deaths
1	Heart diseases	232.1	27.9
2	Cancer	189.3	22.8
3	Cerebrovascular diseases	53.6	6.4
4	Chronic lower respiratory diseases	43.2	5.2
5	Accidents	36.1	4.3
6	Diabetes mellitus	25.2	3.0
7	Pneumonia and influenza	21.9	2.6
8	Alzheimer's disease	21.4	2.6
9	Kidney disease	14.5	1.7
10	Septicemia	11.7	1.4

Source: Monthly Vital Statistics Report, 53(15). Hyattsville, MD: National Center for Health Statistics, 2005.

During the 1990s, total cancer deaths fell about 7%, marking the first decline since cancer statistics were first kept in the 1930s.[1,4,6,7] The decline is expected to continue at about 2% per year and has been attributed to reduced cigarette smoking (and a concomitant decrease in male lung cancer death rates) and improved screening and treatment.[2,6,7]

The American Cancer Society has estimated that the lifetime risk of developing cancer is a staggering 46% for men and 38% for women[1] (see Figure 11.4). About 1.4 million Americans are diagnosed with cancer each year (not including the more than 1 million cases of skin cancer)[1,2] (see Table 11.2). Each year, over a half million Americans die of cancer, about 1,500 each day. Just under one in four deaths

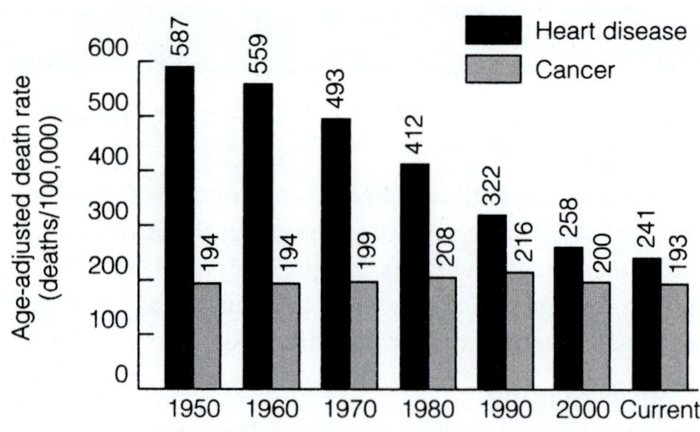

Figure 11.2 Changes in age-adjusted death rates for heart disease and cancer. Death rates for heart disease have fallen sharply since 1950, while those for cancer have stayed about the same. Source: National Center for Health Statistics. *Health, United States, 2004,* Hyattsville, MD: 2004.

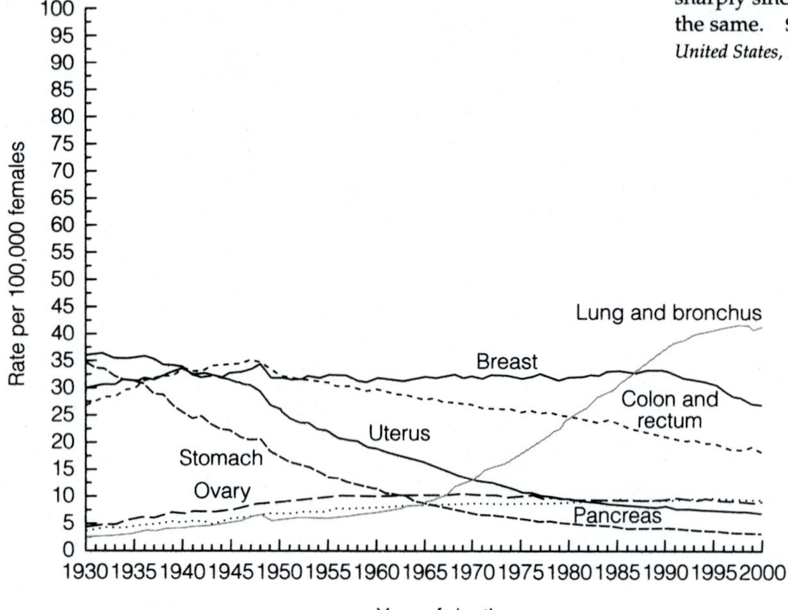

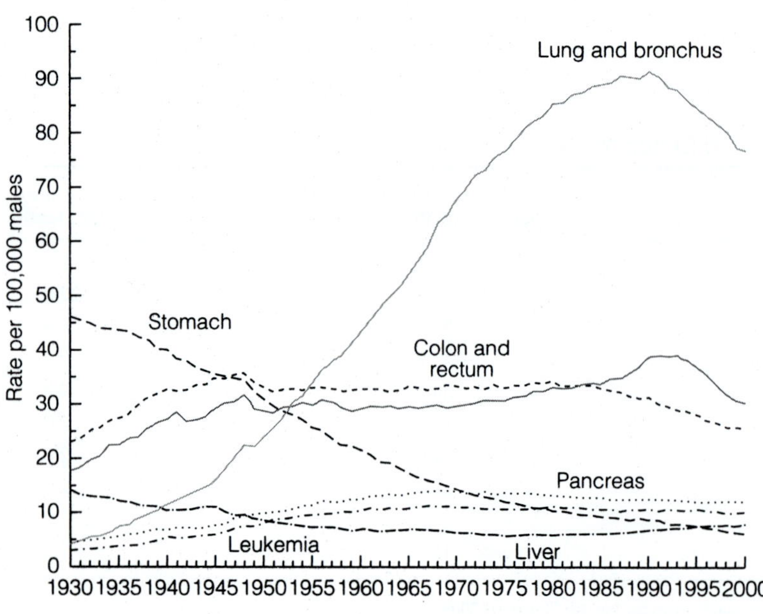

Figure 11.3 Age-adjusted cancer death rates, 1930–2000. Sources: Jemal A, Tiwari RC, Murray T, Ghafoor A, Samuels A, Ward E, Feuer EJ, Thun MJ. Cancer statistics, 2004. *CA Cancer J Clin* 54:8–29, 2004; National Center for Health Statistics. *Health, United States, 2004.* Hyattsville, MD: 2004.

each year in the United States are from cancer. Cancer can strike at any age and, as outlined in Figure 11.5, represents the number one cause of years of potential life lost before age 75.[4] The leading cancer killer for both men and women is lung cancer, followed by prostate or breast cancer, and colorectal cancer.[1,2] (See Figures 11.6 and 11.7.)

A huge interest in and acceptance of alternative and complementary cancer therapies (see Box 11.2) has arisen because of the high lifetime risk for cancer, the absence of significant gains in treatment for the major cancers (despite decades of research and billions of dollars spent since initiation of the war on cancer), the painful side effects of traditional medical treatment for cancer, and widespread public distrust and dissatisfaction with establishment medicine. Unfortunately, most alternative therapies have no proven worth, may delay conventional care, often cost a great deal, can be directly toxic, and raise false hope.

In the early 1900s, few cancer patients had much hope of long-term survival. In the 1930s, fewer than 1 in 5 patients

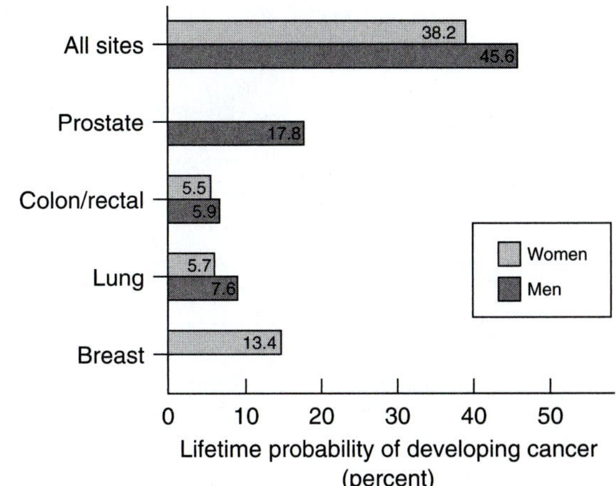

Figure 11.4 Lifetime probability of developing cancer, excluding skin cancer. Source: American Cancer Society. *Cancer Facts & Figures—2005.* Atlanta: Author, 2005.

TABLE 11.2 Basic Cancer Facts and Figures, United States

New cancer cases per year	1,373,000 (plus 1,000,000 skin cancers)
Cancer deaths per year	570,000 (1,500 per day)
Rank as cause of death	Second (behind heart disease)
Percentage of total U.S. deaths	23.0%
Cancer death trends	Steady, slight rise from 1950 to 1990; small decrease since 1990
Lifetime risk of developing cancer	45.6% for males, 38.2% for females
Survival rate for all cancers, 5 years	64%
Americans alive with a history of cancer	9.8 million
Cost of cancer	$190 billion per year, nationwide
Cancer causes	33% poor nutrition 30% tobacco use

Source: American Cancer Society. *Cancer Facts & Figures—2005.* Atlanta: Author, 2005.

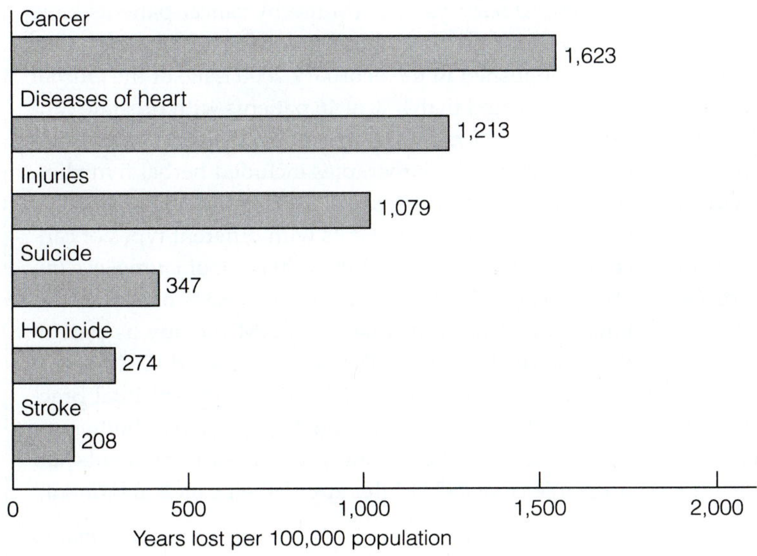

Figure 11.5 Cancer ranks highest as the cause of years of potential life lost before age 75. Source: National Center for Health Statistics. *Health, United States, 2004.* Hyattsville, MD: 2004.

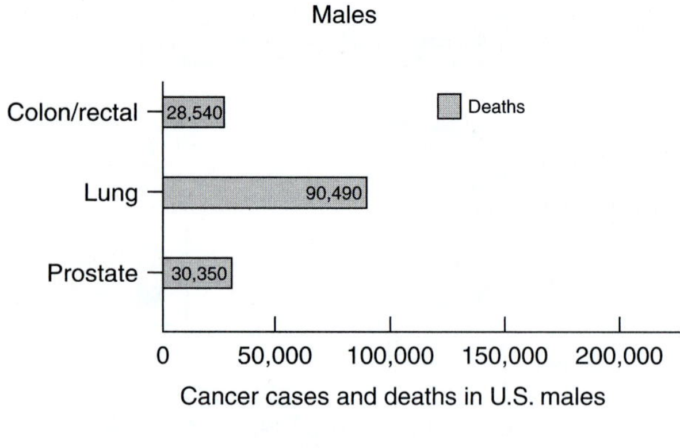

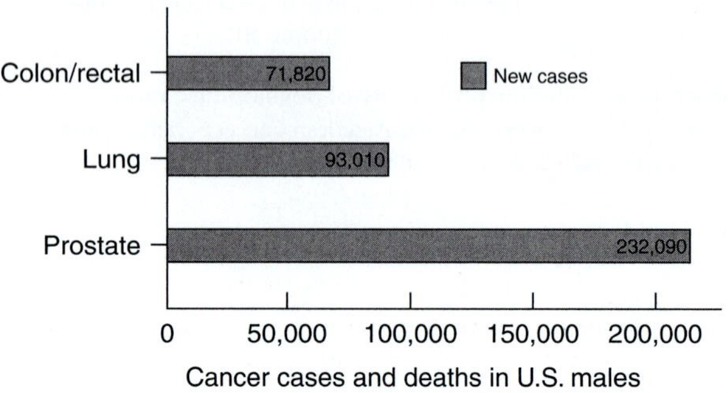

Figure 11.6 Deaths and new cases of the leading cancers in males. Source: American Cancer Society. *Cancer Facts & Figures—*2005. Atlanta: Author, 2005.

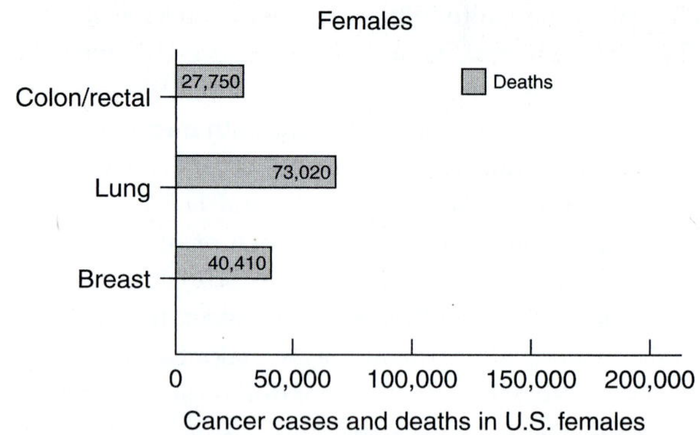

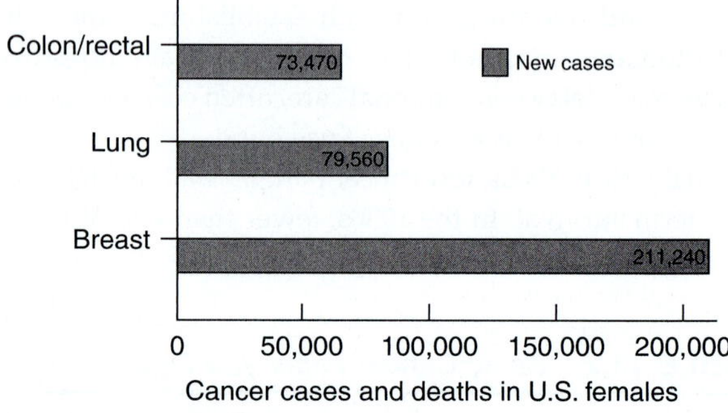

Figure 11.7 Deaths and new cases of the leading cancers in females. Source: American Cancer Society. *Cancer Facts & Figures—2005*. Atlanta: Author, 2005.

Box 11.2

Questions and Answers About Complementary and Alternative Medicine in Cancer Treatment from the National Cancer Institute

What Is Complementary and Alternative Medicine?

Complementary and alternative medicine (CAM)—also referred to as integrative medicine—includes a broad range of healing philosophies, approaches, and therapies. A therapy is generally called complementary when it is used in addition to conventional treatments; it is often called alternative when it is used instead of conventional treatment. (Conventional treatments are those that are widely accepted and practiced by the mainstream medical community.) Depending on how they are used, some therapies can be considered either complementary or alternative.

Complementary and alternative therapies are used in an effort to prevent illness, reduce stress, prevent or reduce side effects and symptoms, or control or cure disease. Some commonly used methods of complementary or alternative therapy include mind/body control interventions such as visualization or relaxation; manual healing, including acupressure and massage; homeopathy; vitamins or herbal products; and acupuncture.

Are Complementary and Alternative Therapies Widely Used?

CAM use among the general public increased from 34% in 1990 to 62% in 2002.

Several surveys of CAM use by cancer patients have been conducted with small numbers of patients. One study published in the February 2000 issue of the journal *Cancer* reported that 37% of 46 patients with prostate cancer used one or more CAM therapies as part of their cancer treatment. These therapies included herbal remedies, old-time remedies, vitamins, and special diets. A larger study of CAM use in patients with different types of cancer was published in the July 2000 issue of *Journal of Clinical Oncology*. That study found that 83% of 453 cancer patients had used at least one CAM therapy as part of their cancer treatment. The study included CAM therapies such as special diets, psychotherapy, spiritual practices, and vitamin supplements. When psychotherapy and spiritual practices were excluded, 69% of patients had used at least one CAM therapy in their cancer treatment.

(continued)

Box 11.2

Questions and Answers About Complementary and Alternative Medicine in Cancer Treatment from the National Cancer Institute *(continued)*

How Are Complementary and Alternative Approaches Evaluated?

It is important that the same scientific evaluation that is used to assess conventional approaches be used to evaluate complementary and alternative therapies. A number of medical centers are evaluating complementary and alternative therapies by developing clinical trials (research studies with people) to test them.

Conventional approaches to cancer treatment have generally been studied for safety and effectiveness through a rigorous scientific process, including clinical trials with large numbers of patients. Often, less is known about the safety and effectiveness of complementary and alternative methods. Some of these complementary and alternative therapies have not undergone rigorous evaluation. Others, once considered unorthodox, are finding a place in cancer treatment—not as cures, but as complementary therapies that may help patients feel better and recover faster. One example is acupuncture. According to a panel of experts at a National Institutes of Health (NIH) Consensus Conference in November 1997, acupuncture has been found to be effective in the management of chemotherapy-associated nausea and vomiting and in controlling pain associated with surgery. Some approaches, such as laetrile, have been studied and found ineffective or potentially harmful.

What Should Patients Do When Considering Complementary and Alternative Therapies?

Cancer patients considering complementary and alternative therapies should discuss this decision with their doctor or nurse, as they would any therapeutic approach, because some complementary and alternative therapies may interfere with their standard treatment or may be harmful when used with conventional treatment.

When Considering Complementary and Alternative Therapies, What Questions Should Patients Ask Their Health-Care Provider?

- What benefits can be expected from this therapy?
- What are the risks associated with this therapy?
- Do the known benefits outweigh the risks?
- What side effects can be expected?
- Will the therapy interfere with conventional treatment?
- Is this therapy part of a clinical trial? If so, who is sponsoring the trial?
- Will the therapy be covered by health insurance?

How Can Patients and Their Health-Care Providers Learn More About Complementary and Alternative Therapies?

Patients and their doctor or nurse can learn about complementary and alternative therapies from the following government agencies:

- The NIH National Center for Complementary and Alternative Medicine (NCCAM) (website: http://nccam.nih.gov) facilitates research and evaluation of complementary and alternative practices, and provides information about a variety of approaches to health professionals and the public.
- The NCI Office of Cancer Complementary and Alternative Medicine (OCCAM) coordinates the activities of the NCI in the area of complementary and alternative medicine. OCCAM supports CAM cancer research and provides information about cancer-related CAM to health providers and the general public. (website: www.cancer.gov/occam/)

Sources: Eisenberg DM, Davis RB, Ettner SL, et al. Trends in alternative medicine use in the United States, 1990–1997. *JAMA* 280(18):1569–1675, 2000; Kao GD, Devine P. Use of complementary health practices by prostate carcinoma patients undergoing radiation therapy. *Cancer* 88(3):615–619, 2000; Richardson MA, Sanders T, Palmer JL, Greisinger A, Singletary SE. Complementary/alternative medicine use in a comprehensive cancer center and the implications for oncology. *J Clin Oncology* 18:2505–2514, 2000; NCHS. *Advance Data from Vital and Health Statistics*, no. 343. Hyattsville, MD, 2004.

was alive 5 years after treatment. Now, 64% of patients who get cancer live 5 or more years after diagnosis.[1,2] With regular screening and self-exams, cancer can often be detected early, greatly enhancing the success of treatment.

Table 11.3 summarizes the American Cancer Society recommendations for the early detection of cancer in the general population.[1] Table 11.4 outlines signs and symptoms for five major cancers. Screening examinations, conducted regularly by a health-care professional can result in the detection of cancers at earlier stages, when treatment is more likely to be successful. More than half of all new cancer cases occur in nine screening-accessible cancer sites (breast, colon, rectum, prostate, tongue, mouth, cervix, testis, and skin). The relative survival rate for these cancers is 80% but could rise to 95% if all Americans participated in regular cancer screenings.[1] As shown in Figure 11.8, 5-year relative survival rates for cancer are much improved when the cancer is diagnosed prior to regional and distant body spread.[1,2]

TABLE 11.3 Summary of American Cancer Society Recommendations for the Early Detection of Cancer in Asymptomatic People

Site	Recommendation
Breast	• Yearly mammograms are recommended starting at age 40. The age at which screening should be stopped should be individualized by considering the potential risks and benefits of screening in the context of overall health status and longevity. • Clinical breast exam should be part of a periodic health exam, about every 3 years for women in their 20s and 30s, and every year for women 40 and older. • Women should know how their breasts normally feel and report any breast change promptly to their health care providers. Breast self-exam is an option for women starting in their 20s. • Women at increased risk (e.g., family history, genetic tendency, past breast cancer) should talk with their doctors about the benefits and limitations of starting mammography screening earlier, having additional tests (i.e., breast ultrasound and MRI), or having more frequent exams.
Colon & rectum	Beginning at age 50, men and women should begin screening with one of the examination schedules below: • A fecal occult blood test (FOBT) or fecal immunochemical test (FIT) every year • A flexible sigmoidoscopy (FSIG) every 5 years • Annual FOBT or FIT and flexible sigmoidoscopy every 5 years* • A double-contrast barium enema every 5 years • A colonoscopy every 10 years ** Combined testing is preferred over either annual FOBT or FIT, or FSIG every 5 years, alone. People who are at moderate or high risk for colorectal cancer should talk with a doctor about a different testing schedule.*
Prostate	The PSA test and the digital rectal examination should be offered annually, beginning at age 50, to men who have a life expectancy of at least 10 years. Men at high risk (African American men and men with a strong family history of 1 or more first-degree relatives diagnosed with prostate cancer at an early age) should begin testing at age 45. For both men at average risk and high risk, information should be provided about what is known and what is uncertain about the benefits and limitations of early detection and treatment of prostate cancer so that they can make an informed decision about testing.
Uterus	**Cervix:** Screening should begin approximately 3 years after a woman begins having vaginal intercourse, but no later than 21 years of age. Screening should be done every year with regular Pap tests or every 2 years using liquid-based tests. At or after age 30, women who have had three normal test results in a row may get screened every 2 to 3 years. Alternatively, cervical cancer screening with HPV DNA testing and conventional or liquid-based cytology could be performed every 3 years. However, doctors may suggest a woman get screened more often if she has certain risk factors, such as HIV infection or a weak immune system. Women 70 years and older who have had 3 or more consecutive normal Pap tests in the last 10 years may choose to stop cervical cancer screening. Screening after total hysterectomy (with removal of the cervix) is not necessary unless the surgery was done as a treatment for cervical cancer. **Endometrium:** The American Cancer Society recommends that at the time of menopause all women should be informed about the risks and symptoms of endometrial cancer, and strongly encouraged to report any unexpected bleeding or spotting to their physicians. Annual screening for endometrial cancer with endometrial biopsy beginning at age 35 should be offered to women with or at risk for hereditary nonpolyposis colon cancer (HNPCC).
Cancer-related checkup	For individuals undergoing periodic health examinations, a cancer-related checkup should include health counseling, and, depending on a person's age and gender, might include examinations for cancers of the thyroid, oral cavity, skin, lymph nodes, testes, and ovaries, as well as for some nonmalignant diseases.

Sources: American Cancer Society. *Cancer Facts & Figures—2005.* Atlanta: American Cancer Society, 2005; American Cancer Society. *Cancer Prevention and Early Detection Facts and Figures 2005.* Atlanta: American Cancer Society, 2005.

TABLE 11.4 Major Risk Factors and Signs and Symptoms for Major Cancer Sites

Lung Cancer	
Risk factors	
Cigarette smoke (causes 87% of all lung cancer)	Air pollution
Exposure to certain industrial substances (e.g., arsenic, asbestos)	Tuberculosis
Radiation exposure	Exposure to environmental tobacco smoke in nonsmokers
Residential radon exposure	
Signs and symptoms	
Persistent cough	Chest pain
Sputum streaked with blood	Recurring pneumonia or bronchitis

TABLE 11.4 *(continued)*

Colorectal Cancer	
Risk factors	
Age	Inflammatory bowel disease
Alcohol consumption	Physical inactivity
Smoking	High-fat and/or low-fiber diet
Personal/family history of colorectal cancer or polyps	Inadequate intake of fruits and vegetables
	Obesity
Signs and symptoms	
Rectal bleeding or blood in the stool	Cramping pain in the lower abdomen
Change in bowel habits	
Breast Cancer	
Risk factors	
Recent use of oral contraceptives or postmenopausal estrogens and progestins	Obesity after menopause
	Personal or family history of breast cancer
Increasing age	Some forms of benign breast disease
Never had children	BRCA1 and BRCA2 gene mutations
First childbirth after age 30	A long menstrual history
Higher education	Higher socioeconomic status
Alcohol consumption (≥1/day)	High dietary fat intake (international contrast)
Physical inactivity	Biopsy-confirmed atypical hyperplasia
	High breast tissue density
Signs and symptoms	
Abnormality that shows up on a mammogram before it can be felt	
Breast changes that persist (lump, thickening, swelling, dimpling, skin irritation, distortion, retraction, scaliness, pain, nipple tenderness)	
Prostate Cancer	
Risk factors	
Age (over 70% are diagnosed after age 65)	Family history
Being African American	Live in North America or northwestern Europe
High dietary fat intake (international contrast)	Obesity
Signs and symptoms	
Weak or interrupted urine flow	Blood in the urine
Inability to urinate or difficulty starting or stopping the urine flow	Pain or burning on urination
	Continuing pain in lower back, pelvis, upper thighs
Need to urinate frequently, especially at night	
Skin Cancer	
Risk factors	
Excessive exposure to ultraviolet radiation; history of sunburns	Multiple or atypical *nevi* (malformed, pigmented skin spots)
Fair complexion	Exposure to tanning booths
Occupational exposure to coal tar, pitch, creosote, arsenic, radium	Sun sensitivity (sunburn easily, difficulty tanning, natural blonde or red hair color)
Family history	
Signs and symptoms	
Any change on the skin, especially size or color of a mole or dark spot	Spread of pigmentation beyond its border
	Change in sensation, itchiness, tenderness, or pain
Scaliness, oozing, bleeding, or change in appearance of a bump or nodule	Sore that does not heal

Source: American Cancer Society. *Cancer Facts & Figures, 2005.* Atlanta: American Cancer Society, 2005.

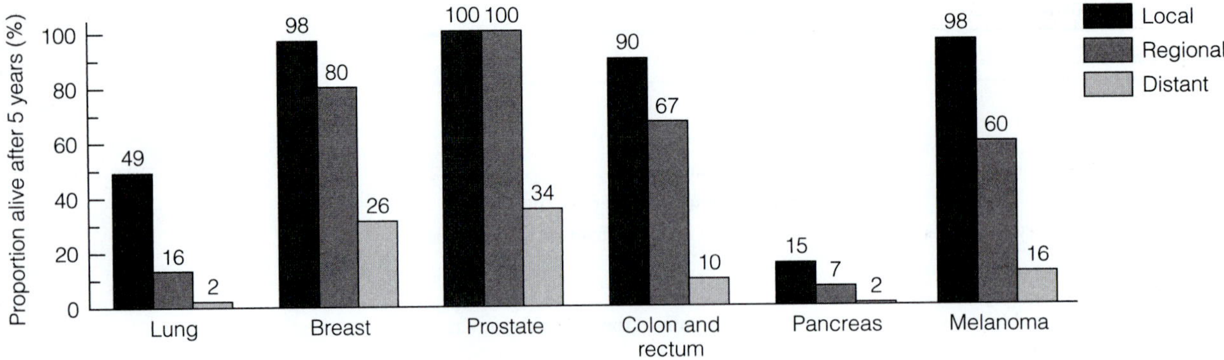

Figure 11.8 Five-year relative survival rates for cancer, by stage at diagnosis. Cancer survival rates are much higher when the cancer is detected early. Source: American Cancer Society. *Cancer Facts & Figures—2005.* Atlanta: Author, 2005.

CANCER PREVENTION

Cancer death rates vary widely throughout the world.[2] For example, colorectal cancer is rare in southwest Asia and equatorial Africa, but common throughout northwestern Europe, the United States, and Canada. Breast cancer rates are four to seven times higher in the United States than in Asia, and this difference is not explained by genetics. Prostate cancer is more common in North America and northwestern Europe and is relatively rare in the Near East, Africa, Central America, and South America. For reasons not fully understood, African Americans have the highest rates for prostate cancer in the world. Prostate cancer rates in China and Japan, for example, are one tenth those of U.S. blacks.

Researchers have reported that when migrants move to a nation with high cancer death rates, their mortality from certain types of cancers, especially colon, breast, and prostate, increase.[8,9] The death rate for colorectal cancer in Japanese immigrants to the United States is three to four times greater than that of Japanese residents in Japan. Puerto Ricans in New York City suffer more colon cancer than those remaining in Puerto Rico. When women migrate from geographic areas with low breast cancer risk to nations such as Australia, Canada, and the United States, their breast cancer risk climbs steeply, even within the lifetime of the migrant. Among older first-generation Japanese American women, for example, incidence of breast cancer is almost seven times higher than that of older Japanese women living in Japan. Chinese Americans and Japanese Americans have prostate cancer rates that are higher than those of their counterparts in Asia. It is widely believed that environmental factors, particularly dietary patterns, account for most of these marked variations in colon, breast, and prostate cancer rates.[9]

Box 11.3 and Table 11.4 list the important risk factors for the leading cancer sites (locations in the body).[1,10] Notice the importance of dietary factors (33% of all cancers) and of tobacco use (30% of all cancers). Other important risk factors include alcohol use, reproductive factors (especially for breast cancer), unsafe sex, environmental factors (e.g., radiation and radon exposure and air pollution), family history, physical inactivity, and obesity. See Box 11.4 for more information on cancer and obesity. Figure 11.9 shows that 80% of all cancers occur at ages 55 and older.[1,4,7,10]

The most common cancer for women is breast cancer. The risk of breast cancer increases with age. Between 40% and 50% of breast cancer can be explained by four well-established risk factors: never had children, late age at first live birth, high education and socioeconomic status, and family history of breast cancer.[1,7,10] Early age at menarche, late age at menopause, and obesity are also important risk factors. Certain types of breast cancer are strongly heritable, and studies with identical twins have shown that if one twin has breast cancer, the risk for the other twin is six times

Box 11.3

Cancer Risk Factors

About 75% of cancers are preventable and are linked to lifestyle. Here are the chief risk factors for cancer:

- Dietary factors (33% of all cancers)
- Tobacco use (30% of all cancers)
- Alcohol use (3–4% of all cancers)
- Reproductive factors (primarily for breast cancer)
- Unsafe sex (exposure to certain types of cancer-promoting viruses)
- Environmental factors (especially sunlight, radiation and radon exposure, and air pollution)
- Family history
- Physical inactivity and obesity

Sources: American Cancer Society. *Cancer Facts & Figures—2005.* Atlanta: American Cancer Society, 2005; American Cancer Society. *Cancer Prevention and Early Detection Facts and Figures 2005.* Atlanta: American Cancer Society, 2005.

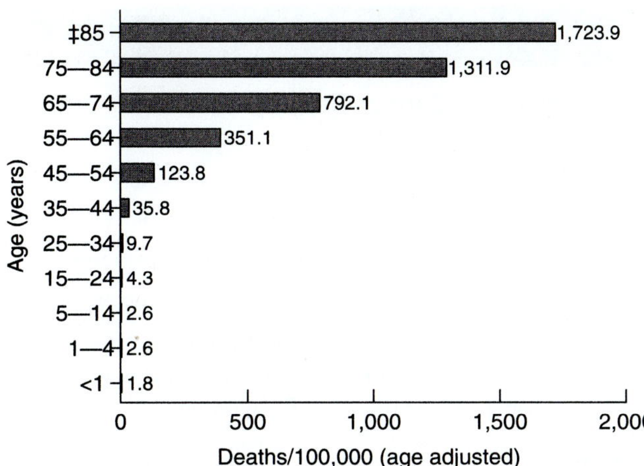

Figure 11.9 Cancer deaths for age groups, United States. Source: National Center for Health Statistics. *Health, United States, 2004.* Hyattsville, MD: 2004.

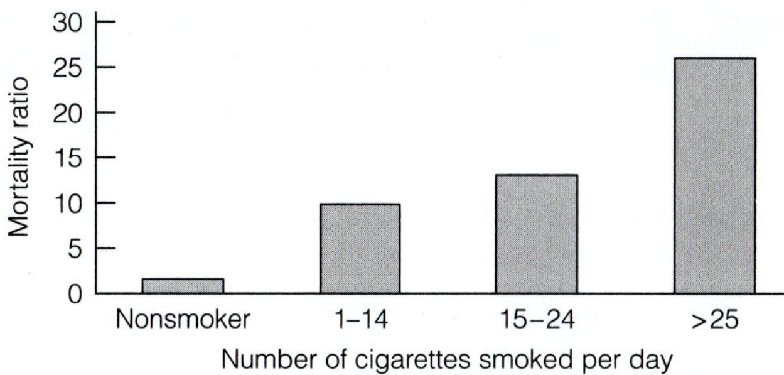

Figure 11.10 Cigarette smoking and lung cancer. A strong dose–response relationship exists between lung cancer death rates and number of cigarettes smoked per day. Source: Carbone D. Smoking and cancer. *Am J Med* 93(1A):13S–17S, 1992.

TABLE 11.5 Lifestyle Habits and Cancer

	Lung	Colon	Breast	Prostate
Smoking	*	†	‡	‡
Low fruit and vegetable intake	*	*	‡	†
Inactivity	‡	*	*	†
Diet fat, red meat	—	*	†	†
Obesity	—	*	*	†
Alcohol	—	†	*	‡

*Solid scientific evidence.
†Many studies suggest link.
‡Few studies to support link.

Source: American Cancer Society guidelines on nutrition and physical activity for cancer prevention: Reducing the risk of cancer with healthy food choices and physical activity. *CA Cancer J Clin* 52:92-119, 2002.

Box 11.4

Obesity and Cancer

- Obesity is related to the following cancers:

  Men. Colon, prostate, liver, pancreas

  Women. Breast (postmenopausal), endometrium, uterine cervix, ovarian, gallbladder, pancreas
- The relative risk of breast cancer in postmenopausal women is 50% higher for the obese
- The relative risk for colon cancer in men is 40% higher for the obese
- Obesity is related to 1 in 7 cancer deaths in men and 1 in 5 in women.

Sources: American Cancer Society. *Cancer Facts & Figures—2005.* Atlanta: American Cancer Society, 2005; American Cancer Society. *Cancer Prevention and Early Detection Facts and Figures 2005.* Atlanta: American Cancer Society, 2005.

greater than normal, and it usually occurs in the same breast (right or left).[1,2] The development of breast cancer is related to female hormones, given that it occurs many times more frequently in women than in men and can be prevented by removal of the ovaries early in life. Any factor that lessens reproductive hormone exposure for a women (e.g., later menarche or early menopause) reduces breast cancer risk.

Prostate cancer is the most common cancer in men. The prostate is a walnut-sized gland tucked away under the bladder and adjacent to the rectum. It provides about a third of the fluid that propels sperm during sex. Prostate cancer rates are about one third higher for black men than for white men. More than 70% of all prostate cancers occur in men over age 65. Studies show that prostate cancer risk is 11 times higher among those who have a brother or a father with prostate cancer.

Lung cancer is the most common cause of cancer death for both men and women. As summarized in Tables 11.4 and 11.5 and Box 11.2, tobacco use is related to lung cancer and many other types of cancers, accounting for about 3 in 10 cancer deaths.[1,2,11–18] Figure 11.10 shows that a strong dose–response relationship exists between lung cancer death rates and the number of cigarettes smoked per day.[11] Smoking is responsible for 87% of all lung cancers.[1,10] Long-term users of smokeless tobacco have a high risk of oral cancer.[1] Each year, about 3,000 nonsmoking adults die of lung cancer as a result of breathing the smoke of other people's cigarettes.[15] New evidence has linked cigarette smoking to prostate, breast, and pancreatic cancers, thus demonstrating that tobacco use is associated with each of the five leading cancer killers.[13–18]

The American Cancer Society has urged that to reduce cancer risk, people should avoid all tobacco use; consume low-fat, high-fiber diets containing plenty of whole grains, fruits, and vegetables; be physically active and maintain a healthy weight; limit consumption of alcoholic beverages; and limit exposure to ultraviolet radiation[1,10] (see Box 11.5). (Visit the American Cancer Society's home page at www.cancer.org.)

Box 11.5

Cancer Prevention Guidelines from the American Cancer Society

One-third of U.S. cancer deaths are due to nutrition and physical activity factors, including excess weight.

A. Recommendations for Individual Choices

1. *Eat a variety of healthy foods, with an emphasis on plant sources.*
   - a. Eat 5 or more servings of vegetables and fruits each day.
   - b. Choose whole grains instead of processed (refined) grains and sugars.
   - c. Limit consumption of red meats, especially high-fat and processed meats.
   - d. Choose foods that help maintain a healthful weight.
2. *Adopt a physically active lifestyle.*
   - a. Adults: Engage in at least moderate activity for 30 minutes or more on 5 or more days of the week; 45 minutes or more of moderate to vigorous activity on 5 or more days per week may further enhance reductions in the risk of breast and colon cancers.
   - b. Children and adolescents: Engage in at least 60 minutes per day of moderate to vigorous physical activity.
3. *Maintain a healthy weight throughout life.*
   - a. Balance caloric intake with physical activity.
   - b. Lose weight if currently overweight or obese.
4. *If you drink alcoholic beverages, limit consumption.*
   - a. People who drink alcohol should limit their intake to no more than 2 drinks per day for men and 1 drink a day for women.

B. Recommendation for Community Action

1. *Increase access to healthy foods in schools, worksites, and communities.*
2. *Provide safe, enjoyable, and accessible environments for physical activity in schools and for transportation and recreation in communities.*

Tobacco Use

A. Health Consequences of Smoking

1. *Smoking accounts for about 30% of all cancer deaths and 87% of lung cancer deaths.*
2. *Smoking is associated with increased risk for at least 15 types of cancer.*

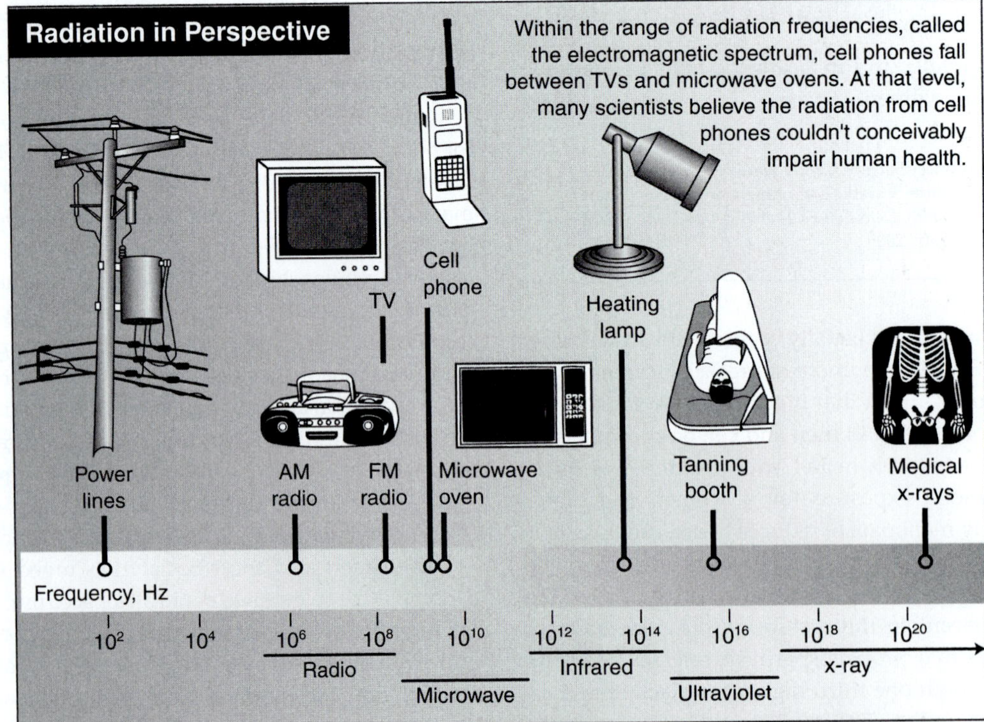

(continued)

Box 11.5

Cancer Prevention Guidelines from the American Cancer Society *(continued)*

B. Reducing Tobacco Use and Exposure

1. *Prevent the initiation of tobacco use among youth, promote quitting among young people and adults, eliminate nonsmokers' exposure to secondhand smoke, and identify and eliminate the disparities related to tobacco use and its effects among different population groups.*

C. Smokeless Tobacco

1. *The use of smokeless tobacco is not a safe substitute for smoking cigarettes, as these products cause various cancers and noncancerous oral conditions, and can lead to nicotine addiction.*

D. Secondhand Smoke

1. *Secondhand smoke, or environmental tobacco smoke (ETS), contains numerous human carcinogens for which there are no safe levels of exposure. Each year, about 3,000 nonsmoking adults die of lung cancer as a result of ETS.*

Avoid Environmental Cancer Risks

1. *Chemicals.* Some chemicals show definite evidence of human carcinogenicity (e.g., benzene, asbestos, vinyl chloride, arsenic, aflatoxin).
2. *Radiation.* Only high-frequency radiation, ionizing radiation (e.g., radon and x-rays), and ultraviolet radiation have been proven to cause human cancer (see the accompanying figure).
3. *Unproven risks.* These include pesticides, nonionizing radiation (e.g., radiowaves, microwaves, radar, and electrical and magnetic fields associated with electric currents), toxic wastes, and nuclear power plants.

Sources: American Cancer Society. *Cancer Facts & Figures—2005.* Atlanta: American Cancer Society, 2005; American Cancer Society. *Cancer Prevention and Early Detection Facts and Figures 2005.* Atlanta: American Cancer Society, 2005; American Cancer Society guidelines on nutrition and physical activity for cancer prevention: Reducing the risk of cancer with healthy food choices and physical activity. *CA Cancer J Clin* 52:92–119, 2002.

Physically active individuals often spend much time outdoors exposed to ultraviolet radiation. Over 1 million skin cancers are diagnosed each year, most of them highly curable basal cell or squamous cell cancers.[1] The most lethal form of skin cancer is melanoma, which is diagnosed in nearly 60,000 persons each year. As outlined in Table 11.4 and Box 11.6, major risk factors for skin cancer include excessive exposure to ultraviolet radiation, fair complexion, family history, and either multiple or atypical *nevi* (malformed, pigmented skin spots). (See Physical Fitness Activities 11.1 and 11.3 at the end of this chapter.)

Of all lifestyle and environmental factors, dietary habits have been most closely linked to cancer[10] (see Tables 11.4 and 11.5 and Box 11.5). Numerous studies have shown that daily consumption of vegetables and fruits is associated with a reduced risk of lung, colon, pancreas, oral cavity and pharynx, esophagus, endometrium, and stomach cancers.[19–29] The types of vegetables or fruits that most often appear to be protective against cancer are raw vegetables, allium vegetables (e.g., onions, garlic, red pepper), carrots, green vegetables, cruciferous vegetables (e.g., broccoli, cabbage, Brussels sprouts), and tomatoes.[19] Vegetables and fruits contain more than 100 beneficial vitamins, minerals, fiber, and other substances. These substances include vitamins (in particular, the antioxidant vitamins A, C, E, and the provitamin beta-carotene), minerals (calcium, selenium), fiber, and nonnutritive constituents (e.g., dithiolthiones, isothiocyanates, isoflavones, protease inhibitors, saponins, phytosterols, lutein, lycopene, and allium compounds).[19,20] These food substances, alone or together, may be responsible for reducing cancer risk. Substances in fruit and vegetables interrupt the cancer process at several different phases.[19]

Intake of a wide variety of fruits and vegetables is recommended, yet surveys indicate that less than one in four Americans eat five or more servings a day.[10,19] The American Cancer Society does not recommend the use of dietary supplements because "the few studies in human populations that have attempted to determine whether supplements can reduce cancer risk have yielded disappointing results."[10] Although there has been some concern about pesticide residues on plant foods, cancer experts have concluded that there is no good evidence that a high ingestion of fruits and vegetables increases pesticide intake enough to enhance risk of cancer.[30]

The antioxidant vitamins in fruits and vegetables appear to improve immune function, scavenge free radicals and singlet oxygen particles (both of which can damage cell membranes), and play a role in numerous biological systems and the synthesis of hormones, neurotransmitters,

Box 11.6

Sunlight and Skin Cancer

- More than 1 million cases of highly curable basal cell or squamous cell cancers occur annually.
- The most serious form of skin cancer is melanoma, with nearly 60,000 new cases and 10,600 deaths a year.
- *Signs and symptoms.* Symptoms of melanoma may include any change on the skin, such as a new spot or one that changes in size, shape, or color. Other important signs of melanoma include changes in size, shape, or color of a mole. Basal cell carcinomas often appear as flat, firm, pale areas or as small, raised, pink or red, translucent, shiny, waxy areas that may bleed following minor injury. Squamous cell cancer may appear as growing lumps, often with a rough surface, or as flat, reddish patches that grow slowly. Another symptom of basal and squamous cell skin cancers is a sore that doesn't heal.
- *Risk factors.* For melanoma, major risk factors include a prior melanoma, one or more family members who had melanoma, and moles (especially if there are many, or if they are unusual or large). Other risk factors for all types of skin cancer include sun sensitivity (sunburn easily, difficulty tanning, natural blonde or red hair color), a history of excessive sun exposure including sunburns, exposure to tanning booths and to diseases that suppress the immune system, a past history of basal cell or squamous cell skin cancers, and occupational exposure to coal tar, pitch, creosote, arsenic compounds, or radium.
- *Prevention.* Limit or avoid exposure to the sun during 10 A.M. to 4 P.M. When outdoors, wear a hat that shades the face, neck, and ears, a long-sleeved shirt, and long pants. Wear sunglasses to protect the skin around the eyes. Use a sunscreen with a sun protection factor (SPF) of 15 or higher. Because severe sunburns in childhood may greatly increase risk of melanoma in later life, children should be protected from the skin.
- *Early detection.* Have a physician evaluate all suspicious skin lesions. Use the ABCD rule for melanoma: A is for asymmetry, one half of the mole does not match the other half; B is for border irregularity, the edges are ragged, notched, or blurred; C is for color, the pigmentation is not uniform, with variable degrees of tan, brown, and black; D is for diameter, greater than 6 millimeters (about the size of a pencil eraser).

collagen, and many other substances.[19–24] As cells use oxygen to "burn" their fuel, one of the by-products is free radicals. *Free radicals* contain one or more unpaired electrons and can be harmful because they attack the vital components of the cell. Beta-carotene can prevent singlet oxygen from producing free radicals, transforming the singlet oxygen into a stable oxygen species lacking the energy to engage in harmful reactions against cells.[22,23] It has been calculated that one molecule of beta-carotene can quench as many as 1,000 molecules of singlet oxygen. Other carotenoids (there are more than 600 in nature) can also participate in this process.[22] Vitamin C is also an important reducing agent and free-radical scavenger and additionally prevents or reduces the formation of certain cancer-causing chemicals, such as nitrosamines.[19–21] Vitamin E is a potent antioxidant and has been related to inhibition of tumors in animal studies.[19,20]

Vitamin C is found in most fruits and vegetables. Beta-carotene, which is partially converted to vitamin A in the body, is plentiful in carrots, green leafy vegetables, sweet potatoes, winter squash, cantaloupe, and tomatoes. Carotenoids are a group of pigments that contribute to the yellow, orange, or red coloration of fruits and vegetables. Beta-carotene is the most plentiful carotenoid found in foods consumed by humans. Vitamin E is available in cereal grains, several vegetable oils, sunflower seeds, nuts, and kale.

Dietary fiber is a term used to cover several types of food components (e.g., cellulose, pectins, hemicellulose, lignins, gums) that are not digested in the human intestinal tract. These substances, abundant in whole grains, fruits, and vegetables, consist largely of complex carbohydrates of diverse chemical composition (see Chapter 9). A large number of studies indicate that colon cancer is low in human populations on other continents, who live on diets of largely unrefined food high in dietary fiber.[10,31,32] Researchers have estimated that if people would increase their fiber intake by 13 grams per day, a 31% reduction in colorectal cancer risk would result.[31] Currently, the average American male and female consumes about half the recommended amount of dietatry fiber (see Chapter 9).

There are several mechanisms whereby fiber may protect against colon cancer.[10,31,32] Fiber has the ability to bind to bile acids, which are released into the intestine from the liver, to aid in digestion of fat. High-fat diets increase bile acid production, ultimately increasing the exposure of the bowel to secondary bile acids, which are produced when colon bacteria degrade the primary bile acids from the liver.

Fiber, however, binds the bile acids, increases stool bulk, dilutes the concentration of secondary bile acids and other cancer-causing chemicals, and speeds up the transit of the fecal mass through the colon. Additionally, some of the water-soluble fibers (from fruits and vegetables) are fermented by the colonic bacteria into volatile free fatty acids, which may be directly anticarcinogenic.

Whether dietary fiber reduces the risk of other cancers is uncertain. It has been hypothesized that dietary fiber may reduce breast cancer risk because fiber reduces the intestinal reabsorption of estrogens excreted with bile acids from the liver.[31,32] Although some animal studies suggest that dietary fiber does reduce breast cancer risk, the evidence in humans is inconclusive. Obesity is strongly related to both colon and breast cancer.[33]

The American Cancer Society recommends reducing total dietary fat intake primarily by decreasing use of animal products.[10] Substantial evidence suggests that excessive fat intake increases the risk of developing cancers of the colon and rectum, prostate, and endometrium.[10,34–38] Several studies have shown a link between consumption of meat, especially red meats, and cancers at several sites, most notably the colon and prostate.[35–37]

There is still controversy regarding the relationship between dietary fat and breast cancer.[39–42] Over 60 years ago, researchers showed that diets high in fat increased the risk of breast tumors in rodents.[33] Around the world, the per capita fat consumption, especially of animal fat, is highly correlated with national breast cancer mortality rates.[42] Breast cancer incidence rates have increased substantially in the United States during the twentieth century, as has per capita fat consumption. However, in various cohort studies where women are followed for 3–20 years, few have found that high fat intake increases the risk of developing breast cancer.[39] Randomized trials of fat reduction have been proposed as a means of resolving the uncertainty about the association between dietary fat and breast cancer.[41]

For colon cancer, the association with dietary fat is much clearer.[10,25,26,28,31,32,36–38] In Western countries, the rates of colon cancer are up to 10 times those of many Far Eastern and developing nations.[1] Rapid increases in rates of colon cancer occur among offspring of migrants from low-risk to high-risk areas.[9] The per capita consumption of meat or animal fat (but not vegetable fat) is highly correlated with national rates of colon cancer worldwide.[9,36–38] As discussed previously, high-fat diets increase the excretion of bile acids, which can then act as tumor promoters in the colon. In one study of 88,751 nurses, intake of animal fat and red meat was positively associated with the risk of colon cancer, with the risk 89% higher for intake of animal fat and 77% higher for red meat intake in women consuming the highest amounts[36] (see Figure 11.11).

A strong correlation between national consumption of fat and national rate of mortality from prostate cancer has been reported.[9,35] As summarized in Figure 11.12, a high intake of animal fat, especially fat from red meat, has been associated with an elevated risk of advanced prostate cancer.[35] These findings support recommendations from the American Cancer Society to lower intake of dietary animal fat and red meat to reduce risk of cancer.[10]

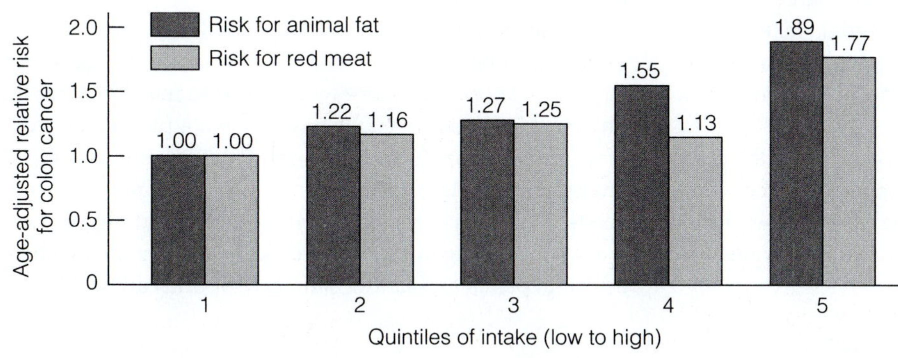

Figure 11.11 Relation of meat and animal fat to risk of colon cancer, 6-year prospective study of women. Colon cancer risk rises with increase in dietary intake of animal fat and red meat. Source: Willett WC, Stampfer MJ, Colditz GA, et al. Relation of meat, fat, and fiber intake to the risk of colon cancer in a prospective study among women. *N Engl J Med* 323:1664–1672, 1990.

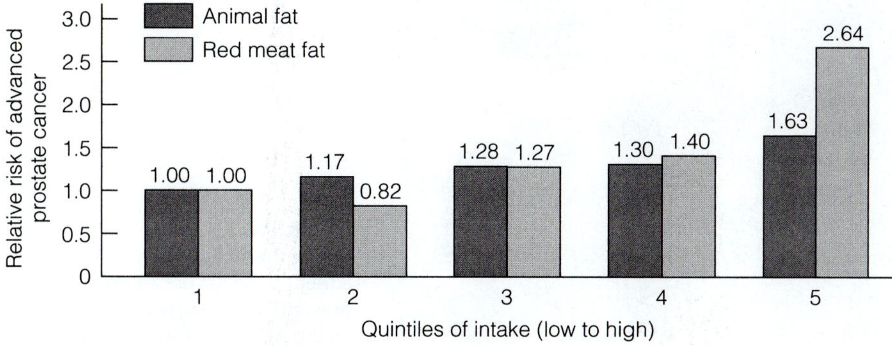

Figure 11.12 Animal fat and risk of prostate cancer, study of 47,855 health professionals. Prostate cancer risk rises with increase in dietary intake of animal fat and red meat. Source: Chao A, Thun MJ, Connell CJ, McCullough ML, Jacobs EJ, Flanders WD, Rodriguez C, Sinha R, Calle EE. Meat consumption and risk of colorectal cancer. *JAMA* 293:172–182, 2005.

Heavy drinkers of alcohol, especially those who are also cigarette smokers, are at unusually high risk for cancers of the oral cavity, larynx, and esophagus.[10] Cancer risk increases with the amount of alcohol consumed and may start to rise with intake of as few as two drinks per day. Some evidence also suggests that regular alcohol consumption increases breast cancer risk in women, perhaps by increasing estrogen levels in the body.[43,44] Heavy alcohol intake can result in liver cirrhosis, which may be associated with liver cancer.[10] There is limited evidence that high alcohol intake also increases the risk for colon and prostate cancers.[45,46] The American Cancer Society advises that people should "limit consumption of alcoholic beverages, if you drink at all."[10]

PHYSICAL ACTIVITY AND CANCER

In 1996, regular physical activity was finally added to the list of cancer-prevention measures advocated by the American Cancer Society[1,10] (see Figure 11.13 and Box 11.5). The American Heart Association also took a long time (until the early 1990s) to add physical inactivity as a risk factor for heart disease (see Chapter 10). The link between chronic disease and inactivity is a difficult one to establish because the relationship is complex, with many other difficult-to-measure lifestyle factors affecting the process.

Evidence is mounting that inactivity does contribute to the development of cancer.[47–50] In 1997, an international panel of cancer experts concluded that as many as 30–40% of all cancer cases worldwide could be avoided if people ate a healthy diet, avoided obesity, and got enough exercise.[51] The panel proposed a rigorous exercise goal: Take a brisk walk for about an hour daily (or the equivalent) and exercise vigorously at least 1 hour total each week if you have a sedentary job.

Although the epidemic of heart disease during the mid-twentieth century diverted the attention of researchers, the fact that cancer deaths now nearly equal those of heart disease has revitalized the nation's determination to wage war against cancer.

Inactivity as a Risk Factor for Cancer

The idea that increased physical exercise may be of benefit in preventing cancer is not a new one.[48] More than 80 years ago, researchers in Australia observed that primitive tribes who labored continuously for food had lower rates of cancer than people from more civilized societies.[52] Other scientists and physicians observed early in this century that most cancer patients had led relatively sedentary lives, and that men who had worked hard physically all their lives had less cancer than those who tended to sit during their day of work.[53]

These findings lay dormant until the mid-1970s, when researchers throughout the world took up the question anew. Since then, many studies have bolstered the evidence of an exercise–cancer connection. Active animals, former athletes, people employed in active occupations, and those who exercise during after-work hours have been compared with their sedentary counterparts. In general, depending on the type of cancer site investigated, they have been found to have a lower risk of cancer.[47–50] The Institute for Aerobics Research in Dallas, for example, showed that over an 8-year period, physically unfit men had four times the overall cancer death rate of the most fit men, with an even wider spread found among the women[54] (see Figure 11.14).

Some investigators have injected animals with certain types of cancer-causing chemicals, divided them into exercise and nonexercise groups, and then measured the size and time of cancer appearance. Results show that exercise tends to retard cancer growth at several different sites.[55–60] The activity of certain cells from the immune system—especially natural killer cells, cytotoxic T cells, and macrophages—appears to be enhanced with exercise, with improved cancer-fighting proficiency.[55,60]

Large groups of people have been followed for extended periods of time to see whether those who exercise regularly have less cancer than those who follow an inactive lifestyle. The most impressive results have shown a protective effect of exercise against three common cancer killers: colon, breast, and prostate cancer.[47–50] Although more research is needed, most experts feel that it is unlikely that physical activity has a strong influence on cancers at other sites such as the lung, pancreas, bladder, stomach, or oral cavity.[48,61]

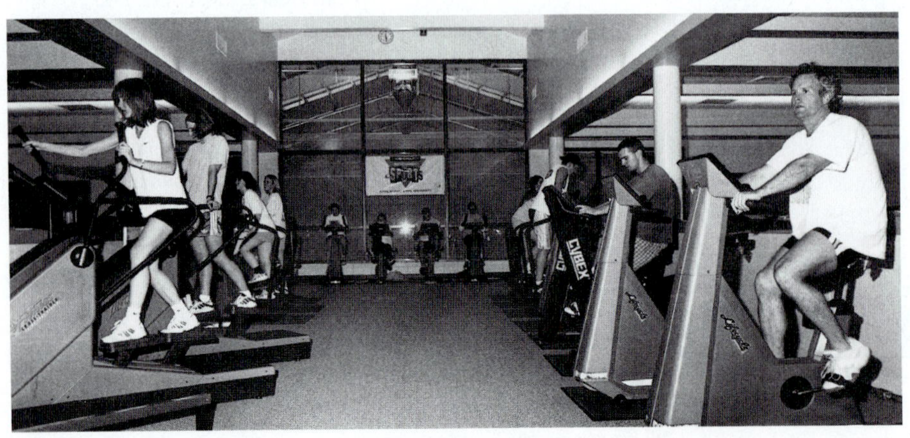

Figure 11.13 In 1996, regular physical activity was finally added to the list of cancer-preventive measures advocated by the American Cancer Society.

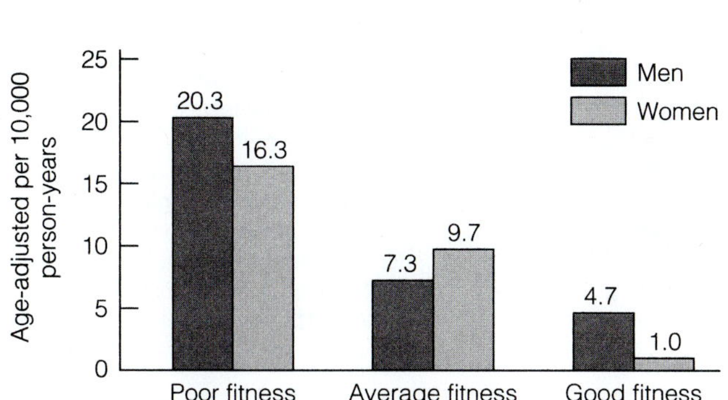

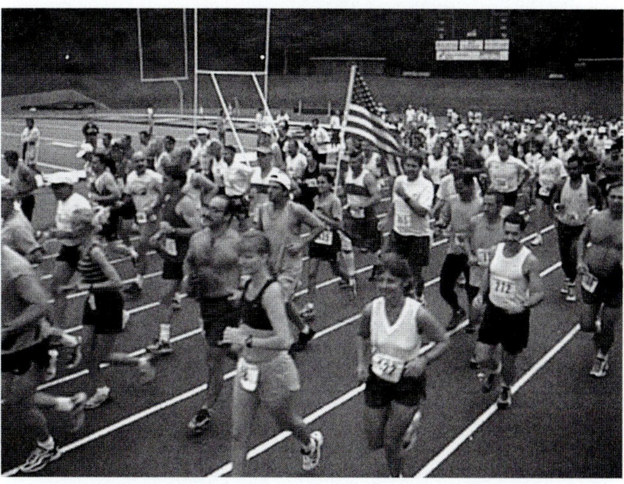

Figure 11.14 Cancer death rates according to fitness status. Cancer death rates were substantially higher in relatively unfit subjects, compared to those with moderate or high levels of fitness. Source: Blair SN, Kohl HW, Paffenbarger RS, et al. Physical fitness and all-cause mortality: A prospective study of healthy men and women. *JAMA* 262:2395–2401, 1989.

Box 11.7

Colon and Rectum Cancer

Risk Factors

- Personal or family history of colorectal cancer or polyps
- Inflammatory bowel disease
- Smoking
- Physical inactivity
- High-fat and/or low-fiber diet
- Alcohol consumption
- Inadequate consumption of fruits and vegetables

Physical Activity

- The epidemiological evidence for a link between activity and lowered risk of colon cancer is convincing.
- Of published studies, about 3 in 4 show a 20–70% decrease in risk of colon cancer among the most physically active men and women (average, 50%).

Potential Mechanisms Mediating Association with Physical Activity

- Exercise has a "fiberlike effect" in decreasing stool transit time, reducing exposure of colon cells to carcinogens (e.g., secondary bile acids).
- Enhancement of imune function.
- Decrease in insulin.
- Enhancement of defense against oxidative stress.

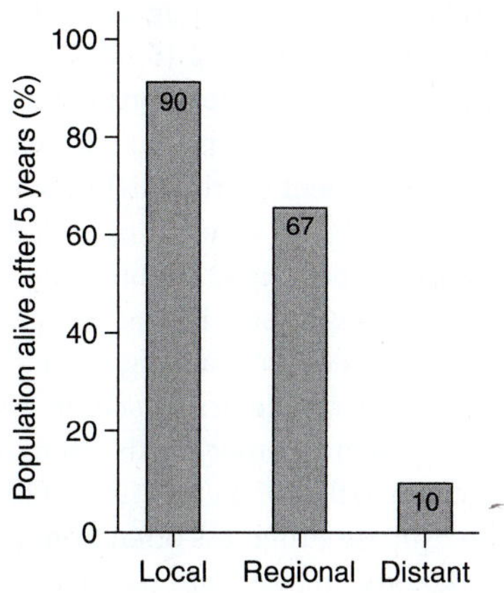

Physical Activity and Colon Cancer

Exercise is most beneficial in preventing cancer of the colon, as compared with other cancer sites.[62] Many studies have been published, looking at both occupational and leisure-time physical activity and the risk of colon cancer.[47,48,63–80] Three fourths of these studies have shown that physically active, compared to inactive, people have a 40–50% decrease in cancer risk, with the best-designed studies showing the strongest relationship.[47,48,50,62] The protective effect of physical activity against colon cancer has been seen in several countries, including China, Sweden, Japan, and the United States. See Box 11.7 for an overview of the risk factors for colon and rectum cancer, and the role of physical activity.

A frequent finding has been that people who tend to sit the majority of their workday or remain inactive in their

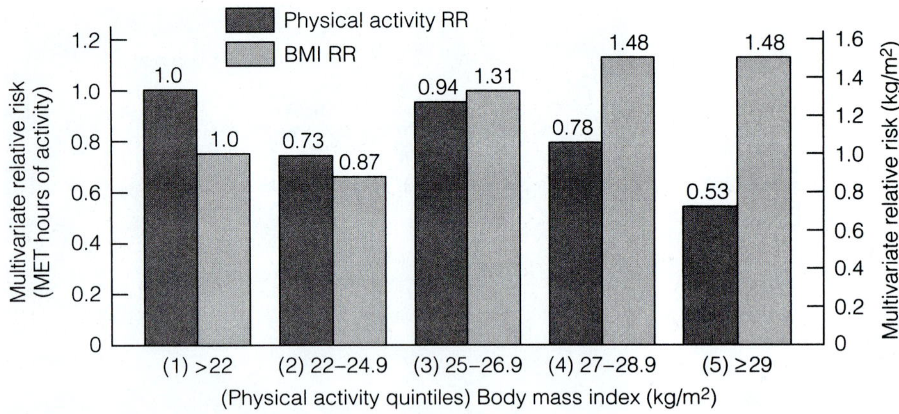

Figure 11.15 Physical activity and risk for colon cancer, 47,723 health professionals, 40–75 years old, 1986–1992 both low activity and high BMI, RR = 4.9 (extreme tertiles). Men who are most active and leanest experience the lowest risk of colon cancer. Source: Giovannucci E, Ascherio A, Rimm EB, Colditz GA, Stampfer MJ, Willett WC. Physical activity, obesity, and risk for colon cancer and adenoma in men. *Ann Intern Med* 122:327–334, 1995.

leisure time have a greater risk of contracting colon cancer.[63–80] For example, researchers at the University of Southern California studied nearly 3,000 men with colon cancer and compared them with the rest of the male population of Los Angeles County.[77] The men who worked at sedentary jobs were found to have a 60% greater colon cancer risk.

In one study of 163 colon cancer patients and 703 controls, 2 hours or more per week of vigorous leisure-time physical activity (e.g., running, bicycling, swimming laps, racquet sports, calisthenics, and rowing) lowered colon cancer risk by 40%.[65] Researchers at Harvard University studied 48,000 male health professionals and showed that colon cancer risk was decreased 50% in the most physically active men, compared to their sedentary peers[64] (see Figure 11.15). The protective effect was most evident in men who exercised on average about 1–2 hours a day. Men who were both physically inactive and obese had a colon cancer risk that was nearly five times higher than that of their active and lean counterparts. A 12-year study of nearly 90,000 nurses has confirmed that the protective effect of regular physical activity against colon cancer also appears in women[63] (see Figure 11.16).

One theory explaining the inverse relationship between physical activity and colon cancer risk is that each exercise bout stimulates muscle movement (peristalsis) of the large intestine.[81–83] In one study, subjects who ran or cycled for 1 hour each day for a week experienced significantly faster mean whole-gut transit times[81] (see Figure 11.17). This shortens the time that various cancer-causing chemicals in the fecal matter (e.g., secondary bile acids) stay in contact with the cells that line the colon. In other words, exercise has a similar effect on the colon to that of dietary fiber. It is well-known that those who exercise suffer less often from constipation than do the sedentary. In one large national survey, people were asked, "Do you have trouble with your bowels that makes you constipated?" Among middle-aged adults, twice as many of those reporting "little exercise" had trouble with constipation, compared to highly active people.[84]

Other theories have been proposed. One of them links exercise, caloric intake, and obesity with colon cancer. In animal studies, when caloric intake is slightly below body needs, cancer risk is lowered.[85] In fact, this is one of the strongest variables controlling cancer incidence in animals. Regular exercise seems to help some people control their diet intakes. As

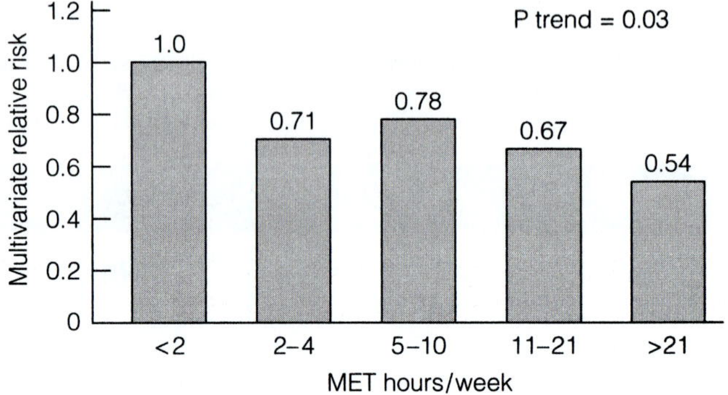

Figure 11.16 Physical activity and risk for colon cancer in women, 12-year study of 89,448 nurses (Nurses Health Study). Colon cancer risk drops by almost half in women who are most active. Source: Martinez ME, Giovannucci E, Spiegelman D, Hunter DJ, Willett WC, Colditz GA. Leisure-time physical activity, body size, and colon cancer in women. *J Natl Cancer Inst* 89:948–955, 1997.

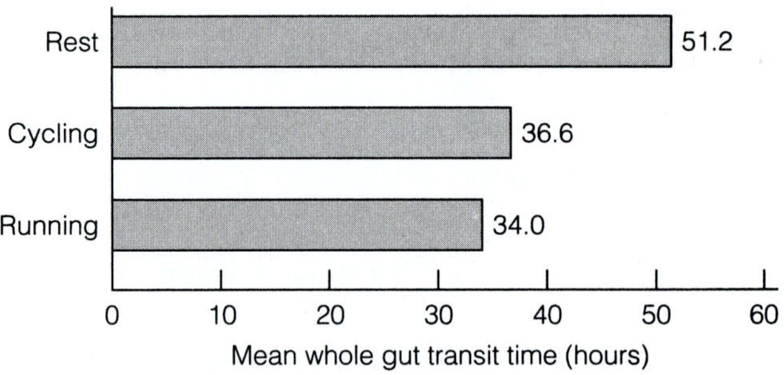

Figure 11.17 Effect of moderate exercise on whole-gut transit time: Subjects either ran, cycled, or rested for 1 hour each day for a week. Exercise intensity = 50% $\dot{V}O_{2max}$; dietary fiber intake the same during each phase. Source: Oettlé GJ. Effect of moderate exercise on bowel habit. *Gut* 32:941–944, 1991.

a result, active people tend to be less obese, which is important because obesity in and of itself promotes several different types of cancer, including colon cancer[63,64,66,86] (see Figures 11.15 and 11.18). Overall energy balance appears to be an important factor related to colon cancer. In one study of 2,073 colon cancer patients and 2,466 controls, those at greatest risk of colon cancer had the most unfavorable energy balance, in that they were physically inactive, had high energy intakes, and were obese.[69] Both obesity and physical inactiv-

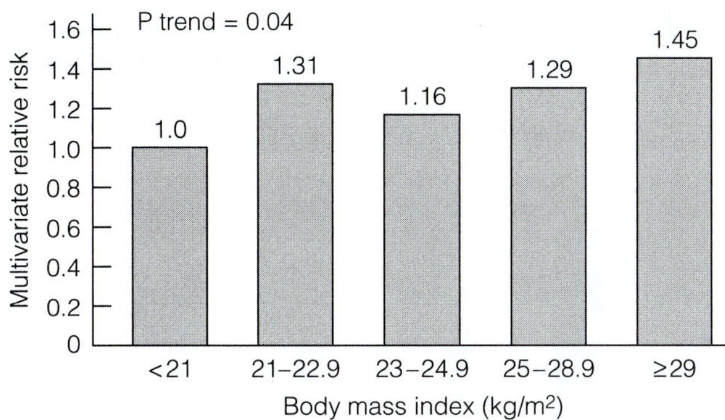

Figure 11.18 Body mass index (BMI) and risk for colon cancer in women, 12-year study of 89,448 nurses (Nurses Health Study). Obesity increases the risk for colon cancer. Source: Martinez ME, Giovannucci E, Spiegelman D, Hunter DJ, Willett WC, Colditz GA. Leisure-time physical activity, body size, and colon cancer in women. *J Natl Cancer Inst* 89:948–955, 1997.

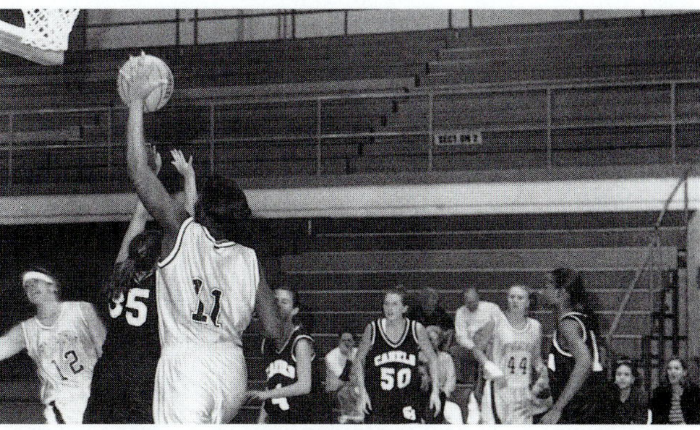

Figure 11.19 There is increasing evidence that women who engage in vigorous exercise from early in life may gain protection against breast cancer.

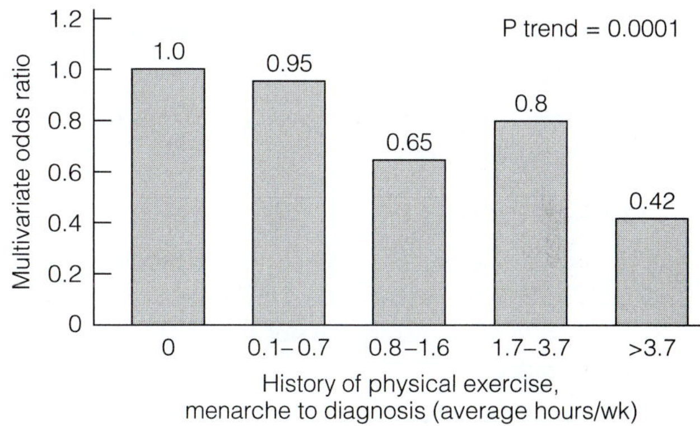

Figure 11.20 Physical exercise and reduced risk of breast cancer, 545 cases (diagnosed under age 40) versus 545 controls. The risk for breast cancer was reduced by more than half in women exercising more than 3.7 hours per week since early in life. Source: Bernstein L, Henderson BE, Hanisch R, Sullivan-Halley J, Ross RK. Physical exercise and reduced risk of breast cancer in young women. *J Natl Cancer Inst* 86:1403–1408, 1994.

ity promote higher levels of insulin in the blood, a hormone that increases the growth rate of cells lining the colon and hence their likelihood of turning cancerous.[33]

Active people may also eat more dietary fiber, enhancing their protection against colon cancer. For example, in the study from Harvard University reviewed earlier, highly active men ate 29 grams of dietary fiber a day, more than double the intake (12 grams) of the inactive men.[64] It should be noted, however, that even after controlling for dietary fiber intake, physical activity, in and of itself, still lowered colon cancer risk.

Other biological mechanisms include enhancement of immune function and defenses against oxidative stress.[49, 68]

Physical Activity and Breast Cancer

There is increasing evidence that women who engage in vigorous exercise from early in life gain protection against breast cancer[48,87–96] (see Figure 11.19). About three in four human studies support a 30–40% protective effect of physical activity against breast cancer. See Box 11.8 for an overview of the risk factors for breast cancer and the role of physical activity. In animal studies, vigorous physical activity has been associated with an inhibition of chemically induced breast cancer.[55,97,98] In humans, risk of breast cancer is lowest in lean and highly active females that have been consistently exercising all their lives.[94, 99, 100]

For example, a review of the death records for some 25,000 women in Washington state revealed that those who had worked in physically demanding jobs had a low breast cancer risk.[78] Another study of 6,888 women with breast cancer and 9,539 controls showed that women who had exercised vigorously on a near-daily basis between the ages of 14 and 22 had a 50% reduction in breast cancer risk.[95]

The lifetime occurrence rate of breast cancer in women was studied in 2,622 former college athletes and 2,776 nonathletes.[92] The nonathletes had an 86% higher risk for breast cancer than the former athletes throughout their lifetimes. Of interest is that the athletes were leaner and had a later age of menarche and an earlier age of menopause than the nonathletes.

The relationship between breast cancer and physical activity was studied in 545 premenopausal women with breast cancer and 545 controls.[88] As shown in Figure 11.20, the risk for breast cancer was reduced by more than half in women exercising more than 3.7 hours per week starting early in life. In a 14-year study of more than 25,000 Norwegian women, regular physical exercise was associated with a 37% reduction in breast cancer risk.[89] If the women were both lean and regularly active, risk was reduced 72% (Figure 11.21). In a case–control study in Australia, a decrease in risk of breast cancer was found with increasing levels of physical activity and was most evident for women who engaged in vigorous exercise.[96]

Exercise might reduce the risk of breast cancer via several mechanisms.[99–103] As discussed earlier, the cumulative exposure to ovarian hormones is an important factor causing breast cancer.[100,102] Women who exercise vigorously from childhood tend to have a later onset of menarche, may experience some missed menstrual cycles, and are generally

Box 11.8

Breast Cancer

Risk Factors

- Age
- Personal or family history
- Biopsy-confirmed atypical hyperplasia
- Long-term menstrual history (early to late in life)
- Recent use of oral contraceptives or postmenopausal estrogens and progestins
- Never had children or first child after age 30
- Consume alcoholic drinks
- Higher education and socioeconomic status
- Obesity after menopause
- Diet factors uncertain; increasing evidence for physical inactivity

Physical Activity

- The epidemiological evidence on link between activity and breast cancer is supportive of a protective relationship, but not as strongly as with colon cancer.
- Of published studies, about 3 in 4 support an inverse association between activity and breast cancer.
- Risk reduction ranges from 10 to 70% (average of 30–40%).

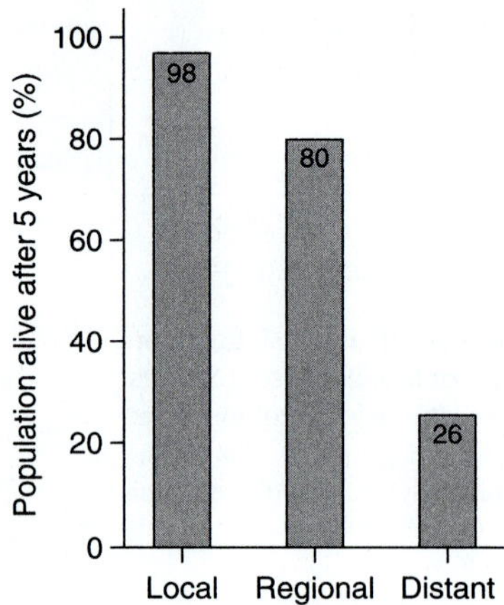

Potential Mechanisms Mediating Association with Physical Activity

- Reductions in endogenous steroid exposure
- Alterations in menstrual cycle patterns
- Delay of age at menarche
- Increase in energy expenditure and reduction in body weight
- Changes in insulin-like and other growth factors
- Enhancement of natural immune mechanisms

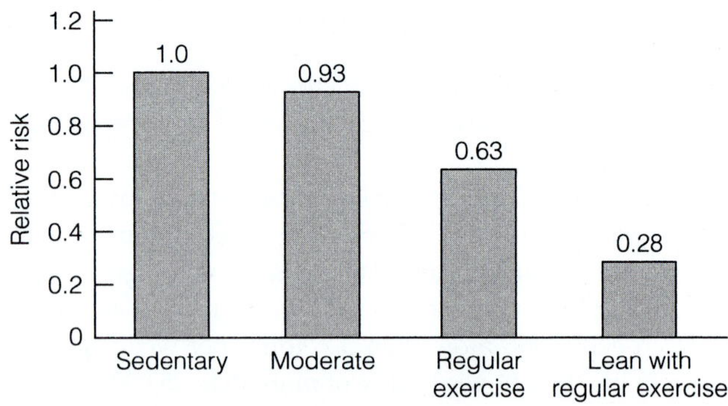

Figure 11.21 Leisure-time physical exercise and reduced risk of breast cancer, 14-year study of 25,624 Norwegian women. Breast cancer risk was lowest in women who were lean and regularly active. Source: Thune I, Brenn T, Lund E, Gaard M. Physical activity and the risk of breast cancer. *N Engl J Med* 336:1269–1275, 1997.

leaner, all of which decrease exposure of the breast tissue to estrogen. However, very strenuous exercise is required before the number of ovulatory cycles is reduced.[103]

Obesity, especially the gynoid type, in which fat accumulates around the waist, increases the risk of breast cancer.[33,99,103] Fat stores provide the substrate for the conversion of androgens to estrogens, increasing the concentration of estrogen in the body.[103] For this reason, some experts feel that reduction of body fat with regular exercise may be one of the chief protective mechanisms against breast cancer. Obesity is also associated with higher blood insulin levels, which promote the growth of breast cancer cells. Thus, active athletic women may be protected from breast cancer because of the indirect effects of exercise on reducing exposure to their own hormones.[103]

The critical role that the female hormone estrogen plays in cancer risk has also been shown for cancer of the uterus.[1] Estrogen stimulates cell division within the lining of the uterus, increasing the risk for cancer cell development. As with breast cancer, uterine cancer risk is increased in women who are obese, who experience a late menopause, or undergo prolonged estrogen therapy. Ovarian cancer risk is elevated in women who have never had children or who have a family history of ovarian cancer. Although more research is needed, there is evidence from several human studies that sedentary women are at substantially greater risk for female reproductive cancers than are those who are moderately to highly physically active.[104–106] In one study, participation in college athletics was related to a reduced lifetime risk of both uterine and ovarian cancer.[92] Nonathletes had more than 2.5 times the risk of female reproductive cancers than did former college athletes. Studies in Europe and the United States have shown that physical inactivity increases the risk for uterine cancer.[104–106] Researchers from the National Cancer Institute have shown that physically inactive women may be at increased risk of endometrial cancer by virtue of their tendency to be obese.[106]

Physical Activity and Prostate Cancer

Prostate cancer is the most frequently diagnosed cancer in men, and physical activity has been studied for its effect on the incidence and mortality due to this cancer.[107–112] About half of studies have found inactivity to be a significant risk factor.[48,110,111] See Box 11.9 for an overview of the risk factors for prostate cancer and the role of physical activity.

Recent studies using the best research designs have generally supported a relationship between physical activity and prostate cancer.[76,79,107–112] Researchers in Norway followed 53,242 men for an average of 16 years and found that risk of prostate cancer was reduced by more than half in those who walked during their work hours and also engaged in regular leisure-time exercise.[109] This protective effect, however, was found only among men older than 60 years of age. These results are similar to those of a well-designed study of 17,719 college alumni, in which risk of prostate cancer was reduced 47% in highly active versus sedentary men age 70 years and older.[107]

At the Cooper Clinic in Dallas, nearly 13,000 men were studied during 1970–1990.[108] All the men were given maximal exercise treadmill tests, divided into various fitness groups, and then tracked for development of prostate cancer over time. As shown in Figure 11.22, men

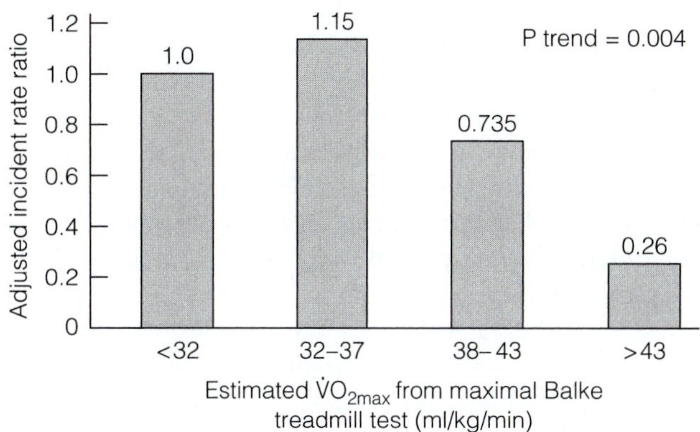

Figure 11.22 Cardiorespiratory fitness and prostate cancer, 12,975 men studied during 1970–1990. Increasing aerobic fitness was related to the lowest risk of prostate cancer.
Source: Oliveria SA, Kohl HW, Trichopoulos D, Blair SN. The association between cardiorespiratory fitness and prostate cancer. *Med Sci Sports Exerc* 28:97–104, 1996.

Box 11.9

Prostate Cancer

Risk Factors

- Age (over 70% diagnosed in those 65 years and older)
- Being African American
- High dietary fat intake
- Family history
- Live in North America or northwestern Europe (rare in Asia, Africa, South America)
- New evidence: inactivity and obesity

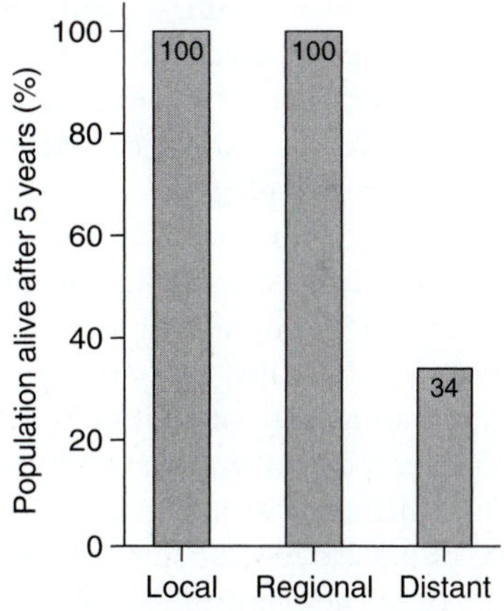

Physical Activity

- The epidemiological evidence suggests only a possible relationship between physical activity and prostate cancer.
- Of published studies, about half show a decrease in risk with an average reduction of 10–30%.

Potential Mechanisms Mediating Association with Physical Activity

- Antitestosterone therapy can often control prostate cancer for prolonged periods by shrinking the size of the tumor, thus relieving pain and other symptoms.
- After a long bout of exercise (>90 minutes), testosterone levels drop in male athletes. The long-term effects are currently unknown as is the exercise threshold linked to this acute decrease.
- Enhancement of natural immunity and defense against oxidative stress.

in the highest versus the lowest fitness group had a 74% reduced risk of developing prostate cancer. The men were also divided into different physical activity groups, and those exercising more than 1,000 Calories per week had less than half the risk of prostate cancer of their more sedentary counterparts.

As with breast cancer, there is an attractive explanation for why regular physical activity may lower prostate cancer risk.[111] Research suggests that higher levels of the male hormone testosterone may contribute to the development of prostate cancer.[1] Animal studies have shown that prostate cancer can be provoked by injecting them with testosterone. As explained earlier, African Americans have the highest prostate cancer incidence rates in the world, which are almost entirely attributed to their higher testosterone levels (15% higher than those of other American males).[1] Antitestosterone therapy is the treatment of choice for advanced prostate cancer.

Most studies have demonstrated that testosterone concentrations are depressed in trained athletes.[113] In other words, repeated bouts of exercise may lower blood levels of testosterone. The net effect is that highly active men may expose their prostate to less testosterone, reducing their risk of prostate cancer. Obesity promotes prostate cancer risk, as depicted in Figure 11.23.[114,115] Thus, regular and vigorous exercise may lower prostate cancer risk by enhancing leanness. Other potential activity–related mechanisms include enhanced immunity and defenses against oxidative stress.[110]

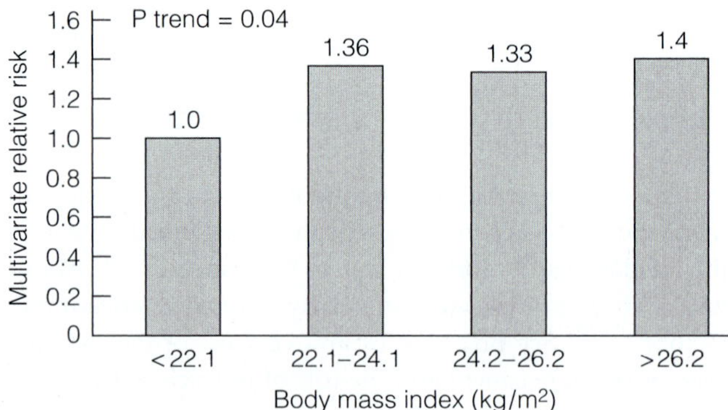

Figure 11.23 Body mass index (BMI) and risk for prostate cancer death, 18-year study of 135,000 male construction workers in Sweden. Obesity was linked to a greater risk of prostate cancer in this large study of men. Source: Andersson SO, Wolk A, Bergstrom R, Adami HO, Engholm G, Englun A, Nyren O. Body size and prostate cancer: A 20-year follow-up study among 135,006 Swedish construction workers. *J Natl Cancer Inst* 89: 385–389, 1997.

SPORTS MEDICINE INSIGHT

Exercise and Cancer Rehabilitation

As reviewed earlier in this chapter, 1.37 million new cancer cases occur each year in the United States, with 64% of these individuals surviving 5 years or more. Nearly 10 million Americans have a history of cancer. Cancer rehabilitation is a burgeoning area of tertiary preventive care, and there is growing evidence for the critical role of physical activity in helping patients cope with cancer treatment.[116–127]

Cancer and its treatments typically cause a significant decrease in quality of life including depression, anxiety, stress, body image concerns, difficulty sleeping, decreased self-esteem, and loss of a sense of control.[117,118] The cancer experience is also associated with many physical symptoms and changes including weakness and debility, decrease in control of muscle movements, weight loss and muscle wasting, reduced aerobic fitness, deep fatigue, nausea, vomiting, and pain. Fatigue occurs in 40–100% of cancer patients during treatment and is the most significant symptom affecting quality of life.[118] Although these side effects peak during treatment, they often persist months or even years following treatment.

Cancer patients need comprehensive care to relieve symptoms of pain, fatigue, and weakness.[121] Cancer rehabilitation includes many interventions such as cognitive-behavioral therapies, educational strategies, individual and group psychotherapy, and other alternative treatments. Until recently, physical exercise was not considered an appropriate intervention for cancer patients or survivors, with concerns raised over exercise-induced decrements in immune function, the likelihood of bone fractures, exacerbation of heart problems related to chemotherapy and radiotherapy, exercise-induced fatigue, and lack of motivation by cancer patients to tolerate physical exercise because of weakness.[117,118] Recent research, however, has dispelled many of these concerns over the safety, efficacy, and feasibility of exercise as an intervention following cancer diagnosis.[117–127]

A growing number of studies have consistently indicated that exercise has beneficial effects on a wide variety of quality-of-life issues, aerobic and muscular fitness, self-concept, mood states, and fatigue.[126] Most studies with cancer patients and survivors show that physical exercise training is associated with less fatigue during and after treatment and improves physical fitness.[118,120] Physical exercise has been found to be a safe, effective, and feasible intervention for most cancer patients and survivors.

(continued)

SPORTS MEDICINE INSIGHT *(continued)*

Exercise and Cancer Rehabilitation

There currently is no evidence that exercise training will influence tumor growth, disease progression, recurrence, and/or survival in cancer patients.[123] Thus exercise following cancer diagnosis should be promoted for its positive influence on fitness and quality of life and not as a means of fighting cancer or improving survival.

EXERCISE TESTING FOR CANCER PATIENTS

Exercise testing is recommended for all cancer patients prior to and periodically during the rehabilitation process. Exercise testing following cancer diagnosis may be used to[117,118]

- Measure and quantify the functional effects of the disease and its treatments.
- Identify comorbid conditions that may influence the type of exercise prescription or prohibit exercise (e.g., advanced cardiovascular disease).
- Develop an appropriate exercise prescription to assist cancer patients in coping with and/or recovering from the disease process and its treatments.
- Determine the functional benefits of the prescribed exercise program.

Exercise testing in cancer patients and survivors requires special considerations in addition to those recommended for healthy middle-aged and older adults. These arise from the significant fatigue, illness, and weakness experienced by cancer patients during and following treatment.

Prior to exercise testing, it is important to have cancer patients and survivors complete a cancer history questionnaire in addition to other exercise and medical history questionnaires that may be indicated (see Chapter 3). The cancer history questionnaire should assess information on important diagnostic and treatment variables such as time since diagnosis, type and stage of disease, type of surgery and adjuvant therapy, and known or suspected side effects of treatment (e.g., unsteady movements, heart and lung complications, orthopedic conditions). The patient's oncology team should be consulted to provide complete and accurate information.

Cancer treatment typically decreases aerobic and muscular fitness, flexibility, and balance in cancer patients. Thus a comprehensive fitness test is recommended that is adapted to the particular cancer patient. Most cancer survivors and early-stage cancer patients with good prognosis can safely perform symptom-limited maximal testing.[117,118]

The battery of exercise tests selected will depend on the specific limitations imposed by the cancer and its treatments. For example, cancer patients that have recently undergone rectal or prostate surgery may prefer a treadmill test to assess aerobic fitness compared to a cycle ergometer test. Cancer patients with limitations in range of motion in the upper extremities following surgery or radiation therapy (e.g., breast, head, and neck) will often be unable to perform tests involving upper body movements (e.g., arm ergometer tests, bench press). Patients that have neurological complications affecting coordination or balance will require stable tests (e.g., cycle ergometer) as opposed to less stable tests (e.g., treadmill test or step test). Some cancer patients will experience severe sickness and fatigue at certain times during chemotherapy and/or radiation therapy and will not tolerate maximal testing. For these patients, submaximal tests should be used.

GUIDELINES FOR EXERCISE PRESCRIPTION FOLLOWING CANCER DIAGNOSIS

Most publications dealing with exercise and cancer rehabilitation have included cancer patients with early-stage disease and good prognoses. Limited data are available for cancer patients with extensive disease.[117,118] Nonetheless, some general guidelines can be drawn from the exercise and cancer literature. The majority of studies on cancer patients and survivors have utilized walking or the cycle ergometer. Walking is preferred and relates to the common activities of daily living. Most studies using cycle ergometry have been laboratory-based and is recommended for patients who have problems with coordination, balance, and upper body movement. The activity mode should consider the acute or chronic physical impairments resulting from medical treatment. Swimming should be avoided by patients with nephrostomy tubes, non-indwelling central venous access catheters, and urinary bladder catheters.[118] High-impact exercises or contact sports should be avoided in cancer patients with primary or metastatic bone cancer. Other contraindications to physical exercise following cancer diagnosis include the following:[117,118]

- Low hemoglobin levels (<8.0 g/dl), neutrophil counts ($\leq 0.5 \times 10^9$/L), or platelet counts (<50×10^9/L) (avoid high-intensity aerobic exercise)

(continued)

SPORTS MEDICINE INSIGHT *(continued)*

Exercise and Cancer Rehabilitation

- High fever (>100°F) (avoid high-intensity exercise)
- Lack of coordination, dizziness, or peripheral sensory neuropathy (avoid activities that require balance, such as treadmill exercise)
- Severe loss of weight and muscle wasting (engage only in mild exercise)
- Difficulty in breathing (investigate cause and exercise to tolerance)
- Bone pain (avoid activities such as contact sports and high-impact exercise)
- Severe nausea (exercise to tolerance and investigate cause)
- Extreme fatigue and muscle weakness (exercise to tolerance)

The optimal rehabilitation program combines aerobic and muscular fitness activities. The frequency, intensity, and duration of aerobic exercise should follow the American College of Sports Medicine (ACSM) guidelines: moderate-intensity exercise performed 3–5 days per week for 20–30 minutes per session. High-intensity exercise should be avoided during cancer treatment because of the potential immunosuppressive effects, but it is not contraindicated in cancer survivors. Few studies are available regarding muscular fitness training programs for cancer patients, but basic ACSM guidelines are recommended until more is known.[117,118] For muscular fitness, the ACSM recommends that individuals perform a minimum of 8–10 separate exercises that train the major muscle groups, perform one set of 8–12 repetitions of each of these exercises to the point of fatigue, and do this at least 2–3 days per week. For flexibility improvement, patients should stretch at least 2–3 days a week and involve at least four repetitions of several stretches that are held 10–30 seconds at a position of mild discomfort.

The ACSM exercise prescription appears appropriate for most cancer patients and survivors but may need to be modified depending on medical treatments, comorbid conditions, and fitness levels. Cancer patients often do not feel like exercising at certain times during their chemotherapy cycles, and the activity program should be modified accordingly. Initially, some cancer patients will not be able to tolerate 30 minutes of continuous exercise, especially if they were previously sedentary. Intermittent activity (i.e., alternating short bouts of exercise and rest until at least 30 minutes is reached) is recommended for patients during chemotherapy treatment or immediately following bone marrow transplantation. For long-term compliance, the cancer patient should engage in physical activity that is enjoyable and social, builds confidence, develops new skills, and takes place in an environment that engages the mind and spirit. Research supports that given an appropriate prescription, exercise is safe and feasible for most cancer patients and survivors.

In summary, the following guidelines can be used for the aerobic exercise prescription of cancer patients and survivors:[118]

- *Mode.* Most exercises involving large muscle groups are appropriate, but walking and cycling are especially recommended because they are safe and tolerable for patients. Exercises are modified based on acute or chronic treatment effects from surgery, chemotherapy, and/or radiotherapy.
- *Frequency.* At least 3–5 sessions each week, but near-daily exercise may be preferable for deconditioned patients who do lighter-intensity and shorter-duration exercises.
- *Intensity.* Moderate, depending on current fitness level and medical treatments. ACSM guidelines recommend 60–80% of maximal heart rate at an RPE of 11–14.
- *Duration.* At least 20–30 minutes of continuous exercise; however, deconditioned patients or those experiencing severe side effects of treatment may need to combine short exercise bouts (e.g., 3–5 minutes) with rest intervals.
- *Progression.* Patients should meet frequency and duration goals before they increase exercise intensity. Progression should be slower and more gradual for deconditioned patients or those who are experiencing severe side effects of treatment.

SUMMARY

1. *Cancer* is defined as the uncontrolled growth and spread of abnormal cells, which can result in death, as vital passageways are blocked and the body's oxygen and nutrient supplies are diverted.
2. Cancer ranks a close second to heart disease as the leading cause of death in the United States. Since 1991, cancer death rates have fallen slightly, due in part to reduced smoking and to improved screening and treatment.
3. Dietary factors are responsible for about one third of all cancers, and cigarette smoking for about 30%. The American Cancer Society has urged that to reduce

cancer risk, people should avoid all tobacco use; consume low-fat, high-fiber diets containing plenty of whole grains, fruits, and vegetables; be physically active and maintain a healthy weight; limit consumption of alcoholic beverages; and limit exposure to ultraviolet radiation.

4. In 1996, regular physical activity was finally added to the list of cancer-prevention measures advocated by the American Cancer Society. The most impressive research results have shown a protective effect of exercise against three common cancer killers: colon, breast, and prostate cancer.
5. Exercise is most beneficial in preventing cancer of the colon, as compared with other cancer sites. Proposed mechanisms include faster movement of fecal material through the large intestine, decreased body fat stores, and improved overall energy balance.
6. There is increasing evidence that women who engage in vigorous exercise from early in life may gain some protection against breast cancer. Proposed mechanisms include reduced estrogen exposure, decreased body fat stores, and lower blood insulin levels.
7. Recent studies using the best research designs have generally supported a relationship between physical activity and prostate cancer. Proposed mechanisms include lower blood levels of testosterone and reduced body fat stores.
8. Exercise does not appear to improve the process of cancer treatment. Nonetheless, exercise for cancer patients is recommended to improve fitness, life quality, and morale.

Review Questions

1. *Which one of the following is* **not** *considered to be a risk factor for skin cancer?*

   A. Hispanic ethnicity
   B. Blonde or red hair
   C. Two or more blistering sunburns as child
   D. Blue, gray, or green eyes
   E. Many moles and freckles

2. *All men should have a blood test for prostate-specific antigen to screen for prostate cancer starting at age ____.*

   A. 30 B. 40 C. 50 D. 65 E. 70

3. *For the early detection of breast cancer, the ACS recommends that women should begin screening mammography at the age of ____.*

   A. 25 B. 30 C. 40 D. 50 E. 60

4. *The ____ is the site with the highest cancer incidence rates among women.*

   A. Lung B. Colon and rectum
   C. Breast D. Prostate
   E. Bladder

5. *Cancer is the abnormal and uncontrolled growth of cells of tissue that leads to death if untreated. About ____ of American women now living will eventually have cancer.*

   A. One fifth B. Four in ten
   C. One third D. Half
   E. Three fourths

6. *The third leading cancer killer among men is*

   A. Lung B. Colon and rectum
   C. Breast D. Prostate
   E. Bladder

7. *Which cancer site listed has the worst 5-year survival rate?*

   A. Breast B. Prostate
   C. Colon and rectum D. Pancreas
   E. Lung

8. *Several factors are most responsible for the high cancer death rates in Western countries. Which one of the following is the most important cause of cancer?*

   A. Alcohol
   B. Environmental factors
   C. Reproductive and sexual behavior
   D. Diet
   E. Tobacco

9. *Staging is the process of describing the extent of the disease or the spread of cancer from the site of origin. In the TNM system, "N" represents*

   A. Primary tumor
   B. Absence or presence of regional lymph node involvement
   C. Absence or presence of distant spread of cells
   D. Advanced stage
   E. Cancer present only in layer of cells where it developed

10. *About ____% of cancer is preventable through a prudent lifestyle.*

    A. 10 B. 25 C. 33 D. 50 E. 75

11. *Which type of cancer arises from epithelial cells (the lining cells of tubes, ducts, etc.)?*

    A. Carcinoma B. Sarcoma
    C. Lymphoma D. Leukemia

12. *The death rate for which type of cancer listed has shown a strong decrease since 1930 (to present)?*

    A. Lung
    B. Breast
    C. Stomach
    D. Colon and rectum
    E. Prostate

13. *There are several risk factors for breast cancer. Which one of the following is* not *included?*

    A. Never had children
    B. Obesity
    C. Family history of breast cancer
    D. Late age at menarche
    E. Late age at menopause

14. *There are several cancer prevention guidelines that the ACS has outlined for reducing the risk of cancer. Which one of the following is* not *included?*

    A. Choose most of the foods you eat from plant sources
    B. Limit intake of high-fat foods, particularly from animal sources
    C. Limit consumption of alcoholic beverages, if you drink at all
    D. Be physically active, and achieve and maintain a healthy weight
    E. Reduce sodium intake to less than 2,400 mg/day

15. *Which of the following is* not *considered to be a major risk factor for prostate cancer?*

    A. Being African American
    B. High intake of dietary fat
    C. Increasing age
    D. Sex at an early age
    E. Family history

16. *Which of the following is considered by the ACS to be a risk factor for colon and rectum cancer?*

    A. Cigarette smoking
    B. High-fat, low-fiber diet
    C. Stomach ulcers
    D. High sodium intake
    E. Male gender

17. *Which one of the following is* not *true regarding potential mechanisms explaining fiber's protective effect against colon cancer?*

    A. Fiber binds bile acids and dilutes the concentration of secondary bile acids and other cancer-causing chemicals
    B. Fiber increases stool bulk
    C. Fiber slows down the transit of fecal mass through the colon
    D. Water-soluble fibers ferment and produce volatile free fatty acids

18. *Dietary fiber is a term used to cover several types of food components that ____ digested in the human intestinal tract.*

    A. Are
    B. Are not

19. *Which one of the following is* not *a risk factor for lung cancer?*

    A. Radiation exposure
    B. Residential radon exposure
    C. Cigarette smoking
    D. Exposure to secondhand cigarette smoke
    E. Obesity

20. *People holding sedentary jobs are at increased risk for what type of cancer?*

    A. Lung
    B. Colon
    C. Brain
    D. Pancreatic
    E. Ovarian

21. *Active athletic women may be protected from breast cancer because of the indirect effects of exercise in reducing ____ exposure.*

    A. Estrogen
    B. Testosterone
    C. Growth hormone
    D. Cortisol
    E. Epinephrine

22. *There is some evidence that exercise may lower the risk for several types of cancers. Which one of the following is* not *included in this list?*

    A. Pancreas
    B. Colon
    C. Breast
    D. Prostate
    E. Endometrial

23. *Most studies have demonstrated that ____ concentrations are decreased in trained athletes, explaining why highly active men may have a reduced risk of prostate cancer (in some studies).*

    A. Estrogen
    B. Glucagon
    C. Insulin
    D. Testosterone
    E. Cortisol

24. *The fourth leading cancer killer among men is*

    A. Lung
    B. Colon and rectum
    C. Pancreas
    D. Prostate
    E. Bladder

25. *The death rate for which type of cancer listed has shown the strongest decrease since 1930 (to present) for women?*

    A. Lung
    B. Breast
    C. Uterus
    D. Colon and rectum
    E. Pancreas

26. *____ out of 10 patients who get cancer live 5 or more years after diagnosis.*

A. 1 **B.** 2 **C.** 3 **D.** 4 **E.** 6

27. *What cancer site has been most closely linked with the beneficial effects of regular physical activity?*

A. Lung
B. Pancreas
C. Colon
D. Brain
E. Uterus

28. *Which one of the following theories is* **not** *linked to physical activity and colon cancer risk?*

A. Activity reduces body fat levels
B. Exercise reduces the risk for constipation
C. Active people may eat more dietary fiber
D. Active people have reduced testosterone and estrogen levels

29. *____ is the number one cause of years of potential life lost before age 75.*

A. Cancer
B. Heart disease
C. Injuries
D. Suicide
E. HIV infection

30. *Which cancer listed for men is linked to obesity?*

A. Lung
B. Brain
C. Liver
D. Pancreas
E. Colon

Answers

1. A	**16.** B
2. C	**17.** C
3. C	**18.** B
4. C	**19.** E
5. B	**20.** B
6. B	**21.** A
7. D	**22.** A
8. D	**23.** D
9. B	**24.** C
10. E	**25.** C
11. A	**26.** E
12. C	**27.** C
13. D	**28.** D
14. E	**29.** A
15. D	**30.** E

REFERENCES

1. American Cancer Society. *Cancer Facts & Figures—2005.* Atlanta: Author, 2005.
2. Jemal A, Tiwari RC, Murray T, Ghafoor A, Samuels A, Ward E, Feuer EJ, Thun MJ. Cancer statistics, 2004. *CA Cancer J Clin* 54:8–29, 2004.
3. Ames BN, Shigenaga MK, Hagen TM. Oxidants, antioxidants, and the degenerative diseases of aging. *Proc Nat Acad Sci* 90:7915–7922, 1993.
4. National Center for Health Statistics. *Health, United States, 2004.* Hyattsville, MD: 2004.
5. Bailar JC, Gornik HL. Cancer undefeated. *N Engl J Med* 336:1569–1574, 1997.
6. Becker N, Muscat JE, Wynder EL. Cancer mortality in the United States and Germany. *J Cancer Res Clin Oncol* 127:293–300, 2001.
7. American Cancer Society. *Cancer Prevention and Early Detection Facts and Figures 2005.* Atlanta: American Cancer Society, 2005.
8. Doll R, Peto R. The causes of cancer: Quantitative estimates of avoidable risks of cancer in the United States today. *J Natl Cancer Inst* 66:1191–1308, 1981.
9. National Research Council. *Diet and Health. Implications for Reducing Chronic Disease Risk.* Washington, DC: National Academy Press, 1989.
10. American Cancer Society guidelines on nutrition and physical activity for cancer prevention: Reducing the risk of cancer with healthy food choices and physical activity. *CA Cancer J Clin* 52:92–119, 2002.
11. Carbone D. Smoking and cancer. *Am J Med* 93(1A):13S–17S, 1992.
12. Colditz GA, Atwood KA, Emmons K, Monson RR, Willett WC, Trichop HDJ. Harvard report on cancer prevention volume 4: Harvard Cancer Risk Index. Risk Index Working Group, Harvard Center for Cancer Prevention. *Cancer Causes Control* 11:477–488, 2000.
13. Rodriquez C, Tatham LM, Thun MJ, Calle EE, Heath CW. Smoking and fatal prostate cancer in a large cohort of adult men. *Am J Epidemiol* 145:466–475, 1997.
14. Couch FJ, Cerhan JR, Vierkant RA, Grabrick DM, Therneau TM, Pankratz VS, Hartmann LC, Olson JE, Vachon CM, Sellers TA. Cigarette smoking increases risk for breast cancer in high-risk breast cancer families. *Cancer Epidemiol Biomarkers Prev* 10:327–332, 2001.
15. U.S. Environmental Protection Agency. *Respiratory Health Effects of Passive Smoking: Lung Cancer and Other Disorders.* U.S. Environmental Protection Agency, Office of Research and Development. Washington, DC: U.S. EPA, 1992.
16. Morabia A, Bernstein M, Heritier S, Khatchatrian N. Relation of breast cancer with passive and active exposure to tobacco smoke. *Am J Epidemiol* 143:918–928, 1996.
17. Fuchs CS, Coldtiz GA, Stampfer MJ, et al. A prospective study of cigarette smoking and the risk of pancreatic cancer. *Arch Intern Med* 156:2255–2260, 1996.
18. Coughlin SS, Neaton JD, Sengupta A. Cigarette smoking as a predictor of death from prostate cancer in 348,874 men screened for the Multiple Risk Factor Intervention Trial. *Am J Epidemiol* 143:1002–1006, 1996.
19. Steinmetz KA, Potter, JD. Vegetables, fruit, and cancer prevention: A review. *J Am Diet Assoc* 96:1027–1039, 1996.

20. Block G, Patterson B, Subar A. Fruit, vegetable, and cancer prevention: A review of the epidemiological evidence. *Nutr Cancer* 18:1–29, 1992.
21. Block G. Epidemiologic evidence regarding vitamin C and cancer. *Am J Clin Nutr* 54:1310S–1314S, 1991.
22. Bendich A. Clinical importance of beta carotene. *Perspect Appl Nutr* 1(1):14–22, 1993.
23. Pool-Zobel BL, Bub A, Muller H, Wollowski I, Rechkemmer G. Consumption of vegetables reduces genetic damage in humans: First results of a human intervention trial with carotenoid-rich foods. *Carcinogenesis* 18:1847–1850, 1997.
24. Ji LL, Peterson DM. Aging, exercise, and phytochemicals: Promises and pitfalls. *Ann NY Acad Sci* 1019:453–461, 2004.
25. Michaud DS, Augustsson K, Rimm EB, Stampfer MJ, Willett WC, Giovannucci E. A prospective study on intake of animal products and risk of prostate cancer. *Cancer Causes Control* 12:557–567, 2001.
26. Sandhu MS, White IR, McPherson K. Systematic review of the prospective cohort studies on meat consumption and colorectal cancer risk: A meta-analytical approach. *Cancer Epidemiol Biomarkers Prev* 10:439–446, 2001.
27. Key TJ, Schatzkin A, Willett WC, Allen NE, Spencer EA, Travis RC. Diet, nutrition and the prevention of cancer. *Public Health Nutr* 7:187–200, 2004.
28. Voorrips LE, Goldbohm RA, Verhoeven DT, van Poppel GA, Sturmans Hermus RJ, van den Brandt PA. Vegetable and fruit consumption and lung cancer risk in the Netherlands Cohort Study on diet and cancer. *Cancer Causes Control* 11:101–115, 2000.
29. Ocke MC, Bueno-de-Mesquita HB, Feskens EJM, van Staveren WA, Kromhout D. Repeated measurements of vegetables, fruits, beta-carotene, and vitamins C and E in relation to lung cancer. *Am J Epidemiol* 145:358–365, 1997.
30. Ritter L. Report of a panel on the relationship between public exposure to pesticides and cancer. *Cancer* 80:2019–2033, 1997.
31. Howe GR, Benito E, Castelleto R, et al. Dietary intake of fiber and decreased risk of cancers of the colon and rectum: Evidence from the combined analysis of 13 case-control studies. *J Natl Cancer Inst* 84:1887–1896, 1992.
32. Potter JD. Reconciling the epidemiology, physiology, and molecular biology of colon cancer. *JAMA* 268:1573–1577, 1992.
33. Calle EE, Rodriguez C, Walker-Thurmond K, Thun MJ. Overweight, obesity, and mortality from cancer in a prospectively studied cohort of U.S. adults. *N Engl J Med* 348:1625–1638, 2003.
34. Kuller LH. Dietary fat and chronic diseases: Epidemiologic overview. *J Am Diet Assoc* 97(suppl):S9–S15, 1997.
35. Giovannucci E, Rimm EB, Colditz GA, Stampfer MJ, Chute CC, Willett WC. A prospective study of dietary fat and risk of prostate cancer. *J Natl Cancer Inst* 85:1571–1579, 1993.
36. Willett WC, Stampfer MJ, Colditz GA, et al. Relation of meat, fat, and fiber intake to the risk of colon cancer in a prospective study among women. *N Engl J Med* 323:1664–1672, 1990.
37. Chao A, Thun MJ, Connell CJ, McCullough ML, Jacobs EJ, Flanders WD, Rodriguez C, Sinha R, Calle EE. Meat consumption and risk of colorectal cancer. *JAMA* 293:172–182, 2005.
38. Martinez ME. Primary prevention of colorectal cancer: Lifestyle, nutrition, exercise. *Recent Results Cancer Res* 166:177–211, 2005.
39. Hunter DJ, Spiegelman D, Adami HO, et al. Cohort studies of fat intake and the risk of breast cancer—a pooled analysis. *N Engl J Med* 334:356–361, 1996.
40. van Gils CH, Peeters PH, Bueno-de-Mesquita HB, et al. Consumption of vegetables and fruits and risk of breast cancer. *JAMA* 293:183–193, 2005.
41. Greenwald P, Sherwood K, McDonald SS. Fat, caloric intake, and obesity: Lifestyle risk factors for breast cancer. *J Am Diet Assoc* 97(suppl):S24–S30, 1997.
42. Sasaki S, Horacsek M, Kesteloot H. An ecological study of the relationship between dietary fat intake and breast cancer mortality. *Prev Med* 22:187–202, 1993.
43. Smith-Warner SA, Spiegelman D, Yaun SS, et al. Alcohol and breast cancer in women. A pooled analysis of cohort studies. *JAMA* 279:535–540, 1998.
44. Longnecker MP, Newcomb PA, Mittendorf R, et al. Risk of breast cancer in relation to lifetime alcohol consumption. *J Natl Cancer Inst* 87:923–929, 1995.
45. Giovannucci E, Rimm EB, Ascherio A, Stampfer MJ, Coldtiz GA, Wsillett WC. Alcohol, low-methionine-low-folate diets, and risk of colon cancer in men. *J Natl Cancer Inst* 87:265–273, 1995.
46. Hayes RB, Brown LM, Schoenberg JB, et al. Alcohol use and prostate cancer risk in US blacks and whites. *Am J Epidemiol* 143:692–697, 1996.
47. Thune I, Furberg AS. Physical activity and cancer risk: Dose-response and cancer, all sites and site specific. *Med Sci Sports Exerc* 33(suppl):S530–S550, 2001.
48. Lee IM. Physical activity and cancer prevention—data from epidemiologic studies. *Med Sci Sports Exerc* 35:1823–1827, 2003.
49. Westerlind KC. Physical activity and cancer prevention—mechanisms. *Med Sci Sports Exerc* 35:1834–1840, 2003.
50. Friedenreich CM. Physical activity and cancer prevention: From observational to intervention research. *Cancer Epidemiol Biomarkers Prev* 10:287–301, 2001.
51. American Institute for Cancer Research. *Food, Nutrition and the Prevention of Cancer: A Global Perspective.* Washington, DC: Author, 1997.
52. Cherry T. A theory of cancer. *Med J Aust* 1:425–438, 1922.
53. Sivertsen I, Dahlstrom AW. The relation of muscular activity to carcinoma. A preliminary report. *J Cancer Res* 6:365–378, 1922.
54. Blair SN, Kohl HW, Paffenbarger RS, et al. Physical fitness and all-cause mortality: A prospective study of healthy men and women. *JAMA* 262:2395–2401, 1989.
55. Hoffman-Goetz L, Husted J. Exercise and breast cancer: Review and critical analysis of the literature. *Can J Appl Physiol* 19:237–252, 1994.
56. Roebuck BD, McCaffrey J, Baumgartner KJ. Protective effects of voluntary exercise during the postinitiation phase of pancreatic carcinogenesis in the rat. *Cancer Res* 50:6811–6816, 1990.
57. Woods JA, Davis JM, Smith JA, Nieman DC. Exercise and cellular innate immune function. *Med Sci Sports Exerc* 31:57–66, 1999.
58. MacNeil B, Hoffman-Goetz L. Chronic exercise enhances in vivo and in vitro cytotoxic mechanisms of natural immunity in mice. *J Appl Physiol* 74:388–395, 1993.
59. Cohen LA, Boylan E, Epstein M, Zang E. Voluntary exercise and experimental mammary cancer. *Adv Exp Med Biol* 322:41–59, 1992.
60. Woods JA, Davis JM. Exercise, monocyte/macrophage function, and cancer. *Med Sci Sports Exerc* 26:147–56, 1994.
61. Thune I, Lund E. The influence of physical activity on lung-cancer risk. A prospective study of 81,516 men and women. *Int J Cancer* 70:57–62, 1997.
62. U.S. Department of Health and Human Services. *Physical Activity and Health: A Report of the Surgeon General.* Atlanta, GA: U.S. Department of Health and Human Services, Centers for Disease Control and Prevention, National Center for Chronic Disease Prevention and Health Promotion, 1996.

63. Martinez ME, Giovannucci E, Spiegelman D, Hunter DJ, Willett WC, Colditz GA. Leisure-time physical activity, body size, and colon cancer in women. *J Natl Cancer Inst* 89:948–955, 1997.

64. Giovannucci E, Ascherio A, Rimm EB, Colditz GA, Stampfer MJ, Willett WC. Physical activity, obesity, and risk for colon cancer and adenoma in men. *Ann Intern Med* 122:327–334, 1995.

65. Longnecker MP, De Verdier MG, Frumkin H, Carpenter C. A case-control study of physical activity in relation to risk of cancer of the right colon and rectum in men. *Int J Epidemiol* 24:42–50, 1995.

66. Giovannucci E, Colditz GA, Stampfer MJ, Willett WC. Physical activity, obesity, and risk of colorectal adenoma in women (United States). *Cancer Causes Control* 7:253–263, 1996.

67. Lee I-M, Paffenbarger RS. Physical activity and its relation to cancer risk: A prospective study of college alumni. *Med Sci Sports Exerc* 26:831–837, 1994.

68. Slattery ML. Physical activity and colorectal cancer. *Sports Med* 34:239–252, 2004.

69. Slattery ML, Potter J, Caan B, Edwards S, Coates A, Ma KN, Berry TD. Energy balance and colon cancer—beyond physical activity. *Cancer Res* 57:75–80, 1997.

70. Marrett LD, Theis B, Ashbury FD. Workshop report: Physical activity and cancer prevention. *Chronic Dis Can* 21:143–149, 2000.

71. Wannamethee G, Shaper AG, Macfarlane PW. Heart rate, physical activity, and mortality from cancer and other noncardiovascular diseases. *Am J Epidemiol* 137:735–748, 1993.

72. Colbert LH, Hartman TJ, Malila N, Limburg PJ, Pietinen P, Virtamo J, Albanes D. Physical activity in relation to cancer of the colon and rectum in a cohort of male smokers. *Cancer Epidemiol Biomarkers Prev* 10:265–268, 2001.

73. Ballard-Barbash R, Schatzkin A, Albanes D, et al. Physical activity and risk of large bowel cancer in the Framingham study. *Cancer Res* 50:3610–3613, 1990.

74. Thun MJ, Calle EE, Namboordiri MM, et al. Risk factors for fatal colon cancer in a large prospective study. *J Natl Cancer Inst* 84:1491–1500, 1992.

75. Fraser G, Pearce N. Occupational physical activity and risk of cancer of the colon and rectum in New Zealand males. *Cancer Causes Control* 4:45–50, 1993.

76. Brownson RC, Zahm SH, Chang JC, Blair A. Occupational risk of colon cancer: An analysis by anatomic subsite. *Am J Epidemiol* 130:675–687, 1989.

77. Garabrant DH, Peters JM, Mack TM, et al. Job activity and colon cancer risk. *Am J Epidemiol* 119:1005–1014, 1984.

78. Vena JE, Graham S, Zielezny M, et al. Lifetime occupational exercise and colon cancer. *Am J Epidemiol* 122:357–365, 1985.

79. Vena JE, Graham S, Zielezny M, Brasure J, Swanson MK. Occupational exercise and risk of cancer. *Am J Clin Nutr* 45:318–327, 1987.

80. Gerhardsson M, Norell SE, Kiviranta H, et al. Sedentary job and colon cancer. *Am J Epidemiol* 123:775–780, 1986.

81. Oettlé GJ. Effect of moderate exercise on bowel habit. *Gut* 32:941–944, 1991.

82. Keeling WF, Martin BJ. Gastrointestinal transit during mild exercise. *J Appl Physiol* 63:978–981, 1987.

83. Peters HP, De Vries WR, Vanberge-Henegouwen GP, Akkermans LM. Potential benefits and hazards of physical activity and exercise on the gastrointestinal tract. *Gut* 48:435–439, 2001.

84. Sandler RS, Jordan MC, Shelton BJ. Demographic and dietary determinants of constipation in the US population. *Am J Public Health* 80:185–189, 1990.

85. Kritchevsky D. Caloric restriction and experimental carcinogenesis. *Toxicol Sci* 52(2 suppl):13–16, 1999.

86. Garfinkel LE. Overweight and cancer. *Ann Intern Med* 103:1034–1036, 1985.

87. McTiernan A, Kooperberg C, White E, Wilcox S, Coates R, Adams-Campbell LL, Woods N, Ockene J. Recreational physical activity and the risk of breast cancer in postmenopausal women: The Women's Health Initiative Cohort Study. *JAMA* 290:1331–1336, 2003.

88. Bernstein L, Henderson BE, Hanisch R, Sullivan-Halley J, Ross RK. Physical exercise and reduced risk of breast cancer in young women. *J Natl Cancer Inst* 86:1403–1408, 1994.

89. Thune I, Brenn T, Lund E, Gaard M. Physical activity and the risk of breast cancer. *N Engl J Med* 336:1269–1275, 1997.

90. Verloop J, Rookus MA, van der Kooy K, van Leeuwen FE. Physical activity and breast cancer risk in women aged 20–54 years. *J Natl Cancer Inst* 92:128–135, 2000.

91. Friedenreich CM, Bryant HE, Courneya KS. Case-control study of lifetime physical activity and breast cancer risk. *Am J Epidemiol* 154:336–347, 2001.

92. Frisch RE, Wyshak G, Albright NL, et al. Lower prevalence of breast cancer and cancers of the reproductive system among former college athletes compared to non-athletes. *Br J Cancer* 52:885–891, 1985.

93. Breslow RA, Ballard-Barbash R, Munoz K, Graubard BI. Long-term recreational physical activity and breast cancer in the National Health and Nutrition Examination Survey I epidemiology follow-up study. *Cancer Epidemiol Biomarkers Prev* 10:805–808, 2001.

94. Dorn J, Vena J, Brasure J, Freudenheim J, Graham S. Lifetime physical activity and breast cancer risk in pre- and postmenopausal women. *Med Sci Sports Exerc* 35:278–285, 2003.

95. Mittendorf R, Longnecker MP, Newcomb PA, et al. Strenuous physical activity in young adulthood and risk of breast cancer (United States). *Cancer Causes Control* 6:347–353, 1995.

96. Friedenreich CM, Rohan TE. Physical activity and risk of breast cancer. *Eur J Cancer Prev* 4:145–151, 1995.

97. Thompson HJ, Westerlind KC, Snedden JR, Briggs S, Singh M. Inhibition of mammary carcinogenesis by treadmill exercise. *J Natl Cancer Inst* 87:453–455, 1995.

98. Thompson HJ. Effect of exercise intensity and duration on the induction of mammary carcinogenesis. *Cancer Res* 54(7 suppl):1960S–1963S, 1994.

99. Friedenreich CM. Physical activity and breast cancer risk: The effect of menopausal status. *Exerc Sport Sci Rev* 32:180–184, 2004.

100. Lagerros YT, Hsieh SF, Hsieh CC. Physical activity in adolescence and young adulthood and breast cancer risk: A quantitative review. *Eur J Cancer Prev* 13:5–12, 2004.

101. Wolk A, Gridley G, Svensson M, Nyren O, McLaughlin JK, Fraumeni JF, Adam HO. A prospective study of obesity and cancer risk (Sweden). *Cancer Causes Control* 12:13–21, 2001.

102. Verkasalo PK, Thomas HV, Appleby PN, Davey GK, Key TJ. Circulating levels of sex hormones and their relation to risk factors for breast cancer: A cross-sectional study in 1092 pre- and postmenopausal women (United Kingdom). *Cancer Causes Control* 12:47–59, 2001.

103. McTiernan A. Exercise and breast cancer—time to get moving? *N Engl J Med* 336:1311–1312, 1997.

104. Moradi T, Weiderpass E, Signorello LB, Persson I, Nyren O, Adami HO. Physical activity and postmenopausal endometrial cancer risk (Sweden). *Cancer Causes Control* 11:829–837, 2000.

105. Levi F, La Vecchia C, Negri E, Franceschi S. Selected physical activities and the risk of endometrial cancer. *Br J Cancer* 67:846–851, 1993.

106. Sturgen SR, Brinton LA, Berman ML, et al. Past and present physical activity and endometrial cancer risk. *Br J Cancer* 68:584–589, 1993.
107. Lee IM, Paffenbarger RS, Hsieh CC. Physical activity and risk of prostatic cancer among college alumni. *Am J Epidemiol* 135:169–179, 1992.
108. Oliveria SA, Kohl HW, Trichopoulos D, Blair SN. The association between cardiorespriatory fitness and prostate cancer. *Med Sci Sports Exerc* 28:97–104, 1996.
109. Thune I, Lund E. Physical activity and the risk of prostate and testicular cancer: A Cohort study of 53,000 Norwegian men. *Cancer Causes Control* 5:549–556, 1994.
110. Torti DC, Matheson GO. Exercise and prostate cancer. *Sports Med* 34:363–369, 2004.
111. Oliveria SA, Lee IM. Is exercise beneficial in the prevention of prostate cancer? *Sports Med* 23:271–278, 1997.
112. Friedenreic CM, Thune I. A review of physical activity and prostate cancer risk. *Cancer Causes Control* 12:461–475, 2001.
113. Hackney AC. The male reproductive system and endurance exercise. *Med Sci Sports Exerc* 28:180–189, 1996.
114. Andersson SO, Wolk A, Bergstrom R, Adami HO, Engholm G, Englund A, Nyren O. Body size and prostate cancer: A 20-year follow-up study among 135,006 Swedish construction workers. *J Natl Cancer Inst* 89:385–389, 1997.
115. Giovannucci E, Rimm EB, Stampfer MJ, Colditz GA, Willett WC. Height, body weight, and risk of prostate cancer. *Cancer Epidemiol Biomarkers Prev* 6:557–673, 1997.
116. Brown JK, Byers T, Doyle C, et al. Nutrition and physical activity during and after cancer treatment: An American Cancer Society guide for informed choices. *CA Cancer J Clin* 53:268–291, 2003.
117. Courneya KS. Exercise interventions during cancer treatment: Biopsychosocial outcomes. *Exerc Sports Sci Rev* 29:60–64, 2001.
118. Courneya KS, Mackey JR, Jones LW. Coping with cancer. Can exercise help? *Physician Sportsmed* 28(5), 2000.
119. Durak E. The use of exercise in the cancer recovery process. A health and sports medicine review. *ACSM's Health & Fitness Journal* 5(1):6–10, 2001.
120. Schwartz AL, Mori M, Gao R, Nail LM, King ME. Exercise reduces daily fatigue in women with breast cancer receiving chemotherapy. *Med Sci Sports Exerc* 33:718–723, 2001.
121. Gerber LH. Cancer rehabilitation into the future. *Cancer* 92(4 suppl):975–979, 2001.
122. Stevinson C, Lawlor DA, Fox KR. Exercise interventions for cancer patients: Systematic review of controlled trials. *Cancer Causes Control* 15:1035–1056, 2004.
123. Rohan TE, Fu W, Hiller JE. Physical activity and survival from breast cancer. *Eur J Cancer Prev* 4:419–424, 1995.
124. Galvao DA, Newton RU. Review of exercise intervention studies in cancer patients. *J Clin Oncol* 23:899–909, 2005.
125. Courneya KS, Keats MR, Turner AR. Physical exercise and quality of life in cancer patients following high dose chemotherapy and autologous bone marrow transplantation. *Psychooncology* 9:127–136, 2000.
126. Courneya KS, Friedenreich CM. Physical exercise and quality of life following cancer diagnosis: A literature review. *Ann Behav Med* 21:171–179, 1999.
127. Pinto BM, Maruyama NC. Exercise in the rehabilitation of breast cancer survivors. *Psychooncology* 8:191–206, 1999.

PHYSICAL FITNESS ACTIVITY 11.1

Test Your Risk from UV Radiation

Your risk of skin cancer is related to your skin type and the amount of time you spend in the sun. How sensitive are you?

	Yes	No
1. I have blonde or red hair.	❑	❑
2. I have light-colored eyes (blue, gray, green).	❑	❑
3. I freckle easily.	❑	❑
4. I have many moles.	❑	❑
5. I had two or more blistering sunburns as a child.	❑	❑
6. I spent lots of time in a tropical climate as a child.	❑	❑
7. There is a family history of skin cancer.	❑	❑
8. I work outdoors.	❑	❑
9. I spend a lot of time in outdoor activities.	❑	❑
10. I like to spend as much time in the sun as I can.	❑	❑

Note: Score 10 points for each "Yes." Add another 10 points if you go to tanning parlors or use a sun lamp.

Score

80–110 *High-risk zone*
Limit time in the sun, always wear a sunscreen outdoors, and use protective clothing and a hat.

40–70 *Increased risk*
Use a sunscreen and hat regularly. Avoid exposure at midday, when the sun is most intense.

10–30 *Still at risk*
Use a sunscreen regularly.

Source: FDA Consumer, July/August 1995.

PHYSICAL FITNESS ACTIVITY 11.2

Eating Smart for Cancer Prevention

How Do You Rate?

Following is a quick, simple eating quiz for all ages that looks at how your diet compares to the American Cancer Society's guidelines. Below each category of food are examples. When rating yourself, think of foods similar to those listed that are in your diet. Circle the points for the answer you choose, and then total your points. Compare your score with the analysis at the end of the quiz. Remember: A poor score does not mean that you will get cancer, nor does a high score guarantee that you will not. Nonetheless, your score will give you a clue to how you eat now and where you need to improve to reduce your cancer risks.

Important: This eating quiz is really for self-information and does not evaluate your intake of essential vitamins, minerals, protein, or calories. If your diet is restricted in some ways (e.g., you are a vegetarian or have allergies) you may want to get professional advice.

Food Category		Points
Oils and Fats		
(Butter, margarine, shortening, mayonnaise, sour cream, lard, oil, salad dressing)	I always add these to foods in cooking and/or at the table.	0
	I occasionally add these to foods in cooking and/or at the table.	1
	I rarely add these to foods in cooking and/or at the table.	2
	I eat fried foods 3 or more times a week.	0
	I eat fried foods 1 to 2 times a week.	1
	I rarely eat fried foods.	2
Dairy Products		
	I drink whole milk.	0
	I drink 1%, 2% milk.	1
	I drink nonfat milk.	2
	I eat ice cream almost every day.	0
	Instead of ice cream, I eat ice milk, low-fat frozen yogurt, and sherbet.	1
	I eat only fruit ices, seldom eat frozen dairy desserts.	2
	I eat mostly high-fat cheese (jack, cheddar, colby, swiss, cream).	0
	I eat both low- and high-fat cheeses.	1
	I eat mostly low-fat cheese (pot, 2% cottage, skim-milk mozzarella).	2
Snacks		
(Potato/corn chips, buttered popcorn, candy bars)	I eat these every day.	0
	I eat some occasionally.	1
	I seldom or never eat these snacks.	2

Baked Goods		
(Pies, cakes, cookies, sweet rolls, doughnuts)	I eat them 5 or more times a week.	0
	I eat them 2 to 4 times a week.	1
	I seldom eat baked goods or eat only low-fat baked goods.	2

Poultry and Fish*		
	I rarely eat these foods.	0
	I eat them 1 to 2 times a week.	1
	I eat them 3 or more times a week.	2

Low-Fat Meats*		
(Extra-lean hamburger, round steak, pork loin roast, tenderloin, chuck roast)	I rarely eat these foods.	0
	I eat these foods occasionally.	1
	I eat mostly fat-trimmed red meats.	2

High-Fat Meats*		
(Luncheon meats, bacon, hot dogs, sausage, steak, regular and lean ground beef)	I eat these every day.	0
	I eat these foods occasionally.	1
	I rarely eat these foods.	2

Cured and Smoked Meat and Fish*		
(Luncheon meats, hot dogs, bacon, ham, and other smoked or pickled meats and fish)	I eat these foods 4 or more times a week.	0
	I eat these foods 1 to 3 times a week.	1
	I seldom eat these foods.	2

Legumes		
(Dried beans and peas: kidney, navy, lima, pinto, garbanzo, split pea, lentil)	I eat legumes less than once a week.	0
	I eat these foods 1 to 2 times a week.	1
	I eat them 3 or more times a week.	2

Whole Grains and Cereals		
(Whole-grain breads, brown rice, pasta, whole-grain cereals)	I seldom eat such foods.	0
	I eat them 2 to 3 times a day.	1
	I eat them 4 or more times daily.	2

Vitamin C–Rich Fruits and Vegetables		
(Citrus fruits and juices, green peppers, strawberries, tomatoes)	I seldom eat them.	0
	I eat them 3 to 5 times a week.	1
	I eat them 1 to 2 times a day.	2

Dark Green and Deep Yellow Fruits and Vegetables†		
(Broccoli, greens, carrots, peaches)	I seldom eat them.	0
	I eat them 1 to 2 times a week.	1
	I eat them 3 to 4 times a week.	2

Vegetables of the Cabbage Family		
(Broccoli, cabbage, Brussels sprouts, cauliflower)	I seldom eat them.	0
	I eat them 1 to 2 times a week.	1
	I eat them 3 to 4 times a week.	2

Alcohol		
	I drink more than 2 oz. daily.	0
	I drink alcohol every week but not daily.	1
	I occasionally or never drink alcohol.	2

Personal Weight		
	I'm more than 20 lb over my ideal weight.	0
	I'm 10 to 20 lb over my ideal weight.	1
	I am within 10 lb of my ideal weight.	2

Total Score

*If you do not eat meat, fish, or poultry, give yourself a 2 for each meat category.

†Dark green and yellow fruits and vegetables contain beta-carotene, which your body can turn into vitamin A, which helps protect you against certain types of cancer-causing substances.

Scoring

0–12 A Warning Signal: Your diet is too high in fat and too low in fiber-rich foods. It would be wise to assess your eating habits to see where you could make improvements.

13–17 Not bad! You're partway there, but you still have a way to go. Review the food guide pyramid (see Chapter 9). This will help you determine where you can make a few improvements.

18–36 Good for you! You're eating smart. You should feel very good about yourself. You have been careful to limit your fats and eat a varied diet. Keep up the good habits and continue to look for ways to improve.

Source: The American Cancer Society.

PHYSICAL FITNESS ACTIVITY 11.3

Estimating Your Cancer Risk

The Harvard Center for Cancer Prevention has produced an Internet program that estimates cancer risk for a number of sites including breast, prostate, lung, colon, bladder, skin, uterus, kidney, pancreas, ovary, stomach, and cervix. This program is based on solid research and, in addition to estimating the risk of cancer, provides personalized tips for prevention.* Go to this Internet site and calculate your cancer risk for breast (females), prostate (males), lung, colon, and melanoma: *www.yourcancerrisk.harvard.edu*. Summarize your estimated cancer risk and tips for prevention in the space provided.

Breast (females) ____

____

____

Prostate (males) ____

____

____

Lung ____

____

____

Colon ____

____

____

Melanoma ____

____

____

*Colditz GA, Atwood KA, Emmons K, Monson RR, Willett WC, Trichop HDJ. Harvard report on cancer prevention. Vol. 4: Harvard Cancer Risk Index. Risk Index Working Group, Harvard Center for Cancer Prevention. *Cancer Causes Control* 11:477–488, 2000.

chapter 12

Diabetes

There is a strong link between type 2 diabetes and sedentary living. The biggest benefits appear to be found among those who incorporate some level of regular physical activity into their daily lives. Physical activity, as recommended by the Surgeon General, would seem to be a prudent strategy for all people, especially those who are at risk or have type 2 diabetes.

—Andrea Kriska, University of Pittsburgh, Graduate School of Public Health

"Diabetes mellitus" gets it name from the ancient Greek word for "siphon" (a kind of tube) because early physicians noted that diabetics tend to be unusually thirsty and to urinate a lot. The "mellitus" part of the term is from the Latin version of the ancient Greek word for honey, used because doctors in centuries past diagnosed the disease by the sweet taste of the patient's urine.

Diabetes impairs the body's ability to burn the fuel or glucose it gets from food for energy. Glucose is carried to the body's cells by the blood, but the cells need insulin, which is made by the pancreas, to allow glucose to move inside. Without insulin, glucose accumulates in the blood and then is dumped into the urine by the kidneys (see Figure 12.1).

This sometimes happens because the cells of the pancreas that make insulin—the beta cells—are mostly or entirely destroyed by the body's own immune system. The patient then needs insulin injections to survive and is diagnosed with type 1 diabetes. In type 2 diabetes, the person's beta cells do make insulin, but the patient's tissues are not sensitive enough to the hormone and use it inefficiently.

PREVALENCE AND INCIDENCE OF DIABETES MELLITUS

Approximately 18.2 million Americans (6.3% of the total population, 8.7% of adults 20 and older) have diabetes.[1–5] Of these, 13 million are diagnosed and 5.2 million are undiagnosed. It is estimated that 41 million persons ages 40–74 have pre-diabetes (40% of the population), placing them at high risk for the development of diabetes.[2,4] Each year, 1.3 million new cases of diabetes are diagnosed. Forty percent of all diabetics are age 65 years or older, and among the elderly, nearly one in five has diabetes (see Figure 12.2). The prevalence of diabetes rose from 4.9% in 1990 to about 6.3% by the year 2000, an increase of 29%. The largest increase occurred among people aged 30–39. American Indians and Alaska Natives are 2.8 times more likely to have diabetes than non-Hispanic whites. African Americans are two times more likely than whites to die of diabetes. See Figure 12.3 for a state-by-state comparison. There are approximately 210,000 cases of diabetes in U.S. children and teenagers. Type 1 diabetes accounts for 5–10% of all diagnosed cases, with type 2 diabetes accounting for 90–95%.[2,4]

Type 2 diabetes mellitus, once considered a disease only of adults, is now being diagnosed at an increasingly alarming rate in children.[2,6] Incidence rates among children are highest in ethnic minority populations.[2] Risk factors for type 2 diabetes mellitus among youth include being overweight and family history of the disease.[6] Prevention is essential, and health-care professionals and parents need to be educated about the potential for type 2 diabetes in children.

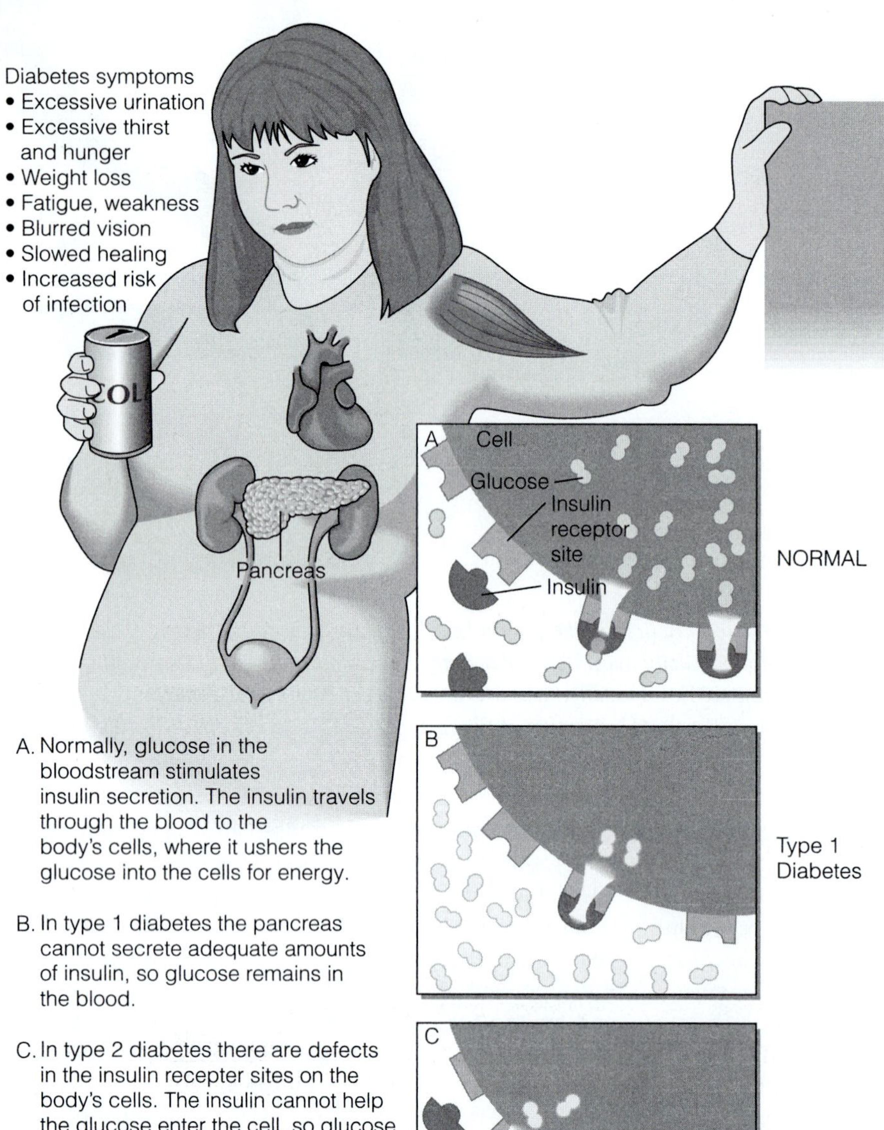

Diabetes symptoms
• Excessive urination
• Excessive thirst and hunger
• Weight loss
• Fatigue, weakness
• Blurred vision
• Slowed healing
• Increased risk of infection
Pancreas
A Cell
Glucose
Insulin receptor site
Insulin
NORMAL
B
Type 1 Diabetes
C
Type 2 Diabetes
A. Normally, glucose in the bloodstream stimulates insulin secretion. The insulin travels through the blood to the body's cells, where it ushers the glucose into the cells for energy.
B. In type 1 diabetes the pancreas cannot secrete adequate amounts of insulin, so glucose remains in the blood.
C. In type 2 diabetes there are defects in the insulin recepter sites on the body's cells. The insulin cannot help the glucose enter the cell, so glucose remains in the bloodstream. Thus, the body fails to use insulin properly. In some patients, the pancreas makes some insulin, but not enough.

Figure 12.1 Symptoms and effects of diabetes. The cells need insulin to allow glucose to move inside. Diabetes mellitus is a group of diseases characterized by high levels of blood glucose resulting from defects in insulin secretion, insulin action, or both.

DEFINITION AND DESCRIPTION OF DIABETES MELLITUS

Diabetes mellitus is defined as a group of metabolic diseases characterized by high blood glucose (i.e., hyperglycemia) resulting from defects in insulin secretion, insulin action, or both[2] (see Box 12.1). The chronic hyperglycemia of diabetes is associated with long-term damage, dysfunction, and failure of various organs, especially the eyes, kidneys, nerves, heart, and blood vessels.

Symptoms of hyperglycemia include excessive urination (*polyuria*), excessive and prolonged thirst (*polydipsia*), weight loss, sometimes with excessive eating (*polyphagia*), and blurred vision[1–4] (see Box 12.2). Impairment of growth and susceptibility to certain infections may also occur. Acute, life-threatening consequences of diabetes include hyperglycemia with *ketoacidosis* (acidosis caused by production of ketone bodies in uncontrolled diabetes).

Complications of Diabetes

Diabetes mellitus is related to many health problems, costing society nearly $132 billion each year in direct and indirect costs.[1,4] Over the past decade, diabetes has remained

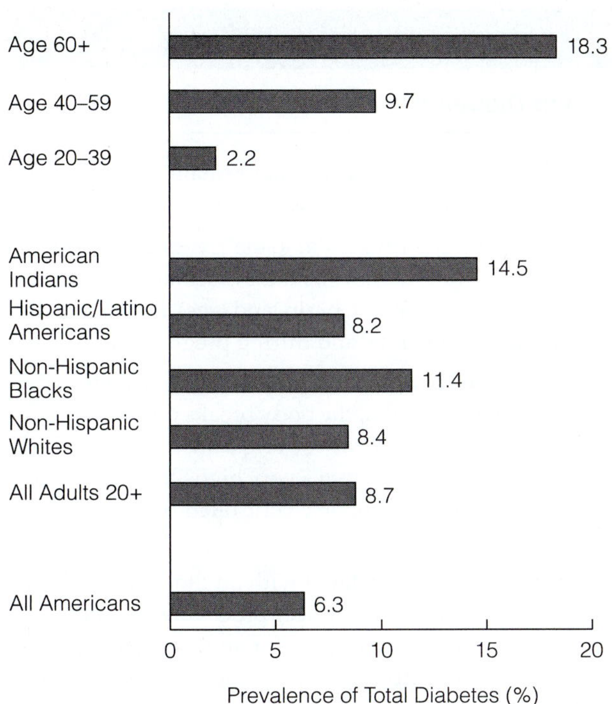

Figure 12.2 Prevalence of total diabetes (both diagnosed and nondiagnosed) in the United States. Sources: Centers for Disease Control and Prevention. *National Diabetes Fact Sheet: General Information and National Estimates on Diabetes in the United States, 2002.* Atlanta, GA: U.S. Department of Health and Human Services; Centers for Disease Control and Prevention, 2003. www.diabetes.org/. See also: CDC. Prevalence of diabetes and impaired fasting glucose in adults—United States, 1999–2000. *MMWR* 52:833–837, 2003.

Prevelance of Diabetes Among U.S. Adults*

1990

NJ
CT DE MD NH RI
MA VT

1993–1994

CT DE MA MD NJ NH RI VT

1997–1998

CT DE MA NH VT
MD NJ RI

2000

NH VT

Not available | Less than 4% | 4%–6% | Above 6%

*Includes gestational diabetes.

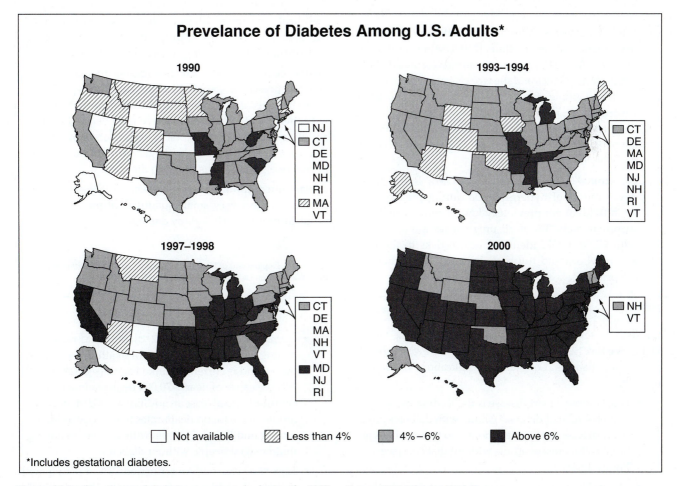

Figure 12.3 Prevalence of diabetes rose strongly during the 1990s. Source: CDC, Behavioral Risk Factor Surveillance System.

Box 12.1

Glossary of Terms Used in Diabetes

comorbidity: The presence of serious health conditions in addition to the one being examined, for example, high blood pressure in people with diabetes mellitus.

diabetes mellitus (diabetes): A chronic disease due to either or both insulin deficiency and resistance to insulin action and associated with hyperglycemia (elevated blood glucose levels). Over time, without proper preventive treatment, organ complications related to diabetes develop, including heart, nerve, foot, eye, and kidney damage; problems with pregnancy also occur. Diabetes is classified into four major categories:

type 1 diabetes: (Previously called insulin-dependent diabetes mellitus [IDDM] or juvenile-onset diabetes [JODM].) Represents clinically about 5% of all persons with diagnosed diabetes. Its clinical onset is typically at ages under 30 years. Most often this type of diabetes represents an autoimmune destructive disease in beta (insulin-producing) cells of the pancreas in genetically susceptible individuals. Insulin therapy always is required to sustain life and maintain diabetes control.

type 2 diabetes: (Previously called non–insulin-dependent diabetes mellitus [NIDDM] or adult-onset diabetes [AODM].) The most common form of diabetes in the United States and the world, especially in certain racial and ethnic groups and in elderly persons. In the United States, approximately 95% of all persons with diagnosed diabetes (10.5 million) and almost 100% of all persons with undiagnosed (5.5 million) diabetes probably have type 2 diabetes.

gestational diabetes mellitus (GDM): Refers to the development of hyperglycemia during pregnancy in an individual not previously known to have diabetes. Approximately 3% of all pregnancies are associated with GDM. GDM identifies health risks to the fetus and newborn and future diabetes in the mother and offspring.

other types: Include genetic abnormalities, pancreatic diseases, and medication use.

complications: Microvascular (small vessel abnormalities in the eyes and kidneys), macrovascular (large vessel abnormalities in the heart, brain, and legs), and metabolic (abnormalities in nerves and during pregnancy).

diabetic acidosis: A severe condition of diabetes. Because of a lack of insulin, the body breaks down fat tissue and converts the fat to very strong acids. The condition most often is associated with a very high blood sugar and happens most often in poorly controlled or newly diagnosed type 1 diabetes.

direct costs: Costs associated with an illness that can be attributed to a medical service, procedure, medication, etc. Examples include payment for an x-ray; pharmaceutical drugs, for example, insulin; surgery; or a clinic visit.

formal diabetes education: Self-management training that includes a process of initial individual patient assessment; instruction provided or supervised by a qualified health professional; evaluation of accumulation by the diabetic patient of appropriate knowledge, skills, and attitudes; and ongoing reassessment and training.

thrifty gene: An idea which suggests that a "thrifty gene" is present in people likely to develop type 2 diabetes. It is speculated that thousands of years ago, people with this "thrifty gene" could store food very efficiently and thus survive long periods of starvation. Now, when starvation is unusual, this thrifty gene tends to make people overweight and thus prone to diabetes.

urinary microalbumin measurement: A laboratory procedure to detect very small quantities of protein in the urine, indicating early kidney damage.

Source: U.S. Department of Health and Human Services. *Healthy People 2010.* Washington DC: 2000. www.health.gov/healthypeople.

the sixth or seventh leading cause of death in the United States. See Box 12.3 for a summary of *Healthy People 2010* objectives for diabetes. Long-term complications of diabetes include:[1–7]

- *Heart disease.* Heart disease is the leading cause of diabetes-related deaths.[6] Adults with diabetes have heart disease death rates about two to four times as high as the rates of adults without diabetes (see Figure 12.4).
- *Stroke.* The risk of stroke is two to four times higher in people with diabetes[6] (Figure 12.4).
- *Overall mortality.* Since 1932, diabetes has ranked among the 10 leading causes of death in the United States, and is currently ranked sixth (see Table 11.1).[5] It is the cause of nearly 70,000 deaths annually and contributes to at least an additional 213,000 deaths. Studies have found death rates to be twice as high among middle-aged people with diabetes as among middle-aged people without diabetes.
- *High blood pressure.* An estimated 73% of people with diabetes have blood pressure greater than or equal to 130/80 mm Hg or use medications.[4,6]

Box 12.2

The Symptoms of Diabetes

The symptoms of type 1 diabetes differ somewhat from those of type 2 diabetes.

Type 1

- Frequent urination
- Unusual thirst
- Extreme hunger
- Unusual weight loss
- Extreme fatigue
- Irritability

Type 2

- Any type 1 symptoms
- Frequent infections
- Blurred vision
- Cuts or bruises that are slow to heal
- Tingling or numbness in the hands or feet
- Recurring skin, gum, or bladder infections

Box 12.3

Healthy People 2010 Objectives for Diabetes (Selected)

Objective 5-1. Increase the proportion of persons with diabetes who receive formal diabetes education. Target: 60%. Baseline: 45%.

Objective 5-2. Prevent diabetes. Target: 2.5 new cases per 1,000 population per year. Baseline: 3.5 new cases per 1,000 population (3-year average).

Objective 5-3. Reduce the overall rate of diabetes that is clinically diagnosed. Target: 25 overall cases per 1,000 population. Baseline: 40 overall cases of diabetes per 1,000 population.

Objective 5-4. Increase the proportion of adults with diabetes whose condition has been diagnosed. Target: 80%. Baseline: 68%.

Objective 5-5. Reduce the diabetes death rate. Target: 45 deaths per 100,000 population. Baseline: 75 deaths per 100,000 population.

Objective 5-7. Reduce deaths from cardiovascular disease in persons with diabetes. Target: 309 deaths per 100,000 persons with diabetes. Baseline: 343 deaths from cardiovascular disease per 100,000 persons with diabetes.

Objective 5-12. Increase the proportion of adults with diabetes who have a glycosylated hemoglobin measurement at least once a year. Target: 50%. Baseline: 24%.

Objective 5-17. Increase the proportion of adults with diabetes who perform self blood-glucose monitoring at least once daily. Target: 60%. Baseline: 42%.

Source: U.S. Department of Health and Human Services. *Healthy People 2010.* Washington DC: 2000. www.health.gov/ healthypeople.

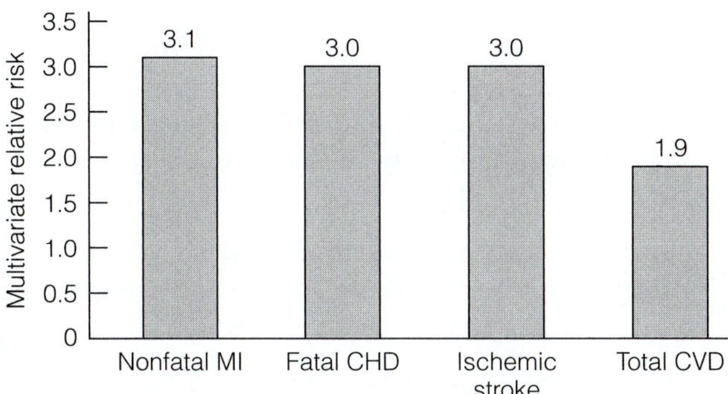

Figure 12.4 Diabetes and risk of cardiovascular disease in women: Relative risk after control for other known risk factors. Risk of nonfatal and fatal heart disease and stroke for diabetics was tripled in this large 8-year study of U.S. nurses. Source: Data from Manson JE, Colditz GA, Stampfer, MJ, et al. A prospective study of maturity-onset diabetes mellitus and risk of coronary heart disease and stroke in women. *Arch Intern Med* 151:1141–1147, 1991.

- *Blindness.* Diabetes is the leading cause of new cases of blindness in adults 20–74 years old. Diabetic retinopathy causes 12,000–24,000 new cases of blindness each year.
- *Kidney disease.* Diabetes is the leading cause of end-stage renal disease, accounting for about 43% of new cases. About 41,000 people with diabetes develop end-stage renal disease each year, with about 129,000 receiving dialysis or kidney transplantation.
- *Nervous system disease.* About 60–70% of people with diabetes have mild to severe forms of nervous system damage (which often includes impaired sensation or pain in the feet or hands, slowed digestion of food in the stomach, carpal tunnel syndrome, and other nerve problems). Severe forms of diabetic nerve disease are a major contributing cause of lower-extremity amputations.
- *Amputations.* More than 60% of lower-limb amputations in the United States occur among people with diabetes. About 82,000 amputations are performed each year among people with diabetes.

- *Dental disease. Periodontal disease* (a type of gum disease that can lead to tooth loss) occurs with greater frequency and severity among people with diabetes. Periodontal disease has been reported to occur among 30% of people age 19 years or older with type 1 diabetes.
- *Complications of pregnancy.* Poorly controlled diabetes before conception and during the first trimester of pregnancy can cause major birth defects in 5–10% of pregnancies and spontaneous abortions in 15–20%.
- *Other complications.* Diabetes can directly cause acute life-threatening events, such as diabetic ketoacidosis and hyperosmolar nonketotic coma. People with diabetes are more susceptible to many other illnesses. For example, they are more likely to die of pneumonia or influenza than people who do not have diabetes.
- *Psychosocial dysfunction.* Psychological problems, depression, and anxiety often arise in patients and their families due to the emotional and social impact of diabetes and to the demands of therapy.[7] Type 2 diabetics have been reported to be at increased risk for the development of dementia such as Alzheimer's disease.[8]

Classification of Diabetes Mellitus

There are four categories of diabetes mellitus:[2]

- Type 1 diabetes
- Type 2 diabetes
- Gestational diabetes (develops during the pregnancy, but disappears afterward)
- Other specific types of diabetes (result from specific genetic syndromes, surgery, drugs, malnutrition, infections, and other illnesses)

Since 1997, diabetes experts have recommended eliminating the old categories of "insulin-dependent diabetes mellitus" (IDDM) and "non–insulin-dependent diabetes mellitus" (NIDDM) because they are based on treatment, which can vary considerably, and do not indicate the underlying problem.[2] Further, in discussing the types of diabetes, the use of Arabic (type 1 and type 2) rather than Roman (type I and type II) numerals is recommended, to prevent confusion (e.g., type II being read as "type eleven"). (Box 12.4 provides a listing of websites where updated information on diabetes is available.)

Type 1 Diabetes Mellitus

Approximately 700,000 Americans have type 1 diabetes, a disease characterized by destruction of the pancreatic beta cells that produce insulin, usually leading to absolute insulin deficiency—that is, a total failure to produce in-

Box 12.4

Directory of Diabetes Organizations

National Institute of Diabetes and Digestive and Kidney Diseases (NIDDK) (www.niddk.nih.gov)
The NIDDK is the government's lead agency for diabetes research. It operates three information clearinghouses of potential interest to people seeking diabetes information and funds six diabetes research and training centers and eight diabetes endocrinology research centers.

National Diabetes Information Clearinghouse (NDIC) (http://diabetes.niddk.nih.gov)
Mission: To serve as a diabetes information, educational, and referral resource for health professionals and the public. NDIC is a service of the NIDDK.

Centers for Disease Control and Prevention (CDC), National Center for Chronic Disease Prevention and Health Promotion, Division of Diabetes Translation (www.cdc.gov/diabetes)
Mission: To reduce the burden of diabetes in the United States by planning, conducting, coordinating, and evaluating federal efforts to translate promising results of diabetes research into widespread clinical and public health practice.

American Association of Diabetes Educators (AADE) (www.aadenet.org)
Mission: To advance the role of the diabetes educator and improve the quality of diabetes education and care.

American Diabetes Association (ADA) (www.diabetes.org)
Mission: To prevent and cure diabetes and to improve the lives of everyone affected by diabetes.

Diabetes Exercise and Sports Association (DESA) (www.diabetes-exercise.org)
Mission: To enhance the quality of life for people with diabetes through exercise.

Juvenile Diabetes Research Foundation International (JDRF) (www.jdf.org)
Mission: To support and fund research to find a cure for diabetes and its complications. The JDRF is a nonprofit, voluntary health agency.

National Certification Board for Diabetes Educators (NCBDE) (www.ncbde.org)
Mission: To promote excellence in the field of diabetes education through the development, maintenance, and protection of the Certified Diabetes Educator (CDE) credential and the certification process.

sulin.[1–4] People with type 1 diabetes are prone to ketoacidosis (a life-threatening acidosis of the body due to the production of ketone bodies during fatty acid breakdown). Risk factors are less well defined for type 1 diabetes than for type 2 diabetes, but autoimmune, genetic, and environmental factors are involved. There are two major forms of type 1 diabetes:[2]

1. *Immune-mediated diabetes.* Results from an autoimmune destruction of the beta cells; it typically starts in children or young adults who are slim but can arise in adults of any age. In this form of diabetes, the rate of beta cell destruction is quite variable, being rapid in some individuals (mainly infants and children) and slow in others (mainly adults). Immune-mediated diabetes commonly occurs in childhood and adolescence, but it can occur at any age, even in the eighth and ninth decades of life. Autoimmune destruction of beta cells has multiple genetic predispositions and is also related to environmental factors that are still poorly defined.
2. *Idiopathic diabetes.* Refers to rare forms of the disease that have no known cause. This form of diabetes is strongly inherited and lacks immunological evidence for beta cell destruction.

Type 2 Diabetes Mellitus

Type 2 diabetes usually arises because of insulin resistance, in which the body fails to use insulin properly, combined with relative (rather than absolute) insulin deficiency.[2,9] People with type 2 can range from predominantly insulin resistant with relative insulin deficiency to predominantly deficient in insulin secretion with some insulin resistance. More than 17 million Americans have type 2 diabetes, making this the most common type.[4]

Chief characteristics of type 2 diabetes include the following:[2]

- *Type 2 diabetes develops gradually.* For a long period of time before type 2 is detected or noticed, blood glucose levels are often high enough to cause pathological changes in various organs and tissues, without clinical symptoms.[9]
- *Most do not need insulin.* At least initially, and often throughout their lifetime, type 2 diabetics do not need insulin treatment to survive.
- *Not ketosis prone.* Ketoacidosis seldom occurs spontaneously in type 2 diabetics.
- *Has multiple risk factors.* Type 2 diabetes typically occurs in people who are over 45 years old, overweight, and sedentary, and who have a family history of diabetes. Most patients with type 2 diabetes are obese, and obesity itself causes some degree of insulin resistance. Type 2 diabetes occurs more frequently in women with prior gestational diabetes mellitus, and in individuals with high blood pressure and high blood LDL cholesterol and triglycerides. African Americans, Hispanic/Latino Americans, Native Americans, and some Asian Americans and Pacific Islanders are at particularly high risk for type 2 diabetes.[1–4,10] (See Physical Fitness Activity 12.1 at the end of this chapter.) Many type 2 diabetics have the metabolic syndrome, which includes obesity, high blood pressure, high blood insulin levels, and dyslipidemia. This syndrome is strongly associated with high morbidity and mortality rates[10] (see Chapter 10).
- *Has a genetic link.* Type 2 diabetes is often associated with a strong genetic predisposition, but the genetics of this form of diabetes are complex and not clearly defined.

Testing and Diagnosis

In 1997, an international expert committee recommended lowering the number for diagnosis on the most commonly used test for diabetes and has urged that consideration be given to wide-scale screening and testing in order to detect diabetes at an earlier stage and help prevent or delay the onset of serious and costly complications.[2] The expert committee was convened under the auspices of the American Diabetes Association. The expert committee's work is an update of a similar process last undertaken in 1979 by the National Diabetes Data Group, and its recommendations are based on a 2-year review of more than 15 years of research. Additional revisions were published in 2003.[2]

The new recommendations are based on data from population-based research showing that serious complications of diabetes begin earlier than previously thought.

Diabetes can be diagnosed in any one of the following three ways, confirmed on a different day (by any one of the three methods):[2,11]

- A *fasting plasma glucose* that is equal to or greater than 126 mg/dl (after no caloric intake for at least 8 hours).
- A *casual plasma glucose* (taken at any time of day, without regard to time of last meal) that is equal to or greater than 200 mg/dl, with the classic diabetes symptoms of increased urination, increased thirst, and unexplained weight loss.
- An *oral glucose tolerance test* (OGTT) value that is equal to or greater than 200 mg/dl in the 2-hour sample. (For the OGTT, the glucose load should contain 75 grams of anhydrous glucose dissolved in water.)

The fasting plasma glucose is the preferred test and is recommended for testing and diagnosis because of its ease of administration, convenience, acceptability to patients, and lower cost (compared to the OGTT).[2] The categories of fasting plasma glucose values are as follows:

- <100 mg/dl = normal fasting glucose
- 100–125 mg/dl = impaired fasting glucose or "pre-diabetes"
- ≥126 mg/dl = diagnosis of diabetes (after confirmation on a separate day)

It should also be noted that the finger-prick test used by people with diabetes to monitor their blood glucose levels, and sometimes used at health fairs and diabetes risk assessments among the general public, is not considered a diagnostic procedure.[2]

Impaired Fasting Glucose or Pre-Diabetes

A fasting plasma glucose value of <100 mg/dl is the upper limit of normal blood glucose. There are two categories of impaired glucose metabolism (or impaired glucose homeostasis) that are considered risk factors for future diabetes and cardiovascular disease:[2]

1. *Impaired fasting glucose (IFG).* A new category, when fasting plasma glucose is 100–125 mg/dl; about 41 million persons between the ages of 40 and 74 are estimated to have impaired fasting glucose.
2. *Impaired glucose tolerance (IGT).* When results of the more complicated oral glucose tolerance test are ≥140 but <200 mg/dl (in the 2-hour sample).

A plasma glucose value of 60–99 mg/dl is normal. Many people feel they are afflicted with hypoglycemia or low blood sugar, a condition popularized in several books devoted to this topic. However, true hypoglycemia is a rare condition seen in less than 1% of the general population.[12] Hypoglycemia is diagnosed when the plasma glucose level drops below 50 mg/dl within a few hours of eating a regular meal, while the patient is experiencing symptoms (weakness, fatigue, stress, headache, trembling, etc.). If the symptoms and low plasma glucose level appear together after the meal, and if the symptoms are relieved soon after eating, hypoglycemia is diagnosed. Hypoglycemia is actually more common among diabetics who use too high a dose of insulin or use it at the wrong time in relationship to dietary and exercise habits.

Risk Factors and Screening for Diabetes

Type 2 diabetes is frequently not diagnosed until complications appear, and close to one third of people with diabetes are undiagnosed.[1,2] The American Diabetes Association recommends that individuals at high risk should be screened for diabetes and pre-diabetes (see Figure 12.5).[1] As summarized in Box 12.5, testing for diabetes should be considered in all individuals at age 45 years and above, especially in those with a BMI of 25 kg/m^2 and higher. If the test is normal, screening for diabetes should be repeated at 3-year intervals. Testing should be considered at a young age or be carried out more frequently in individuals who are overweight and have additional risk factors as listed in Box 12.5. Screening should be carried out within the health-care setting.[1,2] The fasting plasma glucose test is recommended for diabetes screening.

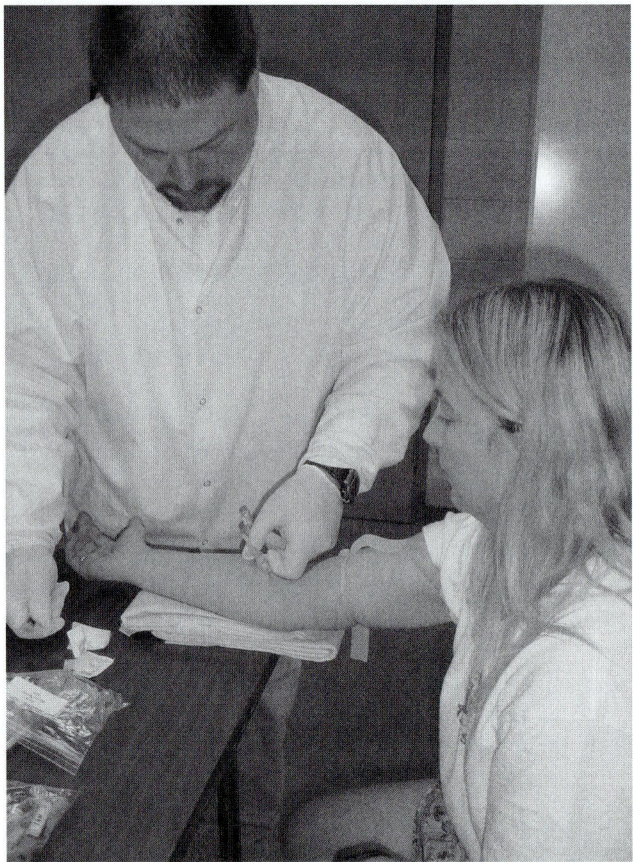

Figure 12.5 Adults at high risk of diabetes should be screened before age 45.

The incidence of type 2 diabetes in children and adolescents has increased strongly in the last decade.[1,6] The American Diabetes Association recommends that youth be screened if they are overweight and have two or more of the risk factors listed in Box 12.5.

Special Recommendations for Pregnant Women

Gestational diabetes mellitus (GDM) is a form of glucose intolerance that is diagnosed in some women during pregnancy.[1] GDM occurs more frequently among African Americans, Hispanic/Latino Americans, Native Americans, obese women, and those with a family history of diabetes.[2] During pregnancy, patients with GDM require treatment to normalize maternal blood glucose levels to avoid complications in the infant. After pregnancy, 5–10% of women with GDM are found to have type 2 diabetes,

Box 12.5

Screening and Risk Factors for Diabetes in Adults and Children

1. *Criteria for testing for diabetes in asymptomatic adult individuals:*

   Testing for diabetes should be considered in all individuals age 45 years and above, especially in those with a BMI of 25 kg/m^2 and higher. If the test is normal, screening for diabetes should be repeated at 3-year intervals. Testing should be considered at a young age or be carried out more frequently in individuals who are overweight (BMI of 25 and higher) and have additional risk factors listed as follows:

   a. Are habitually physically inactive
   b. Have a first-degree relative with diabetes
   c. Are members of a high-risk ethnic population (e.g., African American, Latino, Native American, Asian American, Pacific Islander)
   d. Have delivered a baby weighing more than 9 pounds or have been diagnosed with gestational diabetes mellitus
   e. Are hypertensive (≥ 140/90 mm Hg)
   f. Have an HDL cholesterol level <35 mg/dl and/or a triglyceride level > 250 mg/dl
   g. Have polycystic ovary syndrome
   h. On previous testing, had IGT or IFG (pre-diabetes)
   i. Have other clinical conditions associated with insulin resistance (acanthosis nigricans)
   j. Have a history of vascular disease

2. *Criteria for testing for type 2 diabetes in children:*

   Only children and youth at increased risk for the presence or the development of type 2 diabetes should be tested at age 10 (and then every 2 years), using these criteria:

   a. Overweight (BMI > 85th percentile for age and sex), *plus any two* of the following risk factors:
   b. Family history of type 2 diabetes in first- or second-degree relative
   c. Race/ethnicity (Native American, African American, Latino, Asian American, Pacific Islander)
   d. Signs of insulin resistance or conditions associated with insulin resistance (acanthosis nigricans, hypertension, dyslipidemia, or polycystic ovary syndrome)

Sources: American Diabetes Association. Standards of medical care in diabetes. *Diabetes Care* 28(suppl 1):S4–S36, 2005; The Expert Committee on the Diagnosis and Classification of Diabetes Mellitus. Follow-up report on the diagnosis of diabetes mellitus. *Diabetes Care* 20:1183–1197, 1997; 26:3150–3167, 2003.

and risk of developing diabetes during the next 5–10 years is 20 to 50% higher than normal.[1,2]

Risk assessment for GDM should be undertaken at the first prenatal visit.[1] Women at high risk for GDM (marked obesity, personal history of GDM, glucose in the urine, or a strong family history of diabetes) should have a glucose test (a fasting plasma glucose ≥ 126 mg/dl indicates diabetes). Average-risk women and high-risk women not found to have GDM at the initial screening should be tested between 24 and 28 weeks of gestation using a 100-gram oral glucose tolerance test (OGTT). The OGTT should be conducted in the morning after an overnight fast of 8 to 14 hours. Diagnostic criteria for the 100-gram OGTT are as follows, with a positive diagnosis given when two or more of these values are met or exceeded:

- ≥ 95 mg/dl fasting
- ≥ 180 mg/dl at 1 hour
- ≥ 155 mg/dl at 2 hours
- ≥ 140 mg/dl at 3 hours

Low-risk status requires no glucose testing, but this category is limited to those women meeting all of the following characteristics:[1]

- Age less than 25 years.
- Weight normal before pregnancy.
- Member of an ethnic group with a low prevalence of GDM.
- No known diabetes in first-degree relatives.
- No history of abnormal glucose tolerance.
- No history of poor obstetric outcome.

Women with GDM should be screened for diabetes at 6 weeks postpartum and should be followed up with subsequent screening for the development of diabetes or pre-diabetes.

LIFESTYLE AND RISK OF TYPE 2 DIABETES

Rates for type 2 diabetes rise dramatically as the modernized lifestyle is adopted by people from developing societies. For example, in China, the prevalence of diabetes rose threefold during a recent 10-year period, as changes were made from a traditional to a modernized lifestyle.[13] Among Japanese American men, those retaining a more traditional Japanese lifestyle experienced a reduced prevalence of diabetes.[14] There is growing evidence that 90% of type 2 diabetes can be attributed to poor lifestyles, in particular, obesity, physical inactivity, an unhealthy diet, and smoking.[15–25]

In the United States, approximately 85% of patients with type 2 diabetes are obese at the time of diagnosis. About 70% of type 2 diabetes risk in the United States is attributable to obesity. As shown in Figures 12.6 and 12.7, the risk for developing type 2 diabetes rises in direct relationship to the degree of obesity for both men and women.[15–17] In one 5-year study of more than 20,000 U.S. male physicians, risk of type 2 diabetes tripled when the body mass index rose above 26.4 kg/m^2 (see Figure 12.6).[16] In a 14-year study of more than 114,000 female nurses, after adjustment for age, body mass index was the dominant predictor of risk for type 2 diabetes (see Figure 12.7).[17] Women who gained weight during the study increased their risk for type 2 diabetes, while those who lost weight decreased their risk. These data indicate that women can minimize the risk for diabetes by achieving a lean body build as a young adult and avoiding even modest weight gain throughout life. Another study showed that for both men and women, gaining just 10 pounds increased the risk for developing diabetes by about 25%.[18]

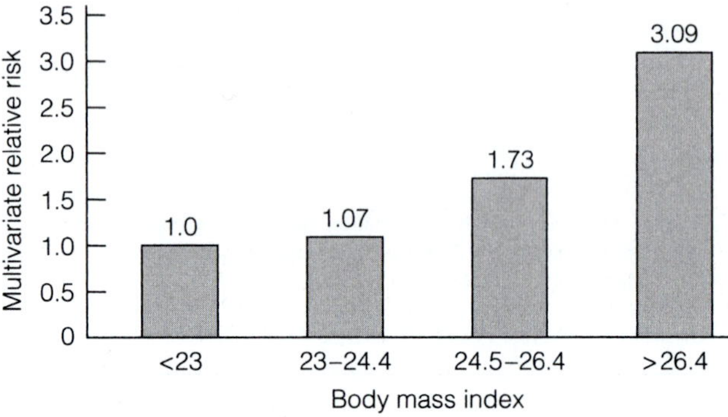

Figure 12.6 Body mass index as a predictor of diabetes: Relative risk of type 2 diabetes. Source: Manson JE, Nathan DM, Krolewski AS, et al. A prospective study of exercise and incidence of diabetes among U.S. male physicians. *JAMA* 268:63–67, 1992.

In severely obese populations, such as the Pima Indians and Nauruans, the prevalence of type 2 diabetes is the highest worldwide.[19] Obesity, especially upper-body or abdominal obesity, is associated with insulin resistance (a decreased ability of the body to respond to the action of insulin, and a reduced number of insulin receptors). A growing number of studies have shown that the risk of type 2 diabetes climbs in direct proportion to the increase in waist circumference or the waist-to-hip ratio (i.e., when the abdominal girth approaches or exceeds the hip girth).[19–21] As shown in Figure 12.8, a 10-inch difference in the waist circumference (e.g., 28 versus 38 inches) increases the risk of type 2 diabetes sixfold.[21] Several other studies have shown that when body weight, especially abdominal fat, is lost, insulin resistance is reduced, and blood glucose levels either improve or often return to normal.[18–21]

The estimated reduction in the risk of type 2 diabetes associated with maintaining desirable body weight compared with being obese is 50–75%, considerably higher than the 30–50% reduction in risk associated with regular, moderate, or vigorous exercise versus a sedentary lifestyle.[19] Thus, avoidance of weight gain with increasing age is the most important prevention measure for type 2 diabetes. The important role of physical activity in preventing diabetes will be reviewed later in this chapter.[15–23]

Few studies have been conducted on the role of diet in the development of type 2 diabetes. In one 6-year study of more than 65,000 nurses, researchers from the Harvard School of Public Health showed that the risk of developing diabetes was 2.5 times greater in those using refined and

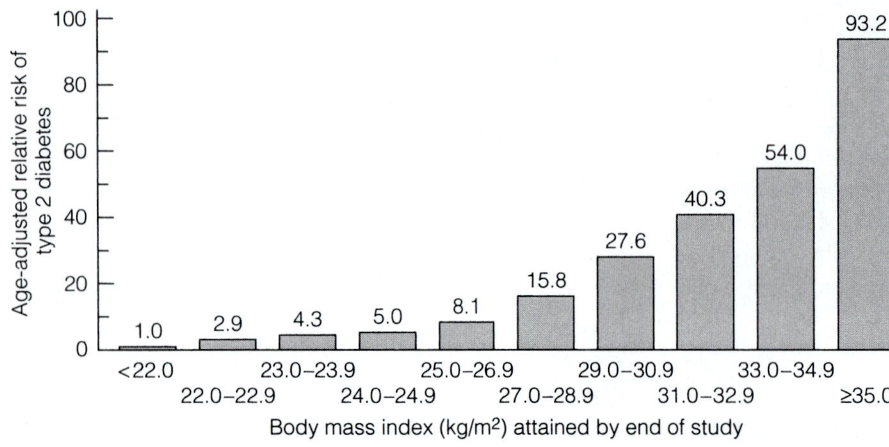

Figure 12.7 Attained body mass index and risk of diabetes, in 114,834 U.S. women age 30–55 years in 1976 and followed for 14 years. Source: Colditz GA, Willett WC, Rotnitzky A, Manson JE. Weight gain as a risk factor for clinical diabetes mellitus in women. *Ann Intern Med* 122:481–486, 1995.

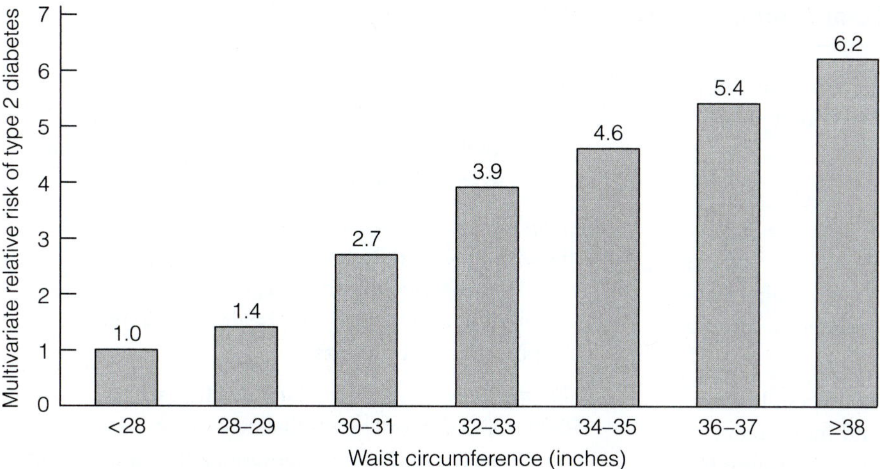

Figure 12.8 Waist circumference and risk of type 2 diabetes, 8-year study of 43,581 nurses. Source: Carey VJ, Walters EE, Colditz GA, et al. Body fat distribution and risk of non–insulin-dependent diabetes mellitus in women. The Nurses' Health Study. *Am J Epidemiol* 145:614–619, 1997.

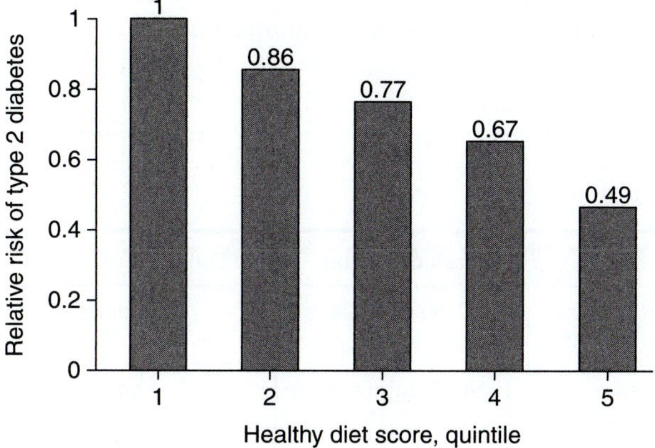

Figure 12.9 Risk of developing diabetes during a 16-year period in 85,000 women according to diet. Diet score based on low *trans* fat and glycemic load, high cereal fiber, and a high ratio of polyunsaturated to saturated fat. Source: Hu FB, Manson JE, Stampfer MJ, Colditz G, Liu S, Solomon CG, Willett WC. Diet, lifestyle, and the risk of type 2 diabetes mellitus in women. *N Engl J Med* 345:790–797, 2001.

processed grain products (low in dietary fiber), compared to those using grains in a minimally refined form (high in fiber).[24] These same results were confirmed in a cohort of 42,759 men.[25] In a 16-year study of 85,000 nurses, risk of developing diabetes was 51% lower in those eating the healthiest diet (see Figure 12.9).[15] The diet score in this study was based on a low intake of *trans* fat, a low glycemic load, high cereal fiber, and a high ratio of polyunsaturated to saturated fat. When this diet score was combined with a low body mass index, 30 or more minutes of daily exercise, and avoidance of tobacco, risk of developing diabetes was nearly 90% lower when compared to the worst-quintile group. These studies suggest that grains should be consumed in a minimally refined form to reduce the risk of type 2 diabetes. It should be noted that while there are few data on dietary habits and risk of developing type 2 diabetes, substantial evidence exists in support of a diet high in carbohydrate and fiber and low in fat in the treatment of type 2 diabetes. (See Sports Medicine Insight at the end of this chapter.) Box 9.5 in Chapter 9 provides more information on the glycemic index.

TREATMENT OF TYPE 1 AND TYPE 2 DIABETES

Treatment for either type of diabetes seeks to accomplish what the human body normally does naturally: maintain a proper balance between glucose and insulin. Food makes the blood glucose level rise, while insulin and exercise make it fall. The challenge is to manage these three factors to keep the blood glucose within a narrow range and prevent diabetes-related complications (see Box 12.6). Training in self-management is integral to the treatment of diabetes. Treatment must be individualized and must address medical, psychosocial, and lifestyle issues.[26–28]

Lack of insulin production by the pancreas makes type 1 diabetes particularly difficult to control. Because there is no cure for type 1 diabetes, treatment is lifelong. For the individual with type 1 diabetes, to keep the blood glucose within narrow limits and avoid the medical complications, a regular and consistent lifestyle must be followed.[1,10,11] Eating times, amounts and types of foods, and physical activity should be consistent from one day to the next. Blood glucose should be measured several times a day, and multiple insulin injections or treatment with an insulin pump is necessary. See Table 12.1 for a list of insulin drugs. Periodic measurement of glycosylated hemoglobin (A1C) is important to monitor long-term glycemic control (see Box 12.7).[10,29]

Results from a major multicenter study by the Diabetes Control and Complications Trial (DCCT) Research Group have shown that when type 1 diabetes patients keep their blood glucose levels under tight control through intensive care, fewer medical complications develop.[30,31] The study showed that keeping blood glucose levels as close to normal as possible slowed the onset and progression of eye, kidney, and nerve diseases caused by diabetes. In fact, it demonstrated that *any* sustained lowering of blood glucose

Box 12.6

Many Complications of Diabetes Can Be Prevented

Early detection, improved delivery of care, and better self-management are key strategies for preventing the following diabetes-related complications:

Eye disease and blindness. Each year, an estimated 12,000–24,000 people become blind because of diabetic eye disease. Appropriate screening and care could prevent 50–60% of diabetes-related blindness. However, only 60% of people with diabetes receive annual dilated eye exams.

Kidney disease. Each year, about 41,000 people with diabetes develop kidney failure, and more than 129,000 are treated for this condition. Treatment to better control blood pressure and blood glucose levels could reduce diabetes-related kidney failure by 30–70%.

Amputations. About 82,000 people undergo diabetes-related lower-extremity amputations each year. About 45–85% of these amputations could be prevented with regular examinations and patient education.

Complications of pregnancy. Women with preexisting diabetes give birth to more than 18,000 babies each year. Preconception diabetes care for these mothers can prevent diabetes-related health problems for both mothers and infants.

Flu- and pneumonia-related death. Each year, 10,000–30,000 people with diabetes die of complications of flu and pneumonia; they are roughly three times more likely to die of these complications than people without diabetes. However, only 54% of people with diabetes get an annual flu shot.

Source: Centers for Disease Control and Prevention. www.cdc.gov/diabetes.

TABLE 12.1 Insulin Drugs

Type of Insulin	Examples	Onset of Action	Peak of Action	Duration of Action
Rapid-acting	Humalog (lispro) Eli Lilly	15 minutes	30–90 minutes	3–5 hours
	NovoLog (aspart) Novo Nordisk	15 minutes	40–50 minutes	3–5 hours
Short-acting (Regular)	Humulin R Eli Lilly Novolin R Novo Nordisk	30–60 minutes	50–120 minutes	5–8 hours
Intermediate-acting (NPH)	Humulin N Eli Lilly Novolin N Novo Nordisk	1–3 hours	8 hours	20 hours
	Humulin L Eli Lilly Novolin L Novo Nordisk	1–2.5 hours	7–15 hours	18–24 hours
Intermediate- and short-acting mixtures	Humulin 50/50 Humulin 70/30 Humalog Mix 75/25 Humalog Mix 50/50 Eli Lilly Novolin 70/30 Novolog Mix 70/30 Novo Nordisk	The onset, peak, and duration of action of these mixtures would reflect a composite of the intermediate and short- or rapid-acting components, with one peak of action.		
Long-acting	Ultralente Eli Lilly	4–8 hours	8–12 hours	36 hours
	Lantus (glargine) Aventis	1 hour	none	24 hours

Source: Lewis C. Diabetes: A growing public health concern. *FDA Consumer* Jan/Feb 2002, pp. 26–33.

Box 12.7

Steps to Control Diabetes for Life

Step 1 Complete Medical Evaluation and Care

- A complete initial medical evaluation should be performed to detect the presence or absence of diabetes complications.
- People with diabetes should receive ongoing medical care from a physician-coordinated team. Individuals with diabetes should assume an active role in their care and learn all they can about diabetes management.
- See the health-care team at least twice a year to find and treat problems early.
- At each visit obtain measurements of blood pressure and weight, and have the feet checked.
- At least two times a year have the A1C checked (check more often if level is over 7%), and have dental exams.
- Once each year have cholesterol measured, and have a dilated eye exam, complete foot exam, urine and blood tests for kidney problems, and a flu shot.
- Get a pneumonia shot at least once a year.

Step 2 Know the ABCs of Diabetes Care

- Individuals with diabetes should manage their **A**1C, **B**lood pressure, and **C**holesterol. This will help lower risk of having a heart attack, stroke, or diabetes problems. These are called the ABCs of diabetes.
  - **A** is for the A1C test (glycosylated hemoglobin, defined as one of four hemoglobin A fractions to which glucose binds). A1C shows how well the blood glucose has been controlled over the last 3 months, and should be checked at least twice a year. The goal for most people is less than 7.0% (most nondiabetic individuals are 4.0–6.0%). Capillary plasma glucose levels before meals should be 90–130 mg/dl, with a peak of less than 180 mg/dl after meals. Self-monitoring of blood glucose should be carried out three or more times daily, especially for patients using multiple insulin injections.
  - **B** is for blood pressure. The goal for most people is <130/80 mm Hg.
  - **C** is for cholesterol. The LDL-cholesterol goal for most people is less than 100 mg/dl. Also try to keep HDL-cholesterol above 40 mg/dl, and triglycerides under 150 mg/dl.

Step 3 Manage Diabetes

- Many individuals with diabetes avoid long-term problems of diabetes by taking good care of themselves and by applying the ABCs of diabetes.
- *Follow the diabetes food plan.* (See Sports Medicine Insight at the end of this chapter.)
- *Eat the right portions of healthy foods.*
- *Eat foods that have less salt and fat.*
- *Get 30–60 minutes of activity on most days of the week.*
- *Stay at a healthy weight by being active and controlling food intake.*
- *Stop smoking and seek help to quit.*
- *Take medicines as medically prescribed.*
- *Check your feet every day for cuts, blisters, red spots, and swelling.*
- *Brush your teeth and floss every day to avoid problems with the mouth, teeth, and gums.*
- *Check blood glucose according to directions given by the medical care team.*

Sources: American Diabetes Association. Standards of medical care in diabetes. *Diabetes Care* 28(suppl 1):S4–S36, 2005; American Diabetes Association, National Institute of Diabetes and Digestive and Kidney Diseases. Prevention or delay of type 2 diabetes. *Diabetes Care* 27(suppl 1):S47–S54, 2004; www.ndep.nih.gov.

helps, even if the person has a history of poor control. Elements of intensive management in the DCCT included the following:[30]

- Testing blood glucose levels four or more times a day
- Four daily insulin injections or use of an insulin pump
- Adjustment of insulin doses according to food intake and exercise
- A diet and exercise plan
- Regular visits to a health-care team composed of a physician, nurse educator, dietitian, and behavioral therapist

Box 12.7 summarizes the principles of diabetic care according to the National Diabetes Education Program and the American Diabetes Association.[1] One problem with intensive therapy is poor patient compliance and acceptance. In the DCCT, the most significant side effect of intensive treatment was an increase in the risk for low blood glucose episodes severe enough to require assistance from another person (severe hypoglycemia). Thus, careful cooperation with a medical care team is critical. DCCT researchers estimated that intensive management doubled the cost of managing diabetes. However, this cost appears to be offset by the reduction in medical expenses related to long-term complications and by the improved quality of life of people with type 1 diabetes.

Implantable, programmable insulin pumps are gaining favor with many diabetes experts.[32,33] Although first considered primarily for type 1 diabetic patients, research data also suggest that type 2 diabetics requiring insulin therapy can also gain benefit.[33] The devices weigh about ½ pound and are surgically implanted just under the skin in the abdomen. A catheter delivers insulin into the abdominal cavity. Insulin refills are performed transcutaneously with a syringe every 4–12 weeks. Long-term studies show that glycemic control is improved with pump therapy.[32,33] Severe hypoglycemia and weight gain are relatively rare, and patients report high satisfaction and improved quality of life.

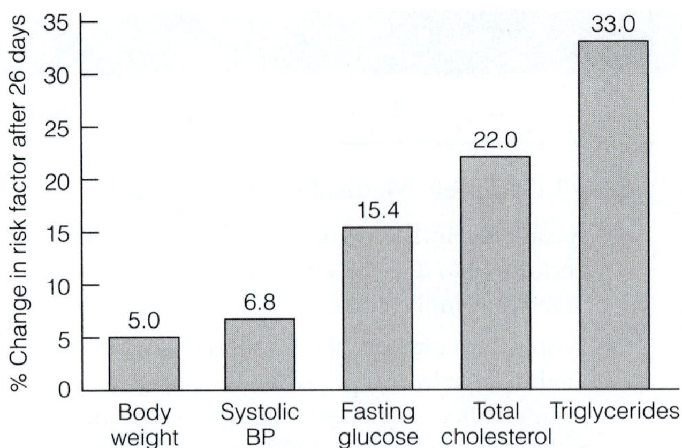

Figure 12.10 Effects of diet and exercise on CHD risk factors in 652 type 2 patients, percentage change after 26-day Pritikin Program (<10% fat, high fiber and carbohydrate diet, 1–2 hours walking/day), in which 71% of subjects taking oral hypoglycemic agents and 39% of those taking insulin discontinued their medication. Source: Barnard RJ, Jung T, Inkeles SB. Diet and exercise in the treatment of NIDDM. *Diabetes Care* 17:1469–1472, 1994.

PREVENTION, DELAY, AND TREATMENT OF TYPE 2 DIABETES

Treatment of type 2 diabetes usually includes diet control, exercise, home blood glucose testing, and in some cases, oral medication and/or insulin.[1,26–28] Most experts recommend that a staged approach to diabetic treatment be followed for type 2 diabetes patients.[10,26,27] Because the vast majority are obese, weight loss through a healthy diet (i.e., low in fat, with an emphasis on carbohydrates and fiber) and exercise is first recommended. If diet, exercise, and weight loss fail to lower blood glucose levels (most often due to patient noncompliance with the recommended lifestyle changes), the doctor may decide to add a diabetes drug, insulin, or both. See Table 12.2 for a list of drugs used to treat type 2 diabetes. Insulin is the usual choice for advanced type 2 diabetes cases. Long-term studies indicate that the majority of type 2 diabetics need multiple lifestyle and drug therapies to achieve glycemic targets.[34]

Type 2 diabetes is regarded as largely preventable and treatable through improved lifestyle habits.[19] The single most important objective for the obese individual with type 2 diabetes is to achieve and maintain a desirable body weight.[19,35–39] Weight reduction reduces serum glucose and improves insulin sensitivity, while also favorably influencing several heart disease risk factors. Diabetics who are at high risk for death from heart disease, and who face a future laden with medical complications from high blood glucose levels, have much to gain from losing weight. Unfortunately, various studies have reported that individuals with type 2 diabetes have a poor history of attaining and then maintaining a desirable body weight despite the motivation that comes from having diabetes and seeing improvements in glycemic control with weight loss.[36,38]

Figure 12.10 summarizes how quickly weight loss through a healthy diet and exercise program can influence type 2 diabetes and heart disease risk factors.[35] In this study, 652 type 2 diabetes patients attended the Pritikin Longevity Center 26-day residential program. The group included 212 patients taking insulin and 197 taking oral hypoglycemic agents. The remaining 243 were taking no diabetic medication but had a fasting glucose level above 140 mg/dl. During the 26-day program, the type 2 diabetes patients were involved in daily aerobic exercise, primarily walking (building up to two 1-hour walks each day). Patients were also placed on a high-carbohydrate, high-fiber, low-fat, low-cholesterol, and low-salt diet. Of dietary calories, less than 10% were obtained from fat. The diet contained 35–40 grams of dietary fiber per 1,000 calories, a very high amount according to most standards. During the program, the average patient lost about 10 pounds and experienced reductions in blood pressure and blood levels of fasting glucose, total cholesterol, and triglycerides. Of patients on insulin, 39% were able to stop therapy, and 71% of patients on oral agents also had their medication discontinued.

Because of the way this study was designed, it is not possible to sort out which lifestyle factor—exercise, weight loss, or improved diet—was most responsible for the impressive results.[35] Although the Pritikin diet has been criticized as being unusually restrictive (and hard to continue once the program stops), the results of this study support a strong emphasis on lifestyle modification consisting of both diet and exercise in the treatment of type 2 diabetes.

TABLE 12.2 Diabetes Drugs*

Oral Antidiabetes Medications*						
Category	**Action**	**Generic Name**	**Brand Name**	**Manufacturer**	**Approval Date**	**Comments**
Sulfonylurea	Stimulates beta cells to release more insulin	Chlorpropamide	Diabinese	Pfizer	10/58	Generally taken one to two times daily, before meals; can have interactions with other drugs, first-generation sulfonylurea (older drug)
		Glipizide	Glucotrol	Pfizer	5/84	Second generation used in smaller doses than first generation
		Glyburide	DiaBeta/Micronase/ Glynase	Aventis, Pharmacia and Upjohn	5/84	
		Glimepiride	Amaryl	Aventis	11/95	
Meglitinide	Works with similar action to sulfonylureas	Repaglinide	Prandin	Novo Nordisk	12/97	Taken before each of three meals
Nateglinide	Works with similar action to sulfonylureas	Nateglinide	Starlix	Novartis	12/00	Taken before each of three meals
Biguanide	Sensitizes the body to the insulin already present	Metformin	Glucophage	Bristol Myers Squibb	3/95	Taken two times daily with food for best results
		Metformin (long lasting)	Glucophage XR	Bristol Myers Squibb	10/00	
		Metformin with glyburide	Glucovance	Bristol Myers Squibb	7/00	
Thiazolidinedione (Glitazone)	Helps insulin work better in muscle and fat; lowers insulin resistance	Rosiglitazone	Avandia	SmithKline Beecham (now GlaxoSmithKline)	5/99	Taken once or twice daily with food; very rare but serious effect on liver
		Pioglitazone	Actos	Takeda Pharmaceuticals	7/99	
Alpha-Glucose Inhibitor	Slows or blocks the breakdown of starches and certain sugars; action slows the rise in blood sugar levels following a meal	Acarbose	Precose	Bayer	9/95	Should be taken with first bite of meal
		Miglitol	Glyset	Pharmacia and Upjohn	12/96	

* Pills to treat diabetes—antidiabetic agents—are used only in type 2 treatment.

Source: Lewis C. Diabetes: A growing public health concern. *FDA Consumer* January–February 2002, pp. 26–33.

Since the 1950s, there has been considerable debate regarding the diet best suited for the diabetic. As is reviewed in the Sports Medicine Insight at the end of this chapter, there has been a progression toward less and less dietary fat and more and more carbohydrate, with an emphasis today on individualizing the diet for each patient.[38] The primary goals of the diabetic diet for type 2 diabetes patients are to lower blood glucose and lipids, blood pressure, and body weight (when necessary). For these reasons, type 2 diabetes patients should follow a healthy and varied diet, with an emphasis on controlling saturated fats.

Prevention/Delay of Type 2 Diabetes

Several randomized controlled trials have tested whether the progression from pre-diabetes to diabetes can be delayed or prevented by intensive lifestyle modification (weight loss, change in diet, and physical activity) or by the use of commercially available glucose-lowering drugs such as metformin or acarbose.[1,10,20,26,36,39,40] All of these interventions were effective to variable degrees. In the lifestyle modification studies, it is noteworthy that these results were obtained by a modest reduction in body weight and moderate exercise such as walking. As summarized in Figure 12.11, risk of developing type 2 diabetes was reduced 31%, 46%, and 42% in subjects randomized to diet only, exercise only, and diet plus exercise interventions, respectively.[40]

In the Diabetes Prevention Program (DPP), subjects with pre-diabetes were randomized to one of three intervention groups: the intensive nutrition and exercise counseling group, the biguanide metformin group, or the placebo group.[39] After about 3 years, a 58% reduction in the progression to diabetes was observed in the lifestyle group compared to a 31% reduction in the metformin group. About 50% of the lifestyle group achieved the goal of 7% or more weight reduction, and 74% maintained at least 150 minutes per week of moderately intense exercise. The greater benefit of weight loss and physical activity strongly suggests that lifestyle modification should be the first choice to prevent or delay diabetes.[1] Lifestyle interventions also have a variety of other health benefits. When all factors are considered, there is insufficient evidence to support the use of drug therapy as a substitute for, or its routine use in addition to, lifestyle modification to prevent diabetes.

Based on the results of these studies, the American Diabetes Association has made these recommendations regarding the prevention/delay of type 2 diabetes:[1]

- Individuals at high risk for developing diabetes need to become aware of the benefits of modest weight loss (goal of 5–10%) and participating in regular physical activity (goal of 30 minutes or more daily).
- Drug therapy should not be routinely used to prevent diabetes until more information is known about its cost-effectiveness.

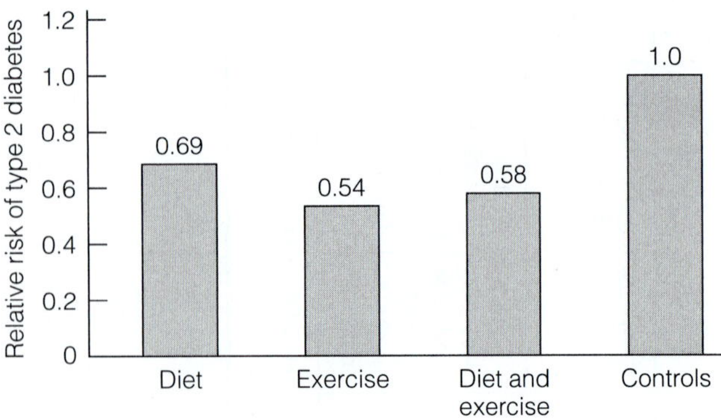

Figure 12.11 Effects of diet and exercise in preventing type 2 diabetes in people with impaired fasting glucose, 6-year study of 530 men and women in China. Source: Pan XR, Li GW, Hu YH, et al. Effects of diet and exercise in preventing NIDDM in people with impaired glucose tolerance. The Da Qing IGT and Diabetes Study. *Diabetes Care* 20:537–544, 1997.

EXERCISE AND DIABETES

Researchers have established that type 2 diabetes is less common in physically active, compared to inactive, societies.[15,19,21,23,40–50] Also, as populations have become more sedentary, the incidence of type 2 diabetes has been observed to increase[13,14,42] (see Figure 12.12). Type 2 diabetes, for example, is unusually common among some South Pacific and Native American peoples who have adopted the sedentary habits of the western world.[19,42] However, ex-

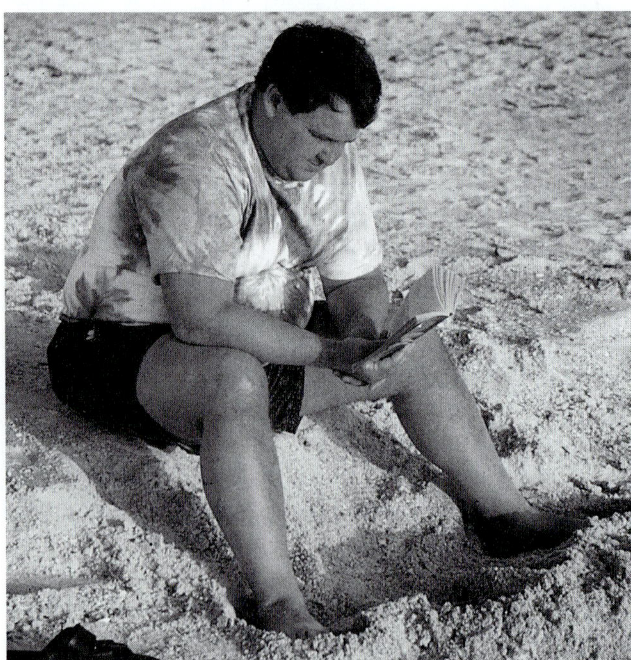

Figure 12.12 Risk of type 2 diabetes is elevated in sedentary societies. (© Myrleen Ferguson/PhotoEdit)

perts point out that other environmental and lifestyle factors are probably involved, including changes in body weight and dietary habits.[19]

Physical Activity and Risk of Developing Diabetes

Several major studies have followed large groups of men and women for extended periods of time, measuring the influence of physical activity and inactivity on the risk of developing type 2 diabetes.[15,23,41–50] The studies have provided convincing support for the role of regular physical activity in the prevention of type 2 diabetes.

Data from a 14-year study of nearly 6,000 male alumni of the University of Pennsylvania were published in 1991.[45,51] Leisure-time physical activity was measured and expressed as Calories expended per week for walking, stair climbing, and sports. Type 2 diabetes developed in 202 men, and the important finding was that for each 500-Calorie-per-week increase in activity expenditure, the risk of type 2 diabetes was reduced by 6%. For men who were both obese and inactive, the likelihood of developing type 2 diabetes was four times greater than for lean and active men. The protective effect of physical activity was especially strong for men at highest risk for type 2 diabetes, as shown in Figure 12.13. In other words, regular physical activity is an important component of a healthy lifestyle for all adults, but it may be particularly important for those at increased risk for chronic diseases.

These results are very similar to a 5-year study of 21,271 male physicians[16] (see Figure 12.14). Subjects who exercised regularly experienced a 36% reduction in risk of type 2 diabetes, with risk found to be lowest among those exercising most frequently. The benefits of exercise were most pronounced among the obese or those at the highest risk of developing type 2 diabetes.

In Finland, men at high risk for type 2 diabetes who exercised at a moderately intense level for more than 40 minutes per week reduced their risk of developing type 2 diabetes by 64%, compared to men who did not exercise.[41] In Hawaii, a 6-year study of 6,815 Japanese American men came to a similar conclusion.[44] As shown in Figure 12.15, the rate of developing type 2 diabetes was lowest among the most active men, even after adjustment for age, obesity, family history, and other factors known to influence the risk of diabetes. A 10-year study of nearly 3,000 men and women in Finland showed that risk of developing type 2 diabetes was highest among those exercising the least[46] (see Figure 12.16).

These epidemiologic studies indicate that physical activity is linked to reduced risk of type 2 diabetes in men.

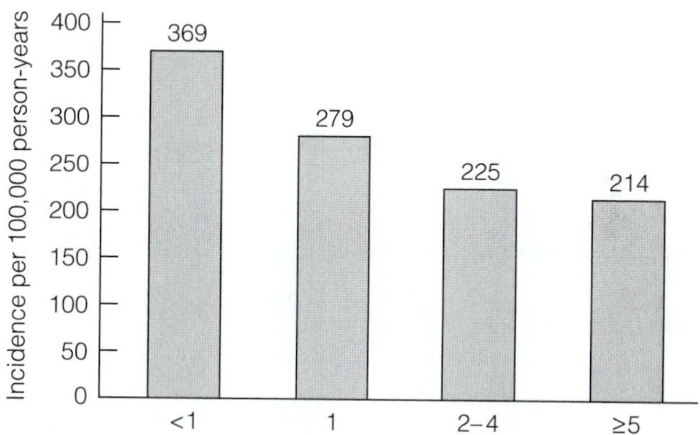

Figure 12.14 Incidence of diabetes among U.S. male physicians, age-adjusted incidence rates of type 2 diabetes. The age-adjusted incidence rate of type 2 diabetes was lower in subjects who exercised vigorously ("enough to work up a sweat") and most frequently in this 5-year study of U.S. physicians. Source: Manson JE, Nathan DM, Krolewski AS, et al. A prospective study of exercise and incidence of diabetes among U.S. male physicians. *JAMA* 268:63–67, 1992.

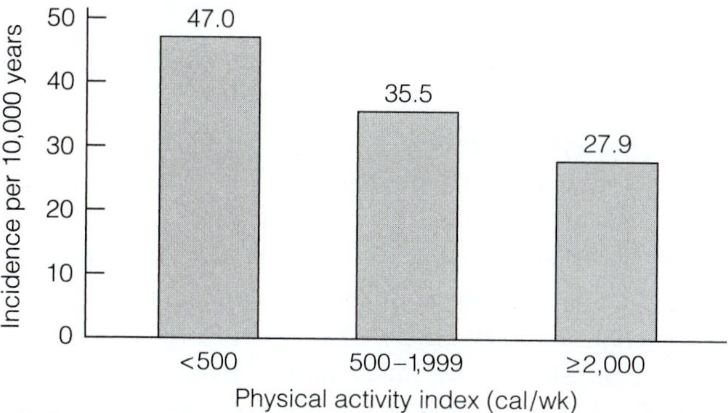

Figure 12.13 Incidence of diabetes among high-risk men, age-adjusted incidence rates of type 2 diabetes. Age-adjusted incidence rates for type 2 diabetes were lowest among the more active "high risk" men (those with obesity, hypertension, or a family history). Source: Helmrich SP, Rogland DR, Leung RW, Paffenbarger RS. Physical activity and reduced occurrence of noninsulin-dependent diabetes mellitus. *N Engl J Med* 325:147–152, 1991.

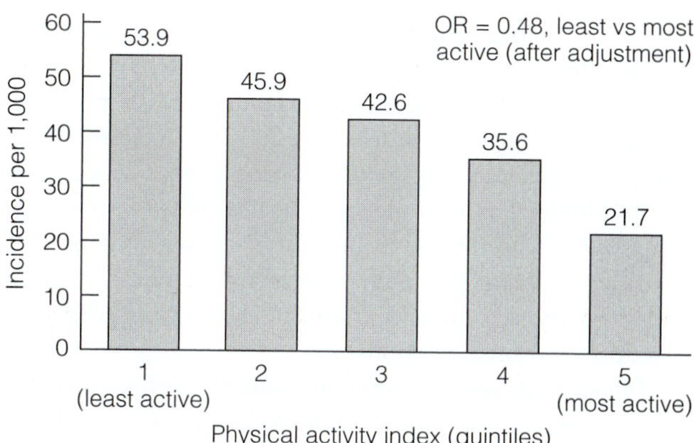

Figure 12.15 Incidence of diabetes among Japanese American men, odds ratio = 0.48, least versus most active (after adjustment). Source: Burchfiel CM, Sharp DS, Curb JD, Rodriguez BL, Hwang L-J, Marcus EB, Yano K. Physical activity and incidence of diabetes: The Honolulu Heart Program. *Am J Epidemiol* 141:360–368, 1995.

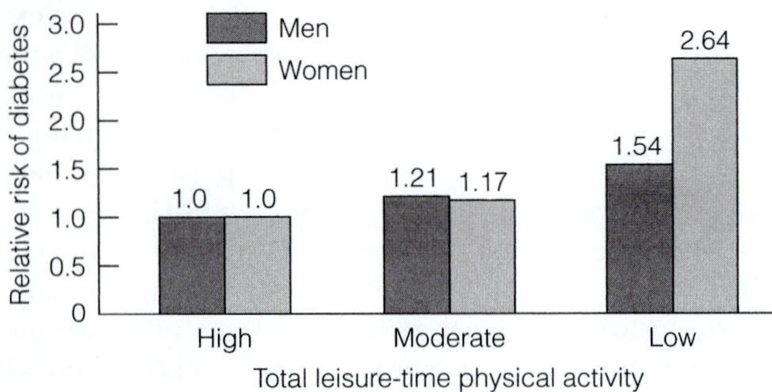

Figure 12.16 Physical activity and risk of type 2 diabetes, 10-year study of 1,340 men and 1,500 women in Finland.
Source: Haapanen N, Miilunpalo S, Vuori I, Oja P, Pasanen M. Association of leisure time physical activity with the risk of coronary heart disease, hypertension and diabetes in middle-aged men and women. *Int J Epidemiol* 26:739–747, 1997.

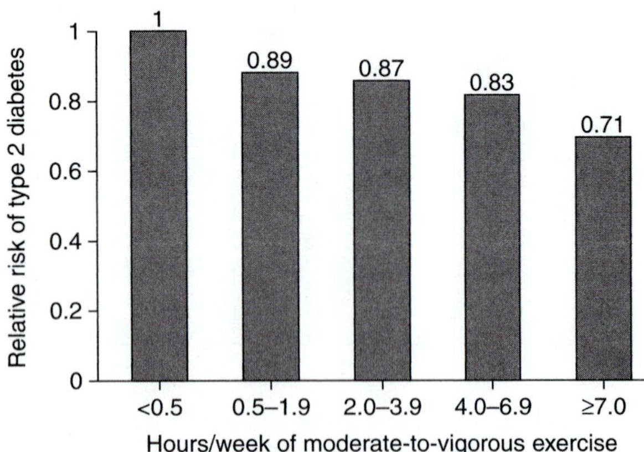

Figure 12.17 In this study of 85,000 women, risk of developing diabetes was lowest in the most active.
Source: Hu FB, Manson JE, Stampfer MJ, Colditz G, Liu S, Solomon CG, Willett WC. Diet, lifestyle, and the risk of type 2 diabetes mellitus in women. *N Engl J Med* 345:790–797, 2001.

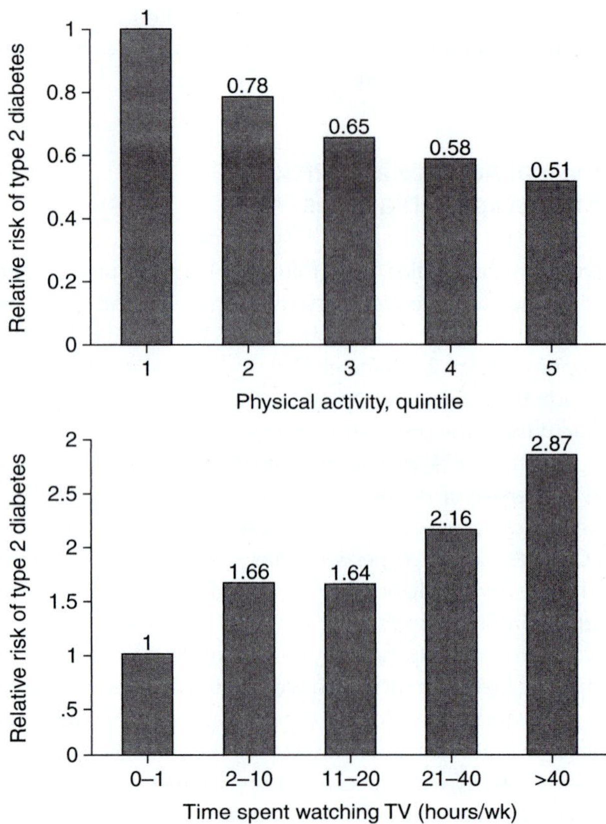

Figure 12.18 Physical activity and TV watching in relation to risk for type 2 diabetes in 38,000 men during a 10-year period. Source: Hu FB, Leitzmann MF, Stampfer MJ, Colditz GA, Willett WC, Rimm EG. Physical activity and television watching in relation to risk for type 2 diabetes mellitus in men. *Arch Intern Med* 161:1542–1548, 2001.

Increasing evidence indicates that regular physical activity also predicts lower risk of type 2 diabetes in women. Several reports from the Nurses' Health Study, a prospective cohort study of more than 120,000 women, have demonstrated that risk of developing type 2 diabetes is 40–50% lower among the most physically active (see Figure 12.17).[15,47,48] These studies have shown that greater leisure-time physical activity, in terms of both duration and intensity, was linked to reduced risk of type 2 diabetes in a dose–response relationship.

Physical fitness is easier to measure than physical activity. In a large cohort study conducted by the Cooper Institute for Aerobics Research, risk of developing diabetes was 3.7-fold higher among men in the low-fitness group (the least fit 20% of the cohort) compared to the high-fitness group (the most fit 40% of the cohort).[49]

Television watching, a major sedentary behavior in the United States, has been associated with obesity and low physical fitness. In a cohort of 38,000 men, the risk of developing type 2 diabetes was significantly higher among those spending more hours watching television, and lower among those exercising the most (see Figure 12.18).[50] In general, low physical fitness and activity and more time spent watching television predict increased risk of developing type 2 diabetes.

The Role of Exercise in Treatment of Diabetes

The concept that physical activity is beneficial for the diabetic is not new. It was promoted as a valuable adjunct to diabetic control in 600 A.D. by Chao Yuan-Fang, a prominent Chinese physician of the Sui Dynasty.[52] Even after the isolation of insulin in 1922, exercise was considered one of the three cornerstones of therapy for persons with type 1 diabetes, along with diet and insulin. Although the concept that physical activity is beneficial for diabetics is centuries old, there is still considerable controversy regarding its value.

The pancreas secretes two hormones, insulin and glucagon, to help maintain blood glucose levels[53,54] (see Figure 12.19). During rest, when blood glucose levels rise after a meal, insulin is secreted to help move the glucose into the body cells.

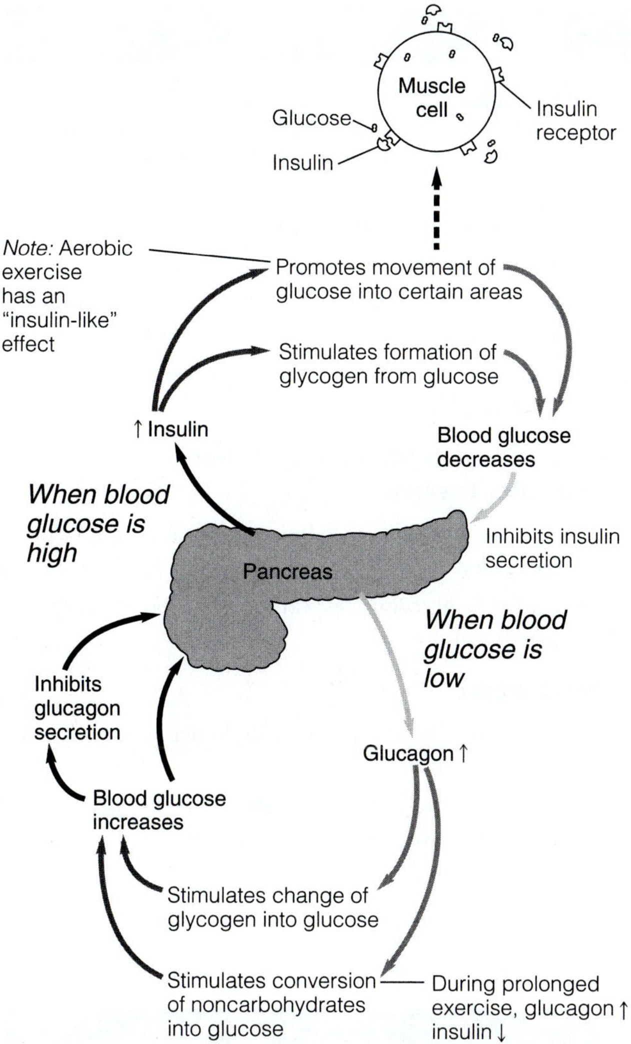

Figure 12.19 Actions of normal pancreas. The pancreas secretes two hormones, insulin and glucagon, to control blood glucose levels. During exercise, glucagon rises while insulin falls to counterbalance the "insulin-like" effect of muscle contraction and the large glucose demands of the working muscle.

Receptors on the body cells require that insulin be present before glucose can enter. On the other hand, when blood glucose levels drop, glucagon is secreted to increase blood glucose levels by stimulating the breakdown of liver glycogen.

During exercise, blood insulin levels drop, while blood glucagon levels increase. These changes take place to counterbalance the insulin-like effect of muscle contraction.[53] As the muscles contract during exercise, they do not require as much insulin to transport glucose into the working cells. The exercising muscle may increase the uptake of glucose 7- to 20-fold during the first 30–40 minutes, depending on the intensity of the exercise. In addition, the insulin receptors become more sensitive to the lower amount of insulin present during exercise.[53–57] This improvement in insulin receptor sensitivity can last for many hours after the exercise bout is over, even for as long as 2 days if the exercise was of long duration and high intensity (see Figure 12.20).

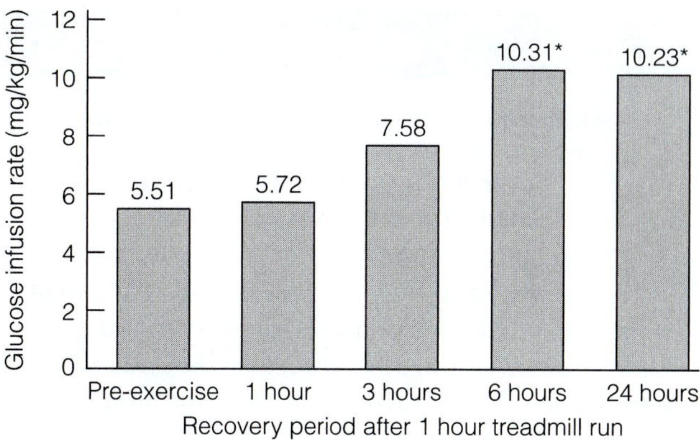

*p < 0.05 vs pre-exercise
Insulin sensitivity defined as glucose infusion rate using the insulin clamp technique

Figure 12.20 Insulin sensitivity after 1 hour of running. Improvements in insulin sensitivity occur within 6 hours of exercise and remain for at least 1 day. Source: Oshida Y, Kamanouchi K, Hayamiru S, et al. Effect of training and training cessation on insulin action. *Int J Sports Med* 12:484–486, 1991.

Type 1 Diabetes and Exercise

For nearly 50 years, researchers have known that regular exercise will reduce the insulin requirements of well-controlled type 1 diabetes patients by 30–50%. Each bout of exercise leads to an improvement in insulin sensitivity that lasts for 1 or 2 days before falling back to pre-exercise levels. The muscles need regular exercise to maintain an enhanced insulin sensitivity. Bed rest and detraining studies have shown that insulin resistance and impaired glucose tolerance develop quickly, indicating that regular physical activity is required for normal insulin action.[53,54]

A given amount of insulin following exercise is more effective in causing glucose uptake by the cells.[58] The patient with type 1 diabetes who exercises regularly will need smaller than normal insulin doses or will have to increase food intake. Although regular exercise leads to reduced insulin requirements for individuals with type 1 diabetes, studies have failed to show that long-term glucose control is improved.[59] People with type 1 diabetes still have much to gain from exercising regularly because of the potential to improve cardiovascular fitness and psychological well-being, and for social interaction and recreation.

Exercise Precautions for Individuals with Type 1 Diabetes

Safe participation in all forms of exercise, consistent with an individual's lifestyle, should be a primary goal for people with type 1 diabetes.[59] However, physical exercise is not without risks to individuals with type 1 diabetes. Before beginning an exercise program, the individual with diabetes should undergo a detailed medical evaluation in accordance with guidelines listed in Box 12.8.[59] While nondiabetic individuals usually experience little change in blood glucose levels during exercise, type 1 diabetes patients may experience

Box 12.8

American College of Sports Medicine and American Diabetes Association General Guidelines for Medical Evaluation Before Exercise

Before beginning an exercise program, the individual with diabetes mellitus should undergo a detailed medical evaluation with appropriate diagnostic studies. This examination should carefully screen for the presence of macro- and microvascular complications which may be worsened by the exercise program. A careful medical history and physical examination should focus on the symptoms and signs of disease affecting the heart and blood vessels, eyes, kidneys, and nervous system.

A graded exercise test may be helpful if the individual with diabetes is about to embark on a moderate- to high-intensity exercise program and is at high risk for underlying cardiovascular disease, based on one of the following criteria:

- Age > 35 years
- Type 2 diabetes of >10 years duration
- Type 1 diabetes of >15 years duration
- Presence of any additional risk factor for coronary artery disease
- Presence of microvascular disease (retinopathy or nephropathy, including microalbuminuria)
- Peripheral vascular disease
- Autonomic neuropathy

Source: American Diabetes Association. Clinical practice recommendations, 2000: Diabetes mellitus and exercise. *Diabetes Care* 23(suppl 1):S50–S54, 2000.

an increase (i.e., hyperglycemia) or a decrease (hypoglycemia), depending on their initial levels.[60] Type 1 diabetes patients who have very high blood glucose levels (above 250 mg/dl), with ketones in their urine, can experience a rapid rise in blood glucose upon starting exercise and can develop ketosis. For this reason, individuals with type 1 diabetes should postpone exercise until they have gotten their blood glucose under control through proper diet and insulin therapy (see Boxes 12.9 and 12.10).[59]

For most patients with type 1 diabetes who begin exercising, the principal risk is hypoglycemia.[59–61] Many variables, including fitness, duration and intensity of exercise, and time of exercise regarding insulin administration and meals will affect the metabolic response to exercise.[59] Hypoglycemia is most likely to occur when the exercise is prolonged or intense and when the blood glucose prior to exercise was near normal.

To avoid hypoglycemia during or after exercise, a regular pattern of exercise and diet should be adopted, with fre-

Box 12.9

American College of Sports Medicine and American Diabetes Association General Guidelines for Exercise and Type 1 Diabetes

Metabolic Control Before Exercise

- Avoid exercising if fasting glucose levels are >250 mg/dl and ketosis is present; use caution if glucose levels are >300 mg/dl and no ketosis is present.
- Ingest added carbohydrates if glucose levels are <100 mg/dl.

Blood Glucose Monitoring Before and After Exercise

- Identify when changes in insulin or food intake are necessary.
- Learn the glycemic response to different exercise conditions.

Food Intake

- Consume added carbohydrate as needed to avoid hypoglycemia.
- Carbohydrate-based foods should be readily available during and after exercise.

Source: American Diabetes Association. Clinical practice recommendations, 2000: Diabetes mellitus and exercise. *Diabetes Care* 23(suppl 1):S50–S54, 2000.

Box 12.10

Exercise Recommendations for Type 1 Diabetes Based on Pre-Exercise Blood Glucose Levels

Glucose Level	Ketones	Exercise Advised?
<100 mg/dl	—	Yes, but carbohydrate snack may be needed first (allows for individual variation in response)
100–250 mg/dl	—	Yes
>250 mg/dl	No	Yes (individuals may choose to inject a small dose of short-acting insulin prior to intensive exercise)
>250 mg/dl	Yes	No
>300 mg/dl	No	Use caution (individuals may choose to inject a small dose of short-acting insulin prior to intensive exercise)
>300 mg/dl	Yes	No

Source: Coberg S. Use of clinical practice recommendations for exercise by individuals with type 1 diabetes. *Diabetes Educator* 26:265–271, 2000.

quent blood glucose measurements to test the body's response[59,60] (see Boxes 12.9 and 12.10). Each individual with type 1 diabetes is unique and will need to discover for her- or himself the best schedule to follow to keep the blood glucose under tight control.[61] Exercise should be performed at the same convenient time every day, at approximately the same intensity, and for the same amount of time.

Exercise should not be performed at the time of peak insulin effect (i.e., within 1 hour after an injection of short-acting insulin).[60] Because of the insulin-like effect of exercise, the person with type 1 diabetes initiating an exercise program will have to reduce insulin (by about one third) dosage and/or increase food intake.[59,60] Insulin injections should not be at sites of the body that will be exercised soon thereafter (e.g., thighs that will be used in running or cycling).

During prolonged physical activity, 60–120 calories of carbohydrate (i.e., the amount found in 1–2 cups of most sports drinks) is recommended for each 30 minutes of activity.[60] A meal 1–3 hours before exercise is recommended, and fluids should be taken during and after exercise to avoid dehydration. A carbohydrate snack is recommended soon after unusually strenuous exercise.

Not long ago, the terms "diabetic" and "athlete" seemed mutually exclusive. Today, partly because of the advent of blood glucose self-monitoring and the recognition that exercise brings multiple benefits, many diabetics have entered the sporting arena with the approval and support of their physicians.[59–63] Nationally known athletes with diabetes have included Ty Cobb, Jackie Robinson, Catfish Hunter, Bobby Clarke, Scott Verplank, and Wade Wilson. Most experts feel that as long as diabetic athletes understand the interactions among diet, exertion, and insulin and are aware of their unique reactions to exercise, they can safely engage in almost any sport or activity.[61–63] Participation in sports during childhood may enhance self-image, provide a sense of accomplishment, and lead to social interactions that are conducive to optimal emotional development. Exercise can also serve as an incentive for children and adolescents to attain tighter control of their blood glucose.[61–63]

No two diabetics respond to exercise in exactly the same way. With the guidance of a physician, athletes with type 1 diabetes, through a process of trial and error, can discover what adjustments in carbohydrate, insulin dosage, or a combination of the two work best. This process requires frequent blood glucose monitoring and correction.[60] The most appropriate exercises for diabetic patients involve predictable levels of physical expenditure. Competitive cyclists, marathon runners, cross-country skiers, and triathletes can all maintain glycemic control by frequent self-testing and adjustment before, during, and after training sessions and events. These sports are compatible with good diabetic control because they involve predetermined distance, duration, and intensity of competition, as well as predictable frequency. Therefore, these activities permit the athlete to anticipate his or her physical needs.

Several of the long-term complications of diabetes may be worsened by exercise[59,60,64,65] (see Box 12.11). Vigorous exercise may precipitate heart attack when there is underlying coronary heart disease, a common medical problem in diabetics. Type 1 diabetes patients over 40 years of age, individuals who have had diabetes for 10 years or more, or those with established complications should first undergo a thorough medical exam that includes a graded exercise stress test (see Box 12.8). For the majority of type 1 diabetics, however, exercise is safe and improves their quality of life. Disease risk factors are generally under better control in physically active compared to inactive type 1 diabetic patients.[66] A survey of 2,800 U.S. adults with diabetes showed that regular exercise was the only self-management behavior to predict improved quality of life.[67]

There is some concern that large and sustained increase in blood pressure during heavy exertion may accelerate the development of eye or kidney problems in type 1 diabetes patients.[65] Until more is known, diabetics with these complications are cautioned to avoid sustained heavy exercise such as vigorous weight lifting or prolonged, intense aerobic activity. Diabetics with nerve and blood vessel damage in their feet and legs should be particularly careful to avoid cuts, blisters, and pounding exercises of the lower extremities (e.g., running, high-impact aerobic dance).[59,60] Good footwear, careful foot hygiene, and regular inspection is necessary (see Box 12.11).

Type 2 Diabetes and Exercise

The major aim of therapy for patients with type 2 diabetes is to improve insulin sensitivity through appropriate use of diet, exercise, and weight reduction. In contrast to results with type 1 diabetes patients, regular exercise by persons with type 2 diabetes does lead to improved long-term diabetic control.[59,68–77] One meta-analysis of controlled clinical trials concluded that exercise training, especially at higher intensities, reduces H1C by a significant amount, enough to decrease the risk of diabetic complications.[75] For obese type 2 diabetes patients on insulin, a combination of exercise and weight reduction can reduce insulin requirements by up to 100%. Improved glucose control has been shown for both middle-aged and elderly type 2 diabetes patients who exercise regularly, due in part to the frequent lowering of the blood glucose level and enhancement of insulin sensitivity with each exercise session.[70,74] Insulin resistance was once thought to be an inevitable part of the aging process, but now there is evidence that age-related declines in physical activity and changes in body composition are largely responsible.[54,70,74]

According to the ADA, patients who are most likely to respond favorably are those with mildly to moderately impaired glucose tolerance and hyperinsulinemia.[59] The ADA cautions that the benefits of exercise typically outweigh the risks if attention is paid to minimizing potential exercise complications. All individuals with type 2 diabetes who are about to start an exercise program should have a thorough

Box 12.11

Benefits and Risks of Exercise for Individuals with Diabetes

Diabetics must be cautious about the possible risks of exercise, but there are also potential benefits.

Potential Benefits

1. Improved control of blood glucose
2. Increased insulin sensitivity
3. Improved blood lipoprotein profile and lowered blood pressure
4. Improved aerobic and muscular fitness
5. Usefulness as adjunct to diet for weight reduction
6. Increased sense of well-being and quality of life
7. Reduced risk of heart disease and stroke

Potential Risks and Precautions

1. Hypoglycemia during or after exercise
2. Increased blood glucose values among poorly controlled patients
3. Complications of atherosclerotic cardiovascular disease
4. Degenerative joint disease
5. Worsening of diabetic complications
   a. *Retinopathy.* Avoid strenuous, high-intensity activities that involve breath holding (e.g., weight lifting and isometrics). Avoid activities that lower the head (e.g., yoga, gymnastics) or that risk jarring the head.
   b. *Hypertension.* Avoid heavy weight lifting or breath holding. Perform primarily dynamic exercise that uses large muscle groups, such as walking and cycling, at a moderate intensity.
   c. *Autonomic neuropathy.* Likelihood of hypoglycemia and hypertension is present as is elevated resting heart rate and reduced maximal heart rate. Use of the RPE is recommended. Prone to dehydration and hypothermia.
   d. *Peripheral neuropathy.* Avoid exercise that may cause trauma to the feet (e.g., prolonged hiking, jogging, or walking on uneven surfaces). Non-weight-bearing activities are best (e.g., cycling and swimming). Swimming is not recommended if active ulcers are present. Regular assessment of the feet is recommended. The feet should be kept clean and dry. Choose shoes for proper fit. Activities requiring a great deal of balance should be avoided.
   e. *Nephropathy.* Avoid exercises that raise blood pressure such as weight lifting, high-intensity aerobic exercises, and breath holding.
   f. *All patients.* Carry identification with diabetes information. Rehydrate carefully (drink fluids before, during, and after exercise). Avoid exercise in the heat of the day and in direct sunlight as this tends to be dehydrating. When exercising outdoors, wear a hat and sunscreen.

Source: Campaigne BN. Exercise and type 1 diabetes. *ACSM's Health & Fitness Journal* 2(4):35–42, 1998.

medical exam to uncover previously undiagnosed complications due to diabetes.

For most individuals with type 2 diabetes who have been given medical clearance to begin exercising, near daily physical activity, for 20–45 minutes, at a moderate-to-somewhat-high intensity level, is recommended.[60] See Box 12.12 for a summary of exercise guidelines for individuals with type 2 diabetes.[76] A high frequency of exercise is essential because the residual effects of an acute exercise bout on glucose tolerance last for only 1 or 2 days. Also, for the obese individual with type 2 diabetes, near-daily activity will help ensure that an adequate number of calories are expended to assist in weight loss.

Exercise sessions of less than 20 minutes duration appear to have little benefit for diabetic control, while sessions lasting more than 45 minutes increase the risk of hypoglycemia.[59,60] Low-intensity exercise (50% of $\dot{V}O_{2max}$) is just as effective as high-intensity exercise (75% of $\dot{V}O_{2max}$) in enhancing insulin sensitivity in diabetics, as long as the caloric expenditure is equated by increasing the duration of the low-intensity exercise bouts.[56]

Because persons with type 2 diabetes are often poorly conditioned, an easy start to the exercise program with gradual progression is advised.[60,76] Aerobic, endurance-type activities involving large-muscle groups, such as cycling, brisk walking, and swimming, are recommended. Weight training exercises designed to improve muscle endurance through high repetitions with moderate weight will help avoid high blood pressure responses. Each exercise session should begin with an appropriate warm-up and cool-down period.[76]

Several studies have shown that resistance training is feasible and beneficial for type 2 diabetics.[54,71] Data suggest that both an increase in abdominal fat and a loss of

Box 12.12

American College of Sports Medicine Position Stand on Exercise and Type 2 Diabetes

The American College of Sports Medicine has concluded that physical activity affords significant acute and chronic benefits for those with type 2 diabetes. Unfortunately, physical activity is underutilized in the management of type 2 diabetes. Exercise guidelines include the following:

- Physical activity, including appropriate endurance and resistance training, is a major therapeutic modality for type 2 diabetes.
- Favorable changes in glucose tolerance and insulin sensitivity usually deteriorate within 72 hours of the last exercise session; consequently, regular physical activity is imperative to sustain glucose-lowering effects and improved insulin sensitivity.
- Individuals with type 2 diabetes should strive to achieve a minimum cumulative total of 1,000 Calories per week from physical activities.
- Those with type 2 diabetes generally have a lower level of aerobic fitness than nondiabetic individuals, and therefore exercise intensity should be at a comfortable level (RPE 10–12) in the initial periods of training and should progress cautiously as tolerance for activity improves.
- Resistance training has the potential to improve muscle strength and endurance, enhance flexibility and body composition, decrease risk factors for cardiovascular disease, and result in improved glucose tolerance and insulin sensitivity.
- Modifications to exercise type and/or intensity may be necessary for those who have complications of diabetes. Individuals with type 2 diabetes may develop autonomic neuropathy, which affects the heart rate response to exercise (thus RPE should be used). Although walking may be the most convenient low-impact mode, some persons, because of peripheral neuropathy and/or foot problems, may need to do non-weight-bearing activities.

Source: Albright A, Franz M, Hornsby G, Kriska A, Marrero D, Ullrich I, Verity L. American College of Sports Medicine position stand. Exercise and type 2 diabetes. *Med Sci Sports Exerc* 32:1345–1360, 2000.

muscle mass are highly associated with the development of insulin resistance in type 2 diabetics.[54] Resistance training can help prevent muscle atrophy and stimulate muscle development, improving overall glycemic control. For example, in one 3-month study of type 2 diabetic subjects, a progressive resistance training program (moderate intensity, high volume) twice a week improved muscle size and muscular endurance while lowering glycosylated hemoglobin levels.[71]

Unfortunately, studies have shown that the majority of diabetics do not exercise regularly, and they tend to exercise less than people who do not have diabetes. According to one national survey, only about one in three people with diabetes reported exercising regularly, and less than one in five burned 2,000 Calories or more per week in exercise.[78]

With regular exercise, persons with type 2 diabetes respond to a 100-gram oral glucose load with significantly lower blood glucose and insulin levels.[54] Various mechanisms have been proposed for the beneficial role of physical activity in the treatment of insulin resistance, impaired glucose tolerance, and type 2 diabetes:[54]

- Exercise training results in a preferential loss of fat from the central regions of the body. This is important because abdominal fat accumulation is highly related to the development of insulin resistance.
- Skeletal muscle is the largest mass of insulin-sensitive tissue in the body. Therefore, a reduction in muscle mass could reduce the effectiveness of insulin to clear blood glucose. Exercise training can prevent muscle atrophy and build muscle mass, helping to alleviate insulin resistance.
- With deconditioning, insulin loses its ability to vasodilate skeletal muscle and increase muscle blood flow. With regular exercise, this problem is countered, improving the control of insulin over blood glucose.
- A reduced number of insulin receptors has been reported in obese individuals and those with type 2 diabetes. Exercise training appears to increase insulin receptor numbers.
- With regular exercise, skeletal muscle insulin action is improved and is associated with an increase in the insulin-regulatable glucose transporters, GLUT4 (one type of glucose transporter located within the cell), and enzymes responsible for the phosphorylation, storage, and oxidation of glucose.
- Conditioned muscles have a greater density of oxidative fibers and capillaries that favor improved glucose tolerance.

SPORTS MEDICINE INSIGHT

Nutrition Principles for the Treatment and Prevention of Diabetes

Physical activity and good nutrition are integral components of diabetes management. Yet many misconceptions exist concerning nutrition and diabetes. The American Diabetes Association published evidence-based principles and recommendations for diabetes medical nutrition therapy.[38]

Because of the complexity of these nutrition issues, the American Diabetes Association recommends that a registered dietitian, knowledgeable and skilled in implementing nutrition therapy into diabetes management, be the team member providing medical nutrition therapy. However, all team members, including clinical exercise physiologists and physical therapists, should be knowledgeable about nutrition therapy and provide support for the person with diabetes making lifestyle changes.

GOALS OF MEDICAL NUTRITION THERAPY FOR DIABETES

There are four primary goals of medical nutrition therapy that apply to all individuals with diabetes:[38]

1. Attain and maintain optimal metabolic outcomes, including:
   - Blood glucose levels in the normal range or as close to normal as is safely possible to prevent or reduce the risk for complications of diabetes.
   - A lipid and lipoprotein profile that reduces the risk for macrovascular disease.
   - Blood pressure levels that reduce the risk for vascular disease.
2. Prevent and treat the chronic complications of diabetes. Modify nutrient intake and lifestyle as appropriate for the prevention and treatment of obesity, dyslipidemia, cardiovascular disease, high blood pressure, and kidney disease.
3. Improve health through healthy food choices and physical activity.
4. Address the individual's nutritional needs, taking into consideration personal and cultural preferences and lifestyle while respecting the individual's wishes and willingness to change.

NUTRITION RECOMMENDATIONS FOR INDIVIDUALS WITH DIABETES

Recommendations for medical nutrition therapy for type 1 and type 2 diabetes are classified by the American Diabetes Association according to the strength of evidence: A-, B-, and C-level, with "A" indicating strong scientific support, "B" moderate scientific support, and "C" weak scientific support. These levels of evidence are not available for all nutritional components.

Recommendations by the American Diabetes Association for carbohydrate intake are classified as follows:

1. A-level evidence
   - Foods containing carbohydrates from whole grains, fruits, vegetables, and low-fat milk should be included in a healthy diet.
   - With regard to the glycemic effects of carbohydrates (Table 9.5 in Chapter 9), the total amount of carbohydrate in meals or snacks is more important than the source or type.
   - Sucrose does not increase blood glucose to a greater extent than an equal amount of starch. Thus sucrose and sucrose-containing foods do not need to be restricted by people with diabetes; however, they should be substituted for other carbohydrate sources or, if added, covered with insulin or other glucose-lowering medication.
   - Non-nutritive sweeteners (e.g., aspartame in Equal, saccharin in Sweet N' Low) are safe when consumed within the acceptable daily intake levels established by the Food and Drug Administration.
2. B-level evidence
   - Individuals receiving intensive insulin therapy should adjust their premeal insulin doses based on the carbohydrate content of meals.
   - Although the use of low glycemic index foods may reduce the blood glucose response after meals, there is not sufficient evidence of long-term benefit to recommend use of low glycemic index diets as a primary strategy in food/meal planning.
   - As with the general public, consumption of dietary fiber is encouraged; however, there is no reason to recommend that people with

(continued)

SPORTS MEDICINE INSIGHT *(continued)*

Nutrition Principles for the Treatment and Prevention of Diabetes

diabetes consume a greater amount of fiber than other Americans.

3. C-level evidence
   - Individuals receiving fixed daily insulin doses should try to be consistent in day-to-day carbohydrate intake.

The American Diabetes Association recommends that carbohydrate and monounsaturated fat together provide 60–70% of energy intake for individuals with diabetes. However, the metabolic profile (e.g., blood glucose and lipid levels) and need for weight loss should be considered when determining the monounsaturated fat content of the diet. Sucrose and sucrose-containing foods should be eaten within the context of a healthy diet.

Recommendations for protein intake by individuals with diabetes are classified by the American Diabetes Association as follows:

1. B-level evidence
   - In individuals with type 2 diabetes, ingested protein does not increase plasma glucose concentrations. Protein increases insulin secretion to a similar extent as carbohydrate.
   - For individuals with diabetes, especially those not in optimal glucose control, the protein requirement may be greater than the Recommended Dietary Allowance, but not greater than usual intake.

In general, the American Diabetes Association concludes that there is no evidence to suggest that usual protein intake (15–20% of total daily energy) should be modified if kidney function is normal. The long-term effects of diets high in protein and low in carbohydrate are unknown. These diets may produce short-term weight loss and improve blood glucose levels. There is concern, however, that high protein, low carbohydrate diets may not lead to long-term weight loss, and may negatively influence LDL cholesterol levels.

Recommendations for dietary fat and diabetes include the following:

1. A-level evidence
   - Less than 10% of energy intake should be derived from saturated fats. Some individuals with LDL cholesterol levels ≥ 100 mg/dl may benefit from lowering saturated fat intake to less than 7% of energy intake.
   - Dietary cholesterol intake should be less than 300 mg/day. Some individuals with LDL cholesterol levels ≥ 100 mg/dl may benefit from lowering dietary cholesterol to less than 200 mg/day.

2. B-level evidence
   - To lower LDL cholesterol, energy derived from saturated fat can be reduced if weight loss is desirable or replaced with either carbohydrate or monounsaturated fat when weight loss is not a goal.
   - Intake of *trans*-unsaturated fatty acids should be minimized.
   - Reduced-fat diets, when maintained long-term, contribute to modest loss of weight and improvement in dyslipidemia.

3. C-level evidence
   - Polyunsaturated fat intake should be about 10% of energy intake.

Recommendations from the American Diabetes Association regarding energy balance and obesity include the following:

1. A-level evidence
   - In insulin-resistant individuals, reduced energy intake and modest weight loss improve insulin resistance and blood glucose control in the short-term.
   - Structured programs that emphasize lifestyle changes, including education, reduced fat and energy intake, regular physical activity, and regular participant contact, can produce long-term weight loss on the order of 5–7% of starting weight.
   - Exercise and behavior modification are most useful as adjuncts to other weight loss strategies. Exercise is helpful in maintenance of weight loss.
   - Standard weight reduction diets, when used alone, are unlikely to produce long-term weight loss. Structured intensive lifestyle programs are necessary.

Recommendations regarding micronutrient intake by individuals with diabetes include the following:

1. B-level evidence
   - There is no clear evidence of benefit from vitamin or mineral supplementation in people

(continued)

SPORTS MEDICINE INSIGHT *(continued)*

Nutrition Principles for the Treatment and Prevention of Diabetes

with diabetes who do not have underlying deficiencies. Exceptions include folate for prevention of birth defects and calcium for prevention of bone disease.

- Routine supplementation of the diet with antioxidants is not advised because of uncertainties related to long-term efficacy and safety.

Recommendations for alcohol intake and diabetes include:

1. B-level evidence
   - If individuals choose to drink alcohol, daily intake should be limited to one drink for adult women and two drinks for adult men. One drink is defined as 12 oz beer, 5 oz of wine, or 1.5 oz of ~80 proof spirits.
   - To reduce risk of hypoglycemia, alcohol should be consumed with food.

In general, medical nutrition therapy for people with diabetes should be individualized, and much more research is required before definitive recommendations can be given in all nutritional areas.[38] In other words, consideration should be given for the individual's usual food and eating habits, metabolic profile, treatment goals, and desired outcomes. Metabolic and quality-of-life parameters should be monitored to assess the need for changes in therapy and to ensure successful outcomes. These measurements should include glucose, HbA_{1c}, lipids, blood pressure, body weight, and kidney function.

SUMMARY

1. *Diabetes mellitus* is defined as a group of metabolic diseases characterized by high blood glucose resulting from defects in insulin secretion, insulin action, or both. The chronic hyperglycemia of diabetes is associated with long-term damage, dysfunction, and failure of various organs, especially the eyes, kidneys, nerves, heart, and blood vessels.
2. Of the 18.2 million Americans with diabetes, type 1 accounts for 5–10% and type 2 for 90–95%.
3. There are four categories of diabetes mellitus: type 1, type 2, gestational diabetes, and other specific types. Type 1 diabetes is characterized by destruction of the pancreatic beta cells that produce insulin, usually leading to absolute insulin deficiency. Type 2 diabetes usually arises because of insulin resistance, in which the body fails to use insulin properly, combined with relative insulin deficiency. Type 2 diabetes has multiple risk factors, including age, obesity, physical inactivity, family history, ethnicity, previous gestational diabetes, impaired fasting glucose, hypertension, and dyslipidemia.
4. Diabetes can be diagnosed in any one of three ways and must be confirmed on a different day. A fasting plasma glucose that is ≥126 mg/dl is most commonly used.
5. Approximately 85% of patients with type 2 diabetes are obese at the time of diagnosis. The risk for developing type 2 diabetes rises in direct relationship to the degree of obesity.
6. Treatment for either type of diabetes seeks to accomplish what the human body normally does naturally: maintain a proper balance between glucose and insulin. Food makes the blood glucose level rise, while insulin and exercise make it fall. The challenge is to manage these three factors to keep the blood glucose within a narrow range. Training in self-management is integral to the treatment of diabetes. Treatment must be individualized and must address medical, psychosocial, and lifestyle issues.
7. Type 2 diabetes is less common in physically active, compared to inactive, societies. Several prospective studies have shown that physical activity is protective against type 2 diabetes.
8. Exercise is useful in the treatment of both type 1 and type 2 diabetes. Although regular exercise leads to reduced insulin requirements for individuals with type 1 diabetes, studies have failed to show that long-term glucose control is improved. Regular exercise by persons with type 2 diabetes does lead to improved long-term diabetic control. Several mechanisms were reviewed explaining the beneficial role of physical activity in the treatment of insulin resistance, impaired glucose tolerance, and type 2 diabetes.
9. Physical exercise is not without risk to individuals with type 1 diabetes.

Review Questions

1. *Which one of the following is* **not** *a symptom of type 1 diabetes onset?*

   A. Polyuria
   B. Hypoglycemia
   C. Polydipsia
   D. Polyphagia
   E. Fatigue, weakness

2. *Type I diabetes*

   A. Accounts for 33% of all diabetes in the United States
   B. Is common among obese older adults
   C. Is a problem of deficient insulin receptors
   D. Can occur at any age, but especially in the young during puberty
   E. Has a gradual onset of symptoms

3. *Regarding the diabetic diet guidelines, the emphasis is that*

   A. Dietary fiber should be more than 50 grams a day
   B. The diet should be individualized for each patient
   C. Dietary fat should be less than 15% of Calories
   D. All sugar should be avoided
   E. Carbohydrate content should be greater than 75% of Calories

4. *What percent of American adults have diabetes?*
   A. 2.7
   B. 6.3
   C. 21.2
   D. 27.8
   E. 31.3

5. *Which one of the following is* **not** *a major clinical complication of diabetes?*

   A. End-stage kidney disease
   B. Blindness
   C. Cancer
   D. Heart disease and stroke
   E. Lower-extremity amputations

6. *Which one of the following is* **not** *true regarding type 2 diabetes?*

   A. Found primarily in obese adults
   B. Has an abrupt onset of symptoms
   C. Most common form of diabetes
   D. Typically symptom-free for many years
   E. Not prone to ketosis

7. *In the United States, which subgroup is* **not** *at increased risk for type 2 diabetes?*

   A. Caucasians
   B. African Americans
   C. Asian Americans
   D. Native Americans
   E. Latino/Hispanic

8. *The target for diabetes control in patients is to reduce HbA1c to less than ____%.*

   A. 2 B. 7.0 C. 8.7 D. 10.0 E. 15.0

9. *The prevalence of diabetes is more common among*

   A. The elderly versus the young
   B. Whites versus blacks
   C. Men versus women

10. *If the fasting plasma glucose is ≥ ____ mg/dl on two occasions, diabetes is diagnosed.*

    A. 25 B. 50 C. 75 D. 115 E. 126

11. *For most type 1 patients who exercise, the principal risk is ____.*

    A. Hyperglycemia
    B. Hypoglycemia
    C. Musculoskeletal injury
    D. Heart attack

12. *If a type 1 diabetic in good metabolic balance and control starts an exercise program with no change in insulin dose or dietary intake,*

    A. Hypoglycemia may result.
    B. Hyperglycemia may result.
    C. No change in blood glucose levels would be expected.

13. *The American Diabetes Association published a list of dietary recommendations for diabetics. Which statement does* **not** *agree with ADA recommendations?*

    A. Refined sugars are not acceptable for most diabetics.
    B. Saturated fat should comprise less than 10% of calories.
    C. Distribution of energy from fat and carbohydrate can vary and be individualized.
    D. Dietary fiber should be 20–35 grams a day from a wide variety of foods (same as the general population).
    E. Alcohol can be used in moderate amounts, the same as for nondiabetics.

14. *Which one of the following is* **not** *a risk factor for type 2 diabetes?*

    A. Delivery of baby weighing more than 7.5 pounds
    B. Family history
    C. Overweight
    D. Increased triglycerides and/or low HDL cholesterol
    E. Previously identified impaired glucose tolerance or impaired fasting glucose

15. *Regarding exercise, diabetes, and glucose control:*

    A. When glucose drops, insulin is secreted to increase blood glucose.
    B. Muscle contraction has an insulin-like effect.

C. Insulin sensitivity decreases after each exercise bout.
D. Long-term metabolic control of those with type 1 diabetes who exercise is enhanced.

16. *Among the elderly, one in ____ have diabetes.*

A. Two B. Three C. Four D. Five E. Six

17. *The leading cause of diabetes-related deaths is*

A. Heart disease B. Stroke
C. Kidney disease D. Retinopathy
E. COPD

18. *Which one of the following is* **not** *a method for diagnosing diabetes?*

A. A fasting plasma glucose that is equal to or greater than 126 mg/dl (after >8 hours fasting)
B. A casual plasma glucose greater than 200 mg/dl with classic symptoms
C. An OGTT value that is equal to or greater than 200 mg/dl in the 2-hour sample
D. A glycosylated hemoglobin value of 7% or higher

19. *Impaired fasting glucose is diagnosed when the fasting plasma glucose is*

A. 110–125 mg/dl
B. >140 mg/dl
C. <90 mg/dl
D. 115–140 mg/dl

20. *Hypoglycemia is diagnosed when the plasma glucose level drops below ____ mg/dl within a few hours of eating a regular meal while the patient is experiencing symptoms.*

A. 20 B. 50 C. 100 D. 75 E. 140

21. *The "A" in the ABCs of diabetes care stands for:*
A. A1C B. Acute exercise
C. Apple-shaped obesity D. Average glucose
E. Aerobic exercise

22. *Diabetes ranks ____ as a cause of death in the United States.*

A. First B. Second
C. Third D. Fifth
E. Sixth

23. *About ____% of type 2 diabetes can be attributed to poor lifestyles, in particular, obesity, physical inactivity, an unhealthy diet, and smoking.*

A. 90 B. 75 C. 67 D. 50 E. 25

24. *What lifestyle habit explains the majority of type 2 diabetes in the United States?*

A. Obesity
B. Physical inactivity
C. Diet high in saturated and *trans* fat, low in fiber
D. Smoking
E. High alcohol intake

25. *The majority of individuals with diabetes have type ____.*

A. 1 B. 2 C. 3 D. 4 E. 5

Answers

1. B
2. D
3. B
4. B
5. C
6. B
7. A
8. B
9. A
10. E
11. B
12. A
13. A
14. A
15. B
16. D
17. A
18. D
19. A
20. B
21. A
22. E
23. A
24. A
25. B

REFERENCES

1. American Diabetes Association. Standards of medical care in diabetes. *Diabetes Care* 28(suppl 1):S4–S36, 2005.
2. The Expert Committee on the Diagnosis and Classification of Diabetes Mellitus. Follow-up report on the diagnosis of diabetes mellitus. *Diabetes Care* 20:1183–1197, 1997; 26:3150–3167, 2003.
3. Mokdad AH, Bowman BA, Ford ES, Vinicor F, Marks JS, Koplan JP. The continuing epidemics of obesity and diabetes in the United States. *JAMA* 286:1195–1200, 2001.
4. Centers for Disease Control and Prevention. *National Diabetes Fact Sheet: General Information and National Estimates on Diabetes in the United States, 2002.* Atlanta, GA: U.S. Department of Health and Human Services, Centers for Disease Control and Prevention, 2003. www.diabetes.org/. See also: CDC. Prevalence of diabetes and impaired fasting glucose in adults—United States, 1999–2000. *MMWR* 52:833–837, 2003.
5. National Center for Health Statistics. *Health, United States, 2004.* Hyattsville, MD: 2004.
6. Gaylor AS, Condren ME. Type 2 diabetes in the pediatric population. *Pharmacotherapy* 24:871–878, 2004.
7. Peyrot M, Rubin RR. Levels and risks of depression and anxiety symptomatology among diabetic adults. *Diabetes Care* 20:585–590, 1997.

8. Leibson CL, Rocca WA, Hanson VA, et al. Risk of dementia among persons with diabetes mellitus: A population-based cohort study. *Am J Epidemiol* 145:301–308, 1997.
9. Stumvoll M, Goldstein BJ, van Haeften TW. Type 2 diabetes: Principles of pathogenesis and therapy. *Lancet* 365:1333–1346, 2005.
10. American Diabetes Association, National Institute of Diabetes and Digestive and Kidney Diseases. Prevention or delay of type 2 diabetes. *Diabetes Care* 27(suppl 1):S47–S54, 2004.
11. CDC Diabetes Cost-Effectiveness Study Group. The cost-effectiveness of screening for type 2 diabetes. *JAMA* 280:1757–1763, 1998.
12. Dagogo-Jack S. Hypoglycemia in type 1 diabetes mellitus: Pathophysiology and prevention. *Treat Endocrinol* 3:91–103, 2004.
13. Pan XR, Yang WY, Li GW, Liu J. Prevalence of diabetes and its risk factors in China, 1994. *Diabetes Care* 20:1664–1670, 1997.
14. Huang B, Rodriguez BL, Burchfiel CM, Chyou PH, Curb JD, Yano K. Acculturation and prevalence of diabetes among Japanese-American men in Hawaii. *Am J Epidemiol* 144:674–681, 1996.
15. Hu FB, Manson JE, Stampfer MJ, Colditz G, Liu S, Solomon CG, Willett WC. Diet, lifestyle, and the risk of type 2 diabetes mellitus in women. *N. Engl J Med* 345:790–797, 2001.
16. Manson JE, Nathan DM, Krolewski AS, et al. A prospective study of exercise and incidence of diabetes among U.S. male physicians. *JAMA* 268:63–67, 1992.
17. Colditz GA, Willett WC, Rotnitzky A, Manson JE. Weight gain as a risk factor for clinical diabetes mellitus in women. *Ann Intern Med* 122:481–486, 1995.
18. Ford ES, Williamson DF, Liu S. Weight change and diabetes incidence: Findings from a national cohort of US adults. *Am J Epidemiol* 146:214–222, 1997.
19. Manson JE, Spelsberg A. Primary prevention of non–insulin-dependent diabetes mellitus. *Am J Prev Med* 10:172–184, 1994.
20. Tuomilehto J, Lindstrom J, Eriksson JG, et al. Prevention of type 2 diabetes mellitus by changes in lifestyle among subjects with impaired glucose tolerance. *N Engl J Med* 344:1343–1350, 2001.
21. Carey VJ, Walters EE, Colditz GA, et al. Body fat distribution and risk of non–insulin-dependent diabetes mellitus in women. The Nurses' Health Study. *Am J Epidemiol* 145:614–619, 1997.
22. Torjensen PA, Birkeland KI, Anderssen SA, Hjermann I, Holme I, Urdal P. Lifestyle changes may reverse development of the insulin resistance syndrome. The Oslo Diet and Exercise Study: A randomized trial. *Diabetes Care* 20:26–31, 1997.
23. The Diabetes Prevention Program. Design and methods for a clinical trial in the prevention of type 2 diabetes. *Diabetes Care* 22:623–634, 1999.
24. Salmerón J, Manson JE, Stampfer MJ, Colditz GA, Wing AL, Willett WC. Dietary fiber, glycemic load, and risk of non–insulin-dependent diabetes mellitus in women. *JAMA* 277:472–477, 1997.
25. Salmerón J, Ascherio A, Rimm EB, et al. Dietary fiber, glycemic load, and risk of NIDDM in men. *Diabetes Care* 20:545–551, 1997.
26. Eyre H, Kahn R, Robertson RM. Preventing cancer, cardiovascular disease, and diabetes. A common agenda for the American Cancer Society, the American Diabetes Association, and the American Heart Association. *Diabetes Care* 27:1812–1824, 2004.
27. Warren RE. The stepwise approach to the management of type 2 diabetes. *Diabetes Res Clin Pract* 65(suppl 1):S3–S8, 2004.
28. Knight K, Badamgarav E, Henning JM, Hasselblad V, Gano AD Jr, Ofman JJ, Weingarten SR. A systematic review of diabetes disease management programs. *Am J Manag Care* 11:242–250, 2005.
29. Palta M, Shen G, Allen C, Klein R, D'Alessio D. Longitudinal patterns of glycemic control and diabetes care from diagnosis in a population-based cohort with type 1 diabetes. *Am J Epidemiol* 144:954–961, 1996.
30. The Diabetes Control and Complications Trial Research Group. The effect of intensive treatment of diabetes on the development and progression of long-term complications of insulin-dependent diabetes mellitus. *N Engl J Med* 329:977–986, 1993. See also: *Diabetes* 12:1555–1558, 1993.
31. The Diabetes Control and Complications Trial Research Group. Lifetime benefits and costs of intensive therapy as practiced in the Diabetes Control and Complications Trial. *JAMA* 276:1409–1415, 1996.
32. Dunn FL, Nathan DM, Scavini M, Selam JL, Wingrove TG. Long-term therapy of IDDM with an implantable insulin pump. *Diabetes Care* 20:59–64, 1997.
33. Davidson JA. Treatment of the patient with diabetes: Importance of maintaining target HbA(1c) levels. *Curr Med Res Opin* 20:1919–1927, 2004.
34. Turner RC, Cull CA, Frighi V, Holman RR. Glycemic control with diet, sulfonylurea, metformin, or insulin in patients with type 2 diabetes mellitus. *JAMA* 281:2005–2012, 1999.
35. Barnard RJ, Jung T, Inkeles SB. Diet and exercise in the treatment of NIDDM. *Diabetes Care* 17:1469–1472, 1994.
36. Kriska AM, Delahanty LM, Pettee KK. Lifestyle intervention for the prevention of type 2 diabetes: Translation and future recommendations. *Curr Diab Rep* 4:113–118, 2004.
37. Davis T, Edelman SV. Insulin therapy in type 2 diabetes. *Med Clin North Am* 88:865–895, 2004.
38. American Diabetes Association. Nutrition principles and recommendations in diabetes. *Diabetes Care* 27(suppl 1):S36–S46, 2004.
39. Knowler WC, Barrett-Connor E, Fowler SE, Hamman RF, Lachin JM, Walker EA, Nathan DM. Reduction in the incidence of type 2 diabetes with lifestyle intervention or metformin. *N Engl J Med* 346:393–403, 2002.
40. Pan XR, Li GW, Hu YH, et al. Effects of diet and exercise in preventing NIDDM in people with impaired glucose tolerance. The Da Qing IGT and Diabetes Study. *Diabetes Care* 20:537–544, 1997.
41. Lynch J, Helmrich SP, Lakka TA, Kaplan GA, Cohen RD, Salonen R, Salonen JT. Moderately intense physical activities and high levels of cardiorespiratory fitness reduce the risk of non–insulin-dependent diabetes mellitus in middle-aged men. *Arch Intern Med* 156:1307–1314, 1996.
42. Monterrosa AE, Haffner SM, Stern MP, Hazuda HP. Sex difference in lifestyle factors predictive of diabetes in Mexican-Americans. *Diabetes Care* 18:448–456, 1995.
43. Kelley DE, Goodpaster BH. Effects of exercise on glucose homeostasis in type 2 diabetes mellitus. *Med Sci Sports Exerc* 33(suppl):S495–S501, 2001.
44. Burchfiel CM, Sharp DS, Curb JD, Rodriguez BL, Hwang L-J, Marcus EB, Yano K. Physical activity and incidence of diabetes: The Honolulu Heart Program. *Am J Epidemiol* 141:360–368, 1995.
45. Helmrich SP, Rogland DR, Leung RW, Paffenbarger RS. Physical activity and reduced occurrence of noninsulin-dependent diabetes mellitus. *N Engl J Med* 325:147–152, 1991.
46. Haapanen N, Miilunpalo S, Vuori I, Oja P, Pasanen M. Association of leisure time physical activity with the risk of coronary heart disease, hypertension and diabetes in middle-aged men and women. *Int J Epidemiol* 26:739–747, 1997.

47. Hu FB, Sigal RJ, Rich-Edwards JW, Colditz GA, Solomon CG, Willett WC, Speizer FE, Manson JE. Walking compared with vigorous physical activity and risk of type 2 diabetes in women. *JAMA* 282:1433–1439, 1999.

48. Hu FB, Stampfer MJ, Solomon C, Liu S, Colditz GA, Speizer FE, Willett WC, Manson JE. Physical activity and risk for cardiovascular events in diabetic women. *Ann Intern Med* 134:96–105, 2001.

49. Wei M, Gibbons LW, Mitchell TL, Kampert JB, Lee CD, Blair SN. The association between cardiorespiratory fitness and impaired fasting glucose and type 2 diabetes mellitus in men. *Ann Intern Med* 130:89–96, 1999. Also see: Church TS, Cheng YJ, Earnest CP, Barlow CE, Gibbons LW, Priest EL, Blair SN. Exercise capacity and body composition as predictors of mortality among men with diabetes. *Diabetes Care* 27:83–88, 2004.

50. Hu FB, Leitzmann MF, Stampfer MJ, Colditz GA, Willett WC, Rimm EG. Physical activity and television watching in relation to risk for type 2 diabetes mellitus in men. *Arch Intern Med* 161:1542–1548, 2001.

51. Helmrich SP, Ragland DR, Paffenbarger RS. Prevention of non–insulin-dependent diabetes mellitus with physical activity. *Med Sci Sports Exerc* 26:824–830, 1994.

52. Cantu RC. *Diabetes and Exercise.* Ithaca, New York: Movement Publications, 1982.

53. Ivy JL, Zderic TW, Fogt DL. Prevention and treatment of non–insulin-dependent diabetes mellitus. *Exerc Sport Sci Rev* 27:1–35, 1999.

54. Ivy JL. Muscle insulin resistance amended with exercise training: Role of GLUT4 expression. *Med Sci Sports Exerc* 36:1207–1211, 2004. See also: Ivy JL. Role of exercise training in the prevention and treatment of insulin resistance and non–insulin-dependent diabetes mellitus. *Sports Med* 24:321–336, 1997.

55. Oshida Y, Kamanouchi K, Hayamiru S, et al. Effect of training and training cessation on insulin action. *Int J Sports Med* 12:484–486, 1991.

56. Bruce CR, Hawley JA. Improvements in insulin resistance with aerobic exercise training: A lipocentric approach. *Med Sci Sports Exerc* 36:1196–1201, 2004.

57. Brown MD, Korytkowski MT, Zmuda JM, McCole SD, Moore GE, Hagberg JM. Insulin sensitivity in postmenopausal women: Independent and combined associations with hormone replacement, cardiovascular fitness, and body composition. *Diabetes Care* 23:1731–1736, 2000.

58. Araujo-Vilar D, Osifo E, Kirk M, Garcia-Estevez DA, Cabezas-Cerrato J, Hockaday TD. Influence of moderate physical exercise on insulin-mediated and non–insulin-mediated glucose uptake in healthy individuals. *Metabolism* 46:203–209, 1997.

59. Sigal RJ, Kenny GP, Wasserman DH, Castaneda-Sceppa C. Physical activity/exercise and type 2 diabetes. *Diabetes Care* 27:2518–2539, 2004. See also: American Diabetes Association. Clinical practice recommendations, 2000: Diabetes mellitus and exercise. *Diabetes Care* 23(suppl 1):S50–S54, 2000.

60. Campaigne BN. Exercise and type 1 diabetes. *ACSM's Health & Fitness Journal* 2(4):35–42, 1998.

61. Colberg S. Use of clinical practice recommendations for exercise by individuals with type 1 diabetes. *Diabetes Educator* 26:265–271, 2000.

62. Colberg S. *The Diabetic Athlete.* Champaign, IL: Human Kinetics, 2001.

63. Campaigne BN, Lampman RL. *Exercise in the Clinical Management of Diabetes Mellitus.* Champaign, IL: Human Kinetics, 1994.

64. Colberg SR. Exercise: A diabetes "cure" for many? *ACSM's Health & Fitness Journal* 5(2):20–26, 2001.

65. Albert SG, Bernbaum M. Exercise for patients with diabetic retinopathy. *Diabetes Care* 18:130–132, 1995.

66. Lehmann R, Kaplan V, Bingisser R, Bloch KE, Spinas GA. Impact of physical activity on cardiovascular risk factors in IDDM. *Diabetes Care* 20:1603–1611, 1997.

67. Glasgow RE, Ruggiero L, Eakin EG, Dryfoos, J, Chobanian L. Quality of life and associated characteristics in a large national sample of adults with diabetes. *Diabetes Care* 20:562–569, 1997.

68. Carroll S, Dudfield M. What is the relationship between exercise and metabolic abnormalities? A review of the metabolic syndrome. *Sports Med* 34:371–418, 2004.

69. Agurs-Collins TD, Kumanyika SK, Have TR, Adams-Campbell LL. A randomized controlled trial of weight reduction and exercise for diabetes management in older African-American subjects. *Diabetes Care* 20:1503–1511, 1997.

70. Yamanouchi K, Shinozaki T, Chikada K, et al. Daily walking combined with diet therapy is a useful means for obese NIDDM patients not only to reduce body weight but also to improve insulin sensitivity. *Diabetes Care* 18:775–778, 1995.

71. Eriksson J, Taimela S, Eriksson K, Parvianinen S, Peltonen J, Kujala U. Resistance training in the treatment of non–insulin-dependent diabetes mellitus. *Int J Sports Med* 18:242–246, 1997.

72. Hawley JA. Exercise as a therapeutic intervention for the prevention and treatment of insulin resistance. *Diabetes Metab Res Rev* 20:383–393, 2004.

73. Young JC. Exercise for client with type 2 diabetes. *ACSM's Health & Fitness Journal* 2(3):24–29, 1998.

74. Yamanouchi K, Nakajima H, Shinozaki T, et al. Effects of daily physical activity on insulin action in the elderly. *J Appl Physiol* 73:2241–2245, 1992.

75. Boule NG, Haddad E, Kenny GP, Wells GA, Sigal RJ. Effects of exercise on glycemic control and body mass in type 2 diabetes mellitus. A meta-analysis of controlled clinical trials. *JAMA* 286:1218–1227, 2001. See also: Boule NG, Kenny GP, Haddad E, Wells GA, Sigal RJ. Meta-analysis of the effect of structured exercise training on cardiorespiratory fitness in type 2 diabetes mellitus. *Diabetologia* 46:1071–1081, 2003.

76. Albright A, Franz M, Hornsby G, Kriska A, Marrero D, Ullrich I, Verity L. American College of Sports Medicine position stand. Exercise and type 2 diabetes. *Med Sci Sports Exerc* 32:1345–1360, 2000.

77. Wallberg-Henriksson H, Rincon J, Zierath JR. Exercise in the management of non–insulin-dependent diabetes mellitus. *Sports Med* 25:25–35, 1998.

78. Ford ES, Herman WH. Leisure-time physical activity patterns in the U.S. diabetic population. *Diabetes Care* 18:27–33, 1995.

79. The American Dietetic Association. *Exchange Lists for Meal Planning.* Chicago: Author, 1995.

PHYSICAL FITNESS ACTIVITY 12.1

Assessing Your Diabetes Risk Score*

Diabetes. You Could Be at Risk

Take the Test—Know Your Score!

Diabetes means your blood sugar (glucose) is too high. How would you know? Are you often thirsty, hungry, or tired? Do you urinate often? Do you have sores that heal slowly, tingling in your feet, or blurry eyesight? Even without these signs, you could still have diabetes. Diabetes is a serious disease. It can cause heart attack or stroke, blindness, kidney failure, or loss of feet or legs. But diabetes can be controlled. You can reduce or avoid these health problems. Take the first step. Find out if you are at high risk.

Know your risk of having diabetes now. Answer these quick questions. For each Yes answer, add the number of points listed. All No answers are 0 points.

Question	Yes	No
Are you a woman who has had a baby weighing more than 9 pounds at birth?	1	0
Do you have a sister or brother with diabetes?	1	0
Do you have a parent with diabetes?	1	0
Find your height on the chart. Do you weigh as much as or more than the weight listed for your height? (*See chart below*)	5	0
Are you under 65 years old and get little or no exercise in a typical day?	5	0
Are you between 45 and 64 years old?	5	0
Are you 65 years or older?	9	0
Add Your Score		

At Risk Weight Chart

Height	Weight (Pounds)	Height	Weight (Pounds)
4′10	129	5′8	177
4′11	133	5′9	182
5′0	138	5′10	188
5′1	143	5′11	193
5′2	147	6′0	199
5′3	152	6′1	204
5′4	157	6′2	210
5′5	162	6′3	216
5′6	167	6′4	221
5′7	172		

Know Your Score

10 or more points	High for having diabetes now. **Please bring this form to your health care provider soon.** If you don't have insurance and can't afford a visit to your provider, contact your local health department.
3 to 9 points	Probably low for having diabetes now. Keep your risk low. If you're overweight, lose weight. Be active most days, and don't use tobacco. Eat low-fat meals with fruits, vegetables, and whole-grain foods. If you have high cholesterol or high blood pressure, talk to your health care provider about your risk for diabetes.

*Also see the Diabetes Risk Test at www.diabetes.org.

Source: These questions are from the American Diabetes Association's online "Diabetes Risk Test" (http://www.diabetes.org/info/risk/risktest.jsp).

chapter 13

Obesity

If a company came up with a drug that would help burn fat, allow you to eat more and not gain weight, and had no major side effects, you would probably buy stock. But we already have this in physical activity.

—James Hill

In most Western societies today, the overabundance of fat-rich foods and lack of physical activity have created a socioeconomic environment conducive to obesity among a significant proportion of both men and women.[1–3] As reviewed in previous chapters, the prevalence of some risk factors for chronic disease (e.g., high blood cholesterol) has decreased as of late. In contrast, every indication is that the prevalence of obesity has been steadily increasing throughout most of the twentieth century.[2–12]

As defined in Chapter 5, obesity is a condition of excess body fat (see Figure 13.1). This is difficult to measure when conducting national studies, so the National Center for Health Statistics uses various height and weight measures. These studies of Americans since the late 1940s have shown that many are overweight and obese. Obesity affects about 3 in 10 adults, with the highest rates among the poor and minority groups.[4–8] For both adult men and women, 65% are considered overweight (defined in most national studies as a

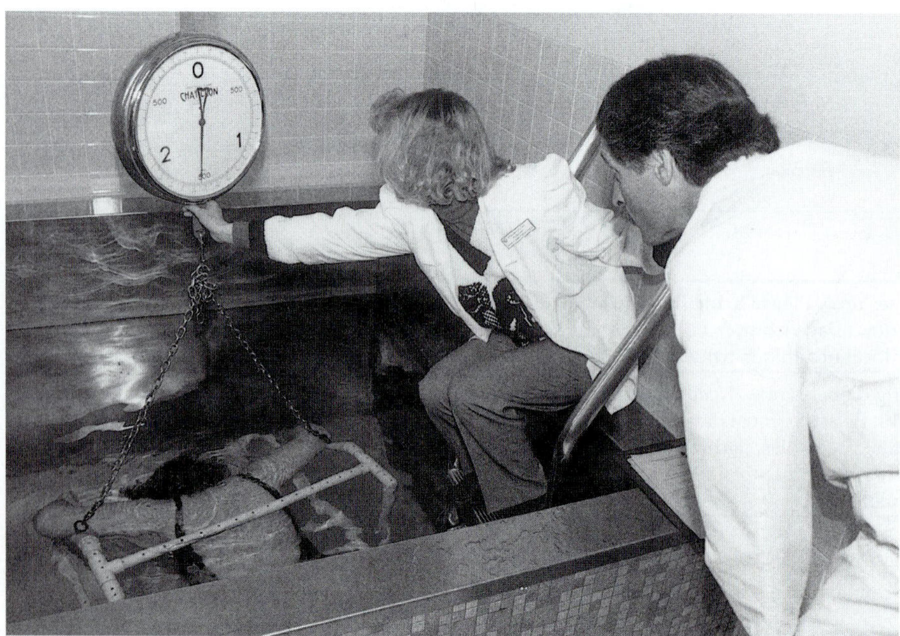

Figure 13.1 Obesity is defined as a condition of excess body fat. This is best measured using underwater weighing techniques, as described in Chapter 5.

body mass index ≥ 25 kg/m^2).[4–8,12] The federal government's year 2010 goal is to reduce the prevalence of obesity in the U.S. adult population to no more than 15%, but trends are in the opposite direction.[12] Figure 13.2 summarizes current estimates of obese people among various groups. Comparisons of these figures with data collected during the 1960s demonstrate significant increases in prevalence of overweight for all segments of the American society[4–7] (see Figure 13.3). Figure 13.4 shows the dramatic increase in prevalence of obesity on a state-by-state basis. Compared to 1960, the average adult now weighs 24 pounds more and the average teenager 15 pounds more.[6] This is despite increasingly thin ideals in physical appearance for both men and women, a marked departure from ancient standards that held obesity in high esteem.[13] Although the causes of the increase in overweight prevalence are hotly debated, most experts feel that Americans are taking in more Calories than in previous decades.[1,12]

The average male adult now weighs 190 pounds at a height of 69 inches (BMI of 28), and the average female adult 163 pounds at 64 inches (BMI of 28).[6]

National surveys also reveal that a growing proportion of U.S. children and teenagers are overweight.[5,9,14–16] As depicted in Figure 13.5, overweight prevalence has more than tripled since the 1960s for both children and adolescents. Defining obesity or overweight for children and adolescents is difficult, but experts recommend a BMI cutoff point equal to or above the 95th percentile for age and sex from the CDC growth charts.[4,9,17] Using this conservative method, approximately 16% of children and 16% of adolescents are overweight.[4]

The increasing number of obese children and youth throughout the United States has led policymakers to rank this trend as a critical threat to public health.[14–16] According to the Institute of Medicine, childhood obesity involves

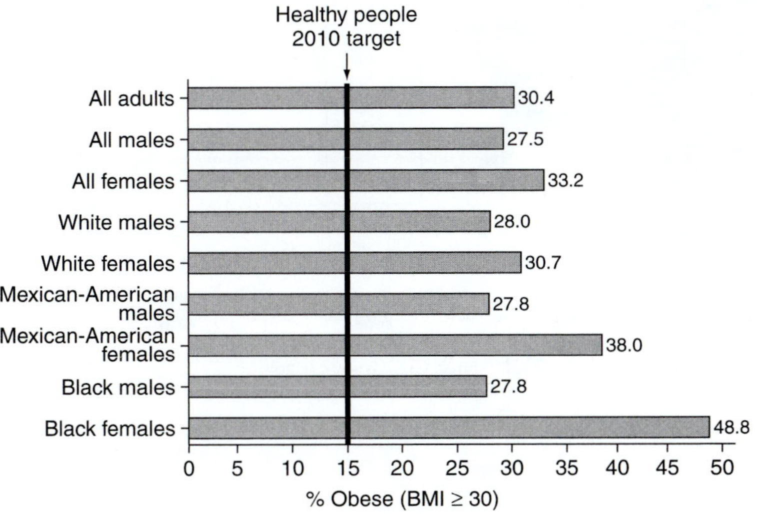

Figure 13.2 Obesity prevalence among U.S. adults, ages 20 years and older. The *Healthy People 2010* target is 15%. Source: National Center for Health Statistics. *Health, United States, 2004.* Hyattsville, MD: 2004.

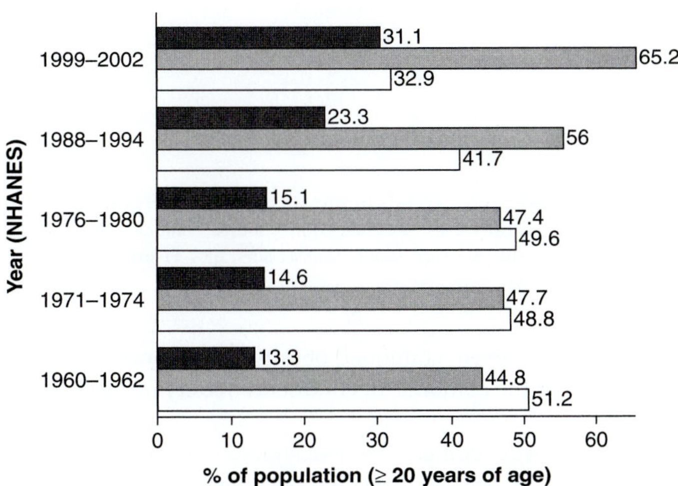

Figure 13.3 Trends in U.S. adult prevalence of healthy weight, overweight or obese, and obese. The prevalence in obesity has more than doubled since 1960. Ages 20–74 years. Source: National Center for Health Statistics. *Health, United States, 2004.* Hyattsville, MD: 2004.

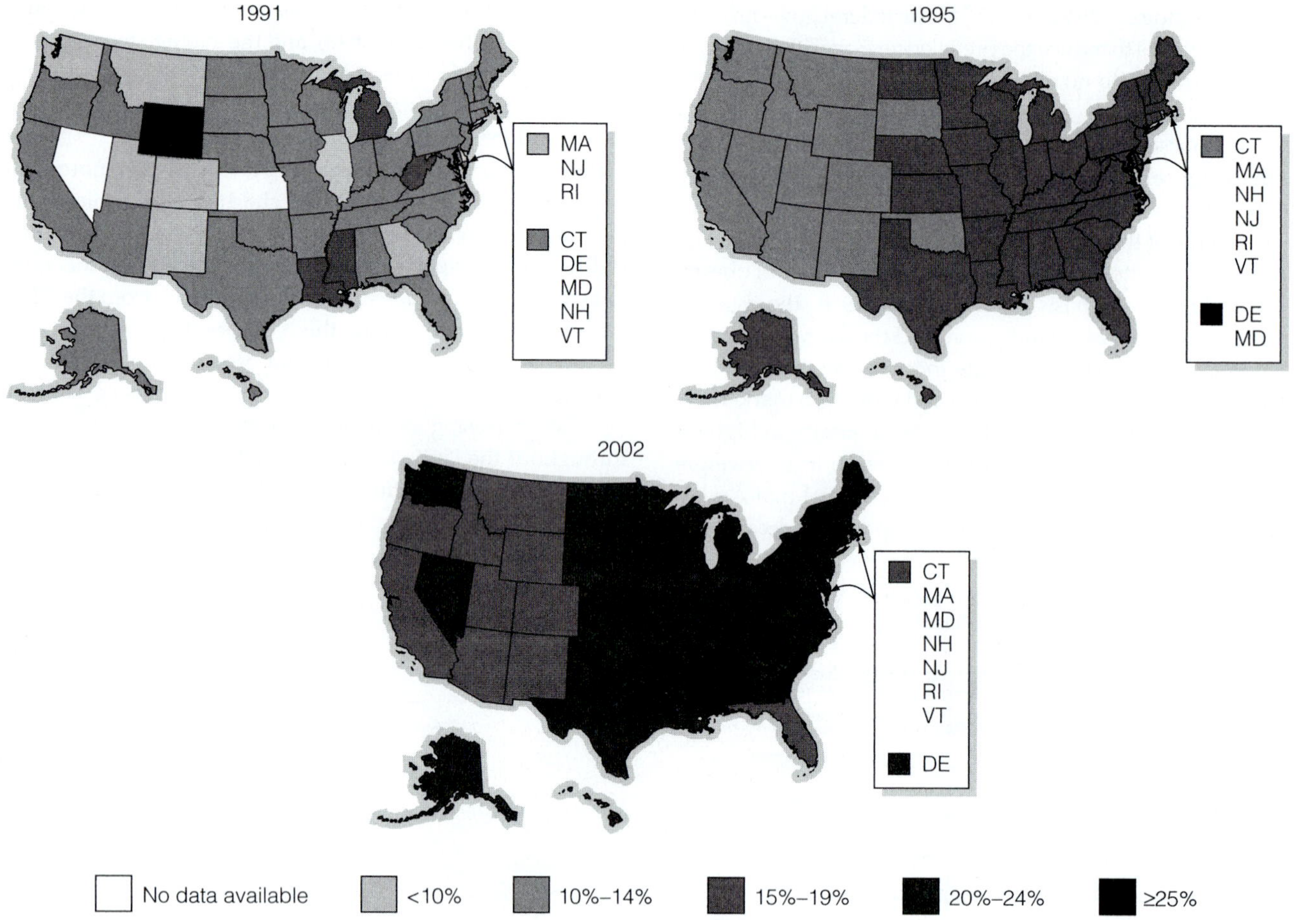

Figure 13.4 Percentage of adults who report being obese, by state, 1991, 1995, 2002. Source: CDC. www.cdc.gov.

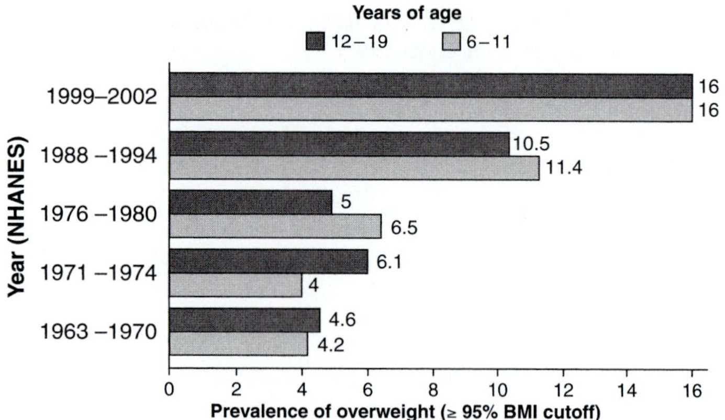

Figure 13.5 Trends in prevalence of overweight for U.S. children and adolescents. Source: National Center for Health Statistics. *Health, United States, 2004*. Hyattsville, MD: 2004.

significant risks to physical and emotional health.[15] About 6 in 10 obese children aged 5 to 10 years have at least one heart disease risk factor, and type 2 diabetes is rapidly becoming a disease of children and adolescents.[15] The rise in childhood obesity is due to complex social, environmental, and policy interactions that have led to excessive eating relative to physical activity and growth energy demands. The Institute of Medicine, the American Academy of Pediatrics, and the American Heart Association are calling for widespread societal changes to support individual efforts by youth to prevent childhood obesity.[14–16] Important steps to confront the epidemic of childhood obesity include:[15]

- The federal government should develop nutrition standards for foods and beverages sold in schools, and develop guidelines regarding advertising and marketing to children and youth.
- Industry and media should develop healthier food and beverage product and packaging innovations, and expand consumer nutrition information.

- State and local governments should expand and promote opportunities for physical activity and access to healthful foods within communities.
- Health-care professionals should routinely track BMI in children and youth and offer appropriate counseling and guidance.
- Schools should improve the nutritional quality of foods and beverages served and sold in schools, and increase opportunities for frequent, more intensive, and engaging physical activity during and after school.
- Parents and families should engage in and promote more healthful dietary intakes and active lifestyles.

HEALTH RISKS OF OBESITY

It has long been suspected that obesity is associated with many health risks, including early death.[18,19] William Shakespeare has written perhaps the most famous description:

> Make less thy body hence, and more thy grace;
> Leave gormandizing; know the grave doth gape
> For thee thrice wider than for other men.
>
> *King Henry IV, Part II*

However, it was not until 1985 that the health hazards of obesity were first officially recognized by the National Institutes of Health.[19] It is now felt that obesity constitutes one of the more important medical and public health problems of our time.

The National Institutes of Health and several other reviewers have summarized the large number of health problems associated with obesity.[18–24]

- *A psychological burden.* Because of the strong pressures from society to be thin, obese people often suffer feelings of guilt, depression, anxiety, and low self-esteem. In terms of suffering, this may be the greatest burden of obesity, especially among adolescents. Severely obese people are often subjected to prejudice and discrimination.[25] The term "fattism" is used to represent this problem. Social and economic consequences of being obese include reduced income and higher rates of poverty, decreased likelihood of getting married, and poorer academic performance and progress.[26]
- *Increased high blood pressure.* High blood pressure is common among the obese.[27,28] As shown in Figure 13.6 the risk of developing hypertension rises sharply with an increase in body mass index.[27] Even among schoolchildren, increases in obesity are associated with corresponding increases in blood pressure.[29] As reviewed in Chapter 10, weight reduction is the single most effective nondrug approach to the control of blood pressure.[28]
- *Increased levels of cholesterol and other lipids in the blood.* The obese, including children, are more likely to have higher blood cholesterol, triglyceride, and LDL-C levels, and lower HDL-C levels.[29–33] Figure 13.7 shows that the ratio of total cholesterol to HDL-C rises with the increase in body mass index.[31] As reviewed in Chapter 10, a high ratio is a strong predictor of heart disease. Weight loss leads to a correction of the negative blood lipid profile, with total cholesterol falling 1 mg/dl for every pound lost.[30]
- *Increased risk of gallstones.* Obesity is a well-recognized risk factor for gallstones, a disease that affects approximately 10–20% of the U.S. population.[34,35] Figure 13.8 shows that the risk for symptomatic gallstones rises sharply with an increase in body mass index.[34]
- *Increased osteoarthritis.* Arthritis and other rheumatic conditions are among the most prevalent diseases in

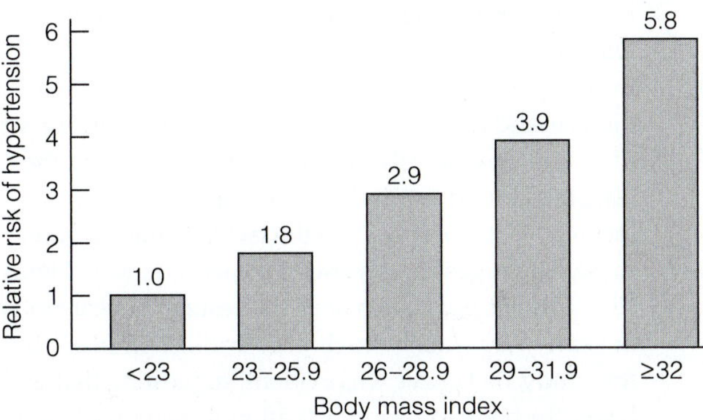

Figure 13.6 BMI and risk of developing hypertension, 8-year study of more than 115,000 nurses. The risk of developing hypertension climbs with the increase in body mass index. Source: Witteman JCM, Willett WC, Stampfer MJ, et al. A prospective study of nutritional factors and hypertension among US women. *Circulation* 80:1320–1327, 1989.

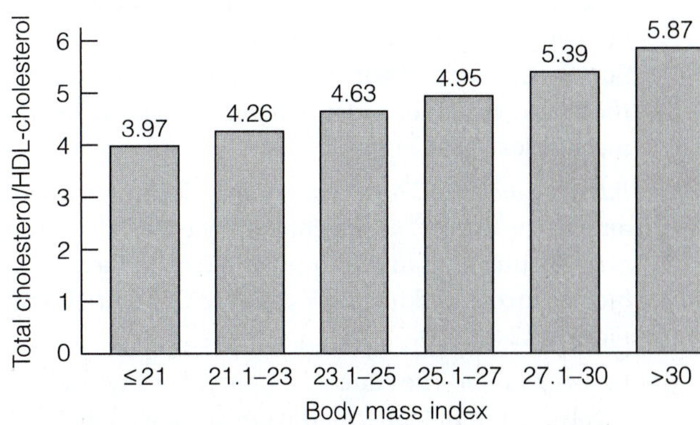

Figure 13.7 Total:HDL-C ratio by body mass index, adult white males, 20–44 years of age, NHANES II. The ratio of total cholesterol to HDL cholesterol rises with an increase in body mass index. Source: Denke MA, Sempos CT, Grundy SM. Excess body weight: An underrecognized contributor to high blood cholesterol levels in white American men. *Arch Intern Med* 153:1093–1103, 1993.

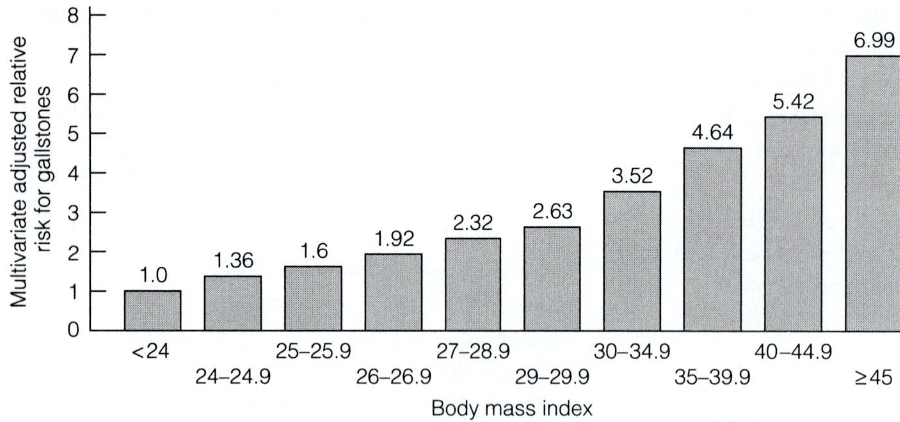

Figure 13.8 Risk of symptomatic gallstones according to obesity status, 8-year study of 90,302 nurses. Risk of gallstones rises sharply with increases in body mass index. Source: Stampfer MJ, Maclure KM, Colditz GA, Manson JE, Willett WC. Risk of symptomatic gallstones in women with severe obesity. *Am J Clin Nutr* 55:652–658, 1992.

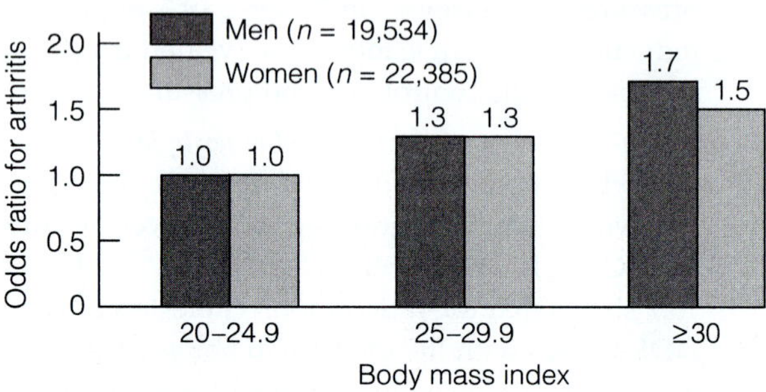

Figure 13.9 Body mass index and odds of arthritis and other rheumatic conditions, National Health Interview Survey, 1989–1991. Source: CDC. Factors associated with prevalent self-reported arthritis and other rheumatic conditions—United States, 1989–1991. *MMWR* 45:487–491, 1996.

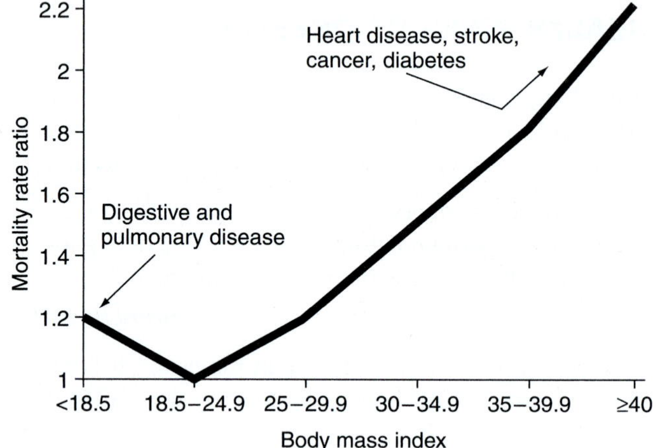

Figure 13.10 Ratios for death from all causes in white men (n = 57,073) and women (n = 240,158) by BMI categories. Source: Stevens J, Cai J, Juhaeri J, Thun MJ, Wood JL. Evaluation of WHO and NHANES II standards for overweight using mortality rates. *J Am Diet Assoc* 100:825–827, 2000.

the United States (see Chapter 15).[36,37] Overweight persons are at high risk of osteoarthritis in the knees and hips. Overweight is among the most potent known risk factors for knee osteoarthritis, with individuals in the upper 20% of weight having 7–10 times the risk of disease of those in the lowest 20% of weight.[37] In the National Health Interview Survey, the odds of self-reported arthritis and other rheumatic conditions rose with an increase in body mass index[36] (see Figure 13.9).

- *Increased diabetes.* The prevalence of diabetes is high among the obese.[38,39] Weight loss by type 2 diabetics often results in dramatic improvements in their blood glucose and insulin levels (see Chapter 12 and Figures 12.6–12.8).
- *Increased cancer.* The American Cancer Society study involving 1 million men and women showed that obese males had a higher mortality rate from cancer of the colon, rectum, prostate, pancreas, liver, and kidney.[40] Obese females had a higher mortality rate from cancer of the gallbladder, breast, uterus, ovaries, colon, rectum, pancreas, liver, and kidney[19,40,41] (see Chapter 11, and Figures 11.16, 11.19, and 11.24).
- *Increased early death.* Hippocrates, the ancient Greek physician, once noted that "sudden death is more common in those who are naturally fat than in the lean." Several modern studies have confirmed the wisdom of Hippocrates. As shown in Figure 13.10, as the body mass increases, mortality from cancer, heart disease, and diabetes increases.[19,23,40,42] The lower part of the curve, where mortality is increased among the lean, has caused much debate. It appears that this increase is due primarily to the fact that smokers and those with digestive diseases die early and lean. Figure 13.11a shows the results of an interesting 26-year study of nearly 9,000 men who did not drink or smoke.[43] In this study, no J curve was evident, suggesting that the lower the body mass index (within reason), the better. This was confirmed in a 16-year study of 115,195 women (see Figure 13.11b).[44] Minimum mortality has been associated with a body weight 10–20% below the average for Americans, after adjustment for cigarette smoking.[44,45] If the American population lost its excess

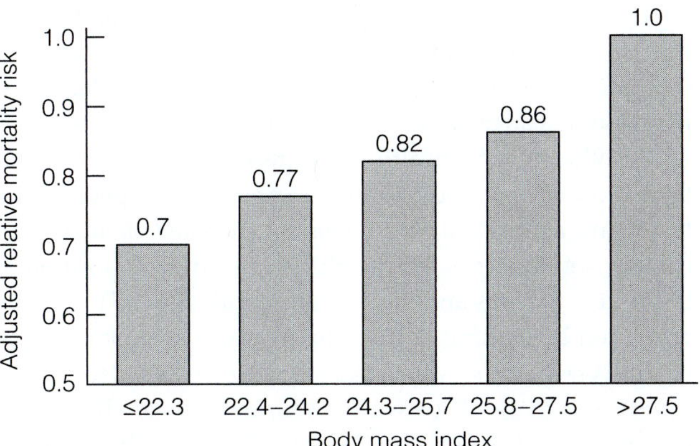

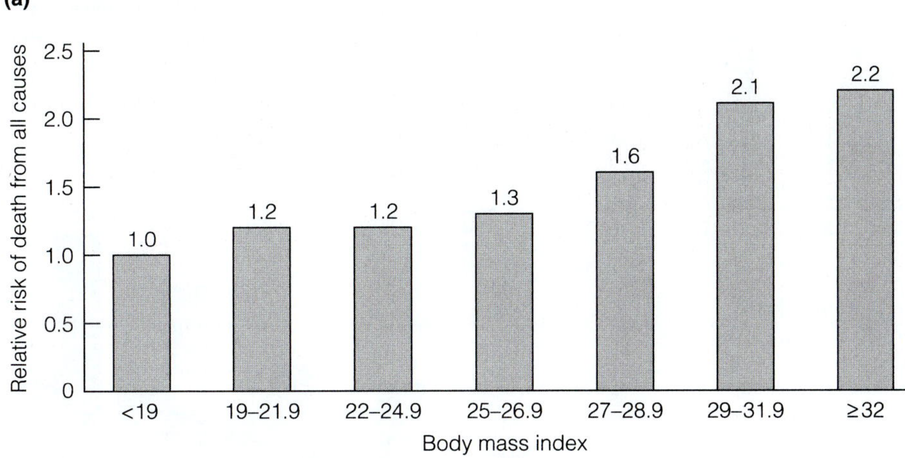

Figure 13.11 (a) Mortality risk according to body mass index, 26-year study of 8,282 nonsmoking, nondrinking males. (b) Mortality risk according to body mass index, 16-year study of 115,195 nonsmoking, weight-stable women; BMI <19.0 vs ≥32.0; risk of cardiovascular disease, 4.1, and cancer, 2.1. Sources: (a) Lindsted K, Tonstad S, Kuzma J. Body mass index and patterns of mortality among Seventh-Day Adventist men. *Int J Obesity* 15:397–406, 1991; (b) Hu FB, Willett WC, Li T, Stampfer MJ, Colditz GA, Manson JE. Adiposity as compared with physical activity in predicting mortality among women. *N Engl J Med* 351:2694–2703, 2004.

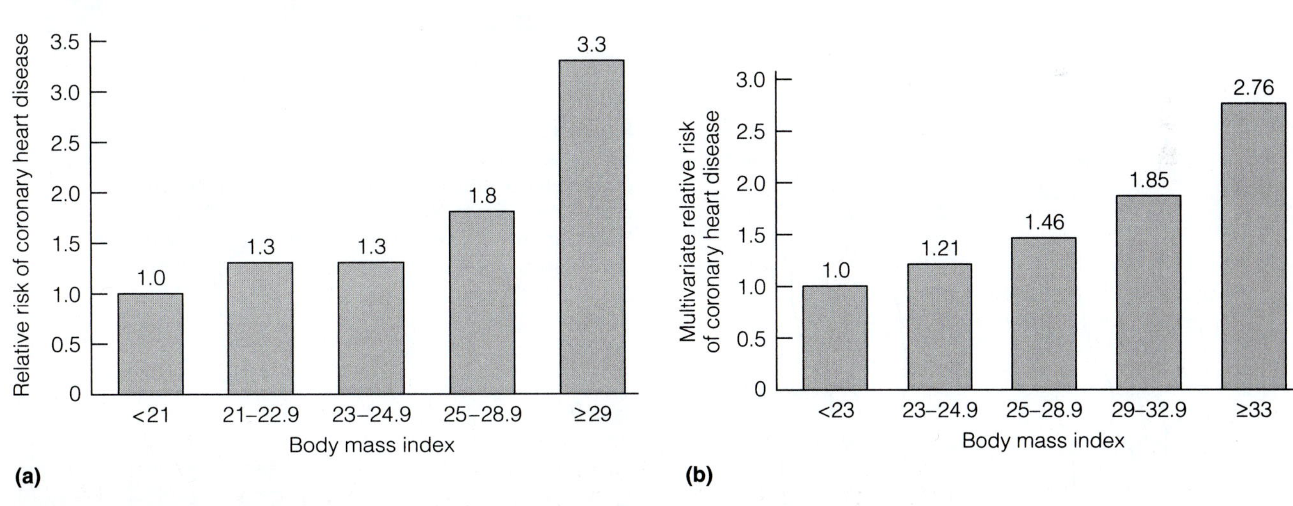

Figure 13.12 (a) BMI and heart disease risk in women, 8-year study of more than 115,000 nurses. Risk of coronary heart disease climbs sharply when the body mass index rises above 29 in women. (b) BMI and risk of coronary heart disease in men, 3-year study of 29,122 U.S. male health professionals. Risk of coronary heart disease rises as the body mass index increases in men. Sources: (a) Manson JE, Colditz GA, Stampfer MJ, et al. A prospective study of obesity and risk of coronary heart disease in women. *N Engl J Med* 322:882–889, 1990; (b) Rimm EB, Stampfer MJ, Giovannucci E, Ascherio A, Spiegelman D, Colditz GA, Willett WC. Body size and fat distribution as predictors of coronary heart disease among middle-aged and older US men. *Am J Epidemiol* 141:1117–1127, 1995.

body mass, mortality would be reduced by 15%, corresponding to 3 years of added life expectancy.

In general, the lowest mortality rates from all diseases combined are found among the lean. Maintaining leanness from early in life to old age is a primary goal.

- *Increased heart disease.* Obese people have more of the typical risk factors for heart disease (high blood pressure and serum cholesterol levels), and as a result, they die from it at a higher rate.[42–50] As shown in Figure 13.12a, in a large 8-year study of nurses, risk of coronary heart disease more than tripled in those with a body mass index greater than 29 versus those with an index less than 21.[48] This has been confirmed in a study of U.S. male health professionals (see Figure 13.12b).[50] Risk of stroke also rises with increase in body mass index (see Figure 13.13).[51]

Recent information is showing that with respect to medical complications, it makes a difference where the excess fat is deposited.[47,50,52–55] The obese people most vulnerable to heart disease, high blood pressure and cholesterol, diabetes, cancers, and early death tend to have more of their fat deposited in abdominal areas rather than the hip and thigh areas.

In other words, health risks are greater for those who have most of their body fat in the upper body, especially the trunk and abdominal areas. This is called *android obesity*, in comparison to *gynoid obesity* (characterized by deposition of body fat in the hips and thighs) (see Figure 13.14). This can be measured by looking at the ratio of waist-to-hip circumferences (WHR) or the waist circumference by itself (see Chapter 5). A high WHR or waist circumference predicts more complications from obesity. Figure 13.15 shows the results of a 5-year study of women where risk of both heart disease and cancer rose as the WHR increased.[53] Figure 13.16 shows that risk of stroke rises with an increase in the WHR.[52] (Also see Figure 12.8, which depicts the relationship between waist circumference and risk of type 2 diabetes.)

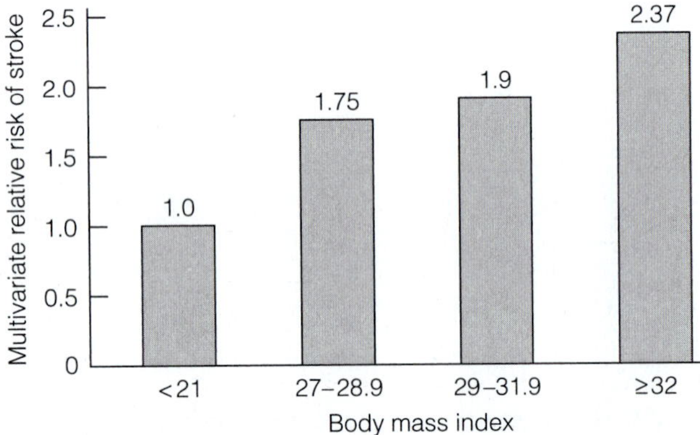

Figure 13.13 Body mass index and risk of ischemic stroke in women, 16-year study of 116,759 women. Risk of ischemic stroke rises with increase in body mass index. Source: Rexrode KM, Hennekens CH, Willett WC, Colditz GA, Stampfer MJ, Rich-Edwards JW, Speizer FE, Manson JE. A prospective study of body mass index, weight change, and risk of stroke in women. *JAMA* 277:1539–1545, 1997.

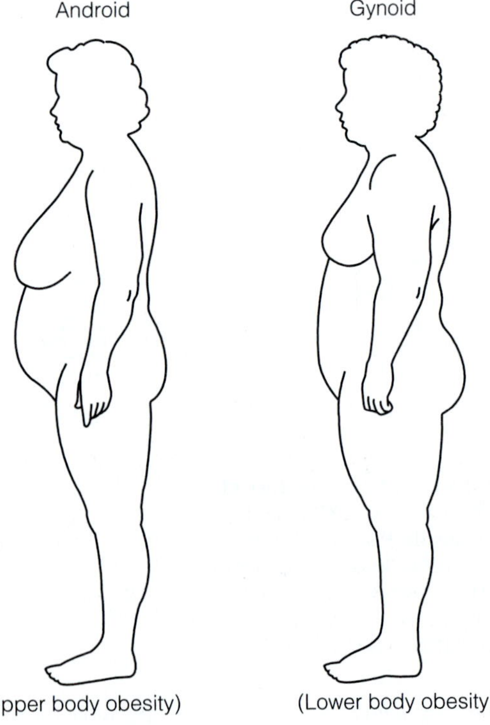

Figure 13.14 *Android obesity* is characterized by high amounts of body fat in the trunk and abdominal areas and is associated with increased medical complications. *Gynoid obesity* is characterized by high amounts of body fat in the hip and thigh areas.

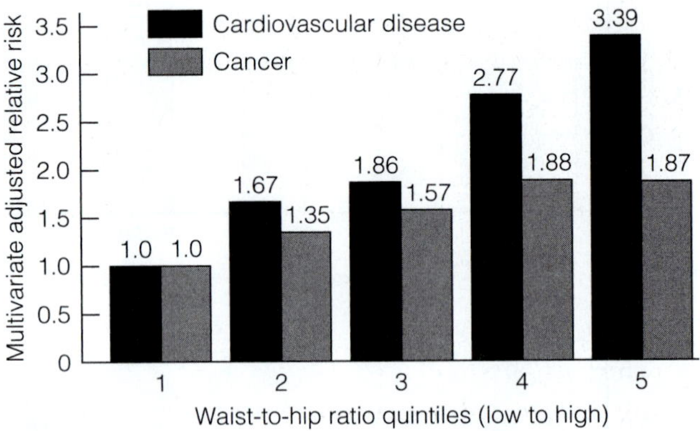

Figure 13.15 Waist-to-hip circumference ratio and disease risk, 5-year-study of 41,837 Iowa women. As the waist-to-hip circumference ratio climbs, risk of both cardiovascular disease and cancer death increases. Source: Folsom AR, Kaye SA, Sellers TA, et al. Body fat distribution and 5-year risk of death in older women. *JAMA* 269:483–487, 1993. See also: *Arch Intern Med* 160:2117–2128, 2000.

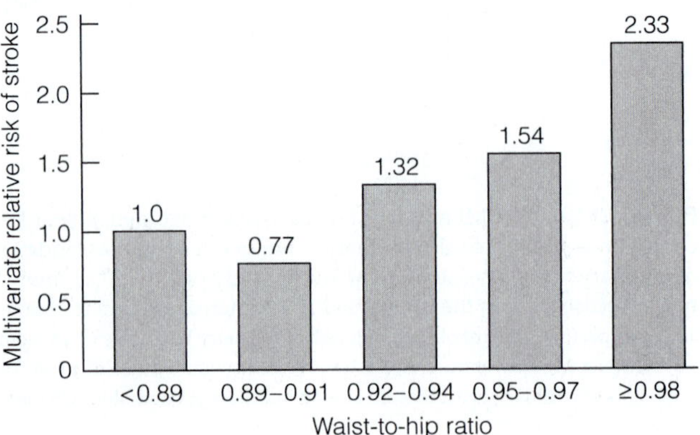

Figure 13.16 Waist-to-hip ratio and risk of stroke, 5-year study of 28,643 U.S. male health professionals. In men, risk of stroke rises with increase in the waist-to-hip ratio. Source: Walker SP, Rimm EB, Ascherio A, Kawachi I, Stampfer MJ, Willett WC. Body size and fat distribution as predictors of stroke among US men. *Am J Epidemiol* 144:1143–1150, 1996.

Fat cells in the abdominal area tend to be more active (releasing and taking up fat molecules) than those in the gluteal and femoral areas.[55] When the supply of abdominal fat is too great, the cells release their fat into the blood vessels that go to the liver; the fat that travels to the liver may be linked to negative health consequences. Various researchers have found that magnetic resonance imaging or computed tomography can image the abdominal fat depot (especially the visceral depot) quite precisely, improving prediction of health risks much better than the WHR (see Chapter 5).

It appears that lifestyle habits have much to do with abdominal fat.[56,57] For example, smoking, alcohol use, and weight cycling appear to preferentially increase abdominal fat stores, whereas exercise decreases them. Weight cycling, or weight fluctuation (i.e., repeated gaining and losing of body weight), has been shown to increase risk of heart disease and death, compared to maintaining a relatively stable weight.[58–60] In general, remaining lean throughout one's lifetime is the safest course to follow to avoid the health risks associated with abdominal obesity, weight cycling, and a high body mass index.[54] For overweight individuals, intentional weight loss, as opposed to unintentional loss of body mass, has been associated with increased longevity and improved quality of life.[61]

THEORIES OF OBESITY

Explaining why so many Americans weigh more than they should has been a source of confusion to researchers and the public alike. Currently, most theories of obesity fall into three categories: genetic and parental influences, high energy intake, and low energy expenditure[62,63] (see Figure 13.17).

Although we know that the development of obesity must involve a prolonged period in which energy intake exceeds energy expenditure, the relative importance of persistent overeating, abnormally low energy expenditure, or the influence of heredity for any particular individual remains controversial.[62]

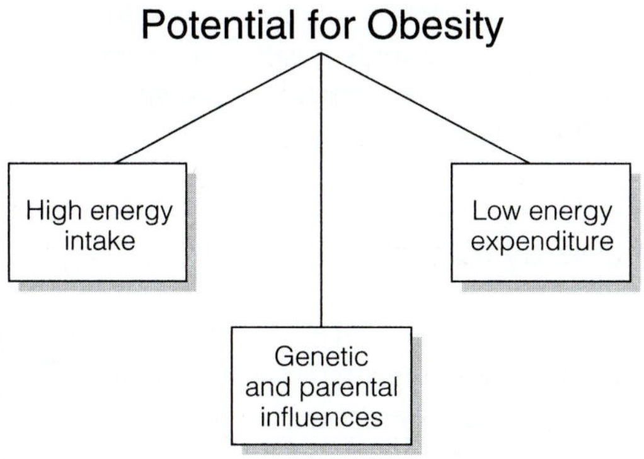

Figure 13.17 The theories of obesity fall into three categories.

Genetic and Parental Influences

Genetic and parental factors are important in explaining why some find it difficult to avoid obesity.[62–65] Jean Mayer reported in 1965 that 80% of the offspring of two obese parents eventually become obese, compared to 40% when one parent is obese and 14% when neither parent is obese.[66] Subsequent research has confirmed the importance of parental obesity in predicting obesity in their offspring, especially when present during the first 10 years of life (see Figure 13.18).

These results, however, gave little indication as to the relative importance of genetics versus the effects of family lifestyle patterns. Researchers have found the study of identical and fraternal twins to be more useful.[67–72] A study comparing adult fraternal and identical twins found that the body weights of the identical twins were much closer together than the body weights of the fraternal twins.[67] When monozygotic twins were reared apart, their body mass indexes were nearly as close as those of monozygotic twins reared together.[69]

A study of adults who had been adopted before the age of 1 year revealed that despite being brought up by their adoptive parents, their body weights were still very similar to those of their biological parents.[68] These studies suggest that shared genes are important in obesity.[71] The heritability of body mass index is about 25–40%.[70] Animal studies support this conclusion. When animals with inherited forms of obesity are paired with lean littermates and fed exactly the same, they gain more weight and fat.[67]

Other factors related to obesity may have a genetic component, including the resting metabolic rate, energy cost of exercise, level of habitual physical activity, tendency to store fat in the abdominal area, response to overfeeding, and relative rate of carbohydrate to lipid oxidation.[64,70,73–75] In one overfeeding experiment, 12 pairs of monozygotic twins were fed 1,000 extra Calories per day for 84 days.[74] Some subjects gained only 9 pounds, while others gained up to 29 pounds (average was 18). Of interest was the finding that there was at least three times more variance in response between twin pairs than within pairs for weight gains, showing that the amount of weight gain has some genetic basis.

In one research project, 1,698 members of 409 families were studied, including spouses, foster parents–adopted children, siblings by adoption, first-degree cousins, uncles/aunts–nephews/nieces, parents–natural children, full siblings, dizygotic twins, and monozygotic twins.[73] Biological inheritance was found to account for 25% of the variance in fat mass (see Figure 13.19). Nongenetic influences such as lifestyle and environmental and cultural factors were shown to be more important. Subsequent research has confirmed that 25–40% of the variability in human obesity has a genetic basis.[62,76]

These studies demonstrate that some people are more prone to obesity than others because of genetic factors. Such people have to be unusually careful with their dietary and exercise habits to counteract these inherited tendencies and may have to accept a body shape and size that is different

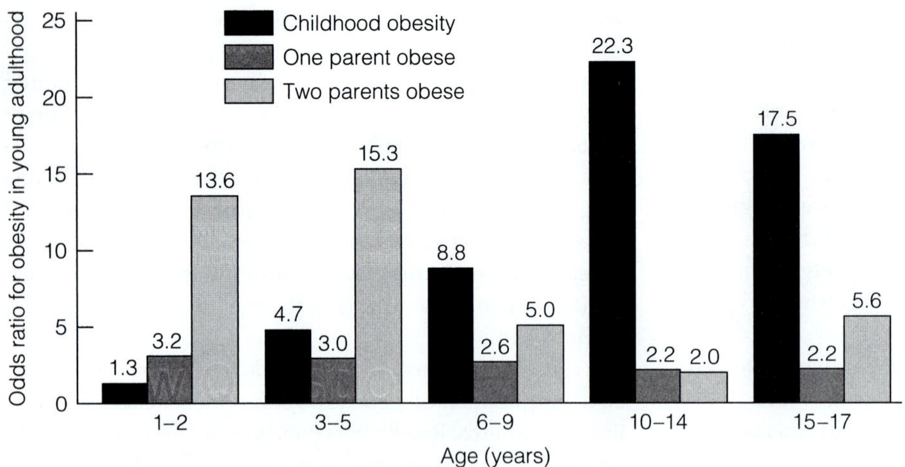

Figure 13.18 Odds for obesity in young adulthood: Parents' versus children's obesity status, retrospective study of 854 U.S. males and females. The odds of obesity in young adulthood are influenced by parental obesity (before the age of 10) and childhood–teenage obesity (especially after the age of 10). Source: Whitaker RC, Wright JA, Pepe MS, Seidel KD, Dietz WH. Predicting obesity in young adulthood from childhood and parental obesity. *N Engl J Med* 337:869–873, 1997.

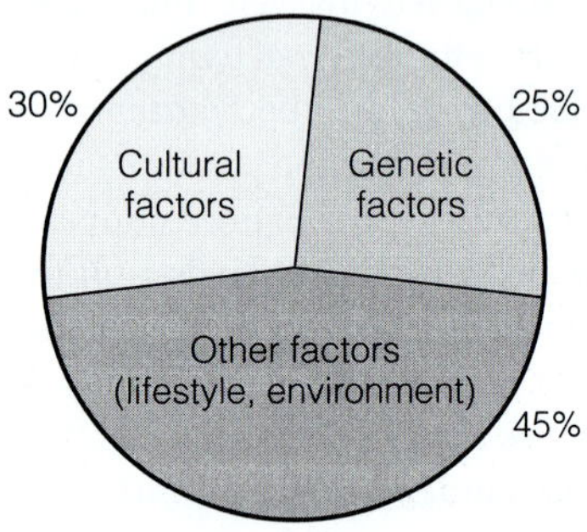

Figure 13.19 Genetic influence of human variation in body fat. Genetic influences on obesity are considered less important than nongenetic influences such as cultural, environmental, and lifestyle factors. Source: Bouchard C, Pérusse L, Leblanc C, et al. Inheritance of the amount and distribution of human body fat. *Int J Obesity* 12:205–215, 1988.

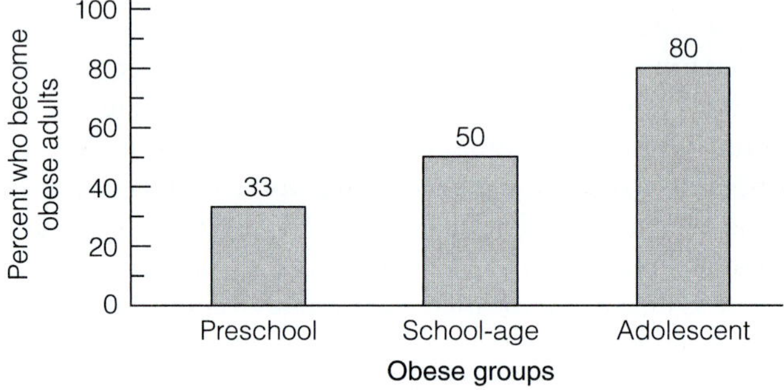

Figure 13.20 Obese children and youths: Percentage of those who become obese adults. The risk of adult obesity is greater for children and youths who are obese at older ages. Source: Serdula MK, Ivery D, Coates RJ, Freedman DS, Williamson DF, Byers T. Do obese children become obese adults? A review of the literature. *Prev Med* 22:167–177, 1993.

than the American ideal portrayed in the media. There is a growing consensus that numerous genes interact with each other and with the environment to express the obesity phenotype.[62–64,76] It is likely that genes that affect both energy intake and energy expenditure are involved. Genes are involved in the regulation of body weight, which is a complex operation involving many different chemical signals, some of which arise from adipose tissue stores and then act in the central nervous system.[62] Leptin, for example, is produced by adipose tissue and acts in the central nervous system through a specific receptor and multiple neuropeptide pathways (under genetic control) to decrease appetite and increase energy expenditure.[62,77]

Most obesity experts feel that obesity is due to both genetic predisposition and environmental circumstances.[62,67,76,78] In other words, a certain genetic makeup can give an individual a predisposition to obesity, and the appropriate environment can cause the expression of it. For example, the Pima Indians in Arizona were once of normal weight, living as farmers near the Gila River.[62] Their lifestyles favored physical activity and a diet high in complex carbohydrates and low in fat. Today, the Pima Indians have high prevalence rates for obesity and diabetes mellitus, live a sedentary existence, and consume a high-fat and high-alcohol diet. Although modern Pima Indians have the same genetic makeup of their predecessors, their environment has been greatly altered, and their biological disposition to obesity is now well expressed.

Although it is widely believed that fat children become fat adults, only about one third of obese preschool children become obese as adults.[65,79,80] However, about half of obese school-age children become obese adults, and more than 80% of obese adolescents remain obese into adulthood.[79] The risk of adult obesity is greater for the fattest children and youths and for those with obese parents and grandparents.[65,79,80] (see Figures 13.18 and 13.20).

High Energy Intake

Do obese people eat more? This has been a controversial issue, with researchers on both sides of the issue.[81–85] In studies indicating that obese people do not eat more than normal-weight people do, subjects were asked to record food intake for 1–14 days using food diaries or memory-

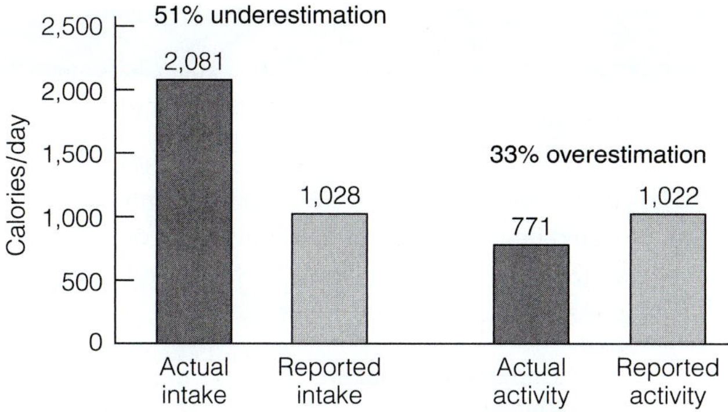

Figure 13.21 Actual versus reported energy intake and expenditure, 14-day study of "diet resistant" subjects. In this study, subjects who claimed they ate little and had a difficult time losing weight were found to underreport caloric intake and to overestimate energy expenditure. Source: Lichtman SW, Pisarska K, Berman ER, et al. Discrepancy between self-reported and actual caloric intake and exercise in obese subjects. *N Engl J Med* 327:1893–1898, 1992.

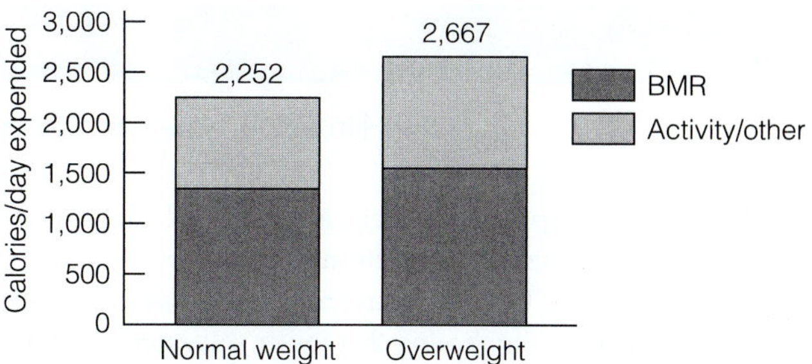

Figure 13.22 Energy expenditure in normal-weight and overweight women, 2-week study using doubly labeled water; body weight, 131 (26% fat) vs 187 (41%) pounds. Obese people expend more energy than normal-weight people and therefore must be eating more to maintain their excess weight. Source: Welle S, Forbes GB, Statt M, Barnard RR, Amatruda JM. Energy expenditure under free-living conditions in normal-weight and overweight women. *Am J Clin Nutr* 55:14–21, 1992.

recall methods. There is now evidence that these methods do not give valid data because obese people tend to underreport their food intake as much as 20–50%.[82,84] Figure 13.21 depicts the result of one study of "diet resistant" subjects who claimed they ate very little, exercised appropriately, yet were obese.[84] When carefully examined by Columbia University researchers during a 2-week period, these subjects were found to be underestimating food intake by about 50% and overestimating physical activity by 33%.

Several researchers have measured energy expenditure using respiratory chambers or doubly labeled water techniques in obese and normal-weight individuals. In these studies, obese people tend to expend and therefore eat about 400–500 Calories more on average each day.[82,86] Figure 13.22 gives the results of a 2-week study of obese and normal-weight women using doubly labeled water, which allowed the subjects to go about their normal duties.[86] Daily energy expenditure was more than 400 Calories higher among the obese women, with half of this due to their higher resting metabolic rates. The investigators concluded that most "overweight subjects must consume more energy than lean subjects to maintain their excess weight."[86] This outcome has also been established in animal studies. For example, fat versus lean rats of the same genetic line have been found to consume significantly more Calories.[87]

There is good reason to believe that the abundance of tasty, calorically rich foods, especially those high in fat, is a major factor in the high prevalence of obesity in Western societies.[88] A consistent finding among many recent studies is that when the intake of dietary fat is high, most adults and children tend to gain weight rather easily and quickly. However, when the intake of dietary fat is low and the intake of carbohydrate and fiber is high, desirable body weight is more readily achieved.[88–98] Cross-cultural studies show that obesity tends to be more prevalent in societies that consume a greater proportion of energy from dietary fat.[90] Within the United States, studies show that portion sizes and energy intake have increased markedly since the 1970s, especially for food consumed at fast food establishments.[89]

There are indications that obese versus lean people tend to choose high-fat and energy-rich foods more often in their day-to-day diets and have different eating behaviors.[88–90] Children from families with obese parents have been found to have a higher preference for fatty foods, a lower liking for vegetables, and a greater tendency to overeat.[97] When the eating behavior of 23 normal-weight and 20 obese children was compared, the obese children were found to eat faster and did not slow down their eating rate toward the end of the meal.[98] Overweight compared to lean teenagers tend to overconsume fast food and are less likely to compensate by adjusting food intake throughout the day.[92] See Box 13.1 for practical tips in lowering saturated fat. One fourth to one half of obese patients who seek weight loss treatment suffer from problems with binge eating.[83] (See discussion of binge eating in the Sports Medicine Insight feature.)

There are several reasons why high-fat diets promote obesity more than those high in carbohydrates.[99–108] Higher-fat foods are often perceived as more palatable, leading to a much greater caloric intake. For example, when eating from a range of either high-fat or high-carbohydrate foods, obese subjects have been found to voluntarily consume twice as much energy from the fat items.[96,101] This finding has led to the theory that the appetite-control system may have only weak inhibitory signals to prevent overconsumption of dietary fat. Researchers believe that while glycogen and protein stores in the body are tightly controlled, fat stores are not, allowing a high degree of expansion.[100,101] This may have served a useful purpose eons ago but now means that obesity can be avoided only if dietary fat intake is low.

Box 13.1

How to Decrease Saturated Fat and Calorie Intake

Overweight people have an elevated risk of heart disease, yet tend to choose foods with high saturated fat content. The table below shows a few practical examples of the differences in the saturated fat content of different forms of commonly consumed foods. Comparisons are made between foods in the same food group (e.g., regular cheddar cheese and low-fat cheddar cheese), illustrating that lower saturated fat choices can be made within the same food group.

Food Category	Portion	Saturated Fat Content (grams)	Calories
Cheese			
☐ Regular cheddar cheese	1 oz	6.0	114
☐ Low-fat cheddar cheese	1 oz	1.2	49
Ground beef			
☐ Regular ground beef (25% fat)	3 oz (cooked)	6.1	236
☐ Extra lean ground beef (5% fat)	3 oz (cooked)	2.6	148
Milk			
☐ Whole milk (3.24%)	1 cup	4.6	146
☐ Low-fat (1%) milk	1 cup	1.5	102
Breads			
☐ Croissant (med)	1 medium	6.6	231
☐ Bagel, oat bran (4″)	1 medium	0.2	227
Frozen desserts			
☐ Regular ice cream	1/2 cup	4.9	145
☐ Frozen yogurt, low-fat	1/2 cup	2.0	110
Table spreads			
☐ Butter	1 tsp	2.4	34
☐ Soft margarine with zero *trans* fats	1 tsp	0.7	25
Chicken			
☐ Fried chicken (leg with skin)	3 oz (cooked)	3.3	212
☐ Roasted chicken (breast no skin)	3 oz (cooked)	0.9	140
Fish			
☐ Fried fish	3 oz	2.8	195
☐ Baked fish	3 oz	1.5	129

Source: Dietary Guidelines for Americans 2005. ARS Nutrient Database for Standard Reference, Release 17. http://www.healthierus.gov/dietaryguidelines/.

Dietary fat also has less of a thermogenic effect than does carbohydrate or protein and can thus be stored as adipose tissue rather easily (see Figure 13.23). Dietary carbohydrate, on the other hand, is not readily converted to body fat, even during periods of high intake.[100,102,104–108] In one study, obese and lean men ingested 50% more energy than normal for 2 weeks.[99] In random order, the additional energy was given as either all fat or all carbohydrate. A whole-room calorimeter determined that carbohydrate overfeeding increased carbohydrate oxidation and total energy expenditure, resulting in 75–85% of the excess energy being stored. Fat overfeeding, however, had minimal effects on fat oxidation and total energy expenditure, leading to storage of 90–95% of excess energy. In other words, excess dietary fat leads to greater fat accumulation in the body than an equal caloric amount of dietary carbohydrate.

A randomized, 11-week crossover study of 16 female subjects by researchers at Cornell University illustrates the importance of keeping dietary fat intake low[93] (see Figure 13.24). Subjects were randomly assigned to either a low-fat diet (22% of calories as fat) or a control diet (37% fat) for 11 weeks, with conditions reversed for another 11 weeks. During the study, subjects were allowed to eat as much food as desired, but they could consume only foods provided by the investigators. The same 41 menu items were offered to the subjects in both groups, but the researchers reduced the quantity of oil, margarine, cream, and so on, used in the preparation of the menu items for subjects on the low-fat diet.

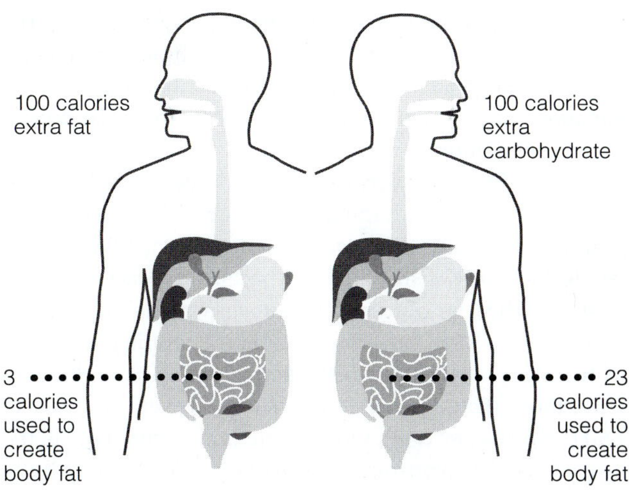

Figure 13.23 Dietary fat versus carbohydrate in body fat formation. The body converts dietary fat into body fat more efficiently than it converts dietary carbohydrate into body fat. Source: Acheson KJ, Schutz Y, Bessard T, Flatt JP, Jequier E. Carbohydrate metabolism and de novo lipogenesis in human obesity. *Am J Clin Nutr* 45:78–85, 1987.

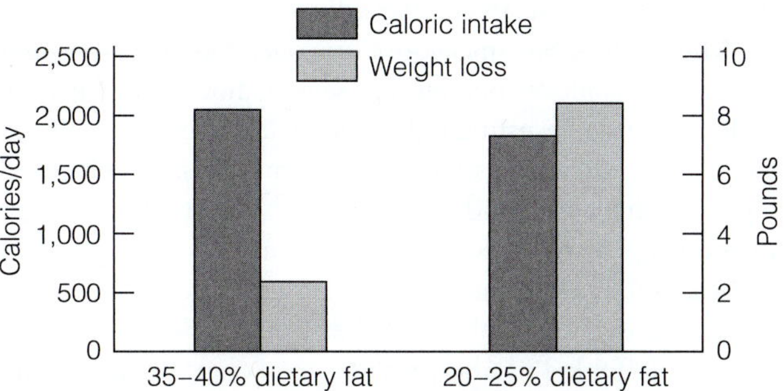

Figure 13.24 Weight loss on a low-fat diet (ad libitum), randomized to low- or high-fat diets for 11 weeks, using the same 41 menu items. Low-fat diets promote more weight loss than high-fat diets. Source: Kendall A, Levitsky DA, Strupp BJ, Lissner L. Weight loss on a low-fat diet: Consequence of the imprecision of the control of food intake in humans. *Am J Clin Nutr* 53:1124–1129, 1991.

While on the low-fat diet, subjects tended to eat less (237 fewer Calories per day) than when on the control diet, and they lost more weight (5.5 pounds). The results of this study clearly demonstrate that when the fat content of the diet is reduced from 37% to 22% of total Calories, people tend to ingest fewer Calories. Also, it seems that some degree of weight loss can be achieved by simply lowering the amount of fat used during food preparation without the necessity of dieting or voluntarily limiting the amount of food consumed.

In another study, 24 women each consumed a sequence of three 2-week dietary treatments in which 15–20%, 30–35%, or 45–50% of the total Calories was derived from fat.[95] The diets consisted of foods that were similar in appearance and taste, but differed in the amount of high-fat ingredients used. The subjects spontaneously consumed 27% fewer Calories when on the low-fat diet versus the high-fat diet, resulting in

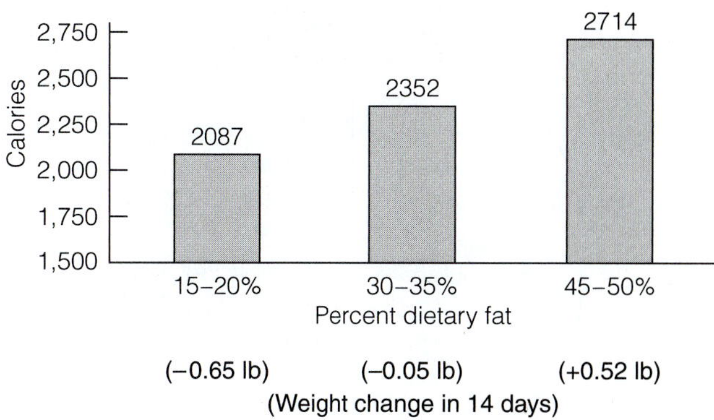

Figure 13.25 Energy intake during 14-day diet, treatments varying in fat content. Reduction in dietary fat is associated with a lower caloric intake and greater weight loss. Source: Lissner L, Levitsky DA, Strupp BJ, et al. Dietary fat and the regulation of energy intake in human subjects. *Am J Clin Nutr* 46:886–892, 1987.

significant changes in body weight (see Figure 13.25). Once again, reduction of habitual fat intake was seen by these researchers as a key element for both the prevention and the treatment of obesity "in that it imposes no strict limitations on the quantity of food consumed, but rather emphasizes the selection of low-fat foods."[95]

Of all the current theories attempting to explain the epidemic of obesity in most Western societies, the "high dietary fat intake" hypothesis is most widely accepted by experts. As emphasized in the medical journal *Lancet* by one team of obesity experts:

> Fat calories represent the only candidate for a sufficient chronic energy imbalance to cause obesity, implying that in addition to an increase in exercise and a restriction of total calories . . . a simple reduction in fat intake will lead to weight loss. This approach . . . could serve as the central strategy for the prevention and treatment of obesity at the individual and population levels. . . . Encouraging the food industry to produce and promote low fat products, and educating consumers to choose these products, are probably the best options for population-wide dietary changes.[107]

Low Energy Expenditure

So far we have seen that some people are more prone to obesity because of genetic tendencies and habitual consumption of high-fat diets. Can obesity also develop because total energy expenditure is lower than normal? Is there some type of metabolic defect that predicts increased obesity because the body is burning fewer Calories than it should? Do obese people burn fewer Calories in physical activity?

All humans expend energy in three ways: through the resting metabolic rate, physical activity, and digesting and metabolizing food (thermic effect of food)[109,110] (see Figure 13.26 and Physical Fitness Activity 13.1).

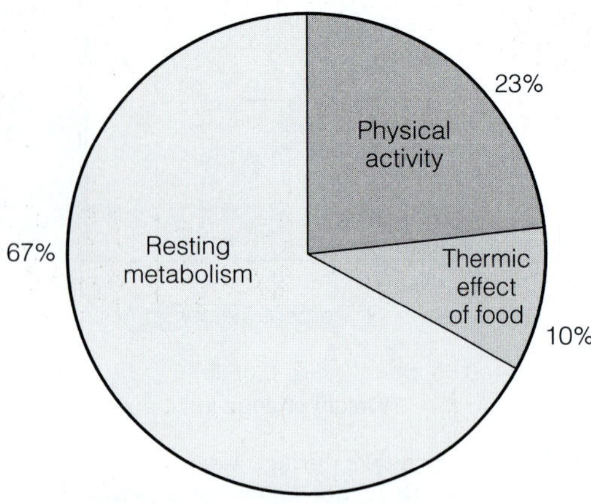

Figure 13.26 Categories of energy expenditure in humans. Approximately 67% of human energy expenditure is from the resting metabolism rate. Sedentary people expend about 23% of their energy in miscellaneous physical activity, and another 10% metabolizing and digesting food. Source: Ravussin E, Bogardus C. A brief overview of human energy metabolism and its relationship to essential obesity. *Am J Clin Nutr* 55:242S–245S, 1992.

Resting Metabolic Rate

The largest number of Calories expended by most people (except for athletes who train several hours a day) is from the *resting metabolic rate* (RMR).[109–115] The basal metabolic rate (BMR) is the rate of energy expenditure when an individual is resting comfortably but awake in a supine position after avoiding food and beverage intake overnight for 12 to 14 hours.[113] The BMR includes the energy expenditure needed to sustain the metabolic activities of cells and tissues, plus the energy to maintain blood circulation, respiration, and gastrointestinal and renal processing (i.e., the basal cost of living). The BMR also includes the energy needed to keep awake, reflecting the fact that the sleeping metabolic rate is about 5–10% lower than the BMR during the morning hours.

The RMR is the energy expenditure under resting conditions when the individual is seated and 4–5 hours postprandial, and tends to be about 10% higher than BMR. Most labs test for RMR instead of BMR because of practical issues related to the ease of testing for subjects and lab personnel. Typically, the RMR is slightly less than 1 calorie per minute in women (or 1,200 to 1,500 calories per day), and somewhat more than 1 calorie per minute in men (or 1,600 to 1,900 calories per day). One calorie per minute equals the heat released by a burning candle or by a 75-watt light bulb. This is a considerable amount of energy, and typically represents (except for athletes) 60–75% of the total daily energy expenditure. The RMR varies up to 20–30% among people of the same age, sex, and body weight, but about 70–80% of this variation is due to differences in body composition, with the RMR higher in those with the greatest fat-free mass (muscle, bone, water, etc.).[109–112] RMR falls about 1–2% per decade of adult life, even after adjusting for fat-free mass.

The RMR is best measured by collecting and analyzing expired air (*indirect calorimetry*) several hours after eating. RMR can also be estimated through the use of equations. Table 13.1 summarizes some of the more commonly used equations for youth and adults.[109,111–115] Because of the tight relationship between RMR and fat-free mass, estimation of RMR is improved especially for obese individuals by using equations 5 and 6 in Table 13.1[111,112] (see Physical Fitness Activity 13.2). Table 13.1 also provides total energy expenditure (TEE) equations from the Institute of Medicine based on age, gender, weight, height, and physical activity level.[113]

TABLE 13.1 Equations for Estimating Resting Metabolic Rate and Total Energy Expenditure

1. Equations by the Institute of Medicine[113]

Institute of Medicine, Basal Energy Expenditure (BEE)*[113]

Adult Males (ages 19 and over)*

BEE = 293 − (3.8 × age) + (456.4 × height) + (10.12 × weight)

Normal-Weight Boys (BMI ≤ 85%, ages 3–18)*

BEE = 68 − (43.3 × age) + (712 × height) + (19.2 × weight)

Overweight/Obese Boys (BMI > 85%, ages 3–18)*

BEE = 419.9 − (33.5 × age) + (418.9 × height) + (16.7 × weight)

Adult Females (ages 19 and over)*

BEE = 247 − (2.67 × age) + (401.5 × height) + (8.6 × weight)

Normal-Weight Girls (BMI ≤ 85%, ages 3–18)*

BEE = 189 − (17.6 × age) + (625 × height) + (7.9 × weight)

Overweight/Obese Girls (BMI > 85%, ages 3–18)*

BEE = 515.8 − (26.8 × age) + (347 × height) + (12.4 × weight)

Institute of Medicine, Total Energy Expenditure (TEE)†[113]

Men 19 years and older:

TEE = 662 − 9.53 × age + PA × (15.91 × weight + 539.6 × height)
PA = 1 for sedentary
PA = 1.11 for low physical activity (equivalent to 1.5–3 miles/day of walking)
PA = 1.25 for moderately active (equivalent to 3–10 miles/day of walking)
PA = 1.48 for very active (equivalent to 10–30 miles/day of walking)

Boys 9 through 18 years:

TEE = 88.5 − 61.9 × age + PA × (26.7 × weight + 903 × height) + 25
PA = 1 for sedentary
PA = 1.13 for low physical activity (equivalent to 1.5–3 miles/day of walking)
PA = 1.26 for moderately active (equivalent to 3–10 miles/day of walking)
PA = 1.42 for very active (equivalent to 10–30 miles/day of walking)

(continued)

TABLE 13.1 ***(continued)***

Women 19 years and older:

TEE = 354 − 6.91 × age + PA × (9.36 × weight + 726 × height)
PA = 1 for sedentary
PA = 1.12 for low physical activity (equivalent to 1.5–3 miles/day of walking)
PA = 1.27 for moderately active (equivalent to 3–10 miles/day of walking)
PA = 1.45 for very active (equivalent to 10–30 miles/day of walking)

Girls 9 through 18 years:

TEE = 135.3 − 30.8 × age + PA × (10.0 × weight + 934 × height) + 25
PA = 1 for sedentary
PA = 1.16 for low physical activity (equivalent to 1.5–3 miles/day of walking)
PA = 1.31 for moderately active (equivalent to 3–10 miles/day of walking)
PA = 1.56 for very active (equivalent to 10–30 miles/day of walking)

2. Harris–Benedict Equations[109]

Males

Resting metabolic rate (Calories/day)
= 66.473 + (13.7516 × kg) + (5.0033 × ht) − (6.755 × age)

Females

Resting metabolic rate (Calories/day)
= 655.0955 + (9.5634 × kg) + (1.8496 × ht) − (4.6756 × age)

3. Revised Harris–Benedict Equations[114]

Males

Resting metabolic rate (Calories/day)
= 88.362 + (4.799 × ht) + (13.397 × kg) − (5.677 × age)

Females

Resting metabolic rate (Calories/day)
= 447.593 + (3.098 × ht) + (9.247 × kg) − (4.330 × age)

4. World Health Organization Equations[115]

Age Range (years)	Equation for Calories Resting Metabolic Rate	Standard Deviation (actual vs predicted)
Males		
18–30	15.3 (kg) + 679	151
30–60	11.6 (kg) + 879	164
>60	13.5 (kg) + 487	148
Females		
18–30	14.7 (kg) + 496	121
30–60	8.7 (kg) + 829	108
>60	10.5 (kg) + 596	108

5. National Institutes of Health, Phoenix, Arizona, Lab[111]

Resting metabolic rate (Calories/day) = 638 + 15.9 (FFM)

6. University of Vermont[112]

Resting metabolic rate (Calories/day) = 418 + 20.3 (FFM)

*Height in meters, weight in kilograms, age in years.

†PA is the physical activity coefficient: at a rate of 3–4 mph or the equivalent energy expenditure in other activities, in addition to the activities that are part of independent living.

Note: kg = body weight in kilograms; ht = height in centimeters; FFM = fat-free mass in kilograms.

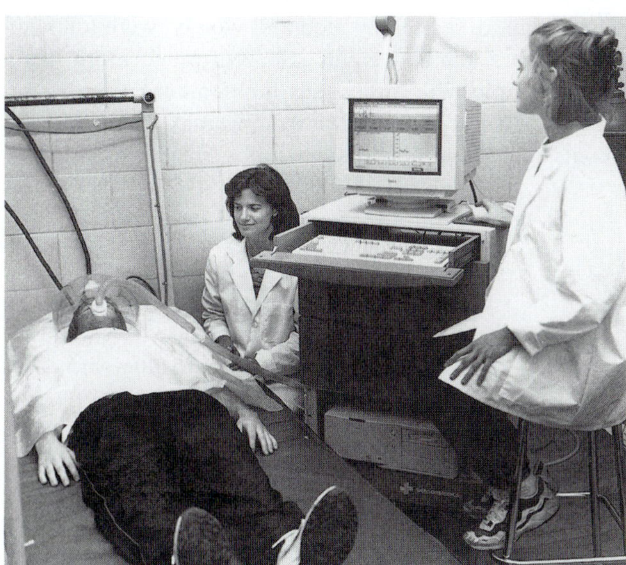

RMR can be measured using a ventilated hood and metabolic cart.

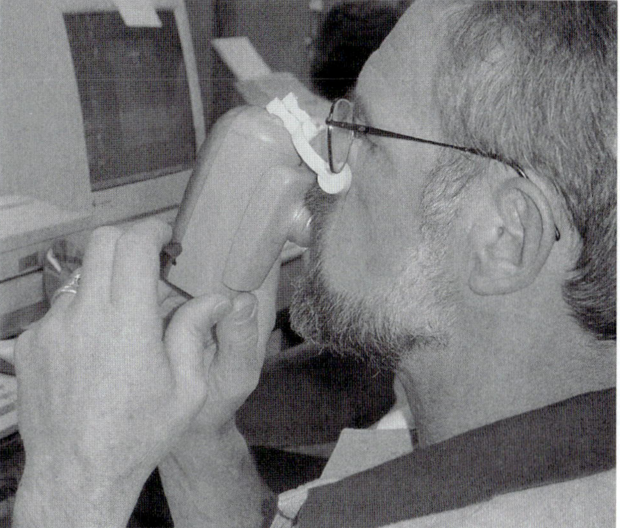

RMR testing is now accurately measured using the handheld BodyGem/MedGem analyzer from HealtheTech (www.healthetech.org).

As would be expected from these equations, an obese person actually has a higher RMR and TEE than a normal-weight person.[111] Obese people, because of the extra weight they carry, have a high fat-free mass—resulting in a higher RMR.

Although obese individuals have elevated RMRs, those levels will fall to normal following achievement of desirable weight.[116,117] The excess weight of mildly and moderately obese people is approximately 25% lean body tissue and 75% fat. With each kilogram of body weight loss, the RMR drops between 10 and 20 Calories per day. A loss of 20 kilograms will reduce RMR by approximately 200–400 Calories per day. As summarized in Figure 13.27, body energy expenditure decreases or increases in parallel with body weight changes.[116]

Although the RMR is closely related to the lean body weight, resting metabolic rate still may vary substantially among people of similar body composition, age, sex, and body weight.[110,111] Heredity may account for as much as 40% of this variation, perhaps by affecting sympathetic nervous activity, which is related to all three major components of energy expenditure.[118] Direct measurement of RMR is thus recommended, and new accurate, and inexpensive devices are now available (e.g., MedGem from Healthetech; www.healthetech.com). Some researchers have determined that a low RMR is a risk factor for future obesity.[118,119] However, others disagree and have not been able to associate low RMR with future weight gain.[120,121] It makes sense, however, that if for a given body weight and fat-free mass the RMR is lower than found in others, that particular individual will have to compensate by exercising more or eating less in order to avoid obesity.

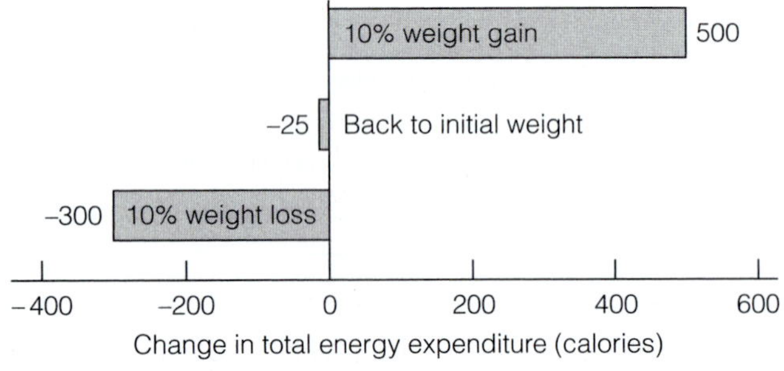

Figure 13.27 Adjustments in body energy expenditure after weight gain or loss, 41 obese and nonobese men and women. Body energy expenditure parallels changes in body weight. Source: Leibel RL, Rosenbaum M, Hirsch J. Changes in energy expenditure resulting from altered body weight. *N Engl J Med* 332:621–628, 1995.

Physical Activity

All physical activity, all muscular movement, expends energy. The average sedentary person usually expends only 300–800 Calories a day in physical activity, most of this from informal, unplanned types of movement. On the other hand, top athletes usually match their RMR energy expenditure through hard, intense exercise. For optimal health, most physical fitness experts recommend burning at least 200–400 Calories per day through planned exercise (see Chapter 8).

It is commonly believed by most obesity experts that the epidemic of obesity in the modern era is in part due to the technological transformations that have made human energy expenditure nearly obsolete during both work and leisure-time pursuits.[122–130] Even when people do exercise during their leisure time, the total daily energy expenditure still falls far short of what was typical during the nineteenth century.[123]

There is some indication that long-term physical activity is related to a lower risk of gaining weight.[124–130] Researchers from the American Cancer Institute followed over 79,000 people for 10 years and found that those engaging in vigorous exercise 1–3 hours a week, or walking for more than 4 hours a week, were better able to ward off weight gain than their more sedentary counterparts.[128] When a group of more than 9,000 men and women were followed for 10 years, major weight gain was much more likely among people with low versus high amounts of physical activity[125] (see Figure 13.28). Among male health professionals, just 30 minutes a day of moderate physical activity

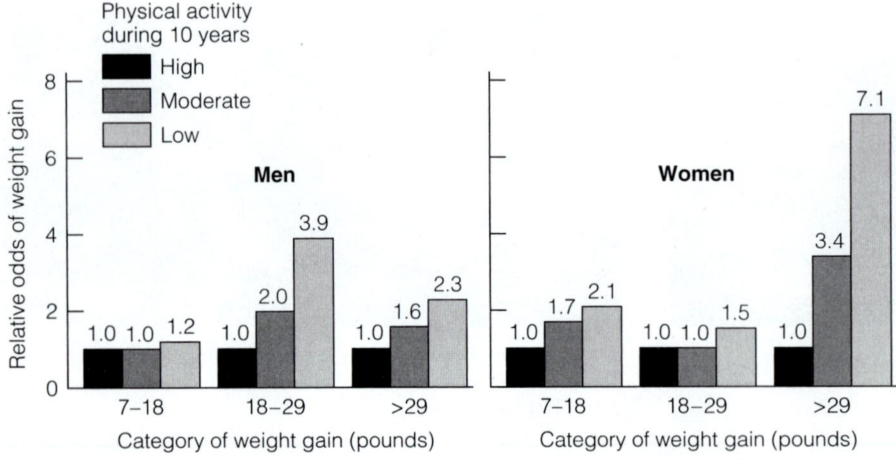

Figure 13.28 Recreational physical activity and 10-year weight change: NHANES I epidemiologic follow-up study of 3,515 men and 5,810 women. For both men and women who engaged in low amounts of physical activity, weight gain over a 10-year period was much more likely than for those who engaged in high levels of activity. Source: Williamson DF, Madans J, Anda RF, et al. Recreational physical activity and ten-year weight change in a US national cohort. *Int J Obesity* 17:279–286, 1993.

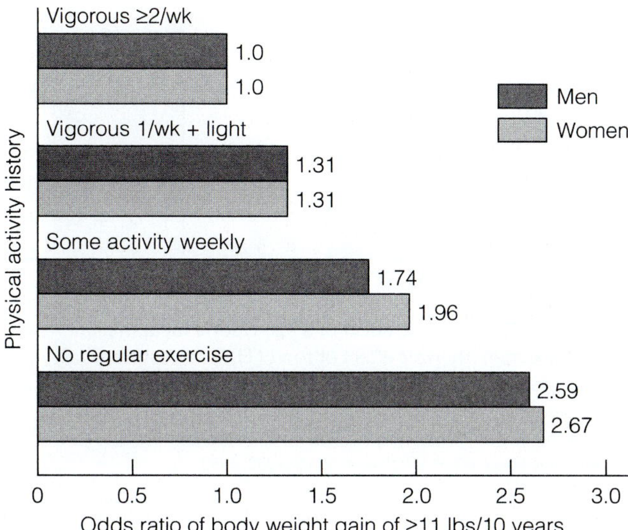

Figure 13.29 Odds for weight gain over 10 years according to physical activity, 10-year study of 5,259 Finnish men and women. The odds of significant weight gain are highest in men and women reporting no regular exercise during a 10-year period. Source: Haapanen N, Miilunpalo S, Pasanen M, Oja P, Vuori I. Association between leisure time physical activity and 10-year body mass change among working-aged men and women. *Int J Obesity* 21:288–296, 1997.

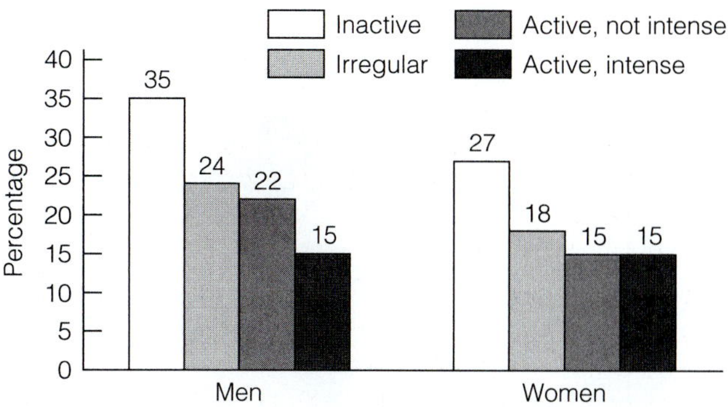

Figure 13.30 Prevalence of overweight by physical activity pattern, CDC BRFSS, 6,125 men, 12,557 women. In cross-sectional studies, the prevalence of obesity has consistently been found to be highest in those reporting no regular physical activity. Source: DiPietro L, Williamson DF, Caspersen CJ, Eaker E. The descriptive epidemiology of selected physical activities and body weight among adults trying to lose weight. The Behavioral Risk Factor Surveillance System Survey, 1989. *Int J Obesity* 17:69–76, 1993.

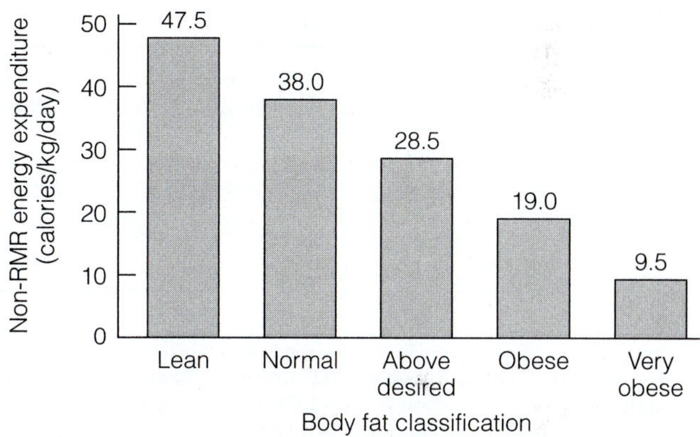

Figure 13.31 Relationship between body fatness and non-RMR energy expenditure, 300 obese and nonobese males and females, measured with the doubly labeled water method. Energy expenditure (non-RMR) is lowest (weight adjusted) in the very obese. Source: Schulz LO, Schoeller DA. A compilation of total daily energy expenditures and body weights in healthy adults. *Am J Clin Nutr* 60:676–681, 1994.

was sufficient to reduce the risk of becoming overweight during a 2-year period.[127] In a 10-year study of more than 5,000 Finnish men and women, the odds of significant weight gain were 2.6-fold greater in those reporting no regular exercise, compared to their peers who engaged in regular vigorous exercise[124] (see Figure 13.29). Prospective studies of young children have demonstrated that those with low, compared to high, levels of physical activity gain more body fat.[129,130] Together, these studies indicate that regular physical activity is associated with a reduced risk of body weight gain over the long term.

Do the obese exercise more or less than normal-weight people? Although measurement of physical activity is extremely difficult and has hampered our understanding of this issue, most studies show that both obese children and obese adults are less active than normal-weight people.[129–144] Overweight girls have been found to be less active than lean ones while playing sports.[131] For example, when swimming, obese adolescent girls spend less time actually moving their arms and legs and more time standing and floating than normal-weight girls. While playing tennis, obese girls have been found to be inactive 77% of the time, compared with 56% of the time for normal-weight girls. In general, obese children spend up to 40% less time in physical activity than lean children.[131]

Obese men informally walk an average of 3.7 miles per day, compared to 6 miles per day for men of normal weight; obese women walk 2 miles per day, compared to 4.9 miles per day for normal-weight women.[133] The obese stay in bed longer and spend 17% less time on their feet than normal-weight people do.[134] When given a choice of an escalator or stairs, the obese are more likely than the lean to take the escalator.

In general, there is good data to indicate that physical activity decreases in direct relationship to the degree of obesity.[135,139,140] In cross-sectional studies, the prevalence of obesity is consistently highest in those reporting the least amount of physical activity[140] (see Figure 13.30). As depicted in Figure 13.31, energy expended in activity (Calories/kg/day) falls in direct relationship to the degree of obesity.[139] It has been difficult to know, however, whether inactivity causes obesity or if obesity leads to inactivity.[126] Some researchers feel that because aerobic fitness levels are lower among the obese, exercise is more difficult, and inactivity is then a result of the increase in body fat stores.[137,138]

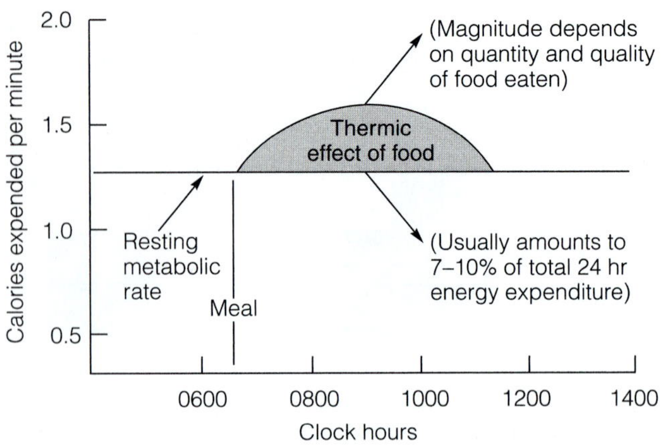

Figure 13.32 Thermic effect of food. The thermic effect of food (TEF) is the energy expended for the digestion, absorption, transport, metabolism, and storage of food. Source: Reed GW, Hill JO. Measuring the thermic effect of food. *Am J Clin Nutr* 63:164–169, 1996.

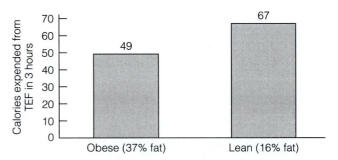

Figure 13.33 Thermic effect of a 720-calorie meal in lean and obese men, thermic effect of food (TEF) = postprandial − postabsorptive RMR. The thermic effect of food is slightly lower among obese, compared to lean, men. Source: Segal KR, Edano A, Tomas MB. Thermic effect of a meal over 3 and 6 hours in lean and obese men. *Metabolism* 39:985–992, 1990.

TABLE 13.2 Energy Expenditure in 177 Humans (Obese and Nonobese) Studied in a Respiratory Chamber

Variable	Average (Calories/day)	Range (Calories/day)	Obese vs Lean
24-hour energy expenditure	2,292	1,371–3,615	Increased*
All types of physical activity	348	138–685	Decreased
Resting metabolic rate	1,813	1,102–2,935	Increased*
Thermic effect of food	165	50–476	Little difference

Note: Average weight = 97 kg; range = 47–178 kg.
*Increased in an obese person, in comparison to a lean person.
Source: Ravussin E, Lillioja S, Anderson TE, Christin L, Bogardus C. Determinants of 24-hour energy expenditure in man. *J Clin Invest* 78:1568–1578, 1986. See also: Ravussin E, Gautier JF. Metabolic predictors of weight gain. *Int J Obesity* 23(suppl 1):37–41, 1999.

Thermic Effect of Food

The *thermic effect of food* (TEF) is the increase in energy expenditure above the RMR that can be measured for several hours after a meal[145–150] (see Figure 13.32). Energy is expended as the body digests, absorbs, transports, metabolizes, and stores the food eaten. The average person's TEF is about 10% of total ingested Calories, or about 200–250 Calories per day for women and about 250–300 Calories per day for men.[145,146] For example, after a meal containing 800 Calories, the body uses about 80 Calories just to process the meal.

The TEF has been found to be higher with larger meals.[147] For normal-weight people, the TEF raises the energy expenditure of the body 40–45% over the RMR 1 hour after a 1,500-Calorie meal; after a 1,000-Calorie meal, there is a 25% increase over the RMR. As depicted in Figure 13.32, the TEF peaks about 60–120 minutes following a meal and lasts up to 4–6 hours.

Do the obese expend fewer Calories in digesting and metabolizing their food than normal-weight people? Most researchers have concluded that obese adults and children have a slightly lower TEF, especially if they are diabetic[145–150] (see Figure 13.33). However, the difference is too small in terms of actual Calories to be important. In addition, most obese people have higher RMRs, due to their increased fat-free mass, more than making up for the small decrease in TEF.[146]

Table 13.2 summarizes information on energy expenditure, comparing obese and nonobese people. The 177 people in this study varied widely in weight and degree of obesity. In general, obese people were found to expend more energy each day than nonobese people, despite lower levels of physical activity. This was due primarily to higher RMRs.[119]

TREATMENT OF OBESITY

As we have seen thus far in this chapter, about two thirds of adults in the United States are classified as overweight and obese. The prevalence of overweight has increased during the twentieth century and is disproportionately high in many subpopulations, including the poor and members of some ethnic groups.[7,11,12,151] Being overweight can seriously affect health and longevity and is a contributing factor to the two leading causes of death in the United States: heart disease and

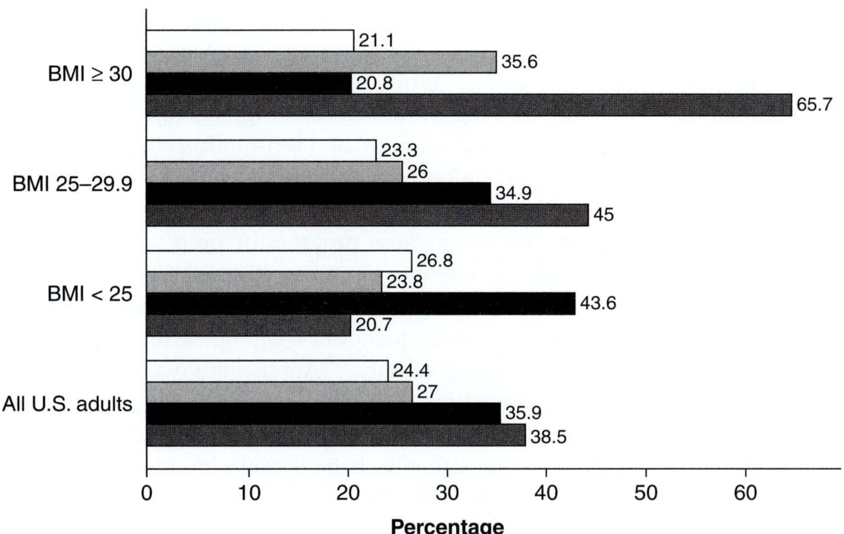

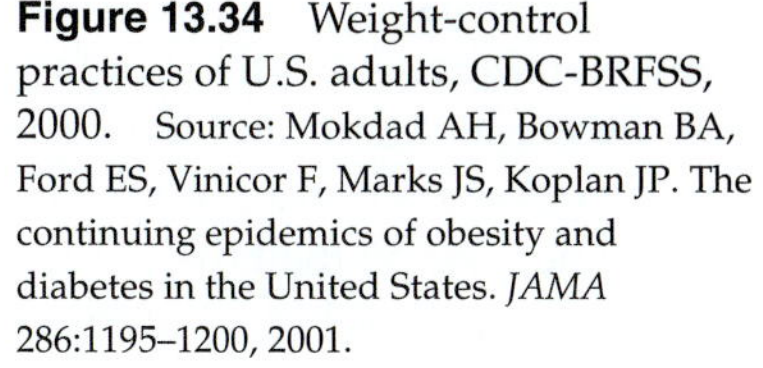

Figure 13.34 Weight-control practices of U.S. adults, CDC-BRFSS, 2000. Source: Mokdad AH, Bowman BA, Ford ES, Vinicor F, Marks JS, Koplan JP. The continuing epidemics of obesity and diabetes in the United States. *JAMA* 286:1195–1200, 2001.

cancer. Although experts still debate the underlying causes, all agree that the basic mechanism is an imbalance between caloric intake and energy expenditure. Evidence suggests that obesity is multifactorial in origin, reflecting genetic, lifestyle, cultural, socioeconomic, and psychological conditions.

Americans are preoccupied with plans and aspirations to lose body weight.[6,151–154] As shown in Figure 13.34, nearly 4 in 10 U.S. adults are trying to lose weight at any given time, with this proportion rising to 66% among the obese.[154] Among adults attempting to lose or maintain weight, only 18% follow the two key recommendations: to eat fewer Calories and to increase physical activity.[154] Only 43% of obese adults have been advised in any given year by their doctor to lose weight.[154]

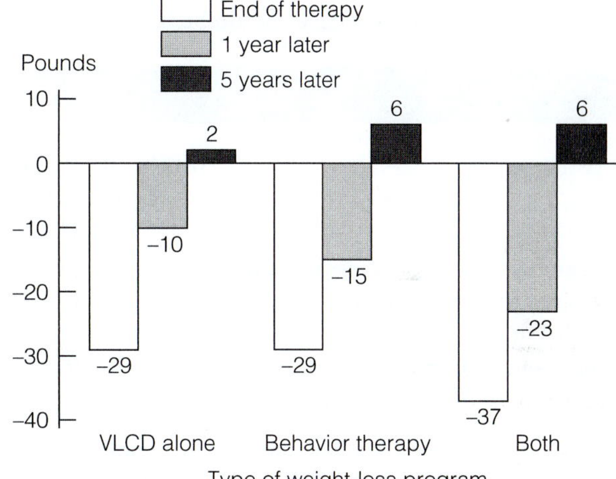

Figure 13.35 Maintenance of weight loss over 5 years, 76 obese women (mean weight 233 lb) treated for 4–6 months and followed 5 years. Long-term success in maintaining the body weight lost during treatment for obesity has been found in this study and others to be poor. Source: Wadden TA, Sternberg JA, Letizia KA, Stunkard AJ, Foster GD. Treatment of obesity by very low calorie diet, behavior therapy, and their combination: A five-year perspective. *Int J Obesity* 13(suppl 2):13:39–46, 1989.

Treatment Is Challenging

Treatment of obesity has proven to be one of the greatest challenges facing health professionals. Many obese people will not stay in treatment. Of those who do, most will not achieve ideal body weight, and of those who lose weight, most will regain it. For most weight loss methods, there are few scientific studies evaluating their effectiveness and safety.[151] Studies that are available indicate that people can be quite successful losing weight in the short term, but after completing the program or weight loss scheme, they tend to regain the weight over time.

For example, in a 4-year study of 152 men and women who had participated in a 15-week behaviorally oriented weight loss program including diet, exercise, and behavior modification, less than 3% of subjects were able to maintain posttreatment weights throughout the 4 years of follow-up observation.[155] Data from a 5-year study of 76 obese women (mean weight 233 pounds) are given in Figure 13.35.[156] At baseline, subjects were randomly assigned to one of three weight loss programs:

1. A very-low-calorie diet (VLCD) of 400–500 Calories per day for 2 months followed by a 1,000- to 1,200-Calorie-per-day diet for 2 more months (designated as "VLCD alone" in Figure 13.35).
2. A 1,200-Calorie-per-day diet plus behavior modification training for 6 months (behavior therapy).
3. Same as group 1, but behavior modification training was included for 6 months ("Both" in the figure).

The data in Figure 13.35 show that although the end-of-treatment and 1-year data are quite impressive, 5 years after treatment, nearly all subjects in each group had returned to their pretreatment weight, with group means actually above starting body weights. Overall, only 5% of subjects maintained all of their weight loss after 5 years, and only 18% maintained a loss greater than 11 pounds, with 64% of subjects regaining all of, or more than, what they had once lost.

Weight Loss Maintenance

These researchers and others have urged that more vigorous efforts should be put forth to help patients maintain the weight they do lose.[156–162] They recommend that patients participate in at least a 6- to 12-month program of weight loss maintenance immediately after losing weight (no matter what the method) and that they be prepared to reenter therapy whenever they show a gain of 10 pounds or more that they cannot lose on their own. During the maintenance program, group and individual counseling with health professionals (especially physicians, who appear to have the most influence with obese patients) and an emphasis on a low-fat diet and regular exercise should be integrated. Behavior treatment should continue after the weight loss program, by which patients are made aware of their current lifestyle habits through various techniques, including record keeping, problem solving, change in thinking processes, social support, and self-reinforcement.

Several studies have attempted to measure factors that predict long-term maintenance of weight loss after participation in a weight loss program or process.[162–165] In one study of 509 obese subjects, predictors of success after 2 years were feeling in control of eating habits, success during actual treatment, frequency of weight measurement, and increase in physical activity.[164] Another study of 118 obese patients followed for more than 3 years showed that weight loss was maintained best in those who reported eating fewer high-fat foods, using the behavioral techniques taught in the program, and exercising more.[165] In the National Weight Control Registry study, a low-fat diet, consistency in the day-to-day diet, and high levels of physical activity were reported by the majority of subjects who had been successful at long-term maintenance of weight loss[161,162] (see Box 13.2 for more information).

Several other studies have found that exercise is one of the best markers for long-term success.[166–170] In one study, 90% of women who had lost weight and maintained their

Box 13.2

Habits of Those Achieving Success in Weight Loss and Management

Researchers at the University of Pittsburgh and University of Colorado have formed a national registry of people who have lost more than 30 pounds and kept it off for more than a year. Several hundred people are now in this registry, and interesting findings have emerged:

- 94% of successful losers increased their physical activity level to accomplish their weight loss, with walking the most common activity reported.
- 92% report that they are continuing to exercise to maintain weight loss. Those most successful in fighting back weight regain typically exercise for at least 1 hour a day, burning at least 400 Calories each day.
- 98% decreased their food intake in some way.
- 57% received professional help from doctors, registered dietitians, Weight Watchers, and others.

Nationwide, about 20% of overweight and obese individuals are able to lose 10% of initial body weight and keep it off for at least 1 year. Weight loss maintenance gets easier over time. Once weight loss has been maintained for 2–5 years, the chances of longer success greatly increase.

Source: Wing RR, Hill JO. Successful weight loss maintenance. *Annu Rev Nutr* 21:323–341, 2001. www.nwcr.ws.

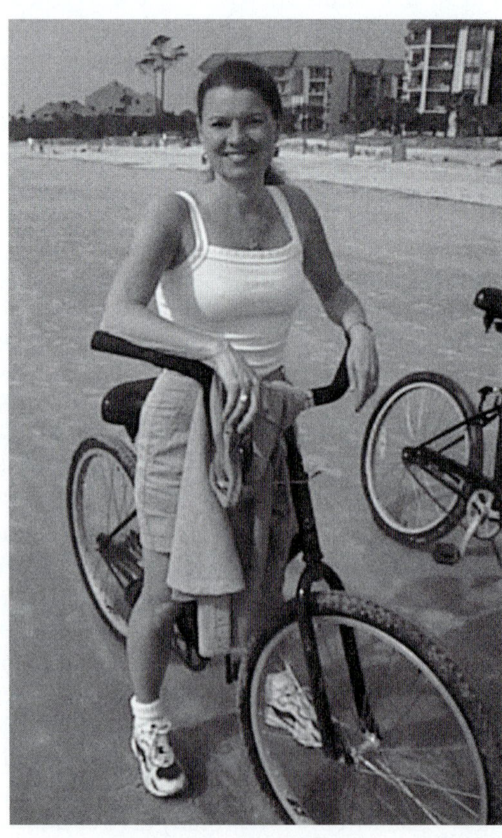

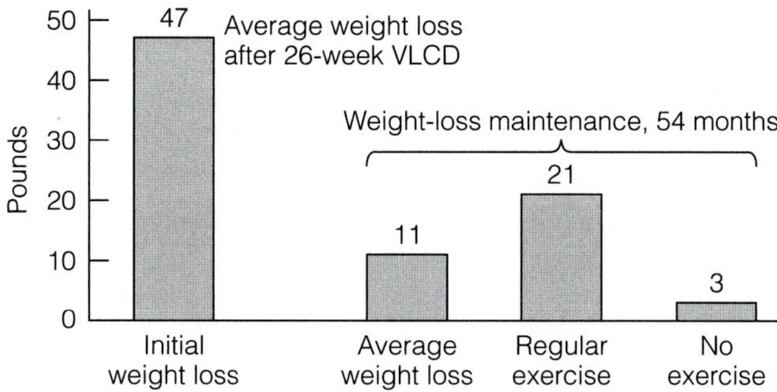

Figure 13.36 Weight loss maintenance following a very-low-calorie diet program, 54 months of follow-up. Regular exercise over a 4.5-year period following a 26-week VLCD program significantly improved weight loss maintenance.
Source: Walsh MF, Flynn TJ. A 54-month evaluation of a popular very low calorie diet program. *J Fam Pract* 41:231–236, 1995.

losses for more than 2 years reported regular exercise, compared with only 34% of the women who had regained their weight losses.[169] Figure 13.36 shows that weight loss maintenance was significantly enhanced in subjects who exercised regularly for 4.5 years after a VLCD program, compared to those who avoided exercise.[166]

Weight regain is probably related to several powerful factors, including genetic influences to retain high fat stores, an innate propensity of the human body in general to defend body fat reserves, and failure on the part of the individual to apply new behavioral skills (especially exercise and eating a low-fat diet) because of barriers imposed by family and societal forces. A tremendous amount of support from several sources is necessary for a prolonged time following treatment of obesity to ensure any type of reasonable success.

There are many health benefits associated with weight loss.[151,171,172] Weight loss reduces many of the health hazards associated with obesity, including insulin resistance, diabetes mellitus, hypertension, dyslipidemia (e.g., high cholesterol, low HDL, and high triglycerides), sleep apnea, and osteoarthritis. Among very obese individuals, weight loss has been followed by greater functional status, reduced work absenteeism, less pain, and greater social interaction.[151] However, there are adverse effects of weight loss when it is too rapid (e.g., during fasting or VLCDs), including a greater risk for gallstone formation and cholecystitis, excessive loss of lean body mass, water and electrolyte problems, mild liver dysfunction, and elevated uric acid levels.

Conservative Treatment Guidelines

Obesity has typically been treated as if it is an acute illness, when it is more appropriately viewed as a chronic condition much like heart disease or diabetes.[151,173] Obesity treatment should include efforts not only at the individual but also at community and national levels. Community interventions could include educational and media programs to lower dietary fat consumption and increase physical activity. National policies to improve food-label information or to provide economic support for local community efforts are examples of what could be done to enhance environmental support for individuals struggling to maintain ideal body weight.

Because the ultimate goal of a weight-reduction program is to lose weight and maintain the loss, a nutritionally balanced, low-calorie diet that is applicable to the patient's lifestyle is most appropriate.[7,11] A comprehensive weight-reduction program that incorporates diet, exercise, and behavior modification is more likely to lead to long-term weight control.[7,11,174,175,176]

1. *Diet.* The caloric intake should be reduced, preferably by reducing the fat content of the diet, while increasing the complex carbohydrates (see Physical Fitness Activity 13.3). In 1998, the National Heart, Lung, and Blood Institute (NHLBI) advised that for most overweight and obese clients, a decrease of 300–1,000 Calories per day will lead to weight losses of ½–2 pounds per week, and a 10% weight loss in 6 months (the initial goal).[7,11] (See Box 13.3 for more information.)
2. *Exercise.* Energy expenditure should be increased at least 200–400 Calories per day by increasing all forms of physical activity.
3. *Behavior modification* (see Box 13.4). Several techniques should be employed, including
   - *Self-monitoring.* Such as keeping diet diaries, emphasizing the recording of food amounts consumed and circumstances surrounding the eating episode (see Physical Fitness Activity 13.4)
   - *Control of the events that precede eating.* Identification of the circumstances that elicit eating and overeating
   - *Development of techniques to control the act of eating.* Typical behavioral modification techniques
   - *Reinforcement through use of rewards.* Involving a system of formal rewards that facilitate progress

Although the majority of obese patients will benefit from these guidelines, there are some who carry substantial amounts of body fat, and may need additional forms of therapy to be successful, including drug therapy, and/or gastric-reduction surgery. Box 13.5 summarizes the treatment scheme advocated by the NHLBI.[7,11] Notice that gastric-reduction surgery is reserved for the most severely obese, while drug therapy is recommended as a consideration for moderately obese patients. These methods have evoked considerable discussion, and a brief review follows.

Gastric-Reduction Surgery

The NHLBI Obesity Education Initiative promotes weight loss surgery as an option for weight reduction in patients with clinically severe obesity, defined as a BMI ≥40, or a BMI ≥35 with comorbid conditions[7,11] (see Box 13.5). Weight loss surgery should be reserved for clinically severe obese patients in whom other methods of treatment have failed.

Box 13.3

How to Lose Weight: The NHLBI Obesity Education Initiative

In 1998, the first federal guidelines for the treatment of overweight and obesity in adults were released by the National Heart, Lung, and Blood Institute (NHLBI) as a part of its nationwide Obesity Education Initiative. With nearly 100 million overweight Americans, the NHLBI has made education about overweight and obesity a major priority. Key diet recommendations from this initiative include the following:

- The initial goal of a weight loss regimen should be to reduce body weight by about 10%. With success, further weight loss can be attempted, if needed.
- Weight loss should be about 1–2 pounds per week for a period of 6 months, with additional plans based on the amount of weight loss. Seek to create a deficit of 500–1,000 Calories per day through a combination of decreased caloric intake and increased physical activity.
- Reducing dietary fat intake is a practical way to reduce Calories. But reducing dietary fat alone without reducing Calories is not sufficient for weight loss.

Each pound of body fat represents about 3,500 Calories. To follow the NHLBI for weight loss, one must expend 500–1,000 Calories more than the amount taken in through the diet. This can be accomplished by increasing energy expenditure 200–400 Calories a day through physical activity, and reducing dietary fat intake by 300–600 Calories. Each tablespoon of fat represents about 100 Calories, so an emphasis on low-fat dairy products and lean meats, and a low intake of visible fats (oils, butter, margarine, salad dressings, sour cream, etc.) is the easiest way to reduce caloric intake without reducing the volume of food eaten.

The NHLBI recommends this diet for weight loss:

- Eat 500–1,000 Calories a day below usual intake.
- Keep total dietary fat intake below 30% of Calories, and carbohydrate at 55% or more of total Calories.
- Emphasize a heart-healthy diet by keeping saturated fats under 10% of total Calories, cholesterol under 300 mg/day, and sodium less than 2,400 mg/day.
- Choose foods high in dietary fiber (20–30 grams/day).

This diet starts in the grocery store. Another challenge is eating healthfully when dining out. Learn to ask for salad dressing on the side and to leave all butter, gravy, or sauces off the dish. Select foods that are steamed, garden fresh, broiled, baked, roasted, poached, or lightly sauteed or stir-fried.

Source: www.nhlbi.nih.gov/.

Box 13.4

Losing Weight by Changing Your Behavior

Any diet will help one lose weight, but to achieve permanent weight control, a program should be selected that focuses on eating and exercise behaviors. If the problem behaviors have not been addressed, the weight will likely return.

Eating habits lie at the very core of one's being. Changing them is hard work and means taking a look at every aspect of the lifestyle including food use during social and cultural events, family meal patterns, shopping and cooking techniques, and how one uses food when stressed or depressed. Several useful behavior change principles can be followed:

- *Self-monitor dietary habits.* Keep a diet diary, recording the amount of food consumed and circumstances surrounding each eating episode. For example, one may find that high-calorie snacks are ingested when studying or that overeating occurs when dining out with friends. The food record is a valuable tool to increase awareness of personal eating behaviors. Once the problem areas are identified, seek support from friends, family, and professionals to make positive changes in these areas.
- *Control the events that precede eating.* Identify and control the circumstances that elicit eating and overeating (e.g., avoid reading or watching television while eating or stay away from food when depressed or stressed); shop wisely (shop from a list, and avoid going to a store when hungry); plan meals (eat at scheduled times and according to an overall plan); reduce temptation (store food out of sight, eat all food in the same place, keep serving dishes off the table, and use smaller dishes); plan for parties (practice polite ways to decline food, and eat a low-calorie snack before parties).
- *Develop techniques to control the act of eating.* Slow down the eating process by putting the fork down between bites; keep serving sizes moderate and don't go back for seconds; avoid unscheduled snacks; chew thoroughly before swallowing.
- *Be wise and think positively.* Avoid setting unreasonable goals; think about progress and not shortcomings; avoid imperatives such as "always" and "never"; counter negative thoughts with reason.
- *Reinforce success with rewards.* A system of formal rewards facilitates progress. For example, close friends or family members could arrange for a special gift, trip, or award for meeting established goals.

Box 13.5

Identification, Evaluation, and Treatment of Overweight and Obesity in Adults. Practical Guide from the National Health, Lung, and Blood Institute, National Institutes of Health

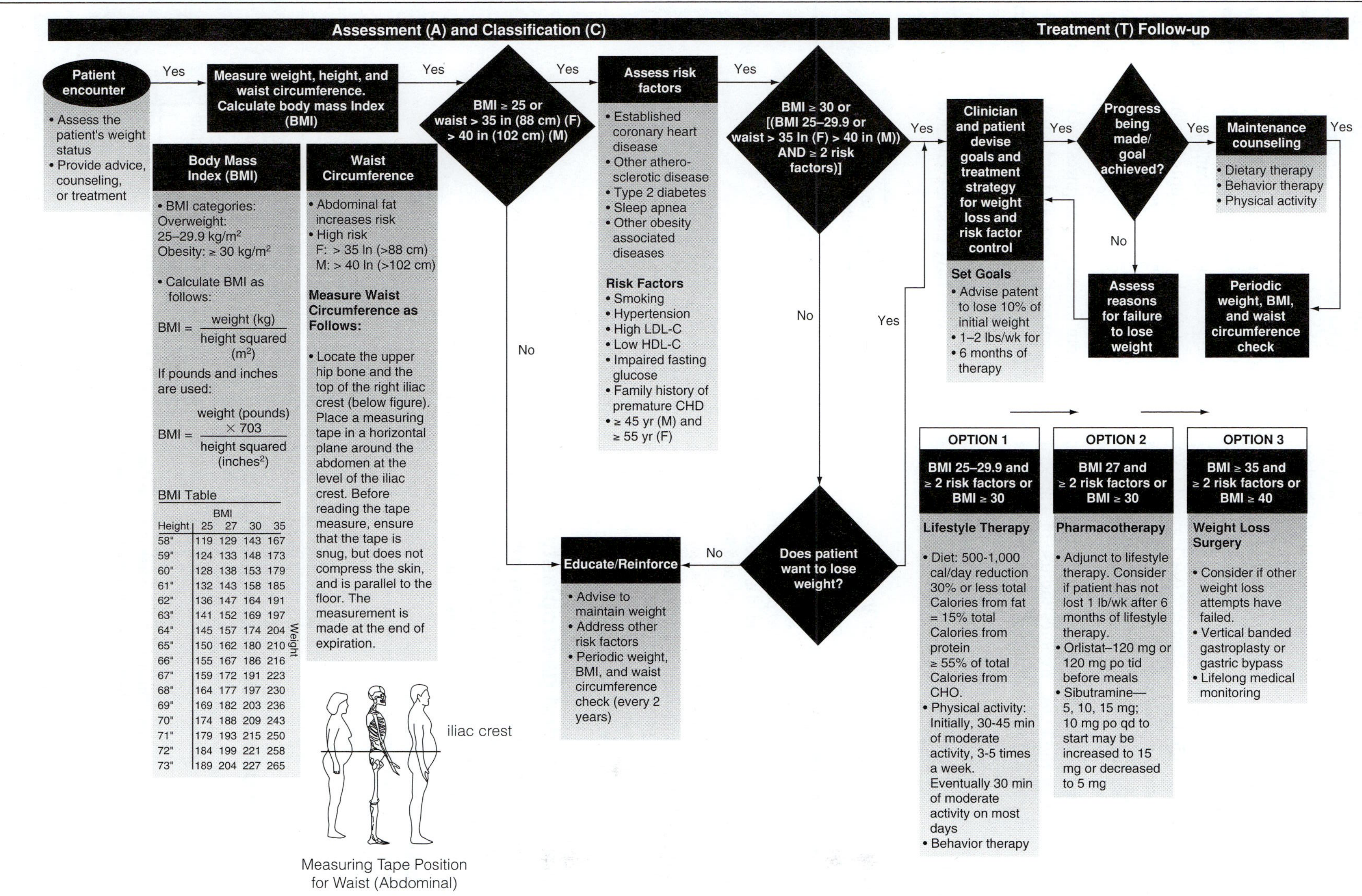

BMI Table

Height	BMI 25	27	30	35
	Weight			
58"	119	129	143	167
59"	124	133	148	173
60"	128	138	153	179
61"	132	143	158	185
62"	136	147	164	191
63"	141	152	169	197
64"	145	157	174	204
65"	150	162	180	210
66"	155	167	186	216
67"	159	172	191	223
68"	164	177	197	230
69"	169	182	203	236
70"	174	188	209	243
71"	179	193	215	250
72"	184	199	221	258
73"	189	204	227	265

Source: National Health, Lung, and Blood Institute.*The Practical Guide. Identification, Evaluation, and Treatment of Overweight and Obesity in Adults.* Bethesda, MD: NIH Publication Number 00-4084, October 2000. www.nhlb.nih.gov.

Until recently, severely obese people were rarely able to lose weight and keep it off using traditional methods. The advent of surgical treatments for obesity in the 1940s dramatically changed this picture. Large amounts of weight (up to 200 pounds) can be lost, with up to half of the loss maintained over the long term.[177]

One type of surgery involves radically reducing the volume of the stomach to less than 50 ml by constructing a pouch with a restricted outlet along the lesser curvature of the stomach (called vertical banded gastroplasty)[178] (see Figure 13.37). Another type of surgery is gastric bypass, which involves stapling shut a small portion of the stomach and then connecting it to the small intestine, bypassing the stomach, duodenum, and first portion of the jejunum. A third procedure, newly approved by the FDA, involves the use of a special band that is placed around the upper stomach to create a small pouch with a narrow outlet (see Figure 13.37).

These surgical procedures are major operations, and a decision to use surgery requires assessing the risk–benefit ratio in each case. Only certain people are qualified to undertake this type of surgery.[177,178] To be cleared for surgery, the patient must show a history of repeated failures to lose weight by acceptable nonsurgical methods, must be experiencing some medical complications from the obesity, and must be highly motivated and well informed about the procedure. There must be a commitment by the patient, surgeon, and hospital for a comprehensive lifelong follow-up.[7,11]

Weight reduction is dramatic and long term. At 5 years postsurgery, half of patients lose more than half of their excess weight, 30% lose 25–50%, while 20% fail to lose significant amounts of weight.[178] Patients go through drastic forced changes in eating habits. The 50-ml stomach resulting from the surgery requires people to eat less during each meal, eat more often, and not have any liquids at mealtime.

The loss in weight and the improvement in eating habits lead to an improvement in blood lipids, glucose, psychological mood state, and overall health in the most morbidly obese subjects who have gastric-reduction surgery.[177–182] However,

Gastric bypass surgery

Done by open surgery or laparoscopically. The stomach is divided into two compartments, each closed by several rows of staples, creating a thumb-size pouch at the top. A small outlet is created in the smaller portion of the stomach, and the small intestine is connected to it. Food entering the small stomach causes a sensation of fullness, and then slowly empties into the intestine through the small outlet.

Risks: One of 200 patients dies as a consequence of surgery. Possible hernia or ulcer. Failure of weight loss can occur if the staple line is disrupted or the patient nibbles high-calorie junk food such as chips.

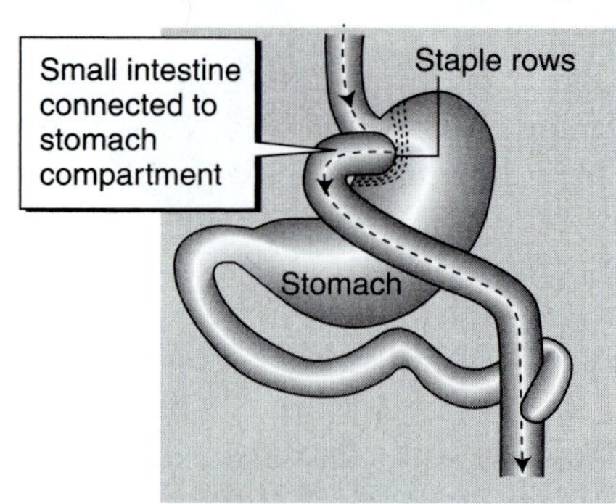

Vertical banded gastroplasty

Four rows of staples are placed vertically in the upper part of the stomach. The outlet at the lower end of the pouch created by these staples is restricted by a ring that limits the passage of food into the rest of stomach. The person feels full after a few bites of food.

Risks: Similar to those for gastric bypass surgery. Patients can fail to lose weight if they eat—or especially drink—too many high-calorie foods.

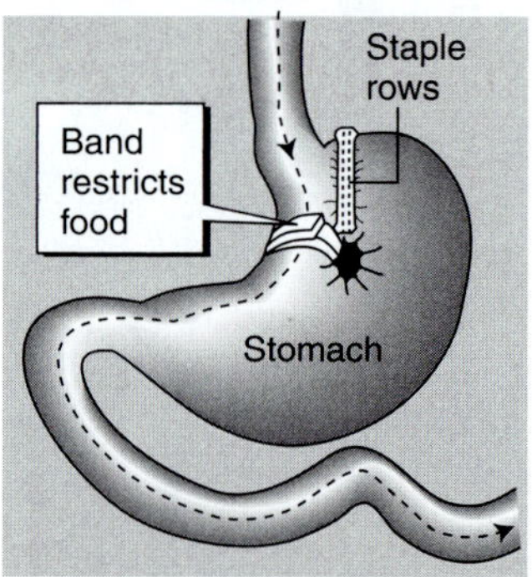

Laparoscopic adjustable gastric banding

A band is placed around the outside of the upper stomach to create a small (golf-ball size) pouch with a narrow outlet.

Risks: The band could slip or erode. Studies indicate the weight loss is much less than with gastric bypass surgery.

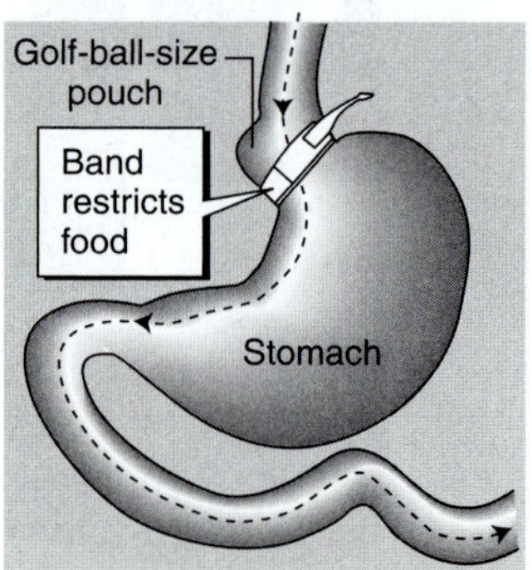

Figure 13.37 Description of three FDA-approved methods for weight loss surgery. Source: National Health, Lung, and Blood Institute. *The Practical Guide. Identification, Evaluation, and Treatment of Overweight and Obesity in Adults.* Bethesda, MD: NIH Publication Number 00-4084, October 2000. www.nhlbi.nih.gov.

a subgroup of patients respond poorly to the surgery in terms of failure to lose substantial weight, moderate to life-threatening medical complications, and emotional trauma.[183] Complications occur in 5–10% of cases, but mortality is very rare (0.1%). The most common complications are respiratory problems, severe vomiting, nutritional deficiencies, and wound infections, with the most severe complications being deep venous thrombosis and gastrointestinal leakage.[177,178]

Drug Therapy

The NHLBI Obesity Education Initiative promotes FDA-approved weight loss drugs for long-term use as an adjunct to diet and physical activity for patients with a BMI ≥30 and without concomitant obesity-related risk factors or disease[7,11] (see Box 13.5). Drug therapy may also be useful for patients with a BMI ≥27 who also have concomitant obesity-related risk factors or diseases.

Appetite-suppressant drugs (also called anorectic or anorexiant medications) have been available for several decades, and although there has been some stigma in their use, recent studies are showing that they may have a role in the treatment of some patients.[184–190] The majority of weight loss medications prescribed in the 1950s and 1960s were amphetamines and had widespread and indiscriminate use. Between 1970 and 1990, medication usage for the treatment of obesity decreased, and no new medication was approved by the Food and Drug Administration (FDA) for the treatment of obesity until 1996.

In the late 1980s and early 1990s, a series of reports showing sustained weight loss with the use of a combination of fenfluramine hydrochloride and phentermine resin (nicknamed fen-phen) fueled widespread interest from patients, health professionals, and the media.[187] The number of prescriptions written for fenfluramine increased from about 60,000 in 1992 to over 1 million in 1995. In 1996, the FDA approved dexfenfluramine (a more potent form of fenfluramine, with the trade name of Redux) for use up to 1 year in the treatment of obesity.

The explosion of interest led to the development of clinics devoted to the prescription of weight loss medications. Despite little training or expertise in obesity, many physicians established overnight fen-phen treatment programs with the promise of long-term cure. In the fall of 1997, all this came crashing down when fenfluramine and dexfenfluramine were withdrawn from the market because a high incidence of heart valve defects was found in patients who used them.[189] Redux was also linked to an increased risk of primary pulmonary hypertension, a rare but potentially deadly lung disorder.[187] No drug approved by the FDA for beyond 3 months remained available until November 1997, when the FDA approved sibutramine for long-term use in obesity.[7,11] In April 1999, the FDA approved orlistat for long-term use (see Figure 13.38 and Table 13.3).

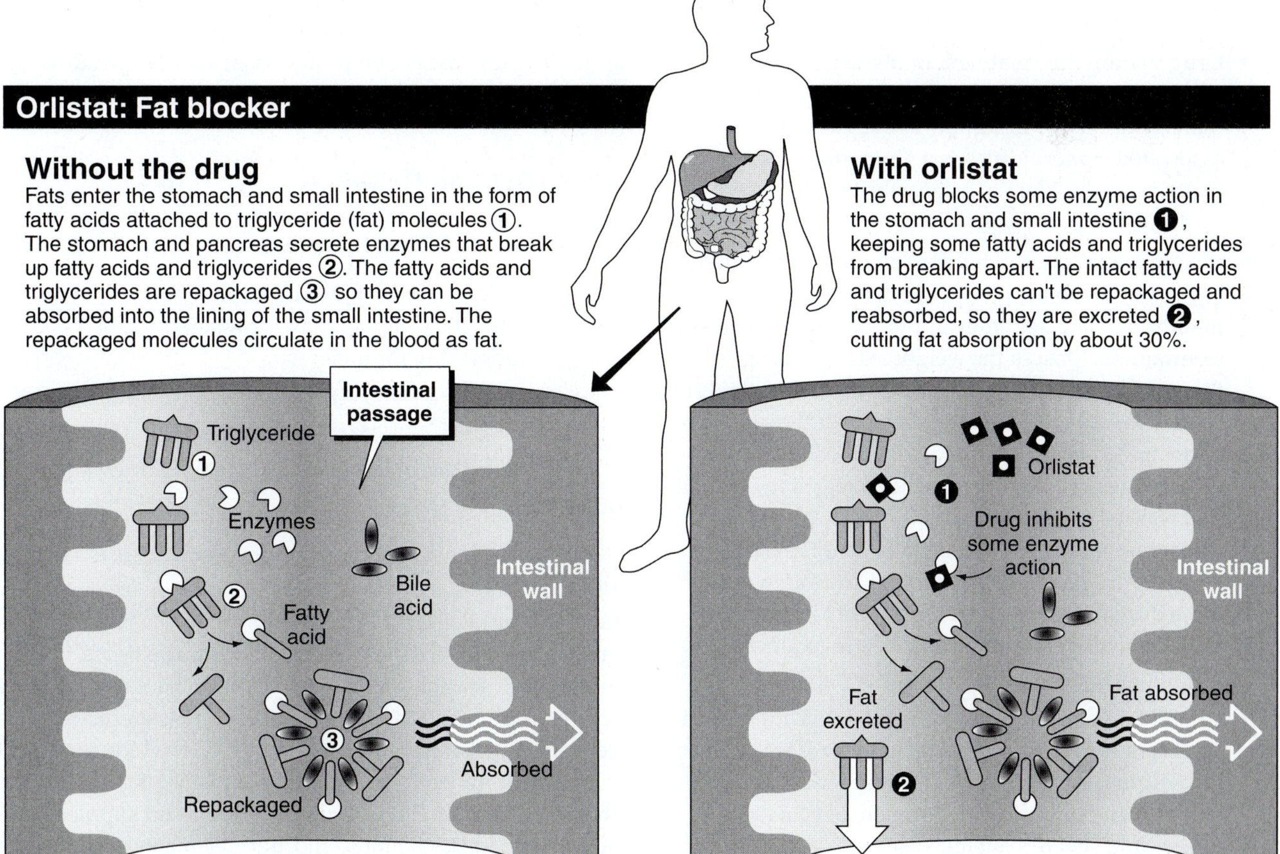

Figure 13.38 Description of how orlistat decreases fat absorption.

TABLE 13.3 Weight Loss Drugs*

Drug	Dose	Action	Adverse Effects
Sibutramine (Meridia)	5, 10, 15 mg; 10 mg po qd to start; may be increased to 15 mg or decreased to 5 mg	Norepinephrine, dopamine, and serotonin reuptake inhibitor	Increase in heart rate and blood pressure
Orlistat (Xenical)	120 mg 120 mg po tid before meals	Inhibits pancreatic lipase, decreases fat absorption	Decrease in absorption of fat-soluble vitamins; soft stools and anal leakage

* Ephedrine plus caffeine, and fluoxetine have also been tested for weight loss but are not approved for use in the treatment of obesity. Mazindol, diethylpropion, phentermine, benzphetamine, and phendimetrazine are approved for only short-term use for the treatment of obesity. Herbal preparations are not recommended as part of a weight loss program. These preparations have unpredictable amounts of active ingredients and unpredictable, and potentially harmful, effects.

po = by mouth; qd = 4 times daily; tid = 3 times daily.

Source: National Health, Lung, and Blood Institute. *The Practical Guide. Identification, Evaluation, and Treatment of Overweight and Obesity in Adults.* Bethesda, MD: NIH Publication No. 00-4084, October 2000. www.nhlbi.nih.gov.

Sibutramine is an anorexiant, or appetite suppressant, and affects neurotransmitters in the brain.[185,188,190] This drug inhibits the reuptake of norepinephrine and serotonin in the synaptic neural cleft, suppressing appetite. Orlistat is not an appetite suppressant and has a different mechanism of action. Orlistat is a gastrointestinal lipase inhibitor, blocking one third of fat absorption in the small intestine (Figure 13.38).[11,184]

Many new obesity drugs are under development. Based on the events that took place in the 1990s, several guidelines were developed for practitioners regarding the use of obesity medications:[7,11,187]

- Pharmacological agents are a useful adjunct to, but not a substitute for, the necessary changes in dietary and exercise habits.
- Drug therapy for treatment of obesity should be reserved for patients with a body mass index greater than 30 kg/m^2, or 27 kg/m^2 in the presence of associated comorbidities (e.g., hypertension, type 2 diabetes, dyslipidemia, osteoarthritis, and cardiovascular disease).[7,11]
- Moderately obese patients lose about 5–10% of their body weight (about 10–20 pounds) within 4–6 months of using appetite-suppressant drugs such as sibutramine. Most of the weight loss with drug therapy occurs within 6 months. Weight then tends to be maintained or to increase slightly for the duration of treatment. When the weight loss medications are discontinued, most patients tend to regain the weight that was lost, and several months after discontinuation, there is generally no difference between drug and placebo groups. In other words, these drugs produce a modest weight loss, and the achievement of desirable body weight requires a healthy lifestyle of proper dietary and exercise habits.
- Anorexiant agents should be used with caution and careful monitoring in patients with cardiac arrhythmias, symptomatic cardiovascular disease, diabetes, hypertension, depression, psychiatric illness, and severe systemic disease, such as liver or kidney failure. Anorexiant agents are contraindicated in patients taking monoamine oxidase inhibitors, in patients with glaucoma, and in pregnant and lactating women.
- Adverse effects noted for sibutramine therapy include increases in blood pressure and pulse.[185,188,190] With orlistat, a possible decrease in the absorption of fat-soluble vitamins, and oily and loose stools are side effects; a multivitamin supplement is recommended when taking this drug (see Table 13.3).[7,11,184]

In general, drugs should be used only as part of a comprehensive program that includes behavior therapy, diet, and physical activity.[7,11] Appropriate monitoring for side effects must be continued while drugs are part of the regimen. Since obesity is a chronic disease, the short-term use of drugs is not helpful. The health professional should include drugs only in the context of a long-term treatment strategy.[7,11]

Very-Low-Calorie Diets

Reducing diets fall into one of four categories:

- *Moderate deficit diet* (NHLBI recommended level).[7,11] 1,000–1,200 Calories/day for women, 1,200–1,600 Calories/day for men
- *Low-calorie diet.* 800–1,000 Calories/day for women, 800–1,200 Calories/day for men
- *Very-low-calorie diet* (VLCD). <800 Calories/day
- *Fasting.* <100 Calories/day

Formerly called the protein-sparing modified fast, the VLCD provides 400–800 Calories per day, or fewer than 12 Calories per kilogram of ideal body weight.[165–170,191–202] Protein is emphasized to help avoid loss of muscle tissue, with an intake of at least 1 gram of protein per kilogram of body weight recommended. Patients can use either special-formula beverages or natural foods such as fish, fowl, or lean meat (along with mineral and vitamin supplements). All subjects should receive 1.5 liters of water per day and supplementation of minerals, vitamins, and trace elements according to RDA. Carbohydrates are added to diminish ketosis.

In the 1970s, some very-low-calorie commercial preparations were made largely from collagen, a protein of low biological value.[195,196] Reports of sudden deaths and fatal heart arrhythmias led to a formal Public Health Service investigation. Fifty-eight cases of sudden, unexpected death were attributed to the low quantity and quality of the protein in the liquid preparations and to inadequate medical supervision. This report led to a more conservative use and attempts to improve the quality and balance of the nutrients. Most VLCDs now provide 45–100 grams of high-quality protein, carbohydrates, essential fatty acids, vitamins, minerals, and more Calories than initially used (420–800 Calories per day in most preparations). The amount of weight lost over 12–16 weeks with VLCDs providing 800 Calories a day is little different from those providing 420–600, probably the result of improved compliance on the part of the patient.[195] Serious complications of modern VLCDs are unusual.

The primary benefit of VLCDs is that they can produce large weight losses in a large proportion of patients.[194–195] Patients tend to lose 3–5 pounds a week on the VLCD, with the total loss after 12–16 weeks averaging 40–45 pounds. In contrast to fasting, for every 20 pounds lost on the VLCD, 5 of them (25%) are from the lean body mass and 15 (75%) from the fat tissue.[195] In that excess body weight is about one fourth lean body mass, this loss during the VLCD is to be expected. During the first 3–4 days, weight loss is rapid, with weight change due primarily to loss of body water and glycogen. After this, weight loss is slower and is related more to changes in the fat stores, with some loss of protein.[198] The resting metabolic rate falls 15–20% after just 2 weeks on the VLCD, partially negating the expected weight loss.[199] Upon refeeding, the metabolic rate when adjusted for the loss of fat-free mass is usually reported to be normal.

As with severe obesity, weight loss during the VLCD for moderately obese patients leads to improvement in blood lipids, blood pressure, glycemic control for diabetics, and psychological mood state.[195] Minor side effects during VLCD include fatigue, weakness, dizziness, constipation, hair loss, dry skin, brittle nails, nausea, diarrhea, changes in menses, edema, and cold intolerance. More significant side effects are gout and gallstones. Serum levels of uric acid may rise during VLCDs and lead to a gallbladder attack, especially in patients with a history of gout. Dieting with rapid weight loss appears to increase the risk of gallstone disease. Cardiac complications are considered extremely rare on modern VLCDs when appropriate screening and surveillance procedures are followed. A disadvantage of VLCD programs, as currently conducted, is their high cost (about $3,000 per program).[195] Over the long term, VLCD programs have been estimated to cost $630 per pound lost and maintained.[166]

Unfortunately, about half of patients do not complete VLCD programs, and for those who do, losses are poorly maintained unless unusual effort is expended by a team of dietitians, psychologists, exercise physiologists, and medical personnel for years following the initial program[197] (see Figures 13.35, 13.36, 13.39). In one study of 400 patients, half of the patients who started the VLCD program did not complete the treatment.[200] Patients who completed the treatment lost a mean of 84% of their excess weight but regained an average of 59–82% of their initial excess weight by 30 months follow-up. In another study of 4,026 obese patients in the Optifast (420 Calories protein supplement) treatment program, 25% of patients dropped out within the first 3 weeks.[201] Of the patients remaining in the program, 68% lost weight but did not reach their goal. Of this group, recidivism was extremely high, with only 5–10% maintaining weight loss after 18 months. Thirty-two percent of the patients successfully attained their goal weight. Of this group, 30% of women and 58% of men maintained weight loss to within 10 pounds of posttreatment weight for at least 18 months. Figure 13.39 shows that 3 years after a VLCD program, the average weight of the group differed little from the initial weight, and only 12% were able to maintain more than three fourths of the weight loss.[170]

VLCDs are not appropriate for everyone.[192,195] Selection criteria for VLCD candidates include failure at more conservative approaches to weight loss; a body mass index greater than 30 kg/m^2 (or indices of 27–30 kg/m^2 who have medical conditions that might respond to rapid weight loss); no serious medical conditions (recent heart attack, stroke, history of heart conduction problems, kidney or liver problems, cancer, type 1 diabetes, or significant psychiatric problems); high motivation; and willingness to commit to establishing new eating behaviors after therapy. The VLCD should be preceded by 2–4 weeks of a well-balanced 1,200 Calorie diet, should last 12–16 weeks, and should then be followed by a gradual refeeding period of 2–4 weeks with foods slowly introduced. During the VLCD, weekly medical exams, with serum electrolytes

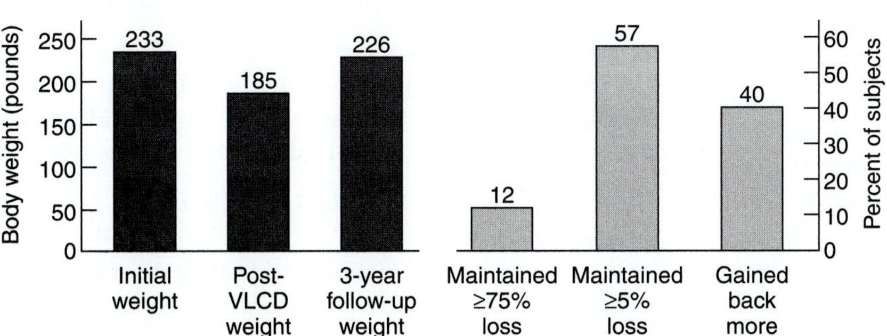

Figure 13.39 Three-year follow-up of 192 participants in a VLCD program. Three years after a VLCD program, average weight differed little from the initial weight, and only 12% were able to maintain more than three fourths of the weight loss. Source: Grodstein F, Levine R, Troy L, Spencer T, Colditz GA, Stampfer MJ. Three-year follow-up of participants in a commercial weight loss program. Can you keep it off? *Arch Intern Med* 156:1302–1306, 1996.

checked every 2 weeks, are recommended. All VLCD clients should continue in some type of maintenance program to avoid relapse. Behavior modification and aerobic exercise should be included during and after the VLCD.[202]

In 1998, the NHLBI recommended that VLCDs not be used routinely for weight loss therapy for several reasons:[7,11]

1. Energy deficits are too great.
2. Nutritional inadequacies will occur unless nutrient supplements are used.
3. Moderate energy restriction is just as effective as the VLCD in producing long-term weight loss.
4. Rapid weight reduction does not allow for gradual acquisition of changes in eating behavior.
5. Clients using VLCDs are at increased risk for gallstones.
6. They require special monitoring.

Weight Loss Programs and Methods

In their attempts to lose weight, American adults use many methods, including low-calorie foods and beverages, exercise, weight loss classes, medication, meal substitution, and self-imposed fasting.[203,204] Although many people attempt to lose weight on their own, a significant proportion use commercial products or join commercial weight loss programs.

People seeking help from commercial programs are urged to ask for valid and reliable data backing up claims and for additional information on program characteristics. Box 13.6 provides a listing of Internet sites that offer good information and programs for the treatment of obesity.

There are several characteristics of desirable weight loss programs for obese individuals.[203–207] These are described in Box 13.7.

As has been emphasized thus far in this chapter, a fundamental principle of weight loss and control is that for almost all people, a lifelong commitment to a change in lifestyle, behavioral responses, and dietary practices is necessary.[7,11,151] For most mildly obese people, modest goals and a slow course will maximize the probability of both losing the weight and keeping it off.

The whole concept of dieting can be criticized on psychological grounds, for going on a diet implies going off it and the resumption of old eating habits. For this reason, one can argue that the most effective diet is not a diet at all but rather a gradual change in eating patterns and a shift to foods that the person can continue to eat indefinitely. This means increasing the intake of complex carbohydrates, particularly in fruits, vegetables, legumes, and cereals, and decreasing the intake of fats and refined sugars. This course of action probably gives the best chance of maintaining the weight that is lost, and it is an eminently safe one. One should not lose weight by any method that cannot be included permanently within a healthy lifestyle.

In other words, the same diet that is being recommended for the treatment and prevention of heart disease, cancer, and diabetes is the same diet that should be used in preventing and treating obesity. This diet is high in carbohydrate, but low in fat. Complex carbohydrates as found in whole grains, vegetables, and fruits are emphasized, and only low-fat meats and dairy products are used. See Box 13.8 for a review of high-protein diets.

The Role of Exercise during Weight Loss

Thus far, this chapter has emphasized that regular exercise has proven to be a consistent indicator of the ability to maintain weight loss over the long term following periods of caloric restriction. Also, many studies have shown that obese people tend to exercise less than normal-weight individuals and that active people are leaner.

Box 13.6

Weight Management Internet Sites

National Heart, Lung, and Blood Institute (NHLBI) (www.nhlbi.nih.gov)
Includes consumer information on weight management and clinical guidelines on overweight and obesity for professionals.

Weight-Control Information Network (WIN) (www.niddk.nih.gov)
A reliable source of weight control, obesity, and nutrition information for consumers and health professionals. A service of the National Institute of Diabetes and Digestive and Kidney Diseases, National Institutes of Health, and U.S. Department of Health and Human Services.

Weightfocus.com (www.weightfocus.com)
Offers visitors a wide variety of webcast programming featuring weight management experts, complemented by in-depth articles on weight loss strategies, diet myths, and health issues.

Shape Up America! (www.shapeup.org)
Provides information on safe weight management, healthy eating, and physical fitness.

Diettalk (www.diettalk.com)
A comprehensive source of information on obesity, nutrition, physical activity, diets, and eating disorders.

Cyberdiet (www.cyberdiet.com)
A complete source of information on diet and nutrition, exercise and fitness, weight loss, and self-assessment of body fat distribution and disease risk.

American Anorexia Bulimia Association, Inc. (www.aabainc.org)
Gives complete information about eating disorders for sufferers, family and friends, and professionals.

Box 13.7

Choosing a Safe and Successful Weight Loss Program

Many overweight people lose weight on their own without entering a weight loss program. Others need the social and professional support that commercial weight loss programs provide. Almost any of the commercial weight loss programs can work on the short term, but they may not promote safe and healthy habits that can be followed over the long term.

What elements of a weight loss program should one look for in judging its potential for safe and successful weight loss? Look for these features:

- *Provides or encourages food intake that exceeds 1,200 Calories per day for a woman and 1,600 Calories per day for a man.* Diets lower than this amount are not recommended for most overweight and obese individuals because they are typically low in essential vitamins and minerals and can lead to excess muscle loss and lower metabolism.
- *The diet is nutritionally safe.* It should include all the vitamins and minerals at recommended intake levels. Although low in Calories, it should be based on the food guide pyramid, providing servings from all the recommended food groups. High-protein diets are not recommended. Weight loss diets should promote health, not harm it.
- *Promotes a safe and realistic weight loss of 1–2 pounds per week.* Good weight-management programs don't promise or imply dramatic, rapid weight loss. Don't seek a "quick fix" because the quicker the weight comes off, the quicker it goes back on. Although not as appealing, slow and gradual weight loss is more effective.
- *Does not attempt to make one dependent on special products that are sold for a profit.* The best programs emphasize wise choices from the traditional food supply and feature supermarket and restaurant tours and cooking schools to teach you how to improve food selection and meal preparation. Learn how to improve eating habits within the context of one's own social, cultural, and income background.
- *Does not promote or sell products that are unproven or spurious.* Companies sell a wide array of weight loss products that have little if any value, including starch blockers, grapefruit pills, sauna belts, body wraps, ear staples, and hormone releasers.
- *Is led by a qualified instructor.* Health-promotion professionals, registered dietitians, and physicians specializing in weight control are qualified to direct weight-control programs. Check out the experience and credentials of the weight-control program leaders before signing up.
- *Includes a maintenance phase.* It is difficult to change behaviors that have formed over many years. Relapse often occurs during stressful life events. Weight-control programs should provide support on a regular basis for at least 1 year after one has lost weight.
- *Emphasizes a lifestyle approach.* Good programs include guidance on exercise, diet, and behavior change that are continued for a lifetime, not just the duration of the program.

Although it is often accepted that physical activity is a powerful tool in the treatment of obesity, the best-designed research studies have failed to support this belief. In fact, most researchers in this area now regard exercise as a relatively weak weapon in the "battle of the bulge," with control of caloric intake representing the real power behind weight loss efforts.[208–214]

There are several misconceptions regarding the role of exercise in the treatment of obesity. These are summarized in Box 13.9. Each of these is explained in turn, with the true benefits reviewed later in this chapter.

Misconception 1: Aerobic Exercise Accelerates Weight Loss Significantly, When Combined with a Reducing Diet

Some obese people have been led to believe that if they start brisk walking 2–3 miles a day, significant amounts of body weight will be lost quickly. Most research does not support this idea, even when the exercise program lasts several months. For example, in a randomized, controlled, 1-year study of 160 females and 197 males, three or five 30- to 40-minute exercise sessions per week had no significant effect on body weight despite a 5–8% improvement in cardiorespiratory endurance.[215] Many other studies have come to the same conclusion that when young and old alike exercise moderately in a free-living condition (with no diet control), this amount of exercise ends up being an insufficient stimulus to affect body weight significantly.[208–214,216–220]

It has been argued that when people begin exercising, they may start eating more, negating the increased energy expenditure from initiation of regular exercise. Instead, perhaps they may alter other areas of their lifestyle (e.g., resting more than normal during the remainder of the day after exercise), diluting the effect of added exercise. For these reasons, researchers have tested the effects of exercise under controlled dietary conditions, where all subjects are fed the same amount of food, while some exercise and others remain

Box 13.8

An Evaluation of Low-Carbohydrate, High-Protein Diets

Low-carbohydrate, high-protein diets are back. These diets have been around since the 1930s, but were first popularized in the 1970s when liquid protein diets and Dr. Atkins' first book on the high-protein diet hit the market. The liquid protein diets were made of poor-quality protein and provided only 300–500 Calories per day. By the late 1970s, 58 deaths were related to the liquid protein diet. Dr. Atkins promoted a low-carbohydrate, high-protein diet as the best way to lose weight quickly. Several studies refuted the usefulness and healthfulness of this diet and other similar plans, and the public moved on to other schemes.

Well, they're back. Today, most best-selling diet books push low-carbohydrate, high-protein diets as the superior method to lose weight. These low-carbohydrate diets (less than 30% of Calories) are higher in fat (30–80% of Calories) and protein (30–40% of Calories) than is recommended for health.

These books all recommend building breakfast, lunch, and dinner around eggs, meat, or fish. High-carbohydrate foods such as pasta, bread, rice, potatoes, sugar-rich desserts, and most fruits are restricted. If you follow these rules, the authors say, one can eat more than normal while losing body fat.

Despite lack of support from reputable health professionals, low-carbohydrate, high-protein and high-fat diets are extremely popular. During the past decade, most of the top-selling diet books emphasized carbohydrate restriction or "bad carbs" versus "good carbs." Leading the charge is the Atkins diet plan. The Atkins group food guide pyramid has protein sources such as beef, pork, and poultry at the foundation, with the rest of the pyramid plan devoted to helping people follow a restricted carbohydrate lifestyle.

What about studies showing that the Atkins diet is not only effective at weight loss, but helps decrease blood cholesterol and levels of other heart disease risk factors? Here is a summary of results from these studies comparing low-carbohydrate diets with conventional diets (low-fat, moderate-to-high carbohydrate)[203–207]:

- Weight loss is similar, especially when subjects are studied for 1 year or longer.
- Both types of diets suffer from high attrition rates and poor adherence.
- Improvements in disease risk factors are also similar, supporting the adage that weight loss by any means is a good thing, but only for the short term.
- Low-carbohydrate diets are high in cholesterol and saturated fat, and deficient in dietary fiber and some nutrients, especially calcium, folic acid, antioxidants, and phytochemicals.

Most long-term epidemiological studies indicate that the low-carbohydrate, high-fat dietary pattern promotes heart disease, colon cancer, and osteoporosis. Populations with high-carbohydrate diets have low heart disease and cancer death rates, along with high life expectancy. Case examples include the Japanese with their rice-based diets supplemented with fish and vegetables, and people living along the Mediterranean basin who enjoy their pasta, fruits, vegetables, legumes, olives, nuts, and olive oil, while largely avoiding red meats.

The cause of the U.S. obesity epidemic is simple—Americans are eating too much and exercising too little. Fad diets such as the Atkins diet are not the solution because they postpone the ultimate decision to get diet and exercise habits under control. People can't live on the Atkins diet for the rest of their lives because of the elevated heart disease and cancer risk. In general, obese individuals should not lose weight by any method that they cannot live with healthfully for the rest of their lives.

---

sedentary. Even under these conditions, exercise has been found to add little to the weight loss.[221–230]

Figures 13.40 and 13.41 portray the typical findings of researchers who have tested the effect of moderate exercise in accelerating weight loss during a reducing diet.[224,229] In the study summarized in Figure 13.40, 91 obese women were randomized into one of four groups for the 12-week study: control (no exercise or special diet), walking (five 45-minute walking sessions per week at 75% maximum heart rate), diet (1,300 Calories/day), and both diet and walking.[224] In this well-controlled study, walking alone was an insufficient stimulus to decrease body weight compared to the control group. Subjects in the two diet groups lost between 17 and 18 pounds on average (about 1.5 pounds of weight loss per week), with walking providing no added benefit. For the two diet groups, 80–90% of the weight loss was body fat, and walking did not affect this proportion.

Results shown in Figure 13.41 are from a 90-day study of 69 moderately obese females who each were put on a VLCD of 520 Calories a day.[229] Subjects were randomized into four groups: diet only, diet plus aerobic training, diet plus weight training, and diet plus aerobic and weight training. Aerobic training consisted of four sessions a week, with duration increasing from 20 minutes up to 60 minutes per session by the end of the study, at 70% of the heart rate reserve. The weight trainers exercised four times a week, engaging in two to three sets, 6–8 repetitions of several exercises at 70–80% of their one-repetition maximum. As shown in Figure 13.41, exercise had no significant effect on weight loss, with each group losing about 46 pounds, with three fourths of the loss

Box 13.9

Misconceptions Regarding the Role of Exercise in the Treatment of Obesity

Following are some of the most common misconceptions about the role of exercise in weight loss.

1. Accelerates weight loss significantly when combined with a reducing diet
2. Causes the resting metabolic rate to stay elevated for a long time after the bout, burning extra Calories
3. Counters the diet-induced decrease in resting metabolic rate
4. Counters the diet-induced decrease in fat-free mass

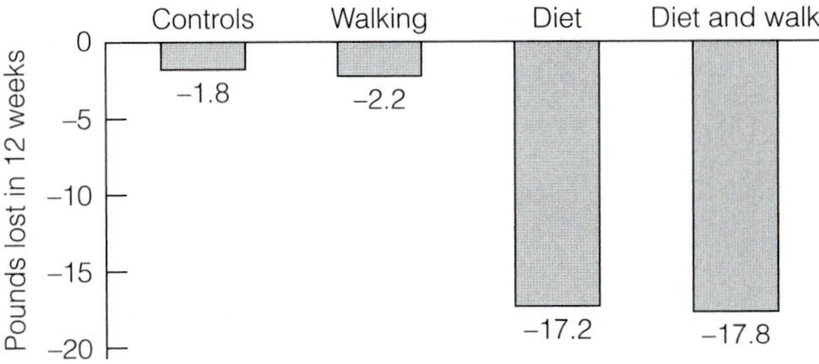

Figure 13.40 Body weight changes in response to diet and/or exercise, 12-week study of 91 obese women; diet = 1,300 Calories/day; exercise = five 45-minute walk session/week, 75% MHR. Exercise alone had little effect on weight loss and did not accelerate weight loss significantly beyond the effects due to the reducing diet. Source: Utter AC, Nieman DC, Shannonhouse EM, Butterworth DE, Nieman CN. Influence of diet and/or exercise on body composition and cardiorespiratory fitness in obese women. *Int J Sport Nutr* 8:213–222, 1998.

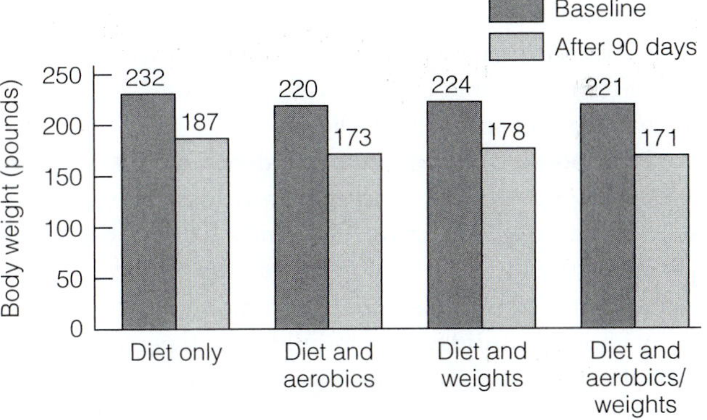

Figure 13.41 Moderate exercise does not enhance weight loss during dieting; 90-day study of 69 obese females, all on 520-Calorie/day formula: Exercise had no effect on RMR (10% decrease) or LBW (¼ of 46-pound loss). Source: Donnelly JE, Pronk NP, Jacobsen DJ, Pronk SJ, Jakicic JM. Effects of a very-low-calorie diet and physical training regimens on body composition and resting metabolic rate in obese females. *Am J Clin Nutr* 54:56–61, 1991.

being fat mass and the other fourth, lean body weight (LBW). Exercise also had no effect on the fall in resting metabolic rate (RMR), which averaged about 10% for all groups.

These and other studies demonstrate that in obesity treatment programs lasting 12–20 weeks, only a few extra pounds, at best, will be lost when moderate amounts of aerobic exercise (2–7 hours per week) are combined with a reducing diet.[208–234] Figure 13.42 shows a summary graph of a meta-analysis of 493 studies conducted over a 25-year period.[212] During a typical 15-week program, the combination of diet and exercise can be expected to cause a 24.2-pound weight loss, little different than the 23.5 pounds from diet alone. It appears that in order for aerobic exercise to have a major effect on reduction of body weight, daily exercise sessions need to be unusually long in duration (more than 1 hour) and high in intensity, something that most obese people cannot do.[228,234,235]

There are several reasons for the weak effect of moderate exercise on weight loss, the primary one being that the net energy expenditure of such exercise sessions is small. From a quantitative point of view, the energy cost of formal exercise is much less than most people believe.[210] The net energy cost of exercise equals the Calories expended during the exercise session minus the Calories expended for the resting metabolic rate and other activities that individuals would have been doing had they not been formally exercising.[231]

For example, the net energy cost of a 3-mile, 45-minute walk for a 70-kg obese woman is only about 130–140 Calories (215 total Calories minus 50 Calories for the RMR and 25 to 35 for incidental activity) (see Figure 13.43). One pound of human fat contains approximately 3,500 calories, which means that if all else stayed exactly the same, it would take nearly one month of daily brisk walking (3 miles each session) to lose 1 pound of fat. Many obese people find walking 2–3 miles a day to be the most they can handle without injury, yet much more than this is necessary if significant weight loss is to be achieved.[234,235]

As emphasized by University of Vermont obesity researchers, "The types and intensities of exercise that carry a high energy expenditure for a single bout are basically confined to those that can be undertaken by elite athletes or subjects with an excellent level of physical fitness. On a clinical basis, and especially for the obese patient, it would be unrealistic (even dangerous) to expect [such] a level of exercise performance."[210]

Also, some people may "reward" themselves with extra food (in free-living conditions) or by resting and sitting more after exercising, negating the energy expenditure of the entire exercise bout. A team of researchers from Loughborough University in England had women walk 2.5 hours a week for a whole year and were unable to measure any decrease in body fat, even though the women did not change their diets. The researchers concluded that the walkers may have rested more throughout the day after their walk, thereby erasing the effects of the walking session.[220]

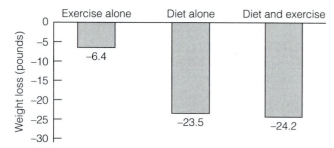

Figure 13.42 Average weight loss during 15-week interventions with diet and/or exercise, meta-analysis of 493 studies over a 25-year period. Exercise alone has a relatively minor effect on weight loss and does not add much to the weight loss effects of a reducing diet. Source: Miller WC, Koceja DM, Hamilton EJ. A meta-analysis of the past 25 years of weight loss research using diet, exercise or diet plus exercise intervention. *Int J Obes Relat Metab Disord* 21:941–947, 1997.

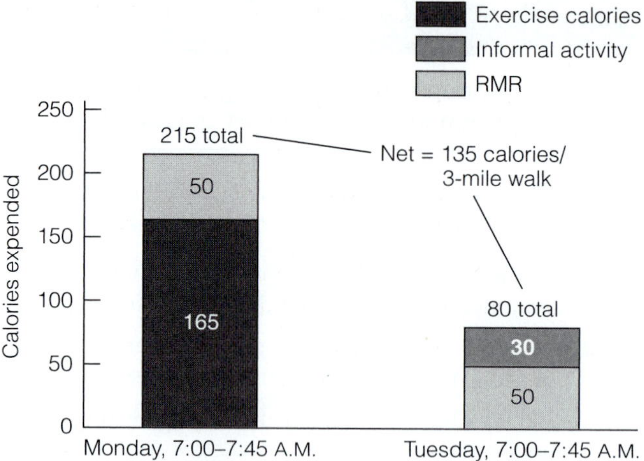

Figure 13.43 The concept of net energy expenditure: Net energy expenditure = gross energy expended − RMR − informal exercise Calories. The net caloric expenditure of moderate exercise is much smaller than many people realize—in this example, only 135 Calories.

The practical advice from these studies is that exercise alone must not be seen as a major weapon in the treatment of obesity. Instead, improvements in the quality and quantity of the diet should take the lead, with exercise relegated to an important supporting role.

In response to accumulating evidence, the 2005 *Dietary Guidelines for Americans* recommends increasing exercise for some adults to as much as an hour and a half a day to maintain a healthy weight.[226] Following are the physical activity recommendations. Notice that the amount of physical activity varies according to the individual and personal goals, with the greatest duration reserved for adults trying to sustain weight loss:

- To reduce the risk of chronic disease in adulthood, engage in at least 30 minutes of moderate-intensity physical activity, above usual activity, at work or home on most days of the week.
- For most people, greater health benefits can be obtained by engaging in physical activity of more vigorous intensity or longer duration.
- To help manage body weight and prevent gradual, unhealthy body weight gain in adulthood, engage in approximately 60 minutes of moderate- to vigorous-intensity activity on most days of the week while not exceeding caloric intake requirements.
- To sustain weight loss in adulthood, participate in at least 60 to 90 minutes of daily moderate-intensity physical activity while not exceeding caloric intake requirements. Some people may need to consult with a health-care provider before participating in this level of activity.

Misconception 2: Exercise Causes the Resting Metabolic Rate to Stay Elevated for a Long Time After the Bout, Burning Extra Calories

Another common misconception is that aerobic exercise causes the resting metabolic rate (RMR) to stay elevated for a long time after the bout, burning extra Calories. In general, most researchers have found that the energy expended after aerobic exercise is small unless a great amount of high-intensity exercise is engaged in.[236–241] For example, jogging (12 minutes per mile), walking, or cycling at moderate intensities (40–60% aerobic capacity) for about one half hour causes the RMR to stay elevated for 20–30 minutes, burning 10–12 extra Calories.[236,240] When the intensity is increased to about 75%, RMR is increased for about 35–45 minutes, with 15–30 extra Calories expended. Obviously, this amount of caloric expenditure following exercise is too little to have any significant effect on body weight loss. Even when the duration is quite long (e.g., 80 minutes), the amount of Calories expended afterward through elevation of the RMR is low unless the intensity is high during the entire exercise bout[237–239] (see Figures 13.44 and 13.45). For the obese individual who takes a 20- to 30-minute walk, at most, about 10 extra Calories will be burned afterward, hardly enough to be meaningful when balanced against other diet and energy expenditure factors.[210,239]

Is there a chronic effect of exercise training on the RMR beyond that expected with increase in fat-free mass? Potentially, any effect of exercise on the RMR could be important because it represents such a large percentage of the total energy expenditure.[210] There has been some disagreement among researchers on this issue, with some concluding that trained individuals (especially elite athletes) have higher RMRs than sedentary people (when adjusted for differences in lean body weight[242–244]), while others have been unable to establish significant differences.[245–247] However, there is a growing consensus that when differences in RMR between active and inactive individuals have been found, this has been due more to the acute effect of the previous day's exercise bout (in athletes) than to any real chronic adaptation.[248–250] When athletes

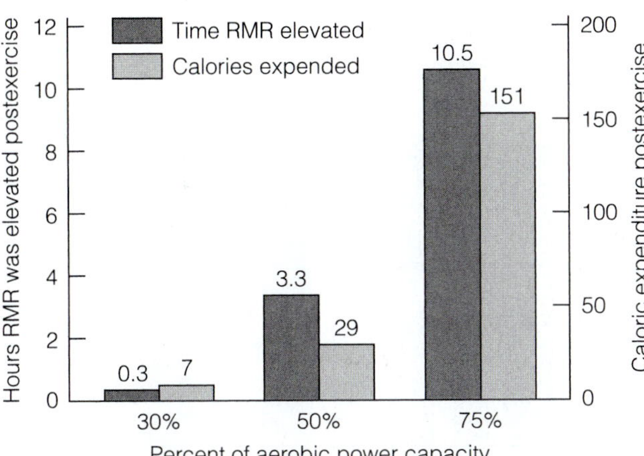

Figure 13.44 Calories burned after 80 minutes of cycling at different intensities, subjects rested in bed for 14 hours postexercise. This study shows the importance of intensity for postexercise RMR elevation. Eighty minutes of high-intensity cycling resulted in 151 extra Calories being burned after exercise. However, most obese individuals are incapable of this amount of exercise. Source: Bahr R, Sejersted OM. Effect of intensity of exercise on excess postexercise oxygen consumption. *Metabolism* 40:836–841, 1991.

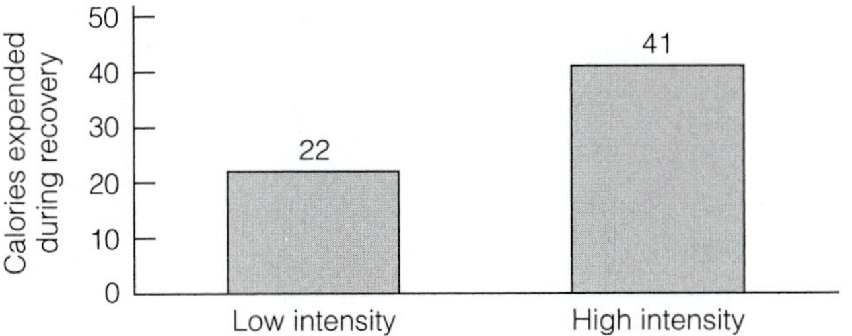

Figure 13.45 Postexercise energy expenditure in women, low-intensity cycling (80 minutes, 50% $\dot{V}O_{2max}$) versus high-intensity (50 minutes, 70% $\dot{V}O_{2max}$). High-intensity exercise for 50 minutes results in a higher postexercise energy expenditure than low-intensity exercise for 80 minutes. Source: Phelain JF, Reinke E, Harris MA, Melby CL. Postexercise energy expenditure and substrate oxidation in young women resulting from exercise bouts of different intensity. *J Am College Nutr* 16:140–146, 1997.

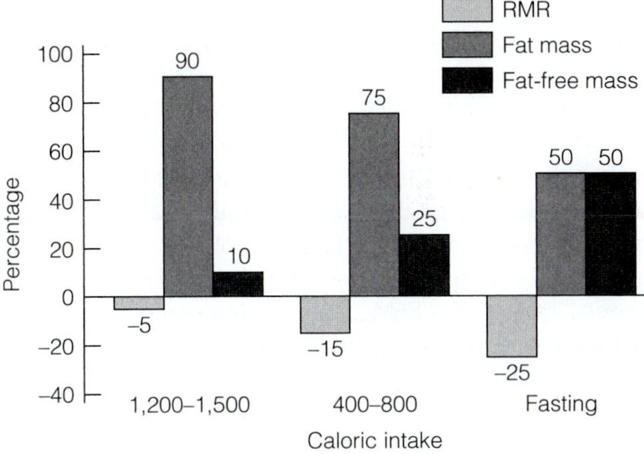

Figure 13.46 Caloric restriction, effect on resting metabolic rate, fat mass, and fat-free mass. Both the resting metabolic rate and the fat-free mass are decreased in parallel with the degree of caloric restriction.

have been tested 2 days after hard exercise, no difference in RMR has been found.[248,250] These researchers have suggested that when athletes don't exercise, they also don't eat as much, which means they have a lower caloric turnover and therefore normal RMRs. When training is heavy and food intake is higher, caloric turnover is elevated, along with the RMR. Although these findings are interesting to academicians and researchers, for obese individuals, they have no practical significance because the amount of exercise they can engage in will be too little to have any true chronic effect on RMR beyond that achieved by their higher fat-free mass.

Misconception 3: Exercise Counters the Diet-Induced Decrease in Resting Metabolic Rate

During caloric restriction, the resting metabolic rate drops substantially and is related to the rate of weight loss, averaging 10–20% for VLCDs and up to 20–30% for long-term fasting (see Figure 13.46). Can exercise during caloric restriction counter this diet-induced decrease in the RMR?

Most studies do not support this idea, and when a protective effect of exercise training on RMR is found, it is rather small.[210,211,226–229,251–255] For example, in one study, 12 mildly obese women were put onto 530-Calorie/day diets for 28 days and an exercise program (three sessions per week, 30–45 minutes at 60% $\dot{V}O_{2max}$). RMR dropped 16% despite the exercise program.[252] In another study, half of 13 mildly obese subjects on a 4-week VLCD (720 Calories/day) exercised a total of 27 hours at 50% $\dot{V}O_{2max}$.[251] RMR dropped more in the exercise group than in the sedentary group (10% for both groups in the first week, but then a further 17% drop in the exercise group). Apparently, the exercise session prompted energy conservation in the dieting obese subjects, decreasing the RMR.[254] Figure 13.47 suggests that even when obese subjects are on a mild energy-deficit diet (1,200 Calories/day), aerobic or weight training is an insufficient stimulus to counter the drop in RMR.[253]

Figure 13.48 shows the results of a study reviewed previously[213] (Figure 13.41). Notice that neither aerobic nor resistive training had any effect on the drop in RMR induced by the 520-Calorie/day diet. This may have been because the fat-free mass dropped equally in all groups, important because the RMR is so tightly connected to it.

Misconception 4: Exercise Counters the Diet-Induced Decrease in Fat-Free Mass

During weight loss, the percentage lost as fat-free mass (FFM) increases in proportion to the severity of the caloric deficit. With total fasting, the body weight loss is close to 50% fat and 50% FFM.[256] During a VLCD (with appropriate protein intake), the proportions improve to 75% fat and 25% FFM.[213,229] While on a 1,200–1,500-Calorie diet, the proportions improve even more to 90% fat and 10% fat-free

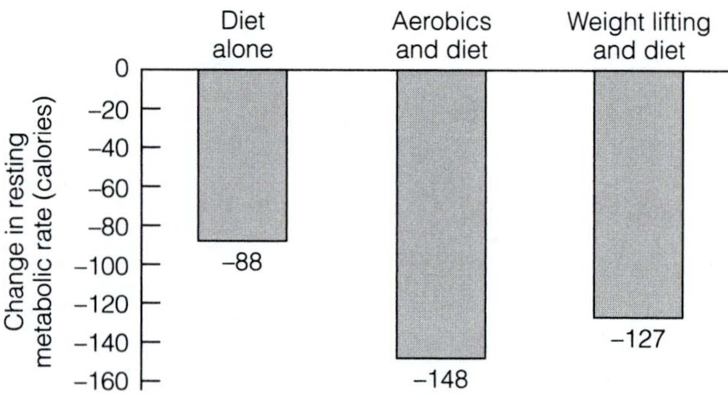

Figure 13.47 Change in resting metabolic rate with diet and/or exercise, 65 moderately obese subjects, 8-week intervention; all on formula diet, 70% RMR (1,200 Calories/day), with exercise three times/week; weight training = three sets, 6 reps, eight stations; aerobics = leg and arm cycling, 70% MHR. Aerobic and weight training were not sufficient to counter diet-induced decrements in RMR. Source: Geliebter A, Maher MM, Gerace L, Gutin B, Heymsfield SB, Hashim SA. Effects of strength or aerobic training on body composition, resting metabolic rate, and peak oxygen consumption in obese dieting subjects. *Am J Clin Nutr* 66:557–563, 1997.

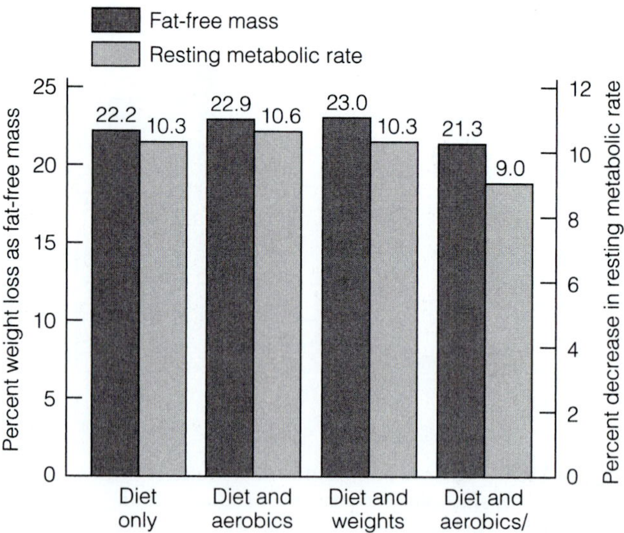

Figure 13.48 Exercise does not counter diet-induced decreases in RMR and FFM; 90-day study of 69 obese females, all on 520-Calorie/day formula, aerobic exercise = 4 days/week, 20 minutes, progressing to 60 minutes/session; weights = 4 days/week, 2–3 sets, 6–8 repetitions. Source: Donnelly JE, Pronk NP, Jacobsen DJ, Pronk SJ, Jakicic JM. Effects of a very-low-calorie diet and physical training regimens on body composition and resting metabolic rate in obese females. *Am J Clin Nutr* 54:56–61, 1991.

mass[221] (see Figure 13.46). Thus the degree of caloric deprivation appears to be the major controlling factor in determining the magnitude of loss from FFM. As explained earlier in this chapter, excess weight in obese individuals is about 75% fat, 25% FFM. Thus, during weight reduction, some loss of FFM is expected and probably desirable.[257]

Can exercise counter the diet-induced decrease in FFM (if this is the desire of the patient)? In general, both moderate aerobic and strength training programs have been found to have little effect (see reviews[211,213,214,257]). As depicted in Figure 13.48, despite fairly rigorous aerobic and resistive training programs by moderately obese females, FFM still represented about 22% of the 46 pounds that were lost by each group.[213] In another 90-day study, FFM represented one fourth the weight loss in moderately obese females who were on an 800-Calorie diet, despite engaging in strength training three times a week and showing significant improvements in strength (see Figure 13.49).[258]

In general, it appears that the caloric deficit is dominant in its effects on the FFM, with moderate amounts of exercise representing an insufficient stimulus to alter the decrease.

Some individuals trying to lose body fat have been led to believe that the optimal exercise intensity for fat burning is low intensity (e.g., moderate walking). Figure 13.50 shows that when the same individuals exercise moderately (50% $\dot{V}O_{2max}$) or very intensely (80% $\dot{V}O_{2max}$) for 45 minutes, the proportion of fat Calories expended is three times greater with moderate exercise (49% versus 16%).[259] However, the moderate exercise bout burns about 40% fewer total Calories. Because 1 pound of body fat is about 3,500 Calories, and any type of food Calorie can be turned into body fat (carbohydrate, protein, or fat); what really matters is energy balance—expending more energy than what is consumed.

Several studies have now confirmed that vigorous and intense, compared to moderate, exercise is associated with a greater reduction in body fat, especially from the abdominal area.[260–264] For example, in a large study of more than 2,000 middle-aged and elderly men and women in the Netherlands, intensive physical activity such as playing sports was negatively associated with abdominal fat.[262] Another study of more than 2,500 men and women in Canada showed that higher-intensity exercise was associated with a preferential reduction in abdominal fat.[263] There is some evidence that fat in the abdominal, compared to the gluteal, area is more responsive to lipolysis or breakdown from epinephrine (which is elevated during vigorous but not moderate exercise).[264] Thus, brisk activity is recommended for overweight individuals when possible because physical training is viewed as an important nonpharmacological tool in the treatment of abdominal obesity and associated metabolic disorders.[261] However, moderately and severely obese subjects should first bring their body mass index below 30 kg/m^2 before concerning themselves with exercise intensity, due to the injury potential (see section on precautions).

Benefits of Exercise for Weight Loss

If exercise training has relatively little effect during weight loss programs in accelerating weight loss, or in protecting diet-induced decreases in the RMR and the FFM, then why should obese patients exercise? The main reason is to improve their health. Moderate exercise may be a weak weapon in promoting a great deal of weight loss, but it has much greater power in enhancing health (see Figure 13.51). As outlined in Box 13.10, there are at least five health-related benefits of exercise for obese patients.

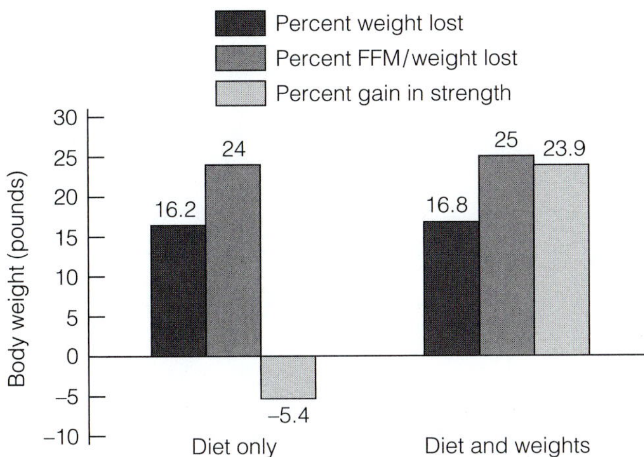

Figure 13.49 Effect of resistance training during weight loss, 14 obese females on 800-VLCD formula for 90 days, three session/week, eight exercises, 3–4 sets, 70–80% 1-RM. During 800-Calorie diets, obese women who lift weights increase their strength but do not experience greater weight loss or protection of their fat-free mass. Source: Donnelly JE, Sharp T, Houmard J, et al. Muscle hypertrophy with large-scale weight loss and resistance training. *Am J Clin Nutr* 58:561–565, 1993.

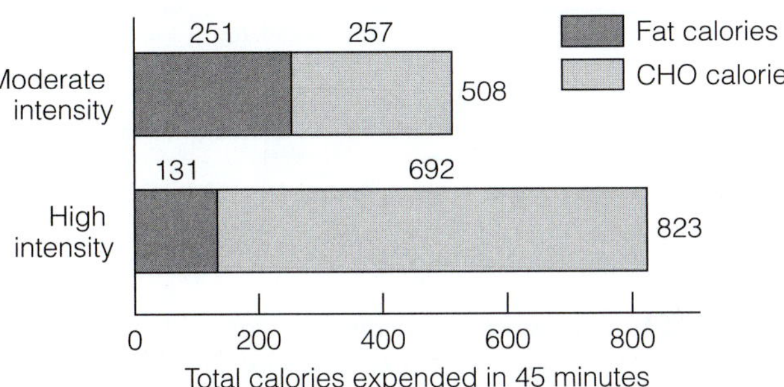

Figure 13.50 Calories from fat and carbohydrate during exercise, 45 minutes of high- (80% $\dot{V}O_{2max}$) versus moderate- (50% $\dot{V}O_{2max}$) intensity exercise. Although moderate exercise may burn more fat Calories than high-intensity exercise, the total Calories expended per unit of time is far less.
Source: Nieman DC, Miller AR, Henson DA, Warren BJ, Gusewitch G, Johnson RL, David JM, Butterworth DE, Herring JL, Nehlsen-Cannarella SL. The effects of high versus moderate-intensity exercise on lymphocyte subpopulations and proliferative response. *Int J Sports Med* 15:199–206, 1994.

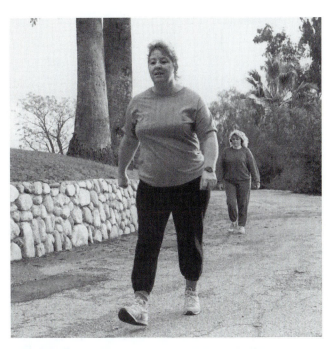

Figure 13.51 Regular aerobic exercise such as brisk walking is associated with several important health benefits for the obese.

Box 13.10

Benefits of Moderate Aerobic Exercise for the Obese Individual

Regular exercise by the obese individual is associated with:

1. Improved cardiorespiratory endurance $\dot{V}O_{2max}$
2. Improved blood lipid profile, in particular decreased triglycerides and increased HDL-C, with weight loss more responsible for decreases in total cholesterol and LDL-C
3. Improved psychological state, especially increased general well-being and vigor and decreased anxiety and depression
4. Enhanced group social support, which may improve long-term maintenance of weight loss
5. Decreased risk of obesity-related diseases (e.g., diabetes, heart disease, cancer, hypertension)

Each of these benefits is reviewed in detail elsewhere in this textbook and is perhaps even more important for obese individuals. The improvement in $\dot{V}O_{2max}$ by obese individuals following moderate aerobic exercise programs has been found to vary from 10% to 25% after 5–15 weeks of exercise[224] (see Figures 13.52 and 13.53).

As reviewed in Chapter 10, weight loss is associated with a dramatic improvement in the blood lipid profile. A consistent finding is that with weight loss, total cholesterol, LDL-C, and triglycerides decrease, while HDL-C increases.[265] The independent effect of aerobic exercise, however, is limited to improving the magnitude of change in the triglycerides and HDL-C, but not total cholesterol and LDL-C.

In addition to the physiological benefits, exercise is associated with feelings of well-being, a reduction in anxiety and depression, and a positive self-concept and elevated mood (see Chapter 14). The strong evidence in this area provides additional support for including exercise within weight loss programs.[227,253] During weight loss, many individuals experience feelings of depression and irritability, which exercise can help counter. Figure 13.54 shows that exercise and diet together improved depression scores more than diet alone did.[253]

In most obesity studies, subjects exercise together. The social interaction during the weeks of exercising may

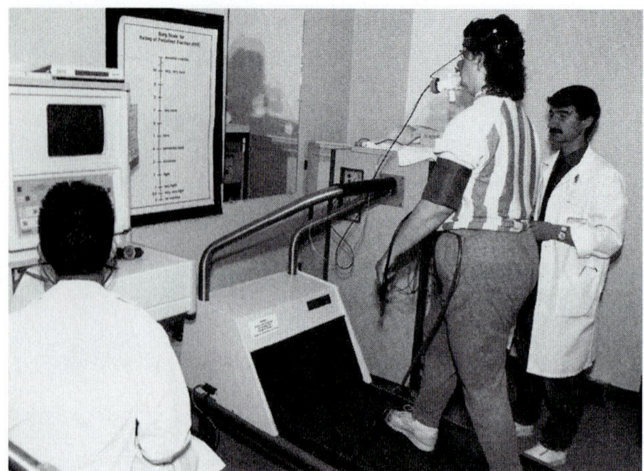

Figure 13.52 Most studies show that a brisk walking program increases $\dot{V}O_{2max}$ in obese subjects.

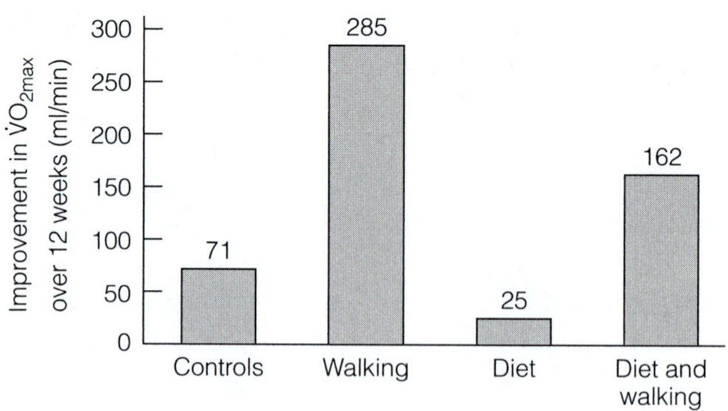

Figure 13.53 $\dot{V}O_{2max}$ changes in response to diet and/or exercise, 12-week study of 91 obese women; diet = 1,300 Calories/day; exercise = five 45-minute walk sessions/week, 75% MHR. Regular brisk walking significantly improves $\dot{V}O_{2max}$ in obese women, whether they are on or off of a reducing diet. Source: Utter AC, Nieman DC, Shannonhouse EM, Butterworth DE, Nieman CN. Influence of diet and/or exercise on body composition and cardiorespiratory fitness in obese women. *Int J Sport Nutr* 8:213–222, 1998.

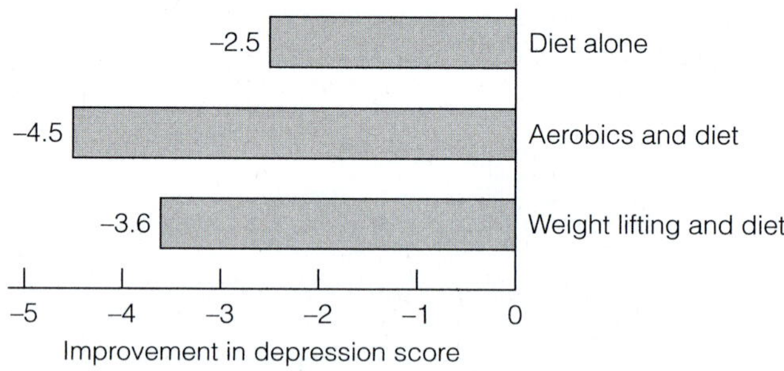

Figure 13.54 Improvement in depression score with diet and/or exercise, in 65 moderately obese subjects, 8-week intervention; all on formula diet, 70% RMR (1,200 Calories/day), with exercise three times/week: weight training = three sets, 6 reps, eight stations; aerobics = leg and arm cycling, 70% MHR. Source: Geliebter A, Maher MM, Gerace L, Gutin B, Heymsfield SB, Hashim SA. Effects of strength or aerobic training on body composition, resting metabolic rate, and peak oxygen consumption in obese dieting subjects. *Am J Clin Nutr* 66:557–563, 1997.

enhance long-term maintenance of the weight loss. As reviewed earlier in this chapter, exercise has emerged as one of the best predictors of weight loss maintenance (see Box 13.11). Exercise may also provide ancillary benefits such as increased group cohesiveness, communication, and opportunities for information passage that persist for months after the program is over.

As discussed at the beginning of this chapter, obesity is associated with many complications, such as heart disease, diabetes, high blood pressure, and high blood cholesterol levels. There is strong evidence that exercise can help to counter each of these complications (see Chapters 10 through 15). As reviewed earlier, there is some evidence that people who exercise regularly accumulate less fat in the abdominal area than inactive people, promoting a more favorable fat distribution.[266,267] This may be one reason why active people tend to be protected against various chronic diseases and have fewer risk factors for them.

In summary, then, moderate aerobic exercise during weight reduction helps to improve the health status of the individual, while the real power behind weight loss comes from a reduction in the amount of Calories (in particular, the dietary fat) consumed. A moderate reduction in Calories (to about 1,200–1,500/day for mildly obese individuals) promotes loss of fat weight while sparing the lean body weight, whereas aerobic exercise improves the fitness and health status of the dieting individual. As summarized in Box 13.11, physical activity has stronger effects on preventing weight gain and maintaining weight loss than in treating obesity.

Exercise Prescription and Precautions for the Obese

According to the NHLBI Obesity Education Initiative, physical activity should be an integral part of weight loss therapy and weight maintenance. Initially, moderate levels of physical activity for 30–45 minutes, 3–5 days per week, should be encouraged.[7,11]

Many obese people live sedentary lives, have little training or skills in physical activity, and are difficult to motivate toward increasing their activity. For these reasons, some people may require supervision when starting a physical activity regimen. The need to avoid injury during physical activity is a high priority.

Extremely obese persons may need to start with simple exercises that can be intensified gradually. For most obese patients, physical activity should be initiated slowly, and the intensity should be increased gradually. Initial activities may be increasing small tasks of daily living such as taking the stairs or walking or swimming at a slow pace. With time, depending on progress, the amount of weight lost, and functional capacity, the patient may engage in more strenuous activities.

A regimen of daily walking is an attractive form of physical activity for many people, particularly those who are overweight or obese. The patient can start by walking 10 minutes, 3 days a week, and can build to 30–45 minutes of more intense

Box 13.11

Role of Physical Activity in Weight Management

Physical activity is a critical strategy in the "battle of the bulge." It makes sense that if 1 pound of fat contains 3,500 surplus Calories, one has to burn these Calories through extra activity to lose the fat.

Physical activity can influence body weight in three different ways:

- Prevent weight gain in the first place. Near-daily physical activity that is continued month after month, year after year, lowers the risk of weight gain with age. Most adults gain weight slowly, about 1 pound a year on average according to most estimates. At the same time, muscle mass is slowly lost while body fat increases. This slow change in the quality and quantity of body weight is countered by regular physical activity if the diet is also kept under good control. In other words, one of the chief benefits of near-daily physical activity is the capacity to fight off the "creeping obesity" that most adults experience from ages 25 to 65.
- Help one lose weight if overweight or obese. Does aerobic exercise accelerate weight loss significantly when combined with a reducing diet? The answer is "yes," but for most overweight and obese people, the extra weight lost is small when compared to that caused by the diet. Because most overweight people can only exercise moderately, the actual amount of energy expended tends to be lower than expected, and has a rather small impact on weight loss during a 2–4 month reducing diet. The practical advice is that exercise alone must not be seen as the major weapon in the treatment of obesity. Instead, improvements in the quality and quantity of the diet should take the lead, with exercise relegated to an important supporting role. Regular exercise has many other more important benefits, especially those related to health.
- Maintain a good body weight after the excess weight is lost. Vigorous efforts should be put forth to maintain weight loss. Losing weight and then keeping it off is hard work, and relapse occurs in 95 of 100 people attempting to achieve a healthy weight. In general, one should seek to redouble lifestyle efforts and obtain professional help whenever 10 or more pounds are regained. Regular physical activity is one of the best predictors of those who are able to maintain weight loss over the long term.

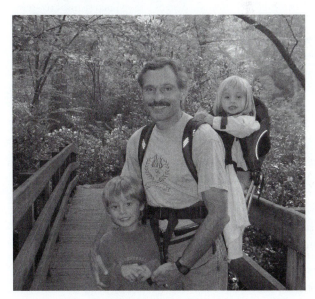

walking at least 3 days a week and increase to most, if not all, days. All adults should set a long-term goal to accumulate at least 30 minutes or more of moderate-intensity physical activity on most, and preferably all, days of the week. With time, a larger weekly volume of physical activity (60 minutes) can be performed that would normally cause a greater weight loss if it were not compensated by a higher caloric intake.

Reducing sedentary time, i.e., time spent watching television or playing video games, is another approach to increasing activity. Obese individuals should be encouraged to build physical activities into each day.

There are several exercise precautions for the obese, and their importance increases with the increasing degree of obesity.[268] These include providing for heat intolerance, difficulty breathing, movement restriction, musculoskeletal pain and injury, local muscular weakness, and balance anxiety.

In addition, the obese are at higher risk for cardiovascular disease, diabetes, and hypertension. However, if the exercise leader is careful to follow appropriate American College of Sports Medicine screening procedures (Chapter 3), has adequately prepared for emergencies, and emphasizes low-to-moderate intensity *non-weight-bearing activities* (such as bicycling, swimming, water exercises, and brisk walking), exercise programs for the severely obese can be conducted safely.

Social reinforcement and compliance are enhanced through group participation in activities that are recreational, fun, and varied, and which offer the participant a feeling of personal success.[269,270] Regimented calisthenics are not generally advisable. On the other hand, music, games, and social interaction will improve compliance.

Another key principle is that exercise need not be formal to be beneficial. It can take place at different times of the day, as a part of regular daily activities (such as climbing stairs or walking to a neighbor's house), and as such is often more attractive to the obese, who may want to avoid being noticed during exercise.

SPORTS MEDICINE INSIGHT

Eating Disorders: Bulimia and Anorexia Nervosa

It is an ongoing paradox that our food-laden, sedentary society equates thin with beautiful. On the one hand, our magazine covers, movie stars, and athletic heroes advance the concept that thin is in. On the other hand, we are led (often through advertising) to believe that technological labor-saving devices and sumptuous foods rich in fats and sugars are desirable rewards of a successful society.

It is perhaps not surprising that one sector of our population finds itself extremely disordered in its eating habits—the bulimics and the anorexics. The characteristics of bulimia and anorexia nervosa have been summarized by the American Psychiatric Association.[271] People with bulimia, known as bulimics, indulge in *binge eating* (episodes of eating large quantities of food) and *purging* (getting rid of food by vomiting or using laxatives). Key diagnostic criteria for bulimia nervosa include:[271]

- Recurrent episodes of binge eating (defined as eating a large amount of food within 2 h while feeling a lack of control).
- Recurrent inappropriate compensatory behavior to prevent weight gain (vomiting, laxatives, diuretics, enemas, medications, fasting, excessive exercise).
- Binge eating and purging occur on average at least 2x/wk for 3 months.
- Body image disturbance.

Some bulimics may consume up to 20,000 Calories in 8 hours, sometimes resorting to stealing food or money to support their obsession. The average bulimic binge is 1,200–4,500 Calories, and total daily energy intake averages over 10,000 Calories.[272–274] People with anorexia, known as anorexics or anorectics, severely limit their food intake. Key diagnostic criteria for anorexia nervosa include:[271]

- Refusal to maintain normal body weight (<85% of expected).
- Intense fear of gaining weight or becoming fat, even though underweight.
- Body image disturbance.
- Amenorrhea (3 consecutive cycles).

An estimated 0.5 to 3.7% of females suffer from anorexia nervosa, and 1.1 to 4.2% in their lifetime.[275,276] Eating disorders frequently co-occur with other psychiatric disorders such as depression, substance abuse, and anxiety disorders.[276] It is estimated that 85% of eating disorders have their onset during the adolescent age period.[272–285] Symptoms of bulimia and anorexia, such as binge eating, induced vomiting, and an extreme fear of gaining weight are present in significant numbers of college students and obese individuals. Among the obese, 20–40% report significant problems with binge eating. There are indications that the incidence and prevalence of eating disorders are rising.[277]

There are published reports of abnormal weight-control behaviors in athletes, especially ballet dancers, gymnasts, runners, and swimmers.[278,285] At one competitive-swimming camp, researchers found that of the 900 swimmers ages 9 to 18, 15.4% of the girls and 3.6% of the boys used a variety of abnormal weight loss techniques to meet the demands of their sport. Girls in particular were likely to misperceive themselves as overweight.[285] Among 93 elite women runners, 13% reported a history of anorexia nervosa, 25% binge eating, 9% bingeing and purging, and 34% abnormal eating practices.[286] In general, athletes are considered to be at increased risk for eating disorders but at least one study showed that female collegiate athletes did not exhibit more disordered-eating symptoms than nonathletes[287–289] (see Chapter 16).

Weight patterns of athletes can be grouped into three categories.[290] First, there are sports such as baseball, where maintenance of low weight is not important. The second category involves sports with specific weight divisions, such as wrestling or boxing. Weight fluctuations can be rapid, frequent (15 times per season), and large (one survey found that the weight of 41% fluctuated 11–20 pounds every week of the season, with an average end-of-season weight gain of 4–5 pounds). The third category involves sports in which low weights are the norm, such as distance running, gymnastics, figure skating, and ballet. Low weights in this category are necessary for optimal performance and appearance, and participants are often willing to utilize bizarre and unhealthy weight-control measures to attain the necessary weight for competition.

Signs to watch for if someone is suspected of having an eating disorder are summarized in Box 13.12.

Risk factors for anorexia and bulimia are listed in Table 13.4.[272,273,291–294] Eating disorders are associated with multiple risk factors that represent a complex interplay among genetic, psychological, and social processes.[292] Eating disorders are commonly understood to reflect a failed adaptation to the developmental challenges associated with

(continued)

SPORTS MEDICINE INSIGHT *(continued)*

Eating Disorders: Bulimia and Anorexia Nervosa

TABLE 13.4 Risk Factors for Anorexia Nervosa and Bulimia Nervosa

Anorexia Nervosa	Bulimia Nervosa
High parental education and income	Childhood obesity
Early feeding problems	Early onset of menarche
Low self-esteem	Weight concern
High neuroticism	Perfectionism
Maternal over-protectiveness	Low self-esteem
Eating disorders among family members	Social pressure about weight/eating
	Family dieting
	Eating disorders among family members
	Inadequate parenting
	Parental discord
	Parental psychopathology
	Childhood sexual abuse
	Chronic illness (diabetes, asthma, physical disabilities, etc.)

Sources: Neumark-Sztainer D, Story M, Resnick MD, Garwick A, Blum RW. Body dissatisfaction and unhealthy weight-control practices among adolescents with and without chronic illness: A population-based study. *Arch Pediatr Adolesc Med* 149:1330–1335, 1995; Striegel-Moore RH. Risk factors for eating disorders. *Ann N Y Acad Sci* 817:98–109, 1997; Wonderlich SA, Wilsnack RW, Wilsnack SC, Harris RH. Childhood sexual abuse and bulimic behavior in a nationally representative sample. *Am J Public Health* 86:1082–1086, 1996. See also: *J Am Acad Child Adolesc Psychiatry* 36:1107–1115, 1997.

female adolescence. Physical Fitness Activity 13.5 can be used to help detect people with an eating disorder.

Binge eating and the various forms of purging (vomiting, laxative and diuretic use) can cause serious medical problems, including stomach dilation and rupture, infection of the lung from vomitus, low body levels of chloride and potassium ions, infection and rupture of the esophagus, enlargement of the salivary glands, and tooth erosion and loss[295–297] (see Box 13.12). Gastrointestinal complaints are the most common medical complaint of eating-disordered patients and include slow gastric emptying, bloating, constipation, and abdominal discomfort.[296] Death is possible among anorexics—who can literally starve themselves to death. Karen Carpenter, a famous pop singer of the 1970s, died from complications related to her battles with anorexia. She used syrup of ipecac to induce vomiting and died after buildup of the drug irreversibly damaged her heart.[272] Each year, in the United States, approximately 70 people die from anorexia. The mortality rate among people with anorexia is 12 times higher than for female peers without eating disorders.[276] The resting metabolic rate can fall substantially in anorexics, as noted in Figure 13.55.[298]

What can be done to help the anorexic or bulimic?[272,299] Generally, they find it difficult to stop on their own, and most experts feel they need specialized professional help—generally in eating disorder clinics. These clinics usually have a staff of professionals, including physicians, psychologists, dietitians, and nurses to meet the varied needs of people with eating disorders. Often, bulimics and anorexics have deep-seated emotional problems at the foundation of their eating problems. Long-term professional care is necessary but can have mixed results. One study of teenagers with anorexia and/or bulimia showed that 5–8 years after treatment, 86% had returned to normal weight and menstrual function.[300] However, a 12-year study of 84 anorexia nervosa patients showed that 11% died, 11% remained anorexic, whereas the rest varied between moderate and good improvement[301] (see Figure 13.56).

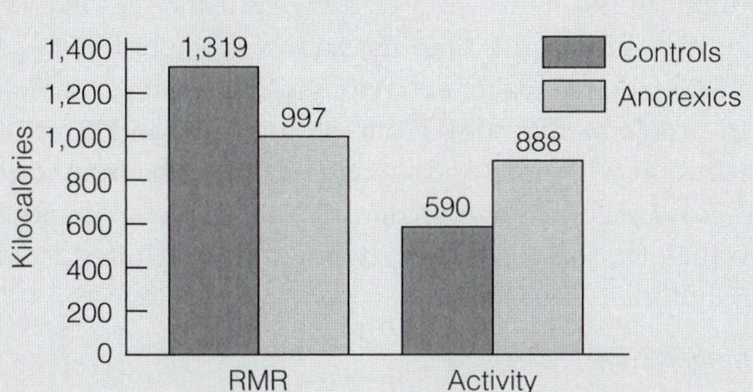

Figure 13.55 Energy expenditure in anorexics versus controls: Anorexics = 94 lb, 11% fat; controls = 124 lb, 25% fat. In this study, females with anorexia nervosa experienced a 25% reduction in their resting metabolic rates due to their low body weights (94 pounds). They partially compensate for this by exercising more. Source: Casper RC, Schoeller DA, Kushner R, Hnilicka J, Gold ST. Total daily energy expenditure and activity level in anorexia nervosa. *Am J Clin Nutr* 53:1143–1150, 1991.

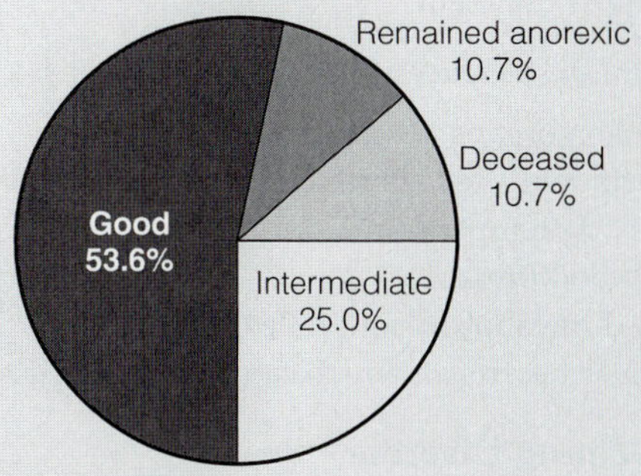

Figure 13.56 Twelve-year follow-up of 84 anorexia nervosa patients: Purging, physical symptoms, older age, and high social status predicted unfavorable course. In this follow-up study, nearly one out of four patients had an unfavorable outcome, while only about one in two had "good" progress.[284] Source: Deter HC, Herzog W. Anorexia nervosa in a long-term perspective: Results of the Heidelberg–Mannheim study. *Psychosom Med* 56:20–27, 1994.

Box 13.12

Danger Signs and Medical Consequences of Eating Disorders

Anorexia Nervosa

Anorexia nervosa is a disorder in which preoccupation with dieting and thinness leads to excessive weight loss. Anorexics have an intense fear of fat, and their preoccupation with food and weight often masks other underlying psychological problems. The individual may not acknowledge that his or her weight loss or restrictive eating is a problem. One percent of teenage girls in the United States develop anorexia nervosa and up to 10% of those may die as a result.

Danger Signs

Loss of a significant amount of weight
Continuing to diet although thin
Feeling fat, even after losing weight
Intense fear of weight gain
Loss of monthly menstrual periods
Preoccupation with food, calories, fat contents, and nutrition
Preferring to diet in isolation
Cooking for others
Hair loss
Cold hands and feet
Fainting spells
Exercising compulsively
Lying about food
Depression, anxiety
Weakness, exhaustion
Periods of hyperactivity
Constipation
Growth of fine body hair on arms, legs, and other body parts
Heart tremors
Dry, brittle skin
Shortness of breath

Medical Consequences

Shrunken organs
Bone mineral loss, which can lead to osteoporosis
Low body temperature
Low blood pressure
Slowed metabolism and reflexes
Irregular heartbeat, which can lead to cardiac arrest

Binge-Eating Disorder

Binge-eating disorder, or compulsive overeating, involves uncontrolled eating usually kept secret. People with this condition engage in frequent binges, but unlike bulimics, they do not purge afterward. Binges are usually followed by intense feelings of guilt and shame. Again, food is used as a dysfunctional means of coping with psychological problems. The individual often experiences depression and other psychological problems. Up to 40% of people who are obese may be binge eaters.

Danger Signs

Episodes of binge eating
Eating when not physically hungry
Frequent dieting
Feeling unable to stop eating voluntarily
Awareness that eating patterns are abnormal
Weight fluctuations
Depressed mood
Feeling ashamed
Antisocial behavior
Obesity

Medical Consequences

High blood pressure
High cholesterol
Gallbladder disease
Diabetes
Heart disease
Certain types of cancer

Bulimia Nervosa

Bulimia nervosa is described as a disorder in which frequent episodes of binge eating (rapid consumption of food in one sitting) are almost always followed by purging (ridding the body of food). Purging can involve vomiting, abusing laxatives and/or diuretics, exercising compulsively, and/or fasting. Binging and purging is often followed by intense feelings of guilt and shame. The bulimic may not be visibly underweight and may even be slightly overweight. Like the anorexic, the bulimic uses self-destructive eating behaviors to deal with psychological problems that may go much deeper than her or his obsession with food and weight. Usually, the individual feels out of control and recognizes that the behavior is not normal. Up to 5% of college women in the United States are bulimic.

Danger Signs

Binging, or eating uncontrollably
Purging by strict dieting, fasting, vigorous exercise, vomiting, or abusing laxatives or diuretics in an attempt to lose weight

(continued)

Box 13.12

Danger Signs and Medical Consequences of Eating Disorders *(continued)*

Danger Signs (continued)

Using the bathroom frequently after meals
Preoccupation with body weight
Depression
Mood swings
Feeling out of control
Swollen glands in neck and face
Heartburn
Bloating
Irregular periods
Dental problems
Constipation
Indigestion
Sore throat
Vomiting blood
Weakness, exhaustion
Bloodshot eyes

Medical Consequences

Dehydration
Damage to bowels, liver, and kidney
Electrolyte imbalance, which leads to irregular heartbeat, and in some cases, cardiac arrest

Source: The American Anorexia Bulimia Association. www.aabainc.org.

SUMMARY

1. This chapter placed emphasis on describing the various theories of obesity and how this major health problem can be treated.
2. The majority of American adults weigh more than they should. Sixeen percent of children and adolescents are overweight.
3. There are many disadvantages associated with obesity, including several diseases such as cancer, diabetes, and heart disease. Obesity is associated with early death.
4. Three major theories of obesity were discussed, with emphasis placed on the importance of genetic and parental influences, dietary factors (especially excess dietary fat), and insufficient energy expenditure.
5. Some people are more prone to obesity due to genetic influences than are others, and they need to be unusually careful in their dietary and exercise habits.
6. When humans eat diets high in fat, excess body fat is formed more easily than it is with a high-carbohydrate, high-fiber diet. Including more fruits, vegetables, legumes, and whole grains in the diet while moderating high-fat, low-fiber foods such as oils, margarine, butter, cheese, and fatty meats is probably the most important measure for controlling obesity.
7. Although obese people have higher resting metabolic rates than normal-weight people because of their greater lean body weight, they tend to exercise less than lean people. However, most studies have found that overeating is more prominent than underexercising in explaining obesity.
8. Following a meal, energy is expended by the body to process the food. This is the *thermic effect of food.* Some obese people may have a slightly lower than average thermic effect of food, but this does not appear to be a major factor explaining why people gain excess weight.
9. The NHLBI Obesity Education Initiative recommends that for most overweight and obese clients, a decrease of 300–1,000 Calories per day will lead to weight losses of 0.5–2 pounds per week, and a 10% weight loss in 6 months (the initial goal). Energy expenditure should be increased to at least 200–400 Calories per day. These efforts should be combined with several behavior modification techniques.
10. The NHLBI Obesity Education Initiative promotes FDA-approved weight loss drugs for long-term use as an adjunct to diet and physical activity for patients with a BMI $\geq$ 30 and without concomitant obesity-related risk factors or disease. Drug therapy may also be useful for patients with a BMI $\geq$ 27 who also have concomitant obesity-related risk factors or diseases.
11. The NHLBI Obesity Education Initiative promotes weight loss surgery as an option for weight reduction in patients with clinically severe obesity, defined as a BMI $\geq$ 40, or a BMI $\geq$ 35 with comorbid conditions. Weight loss surgery should be reserved for clinically severe obese patients in whom other methods of treatment have failed.
12. Four misconceptions regarding the role of physical activity in weight reduction were reviewed, including the theories that aerobic exercise accelerates weight loss significantly when combined with a reducing diet; causes the resting metabolic rate to stay elevated for a long time after the exercise bout, burning extra Calories; counters the diet-induced decrease in resting metabolic rate; and counters the diet-induced decrease in fat-free mass.
13. There are several important benefits of exercise for the obese, including these effects of moderate aerobic activity: improved cardiorespiratory endurance;

improved blood lipid profile; improved psychological state; group social support, which may enhance long-term maintenance of weight loss; and decreased risk of obesity-related diseases.

14. Moderate aerobic exercise during weight reduction helps to improve one's general health status, but the real power behind weight loss comes from a reduction in dietary Calories. The success of a weight loss program should be measured not only by the total amount of weight lost but also by the quality of the weight loss and final health status.
15. Bulimia and anorexia nervosa are two unhealthy and sometimes life-threatening eating disorders. Bulimics consume large amounts of food within short periods of time and then engage in various purging techniques. People with anorexia nervosa have disturbed perceptions of their body images, which tend to prompt excessive weight loss. Long-term professional care is necessary for both disorders.

Review Questions

1. *Which of the statements regarding obesity in America is true?*

   A. The percentage of obese children and teenagers has decreased since the 1960s.
   B. Approximately three fourths of adults are considered obese.
   C. Obesity is more prevalent among the poor and minority groups.
   D. The prevalence of obesity decreases between the ages of 25 and 55 years.

2. *There are many disadvantages associated with obesity. Which one of the following is* **not** *included?*

   A. Increased levels of serum cholesterol
   B. Increased prevalence of high blood pressure
   C. Increased diabetes
   D. Increased lung cancer
   E. Increased mortality rates, resulting in earlier death

3. *What percent of the variability in human obesity has a genetic basis?*

   A. 25–40% **B.** 90–100%
   C. 10–20% **D.** 50–75%

4. *Which of the statements regarding the resting metabolic rate (RMR) is true?*

   A. The RMR for the average person amounts to one third of daily energy expenditure.
   B. The RMR is higher in lean people than obese people.
   C. The RMR increases as the body weight of an individual increases.
   D. The RMR is the major factor explaining obesity in the United States.

5. ____ *obesity is characterized by high amounts of body fat in the hip and thigh areas and is associated with fewer of the medical complications that excess body fat brings.*

   A. Android **B.** Gynoid

6. *About* ____% *of Americans are considered obese using conservative government criteria.*

   A. 10 **B.** 17 **C.** 30 **D.** 35 **E.** 40

7. *Which statement is* **false?**

   A. Three miles of walking a day does not accelerate weight loss significantly (many extra pounds lost each month) when eating 1,200–1,500 Calories a day.
   B. Moderate exercise causes the metabolic rate to stay elevated for a long time after the bout, burning many extra Calories.
   C. During a diet of 1,200–1,500-Calories per day, about 90% of the weight loss is from the fat weight and 10% is from the fat-free mass.
   D. Moderate aerobic exercise during weight loss does not protect the fat-free mass.

8. *Which one of the following is* **not** *regarded as a benefit of moderate aerobic exercise for mildly obese subjects?*

   A. Improved heart and lung fitness
   B. Improved psychological state, especially general well-being
   C. Decreased serum triglycerides, increased HDL-C
   D. Substantial decrease in body fat, increase in fat-free mass
   E. Decreased risk of heart disease and diabetes

9. **The Healthy People 2010** *goal is to reduce obesity prevalence to below* ____%.

   A. 10 **B.** 15 **C.** 20 **D.** 30 **E.** 40

10. *When the body mass index rises above the threshold of* ____ *kg/m^2, mortality from heart disease, cancer, and diabetes also increases.*

    A. 15 **B.** 20 **C.** 25 **D.** 35

11. *There are three major theories of obesity. Which one of the following is* **not** *included?*

    A. High energy intake
    B. Genetic and parental influences
    C. Low energy expenditure
    D. High carbohydrate intake

12. *Which factor appears to be most important in explaining the high prevalence of obesity in the United States?*

    A. High energy and fat content of the diet
    B. Genetic and parental influences
    C. Excess body fat cells
    D. High-fiber, high-carbohydrate diet
    E. Inactivity

13. *Obese people tend to expend more energy than normal-weight people for which category?*

    A. Resting metabolic rate
    B. Total physical activity
    C. Thermic effect of food

14. *If an obese person has 40 extra pounds of body weight, approximately ____ of these pounds are fat-free mass and ____ of these pounds are fat weight.*

    A. 15/25 **B.** 5/35
    C. 30/10 **D.** 10/30
    E. 20/20

15. *Which statement listed would indicate to you that the weight loss program is probably fraudulent?*

    A. Promotes a diet of 1,250 Calories a day
    B. Attempts to make a client dependent on a special product
    C. Promotes a plan that will lead to a weight loss of 1–2 pounds a week
    D. Promotes a high-carbohydrate, high-fiber, low-fat dietary regimen
    E. All of these

16. *For each kilogram of body weight loss, the RMR drops about ____ Calories per day.*

    A. 100–200 **B.** 200–400
    C. 10–20 **D.** 5–10
    E. 80–100

17. *The RMR falls about ____% per decade of adult life, even after adjusting for fat-free mass.*

    A. 1–2 **B.** 3–8
    C. 5–15 **D.** 15–20
    E. 30–40

18. *Effective treatment for obesity involves three elements. Which one of the following is* **not** *included?*

    A. Diet of 400–800 Calories per day
    B. Behavior modification
    C. Physical activity

19. *Moderate-intensity aerobic exercise causes the RMR to stay elevated 20–30 minutes, burning ____ extra Calories.*

    A. 100–200 **B.** 50–100
    C. 25–40 **D.** 10–12
    E. 2–5

20. *When on an VLCD, about 75% of the weight loss is ____.*

    A. Water **B.** Fat
    C. Muscle **D.** Bone

21. *Which criteria listed is used to determine if a person is anorexic?*

    A. Minimum average of two binge-eating episodes per week for at least 3 months
    B. Regularly engages in self-induced vomiting, use of laxatives, or other purging techniques to counteract the effects of the binge eating
    C. Weight loss so severe that weight is more than 15% below normal

22. *What cohort is more likely to produce obese adults?*

    A. Obese infants **B.** Obese children
    C. Obese adolescents

23. *Using the best current methodology, it appears that obese people eat ____ normal-weight individuals.*

    A. Less than
    B. More than
    C. About the same as

24. *Obesity prevalence is greatest among what subgroup?*

    A. Black females **B.** White females
    C. Black males **D.** Mexican-American females
    E. White women

25. *About 80% of variation in RMR is due to differences in ____.*

    A. Fat-free mass **B.** Genetics
    C. Race **D.** Gender
    E. Activity level

26. *The average male engaging in light-to-moderate daily activity should multiply his RMR times ____ to obtain 24-h energy expenditure.*

    A. 1.25 **B.** 1.45 **C.** 1.60 **D.** 2.05 **E.** 2.25

27. *About ____% of American adults are overweight.*

    A. 10 **B.** 20 **C.** 33 **D.** 65 **E.** 48

28. *The VLCD provides about ____ Calories a day through special-formula beverages.*

    A. 200–400 **B.** 400–800
    C. 800–1,000 **D.** 1,000–1,200

29. *The net energy cost of exercise equals the Calories expended during the exercise bout minus the Calories expended for ____ and other activities that the individual would have been engaging in.*

    A. TEF **B.** RMR
    C. Formal exercise **D.** Adaptative thermogenesis

30. ***Among women, about ____% will have bulimia within their lifetime.***

A. 0.2–1 **B.** 1.1–4.2 **C.** 4.3–5.0
D. 9.5–12.0 **E.** 10.1–15.2

31. ***For bulimia nervosa to be diagnosed, the binge eating and inappropriate compensatory behaviors need to both occur, on average, at least ____ time(s) a week for 3 months.***

A. 1 **B.** 2 **C.** 3 **D.** 4 **E.** 5

32. ***Drug therapy for treatment of obesity should be used as an adjunct to lifestyle therapy and reserved for selected patients with a body mass index greater than a threshold of ____.***

A. 25 **B.** 30 **C.** 40 **D.** 50

33. ***The resting metabolic rate typically represents ____% of total energy expenditure in a given day.***

A. 23 **B.** 67 **C.** 10 **D.** 35 **E.** 88

34. ***During a diet of 1,200–1,300 Calories per day, ____% of the weight loss is from the fat-free mass.***

A. 25 **B.** 10 **C.** 50 **D.** 90 **E.** 75

35. ***One of the best markers for long-term success in keeping weight off is***

A. Regular exercise
B. Use of diet pills
C. Use of diet soft drinks
D. Use of nutrient supplements
E. Skipping meals

36. ***The NHLBI Obesity Education Initiative promotes weight loss surgery as an option for weight reduction in patients with clinically severe obesity, defined as a BMI ≥ ____, or a BMI ≥ ____ with comorbid conditions and disease risk factors.***

A. 30/40 **B.** 40/35
C. 25/35 **D.** 50/40
E. 20/40

37. ***According to the NHLBI Obesity Education Initiative, the initial goal of a weight loss regimen should be to reduce body weight by about ____%.***

A. 1 **B.** 5 **C.** 10 **D.** 20 **E.** 30

38. ***Regular physical activity is* least *effective in***

A. Preventing weight gain
B. Maintaining weight loss
C. Treatment of obesity

Answers

1. C
2. D
3. A
4. C
5. B
6. C
7. B
8. D
9. B
10. C
11. D
12. A
13. A
14. D
15. B
16. C
17. A
18. A
19. D
20. B
21. C
22. C
23. B
24. A
25. A
26. C
27. D
28. B
29. B
30. B
31. B
32. B
33. B
34. B
35. A
36. B
37. C
38. C

REFERENCES

1. Hill JO, Wyatt HR, Reed GW, Peters JC. Obesity and the environment: Where do we go from here? *Science* 299:853–855, 2003.
2. Office of the Surgeon General. *The Surgeon General's Call to Action to Prevent and Decrease Overweight and Obesity.* Rockville, MD: USDHHS, PHS, 2001.
3. U.S. Department of Health and Human Services. *Physical Activity and Health: A Report of the Surgeon General.* Atlanta, GA: U.S. Department of Health and Human Services, Centers for Disease Control and Prevention, National Center for Chronic Disease Prevention and Health Promotion, 1996.
4. National Center for Health Statistics. *Health, United States, 2004.* Hyattsville, MD: 2004.
5. Hedley AA, Ogden CL, Johnson CL, Carroll MD, Curtin LR, Flegal KM. Prevalence of overweight and obesity among US children, adolescents, and adults, 1999–2002. *JAMA* 291:2847–2850, 2004.
6. Ogden CL, Fryar CD, Carroll MD, Flegal KM. Mean body weight, height, and body mass index, United States 1960–2002. *Advance Data from Vital and Health Statistics,* no. 347. Hyattsville, MD: National Center for Health Statistics, 2004.
7. Expert Panel on the Identification, Evaluation, and Treatment of Overweight in Adults. Clinical guidelines on the identification, evaluation, and treatment of overweight and obesity in adults: Executive summary. *Am J Clin Nutr* 68:899–917, 1998. www.nhlbi.nih.gov.
8. Flegal KM, Carroll MD, Ogden CL, Johnson CL. Prevalence and trends in obesity among US adults, 1999–2000. *JAMA* 288:1723–1727, 2002.
9. Ogden CL, Flegal KM, Carroll MD, Johnson CL. Prevalence and trends in overweight among US children and adolescents, 1999–2000. *JAMA* 288:1728–1732, 2002.
10. Basjub NKm Ard J, Franklin F, Allison DB. Prevalence of obesity in the United States. *Obes Rev* 6:5–7, 2005.

11. National Health, Lung, and Blood Institute. *The Practical Guide. Identification, Evaluation, and Treatment of Overweight and Obesity in Adults.* Bethesda, MD: NIH Publication Number 00–4084, October 2000. www.nhlbi.nih.gov.

12 U.S. Department of Health and Human Services. *Healthy People 2010.* Washington DC: January, 2000. www.health.gov/healthypeople/.

13. Rodin J. Cultural and psychosocial determinants of weight concerns. *Ann Intern Med* 119:643–645, 1993.

14. Daniels SR, Arnett DK, Eckel RH, et al. Overweight in children and adolescents: Pathophysiology, consequences, prevention, and treatment. *Circulation* 111:1999–2012, 2005.

15. Food and Nutrition Board, Institute of Medicine. *Preventing Childhood Obesity: Health in the Balance.* Washington, DC: The National Academies Press, 2005.

16. American Academy of Pediatrics. Prevention of pediatric overweight and obesity. *Pediatrics* 112:424–430, 2003.

17. Zimmermann MB, Gubeli C, Puntener C, Molinari L. Detection of overweight and obesity in a national sample of 6–12-y-old Swiss children: Accuracy and validity of reference values for body mass index from the US Centers for Disease Control and Prevention and the International Obesity Task Force. *Am J Clin Nutr* 79:838–843, 2004.

18. Must A, Spadano J, Coakley EH, Field AE, Colditz G, Dietz WH. The disease burden associated with overweight and obesity. *JAMA* 282:1523–1529, 1999.

19. National Institutes of Health. Consensus development conference statement. Health implications of obesity. *Ann Intern Med* 103:981–1077, 1985.

20. Klein S, Burke LE, Bray GA, Blair SN, Allison DB, Pi-Sunyer X, Hong Y, Eckel RH. Clinical implications of obesity with special focus on cardiovascular disease. A statement for professionals from the American Heart Association Council on Nutrition, Physical Activity, and Metabolism. *Circulation* 110:2952–2967, 2004.

21. Peeters A, Barendregt JJ, Willekens F, Mackenbach JP, Mamun AA, Bonneux L. Obesity in adulthood and its consequences for life expectancy: A life-table analysis. *Ann Intern Med* 138:24–32, 2003.

22. Field AE, Coakley EH, Must A, Spadano JL, Laird N, Dietz WH, Rimm E, Colditz GA. Impact of overweight on the risk of developing common chronic diseases during a 10–year period. *Arch Intern Med* 161:1581–1586, 2001.

23. Fontaine KR, Redden DT, Wang C, Westfall AO, Allison DB. Years of life lost due to obesity. *JAMA* 289:187–193, 2003.

24. Thompson D, Edelsberg J, Colditz GA, Bird AP, Oster G. Lifetime health and economic consequences of obesity. *Arch Intern Med* 159:2177–2183, 1999.

25. Stunkard AJ, Wadden TA. Psychological aspects of severe obesity. *Am J Clin Nutr* 55:524S–532S, 1992.

26. Gortmaker SL, Must A, Perrin JM, Sobol AM, Dietz WH. Social and economic consequences of overweight in adolescence and young adulthood. *N Engl J Med* 329:1008–1012, 1993.

27. Witteman JCM, Willett WC, Stampfer MJ, et al. A prospective study of nutritional factors and hypertension among US women. *Circulation* 80:1320–1327, 1989.

28. McCarron DA, Reusser ME. Body weight and blood pressure regulation. *Am J Clin Nutr* 63(suppl):423S–425S, 1996.

29. McMurray RG, Harrell JS, Levine AA, Gansky SA. Childhood obesity elevates blood pressure and total cholesterol independent of physical activity. *Int J Obesity Relat Metab Disord* 19:881–886, 1995.

30. Dattilo Am, Kris-Etherton PM. Effects of weight reduction on blood lipids and lipoproteins: A meta-analysis. *Am J Clin Nutr* 56:320–328, 1992.

31. Denke MA, Sempos CT, Grundy SM. Excess body weight: An underrecognized contributor to high blood cholesterol levels in white American men. *Arch Intern Med* 153:1093–1103, 1993.

32. Gregg EW, Cheng YJ, Cadwell BL, Imperatore G, Williams DE, Flegal KM, Narayan KM, Williamson DF. Secular trends in cardiovascular disease risk factors according to body mass index in US adults. *JAMA* 293:1868–1874, 2005.

33. Whitelaw DC, O'Kane M, Wales JK, Barth JH. Risk factors for coronary heart disease in obese non-diabetic subjects. *Int J Obesity* 25:1042–1046, 2001.

34. Stampfer MJ, Maclure KM, Colditz GA, Manson JE, Willett WC. Risk of symptomatic gallstones in women with severe obesity. *Am J Clin Nutr* 55:652–658, 1992.

35. Utter A, Goss F. Exercise and gall bladder function. *Sports Med* 23:218–227, 1997.

36. CDC. Factors associated with prevalent self-reported arthritis and other rheumatic conditions—United States, 1989–1991. *MMWR* 45:487–491, 1996.

37. Felson DT. Weight and osteoarthritis. *Am J Clin Nutr* 63(suppl):430S–432S, 1996.

38. Colditz GA, Willett WC, Rotnitzky A, Manson JE. Weight gain as a risk factor for clinical diabetes mellitus in women. *Ann Intern Med* 122:481–486, 1995.

39. Carey VJ, Walters EE, Colditz GA, et al. Body fat distribution and risk of non–insulin-dependent diabetes mellitus in women. The Nurses' Health Study. *Am J Epidemiol* 145:614–619, 1997.

40. Calle EE, Rodriguez C, Walker-Thurmond K, Thun MJ. Overweight, obesity, and mortality from cancer in a prospectively studied cohort of U.S. adults. *N Engl J Med* 348:1625–1638, 2003. See also: Lew EA. Mortality and weight: Insured lives and the American Cancer Society studies. *Ann Intern Med* 103:1024–1029, 1985.

41. Ballard-Barbash R, Swanson CA. Body weight: Estimation of risk for breast and endometrial cancers. *Am J Clin Nutr* 63(suppl):437S–441S, 1996.

42. Stevens J, Cai J, Juhaeri J, Thun MJ, Wood JL. Evaluation of WHO and NHANES II standards for overweight using mortality rates. *J Am Diet Assoc* 100:825–827, 2000.

43. Lindsted K, Tonstad S, Kuzma J. Body mass index and patterns of mortality among Seventh-Day Adventist men. *Int J Obesity* 15:397–406, 1991.

44. Must A, Jacques PF, Dallal GE, Bajema CJ, Dietz WH. Long-term morbidity and mortality of overweight adolescents: A follow-up of the Harvard Growth Study of 1922 to 1935. *N Engl J Med* 327:1350–1355, 1992.

45. Lee IM, Manson JE, Hennekens CH, Paffenbarger RS. Body weight and mortality. A 27–year follow-up of middle-aged men. *JAMA* 270:2823–2828, 1993.

46. Hu FB, Willett WC, Li T, Stampfer MJ, Colditz GA, Manson JE. Adiposity as compared with physical activity in predicting mortality among women. *N Engl J Med* 351:2694–2703, 2004.

47. Rexrode KM, Buring JE, Manson JE. Abdominal and total adiposity and risk of coronary heart disease in men. *Int J Obesity* 25:1047–1056, 2001.

48. Manson JE, Colditz GA, Stampfer MJ, et al. A prospective study of obesity and risk of coronary heart disease in women. *N Engl J Med* 322:882–889, 1990.

49. Jousilahti P, Tuomilehto J, Vartiainen E, Pekkanen J, Puska P. Body weight, cardiovascular risk factors, and coronary mortality. *Circulation* 93:1372–1379, 1996.

50. Rimm EB, Stampfer MJ, Giovannucci E, Ascherio A, Spiegelman D, Colditz GA, Willett WC. Body size and fat distribution as predictors of coronary heart disease among middle-aged and older US men. *Am J Epidemiol* 141:1117–1127, 1995.

51. Rexrode KM, Hennekens CH, Willett WC, Colditz GA, Stampfer MJ, Rich-Edwards JW, Speizer FE, Manson JE. A prospective study of body mass index, weight change, and risk of stroke in women. *JAMA* 277:1539–1545, 1997.
52. Walker SP, Rimm EB, Ascherio A, Kawachi I, Stampfer MJ, Willett WC. Body size and fat distribution as predictors of stroke among US men. *Am J Epidemiol* 144:1143–1150, 1996.
53. Folsom AR, Kaye SA, Sellers TA, et al. Body fat distribution and 5-year risk of death in older women. *JAMA* 269:483–487, 1993. See also: *Arch Intern Med* 160:2117–2128, 2000.
54. Tanko LB, Bagger YZ, Qin G, Alexandersen P, Larsen PJ, Christiansen C. Enlarged waist circumference with elevated triglycerides is a strong predictor of accelerated atherogenesis and related cardiovascular mortality in postmenopausal women. *Circulation* 111:1883–1890, 2005. See also: Van Pelt RE, Evans EM, Schechtman KB, Ehsani AA, Kohrt WM. Waist circumference vs body mass index for prediction of disease risk in postmenopausal women. *Int J Obesity* 25:1183–1188, 2001.
55. Rebuffé-Scrive M, Anderson B, Olbe L, Björntorp P. Metabolism of adipose tissue in intraabdominal depots in severely obese men and women. *Metabolism* 39:1021–1025, 1990.
56. Trosis RJ, Heinold JW, Vokonas PS, Weiss ST. Cigarette smoking, dietary intake, and physical activity: Effects on body fat distribution. The Normative Aging Study. *Am J Clin Nutr* 53:1104–1111, 1991.
57. Rodin J. Determinants of body fat localization and its implications for health. *Ann Behav Med* 14:275–281, 1992.
58. French SA, Folsom AR, Jeffery RW, Zheng W, Mink PJ, Baxter JE. Weight variability and incident disease in older women: The Iowa Women's Health Study. *Int J Obesity* 21:217–223, 1997.
59. Lee I-M, Paffenbarger RS. Change in body weight and longevity. *JAMA* 268:2045–2049, 1992.
60. Harris TB, Ballard-Barbasch R, Madans J, Makuc DM, Feldman JJ. Overweight, weight loss, and risk of coronary heart disease in older women: The NHANES I Epidemiologic Follow-up Study. *Am J Epidemiol* 137:1318–1327, 1993.
61. Dietz WH, Robinson TN. Clinical practice. Overweight children and adolescents. *N Engl J Med* 352:2100–2109, 2005.
62. Speakman JR. Obesity: The integrated roles of environment and genetics. *J Nutr* 134(8 Suppl):2090S–2105S, 2004.
63. Bray G, Bouchard C. Genetics of human obesity: Research directions. *FASEB* J 11:937–945, 1997.
64. Bouchard C, Tremblay A. Genetic influences on the response of body fat and fat distribution to positive and negative energy balances in human identical twins. *J Nutr* 127(suppl 5):943S–947S, 1997.
65. Whitaker RC, Wright JA, Pepe MS, Seidel KD, Dietz WH. Predicting obesity in young adulthood from childhood and parental obesity. *N Engl J Med* 337:869–873, 1997.
66. Mayer J. Genetic factors in human obesity. *Ann NY Acad Sci* 131:412–421, 1965.
67. Stunkard AJ, Foch TT, Hrubec Z. A twin study of human obesity. *JAMA*; 256:51–54, 1986.
68. Stunkard AJ, Sorensen TIA, Hanis C, et al. An adoption study of human obesity. *N Engl J Med* 314:193–198, 1986.
69. Stunkard AJ, Harris JR, Pedersen NL, McClearn GE. The body-mass index of twins who have been reared apart. *N Engl J Med* 322:1483–1487, 1990.
70. Bouchard C. Human variation in body mass: Evidence for a role of the genes. *Nutr Rev* 55:S21–S30, 1997.
71. Sorensen TIA, Holst C, Stunkard AJ. Adoption study of environmental modifications of the genetic influences on obesity. *Int J Obesity* 22:73–81, 1998.
72. Sorensen TIA, Holst C, Stunkard AJ, Skovgaard LT. Correlations of body mass index of adult adoptees and their biological and adoptive relatives. *Int J Obesity* 16:227–236, 1992.
73. Bouchard C, Pérusse L, Leblanc C, et al. Inheritance of the amount and distribution of human body fat. *Int J Obesity* 12:205–215, 1988.
74. Bouchard C, Tremblay A, Després JP, et al. The response to long-term overfeeding in identical twins. *N Engl J Med* 322:1477–1482, 1990.
75. Loos RJ, Rankinen T. Gene-diet interactions on body weight changes. *J Am Diet Assoc* 105:29–34, 2005.
76. Bouchard C. Genetics of human obesity: Recent results from linkage studies. *J Nutr* 127:1887S–1890S, 1997.
77. Lafontan M. Fat cells: Afferent and efferent messages define new approaches to treat obesity. *Annu Rev Pharmacol Toxicol* 45:119–146, 2005.
78. Cutting TM, Fisher JO, Grimm-Thomas K, Birch LL. Like mother, like daughter: Familial patterns of overweight are mediated by mothers' dietary disinhibition. *Am J Clin Nutr* 69:608–613, 1999.
79. Serdula MK, Ivery D, Coates RJ, Freedman DS, Williamson DF, Byers T. Do obese children become obese adults? A review of the literature. *Prev Med* 22:167–177, 1993.
80. Guo SS, Chumlea WC. Tracking of body mass index in children in relation to overweight in adulthood. *Am J Clin Nutr* 70(suppl):145S–148S, 1999.
81. Briefel RR, Sempos CT, McDowell MA, Chien SCY, Alaimo K. Dietary methods research in the Third National Health and Nutrition Examination Survey: Underreporting of energy intake. *Am J Clin Nutr* 65(suppl):1203S–1209S, 1997.
82. Heymsfield SB, Darby PC, Muhlheim LS, Gallagher D, Wolper C, Allison DB. The calorie: Myth, measurement, and reality. *Am J Clin Nutr* 62(suppl):1034S–1041S, 1995.
83. Bruce B, Wilfley D. Binge eating among the overweight population: A serious and prevalent problem. *J Am Diet Assoc* 96:58–61, 1996.
84. Lichtman SW, Pisarska K, Berman ER, et al. Discrepancy between self-reported and actual caloric intake and exercise in obese subjects. *N Engl J Med* 327:1893–1898, 1992.
85. Black AE, Cole TJ. Biased over- or under-reporting is characteristic of individuals whether over time or by different assessment methods. *J Am Diet Assoc* 101:70–80, 2001.
86. Welle S, Forbes GB, Statt M, Barnard RR, Amatruda JM. Energy expenditure under free-living conditions in normal-weight and overweight women. *Am J Clin Nutr* 55:14–21, 1992.
87. Scotellaro PA, Gorski LLJ, Oscai LB. Body fat accretion: A rat model. *Med Sci Sports Exerc* 23:275–279, 1991.
88. Golay A, Bobbioni E. The role of dietary fat in obesity. *Int J Obes Relat Metab Disord* 21(suppl 3):S2–S11, 1997.
89. Nielsen SJ, Popkin BM. Patterns and trends in food portion sizes, 1977–1998. *JAMA* 289:450–453, 2003.
90. Gray GA, Popkin BM. Dietary fat intake does affect obesity! *Am J Clin Nutr* 68:1157–1173, 1998.
91. Carmichael HE, Swinburn BA, Wilson MR. Lower fat intake as a predictor of initial and sustained weight loss in obese subjects consuming an otherwise ad libitum diet. *J Am Diet Assoc* 98:35–39, 1998.
92. Ebbeling CB, Sinclair KB, Pereira MA, Garcia-Lago E, Feldman HA, Ludwig DS. Compensation for energy intake from fast food among overweight and lean adolescents. *JAMA* 291:2828–2833, 2004.
93. Kendall A, Levitsky DA, Strupp BJ, Lissner L. Weight loss on a low-fat diet: Consequence of the imprecision of the control of food intake in humans. *Am J Clin Nutr* 53:1124–1129, 1991.

94. Lissner L, Habicht JP, Strupp BJ, et al. Body composition and energy intake: Do overweight women overeat and underreport? *Am J Clin Nutr* 49:320–325, 1989.

95. Lissner L, Levitsky DA, Strupp BJ, et al. Dietary fat and the regulation of energy intake in human subjects. *Am J Clin Nutr* 46:886–892, 1987.

96. Lawton CL, Burley VJ, Wales JK, Blundell JE. Dietary fat and appetite control in obese subjects: Weak effects on satiation and satiety. *Int J Obesity* 17:337–342, 1993.

97. Wardle J, Guthrie C, Sanderson S, Birch L, Plomin R. Food and activity preferences in children of lean and obese parents. *Int J Obesity* 25:971–977, 2001.

98. Barkeling B, Ekman S, Rössner S. Eating behavior in obese and normal weight 11–year-old children. *Int J Obesity* 16:355–360, 1992.

99. Horton TJ, Drougas H, Brachey A, Reed GW, Peters JC, Hill JO. Fat and carbohydrate overfeeding in humans: Different effects on energy storage. *Am J Clin Nutr* 62:19–29, 1995.

100. Swinburn B, Ravussin E. Energy balance or fat balance. Am J Clin Nutr 57(suppl):766S–771S, 1993.

101. Blundell JE, Burley VJ, Cotton JR, Lawton CL. Dietary fat and the control of energy intake: Evaluating the effects of fat on meal size and postmeal satiety. *Am J Clin Nutr* 57(suppl):772S–778S, 1993.

102. Rising R, Alger S, Boyce V, et al. Food intake measured by an automated food-selection system: Relationship to energy expenditure. *Am J Clin Nutr* 55:343–349, 1992.

103. Proserpi C, Sparti A, Schutz Y, Vetta VD, Milon H, Jequier E. Ad libitum intake of a high-carbohydrate or high-fat diet in young men: Effects on nutrient balances. *Am J Clin Nutr* 66:539–545, 1997.

104. Sims EAH, Danforth E. Expenditure and storage of energy in man. *J Clin Invest* 79:1019–1025, 1987.

105. Acheson KJ, Schutz Y, Bessard T, Flatt JP, Jequier E. Carbohydrate metabolism and de novo lipogenesis in human obesity. *Am J Clin Nutr* 45:78–85, 1987.

106. Marin P, Rebuffé-Scrive dM, Björntorp dP. Glucose uptake in human adipose tissue. *Metabolism* 36:1154–1160, 1987.

107. Ravussin E, Swinburn BA. Pathophysiology of obesity. *Lancet* 340:404–408, 1992.

108. Schutz Y, Flatt JP, Jéquier E. Failure of dietary fat intake to promote fat oxidation: A factor favoring the development of obesity. *Am J Clin Nutr* 50:307–314, 1989.

109. Frankenfield DC, Muth ER, Rowe WA. The Harris-Benedict studies of human basal metabolism: History and limitations. *J Am Diet Assoc* 98:439–445, 1998.

110. Wang Z, Heshka S, Zhang K, Boozer CN, Heymsfield SB. Resting energy expenditure: Systematic organization and critique of prediction methods. *Obes Res* 9:331–336, 2001.

111. Tataranmi PA, Ravussin E. Variability in metabolic rate: Biological sites of regulation. *Int J Obesity* 19(suppl 4):S102–S106, 1995.

112. Arciero PJ, Goran MI, Poehlman ET. Resting metabolic rate is lower in women than in men. *J Appl Physiol* 75:2514–2520, 1993.

113. Food and Nutrition Board, Institute of Medicine. *Dietary Reference Intakes for Energy, Carbohydrate, Fiber, Fat, Fatty Acids, Cholesterol, Protein, and Amino Acids (Macronutrients).* Washington, DC: The National Academies Press, 2002.

114. Roza AM, Shizgal HM. The Harris Benedict equation reevaluated: Resting energy requirements and the body cell mass. *Am J Clin Nutr* 40:168–182, 1984.

115. Report of a Joint FAO/WHO/UNU Expert Consultation. *Energy and Protein Requirements.* World Health Organization, 1985.

116. Leibel RL, Rosenbaum M, Hirsch J. Changes in energy expenditure resulting from altered body weight. *N Engl J Med* 332:621–628, 1995.

117. Wyatt HR, Grunwald GK, Seagle HM, Klem ML, McGuire MT, Wing RR, Hill JO. Resting energy expenditure in reduced-obese subjects in the National Weight Control Registry. *Am J Clin Nutr* 69:1189–1193, 1999.

118. Ravussin E. Low resting metabolic rate as a risk factor for weight gain: Role of the sympathetic nervous system. *Int J Obesity* 19(suppl 7):S8–S9, 1995.

119. Ravussin E, Lillioja S, Anderson TE, Christin L, Bogardus C. Determinants of 24-hour energy expenditure in man. *J Clin Invest* 78:1568–1578, 1986. See also: Ravussin E, Gautier JF. Metabolic predictors of weight gain. *Int J Obesity* 23(suppl 1):37–41, 1999.

120. Davies PSW, Day JME, Lucas A. Energy expenditure in early infancy and later body fatness. *Int J Obesity* 15:727–731, 1991.

121. Seidell JC, Muller DC, Sorkin JD, Andres R. Fasting respiratory exchange ratio and resting metabolic rate as predictors of weight gain: The Baltimore Longitudinal Study on Aging. *Int J Obesity* 16:667–674, 1992.

122. Hu FB, Li TY, Colditz GA, Willett WC, Manson JE. Television watching and other sedentary behaviors in relation to risk of obesity and type 2 diabetes mellitus in women. *JAMA* 289:1785–1791, 2003.

123. Park RJ. Human energy expenditure from Australopithecus Afarensis to the 4–minute mile: Exemplars and case studies. *Exerc Sport Sci Rev* 20:185–220, 1992.

124. Haapanen N, Miilunpalo S, Pasanen M, Oja P, Vuori I. Association between leisure time physical activity and 10–year body mass change among working-aged men and women. *Int J Obesity* 21:288–296, 1997.

125. Williamson DF, Madans J, Anda RF, et al. Recreational physical activity and ten-year weight change in a US national cohort. *Int J Obesity* 17:279–286, 1993.

126. DiPietro L, Kohl HW, Barlow CE, Blair SN. Improvements in cardiorespiratory fitness attenuate age-related weight gain in healthy men and women: The Aerobics Center Longitudinal Study. *Int J Obesity* 22:55–62, 1998.

127. Ching PLYH, Willett WC, Rimm EB, Colditz GA, Gortmaker SL, Stampfer MJ. Activity level and risk of overweight in male health professionals. *Am J Public Health* 86:25–30, 1996.

128. Kahn HS, Tatham LM, Rodriguez C, Calle EE, Thun MJ, Heath CW. Stable behaviors associated with adults' 10–year change in body mass index and likelihood of gain at the waist. *Am J Public Health* 87:747–754, 1997.

129. Moore LL, Nguyen USDT, Rothman KJ, Cupples LA, Ellison RC. Preschool physical activity level and change in body fatness in young children. *Am J Epidemiol* 142:982–988, 1995.

130. Klesges RC, Klesges LM, Eck LH, Shelton ML. A longitudinal analysis of accelerated weight gain in preschool children. *Pediatrics* 95:126–130, 1995.

131. Bullen BA, Reed RB, Mayer J. Physical activity of obese and nonobese adolescent girls appraised by motion picture sampling. *Am J Clin Nutr* 14:211–223, 1964.

132. Styne DM. Obesity in childhood: What's activity got to do with it? *Am J Clin Nutr* 81:337–338, 2005.

133. Chirico AM, Stunkard AJ. Physical activity and human obesity. *N Eng J Med* 263:935–940, 1960.

134. Bloom WL, Eidex MF. Inactivity as a major factor in adult obesity. *Metabolism* 16:679–684, 1967.

135. Tryon WW, Goldberg JL, Morrison DF. Activity decreases as percentage overweight increases. *Int J Obesity* 16:591–595, 1992.

136. Ferraro R, Boyce VL, Swinburn B, De Gregorio M, Ravussin E. Energy cost of physical activity on a metabolic ward in relationship to obesity. *Am J Clin Nutr* 53:1368–137, 1991.
137. Rowland TW. Effects of obesity on aerobic fitness in adolescent females. *AJDC* 145:764–768, 1991.
138. Voorrips LE, Meijers JHH, Sol P, Seidell JC, van Staveren WA. History of body weight and physical activity of elderly women differing in current physical activity. *Int J Obesity* 16:199–205, 1992.
139. Schulz LO, Schoeller DA. A compilation of total daily energy expenditures and body weights in healthy adults. *Am J Clin Nutr* 60:676–681, 1994.
140. DiPietro L, Williamson DF, Caspersen CJ, Eaker E. The descriptive epidemiology of selected physical activities and body weight among adults trying to lose weight. The Behavioral Risk Factor Surveillance System Survey, 1989. *Int J Obesity* 17:69–76, 1993.
141. CDC. Prevalence of leisure-time physical activity among overweight adults. United States, 1998. *MMWR* 49(15):326–330, 2000.
142. Hill JO, Melanson EL. Overview of the determinants of overweight and obesity: Current evidence and research issues. *Med Sci Sports Exerc* 31(suppl):S515–S521, 1999.
143. Rising M, Harper IT, Fontvielle AM, Ferraro RT, Spraul M, Ravussin E. Determinants of total daily energy expenditure: Variability in physical activity. *Am J Clin Nutr* 59:800–804, 1994.
144. Saris WHM. Fit, fat and fat free: The metabolic aspects of weight control. *Int J Obesity* 22(suppl 2):S15–S21, 1998.
145. Reed GW, Hill JO. Measuring the thermic effect of food. *Am J Clin Nutr* 63:164–169, 1996.
146. Tataranni PA, Larson DE, Snitker S, Ravussin E. Thermic effect of food in humans: Methods and results from use of a respiratory chamber. *Am J Clin Nutr* 61:1013–1019, 1995.
147. Tai MM, Castillo P, Pi-Sunyer FX. Meal size and frequency: Effect on the thermic effect of food. *Am J Clin Nutr* 54:783–787, 1991.
148. Granata GP, Brandon LJ. The thermic effect of food and obesity: Discrepant results and methodological variations. *Nutr Rev* 60:223–233, 2002.
149. Rothwell N. Thermogenesis: Where are we and where are we going? *Int J Obesity* 25:1272–1274, 2001.
150. Schoeller DA. The importance of clinical research: The role of thermogenesis in human obesity. *Am J Clin Nutr* 73:511–516, 2001.
151. Tsai AG, Wadden TA. Systematic review: An evaluation of major commercial weight loss programs in the United States. *Ann Intern Med* 142:56–66, 2005. See also: NIH Technology Assessment Conference Panel. Methods for voluntary weight loss and control. *Ann Intern Med* 119(7 pt 2):764–770, 1993.
152. Levy AS, Heaton AW. Weight control practices of US adults trying to lose weight. *Ann Intern Med* 119(7 pt 2):661–666, 1993.
153. Serdula MK, Mokdad AH, Williamson DF, Galuska DA, Mendlein JM, Heath GW. Prevalence of attempting weight loss and strategies for controlling weight. *JAMA* 282:1353–1358, 1999.
154. Mokdad AH, Bowman BA, Ford ES, Vinicor F, Marks JS, Koplan JP. The continuing epidemics of obesity and diabetes in the United States. *JAMA* 286:1195–1200, 2001.
155. Kramer FM, Jeffery RW, Forster JL, Snell MK. Long-term follow-up of behavioral treatment for obesity: Patterns of weight regain among men and women. *Int J Obesity* 13:123–136, 1989.
156. Wadden TA, Sternberg JA, Letizia KA, Stunkard AJ, Foster GD. Treatment of obesity by very low calorie diet, behavior therapy, and their combination: A five-year perspective. *Int J Obesity* 13(suppl 2):13:39–46, 1989.
157. Hill JO, Thompson H, Wyatt H. Weight maintenance: What's missing? *J Am Diet Assoc* 105(5 Pt 2):63–66, 2005.
158. Mustajoki P, Pekkarinen T. Maintenance programs after weight reduction. How useful are they? *Int J Obesity* 23:553–555, 1999.
159. McGuire MT, Wing RR, Hill JO. The prevalence of weight loss maintenance among American adults. *Int J Obes Relat Metab Disord* 23:1314–1319, 1999.
160. Berkel LA, Carlos Poston WS, Reeves RS, Foreyt JP. Behavioral interventions for obesity. *J Am Diet Assoc* 105(5 Pt 2):35–43, 2005.
161. Wing RR, Hill JO. Successful weight loss maintenance. *Annu Rev Nutr* 21:323–341, 2001.
162. Gorin AA, Phelan S, Wing RR, Hill JO. Promoting long-term weight control: Does dieting consistency matter? *Int J Obes Relat Metab Disord* 28:278–281, 2004. See: http://www.nwcr.ws/.
163. Lyznicki JM, Young DC, Riggs JA, Davis RM. Obesity: Assessment and management in primary care. *Am Fam Physician* 63:2185–2196, 2001.
164. Lavery MA, Loewy JW. Identifying predictive variables for long-term weight change after participation in a weight loss program. *J Am Diet Assoc* 93:1017–1024, 1993.
165. Holden JH, Darga LL, Olson SM, et al. Long-term follow-up of patients attending a combination very-low calorie diet and behavior therapy weight loss program. *Int J Obesity* 16:605–613, 1992.
166. Walsh MF, Flynn TJ. A 54–month evaluation of a popular very low calorie diet program. *J Fam Pract* 41:231–236, 1995.
167. Saris WHM, Koenders MC, Pannemans DLE, van Baak MA. Outcome of a multicenter outpatient weight-management program including very-low-calorie diet and exercise. *Am J Clin Nutr* 56:294S–296S, 1992.
168. Phinney SD. Exercise during and after very-low-calorie dieting. *Am J Clin Nutr* 56:190S–194S, 1992.
169. Kayman S, Bruvold W, Stern JS. Maintenance and relapse after weight loss in women: Behavioral aspects. *Am J Clin Nutr* 52:800–807, 1990.
170. Grodstein F, Levine R, Troy L, Spencer T, Colditz GA, Stampfer MJ. Three-year follow-up of participants in a commercial weight loss program. Can you keep it off? *Arch Intern Med* 156:1302–1306, 1996.
171. Pi-Sunyer FX. Short-term medical benefits and adverse effects of weight loss. *Ann Intern Med* 119(7, pt 2):722–726, 1993.
172. Higgins M, D'Agostino R, Kannel W, Cobb J. Benefits and adverse effects of weight loss: Observations from the Framingham Study. *Ann Intern Med* 119(7 pt 2):758–763, 1993.
173. Atkinson RL. Proposed standards for judging the success of the treatment of obesity. *Ann Intern Med* 119(7 pt 2):677–680, 1993.
174. Brownell KD, Cohen LR. Adherence to dietary regimens 2: Components of effective interventions. *Beh Med* 20:155–163, 1995.
175. Stunkard AJ. Conservative treatments for obesity. *Am J Clin Nutr* 45:1142–1154, 1987.
176. Bray GA. Pathophysiology of obesity. *Am J Clin Nutr* 55:488S–494S, 1992.
177. National Institutes of Health Consensus Development Conference Panel. Gastrointestinal surgery for severe obesity. *Ann Int Med* 115:956–961, 1991.
178. Fobi MA, Lee H, Felahy B, Che K, Ako P, Fobi N. Choosing an operation for weight control, and the transected banded gastric bypass. *Obes Surg* 15:114–121, 2005.
179. Fried M, Peskova M. Gastric banding in the treatment of morbid obesity. *Hepato-Gastroenterology* 44:582–587, 1997.
180. Sjostrom L, Lindroos AK, Peltonen M, Torgerson J, Bouchard C, Carlsson B, Dahlgren S, Larsson B, Narbro K, Sjostrom CD, Sullivan M, Wedel H. Lifestyle, diabetes, and cardiovascular risk factors 10 years after bariatric surgery. *N Engl J Med* 351:2683–2693, 2004.

181. Cooper PL, Brearley LK, Jamieson AC, Ball MJ. Nutritional consequences of modified vertical gastroplasty in obese subjects. *Int J Obesity* 23:382–388, 1999.

182. Ballantyne GH. Measuring outcomes following bariatric surgery: Weight loss parameters, improvement in co-morbid conditions, change in quality of life and patient satisfaction. *Obes Surg* 13:954–964, 2003.

183. Mason EE, Renquist KE, Jiang D. Perioperative risks and safety of surgery for severe obesity. *Am J Clin Nutr* 55:573S–576S, 1992.

184. Heymsfield SB, Segal KR, Hauptman J, Lucas CP, Boldrin MN, Rissanen A, Wilding JP, Sjostrom L. Effects of weight loss with orlistat on glucose tolerance and progression to type 2 diabetes in obese adults. *Arch Intern Med* 8:160:1321–1326, 2000.

185. Wadden TA, Berkowitz RI, Sarwer DB, Prus-Wisniewski R, Steinberg C. Benefits of lifestyle modification in the pharmacologic treatment of obesity. *Arch Intern Med* 161:218–227, 2001.

186. Klein S. Long-term pharmacotherapy for obesity. *Obes Res* 12(suppl):163S–166S, 2004. See also: Waitman JA, Aronne LJ. Pharmacotherapy of obesity. *Obesity Management,* January, 2005, pp. 15–20.

187. National Task Force on the Prevention and Treatment of Obesity. Long-term pharmacotherapy in the management of obesity. *JAMA* 276:1907–1915, 1996.

188. Wirth A, Krause J. Long-term weight loss with sibutramine. A randomized controlled trial. *JAMA* 286:1331–1339, 2001.

189. Weissman NJ, Tighe JF, Gottdiener JS, Gwynne JT. An assessment of heart-valve abnormalities in obese patients taking dexfenfluramine, sustained-release dexfenfluramine, or placebo. *N Engl J Med* 339:725–732, 1998.

190. Berube-Parent S, Prudhomme D, St-Pierre S, Doucet ED, Tremblay A. Obesity treatment with a progressive clinical tri-therapy combing sibutramine and a supervised diet-exercise intervention. *Int J Obesity* 25:1144–1153, 2001.

191. Wadden TA, Van Itallie TB, Blackburn GL. Responsible and irresponsible use of very-low-calorie diets in the treatment of obesity. *JAMA* 263:83–85, 1990.

192. ADA Reports. Position of the American Dietetic Association: Very-low-calorie weight loss diets. *J Am Diet Assoc* 90:722–726, 1990.

193. Pi-Sunyer FX. The role of very-low-calorie diets in obesity. *Am J Clin Nutr* 56:240S–243S, 1992.

194. Wadden TA. Treatment of obesity by moderate and severe caloric restriction: Results of clinical research trials. *Ann Intern Med* 119(7, pt 2):688–693, 1993.

195. National Task Force on the Prevention and Treatment of Obesity. Very low-calorie diets. *JAMA* 270:967–974, 1993.

196. Howard AN. The historical development of very low calorie diets. *Int J Obesity* 13(suppl 2):1–9, 1989.

197. Wadden TA, Foster GD, Letizia KA, Stunkard AJ. A multicenter evaluation of a proprietary weight reduction program for the treatment of marked obesity. *Arch Intern Med* 152:961–966, 1992.

198. Raghuwanshi M, Kirschner M, Xenachis C, Ediale K, Amir J. Treatment of morbid obesity in inner-city women. *Obes Res* 9:342–347, 2001.

199. Foster GD, Wadden TA, Feurer ID, et al. Controlled trial of the metabolic effects of a very-low-calorie diet: Short- and long-term effects. *Am J Clin Nutr* 51:167–172, 1990.

200. Hovell MF, Koch A, Hofstetter R, et al. Long-term weight loss maintenance: Assessment of a behavioral and supplemented fasting regimen. *Am J Public Health* 78:663–666, 1988.

201. Kirschner MA, Schneider G, Ertel NH, Gorman J. An eight-year experience with a very-low-calorie formula diet for control of major obesity. *Int J Obesity* 12:69–80, 1988.

202. Torgerson JS, Lissner L, Lindroos AK, Kruijer H, Sjostrom IL. VLCD plus dietary and behavioral support versus support alone in the treatment of severe obesity. A randomized two-year clinical trial. *Int J Obesity* 21:987–994, 1997.

203. Dansinger ML, Gleason JA, Griffith JL, Selker HP, Schaefer EJ. Comparison of the Atkins, Ornish, Weight Watchers, and Zone diets for weight loss and heart disease risk reduction. *JAMA* 293:43–53, 2005.

204. Avenell A, Brown TJ, McGee MA, Campbell MK, Grant AM, Broom J, Jung RT, Smith WC. What are the long-term benefits of weight reducing diets in adults? A systematic review of randomized controlled trials. *J Hum Nutr Diet* 17:317–335. 2004.

205. Stern L, Iqbal N, Seshadri P, Chicano KL, Daily DA, McGrory J, Williams M, Gracely EJ, Samaha FF. The effects of low-carbohydrate versus conventional weight loss diets in severely obese adults: One-year follow-up of a randomized trial. *Ann Intern Med* 140:778–785, 2004.

206. Yancy WS, Olsen MK, Guyton JR, Bakst RP, Westman EC. A low-carbohydrate, ketogenic diet versus a low-fat diet to treat obesity and hyperlipidemia. *Ann Intern Med* 140:769–777, 2004.

207. Foster GD, Wyatt HR, Hill JO, McGuckin BG, Brill C, Mohammed BS, Szapary PO, Rader DJ, Edman JS, Klein S. A randomized trial of low-carbohydrate diet for obesity. *N Engl J Med* 348:2082–2090, 2003.

208. Garrow JS. Exercise in the treatment of obesity: A marginal contribution. *Int J Obesity* 19(suppl 4):S126–S129, 1995.

209. Ross R, Janssen I. Physical activity, total and regional obesity: Dose–response considerations. *Med Sci Sports Exerc* 33(6 suppl):S521–S527, 2001.

210. Calles-Escandón, Horton ES. The thermogenic role of exercise in the treatment of morbid obesity: A critical evaluation. *Am J Clin Nutr* 55:533S–537S, 1992.

211. Jakicic JM, Gallagher KI. Exercise considerations for the sedentary, overweight adults. *Exerc Sport Sci Rev* 31:91–95, 2003.

212. Miller WC, Koceja DM, Hamilton EJ. A meta-analysis of the past 25 years of weight loss research using diet, exercise or diet plus exercise intervention. *Int J Obes Relat Metab Disord* 21:941–947, 1997.

213. Donnelly JE, Smith B, Jacobsen DJ, Kirk E, Dubose K, Hyder M, Bailey B, Washburn R. The role of exercise for weight loss and maintenance. *Best Pract Res Clin Gastroenterol* 18:1009–1029, 2004.

214. Garrow JS, Summerbell CD. Meta-analysis: Effect of exercise, with or without dieting, on the body composition of overweight subjects. *Eur J Clin Nutr* 49:1–10, 1995.

215. King AC, Haskell WL, Taylor B, Kraemer HC, DeBusk RF. Group- vs home-based exercise training in healthy older men and women: A community-based clinical trial. *JAMA* 266:1535–1542, 1991.

216. Warren BJ, Nieman DC, Dotson RG, Adkins CH, O'Donnell KA, Haddock BL, Butterworth DE. Cardiorespiratory responses to exercise training in septuagenarian women. *Int J Sports Med* 14:60–65, 1993.

217. Hinkleman L, Nieman DC. The effects of a walking program on body composition and serum lipids and lipoproteins in overweight women. *J Sports Med Phys Fit* 33:49–58, 1993.

218. Wing RR. Physical activity in the treatment of the adulthood overweight and obesity: Current evidence and research issues. *Med Sci Sports Exerc* 31(suppl):S547–S552, 1999.

219. Jeffery RW, Wing RR, Sherwood NE, Tate DF. Physical activity and weight loss: Does prescribing higher physical activity goals improve outcome? *Am J Clin Nutr* 78:684–689, 2003.

220. Hardman AE, Jones PRM, Norgan NG, Hudson A. Brisk walking improves endurance fitness without changing body fatness in previously sedentary women. *Eur J Appl Physiol* 65:354–359, 1992.

221. Nieman DC, Haig JL, De Guia ED, et al. Reducing diet and exercise training effects on resting metabolic rates in mildly obese women. *J Sports Med* 28:9–88, 1988.

222. Jakicic JM, Marcus BH, Gallagher KI, Napolitano M, Lang W. Effect of exercise duration and intensity on weight loss in overweight, sedentary women: A randomized trial. *JAMA* 290:1323–1330, 2003.

223. Irwin ML, Yasui Y, Ulrich CM, Bowen D, Rudolph RE, Schwartz RS, Yukawa M, Aiello E, Potter JD, McTiernan A. Effect of exercise on total and intra-abdominal body fat in postmenopausal women: A randomized controlled trial. *JAMA* 289:323–330, 2003.

224. Utter AC, Nieman DC, Shannonhouse EM, Butterworth DE, Nieman CN. Influence of diet and/or exercise on body composition and cardiorespiratory fitness in obese women. *Int J Sport Nutr* 8:213–222, 1998.

225. Fogelholm M, Kukkonen-Harjula K, Nenonen A, Pasanen M. Effects of walking training on weight maintenance after a very-low-energy diet in premenopausal obese women: A randomized controlled trial. *Arch Intern Med* 160:2177–2184, 2000.

226. U.S. Department of Health and Human Services and U.S. Department of Agriculture. Dietary Guidelines for Americans (6th ed). Washington, DC: U.S. Government Printing Office, 2005.

227. Wadden TA, Vogt RA, Anderson RE, et al. Exercise in the treatment of obesity: Effects of four interventions on body composition, resting energy expenditure, appetite, and mood. *J Consult Clin Psyc* 65:269–277, 1997.

228. Whatley JE, Gillespie WJ, Honig J, Walsh MJ, Blackburn AL, Blackburn GL. Does the amount of endurance exercise in combination with weight training and a very-low-energy diet affect resting metabolic rate and body composition? *Am J Clin Nutr* 59:1088–1092, 1994.

229. Donnelly JE, Pronk NP, Jacobsen DJ, Pronk SJ, Jakicic JM. Effects of a very-low-calorie diet and physical training regimens on body composition and resting metabolic rate in obese females. *Am J Clin Nutr* 54:56–61, 1991.

230. Ross R, Dagnone D, Jones PJH, Smith H, Paddags A, Hudson R, Janssen I. Reduction in obesity and related comorbid conditions after diet-induced weight loss or exercise-induced weight loss in men. A randomized, controlled trial. *Ann Intern Med* 133:92–103, 2000.

231. Hill JO, Melby C, Johnson SL, Peters JC. Physical activity and energy requirements. *Am J Clin Nutr* 62(suppl):1059S–1066S, 1995.

232. Poehlman ET, Melby CL, Goran MI. The impact of exercise and diet restriction on daily energy expenditure. *Sports Med* 11:78–101, 1991.

233. Blair SN. Evidence for success of exercise in weight loss and control. *Ann Intern Med* 119(7, pt 2):702–706, 1993.

234. Schoeller DA, Shay K, Kushner RF. How much physical activity is needed to minimize weight gain in previously obese women? *Am J Clin Nutr* 66:551–556, 1997.

235. Mattsson E, Larsson UE, Rossner S. Is walking for exercise too exhausting for obese women? *Int J Obes Relat Metab Disord* 21:380–386, 1997.

236. Sedlock DA, Fissinger JA, Melby CL. Effect of exercise intensity and duration on postexercise energy expenditure. *Med Sci Sports Exerc* 21:662–666, 1989.

237. Bahr R, Sejersted OM. Effect of intensity of exercise on excess postexercise oxygen consumption. *Metabolism* 40:836–841, 1991.

238. Phelain JF, Reinke E, Harris MA, Melby CL. Postexercise energy expenditure and substrate oxidation in young women resulting from exercise bouts of different intensity. *J Am College Nutr* 16:140–146, 1997.

239. Borsheim E, Bahr R. Effect of exercise intensity, duration and mode on post-exercise oxygen consumption. *Sports Med* 33:1037–1060, 2003.

240. Short KR, Sedlock DA. Excess postexercise oxygen consumption and recovery rate in trained and untrained subjects. *J Appl Physiol* 83:153–159, 1997.

241. Speakman JR, Selman C. Physical activity and resting metabolic rate. *Proc Nutr Soc* 62:621–634, 2003.

242. Sullo A, Cardinale P, Brizzi G, Fabbri B, Maffulli N. Resting metabolic rate and post-prandial thermogenesis by level of aerobic power in older athletes. *Clin Exp Pharmacol Physiol* 31:202–206, 2004.

243. Poehlman ET, Gardner AW, Ades PA, et al. Resting energy metabolism and cardiovascular disease risk in resistance-trained and aerobically trained males. *Metabolism* 41:1351–1360, 1992.

244. Toth MJ, Poehlman ET. Resting metabolic rate and cardiovascular disease risk in resistance- and aerobic-trained middle-aged women. *Int J Obesity* 19:691–698, 1995.

245. Meijer GAL, Westerterp KR, Seyts GHP, Janssen GME, Saris WHM, ten Hoor F. Body composition and sleeping metabolic rate in response to a 5-month endurance-training program in adults. *Eur J Appl Physiol* 62:18–21, 1991.

246. Broeder CE, Burrhus KA, Svanevik LS, Wilmore JH. The effects of aerobic fitness on resting metabolic rate. *Am J Clin Nutr* 55:795–801, 1992.

247. Wilmore JH, Stanforth PR, Hudspeth LA, Gagnon J, Daw EW, Leon AS, Rao DC, Skinner JS, Bouchard C. Alterations in resting metabolic rate as a consequence of 20 wk of endurance training: The HERITAGE Family Study. *Am J Clin Nutr* 68:66–71, 1998.

248. Bell C, Day DS, Jones PP, Christou DD, Petitt DS, Osterberg K, Melby CL, Seals DR. High energy flux mediates the tonically augmented beta-adrenergic support of resting metabolic rate in habitually exercising older adults. *J Clin Endocrinol Metab* 89:3573–3578, 2004.

249. Herring JL, Molé PA, Meredith CN, Stern JS. Effect of suspending exercise training on resting metabolic rate in women. *Med Sci Sports Exerc* 24:59–65, 1992.

250. Bullough RC, Gillette CA, Harris MA, Melby CL. Interaction of acute changes in exercise energy expenditure and energy intake on resting metabolic rate. *Am J Clin Nutr* 61:473–481, 1995.

251. Phinney SD, LaGrange BM, O'Connell M, Danforth E. Effects of aerobic exercise on energy expenditure and nitrogen balance during very low calorie dieting. *Metabolism* 37:758–765, 1988.

252. Mathieson RA, Walberg JL, Gwazdauskas FC, et al. The effect of varying carbohydrate content of a very-low-caloric diet on resting metabolic rate and thyroid hormones. *Metabolism* 35:394–398, 1986.

253. Geliebter A, Maher MM, Gerace L, Gutin B, Heymsfield SB, Hashim SA. Effects of strength or aerobic training on body composition, resting metabolic rate, and peak oxygen consumption in obese dieting subjects. *Am J Clin Nutr* 66:557–563, 1997.

254. Westerterp KR, Meijer GAL, Schoffelen P, Janssen EME. Body mass, body composition and sleeping metabolic rate before, during and after endurance training. *Eur J Appl Physiol* 69:203–208, 1994.

255. Kempen KPG, Saris WHM, Westerterp KR. Energy balance during an 8-wk energy-restricted diet with and without exercise in obese women. *Am J Clin Nutr* 62:722–729, 1995.

256. Garrow JS. Energy balance in man—an overview. *Am J Clin Nutr* 45:1114–1119, 1987.

257. Marks BL, Rippe JM. The importance of fat free mass maintenance in weight loss programs. *Sports Med* 22:273–281, 1996.

258. Donnelly JE, Sharp T, Houmard J, et al. Muscle hypertrophy with large-scale weight loss and resistance training. *Am J Clin Nutr* 58:561–565, 1993.

259. Nieman DC, Miller AR, Henson DA, Warren BJ, Gusewitch G, Johnson RL, Davis JM, Butterworth DE, Herring JL, Nehlsen-Cannarella SL. The effects of high versus moderate-intensity exercise on lymphocyte subpopulations and proliferative response. *Int J Sports Med* 15:199–206, 1994.

260. Tremblay A, Simoneau JA, Bouchard C. Impact of exercise intensity on body fatness and skeletal muscle metabolism. *Metabolism* 43:814–818, 1994.

261. Buemann B, Tremblay A. Effects of exercise training on abdominal obesity and related metabolic complications. *Sports Med* 21:191–212, 1996.

262. Visser M, Launer LJ, Deurenberg P, Deeg DJH. Total and sports activity in older men and women: Relation with body fat distribution. *Am J Epidemiol* 145:752–761, 1997.

263. Tremblay A, Despres JP, Leblanc C, et al. Effect of intensity of physical activity on body fatness and fat distribution. *Am J Clin Nutr* 51:153–157, 1990.

264. Wahrenberg H, Bolinder J, Arner P. Adrenergic regulation of lipolysis in human fat cells during exercise. *Eur J Clin Invest* 21:534–541, 1991.

265. Stevenson DW, Darga LL, Spafford TR, et al. Variable effects of weight loss on serum lipids and lipoproteins in obese patients. *Int J Obesity* 12:495–502, 1987.

266. Wong SL, Katzmarzyk PT, Nichaman MZ, Church TS, Blair SN, Ross R. Cardiorespiratory fitness is associated with lower abdominal fat independent of body mass index. *Med Sci Sports Exerc* 36:286–291, 2004.

267. Kohrt WM, Malley MT, Dalsky GP, Holloszy JO. Body composition of healthy sedentary and trained, young and older men and women. *Med Sci Sports Exerc* 24:832–837, 1992.

268. McInnis KJ. Exercise for obese clients. Benefits, limitations, guidelines. *ACSM's Health & Fitness Journal* 4(1):25–31, 2000.

269. Miller WC. Effective diet and exercise treatments for overweight and recommendations for intervention. *Sports Med* 31:717–724, 2001.

270. Zachwieja JJ. Exercise as treatment for obesity. *Endocrinol Metab Clin North Am* 25:965–988, 1996.

271. American Psychiatric Association. *Diagnostic and Statistical Manual for Mental Disorders* (4th edition, text revision). Washington, DC: APA Press, 2000.

272. American Dietetic Association. Position of the American Dietetic Association: Nutrition intervention in the treatment of anorexia nervosa, bulimia nervosa, and eating disorders not otherwise specified (EDNOS). *J Am Diet Assoc* 101:810–819, 2001.

273. Kohn M, Golden NH. Eating disorders in children and adolescents: Epidemiology, diagnosis, and treatment. *Paediatr Drugs* 3:91–99, 2001.

274. Heterington MM, Altemus M, Nelson ML, Bernat AS, Gold PW. Eating behavior in bulimia nervosa: Multiple meal analyses. *Am J Clin Nutr* 60:864–873, 1994.

275. American Psychiatric Association Work Group on Eating Disorders. Practice guidelines for the treatment of patients with eating disorders (revision). *Am J Psychiatry* 157(suppl 1):1–39, 2000.

276. National Institutes of Mental Health. *Eating Disorders: Facts about Eating Disorders and the Search for Solutions.* Bethesda, MD: NIMH, 2001.

277. Wakeling A. Epidemiology of anorexia nervosa. *Psychiatry Res* 62:3–9, 1996.

278. Leon GR. Eating disorders in female athletes. *Sports Med* 12:219–227, 1991.

279. Phillips EL, Pratt HD. Eating disorders in college. *Pediatr Clin North Am* 52:85–96, 2005.

280. Ricciardelli LA, McCabe MP. Children's body image concerns and eating disturbances: A review of the literature. *Clin Psychol Rev* 21:325–344, 2001.

281. Seidenfeld ME, Rickert VI. Impact of anorexia, bulimia and obesity on the gynecologic health of adolescents. *Am Fam Physician* 64:445–450, 2001.

282. Mehler PS. Diagnosis and care of patients with anorexia nervosa in primary care settings. *Ann Intern Med* 134:1048–1059, 2001.

283. Garfinkel PE, Newman A. The eating attitudes test: Twenty-five years later. *Eat Weight Disorder* 6:1–24, 2001.

284. Killen JD, Taylor CB, Telch MJ, et al. Self-induced vomiting and laxative and diuretic use among teenagers. *JAMA* 255:1447–1449, 1986.

285. Dummer GM, Rosen LW, Heusner WW, et al. Pathogenic weight-control behaviors of young competitive swimmers. *Physician Sportsmed* 15(5):75–86, 1987.

286. Clark N, Nelson M, Evans W. Nutrition education for elite female runners. *Physician Sportsmed* 15:75–84, 1987.

287. Sudi K, Ottl K, Payerl D, Baumgartl P, Tauschmann K, Muller W. Anorexia athletica. *Nutrition* 20:657–661, 2004.

288. Reinking MF, Alexander LE. Prevalence of disordered-eating behaviors in undergraduate female collegiate athletes and nonathletes. *J Athletic Train* 40:47–51, 2005.

289. ACSM position stand on the female athlete triad. *Med Sci Sports Exerc* 29:i–ix, 1997.

290. Brownell KD, Steen SN, Wilmore JH. Weight regulation practices in athletes: Analysis of metabolic and health effects. *Med Sci Sports Exerc* 19:546–556, 1987.

291. National Institute of Nutrition. An overview of the eating disorders anorexia nervosa and bulimia nervosa. *Nutrition Today,* May/June, 1989, pp. 27–29.

292. Striegel-Moore RH. Risk factors for eating disorders. *Ann N Y Acad Sci* 817:98–109, 1997.

293. Wonderlich SA, Wilsnack RW, Wilsnack SC, Harris RH. Childhood sexual abuse and bulimic behavior in a nationally representative sample. *Am J Public Health* 86:1082–1086, 1996. See also: *J Am Acad Child Adolesc Psychiatry* 36:1107–1115, 1997.

294. Jacobi C, Haward C, de Zwaan M, Kraemer HC, Agras WS. Coming to terms with risk factors for eating disorders: Application of risk terminology and suggestions for a general taxonomy. *Psychol Bull* 130:19–65, 2004.

295. Mehler PS, Crews C, Weiner K. Bulimia: Medical complications. *J Womens Health (Larchmt)* 13:668–675, 2004.

296. Carney CP, Andersen AE. Eating disorders: Guide to medical evaluation and complications. *Psychiatr Clin North Am* 19:657–679, 1996.

297. Casper RC. The pathophysiology of anorexia nervosa and bulimia nervosa. *Ann Rev Nutr* 6:299–316, 1986.

298. Casper RC, Schoeller DA, Kushner R, Hnilicka J, Gold ST. Total daily energy expenditure and activity level in anorexia nervosa. *Am J Clin Nutr* 53:1143–1150, 1991.

299. Position of The American Dietetic Association. Nutrition intervention in the treatment of anorexia nervosa and bulimia nervosa. *J Am Diet Assoc* 88:68–71, 1988.

300. Churchill BH, Strauss J. Long-term outcome of adolescents with anorexia nervosa. *Am J Dis Children* 143:1322–1327, 1989.

301. Deter HC, Herzog W. Anorexia nervosa in a long-term perspective: Results of the Heidelberg-Mannheim Study. *Psychosom Med* 56:20–27, 1994.

PHYSICAL FITNESS ACTIVITY 13.1

Calculating Your Energy Expenditure

In this physical fitness activity, you will be calculating your average daily Calorie expenditure. As you may remember from your study of this chapter, during any given 24-hour period, the majority of your energy expenditure (if you are no more than moderately active) comes from your resting metabolic rate, with smaller amounts from physical activity and the energy used in digesting and metabolizing your food.

Table 13.5 outlines a method for determining the number of Calories burned each day, combining RMR and physical activity. Notice that Category 1 represents the energy you expend during sleeping or resting in bed, or in other words, your resting metabolic rate. Categories 2 through 9 represent different forms of physical activity, with category 9 being the most intense.

The average female in the United States burns only 1,500–2,000 total Calories per day, and the average male, 2,300–3,000 Calories per day. Those spending more time in categories 6 through 9 will burn more than these amounts.

Estimate the number of Calories you burn in a given day by averaging the number of hours you spend in each activity category. Make sure that your hour total equals 24.

Multiply the number of hours by the Calorie/kg factor and then your weight (in kilograms). The final step is to total the Calories you have estimated in the final column. Your final result should be close to the estimated amount of Calories you consume each day.

TABLE 13.5 Calculating Energy Expenditure

Directions: Estimate the average number of hours you spend in each category. Multiply the Calorie/kg factor times the hours/day and then by your body weight. Put the total number of Calories calculated for each category in the Calorie/Category blank.

Category	Average Hours/Day		Calorie/kg per Hour		Body Wt (kg)		Calorie/ Category
1	____	×	1.00	×	____	=	____
2	____	×	1.35	×	____	=	____
3	____	×	2.00	×	____	=	____
4	____	×	2.50	×	____	=	____
5	____	×	3.00	×	____	=	____
6	____	×	4.25	×	____	=	____
7	____	×	5.00	×	____	=	____
8	____	×	6.00	×	____	=	____
9	____	×	8.00	×	____	=	____
Total	24					=	____ Total (24-hour energy expenditure)

Category 1 Sleeping; resting in bed

Category 2 Sitting; eating; listening; writing; etc.

Category 3 Light activity while standing; washing, shaving, combing hair, cooking

Category 4 Slow walking; driving; dressing; showering

Category 5 Light manual work (floor sweeping, window washing, driving a truck, painting, waiting on tables, nursing chores, house chores, electrical work, walking at moderate pace)

TABLE 13.5 ***(continued)***

Category 6	Leisure activities and sports in a recreational environment (baseball, golf, volleyball, canoeing or rowing, archery, bowling, slow cycling, table tennis, etc.)
Category 7	Manual work at moderate pace (mining, carpentry, house building, snow shoveling, loading and unloading goods)
Category 8	Leisure and sport activities of higher intensity, but not competitive (canoeing, bicycling at less than 10 mph, dancing, skiing, badminton, gymnastics, moderately paced swimming, tennis, brisk walking, etc.)
Category 9	Intense manual work, high-intensity sport activities or sport competition (tree cutting, carrying heavy loads, jogging and running faster than 12 minutes a mile, racquetball, swimming, cross-country skiing, mountain biking, etc.)

Source: Bouchard C, et al. A method to assess energy expenditure in children and adults. *Am J Clin Nutr* 37:461–467, 1983.

PHYSICAL FITNESS ACTIVITY 13.2

Estimating Resting Metabolic Rate and Total Energy Expenditure

The resting metabolic rate (RMR) is the energy expended each day by the body to maintain life and normal body functions such as respiration and circulation. In other words, if one sat or laid down all day, and did not move a muscle, the RMR is the energy expended by the body to keep it alive. The RMR varies according to age, sex, and weight. It falls about 1–2% per decade of life, with the lowest levels measured in the elderly. Heavy people have higher RMR rates than those with low body weight.

Use the formulas listed in the given table to calculate your RMR in Calories per day. Choose the appropriate formula based on your age and sex. Next calculate your body weight in kilograms. Take your weight in pounds and divide it by 2.2. For example, if you weigh 154 pounds, then your weight in kilograms is 154 pounds/2.2 = 70 kg. Finally, multiply your kilogram body weight by the appropriate number listed in the formula and add the constant. For example, if you are a 20-year-old male weighing 70 kg, your RMR would be calculated as follows: (15.3 × 70) + 679 = 1,750 Calories per day.

Your RMR = ______________________________ calories per day

Age Range (years)	Equation for Calories/ Day Resting Metabolic Rate
Males	
18–30	15.3 (kg) + 679
30–60	11.6 (kg) + 879
>60	13.5 (kg) + 487
Females	
18–30	14.7 (kg) + 496
30–60	8.7 (kg) + 829
>60	10.5 (kg) + 596

To determine your total daily energy expenditure, first choose an activity factor using the following guidelines:

- 1.0–1.39 = sedentary (no planned exercise, little work activity)
- 1.4–1.59 = light activity (typical American, with infrequent planned exercise, some work activity)
- 1.6–1.89 = moderate activity (3–5 days/week of planned exercise for 30–45 minutes per session, some work activity)
- 1.9–2.5 = heavy activity (daily planned vigorous exercise lasting 1 hour or more and/or manual labor throughout the day)

Your total daily energy expenditure in Calories per day =*
RMR __________ × activity factor __________ = __________ Calories

*Compare this result with the appropriate TEE equation from Table 13.1.

PHYSICAL FITNESS ACTIVITY 13.3

Counting the Calories and Fat Grams from Fast Food

Most fast foods are high in Calories and fat grams, more than you may think. Visit the Internet site Cyberdiet at www.cyberdiet.com. Go to the section called Diet & Nutrition and click on Fast Food Quest. Use the search engine provided at this Internet site and list the number of Calories and fat grams given for each fast food listed in the table.

Food Description	Calories	Fat grams
McDonald's Big Mac (hamburger)		
McDonald's Quarter Pounder, with cheese		
Burger King Big King (hamburger)		
Burger King Bacon Double Cheeseburger		
Burger King Double Whopper		
Wendy's Big Bacon Classic (hamburger)		
Domino's Pizza, bacon topping, 14 inches		
Domino's Pizza, beef topping, 14 inches		
Papa John's Pizza, All the Meats		
Pizza Hut Cheese Personal		

What is your reaction to this information?

____

____

____

____

____

PHYSICAL FITNESS ACTIVITY 13.4

Monitoring Your Dietary Habits

A key strategy in weight management is to know your personal dietary habits. When do you eat and where are you? How hungry are you when you eat? What else are you doing when you eat? Who do you eat with? What are your feelings before and during eating? This information will help you improve your eating habits, keeping caloric intake under control.

Fill in the food diary for 1 day (the more typical the better). Fill in all the blanks using the given instructions. You will notice that keeping this food diary will make you unusually aware of everything you eat and why.

Instructions

Time	Record the starting time for a meal or snack.
Minutes spent eating	Record the length of each eating episode (no matter how short or long).
Food type and quantity	Describe the type of food eaten and how much.
Hunger scale	Record a "0" if you had no hunger, a "1" if you had some hunger, a "2" if you had much hunger, and a "3" if you had extreme hunger.
Activity while eating	Record any activity that accompanied eating such as watching television, reading, partying with friends, driving your car, walking to class.
Location of eating	Record where you ate the meal or snack, such as your kitchen table, your car, the living room couch, your bed, a restaurant.
Feelings	Record your feelings and mood before and during eating, such as bored, angry, confused, depressed, frustrated, sad, tense.

Time of Day	Minutes spent eating	Food type and quantity	Hunger scale (0 to 3)	Activity while eating	Location of eating	Feelings

FOOD PHYSICAL FITNESS ACTIVITY 13.5*

Eating Disorder Checksheet

As discussed in the Sports Medicine Insight, a significant number of college-age students have eating disorders. This activity will help determine whether you have an eating disorder.

Place an (X) under the column that applies best to each of the numbered statements.

Section One

Always 0	Very Often 0	Often 0	Sometimes 1	Rarely 2	Never 3	
						1. I like eating with other people.
						2. I like my clothes to fit tightly.
						3. I enjoy eating meat.
						4. I have regular menstrual periods.
						5. I enjoy eating at restaurants.
						6. I enjoy trying new, rich foods.

Section Two

Always 3	Very Often 2	Often 1	Sometimes 0	Rarely 0	Never 0	
						7. I prepare foods for others but do not eat what I cook.
						8. I become anxious prior to eating.
						9. I am terrified about being overweight.
						10. I avoid eating when I am hungry.
						11. I find myself preoccupied with food.
						12. I have gone on eating binges where I feel that I may not be able to stop.
						13. I cut my food into small pieces.
						14. I am aware of the Calorie content of foods that I eat.
						15. I particularly avoid foods with a high carbohydrate content (bread, potatoes, rice, etc.)
						16. I feel bloated after meals.
						17. I feel others would prefer that I ate more.
						18. I vomit after I have eaten.
						19. I feel extremely guilty after eating.
						20. I am preoccupied with a desire to be thinner.

Always 3	Very Often 2	Often 1	Some-times 0	Rarely 0	Never 0	
						21. I exercise strenuously to burn off Calories.
						22. I weigh myself several times a day.
						23. I wake up early in the morning.
						24. I eat the same foods day after day.
						25. I think about burning up Calories when I exercise.
						26. Other people think I am too thin.
						27. I am preoccupied with the thought of having fat on my body.
						28. I take longer than others to eat my meals.
						29. I take laxatives.
						30. I avoid foods with sugar in them.
						31. I eat diet foods.
						32. I feel that food controls my life.
						33. I display self-control around foods.
						34. I feel that others pressure me to eat.
						35. I give too much time and thought to food.
						36. I suffer from constipation.
						37. I feel uncomfortable after eating sweets.
						38. I engage in dieting behavior.
						39. I like my stomach to be empty.
						40. I have the impulse to vomit after meals.

Total your points (use the numbers given at the top of each column for the two sections).

Norms	Range (0–120 points)
Eating disorder	>50 points
Borderline eating disorder	30–50 points
Normal[†]	<30 points

[†]Average score among those with normal eating habits = 15.4.

Source: Garner DM, Omstead M, Polivy J. Development and validation of a multidimensional eating disorder inventory for anorexia nervosa and bulimia. *Int J Eating Disorders* 2:15–33, 1983. Reprinted by permission of John Wiley & Sons, Inc.

[*]Go to www.river-centre.org/cgi-bin/test.cfm for an Internet screening program, The Eating Attitudes Test.

chapter 14

Psychological Health

I thought of that while riding my bike.

—Albert Einstein, on his theory of relativity

As discussed in Chapter 1, the promotion of physical activity is public policy in both the United States and Canada. Though directed primarily at the reduction of cardiovascular diseases, obesity, and other chronic diseases, this policy could also have some beneficial effects on the population's mental health. Even a small effect could be significant because mental health problems and stress are so widespread in most Western countries.[1]

MENTAL HEALTH

The surgeon general released a landmark report on mental health in 1999.[2] In this report, emphasis was placed on several key points:

- Mental health is fundamental to overall health.
- Mental disorders are real health conditions that have an immense impact on individuals and families throughout the world.
- People should seek help if they have a mental health problem or think they have symptoms of a mental disorder. The efficacy of mental health treatments is well documented, and a range of treatments exists for most mental disorders including:

  Medications. More medications are available than ever before.

  Psychotherapy. This includes behavioral therapy (focus on changing specific actions and uses several techniques to stop unwanted behaviors), and cognitive-behavioral therapy (teaches people to understand and change their thinking patterns so they can improve reactions).

Mental health is defined in the surgeon general's report as "the successful performance of mental function, resulting in productive activities, fulfilling relationships with other people, and the ability to adapt to change and to cope with adversity; from early childhood until late life, mental health is the springboard of thinking and communication skills, learning, emotional growth, resilience, and self-esteem."[2] Mental illness refers collectively to all mental disorders, which are defined as "health conditions that are characterized by alterations in thinking, mood, or behavior (or some combination thereof) associated with distress and/or impaired functioning."[2]

During any 1-year period, 45 million American adults—about one in five—suffer some form of mental disorder[2–7] (see Figure 14.1). Box 14.1 summarizes some of the key facts on prevalence of mental disorders in the United States. Anxiety and depressive disorders are the primary mental disor-

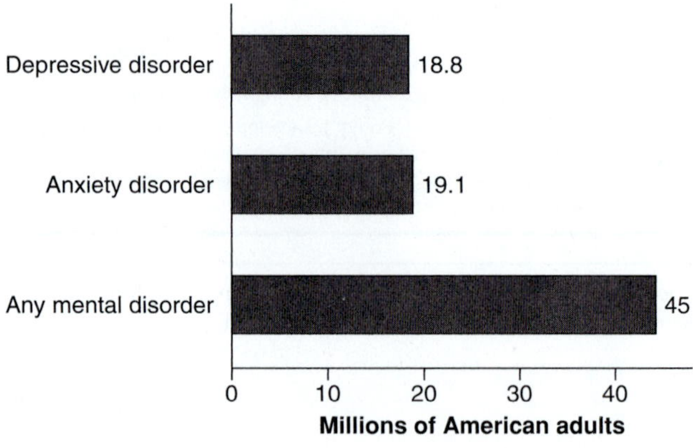

Figure 14.1 Prevalence of mental health disorders in the United States. Source: National Institute of Mental Health. www.nimh.nih.gov.

Box 14.1

Facts on Mental Disorders in America*

- Forty-five million (22.1% of American adults) suffer from a diagnosable mental disorder in a given year.

  Anxiety disorder: 19.1 million (13.3% of adults ages 18–54)

  - Specific phobia: 6.3 million
  - Social phobia: 5.3 million
  - Post traumatic stress disorder: 5.2 million
  - Generalized anxiety disorder: 4.0 million
  - Obsessive-compulsive disorder: 3.3 million
  - Panic disorder: 2.4 million

  Depressive disorder: 18.8 million (9.5% of adults 18 and older)

  - Dysthymic disorder: 10.9 million
  - Major depressive disorder: 9.9 million
  - Bipolar disorder: 2.3 million
- Four of the 10 leading causes of disability in the United States and other developed countries are mental disorders.
- Nearly twice as many women as men are affected by a depressive disorder.
- The average age at onset for major depressive disorder is the middle twenties.
- More than 90% of suicides involve people who have a diagnosable mental disorder.
- Anxiety disorders frequently co-occur with depressive disorders, eating disorders, or substance abuse. Many people have more than one anxiety disorder.
- Approximately twice as many women as men suffer from panic disorder, posttraumatic stress disorder, generalized anxiety disorder, and specific phobia.
- Agoraphobia is the most common specific phobia among Americans (3.2 million American adults aged 18–54), and involves intense fear and avoidance of any place or situation where escape might be difficult or help unavailable in the event of developing sudden panic-like symptoms.

*Many people have more than one type of anxiety or depressive disorder.

Source: National Institute of Mental Health. www.nimh.nih.gov.

ders, and these are described in Boxes 14.2 and 14.3, respectively. The American Psychiatric Association uses specific criteria to diagnose depressive disorders and anxiety. These are listed in Boxes 14.4 and 14.5, respectively.[8]

Box 14.2

Anxiety Disorders

Anxiety, a condition characterized by apprehension, tension, or uneasiness, stems from the anticipation of real or imagined danger. This relatively normal feeling affects almost everyone at some point in their lifetime. If the anxiety becomes excessive and unrealistic, however, it can interfere with normal functioning. Anxiety disorders, including various phobias, panic attacks, posttraumatic stress disorder, and obsessive-compulsive behavior, are the most prevalent of all mental health problems in the United States (19.1 million). Anxiety disorders are two times as prevalent in females as males.

There are five major types of anxiety disorders:

- *Panic disorder.* Repeated episodes of intense fear that strike often and without warning. Physical symptoms include chest pain, heart palpitations, shortness of breath, dizziness, abdominal distress, feelings of unreality, and fear of dying.
- *Obsessive-compulsive disorder.* Repeated, unwanted thoughts or compulsive behaviors that seem impossible to stop or control.
- *Posttraumatic stress disorder.* Persistent symptoms that occur after experiencing a traumatic event such as rape or other criminal assault, war, child abuse, natural disasters, or crashes. Nightmares; flashbacks; numbing of emotions; depression; feeling angry, irritable, or distracted; and being easily startled are common.
- *Phobias.* Two major types of phobias are social phobia and specific phobia. People with social phobia have an overwhelming and disabling fear of scrutiny, embarrassment, or humiliation in social situations, which leads to avoidance of many potentially pleasurable and meaningful activities. People with specific phobia experience extreme, disabling, and irrational fear of something that poses little or no danger; the fear leads to avoidance of objects or situations and can cause people to limit their lives unnecessarily.
- *General anxiety disorder.* Constant, exaggerated worrisome thoughts and tension about everyday routine life events and activities, lasting at least 6 months. Almost always anticipating the worst even though there is little reason to expect it; accompanied by physical symptoms, such as fatigue, trembling, muscle tension, headache, or nausea.

Source: National Institute of Mental Health. www.nimh.nih.gov.

Box 14.3

Depressive Disorders

Depression is a pernicious illness linked with episodes of long duration, relapse, and social and physical impairment. Most people with major depression are misdiagnosed, receive inappropriate or inadequate treatment, or are given no treatment at all. In any given 1-year period, 9.5% of the population (18.8 million American adults) suffer from a depressive illness. The lifetime estimate for major depression is 17% and is most common among females, the elderly, young adults, and people with less than a college education.

A depressive disorder is an illness that involves the body, mood, and thoughts. It affects the way a person eats and sleeps, the way one feels about oneself, and the way one thinks about things. Depression may range in severity from mild symptoms to more severe forms. Three of the most common types of depressive disorders are described here.

- *Major depression.* Manifested by a combination of symptoms that interfere with the ability to work, study, sleep, eat, and enjoy once-pleasurable activities. Symptoms include

  Persistent sad, anxious, or "empty" mood

  Feelings of hopelessness, pessimism

  Feelings of guilt, worthlessness, helplessness

  Loss of interest or pleasure in hobbies and activities that were once enjoyed

  Decreased energy, fatigue, being "slowed down"

  Difficulty concentrating, remembering, making decisions

  Insomnia, early-morning awakening, or oversleeping

  Appetite and/or weight loss or overeating and weight gain

  Thoughts of death or suicide; suicide attempts

  Restlessness, irritability

  Persistent physical symptoms that do not respond to treatment, such as headaches, digestive disorders, and chronic pain

- *Dysthymia.* Involves long-term chronic symptoms that do not disable, but do keep one from functioning well or from feeling good. Many people with dysthymia also experience major depressive episodes at some time in their lives.
- *Bipolar disorder.* Also called manic-depressive illness. Not nearly as prevalent as other forms of depressive disorders, bipolar disorder is characterized by cycling mood changes: severe highs (mania) and lows (depression). Sometimes the mood switches are dramatic and rapid, but most often they are gradual. Symptoms of mania include abnormal or excessive elation, unusual irritability, decreased need for sleep, grandiose notions, increased talking, racing thoughts, increased sexual desire, markedly increased energy, poor judgment, and inappropriate social behavior.

Source: National Institute of Mental Health. www.nimh.nih.gov.

Box 14.4

Diagnosis of Depression

A person who suffers from a major depressive disorder must either have a depressed mood or a loss of interest or pleasure in daily activities consistently for at least a 2-week period. This mood must represent a change from the person's normal mood. Social, occupational, educational, or other important functioning must also be negatively impaired by the change in mood. A depressed mood caused by substances (such as drugs, alcohol, medications) or a general medical condition is not considered a major depressive disorder. Major depressive disorder cannot be diagnosed if a person has a history of manic, hypomanic, or mixed episodes (e.g., a bipolar disorder) or if the depressed mood is better accounted for by schizoaffective disorder and is not superimposed on schizophrenia, a delusion or psychotic disorder.

This disorder is characterized by the presence of a majority of the following symptoms:

- Depressed mood most of the day, nearly every day, as indicated by either subjective report (e.g., feels sad or empty) or observation made by others (e.g., appears tearful). (In children and adolescents, this may be characterized as an irritable mood.)

(continued)

Box 14.4

Diagnosis of Depression *(continued)*

- Markedly diminished interest or pleasure in all, or almost all, activities most of the day, nearly every day.
- Significant weight loss when not dieting or weight gain (e.g., a change of more than 5% of body weight in a month), or decrease or increase in appetite nearly every day.
- Insomnia or hypersomnia nearly every day.
- Psychomotor agitation or retardation nearly every day.
- Fatigue or loss of energy nearly every day.
- Feelings of worthlessness or excessive or inappropriate guilt nearly every day.
- Diminished ability to think or concentrate, or indecisiveness, nearly every day.
- Recurrent thoughts of death (not just fear of dying), recurrent suicidal ideation without a specific plan, or a suicide attempt or a specific plan for committing suicide.

The symptoms are not better accounted for by bereavement, i.e., after the loss of a loved one; the symptoms persist for longer than 2 months or are characterized by marked functional impairment, morbid preoccupation with worthlessness, suicidal ideation, psychotic symptoms, or psychomotor retardation.

Source: Criteria summarized from American Psychiatric Association. *Diagnostic and Statistical Manual of Mental Disorders* (4th ed.). Washington, DC: American Psychiatric Association, 1994.

Box 14.5

Diagnosis of Generalized Anxiety Disorder

Generalized anxiety disorder (GAD) is much more than the normal anxiety people experience day to day. It is chronic and exaggerated worry and tension, even though nothing seems to provoke it. Having this disorder means always anticipating disaster, often worrying excessively about health, money, family, or work. Sometimes, though, the source of the worry is hard to pinpoint. Simply the thought of getting through the day provokes anxiety.

Specific Symptoms of This Disorder

- Excessive anxiety and worry (apprehensive expectation), occurring more days than not for at least 6 months, about a number of events or activities (such as work or school performance).
- The person finds it difficult to control the worry.
- The anxiety and worry are associated with three (or more) of the following six symptoms (with at least some symptoms present for more days than not for the past 6 months; children don't need to meet as many criteria):

  Restlessness or feeling keyed up or on edge

  Being easily fatigued

  Difficulty concentrating or mind going blank

  Irritability

  Muscle tension

  Sleep disturbance (difficulty falling or staying asleep, or restless unsatisfying sleep)
- The anxiety or worry is not about having a panic attack, being embarrassed in public (as in social phobia), being contaminated (as in obsessive-compulsive disorder), being away from home or close relatives (as in separation anxiety disorder), gaining weight (as in anorexia nervosa), having multiple physical complaints (as in somatization disorder), or having a serious illness (as in hypochondriasis), and the anxiety and worry do not occur exclusively during posttraumatic stress disorder (PTSD).
- The anxiety, worry, or physical symptoms cause clinically significant distress or impairment in social, occupational, or other important areas of functioning.
- The disturbance is not due to the direct physiological effects of a substance (e.g., a drug of abuse, a medication) or a general medical condition (e.g., hyperthyroidism) and does not occur exclusively during a mood disorder, a psychotic disorder, or a pervasive developmental disorder.

Source: American Psychiatric Association. *Diagnostic and Statistical Manual of Mental Disorders* (4th ed.). Washington, DC: American Psychiatric Association, 1994.

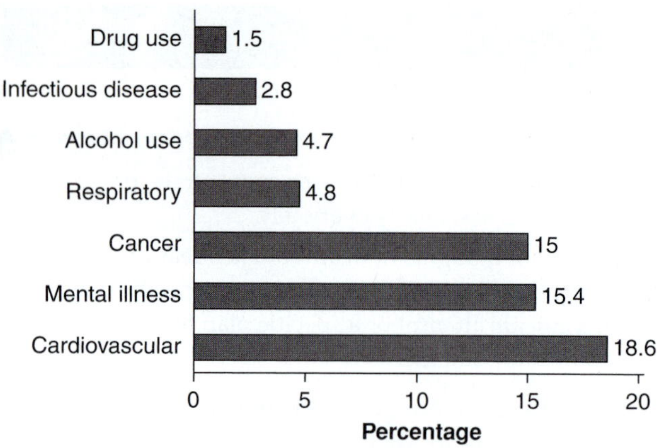

Figure 14.2 Disease burden around the world. Measured in DALYs, an estimate of lost years of healthy life due to premature death and disability. Source: Murray CJL, Lopez AD. *The Global Burden of Disease and Injury*. Cambridge, MA: Harvard School of Public Health on behalf of the World Health Organization and the World Bank, Harvard University Press, 1996.

The World Health Organization, in collaboration with the World Bank and Harvard University, has determined the "burden of disability" associated with the whole range of diseases and health conditions suffered by peoples throughout the world.[9–12] This study showed that the burden of mental disorders has been greatly underestimated. Worldwide, mental illness is the second leading cause of disability and premature mortality, as summarized in Figure 14.2.[9] Five of the 10 leading causes of disability are mental disorders, generating an immense public health burden.[9–13] According to the World Health Organization, one in four people in the world will be affected by mental or neurological disorders at some point in their lives.[10] Around 450 million people currently suffer from such conditions, placing mental disorders among the leading causes of ill health and disability worldwide.

Projections show that with the aging of the world population and the conquest of infectious diseases, mental disorders will increase their share of the total global burden of disease and disability.[9,10] Depressive disorders are expected to rank second as a cause of the global disease burden by the year 2020. Treatments are available, but nearly two thirds of people with a known mental disorder never seek help from a health professional. Stigma, discrimination, and neglect prevent care and treatment from reaching people with mental disorders.

Box 14.6 summarizes the burden of suicide in the United States.[6,7] About 30,000 people die from suicide each year, and of these, 9 in 10 have a mental disorder. Among high school students, 17% have seriously considered suicide and 8.5% have attemped suicide.[7]

Box 14.6

Suicide: Cost to the Nation

- Every 17 minutes another life is lost to suicide. Every day 86 Americans take their own life and over 1,500 attempt suicide.
- Suicide is now the 11th leading cause of death among Americans.
- For every two victims of homicide in the United States there are three persons who take their own lives.
- There are now twice as many deaths due to suicide than due to HIV/AIDS.
- Between 1952 and 1995, the incidence of suicide among adolescents and young adults nearly tripled.
- In the month prior to their suicide, 75% of elderly persons had visited a physician.
- Over half of all suicides occur in adult men, aged 25–65.
- Many who make suicide attempts never seek professional care immediately after the attempt. There are between 8 and 25 attempted suicides for every suicide death.
- Males are four times more likely to die from suicide than are females. Suicide by firearm is the most common method for both men and women (6 of 10 suicides).
- More teenagers and young adults die from suicide than from cancer, heart disease, AIDS, birth defects, stroke, pneumonia and influenza, and chronic lung disease, combined.
- Suicide takes the lives of about 30,000 Americans every year.

Source: National Strategy for Suicide Prevention. www.mentalhealth.org; www.nimh.nih.gov.

THE MEANING OF STRESS

Stress has been defined as any action or situation (stressor) that places special physical or psychological demands on a person—in other words, anything that unbalances one's equilibrium.[14–16] Hans Selye, one of the great pioneers of medicine and the originator of the concept of stress, wrote in his famous 1956 classic, *The Stress of Life*, "In its medical sense, stress is essentially the rate of wear and tear in the body . . . the nonspecific response of the body to any demand."[17]

There are two types of stress: eustress and distress.[14–18] *Eustress* is good stress and appears to motivate and inspire (e.g., falling in love or exercising moderately). *Distress* is considered bad stress and can be *acute* (quite intense, but then disappears quickly) or *chronic* (not so intense, but lingers for prolonged periods of time). (See Physical Fitness Activities 14.1 and 14.2 for two questionnaires used in measuring stress.) Selye observed that whether a situation was perceived as very good (e.g., getting married) or very bad (e.g., getting divorced), demands were placed on the body and mind, forcing them to adapt. According to Selye, the physiological response or arousal was very similar during both good and bad situations, producing a similar physiological response.[17]

Medical research on the effects of stress dates back to the early part of the 1900s, when Walter Cannon of Harvard University first coined the term "fight-or-flight response," now known as the stress response.[18] In this response, the muscles tense and tighten, breathing becomes deep and fast, the heart rate rises and blood vessels constrict, blood pressure rises, the stomach and intestines temporarily halt digestion, perspiration increases, the thyroid gland is stimulated, secretion of saliva slows, blood sugar and fats rise, and sensory perception becomes sharper. These responses are regulated by the nervous system and various hormones, redirecting energy, oxygen, and fuel to allow the body to cope with the physical or emotional stress (see Figure 14.3).

In the 1940s and 1950s, Selye extended Cannon's work, laying the foundation for today's understanding of stress and its medical consequences.[17] Experimenting with rats while using various physical stressors such as cold temperature or random electrical shock, Selye discovered that if the stressor was maintained long enough, the body would go through three stages (termed the "general adaptation syndrome"):[17]

1. *Alarm* reaction (essentially the fight-or-flight response)
2. *Resistance* stage (body functions return to normal as the body adjusts)
3. *Exhaustion* stage (alarm symptoms return, leading to disease and death)

Selye and other stress researchers, however, urged recognizing that not all stress is harmful.[14–18] In fact, it appears that humans need some degree of stress to stay healthy. While the human body needs some sort of balance (*homeostasis,* or physiological calm), it also requires occasional arousal to ensure that the heart, muscles, lungs, nerves, brain, and other tissues stay in good shape.

Ill Effects of High Stress and Poor Mental Health

Mental stress is a common complaint among American adults and has increased in recent years.[2,19] The prevalence of frequent mental distress (FMD), defined by the Centers for Disease Control and Prevention (CDC) as "self-reported

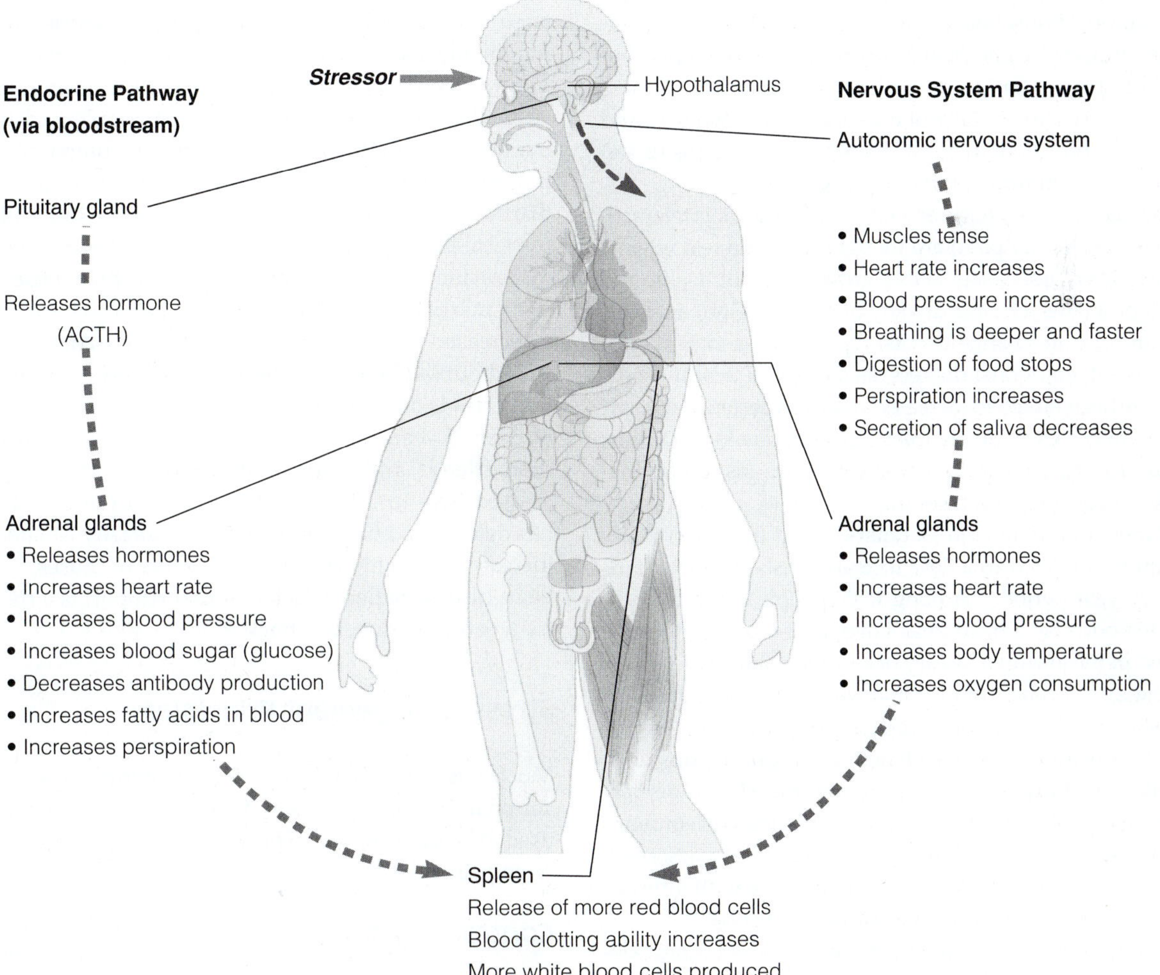

Figure 14.3 The stress response affects the entire body through both hormonal and nerve pathways (RBCs = red blood cells; ACTH = adrenocorticotropic hormone).

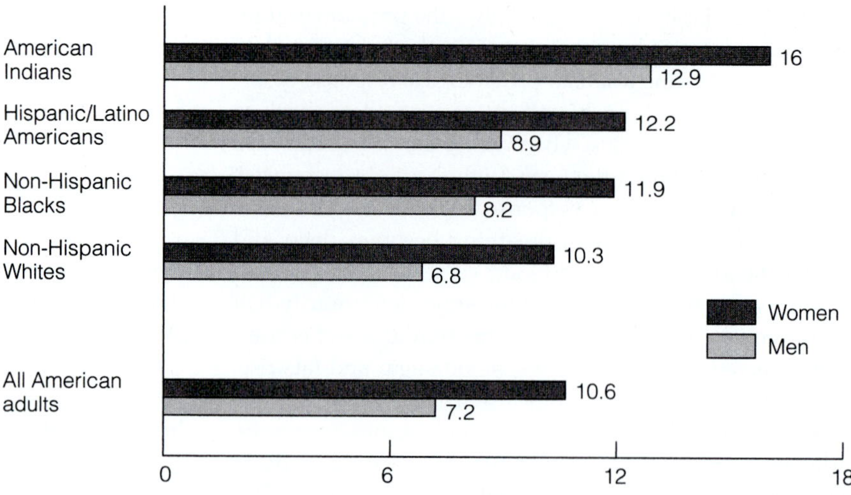

Figure 14.4 Prevalence of frequent mental distress (FMD) among adults by racial/ethnic population and sex. FMD is defined as "self-reported mental health not good (e.g., stress, depression, or emotional problems) on 14 days or more during the preceding 30 days." Source: CDC. Self-reported frequent mental distress among adults—U.S., 1993–2001. *MMWR* 53:963–966, 2004.

mental health not good (e.g., stress, depression, or emotional problems) on 14 or more days during the preceding 30 days," rose from 8.4% in 1993 to 10.1% in 2001.[19] As summarized in Figure 14.4, FMD is most prevalent among women compared to men, and among minority ethnic/racial groups. According to the CDC, FMD was significantly more prevalent in adults who were younger, female, separated or divorced, widowed, unemployed or unable to work, had less than $15,000 annual household income, less than a high school education, and/or had no health insurance.[19] Serious psychological distress (for a definition, see Physical Fitness Activity 14.7) occurs in 2.4% of men and 3.8% of women, and is also more prevalent in adults below poverty status (8.3%) and in various minority ethnic/racial groups.[7]

Chronic stressors (e.g., economic difficulties, intolerable relationships, bodily pain) are thought to be the real villains and have been associated with a growing list of health and disease problems: chronic anxiety and depression, an overabundance of life-change events, repressed feelings of loss, bereavement, emotional distress, lack of social ties, and hostility have been linked to increased risk of hypertension, heart disease, cancer, early death, infection, suppressed immunity, asthma attacks, back pain, chronic fatigue, gastrointestinal distress, headaches, and insomnia.[20–47] For example, a study of 740 men and women in Denmark found that chronic depression was related to a 70% increased risk of heart attack over a 20-year period.[20] Among 1,500 people living in Baltimore, the odds for a heart attack over a 13-year period were doubled in those with a history of *dysphoria* (2 weeks or more of sadness).[21] A cohort of men and women followed for 7–16 years showed that risk of developing hypertension was increased about 80% in those with high anxiety or depression.[22]

A 40-year study of 1,200 men showed that clinical depression more than doubled the risk for development of coronary heart disease.[23] Anger and mental stress have been described as triggers for heart attacks, especially in those with little education or with preexisting coronary artery disease.[24–29]

Among elderly Americans, those with the highest depression scores experienced a 40% increased risk of heart disease and 60% increased risk of early death.[30] A Swedish study, involving nearly a million people, linked stressful jobs—high pressure or little power to make decisions—with a 60% increase in heart attack risk.[31] A meta-analysis of 485 studies showed that job satisfaction is an important factor influencing the health of workers.[42]

Researchers at Carnegie Mellon University injected cold viruses into the noses of some 400 volunteers and reported that the risk of coming down with a cold was directly related to the stress levels of the subjects.[32] Those experiencing the most stress and tension were almost twice as likely to catch a cold as those who reported the least. A study in Australia found that highly stressed people had twice as many days with flu and cold symptoms, compared to those reporting little stress, during a 6-month period.[33] Marital disruption has been linked to depressed immunity and physical illness, with separated partners having about 30% more acute illnesses and physician visits than those who remain married.[34] A lack of social ties has also been linked to a decreased resistance to infection from the common cold.[35]

About 7–12 months following the loss of a spouse, mortality risk is doubled for both men and women.[36,37] Among women 75 years of age and older with no contact from children, friends, and group organizations, mortality risk is increased two- to threefold.[38] A review of published studies has determined that people who are socially isolated are at increased mortality risk from a number of causes.[39] Among heart disease patients, lack of social support is a risk factor for an additional heart attack.[40,41]

Stress Management Principles

Much has been written about controlling stress. Box 14.7 summarizes the basic formats of stress management often used at work settings.[16] There are five basic stress management principles.[14–18]

Control Stressors

Stressors are everywhere. They cannot all be avoided, but much can be done to reduce, modify, or avoid many of them

Box 14.7

Basic Formats of Stress Management Programs Used at Work Settings

Since the late 1970s, a consistent finding among investigators is that the psychosocial factors of high psychological job demands and low control over the work process (i.e., job strain) are associated with excess cardiovascular disease. About one third of employed workers report that exposure to mental stress is the work condition that most endangers their health. About half of workers report that their job is very stressful, with one fourth characterizing their job as the single greatest cause of stress in their lives. Emerging changes in the work environment (e.g., downsizing and reorganization, flexiplace arrangements, total quality management) and changes in workforce demographics (e.g., cultural diversity) indicate that job stress will continue to be a problem for the foreseeable future.

Stress management interventions are defined as techniques designed to help employees modify their appraisal of stressful situations or deal more effectively with the symptoms of stress. There is great variability in the strategies used to manage stress, but in general, a combination of techniques (e.g., muscle relaxation plus cognitive-behavioral skills training) is more effective than a single technique. Stress management interventions can be grouped into four categories:

1. *Progressive muscle relaxation.* This technique involves focusing attention on muscle activity, learning to identify even small amounts of tension in a muscle group, and practicing the release of tension from the muscles. The underlying theory is that because relaxation and muscle tension are incompatible states, reducing muscle tension levels indirectly reduces autonomic nervous activity and, consequently, anxiety and stress levels.
2. *Biofeedback.* In biofeedback training, a person is provided with information or feedback about the status of a physiological function and, over time, learns to control the activity of that function. For example, the electrical activity produced when muscles tense can be recorded and transformed into a tone, the pitch of which rises as muscle activity increases and falls as muscle activity decreases.
3. *Meditation.* There are several types of meditation techniques. Most of them involve finding a quiet place and sitting comfortably for 20 minutes twice a day. While maintaining a passive attitude toward intruding thoughts, the person repeats some neutral word with each exhalation. Meditation is thought to invoke a "relaxation response," which is the opposite of the stress response.
4. *Cognitive-behavioral skills.* Cognitive methods help people restructure their thinking patterns and are often referred to as cognitive restructuring techniques. *Stress inoculation* (a common form of cognitive-behavioral skills training) involves three stages: (1) education (learning about how one has responded to past stressful experiences), (2) rehearsal (learning various coping techniques such as problem solving, relaxation, and cognitive coping), and (3) application (practicing the skills under simulated conditions).

Sources: Johnson JV, Stewart W, Hall EM, Fredlund P, Theorell T. Long-term psychosocial work environment and cardiovascular mortality among Swedish men. *Am J Public Health* 86:324–331, 1996; Murphy LR. Stress management in work settings: A critical review of the health effects. *Am J Health Promot* 11:112–135, 1996.

in a way that will allow one to accomplish goals. For example, in climbing a tall mountain, one can make the trip miserable by hiking too fast with a heavy backpack, or satisfying and pleasurable by walking at a moderate pace with a lighter load. Same goal, same path, but a completely different experience.

Suppose that a college student is taking a heavy academic load in a subject area (e.g., biochemistry) that is too difficult for him at present, working 15 hours a week to help pay for expenses, living in a crowded and noisy apartment with an unbearable roommate, experiencing constant transportation problems because of a car that keeps breaking down, and dealing with crushing family problems due to the divorce of his parents. The first step would be for the student to sit down, make a list of all his major goals, in order of importance, and then catalog each of the stressors, along with plans to either eliminate or modify them. (See Physical Fitness Activity 14.4 at the end of this chapter.)

For example, finishing biochemistry has a high priority because he must do so to have a chance to achieve his major life goal of becoming a physician. He should give it his first attention (he could increase his study time by quitting work and taking out a loan). He could move closer to campus, find more desirable living accommodations, and walk or bicycle for transportation until finances improve.

Just as in climbing a mountain, stressors often can be managed by controlling the pace of life and the load carried. A key is to avoid crowding too much into the schedule, and learning to control circumstances to allow the pace of life to flow with one's psychological makeup. The important objective is to control your circumstances—don't let them control you.

Let the Mind Choose the Reaction

This strategy is also called "stress reaction management." As mentioned, a stress reaction (the fight-or-flight response) stimulates production of various stress hormones, depressing immune function, increasing blood pressure, and so on. Over time, the response has negative health effects, so the goal is to head off stress reactions before they become chronic.

To understand how to do this, one needs to remember that events only cause stress when they are seen, heard, felt, or sensed by the brain. The mind interprets the event, and the type of interpretation governs the reaction. When a stressor presents itself, one can decide what kind of reaction to have. Usually we have "knee-jerk" reactions to potentially stressful events, without taking the opportunity to calmly reason them out. In other words, we are largely responsible for creating our emotional reactions, and we miss our opportunities to control them.

Once again, the strategy is not new. Marcus Aurelius said long ago, "If you are distressed by anything external, the pain is not due to the thing itself but to your estimate of it. This you have the power to revoke at any time."

So when an event takes place (e.g., a flat tire on your way to work or school), one can choose how to react. One can react with the stress response of anger (e.g., cussing and kicking the tire), or one can choose a calm response by considering practical options (I'll call at the first opportunity and work it out with the boss or professor).

Seek the Social Support of Others

About one fourth of the American population feels extremely lonely at some time during any given month—especially divorced parents, single mothers, people who have never married, and housewives.

As reviewed in this chapter, when people are socially isolated (few social contacts with family and friends, neighbors, or the "society at large"), they are more vulnerable to sickness, mental stress, and even early death. One 9-year study (of 7,000 residents of Alameda County, California) found that people with few ties to other people had death rates from various diseases two to five times higher than those with more ties. The researchers measured social ties by looking at whether people were married, the number of close friends and relatives they had and how often they were in contact with them, church attendance, and involvement in informal and formal group associations.[46]

Social support means reaching out to other people, sharing emotional, social, physical, financial, and other types of comfort and assistance. The principle was summarized by the Institute of Medicine (Division of Health Promotion and Disease Prevention): "A lack of family and community supports plays an important role in the development of disease. An absence of social support weakens the body's defenses through psychological stress. Isolated individuals must be identified, and strategies for increasing social contact and diminishing feelings of loneliness must be developed. Clinicians, family, friends, and social institutions bear a responsibility for diminishing social isolation."[48]

Find Satisfaction in Work and Service

Albert Schweitzer once wrote, "I don't know what your destiny will be. But I do know that the only ones among you who will find true happiness are those who find a place to serve." Selye echoed this thought in his book *Stress without Distress*:[17] "My own code is based on the view that to achieve peace of mind and fulfillment through self-expression, most men need a commitment to work in the service of some cause that they can respect."

Keep Physically Healthy

It is far easier to handle stressors when the body is healthy from adequate exercise, sleep, good food and water, clean air and sunshine, and relaxation.

Problems with sleep have become a modern epidemic that is taking an enormous toll on our bodies and minds. Desperately trying to fit more into the hours of the day, many people are stealing extra hours from the night. The result, say sleep researchers, is a sleep deficit that undermines health, sabotages productivity, blackens mood, clouds judgment, and increases the risk of accidents. Sadly, even those who want to sleep more often cannot. In recent surveys, half of the men and women reported that they have trouble sleeping.

The Better Sleep Council and the National Sleep Foundation give several guidelines for improving sleep, including these (see www.bettersleep.org, www.sleepfoundation.org):

1. Maintain a regular schedule for going to bed and waking up, including weekends.
2. Establish a regular, relaxing bedtime routine such as soaking in a hot bath or hot tub and then reading a book or listening to soothing music.
3. Create a sleep-conducive environment that is dark, quiet, comfortable, and cool.
4. Sleep on a comfortable mattress and pillows.
5. Use your bedroom only for sleep and sex. It is best to take work materials, computers, and televisions out of the sleeping environment.
6. Finish eating at least 2 to 3 hours before your regular bedtime.
7. Exercise regularly. It is best to complete your workout at least a few hours before bedtime.
8. Avoid nicotine (e.g., cigarettes, tobacco products). Used close to bedtime, it can lead to poor sleep.
9. Avoid caffeine (e.g., coffee, tea, soft drinks, chocolate) close to bedtime. It can keep you awake.
10. Avoid alcohol close to bedtime. It can lead to disrupted sleep later in the night.

(See the Sports Medicine Insight at the end of this chapter for more information on sleep.)

PHYSICAL ACTIVITY AND STRESS

One of the most important habits a person can acquire to improve mood state and manage stress is the habit of regular exercise. The rest of this chapter describes how regular physical activity can reduce depression, anxiety, and mental stress, while enhancing psychological well-being and a vigorous attitude toward life.

We have seen that poor psychological health is associated with poor physical health. Is there proof for the converse association? Is a healthy and fit body positively associated with psychological health? Were the ancient Greeks right in their assertion that a physically fit and strong body would lead to a sound mind? Surveys and cross-sectional studies of active, compared to inactive, people strongly support this concept.

The part of the brain that enables us to exercise, the motor cortex, lies only a few millimeters away from the part of the brain that deals with thought and feeling. Might this proximity mean that when exercise stimulates the motor cortex, it has a parallel effect on cognition and emotion?

Since the beginning of time, many have believed in the "cerebral satisfaction" of exercise. The Greeks maintained that exercise made the mind more lucid. Aristotle started his "Peripatetic School" in 335 B.C.—so named because of Aristotle's habit of walking up and down (*peripaton*) the paths of the Lyceum in Athens while thinking or lecturing to his students walking with him. Plato and Socrates had also practiced the art of peripatetics, as did the Roman *Ordo Vagorum* or walking scholars. Centuries later, Oliver Wendell Holmes explained that "in walking the will and the muscles are so accustomed to working together and perform their task with so little expenditure of force that the intellect is left comparatively free."

John F. Kennedy echoed the Greek ideal when he said,

> Physical fitness is not only one of the most important keys to a healthy body, it is the basis of dynamic and creative intellectual activity. Intelligence and skill can only function at the peak of their capacity when the body is strong. Hardy spirits and tough minds usually inhabit sound bodies.

There have been several national surveys in the United States and in Canada to study the relationship between physical activity and feelings of mental well-being.[1,49,50] One of the questionnaires used in national studies was the General Well-Being Schedule (GWBS) (see Physical Fitness Activity 14.1). The GWBS is highly regarded as one of the best measures of stress and mental health. It consists of 18 questions, covering such areas as energy level, satisfaction, freedom from worry, and self-control. A high score on the GWBS reflects an absence of bad feelings, an expression of positive mood state, and low stress.[1,51,52]

In these surveys, physical activity was positively associated with good mental health, especially positive mood, general well-being, and less anxiety and depression."[1,49]

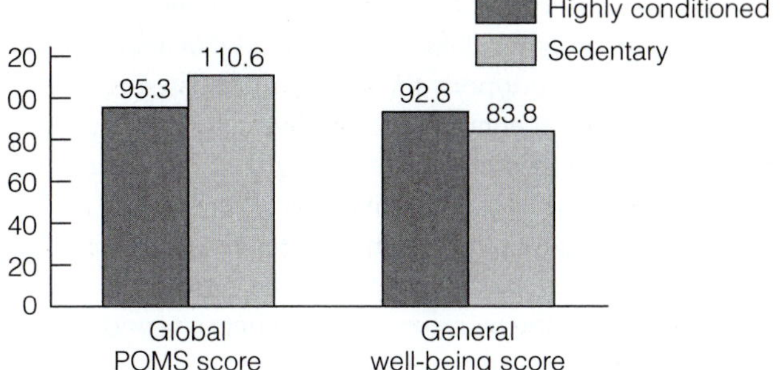

Figure 14.5 Highly conditioned versus sedentary elderly women, mood state and psychological well-being. A comparison of highly conditioned versus sedentary elderly women (mean age = 73 years) revealed superior psychological test scores among the fit subjects. A lower profile of mood states (POMS) score and a higher general well-being score are considered "superior." Source: Nieman DC, Warren BJ, Dotson RG, et al. Physical activity, psychological well-being, and mood state in elderly women. *J Aging Phys Act* 1:22–33, 1993.

This relationship was found to be stronger for the older age group (+40 years of age) than for the younger, and for women than for men. Many other cross-sectional studies of aerobically fit individuals of all ages have found them to have more favorable psychological profiles than their sedentary counterparts.[53–55] In one study of 32 sedentary and 12 highly conditioned elderly women (mean age 73 years), the fit subjects received superior scores on the profile of mood states and the general well-being schedule (see Figure 14.5). (The highly conditioned elderly women were active an average of 1.5 hours a day, and had been exercising for an average of 11 years.[54]) A large study of 5,000 adolescents concluded that emotional well-being was positively associated with the extent of participation in sports and vigorous recreational activity.[55] Among 3,260 elderly individuals, those exercising less than two times a week were more likely to be depressed than those engaging in more physical activity.[53]

There are several problems with cross-sectional studies, however, when evaluating the effect of regular exercise on mental health. Often, the physically active subjects are different from sedentary individuals in many other lifestyle areas (e.g., diet, body weight, genetic endowment), making it difficult to measure the independent role of exercise. The best study design starts with a group of sedentary subjects who are then randomly assigned to exercise and nonexercise groups and followed for several months to study the effects of exercise on depression, anxiety, mood state, self-concept, and other measures of mental health.

CONTROLLED STUDIES ON EXERCISE AND MENTAL HEALTH

Randomized, controlled studies on exercise training and mental health are difficult and expensive to conduct, and few have followed large enough groups of people for long enough periods of time to draw sound conclusions.[56–59] Nonetheless, as is emphasized in the rest of this chapter, growing evidence supports the survey and cross-sectional reports of superior mental health by physically active people, especially when the studies are long term. According to the 1996 surgeon general's report on physical activity and health, a major conclusion of experts in this area was that "physical activity improves mental health."[57] The report goes on to summarize that "the literature reported here supports a beneficial effect of physical activity on relieving symptoms of depression and anxiety and on improving mood."[57]

Cardiovascular Reactivity to Mental Stress

When individuals are subjected to stressful physical or psychological conditions, they experience an increase in heart rate, blood pressure, plasma catecholamine (stress hormones), and other measures of sympathetic nervous system activation.[60] Typical experiments are designed to measure these variables before and after, exposing subjects to behaviorally challenging procedures such as matching geometric shapes and colors, playing color-word games, or solving arithmetic problems with performance-dependent monetary awards. Studies have compared highly fit versus unfit subjects, or followed exercise and nonexercise groups for several weeks.[60–64]

Although not all researchers agree, exercise training is usually associated with a reduction in cardiovascular reactivity to mental stress. In one review of 34 studies with 1,449 subjects, aerobically fit individuals were found to have a significantly reduced stress reactivity to various stressors.[62] If experiments are conducted with careful attention to extraneous factors, exercise training usually leads to a reduction in stress reactivity to behavioral challenges.[60]

This reduction in stress reactivity is felt to be important in day-to-day coping with work and social stressors. (See Physical Fitness Activity 14.5 for a tool to measure life change stress.) Exercise appears to be useful in this regard because as the individual adapts to the increase in heart rate, blood pressure, stress hormones, and other biochemical measures during exercise, the body is strengthened and conditioned to react more calmly when the same responses are elicited during mental stress. For example, a survey of 17,626 Canadians showed that higher levels of participation in physical activity helped workers counter levels of work stress.[63] Also, college students who exercise frequently report less stress-induced physical symptoms than their less-active counterparts.[61]

Depression

National surveys have suggested that sedentary adults are at much higher risk for feeling fatigue and depression than those who are physically active.[1,65] In one study of 1,536 Germans, the odds of being depressed were more than three times higher for sedentary versus physically active adults.[66]

Since 1980, numerous studies and reviews of the literature have concluded that exercise is associated with reduced depression.[1,56,57,67–75] (See Physical Fitness Activity 14.3 for a tool used to measure depression.) Both acute and chronic exercise have been associated with reduced depression, with the greatest improvements seen in clinically depressed subjects who exercise frequently for several months.[70] Two meta-analyses of the literature have shown that all age groups, both men and women, across persons differing in health status, gain strong antidepressant effects from regular, long-term aerobic exercise.[70,74]

In general, depressed patients have been found to be physically sedentary and to experience a reduction in their depressive feelings when they initiate regular exercise. It has been proposed that exercise is as effective as group or individual psychotherapy, or meditative relaxation, in alleviating mild-to-moderate depression.[70–73] However, exercise plus psychotherapy have been shown to be better than exercise alone in reducing depression.[72]

The most frequently used treatment for major depression is antidepressant medication (e.g., sertraline hydrochloride or Zoloft).[5,68] About one third of patients, however, do not respond to treatment, and the medications may induce unwanted side effects, reducing quality of life and compliance to the treatment regimen. Researchers at Duke University have shown in a randomized clinical trial that 16 weeks of aerobic exercise (three supervised group sessions per week, 30 minutes per session, with 15 minutes of warm-up and cool-down) was as beneficial as treatment through medication (Zoloft) in reducing depression scores among 156 male and female patients with major depression[68] (see Figure 14.6). Most of the reduction in depression scores occurred within the first 4–8 weeks of exercise. Six months after treatment concluded, relapse rates were significantly lower in the exercise compared to medication group.[69] These data indicate that aerobic exercise therapy is effective and feasible over the long term in reducing depression among patients with major depression.

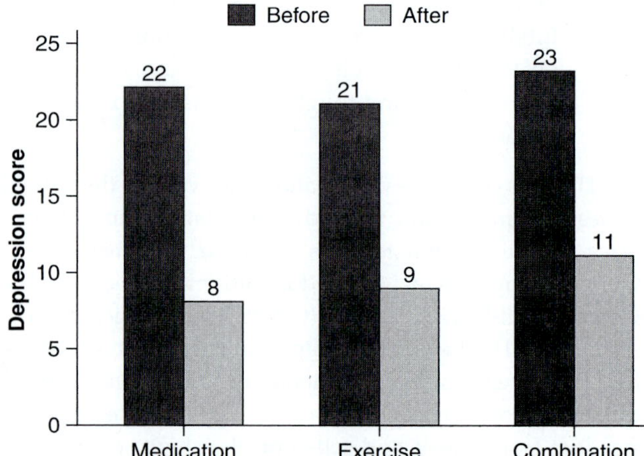

Figure 14.6 Exercise training was as effective as medication (Zoloft) in decreasing depression among patients with major depression. Source: Blumenthal JA, et al. Effects of exercise training on older patients with major depression. *Arch Intern Med* 159:2349–2356, 1999.

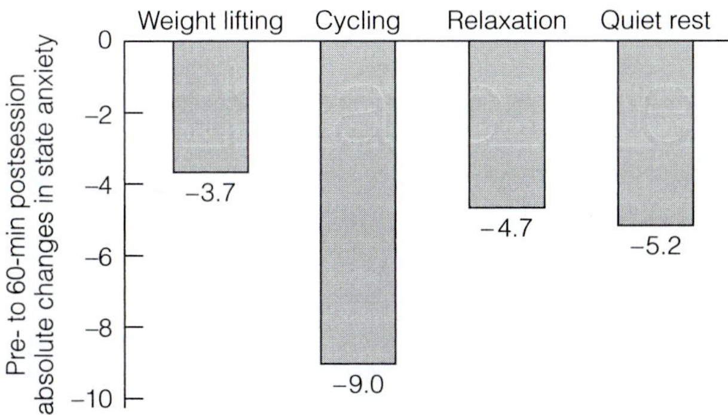

Figure 14.7 Sessions (50 minutes) of cycling, weight lifting, relaxation, and rest, comparative acute effects on state anxiety. State anxiety is decreased most strongly 1 hour following cycling. Source: Garvin AW, Koltyn KF, Morgan WP. Influence of acute physical activity and relaxation on state anxiety and blood lactate in untrained college males. *Int J Sports Med* 18:470–476, 1997.

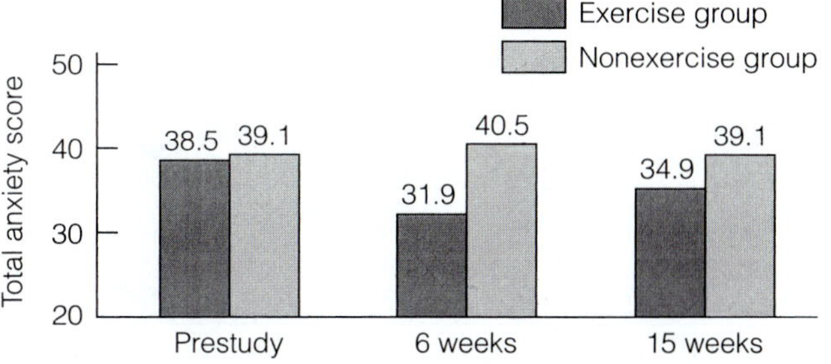

Figure 14.8 Moderate exercise training: Effect on state anxiety. Anxiety scores were significantly reduced in women who walked briskly 5 days a week, 45 minutes per session, for 15 weeks compared to a randomized, nonexercise control group. Source: Cramer SR, Nieman DC, Lee JW. The effects of moderate exercise training on psychological well-being and mood state in women. *J Psychosom Res* 35:437–449, 1991.

Anxiety

Anxiety disorders, including various phobias, panic attacks, and obsessive-compulsive behavior, are the most prevalent of all mental health problems in the United States (see Box 14.1). One of the most common measures of anxiety is the Spielberger State–Trait Anxiety Inventory (STAI).[76] (Also see Physical Fitness Activity 14.6 for a self-test used to screen for common anxiety disorders.)

STAI scores are based on responses to a variety of questions on tension, nervousness, self-confidence, indecisiveness, security, confusion, worry, and so on. Other measures of anxiety include blood pressure, heart rate, skin responses (galvanic, palmar sweating, and skin temperature), central nervous system measures (electroencephalogram [EEG]), and electromyography (e.g., muscular tension of the forehead muscles).

Researchers have studied the effects of *acute* (before and after one bout) and *chronic* (before and after several weeks of training) exercise on anxiety. One of the most frequently reported psychological benefits of acute exercise is a reduction in state anxiety (anxiety the subject feels "right now") following vigorous exercise, an effect that may last up to several hours.[77–84]

Figure 14.7 shows the results of one study of 60 untrained college males who engaged in one of the following activities for 50 minutes: (a) resistance exercise, (b) cycling at 70% of maximum, (c) autogenic relaxation, or (d) resting quietly in a sound chamber.[82] Notice that 1 hour following these sessions, state anxiety was reduced most strongly in the cycling group. In another study, 15 adults completed 20-minute sessions of cycle ergometer exercise on separate days at intensities equal to 40%, 60%, or 70% $\dot{V}O_{2max}$.[81] State anxiety was reduced for 2 hours following all exercise sessions, demonstrating that light-to-heavy intensities are equally effective. The reduction in state anxiety is a consistent finding following aerobic, but not resistance, exercise[84] and occurs during any time of the day.[83]

Exercise training has been linked to a reduction in trait anxiety (anxiety the subject "generally feels"). The reduction in anxiety is most noticeable when exercise is regular, sessions last longer than 30 minutes, and the training programs last several months.[57] Figure 14.8 summarizes the results of one study involving 35 sedentary, mildly obese women (mean age 34 years) who were randomly assigned to exercise or nonexercise groups.[85] Women in the exercise group walked briskly five times a week, 45 minutes per session, for 15 weeks, and they experienced a significant reduction in anxiety relative to the nonexercise group. This study supports the idea that moderate aerobic exercise such as brisk walking is a sufficient stimulus to reduce anxiety and tension.[86]

One meta-analysis of 104 studies of 3,048 subjects on the anxiety-reducing effects of exercise came to several conclusions, including the following:[77]

1. Training programs usually need to exceed 10 weeks before there are significant changes in trait anxiety (the anxiety one generally feels).
2. Exercise of at least 20 minutes duration seems necessary to achieve reductions in both state and trait anxiety.
3. Reductions in both state and trait anxiety occur after aerobic, but not anaerobic, exercise training programs.

Mood State

Psychological mood state is often measured using the Profile of Mood States (POMS)[87] or the General Well-Being Schedule (GWBS).[52] The POMS consists of 65 adjectives rated on a 5-point scale designed to assess mood during the previous week. The six scales of the POMS are tension/anxiety, depression/dejection, anger/hostility, vigor/activity, fatigue/inertia, and confusion/bewilderment. A POMS global score can be calculated, with a lower score indicating a more favorable mood state.

The GWBS consists of 18 items that generate a total score from six subscale scores that include health concern,

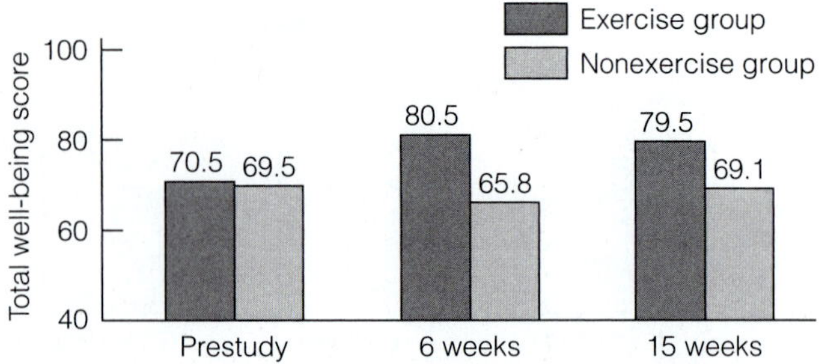

Figure 14.9 Moderate exercise training: Effect on general psychological well-being. General well-being was significantly improved for women who walked briskly for 15 weeks, relative to sedentary controls. Source: Cramer SR, Nieman DC, Lee JW. The effects of moderate exercise training on psychological well-being and mood state in women. *J Psychosom Res* 35:437–449, 1991.

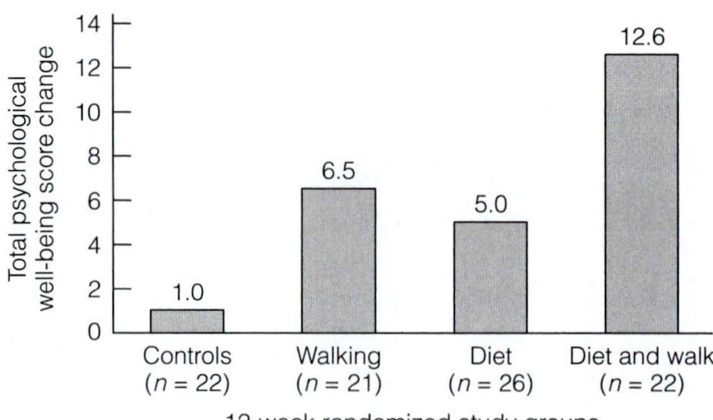

Figure 14.10 Psychological well-being response to diet and/or exercise; controls = mild calisthenics four sessions/week, walking = five 45-minute sessions/week, diet = 1,300 Calories/day. A combination of walking and weight-loss diet was most effective in improving psychological well-being in overweight women. Source: Nieman DC, Custer WF, Butterworth DE, Utter AC, Henson DA. Psychological response to exercise training and/or energy restriction in obese women. *J Psychosom Res* 48:23–29, 2000.

energy level, life satisfaction, cheerfulness/depression, tension/relaxation, and emotional stability. A high score on the GWBS represents an expression of positive well-being and the absence of bad feelings (see Physical Fitness Activity 14.1 at the end of this chapter for norms).

Most studies have shown that psychological mood state as measured by the POMS or GWBS is more favorable for active people and can be improved with regular exercise, especially when mood state is unfavorable prior to initiating training.[1,85,88–91] Figure 14.9 shows the results from the same study described in Figure 14.8.[85] In this study, 15 weeks of moderate exercise training was associated with improved GWBS total scores, with contributions made from each of the six subscales, especially higher energy levels. Figure 14.10 summarizes results from a randomized study of 91 obese women. Notice that GWBS scores improved most in women who both dieted (losing about 17 pounds) and walked regularly.[90]

Self-Esteem

Self-esteem or self-concept is defined as the degree to which individuals feel positive about themselves, and it can be measured by various instruments, including the Rosenberg Self-Esteem Scale.[92] Reviewers have identified self-esteem as the psychological variable with the greatest potential to be improved with exercise training, especially for those with initially low self-esteem.[93–99] A meta-analysis of the literature has shown a strong link between aerobic fitness training and self-concept in adults.[74]

In one study of young men in a juvenile detention center, 2 hours per week of running and hard basketball led to significant improvements in self-esteem and general psychological mood state.[94] The researchers concluded that vigorous aerobic exercise can provide substantial psychological help for delinquent adolescents. A meta-analysis demonstrated a positive effect for physical activity on the self-esteem of children.[99] In a 12-month randomized, controlled trial of 174 older adults, improvements in physical fitness were linked to enhancement of self-esteem.[96] During a 6-month follow-up, self-esteem decreased in parallel with declines in frequency of physical activity.

Weight training leads to measurable improvements in muscular strength and size, providing positive feedback that has been associated in many studies with an improvement in self-esteem. In one 12-week study of 60 women randomly assigned to weight training or brisk walking, body image improved for both groups, but more so for the weight lifters.[95] In cardiac patients, strength training has been associated with enhanced self-efficacy.[98]

Mental Cognition

Does exercise improve mental cognition?[100–111] Animal studies have consistently shown that regular physical exercise enhances learning and both short- and long-term memory.[105,109] Many people report that they feel "mentally alert" shortly after a bout of exercise and can study with greater attentiveness. A large number of studies have evaluated the effect of both acute and chronic exercise on cognition, using various tests involving word recall, memory searches, name retrieval, and so on.[100–111] Although much more research is needed, exercise does appear to have a positive effect on cognitive performance, especially when complex memory tasks are tested.[103,105,108,111] Results indicate that memory and intellectual function may be improved during or shortly after an exercise session, and following long-term training.[104] Several studies also suggest that exercise is effective in reversing or at least slowing certain age-related declines in cognitive performance.[100–103,107,108,111] In a 6-month study of 124 older people, for example, brain function improved 25% compared to controls.[100] In particular, brain function in the frontal and prefrontal areas of the cortex was enhanced. These areas have been linked to decision

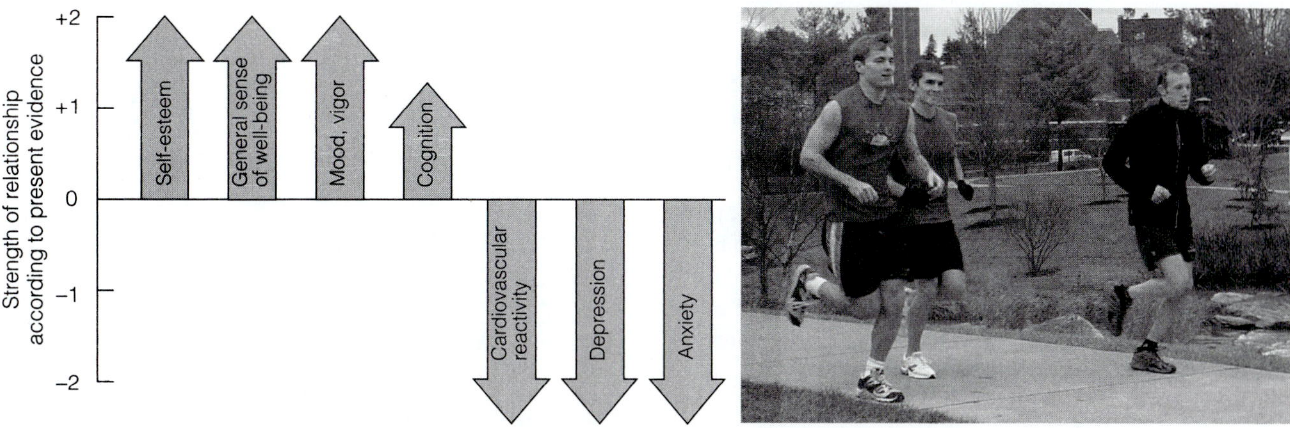

Figure 14.11 Summary of relationship between physical activity and psychological health. This figure summarizes the relationship between physical activity and psychological health, using present evidence. The strength of the relationship is represented on the vertical axis, with "2" representing strong evidence in support and "1" representing preliminary supporting evidence, with more research needed to confirm the association.

making and learning of new skills. Overall, there appears to be some possible influence of exercise on selected measures of cognitive functioning (especially in the elderly), but better-designed studies are needed to confirm this.[100,106]

MECHANISMS: HOW PHYSICAL ACTIVITY HELPS PSYCHOLOGICAL HEALTH

Figure 14.11 summarizes the information reviewed in the previous section. In general, most research is supportive of the Greek ideal of a "strong mind in a strong body." Explaining how and why exercise improves psychological health is a topic of active debate at present. Some of the more tenable hypotheses can be grouped as[70,112,113]

1. Cognitive-behavioral
2. Social interaction
3. Time-out/distraction
4. Cardiovascular fitness
5. Monoamine neurotransmitters
6. Endogenous opioids

Cognitive-Behavioral Hypothesis

Individuals who master something that they perceive as difficult (exercising regularly) may experience a positive change in their psychological health manifested by increased self-confidence, improved self-efficacy (an "I can do it" attitude), ability to cope with personal problems, uplifted vigor and general well-being, and lessening of anxiety and depression. On the other hand, some people may simply report feeling better following exercise because they expect such a change.[77] In the best-designed studies, however, researchers have tried to control for this by using random assignment, the use of mild calisthenic control groups, and concealing the intention of the study from the subjects.[85,112]

Social Interaction Hypothesis

Exercise is often performed with others, leading to improved opportunities for social interaction, pleasure, and personal attention. It has been hypothesized that this could account for the antidepressant and mood elevation effects of exercise. However, in one meta-analysis, exercise was shown to be a significantly better antidepressant than enjoyable group activities alone.[70] In studies that have attempted to control for social interaction, most have concluded that favorable psychological responses to aerobic training were not due to this factor.[85,86,88]

Time-Out/Distraction Hypothesis

This hypothesis maintains that being distracted from stressful stimuli, or taking a "time-out" from the daily routine, is responsible for the mood elevation seen with exercise.[70,77] However, the evidence suggests that the mood elevation experienced after exercise is due to more than simply taking time out from one's daily routine. For example, exercise has been found to reduce depression and anxiety more than relaxation (time-out) or enjoyable activities (distraction).[70] Thus, regular exercise may be a more effective long-term mood elevator than habitual relaxation.

Cardiovascular Fitness Hypothesis

According to this theory, mood elevation and a reduction in anxiety and depression are directly related to the level of aerobic fitness $\dot{V}O_{2max}$. However, several studies have reported that the psychological improvements seen with exercise take place within the first few weeks of treatment before significant increases in aerobic fitness have occurred.[70,85] Also, in some studies, depending on the psychological variable tested, improvement in anaerobic fitness from weight training was just as effective as gains in aerobic fitness.[70,95]

There is some thinking that aerobic exercise may increase oxygen transport to the brain and elevate deep body temperature, inducing an elevation in mood state.[106] However, the research linking these changes to improved mental health is tenuous at best, and further research is needed before conclusions can be made.

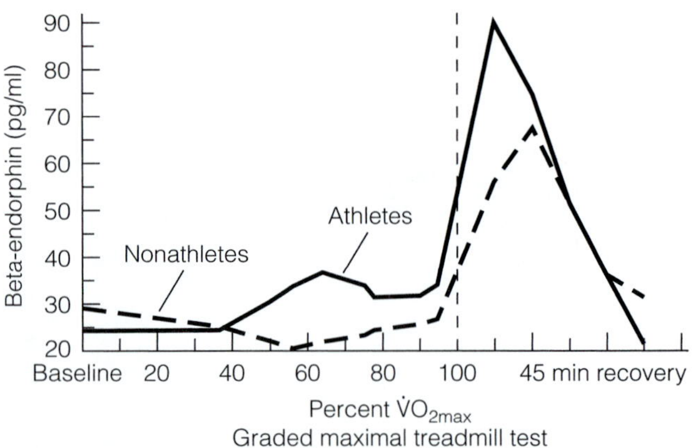

Figure 14.12 Beta-endorphin in athletes versus nonathletes. In this study, sedentary nonathletes and marathon athletes were exercised to exhaustion during a Balke treadmill, graded exercise test. The concentration of β-endorphin in the blood rose sharply during early recovery, in response to near-maximal-intensity exercise.
Source: Author (unpublished data).

Monoamine Neurotransmitter Hypothesis

Disturbances in the brain secretions of three monoamine neurotransmitters—serotonin, dopamine, and norepinephrine—have been implicated in depression and other psychological disorders.[113] There is some evidence that depressed individuals have decreased secretions of these neurotransmitters, and various medications are used to increase their transmission.

In animal studies, an acute bout of exercise increases both dopamine and norepinephrine synthesis and metabolism in various parts of the brain, including the midbrain, cortex, and hypothalamus.[114,115] Exercise could play a role in the treatment and prevention of depression and other mental disorders by promoting optimal neurotransmitter secretions, but this remains uncertain on the basis of available data.[70,113]

Endogenous Opioid Hypothesis

Opiates have been used for centuries to relieve pain and induce euphoria. In 1975, researchers were successful in isolating chemicals from the body that were found to have morphinelike qualities. Since then, many more endogenous opioids have been identified and can roughly be divided into three groups: endorphins, enkephalins, and dynorphins. These endogenous opioids are widely distributed throughout areas of the central nervous system and influence many important systems of the body, including the cardiovascular, respiratory, and immune systems, and metabolism of fuels.[116–122]

Of special interest has been the *β-endorphin system,* which contributes to the regulation of blood pressure, pain perception, and the control of body temperature. β-endorphin has receptors in the hypothalamus and limbic systems of the brain, areas associated with emotion and behavior.

During vigorous exercise, the pituitary increases its production of β-endorphin, leading to an increase in its concentration in the blood. As Figure 14.12 shows, β-endorphin is a late-acting hormone, rising sharply only during and immediately following intense exercise. In this study, the increase in β-endorphin did not differ significantly between athletes and nonathletes when compared on a percent $\dot{V}O_{2max}$ basis. β-endorphin concentrations peaked during recovery at 3–3.5 times resting levels and fell to near-resting levels after 45 minutes of recovery.

Most researchers have found that β-endorphin does not increase unless the exercise intensity exceeds 75% $\dot{V}O_{2max}$ or the duration exceeds 1 hour and the exercise is performed at a steady state between lactate production and elimination.[121]

Although it is widely accepted by the exercising public that endorphins are responsible for exercise-induced euphoria, researchers disagree on the interpretation of the available data. At the center of the debate is whether blood concentrations of β-endorphin actually reflect what is happening in the brain's limbic system, where β-endorphin must activate the central nervous system to produce euphoria.

After the β-endorphin is secreted into the blood by the pituitary gland, it apparently is unable to be able to penetrate the blood–brain barrier to get into the brain. As a result, most researchers have been unable to correlate changes in blood β-endorphin concentrations with reduced tension or pain. Studies show, for example, that although subjects can tolerate more pain than normal during and for 15 minutes after intense exercise, plasma β-endorphin levels do not appear to be related.[122]

However, there is some evidence from animal studies that brain concentrations of β-endorphin increase during exercise.[120] Prolonged, submaximal exercise has been found to increase brain β-endorphin levels and to improve the pain tolerance of rats.

Other animal research suggests that prolonged rhythmic, large-muscle exercise can activate brain opioid systems by triggering certain sensory nerves that go from the muscle to the brain.[120] It is uncertain, however, whether the brain is making its own β-endorphin or whether exercise-induced changes enable β-endorphin to cross the blood–brain barrier and pass into the brain.[121]

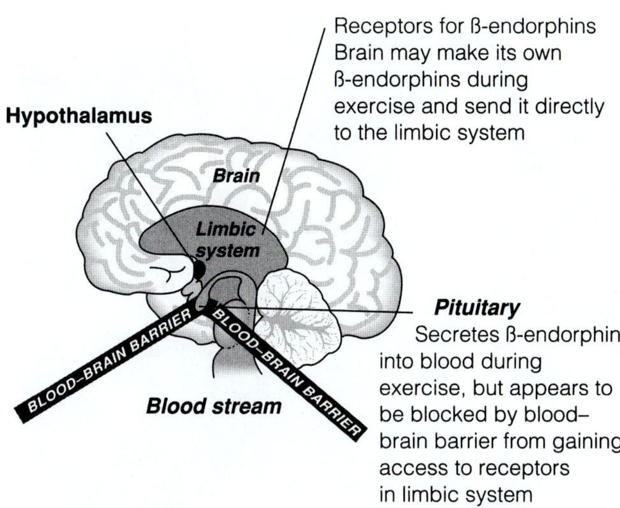

Figure 14.13 Beta-endorphin and the blood–brain barrier. Although it is true that vigorous exercise increases the concentration of β-endorphin in the blood, this complex protein molecule is unable to cross the blood–brain barrier to gain access to the receptors located in the limbic system. However, the brain may be able to make its own β-endorphin during exercise, or this hormone may project into areas of the brain through nerve fibers.

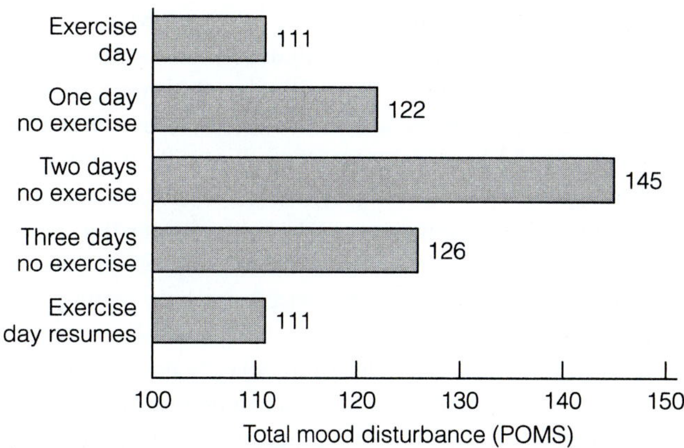

Figure 14.14 Mood disturbance during exercise deprivation in habitual exercisers. Mood disturbance rises sharply within the first 2 days of exercise deprivation in habitual exercisers. Source: Mondin GW, Morgan WP, Piering PN, et al. Psychological consequences of exercise deprivation in habitual exercisers. *Med Sci Sports Exerc* 28:1199–1203, 1996.

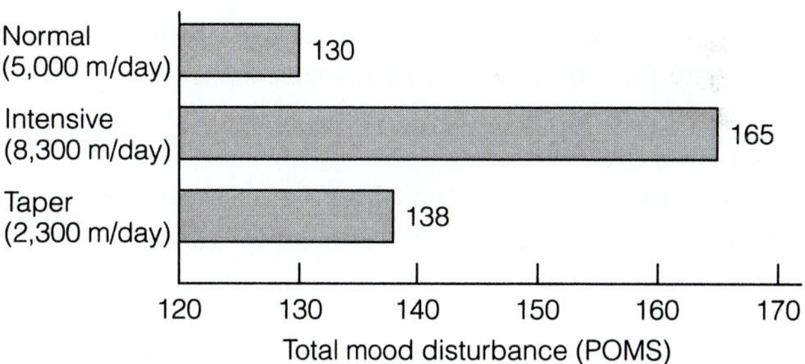

Figure 14.15 Mood disturbance in swimmers during training. Intensive training increases mood disturbance in swim athletes. Source: Raglin JS, Koceja DM, Stager JM, Harms CA. Mood, neuromuscular function, and performance during training in female swimmers. *Med Sci Sports Exerc* 28:372–377, 1996.

Further research is needed to resolve these issues, but there is evidence that intense exercise may activate brain opioid systems, increasing the pain threshold and improving mood state[120] (see Figure 14.13).

It is more than likely that both the physiological and the psychological mechanisms reviewed in this section play a role in explaining the improvements in psychological mood state seen after exercise.

PRECAUTIONS: EXERCISE ADDICTION, MOOD DISTURBANCE, AND SLEEP DISRUPTION

Some individuals are "addicted" to exercise and have such a commitment that obligations to work, family, and interpersonal relationships, and their ability to utilize medical advice, suffer. Such people are also compulsive, use exercise for an escape, are overcompetitive, live in a state of chronic fatigue, are self-centered, and are preoccupied with fitness, diet, and body image. If for any reason exercise has to be discontinued, these individuals experience withdrawal symptoms. Figure 14.14 shows that mood disturbance rises sharply within the first 48 hours of exercise deprivation in habitual exercisers.[123] Bodybuilders who may work out up to 6 hours a day exhibit exercise dependence, an obsession with muscle gain and definition, and a need to train that surpasses family, friends, and work as the focus of their time and energy.[124]

Mood disturbance can increase when training loads are increased too greatly.[125–127] When swimmers increased their daily training distance from 4,000 to 9,000 meters per day during a 10-day period, there were significant increases in muscle soreness, depression, anger, fatigue, and overall mood disturbance, along with a reduced general sense of well-being.[125] Figure 14.15 shows that intensive training periods are associated with mood disturbance in athletes.[126] Intense physical exercise such as a competitive marathon (26.2 miles) has been shown to disrupt both rapid eye movement (REM) sleep and total sleep time[128] (see Sports Medicine Insight at the end of this chapter).

PRACTICAL IMPLICATIONS

Although we are not sure why, the research presented in this chapter has shown that the same amount of exercise that helps the heart also helps the brain. The American College of Sports Medicine has established that three to five, 20–30 minute aerobic exercise sessions per week of moderate-intensity activities such as jogging, swimming, bicycling, or brisk walking are necessary to fully develop the cardiovascular and respiratory systems. Most studies linking exercise and mental health used these same exercise criteria and thus showed that as the heart is strengthened, so is the brain. If exercise is to be effective in alleviating stress, it should be noncompetitive, moderate in intensity, and pursued in pleasant surroundings (see Figure 14.16).

Exercise is a strong weapon to help counter the never-ending onslaught of stress, anxiety, and depression associated with our modern era. Exercise does help, acting as a buffer, reducing the strain of stressful events. Exercise can help to fortify the brain, alleviating anxiety and depression while elevating mood. Stress levels can be reduced by various drugs, but an appropriate program of physical activity is preferred because it has many other positive health effects.

The brain may function better cognitively during exercise. Though we need more research to evaluate the effect of regular exercise on overall mental function, there is evidence that exercise does more than just make people feel better physically.

What this means for busy students and workers everywhere is that time spent in exercise may not be lost in terms of getting the job done. The half-hour exercise session may actually enhance mental functioning to the point of increasing overall time efficiency.

Therefore, the allocation of curricular time to physical education may not hamper academic achievement, as some school boards have thought. Also, exercise breaks for normally sedentary office workers may enhance the productivity of a business. Future research should help to resolve some of these questions.

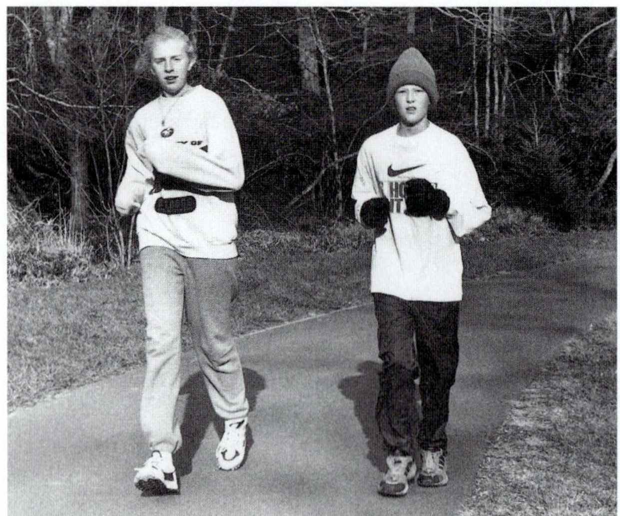

Figure 14.16 If exercise is to be effective in inducing relaxation, it should be noncompetitive, moderate in intensity, and pursued in pleasant surroundings.

SPORTS MEDICINE INSIGHT

Exercise and Sleep

Sleep disorders are common worldwide. According to the National Center on Sleep Disorders Research, as many as 80 million Americans have serious, incapacitating sleep problems, 10–15% have chronic insomnia, and nearly half of older adults say they cannot get a solid night's rest.[129,130] The vast majority of Americans fail to understand what to do about poor sleep and the consequences[131] (see Box 14.8 and Physical Fitness Activity 14.8).

Sleep loss and sleep disturbances are thought to play a major role in 100,000 automobile accidents and 1,500 deaths each year, with as many as 13% of accident-related fatalities caused by falling asleep at the wheel.[130] The loss of 1 hour's sleep when most Americans "spring forward" in April to daylight saving time causes an average increase of 7–8% in traffic accidents. Conversely, the switch back to standard time in the fall causes a 7–8% decrease.

Insomnia is defined by the National Institutes of Health as "the perception or complaint of inadequate or poor-quality sleep"[132] (see Box 14.9). Characteristics of insomnia include[132,133]

- Difficulty falling asleep
- Waking up frequently during the night, with difficulty returning to sleep
- Waking up too early in the morning
- Unrefreshing sleep

Advanced age, being female, marital disruption, lower socioeconomic status, and a history of depression have each been linked to insomnia.[132,133] People with chronic insomnia have a diminished ability to concentrate, memory problems, trouble in carrying out daily tasks, and difficulty in working with and getting along with other people. Poor sleep can result in fatigue, increasing the opportunity for human error and accidents. Shift workers account for 20% of the U.S. workforce, and are two to five times more likely to fall asleep on the job than day workers, while exhibiting more stress and irritability, and experiencing more heart disease and stomach/intestinal ailments.

Sleep requirements vary over the life cycle.[131] Newborns and infants need a lot of sleep and have several periods of sleep throughout a 24-hour time period. Naps are important to them as well as to toddlers, who may nap up to the age of 5. As children enter adolescence, their sleep patterns shift to a later sleep/wake cycle, but they still need around 9 hours of sleep. Throughout adulthood, 7–9

(continued)

SPORTS MEDICINE INSIGHT *(continued)*

Exercise and Sleep

hours of sleep is recommended. Here are the sleep needs over the life cycle:

- Infants/babies (includes naps):
  0–2 months old, 10.5–18.5 hours
  2–12 months old, 14–15 hours
- Toddlers/children (includes naps):
  12–18 months old, 13–15 hours
  18 months to 3 years of age, 12–14 hours
  3–5 years of age, 11–13 hours
  5–12 years of age, 9–11 hours
- Adolescents
  8.5–9.5 hours
- Adults/older persons
  on average, 7–9 hours

Sleep duration is related to length of life.[134,135] In one study of a million Americans, those age 45 years or older who reported sleeping more than 10 hours or fewer than 5 hours per night had higher death rates during follow-up than those sleeping about 7 hours a night.[134] Insomnia early in adult life is a risk factor for the development of clinical depression and psychiatric distress.[136]

SLEEP CYCLES

A night's sleep consists of four or five cycles, each of which progresses through several stages.[136,137] Each stage produces specific brain patterns that can be documented by an electroencephalogram (EEG), a record of the electrical impulses generated in the brain. During each night, a person alternates between non–rapid eye movement (NREM) sleep and rapid eye movement (REM) sleep. The entire cycle of NREM and REM sleep takes about 90 minutes. The average adult sleeps 7.5 hours (five full cycles), with 25% of that in REM. By age 70, total nighttime sleep decreases to about 6 hours (four sleep cycles), but the proportion of REM stays at about 25%. Sleep efficiency is reduced in the elderly, with an increased number of awakenings during the night.

In NREM sleep, brain activity, heart rate, respiration, blood pressure, and metabolism (vital signs) slow down, and body temperature falls, as a deep, restful state is reached. Sleep begins with NREM, during which brain waves gradually lengthen through four distinct stages:[131,137]

1. *Stage 1.* Characterized by lighter sleep, a slowing down of brain activity and vital signs, and dreamlike thoughts
2. *Stage 2.* Characterized by slightly deeper sleep and slower vital signs
3. *Stages 3 and 4 (slow-wave sleep).* Characterized by deep sleep, depressed vital signs, and slow, low-frequency, high-amplitude brain activity known as delta waves

Slow-wave sleep usually terminates with the sleeper changing position. The brain waves now reverse their course as the sleeper heads for the active REM stage. The central nervous system puts on a display of physiology so intense that some have described it as a third stage of earthly existence. In REM sleep, the eyes dart about under closed eyelids, and vivid dreams transpire, which can often be remembered. The even breathing of NREM gives way to halting uncertainty, and the heart rhythm speeds or slows unaccountably. The brain is highly active during REM sleep, and overall brain metabolism may be increased above the level experienced when awake.

BETTER SLEEP

Getting a good night's sleep has proven to be a difficult goal for many people in this modern era. The National Sleep Foundation has published several guidelines for better sleep. Here are 10 guidelines for a better night's sleep:[131]

- Maintain a regular schedule for going to bed and waking up, including weekends.
- Establish a regular, relaxing bedtime routine such as soaking in a hot bath or hot tub and then reading a book or listening to soothing music.
- Create a sleep-conducive environment that is dark, quiet, comfortable, and cool.
- Sleep on a comfortable mattress and pillows.
- Use your bedroom only for sleep and sex. It is best to take work materials, computers, and televisions out of the sleeping environment.
- Finish eating at least 2 to 3 hours before your regular bedtime.
- Avoid nicotine (e.g., cigarettes, tobacco products). Used close to bedtime, it can lead to poor sleep.
- Avoid caffeine (e.g., coffee, tea, soft drinks, chocolate) close to bedtime. It can keep you awake.
- Avoid alcohol close to bedtime. It can lead to disrupted sleep later in the night.
- Exercise regularly. It is best to complete your workout at least a few hours before bedtime.

(continued)

SPORTS MEDICINE INSIGHT *(continued)*

Exercise and Sleep

PHYSICAL ACTIVITY AND SLEEP

The Better Sleep Council and National Sleep Foundation statements on the value of exercise in improving the quality and quantity of sleep are based on relatively few well-designed studies. There is considerable debate on the value of exercise in improving sleep, due in large part to the difficulty researchers have in measuring sleep quality.[137–141]

Compared to those who avoid exercise, physically fit people claim that they fall asleep more rapidly, sleep better, and feel less tired during the day.[137,140] Scientists have confirmed that people who exercise regularly and intensely do indeed spend more time in slow-wave sleep, a measure of sleep quality, than the inactive.[142–146] In one study, researchers compared the total amount of time spent in slow-wave sleep between very fit runners (training an average of 45 miles a week) and sedentary controls.[146] The runners spent 18% more time in slow-wave sleep than the controls (see Figure 14.17). In another study, sleep quality was compared in sedentary and physically active elderly men and women.[145] The exercise group had greater sleep quality in the form of longer sleep duration, shorter time to fall asleep, and better alertness throughout the day. Among 722 adults, both men and women who exercised regularly were at lower risk for sleep disorders.[142]

Some sleep researchers feel that slow-wave sleep helps restore and revitalize people for the next day.[137–141] When people initiate and maintain vigorous exercise programs, it would make sense that during sleep, they would have to increase the amount of slow-wave sleep to compensate. In other words, if there is an increase in energy expenditure through exercise, this requires more restoration time in the form of more sleep overall, especially at the deepest level.

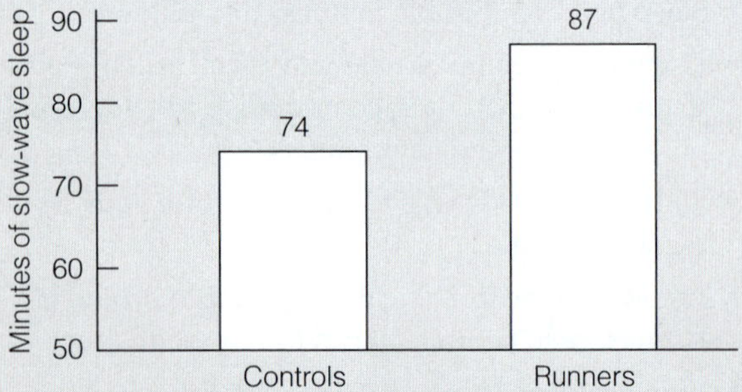

Figure 14.17 Slow-wave sleep in runners and controls. In this study of runners (45 miles/week) and sedentary controls, runners spent 18% more time in slow-wave sleep. Source: Trinder J, Paxton S, Montgomery I, Fraser G. Endurance as opposed to power training: Their effect on sleep. *Psychophysiol* 22:668–673, 1985.

Most studies agree with this "theory of restoration."[140,147] In one comprehensive review of the literature on the effects of exercise on sleep quality, it was concluded that individuals who exercise not only fall asleep faster, but also sleep somewhat longer and deeper than individuals who avoid exercise.[139] An exercise bout has the greatest positive impact on sleep quality for those who are elderly or of low fitness. In other words, those who need it the most gain the greatest sleep benefit from exercise.

The longer the duration of the exercise bout (e.g., beyond 1 hour), the better the sleep quality that night, except for unusually severe and prolonged exercise such as ultramarathon running races, which can actually disrupt sleep.[140,141] For example, wakefulness in runners has been reported to be increased on the night following a marathon race.[128]

There is some evidence that high-intensity exercise leading to sweating has a better effect on sleep quality than does low-intensity exercise.[137,140] However, researchers do caution that exercising and sweating close to bedtime can have an adverse effect on sleep quality for both fit and sedentary subjects. This is why the Better Sleep Council recommends avoiding heavy exercise late in the day.[131] During slow-wave sleep, the body temperature falls. If physical activities that raise body temperature and cause sweating are conducted too close to bedtime, sleep quality is disturbed because the body and brain are not able to reach the cooler temperatures needed for deep sleep. However, some evidence challenges this assumption.[148] In aerobically fit subjects, sleep was not adversely affected by a 1-hour bout of exercise at 60% $\dot{V}O_{2max}$ or by 3 hours of exercise at 70% $\dot{V}O_{2max}$ completed 30 minutes before bedtime.

Most of the studies on exercise and sleep quality have compared fit and unfit individuals, or analyzed the effect of one exercise bout on that night's sleep. There have been very few exercise training studies to determine whether initiating and maintaining an exercise program improves sleep quality.[137–140] In one study of new army recruits, 18 weeks of basic training were found to improve sleep quality by several measures.[143] Most of the sleep quality improvements occurred within the first 9 weeks of training, when the recruits were adapting to the increased exercise.

(continued)

SPORTS MEDICINE INSIGHT *(continued)*

Exercise and Sleep

In a study conducted at Stanford University, physically inactive older adults were assigned to exercise or nonexercise groups for 16 weeks.[149] Subjects in the exercise group engaged in low-impact aerobics and brisk walking for 30–40 minutes, 4 days per week. Exercise training led to improved sleep quality, longer sleep, and a shorter time to fall asleep. The researchers concluded that older adults who often complain of sleep problems can benefit from initiating a regular moderate-intensity endurance exercise program (see Figure 14.18). A yearlong study of postmenopausal women showed that those exercising moderately in the morning for 3–4 hours per week had less trouble falling asleep compared to those exercising less.[144]

SLEEP LOSS AND ABILITY TO EXERCISE

It is well documented that lack of sleep negatively affects mood, vigilance, and ability to accomplish complex mental tasks. In regard to the body, most studies have shown that sleep loss of 4–60 hours does not significantly impair the ability to exercise.[150–156] However, sleep-deprived subjects still report that the exercise feels harder to accomplish than normal. In other words, following sleep loss of one or two nights, physical performance does not appear to be significantly impaired, provided that participants are sufficiently motivated.

A group of researchers from Canada studied the effects of 2 days of sleep deprivation on 33 male volunteers.[155] Although the lack of sleep had no effect on muscle strength, work performance decreased significantly (Figure 14.19). The subjects had a difficult time motivating themselves to do such things as carrying sandbags, walking briskly for 30 minutes, or carrying loads with a wheelbarrow. The researchers concluded that although sleep-deprived individuals may have the physiological capacity to do the work, the interference of mood, perception of effort, or even the repetitive nature of the tasks decreases the ability of individuals to maintain a constant level of work output.

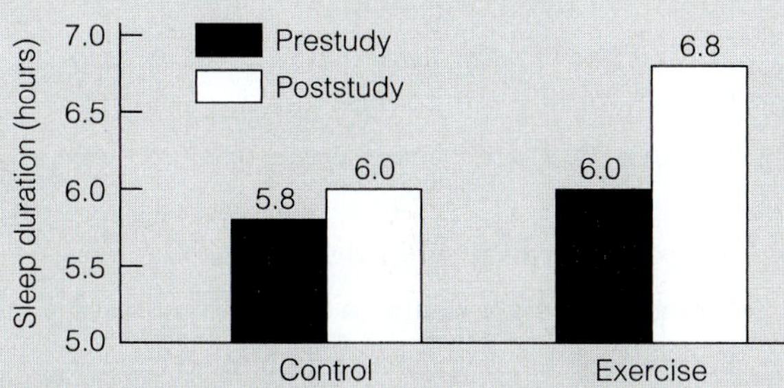

Figure 14.18 Influence of 16 weeks of exercise training on sleep duration in 43 older adults with moderate sleep complaints. Sleep duration increased in older adults exercising four times per week, 30–40 minutes per session, over a 16-week period. Source: King AC, Oman RF, Brassington GS, Bliwise DL, Haskell WL. Moderate-intensity exercise and self-rated quality of sleep in older adults. *JAMA* 277:32–37, 1997.

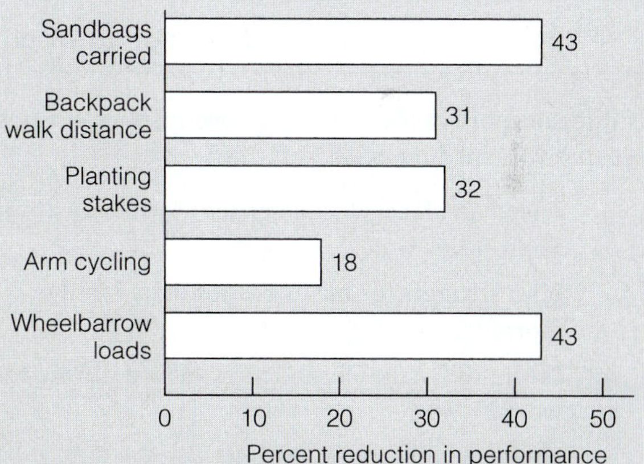

Figure 14.19 Decrease in work/exercise performance after 2 days of sleep deprivation. Sleep deprivation is associated with a decrease in work performance. Source: Rodgers CD, Paterson DH, Cunningham DA, et al. Sleep deprivation: Effects on work capacity, self-paced walking, contractile properties and perceived exertion. *Sleep* 18:30–38, 1995.

Box 14.8

Facts on Sleep in America

- On average, adults sleep 7 hours during a weekday night, 1 hour less than recommended by sleep experts. Only 32% sleep 8 hours or more on weekday nights, and 39% sleep less than 7 hours.
- On weekends, adults sleep an average of 7.5 hours per night.
- One third of Americans say they get less sleep now than 5 years ago, and 74% say they experience frequent sleep problems, though most have not been diagnosed with a sleep disorder.
- A sizable proportion of adults (37%) report that they are so sleepy during the day that it interferes with daily activities at least a few days a month or more. One in five (16%) experience this level of daytime sleepiness a few days per week or more. When they feel sleepy during the day, 65% say they are very likely to accept their sleepiness and keep going.
- More than one half of adults in the United States (51%) report that they have driven while drowsy in the past year, 17% have actually dozed off while driving, and 1% have had an accident because they dozed off or were too tired.
- About one half of adults (51%) report having experienced one or more symptoms of insomnia at least a few nights a week in the past year, and 29% have experienced insomnia nearly every night.
- Almost one half of adults (46%) need an alarm clock to wake up four or more times a week.
- The most common activities within the hour before going to sleep are watching TV (87%), spending time with family and friends (73%), reading (53%), and taking a bath or shower (50%).
- More than 1 in 10 adults (15%) report using prescription and/or over-the-counter medications.

Source: National Sleep Foundation, 2001, 2002 surveys. www.sleepfoundation.org.

Box 14.9

Determining Whether You Are Sleep-Deprived

If three or more of the following describe you, it's possible that you need more sleep:

_____ I need an alarm clock in order to wake up at the appropriate time.

_____ It's a struggle for me to get out of bed in the morning.

_____ I feel tired, irritable, and stressed out during the week.

_____ I have trouble concentrating.

_____ I have trouble remembering.

_____ I feel slow with critical thinking, problem solving, being creative.

_____ I often fall asleep watching television.

_____ I find it hard to stay awake in boring meetings or lectures, or in warm rooms.

_____ I often nod off after heavy meals or after a low dose of alcohol.

_____ I often feel drowsy while driving.

_____ I often sleep extra hours on weekend mornings.

_____ I often need a nap to get through the day.

_____ I have dark circles under my eyes.

Source: National Sleep Foundation, 2005.

SUMMARY

1. Nearly one out of five Americans is affected by one or more mental disorders, especially anxiety and depressive disorders.
2. Stress is defined as any action or situation that places special demands on a person. Five stress management principles were reviewed.
3. Studies have shown that being chronically anxious, depressed, or emotionally distressed is associated with deterioration of health.
4. Active people have a better psychological profile than inactive people. However, a strong self-selection bias may be present when comparing ac-

tive people with the general population. Controlled intervention studies are preferred when looking at the relationship between physical activity and psychological health.

5. In national surveys, physical activity is positively associated with good mental health, defined as positive mood, general sense of well-being, and infrequent symptoms of anxiety and depression.
6. Unfit people show greater cardiovascular and subjective responses to psychological stressors than do those at high levels of aerobic fitness.
7. Depression, anxiety, and mood state are favorably affected by regular aerobic exercise.
8. Both aerobic and nonaerobic exercise have been shown to be helpful in improving self-esteem.
9. Short-term memory and intellectual function may be improved during or shortly after an exercise session. More research is needed to study the long-term effects.
10. β-endorphin rises in the blood during intense exercise, but not during low-intensity exercise. Most researchers have found that despite significant decreases in tension during exercise, the increase in β-endorphin is unrelated to the improvement in mood. It appears that the complex β-endorphin protein molecule is unable to cross the blood–brain barrier to gain access to the receptors located in the limbic system. Nonetheless, the brain may be activated by muscular movement to make its own β-endorphin.
11. Exercise may enhance neurotransmitter activity in the brain, increasing the concentrations of brain norepinephrine and serotonin.
12. In the Sports Medicine Insight, sleep and its relationship to exercise were reviewed.

Review Questions

1. *During any 1-year period, an estimated ____% of individuals suffer from some form of mental disorder.*

   A. 12 B. 22 C. 39 D. 54 E. 87

2. *____ are the most prevalent of all mental disorders.*

   A. Depression disorders
   B. Schizophrenia disorders
   C. Anxiety disorders
   D. Substance abuse disorders
   E. Antisocial personality disorders

3. *Anxiety disorders are ____ times as prevalent in females as males.*

   A. 2 B. 3 C. 4 D. 5 E. 6

4. *When a stressor is perceived by the human mind, the signal is sent to the hypothalamus, then the pituitary gland, and next to the ____, where cortisol is released.*

   A. Spleen B. Adrenal glands
   C. Heart D. Lung
   E. Intestine

5. *More than ____% of suicides involve people who have a diagnosable mental disorder.*

   A. 10 B. 30 C. 50 D. 75 E. 90

6. *The General Well-Being Schedule, a psychological stress test, has been used in several national surveys. In general,*

   A. Scores are highest for physically active people.
   B. Scores are lowest for physically active people.
   C. No difference in scores between active and inactive people has been found.

7. *Being chronically anxious, depressed, or emotionally distressed has been associated with various diseases including*

   A. Cancer B. Heart disease
   C. Infection D. All of the above

8. *Which one of the following does* **not** *occur during the fight-or-flight stress response?*

   A. Blood pressure increases.
   B. Secretion of saliva decreases.
   C. Immune system is suppressed.
   D. Perspiration increases.
   E. Breathing is more shallow and slower.

9. *There are five basic strategies for managing stress. Which of the following statements is* **not** *a recommendation from one of these strategies?*

   A. Manage stressors by controlling the pace of life and daily schedules.
   B. Realize that when stressful events occur, the mind can choose the reaction.
   C. Good health and exercise can help the body deal with stress more easily.
   D. Seek the social support of others.
   E. Allow the fight-or-flight response to occur often so that the body becomes accustomed to it.

10. *Regular physical exercise has* **not** *been associated with*

    A. Increased cardiovascular reactivity to mental stress
    B. Decreased anxiety
    C. Decreased depression
    D. Increased self-concept
    E. Enhanced cognition, especially in the elderly

11. *For diagnosis of depression, a person who suffers from a major depressive disorder must either have a depressed mood or a loss of interest in daily activities consistently for at least a ____-week period.*

A. 1 B. 2 C. 3 D. 4 E. 6

12. *Dr. ____ is the originator of the concept of stress.*

A. Selye
B. Cooper
C. Paffenbarger
D. Haskell
E. Pollock

13. *For diagnosis of generalized anxiety disorder, excessive anxiety and worry about a number of events or activities (such as work or school performance) must occur on more days than not for at least ____ months.*

A. 1 B. 2 C. 3 D. 4 E. 6

14. *The average American adult sleeps ____ hours during the weekday night.*

A. 5 B. 6 C. 7 D. 8 E. 9

15. *Some people have trouble sleeping. The Better Sleep Council has made several recommendations to improve sleep. Which one of the following is* **not** *included?*

A. Keep regular sleeping hours.
B. Exercise regularly.
C. Eat a large meal close to bedtime.
D. Avoid smoking.
E. Cut down on stimulants like coffee.

16. *Slow-wave sleep comes during which of the following stages?*

A. 1 B. 2 C. 3 and 4 D. 5 E. 6

17. *Worldwide, mental illness ranks number ____ as a cause of disability and premature mortality.*

A. 1 B. 2 C. 3 D. 4 E. 6

18. *There are several criteria for diagnosis of depression. Which one of the following is* **not** *included?*

A. Disturbed sleep
B. Suicidal thinking or attempts
C. Feelings of worthlessness, self-reproach
D. Changes in appetite and weight
E. High energy and unusual drive to achieve

19. *Blood levels of β-endorphin would be highest after what type of physical activity?*

A. Walking
B. Half-marathon race
C. Basketball practice
D. Cycling at 10 miles per hour
E. Doubles tennis match

20. *____ is typically increased with exercise training, both aerobic and resistance.*

A. Depression
B. Self-esteem
C. State anxiety
D. Cardiovascular reactivity
E. Intelligence

21. *Projections show that mental disorders will ____ their share of the total global burden of disease and disability during the next several decades.*

A. Increase B. Decrease

22. *There are six potential mechanisms explaining how physical activity helps psychological health. Which one of the following hypotheses is most strongly associated with an increased sense of mastery and self-confidence?*

A. Cognitive-behavioral
B. Social interaction
C. Time-out/distraction
D. Cardiovascular fitness
E. Monoamine neurotransmitter

23. *Most studies have confirmed that favorable psychological responses to aerobic training are ____ to social interaction.*

A. Due B. Not due

24. *Most researchers have found that β-endorphin does not increase unless the exercise intensity exceeds a threshold level of ____% $\dot{V}O_{2max}$ or the duration exceeds 1 hour and the exercise is performed at a steady-state level.*

A. 45 B. 60 C. 75 D. 85 E. 95

25. *After the β-endorphin is secreted into the blood by the pituitary gland, it apparently is ____ to penetrate the blood–brain barrier to get into the brain.*

A. Able B. Unable

26. *The average adult sleeps 7.5 hours (average of weekdays and weekend days), with ____% of that in REM.*

A. 5 B. 50 C. 10 D. 75 E. 25

27. *Sleep begins with ____, during which brain waves gradually lengthen through four distinct stages.*

A. REM B. NREM

28. ***People who exercise regularly and are physically fit tend to spend a greater percent of their time in ____ and tend to sleep longer overall than do the inactive or unfit.***

A. REM sleep **B.** NREM (slow-wave) sleep

29. ***____ is good stress.***

A. Distress **B.** Eustress

Answers

1. B	**9.** E	**17.** B	**24.** C
2. C	**10.** A	**18.** E	**25.** B
3. A	**11.** B	**19.** B	**26.** E
4. B	**12.** A	**20.** B	**27.** B
5. E	**13.** E	**21.** A	**28.** B
6. A	**14.** C	**22.** A	**29.** B
7. D	**15.** C	**23.** B	
8. E	**16.** C		

REFERENCES

1. Stephens T. Physical activity and mental health in the United States and Canada. Evidence from four population surveys. *Prev Med* 17:35–47, 1988.
2. U.S. Department of Health and Human Services. *Mental Health: A Report of the Surgeon General.* Rockville, MD: U.S. Department of Health and Human Services, Substance Abuse and Mental Health Services Administration, Center for Mental Health Services, National Institutes of Health, National Institute of Mental Health, 1999.
3. Narrow WE. One-year prevalence of mental disorders, excluding substance use disorders, in the U.S.: NIMH ECA prospective data. Bethesda, MD: National Institute of Mental Health, 1998. http://www.nimh.nih.gov.
4. National Institute of Mental Health. *Anxiety Disorders.* Bethesda, MD: National Institute of Mental Health, 2004. http://www.nimh.nih.gov.
5. National Institute of Mental Health. *Depression.* Bethesda, MD: National Institute of Mental Health, 2004. http://www.nimh.nih.gov.
6. U.S. Department of Health and Human Services. *Healthy People 2010.* Washington DC: Author, January, 2000. http://www.health.gov/healthypeople/.
7. National Center for Health Statistics. *Health, United States, 2004.* Hyattsville, MD: 2004. http://www.cdc.gov/nchs.
8. American Psychiatric Association. *Diagnostic and Statistical Manual for Mental Disorders* (4th edition, text revision). Washington, DC: APA Press, 2000.
9. Murray CJL, Lopez AD (eds.). *Summary: The Global Burden of Disease—A Comprehensive Assessment of Mortality and Disability from Diseases, Injuries, and Risk Factors in 1990 and Projected to 2020.* Cambridge, MA: Published by the Harvard School of Public Health on behalf of the World Health Organization and the World Bank, Harvard University Press, 1996. http://www.who.int/.
10. World Health Organization. *The World Health Report 2001: Mental Health, New Understanding, New Hope.* Geneva, Switzerland: World Health Organization, 2001. http://www.who.int/.
11. Ustun TB. The global burden of mental disorders. *Am J Public Health* 89:1315–1318, 1999.
12. Andrews G, Sanderson K, Slade T, Issakidis C. Why does the burden of disease persist? Relating the burden of anxiety and depression to effectiveness of treatment. *Bull World Health Organ* 78:446–454, 2000.
13. Sartorius N. The economic and social burden of depression. *J Clin Psychiatry* 62(suppl):15:8–11, 2001.
14. Seward BL. *Managing Stress: Principles and Strategies for Health and Wellbeing* (3rd ed). Boston: Jones and Bartlett Publishers, 2002.
15. Chrousos GP, Gold PW. The concepts of stress and stress system disorders: Overview of physical and behavioral homeostasis. *JAMA* 267:1244–1252, 1992.
16. Murphy LR. Stress management in work settings: A critical review of the health effects. *Am J Health Promotion* 11:112–135, 1996.
17. Selye H. *The Stress of Life.* New York: McGraw-Hill Book Co., Inc., 1956. See also: Selye H. *Stress without Distress.* New York: The New American Library Inc., 1974.
18. Cannon WB. *Bodily Changes in Pain, Hunger, Fear and Rage.* Boston: Charles T. Branford Co., 1953.
19. CDC. Self-reported frequent mental distress among adults—United States, 1993–2001. *MMWR* 53:963–966, 2004.
20. Barefoot JC, Schroll M. Symptoms of depression, acute myocardial infarction, and total mortality in a community sample. *Circulation* 93:1976–1980, 1996.
21. Pratt LA, Ford DE, Crum RM, Armenian HK, Gallo JJ, Eaton WW. Depression, psychotropic medication, and risk of myocardial infarction. Prospective data from the Baltimore ECA follow-up. *Circulation* 94:3123–3129, 1996.
22. Jonas BS, Franks P, Ingram DD. Are symptoms of anxiety and depression risk factors for hypertension? Longitudinal evidence from the National Health and Nutrition Examination Survey I Epidemiologic Follow-up Study. *Arch Fam Med* 6:43–49, 1997.
23. Ford DE, Mead LA, Chang PP, Cooper-Patrick L, Wang NY, Klag MJ. Depression is a risk factor for coronary artery disease in men. *Arch Intern Med* 158:1422–1426, 1998.
24. Everson SA, Kauhanen J, Kaplan GA, Goldberg DE, Julkunen J, Tuomilehto J, Salonen JT. Hostility and increased risk of mortality and acute myocardial infarction: The mediating role of behavioral risk factors. *Am J Epidemiol* 146:142–152, 1997.
25. Mittleman MA, Maclure M, Nachnani M, Sherwood JB, Muller JE. Educational attainment, anger, and the risk of triggering myocardial infarction onset. *Arch Intern Med* 157:769–775, 1997.
26. Kawachi I, Sparrow D, Spiro A, Vokonas P, Weiss ST. A prospective study of anger and coronary heart disease. *Circulation* 94:2090–2095, 1996.
27. Iribarren C, Sidney S, Bild DE, Liu K, Markovitz JH, Roseman JM, Matthews K. Association of hostility with coronary artery calcification in young adults: The CARDIA study. Coronary artery risk development in young adults. *JAMA* 283:2546–2551, 2000.
28. Jiang W, Babyak M, Krantz DS, et al. Mental stress-induced myocardial ischemia and cardiac events. *JAMA* 275:1651–1656, 1996.
29. Knox SS, Adelman A, Ellison RC, Arnett DK, Siegmund K, Weidner G, Province MA. Hostility, social support, and carotid

artery atherosclerosis in the National Heart, Lung, and Blood Institute Family Heart Study. *Am J Cardiol* 86:1086–1089, 2000.

30. Ariyo AA, Haan M, Tangen CM, Rutledge JC, Cushman M, Dobs A, Furberg CD. Depressive symptoms and risks of coronary heart disease and mortality in elderly Americans. *Circulation* 102:1773–1778, 2000.
31. Johnson JV, Stewart W, Hall EM, Fredlund P, Theorell T. Long-term psychosocial work environment and cardiovascular mortality among Swedish men. *Am J Public Health* 86:324–331, 1996.
32. Cohen S, Tyrrell DA, Smith AP. Psychological stress and susceptibility to the common cold. *N Engl J Med* 325:606–612, 1991.
33. Graham HMH, Douglas RM, Ryan P. Stress and acute respiratory infection. *Am J Epidemol* 124:389–395, 1986.
34. Kiecolt-Glaser JK, Glaser R, Cacioppo JT, MacCallum RC, Snydersmith M, Kim C, Malarkey WB. Marital conflict in older adults: Endocrinological and immunological correlates. *Psychosom Med* 59:339–349, 1997.
35. Cohen S, Doyle WJ, Skoner DP, Rabin BS, Gwaltney JM. Social ties and susceptibility to the common cold. *JAMA* 277:1940–1944, 1997.
36. Schaefer C, Quesenberry CP, Wi S. Mortality following conjugal bereavement and the effects of a shared environment. *Am J Epidemiol* 141:1142–1152, 1995.
37. Martikainen P, Valkonen T. Morality after the death of a spouse: Rates and causes of death in a large Finnish cohort. *Am J Public Health* 86:1087–1093, 1996.
38. Yasuda N, Zimmerman SI, Hawkes W, Fredman L, Hebel JR, Magaziner J. Relation of social network characteristics to 5-year mortality among young-old versus old-old white women in an urban community. *Am J Epidemiol* 145:516–523, 1997.
39. Berkman LF. The role of social relations in health promotion. *Psychosom Med* 57:245–254, 1995.
40. Ruberman W. Psychosocial influences on mortality after myocardial infarction. *N Engl J Med* 311:552–559, 1984.
41. Case RB, Moss AJ, Case N, et al. Living alone after myocardial infarction: Impact on prognosis. *JAMA* 267:515–519, 1992.
42. Faragher EB, Cass M, Cooper CL. The relationship between job satisfaction and health: A meta-analysis. *Occup Environ Med* 62:105–112, 2005.
43. Gallo JJ, Armenian HK, Ford DE, Eaton WW, Khachaturian AS. Major depression and cancer: The 13-year follow-up of the Baltimore epidemiologic catchment area sample (United States). *Cancer Causes Control* 11:751–758, 2000.
44. Davidson K, Jonas BS, Dixon KE, Markovitz JH. Do depression symptoms predict early hypertension incidence in young adults in the CARDIA study? Coronary Artery Disease Development in Young Adults. *Arch Intern Med* 160:1495–1500, 2000.
45. Ruo B, Rumsfeld JS, Hlatky MA, Liu H, Browner WS, Whooley MA. Depressive symptoms and health-related quality of life: The Heart and Soul Study. *JAMA* 290:215–221, 2003.
46. Seeman TE, Kaplan GA, Knudsen L, et al. Social network ties and mortality among the elderly in the Alameda County Study. *Am J Epidemiol* 126:714–723, 1987.
47. Orth-Gomer K, Rosengren A, Wilhelmsen L. Lack of social support and incidence of coronary heart disease in middle-aged Swedish men. *Psychosom Med* 55:3743, 1993.
48. Institute of Medicine. *The Second Fifty Years: Promoting Health and Preventing Disability.* Washington, DC: National Academy Press, 1990.
49. Stephens T. Secular trends in adult physical activity: Exercise boom or bust? *Res Quart Exerc Sport* 58:94–105, 1987.
50. Stephens T, Craig CL. The well-being of Canadians: Highlights of the 1988 Campbell's Survey. Ottawa: Canadian Fitness and Lifestyle Research Institute, 1990.
51. Mcdowell I, Newell C. *Measuring Health.* New York: Oxford University Press, 1996.
52. Fazio AF. A concurrent validation study of the NCHS General Well-Being Schedule. *Vital and Health Statistics Series* Vol. 2, No. 73. (DHEW Pub. No. [HRA] 781347). National Center of Health Statistics. Hyattsville, MD: U.S. Public Health Service, 1977.
53. Gazmararian J, Baker D, Parker R, Blazer DG. A multivariate of factors associated with depression: Evaluating the role of health literacy as a potential contributor. *Arch Intern Med* 160:3307–3314, 2000.
54. Nieman DC, Warren BJ, Dotson RG, Butterworth DE, Henson DA. Physical activity, psychological well-being, and mood state in elderly women. *J Aging Phys Act* 1:22–33, 1993.
55. Steptoe A, Butler N. Sports participation and emotional well-being in adolescents. *Lancet* 347:1789–1792, 1996.
56. Scully D, Kremer J, Meade MM, Graham R, Dudgeon K. Physical exercise and psychological well-being: A critical review. *Br J Sports Med* 32:111–120, 1998.
57. U.S. Department of Health and Human Services. *Physical Activity and Health: A Report of the Surgeon General.* Atlanta, GA: U.S. Department of Health and Human Services, Centers for Disease Control and Prevention, National Center for Chronic Disease Prevention and Health Promotion, 1996.
58. Dunn AL, Trivedi MH, O'Neal HA. Physical activity dose-response effects on outcomes of depression and anxiety. *Med Sci Sports Exerc* 33(suppl):S587–S597, 2001.
59. Lawlor DA, Hopker SW. The effectiveness of exercise as an intervention in the management of depression: Systematic review and meta-regression analysis of randomized controlled studies. *BMJ* 322:1–8, 2001.
60. Claytor RP. Stress reactivity: Hemodynamic adjustments in trained and untrained humans. *Med Sci Sports Exerc* 23:873–81, 1991.
61. Carmack CL, Boudreaux E, Amaral-Melendez M, Brantley PJ, de Moor C. Aerobic fitness and leisure physical activity as moderators of the stress-illness relation. *Ann Behav* 21:251–257, 1999.
62. Crews DJ, Landers DM. A meta-analytic review of aerobic fitness and reactivity to psychosocial stressors. *Med Sci Sports Exerc* 19:S114–S120, 1987.
63. Iwasaki Y, Zuzanek J, Mannell RC. The effects of physically active leisure on stress-health relationships. *Can J Public Health* 92:214–218, 2001.
64. Siconolfi SF. Exercise training attenuated the blood pressure response to mental stress. *Med Sci Sports Exerc* 17:281, 1985.
65. O'Connor PJ, Puetz TW. Chronic physical activity and feelings of energy and fatigue. *Med Sci Sports Exerc* 37:299–305, 2005.
66. Weyerer S. Physical inactivity and depression in the community: Evidence from the Upper Bavarian Field Study. *Int J Sports Med* 13:492–496, 1992.
67. Singh NA, Clements KM, Sing MA. The efficacy of exercise as a long-term antidepressant in elderly subjects: A randomized, controlled trial. *J Gerontol A Biol Sci Med Sci* 56:M497–504, 2001.
68. Blumenthal JA, Babyak MA, Moore KA, Craighead WE, Herman S, Khatri P, Waugh R, Napolitano MA, Forman LM, Appelbaum M, Doraiswamy PM, Krishnan R. Effects of exercise training on older patients with major depression. *Arch Intern Med* 159:2349–2356, 1999.
69. Babyak M, Blumenthal JA, Herman S, Khatri P, Doraiswamy M, Moore K, Craighead WE, Baldewicz TT, Krishnan KR. *Psychosom Med* 62:633–638, 2000.
70. North TC, McCullagh P, Tran ZV. Effect of exercise on depression. *Exerc Sport Sci Review* 18:379–415, 1990.
71. Martinsen EW. Benefits of exercise for the treatment of depression. *Sports Med* 9:380–389, 1990.

72. Martinsen EW. Exercise and mental health in clinical populations. In Biddle SJH (ed). *European Perspectives on Exercise and Sport Psychology.* Champaign, IL: Human Kinetics, 1995.

73. Atlantis E, Chow CM, Kirby A, Singh MF. An effective exercise-based intervention for improving mental health and quality of life measures: A randomized controlled trial. *Prev Med* 39:424–434, 2004.

74. McDonald DG, Hodgdon JA. *Psychological Effects of Aerobic Fitness Training.* New York: Springer-Verlag, 1991.

75. Morgan WP. Physical activity, fitness, and depression. In Bouchard C, Shephard RJ, Stephens T (eds.). *Physical Activity, Fitness, and Health.* Champaign, IL: Human Kinetics, 1994.

76. Spielberger CD, Gorsuch RL, Lushene RE. *Manual for the State–Trait Anxiety Inventory.* Palo Alto, CA: Consulting Psychology Press, 1970.

77. Petruzzello SJ, Landers DM, Hatfield BD, Kubitz RA, Salazar W. A meta-analysis on the anxiety-reducing effects of acute and chronic exercise: Outcomes and mechanisms. *Sports Med* 11:143–182, 1991.

78. Breus MJ, O'Connor PJ. Exercise-induced anxiolysis: A test of the "time out" hypothesis in high anxious females. *Med Sci Sports Exerc* 30:1107–1112, 1998.

79. O'Connor PJ, Cook DB. Anxiolytic and blood pressure effects of acute static compared to dynamic exercise. *Int J Sports Med* 19:188–192, 1998.

80. O'Connor PJ, Bryant CX, Veltri JP, Gebhardt SM. State anxiety and ambulatory blood pressure following resistance exercise in females. *Med Sci Sports Exerc* 25:516–521, 1993.

81. Raglin JS, Wilson M. State anxiety following 20 minutes of bicycle ergometer exercise at selected intensities. *Int J Sports Med* 17:467–471, 1996.

82. Garvin AW, Koltyn KF, Morgan WP. Influence of acute physical activity and relaxation on state anxiety and blood lactate in untrained college males. *Int J Sports Med* 18:470–476, 1997.

83. Trine MR, Morgan WP. Influence of time of day on the anxiolytic effects of exercise. *Int J Sports Med* 18:161–168, 1997.

84. Koltyn KF, Raglin JS, O'Connor PJ, Morgan WP. Influence of weight training on state anxiety, body awareness and blood pressure. *Int J Sports Med* 16:266–269, 1995.

85. Cramer SR, Nieman DC, Lee JW. The effects of moderate exercise training on psychological well-being and mood state in women. *J Psychosom Res* 35:437–449, 1991.

86. Moses J, Steptoe A, Mathews A, Edwards S. The effects of exercise training on mental well-being in the normal population: A controlled trial. *J Psychosom Res* 33:47–61, 1989.

87. McNair DM, Lorr M, Droppleman LF. *EDITS Manual: Profile of Mood States.* San Diego: Educational and Industrial Testing Service, 1981.

88. Steptoe A, Edwards S, Moses J, Mathews A. The effects of exercise training on mood and perceiving coping ability in anxious adults from the general population. *J Psychosom Res* 33:537–547, 1989.

89. Nabetani T, Tokunaga M. The effect of short-term (10- and 15-min) running at self-selected intensity on mood alteration. *J Physiol Anthropol Appl Human Sci* 20:231–239, 2001.

90. Nieman DC, Custer WF, Butterworth DE, Utter AC, Henson DA. Psychological response to exercise training and/or energy restriction in obese women. *J Psychosom Res* 48:23–29, 2000.

91. McAuley E, Rudolph D. Physical activity, aging, and psychological well-being. *J Aging Physical Act* 3:67–96, 1995.

92. Wylie RC. *The Self-Concept: A Review of Methodological Considerations and Measuring Instruments.* Lincoln: University of Nebraska Press, 1977.

93. Sonstroem RJ. Physical self-concept: Assessment and external validity. *Exerc Sport Sci Rev* 26:133–160, 1998.

94. MacMahon J, Gross RT. Physical and psychological effects of aerobic exercise in delinquent adolescent males. *Am J Dis Child* 142:1361–1366, 1988.

95. Tucker LA, Mortell R. Comparison of the effects of walking and weight training programs on body image in middle-aged women: An experimental study. *Am J Health Promotion* 8(1):34–42, 1993.

96. McAuley E, Blissmer B, Katula J, Duncan TE, Mihalko SL. Physical activity, self-esteem, and self-efficacy relationships in older adults: A randomized controlled trial. *Ann Behav Med* 22:131–139, 2000.

97. Ekeland E, Heian F, Hagen KB, Abbott J, Nordheim L. Exercise to improve self-esteem in children and young people. *Cochrane Database Syst Rev* (1):CD003683, 2004.

98. Beniamini Y, Rubenstein JJ, Zaichkowsky LD, Crim MC. Effects of high-intensity strength training on quality-of-life parameters in cardiac rehabilitation patients. *Am J Cardiol* 80:841–846, 1997.

99. Gruber JJ. Physical activity and self-esteem development in children: A meta-analysis. In Stull G, Eckert H (eds.). *Effects of Physical Activity on Children: The Academy Papers No. 19.* Champaign, IL: Human Kinetics, 1986.

100. Kramer AF, Hahn S, Cohen NJ, Banich MT, McAuley E, Harrison CR, Chason J, Vakil E, Bardell L, Boileau RA, Colcombe A. Aging, fitness and neurocognitive function. *Nature* 400:418–419, 1999.

101. Laurin D, Verreault R, Lindsay J, MacPherson K, Rockwood K. Physical activity and risk of cognitive impairment and dementia in elderly persons. *Arch Neurol* 58:498–504, 2001.

102. Hassmen P, Koivula N. Mood, physical working capacity and cognitive performance in the elderly as related to physical activity. *Aging (Milano)* 9:136–142, 1997.

103. Chodzko-Zajko WJ, Moore KA. Physical fitness and cognitive functioning in aging. *Exerc Sport Sci Rev* 22:195–220, 1994.

104. Hogervorst E, Riedel W, Jeukendrup A, Jolles J. Cognitive performance after strenuous physical exercise. *Percept Mot Skills* 83:479–488, 1996.

105. Van Praag H, Christie BR, Sejnowski TJ, Gage FH. Running enhances neurogenesis, learning, and long-term potentiation in mice. *Proc Natl Acad Sci USA* 96:13427–13431, 1999.

106. Etnier JL, Landers DM. Brain function and exercise: Current perspectives. *Sports Med* 19:81–85, 1995.

107. Rogers RL, Meyer IS, Mortel KF. After reaching retirement age, physical activity sustains cerebral perfusion and cognition. *J Am Geriat Soc* 38:123–128, 1991.

108. Schuit AJ, Feskens EJM, Launer LJ, Kromhout D. Physical activity and cognitive decline, the role of the apolipoprotein e4 allele. *Med Sci Sports Exerc* 33:772–777, 2001.

109. Radak Z, Kaneko T, Tahara S, Nakamoto H, Pucsok J, Sasvari M, Nyakas C, Goto S. Regular exercise improves cognitive function and decreases oxidative damage in rat brain. *Neurochem Int* 38:17–23, 2001.

110. Weuve J, Kang JH, Manson JE, Breteler MM, Ware JH, Grodstein F. *JAMA* 292:1454–1461, 2004.

111. Van Boxtel MPJ, Paas FGW, Houx PJ, Adam JJ, Teeken JC, Jolles J. Aerobic capacity and cognitive performance in a cross-sectional aging study. *Med Sci Sports Exerc* 29:1357–1365, 1997.

112. Yeung RR. The acute effects of exercise on mood state. *J Psychosom Res* 40:123–141, 1996.

113. Forge RL. Exercise-associated mood alterations: A review of interactive neurobiologic mechanisms. *Med Exerc Nutr Health* 4:17–32, 1995.

114. Mazzeo RS. Catecholamine responses to acute and chronic exercise. *Med Sci Sports Exerc* 23:839–845, 1991.

115. Dishman RK. Brain monoamines, exercise, and behavioral stress: Animal models. *Med Sci Sports Exerc* 29:63–74, 1997.

116. Goldfarb AH, Jamurtas AZ. Beta-endorphin response to exercise. An update. *Sports Med* 24:8–16, 1997.

117. Sforzo GA, Seeger TF, Pert CB, Pert A, Dotson CO. In vivo opioid receptor occupation in the rat brain following exercise. *Med Sci Sports Exerc* 18:380–384, 1986.

118. Goldfarb AH, Hatfield BD, Sforzo GA, et al. Serum beta-endorphin levels during a graded exercise test to exhaustion. *Med Sci Sports Exerc* 19:78–82, 1987.

119. Farrell PA, Gustafson AB, Morgan WP, et al. Enkephalins, catecholamines, and psychological mood alterations: Effects of prolonged exercise. *Med Sci Sports Exerc* 19:347–353, 1987.

120. Thoren P, Floras IS, Hoffmann P, Seals DR. Endorphins and exercise: Physiological mechanisms and clinical implications. *Med Sci Sports Exerc* 22:417–428, 1990.

121. Schwarz L, Kindermann W. Changes in beta-endorphin levels in response to aerobic and anaerobic exercise. *Sports Med* 13:25–36, 1992.

122. Droste C, Greenlee MW, Schreck M, Roskamm H. Experimental pain thresholds and plasma beta-endorphin levels during exercise. *Med Sci Sports Exerc* 23:334–342, 1991.

123. Mondin GW, Morgan WP, Piering PN, et al. Psychological consequences of exercise deprivation in habitual exercisers. *Med Sci Sports Exerc* 28:1199–1203, 1996.

124. Hurst R, Hale B, Smith D, Collins D. Exercise dependence, social physique anxiety, and social support in experienced and inexperienced bodybuilders and weightlifters. *Br J Sports Med* 34:431–435, 2000.

125. Morgan WP, Costill DL, Flynn MG, Raglin JS, O'Connor PJ. Mood disturbance following increased training in swimmers. *Med Sci Sports Exerc* 20:408–414, 1988.

126. Raglin JS, Koceja DM, Stager JM, Harms CA. Mood, neuromuscular function, and performance during training in female swimmers. *Med Sci Sports Exerc* 28:372–377, 1996.

127. Berglund B, Safstrom H. Psychological monitoring and modulation of training load of world-class canoeists. *Med Sci Sports Exerc* 26:1036–1040, 1994.

128. Montgomery I, Trinder J, Paxton S, Fraser G. Sleep disruption following a marathon. *J Sports Med* 25:69–74, 1985.

129. National Center on Sleep Disorders Research and Office of Prevention, Education, and Control, National Heart, Lung, and Blood Institute, National Institutes of Health. *Strategy Development Workshop on Sleep Education.* Bethesda, MD: National Institutes of Health, 1994; *Insomnia: Assessment and Management in Primary Care.* Bethesda, MD: National Institutes of Health, 1998 (NIH Publication No. 98-4088).

130. Dement WC, Mitler MM. It's time to wake up to the importance of sleep disorders. *JAMA* 269:1548–1550, 1993.

131. Better Sleep Council, http://www.betttersleep.org, and the National Sleep Foundation, http://www.sleepfoundation.org.

132. NHLBI Information Center. *Insomnia.* Bethesda, MD: 1995. (NIH Publication No. 95-3801).

133. Kupfer DJ, Reynolds CF. Management of insomnia. *N Engl J Med* 336:341–345, 1997.

134. Hammond EC. Some preliminary findings on physical complaints from a prospective study of 1,064,000 men and women. *Am J Public Health* 54:11–23, 1964.

135. Patel SR, Ayas NT, Malhotra MR, White DP, Schernhammer ES, Speizer FE, Stampfer MJ, Hu FB. A prospective study of sleep duration and mortality risk in women. *Sleep* 27:440–444, 2004.

136. Chang PP, Ford DE, Mead LA, Cooper-Patrick L, Klag MJ. Insomnia in young men and subsequent depression. The Johns Hopkins Precursors Study. *Am J Epidemiol* 146:105–114, 1997.

137. Youngstedt SD. Effects of exercise on sleep. *Clin Sports Med* 24:355–365, 2005.

138. Montgomery P, Dennis J. A systematic review of non-pharmacological therapies for sleep problems in later life. *Sleep Med Rev* 8:47–62, 2004.

139. Kubitz KA, Landers DM, Petruzzello SJ, Han M. The effects of acute and chronic exercise on sleep: A meta-analytic review. *Sports Med* 21:277-291, 1996.

140. Youngstedt SD. Does exercise truly enhance sleep? *Physician Sportsmed* 25(10):72–82, 1997.

141. Youngstedt SD, O'Connor PJ, Dishman RK. The effects of acute exercise on sleep: A quantitative synthesis. *Sleep* 20:203–214, 1997.

142. Sherill DL, Kotchou K, Quan SF. Association of physical activity and human sleep disorders. *Arch Intern Med* 158:1894–1898, 1998.

143. Shapiro CM, Warren PM, Trinder J, et al. Fitness facilitates sleep. *Eur J Appl Physiol* 53:1–4, 1984.

144. Tworoger SS, Yasui Y, Vitiello MV, Schwartz RS, Ulrich CM, Aiello EJ, Irwin ML, Bowen D, Potter JD, McTiernan A. Effects of a yearlong moderate-intensity exercise and a stretching intervention on sleep quality in postmenopausal women. *Sleep* 26:830–836, 2003.

145. Brassington GS, Hicks RA. Aerobic exercise and self-reported sleep quality in elderly individuals. *J Aging Phys Act* 3:120–134, 1995.

146. Trinder J, Paxton S, Montgomery I, Fraser G. Endurance as opposed to power training: Their effect on sleep. *Psychophysiol* 22:668–673, 1985.

147. Taylor SR, Rogers GG, Driver HS. Effects of training volume on sleep, psychological, and selected physiological profiles of elite female swimmers. *Med Sci Sports Exerc* 29:688–693, 1997.

148. Youngstedt SD, Kripke DF, Elliott JA. Is sleep disturbed by vigorous late-night exercise? *Med Sci Sports Exerc* 31:864–869, 1999.

149. King AC, Oman RF, Brassington GS, Bliwise DL, Haskell WL. Moderate-intensity exercise and self-rated quality of sleep in older adults. *JAMA* 277:32–37, 1997.

150. Pilcher JJ, Huffcutt AI. Effects of sleep deprivation on performance: A meta-analysis. *Sleep* 19:318–326, 1996.

151. VanHelder T. Radomski MW. Sleep deprivation and the effect on exercise performance. *Sports Med* 7:235–247, 1989.

152. Mougin F, Simon-Rigaud ML, Davenne D, et al. Effects on sleep disturbances on subsequent physical performance. *Eur J Appl Physiol* 63:77–82, 1991.

153. Chen HI. Effects of 30-h sleep loss on cardiorespiratory functions at rest and in exercise. *Med Sci Sports Exerc* 23:193–198, 1991.

154. Mougin F, Bourdin H, Simon-Rigaud ML, Didier JM, Toubin G, Kantelip JP. Effects of a selective sleep deprivation on subsequent anaerobic performance. *Int J Sports Med* 17:115–119, 1996.

155. Rodgers CD, Paterson DH, Cunningham DA, et al. Sleep deprivation: Effects on work capacity, self-paced walking, contractile properties and perceived exertion. *Sleep* 18:30–38, 1995.

156. Symons JD, VanHelder T, Myles WS. Physical performance and physiological responses following 60 hours of sleep deprivation. *Med Sci Sports Exerc* 20:374–380, 1988.

PHYSICAL FITNESS ACTIVITY 14.1

The General Well-Being Schedule

As described earlier in this chapter, one measure of psychological status that has been used with good success in national surveys is the General Well-Being Schedule (GWBS). The GWBS was designed by the National Center for Health Statistics and consists of 18 items in six subscales covering such constructs as energy level, satisfaction, freedom from worry, and self-control. A high score on the GWBS represents an absence of bad feelings and an expression of positive feelings. Results from national surveys have shown that higher scores for the GWBS are significantly associated with increased amounts of physical activity for all age groups and for both men and women. (See Stephens T. Physical activity and mental health in the United States and Canada: Evidence from four population surveys. *Prev Med* 17:35–47, 1988.)

In this activity, the 18 questions of the GWBS are listed, and an interpretation of results is provided.

The General Well-Being Schedule

Instructions: The following questions ask how you feel and how things have been going for you *during the past month.* For each question, mark an "x" for the answer that most nearly applies to you. Since there are no right or wrong answers, it's best to answer each question quickly without pausing too long on any one of them.

1. How have you been feeling in general?

5 ❑ In excellent spirits

4 ❑ In very good spirits

3 ❑ In good spirits mostly

2 ❑ I've been up and down in spirits a lot

1 ❑ In low spirits mostly

0 ❑ In very low spirits

2. Have you been bothered by nervousness or your "nerves"?

0 ❑ Extremely so—to the point where I could not work or take care of things

1 ❑ Very much so

2 ❑ Quite a bit

3 ❑ Some—enough to bother me

4 ❑ A little

5 ❑ Not at all

3. Have you been in firm control of your behavior, thoughts, emotions or feelings?

5 ❑ Yes, definitely so

4 ❑ Yes, for the most part

3 ❑ Generally so

2 ❑ Not too well

1 ❑ No, and I am somewhat disturbed

0 ❑ No, and I am very disturbed

4. Have you felt so sad, discouraged, hopeless, or had so many problems that you wondered if anything was worthwhile?
   - 0 ❑ Extremely so—to the point I have just about given up
   - 1 ❑ Very much so
   - 2 ❑ Quite a bit
   - 3 ❑ Some—enough to bother me
   - 4 ❑ A little bit
   - 5 ❑ Not at all
5. Have you been under or felt you were under any strain, stress, or pressure?
   - 0 ❑ Yes—almost more than I could bear
   - 1 ❑ Yes—quite a bit of pressure
   - 2 ❑ Yes—some, more than usual
   - 3 ❑ Yes—some, but about usual
   - 4 ❑ Yes—a little
   - 5 ❑ Not at all
6. How happy, satisfied, or pleased have you been with your personal life?
   - 5 ❑ Extremely happy—couldn't have been more satisfied or pleased
   - 4 ❑ Very happy
   - 3 ❑ Fairly happy
   - 2 ❑ Satisfied—pleased
   - 1 ❑ Somewhat dissatisfied
   - 0 ❑ Very dissatisfied
7. Have you had reason to wonder if you were losing your mind, or losing control over the way you act, talk, think, feel, or of your memory?
   - 5 ❑ Not at all
   - 4 ❑ Only a little
   - 3 ❑ Some, but not enough to be concerned
   - 2 ❑ Some, and I've been a little concerned
   - 1 ❑ Some, and I am quite concerned
   - 0 ❑ Much, and I'm very concerned
8. Have you been anxious, worried, or upset?
   - 0 ❑ Extremely so—to the point of being sick, or almost sick
   - 1 ❑ Very much so
   - 2 ❑ Quite a bit
   - 3 ❑ Some—enough to bother me
   - 4 ❑ A little bit
   - 5 ❑ Not at all
9. Have you been waking up fresh and rested?
   - 5 ❑ Every day
   - 4 ❑ Most every day

3 ❑ Fairly often

2 ❑ Less than half the time

1 ❑ Rarely

0 ❑ None of the time

10. Have you been bothered by any illness, bodily disorder, pain, or fears about your health?

0 ❑ All the time

1 ❑ Most of the time

2 ❑ A good bit of the time

3 ❑ Some of the time

4 ❑ A little of the time

5 ❑ None of the time

11. Has your daily life been full of things that are interesting to you?

5 ❑ All the time

4 ❑ Most of the time

3 ❑ A good bit of the time

2 ❑ Some of the time

1 ❑ A little of the time

0 ❑ None of the time

12. Have you felt downhearted and blue?

0 ❑ All of the time

1 ❑ Most of the time

2 ❑ A good bit of the time

3 ❑ Some of the time

4 ❑ A little of the time

5 ❑ None of the time

13. Have you been feeling emotionally stable and sure of yourself?

5 ❑ All of the time

4 ❑ Most of the time

3 ❑ A good bit of the time

2 ❑ Some of the time

1 ❑ A little of the time

0 ❑ None of the time

14. Have you felt tired, worn out, used-up, or exhausted?

0 ❑ All of the time

1 ❑ Most of the time

2 ❑ A good bit of the time

3 ❑ Some of the time

4 ❑ A little of the time

5 ❑ None of the time

Note: For each of the following four scales, the words at each end describe opposite feelings. Circle any number along the bar that seems closest to how you have felt generally *during the past month.*

15. How concerned or worried about your health have you been?

Not concerned at all	10	8	6	4	2	0	**Very concerned**

16. How relaxed or tense have you been?

Very relaxed	10	8	6	4	2	0	**Very tense**

17. How much energy, pep, and vitality have you felt?

No energy at all, listless	0	2	4	6	8	10	**Very energetic, dynamic**

18. How depressed or cheerful have you been?

Very depressed	0	2	4	6	8	10	**Very cheerful**

Directions: Add up all the points from the boxes you have checked for each question. Compare your total score with the norms listed in the following table.

National Norms for the General Well-Being Schedule

Stress State	Total Stress Score	% Distribution U.S. Population
Positive well-being	81–110	55%
Low positive	76–80	10%
Marginal	71–75	9%
Indicates stress problem	56–70	16%
Indicates distress	41–55	7%
Serious	26–40	2%
Severe	0–25	< 1%

Notes: Figure 14.6 gives the scores for the U.S. population by age, gender, and amount of exercise. Notice that all subgroups reporting "much exercise" fell within the "positive well-being" range of 81–110.

Software for analyzing the General Well-Being Schedule is available from: Wellsource, 15431 S.E. 82nd Dr., Suite F, Clackamas, OR 97015.

PHYSICAL FITNESS ACTIVITY 14.2

Life Hassles and Stress

Survey of Recent Life Experiences

Following is a list of experiences that many people have at some time or another. Please indicate for each experience how much it has been a part of your life *over the past month.*

Intensity of Experience over Past Month

1 = not at all part of my life

2 = only slightly part of my life

3 = distinctly part of my life

4 = very much part of my life

____ **1.** Disliking your daily activities

____ **2.** Lack of privacy

____ **3.** Disliking your work

____ **4.** Ethnic or racial conflict

____ **5.** Conflicts with in-laws or boyfriend's/girlfriend's family

____ **6.** Being let down or disappointed by friends

____ **7.** Conflict with supervisor(s) at work

____ **8.** Social rejection

____ **9.** Too many things to do at once

____ **10.** Being taken for granted

____ **11.** Financial conflicts with family members

____ **12.** Having your trust betrayed by a friend

____ **13.** Separation from people you care about

____ **14.** Having your contributions overlooked

____ **15.** Struggling to meet your own standards of performance and accomplishment

____ **16.** Being taken advantage of

____ **17.** Not enough leisure time

____ **18.** Financial conflicts with friends or fellow workers

____ **19.** Struggling to meet other people's standards of performance and accomplishment

____ **20.** Having your actions misunderstood by others

____ **21.** Cash-flow difficulties

____ **22.** A lot of responsibilities

____ **23.** Dissatisfaction with work

____ **24.** Decisions about intimate relationship(s)

____ **25.** Not enough time to meet your obligations

____ **26.** Dissatisfaction with your mathematical ability

____ **27.** Financial burdens

____ **28.** Lower evaluation of your work than you think you deserve

____ **29.** Experiencing high levels of noise

____ **30.** Adjustments to living with unrelated person(s) (e.g., roommate)
____ **31.** Lower evaluation of your work than you hoped for
____ **32.** Conflicts with family member(s)
____ **33.** Finding your work too demanding
____ **34.** Conflicts with friend(s)
____ **35.** Hard effort to get ahead
____ **36.** Trying to secure loan(s)
____ **37.** Getting "ripped off" or cheated in the purchase of goods
____ **38.** Dissatisfaction with your ability at written expression
____ **39.** Unwanted interruptions of your work
____ **40.** Social isolation
____ **41.** Being ignored
____ **42.** Dissatisfaction with your physical appearance
____ **43.** Unsatisfactory housing conditions
____ **44.** Finding work uninteresting
____ **45.** Failing to get money you expected
____ **46.** Gossip about someone you care about
____ **47.** Dissatisfaction with your physical fitness
____ **48.** Gossip about yourself
____ **49.** Difficulty dealing with modern technology (e.g., computers)
____ **50.** Car problems
____ **51.** Hard work to look after and maintain home

Norms

Add up your points, and compare with the following "life hassle and stress score" norms.

Total "Life Hassle and Stress Score"

Very high stress .... ≥136
High stress 116–135
Average stress 76–115
Low stress.................................... 56–75
Very low stress............................... 51–55

Source: Kohn PM, Macdonald JE. The survey of recent life experiences: A decontaminated hassles scale for adults. *J Beh Med* 15:221–236, 1992. Reprinted with permission.

PHYSICAL FITNESS ACTIVITY 14.3

Depression

The National Institute of Mental Health has estimated that 17.6 million Americans suffer from depression. Only a minority of cases are diagnosed and treated, in part because many of the usual symptoms—feelings of hopelessness, despair, lethargy, self-loathing—tend to discourage the depressed individual from reaching out for help. The majority of cases of depression can be successfully treated, usually with medication, psychotherapy, or both. Nonetheless, the condition must first be identified. The Center for Epidemiologic Studies (CES) has developed a tool for measuring depression, known as the CES-D Scale. Take this test to see how you are feeling.

During the past week	**< 1 day**	**1–2 days**	**3–4 days**	**5–7 days**
I was bothered by things that don't usually bother me	0	1	2	3
I did not feel like eating; my appetite was poor	0	1	2	3
I felt that I could not shake off the blues even with the help of my family or friends	0	1	2	3
I felt that I was just as good as other people	3	2	1	0
I had trouble keeping my mind on what I was doing	0	1	2	3
I felt depressed	0	1	2	3
I felt everything I did was an effort	0	1	2	3
I felt hopeful about the future	3	2	1	0
I thought my life had been a failure	0	1	2	3
I felt fearful	0	1	2	3
My sleep was restless	0	1	2	3
I was happy	3	2	1	0
I talked less than usual	0	1	2	3
I felt lonely	0	1	2	3
People were unfriendly	0	1	2	3
I enjoyed life	3	2	1	0
I had crying spells	0	1	2	3
I felt sad	0	1	2	3
I felt that people disliked me	0	1	2	3
I could not get "going"	0	1	2	3

Scoring: A score of 22 or higher indicates possible depression. In general, the higher the score, the greater the mood disturbance—even below that threshold.
Source: Radloff LS. The CES-D Scale: A self-report depression scale for research in the general population. *Appl Psychol Meas* 1:385–401, 1977.

PHYSICAL FITNESS ACTIVITY 14.4

Controlling Stressors

Stressors are everywhere. They cannot all be avoided, but much can be done to reduce, modify, or eliminate them in a way that will allow you to accomplish your goals. Follow these three steps:

Step 1. List top five major life goals, in order of importance.

Step 2. List stressors associated with each goal.

Step 3. Summarize plans to modify or eliminate stressors so that goals can be achieved.

Step 1. Top five goals	**Step 2.** Major stressors associated with goal
Goal 1	
Goal 2	
Goal 3	
Goal 4	
Goal 5	

Step 3. Summarize plans to modify or eliminate stressors so that goals can be achieved.

1. ____________________
2. ____________________
3. ____________________
4. ____________________
5. ____________________
6. ____________________
7. ____________________
8. ____________________
9. ____________________
10. ____________________

PHYSICAL FITNESS ACTIVITY 14.5

Stress and Life Change: Recent Life Changes Questionnaire (RLCQ)

All changes, even desirable events, put demands on one's coping abilities. Such stress can have a strong impact on physical and emotional health. To get a feel for the possible health impact of the various recent changes in your life, think back over the *past year* and circle the "stress points" listed for each of the events that you experienced during that time. Then add up your points. A total score of 250–500 is considered moderate stress, while a score of 500 and above is considered high stress.

Life change event	LCU
Health	
An injury or illness which:	
Kept you in bed a week or more, or sent you to the hospital	74
Was less serious than above	44
Major dental work	26
Major change in eating habits	27
Major change in sleeping habits	26
Major change in your usual type and/or amount of recreation	28
Work	
Change to a new type of work	51
Change in your work hours or conditions	35
Change in your responsibilities at work:	
More responsibilities	29
Fewer responsibilities	21
Promotion	31
Demotion	42
Transfer	32
Troubles at work:	
With your boss	29
With coworkers	35
With persons under your supervision	35
Other work troubles	28
Major business adjustment	60
Retirement	52
Loss of job:	
Laid off from work	68
Fired from work	79
Correspondence course to help you in your work	18
Home and family	
Major change in living conditions	42
Change in residence:	
Move within the same town or city	25
Move to a different town, city, or state	47
Change in family get-togethers	25
Major change in health or behavior of family member	55
Marriage	50
Pregnancy	67
Miscarriage or abortion	65
Gain of a new family member:	
Birth of a child	66
Adoption of a child	65
A relative moving in with you	59
Spouse beginning or ending work	46
Child leaving home:	
To attend college	41
Due to marriage	41
For other reasons	45
Change in arguments with spouse	50
In-law problems	38
Change in the marital status of your parents:	
Divorce	59
Remarriage	50
Separation from spouse:	
Due to work	53
Due to marital problems	76
Divorce	96
Birth of grandchild	43
Death of spouse	119
Death of other family member:	
Child	123
Brother or sister	102
Parent	100
Personal and social	
Change in personal habits	26
Beginning or ending school or college	38
Change of school or college	35
Change in political beliefs	24
Change in religious beliefs	29
Change in social activities	27
Vacation	24
New, close, personal relationship	37
Engagement to marry	45
Girlfriend or boyfriend problems	39
Sexual difficulties	44
"Falling out" of a close personal relationship	47
An accident	48
Minor violation of the law	20
Being held in jail	75
Death of a close friend	70
Major decision regarding your immediate future	51
Major personal achievement	36
Financial	
Major change in finances:	
Increased income	38
Decreased income	60
Investment and/or credit difficulties	56
Loss or damage of personal property	43
Moderate purchase	20
Major purchase	37
Foreclosure on a mortgage or loan	58

Source: Miller MA, Rahe RH. Life changes scaling for the 1990s. *J Psychosom Res* 43:279–292, 1997.

PHYSICAL FITNESS ACTIVITY 14.6

Are You Overly Anxious?

This self-test was developed by the nonprofit organization Freedom From Fear to help screen for common anxiety disorders and depression. Answer each question "yes" or "no" in the space provided; consider seeking professional evaluation and assistance if you are significantly troubled by any of the areas in which you answer "yes."

Panic Disorder

1. During the past month, did you experience a sudden unexplained attack of intense fear, anxiety, or panic for no apparent reason? (If "yes," continue with questions 1a–c; if "no," skip to question 2.) .... ☐

1a. Were you afraid that you might have more of these attacks? .... ☐

1b. Were you worried that these attacks could mean you were losing control, having a heart attack, or "going crazy"? .... ☐

1c. Did these attacks cause changes or avoidance patterns in your behavior?...................... ☐

2. During the past month, have you been afraid of not being able to get help or not being able to escape in certain situations, such as being on a bridge, in a crowded store, or in similar situations?........... ☐

3. During the past month, have you been afraid or unable to travel alone? .... ☐

Generalized Anxiety Disorder

4. During the past month, have you persistently worried about several different things, such as work, school, family, and money? .... ☐

5. During the past month, did you find it difficult to control your worrying? .... ☐

6. During the past month, did persistent worrying or nervousness cause problems with your work or your dealing with people? .... ☐

Obsessive-Compulsive Disorder

7. During the past month, did you have persistent, senseless thoughts you could not get out of your head, such as thoughts of death, illnesses, aggression, sexual urges, contamination, or others? .... ☐

8. During the past month, did you spend more time than necessary doing things over and over again, such as washing your hands, checking things, or counting things? .... ☐

9. During the past month, did you spend more than 1 hour a day involved in your senseless thoughts or your needless checking, washing, or counting?.... ☐

Social Phobia

10. During the past month, were you afraid to do things in front of people, such as public speaking, eating, performing, or teaching? .... ☐

11. During the past month, did you avoid or feel very uncomfortable in situations involving people, such as parties, weddings, dating, dances, and other social events? .... ☐

Posttraumatic Stress Disorder

12. Have you ever had an extremely frightening, traumatic, or horrible experience—such as being the victim of violent crime, being seriously injured in an accident, being sexually assaulted, seeing someone seriously injured or killed, or being the victim of a natural disaster? (If "yes," continue with questions 12a–e; if "no," skip to question 13.) .... ☐

12a. Did you relive the traumatic experience through recurrent dreams, preoccupations, or flashbacks? . . ☐

12b. Did you seem less interested in important things, not "with it," or unable to experience or express emotions? .... ☐

12c. Did you have problems sleeping, concentrating, or keeping your temper?......................... ☐

12d. Did you avoid anything that reminded you of the original horrible event? .... ☐

12e. Did you have some of the above problems for more than 1 month? .... ☐

Depression

13. During the past month, have you often felt sad or depressed? .... ☐

14. During the past month, have you stopped enjoying the same pleasures that you enjoyed in the past? . . ☐

15. During the past month, have you usually felt hopeless about the future?...................... ☐

16. During the past month, have you thought of suicide?....................................... ☐

17. During the past month, have you had difficulty sleeping or staying awake? .... ☐

18. During the past month, have you experienced either a significant weight gain or loss (without dieting)?. ☐

Source: Freedom From Fear. www.freedomfromfear.com.

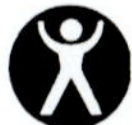

PHYSICAL FITNESS ACTIVITY 14.7

Serious Psychological Distress

The Serious Psychological Distress Scale (K6) is a six-item scale developed to measure serious mental illness. The K6 was used by the CDC in the National Health Interview Survey, and it was determined that 2.4% of males and 3.8% of females had serious psychological distress.[7] Respond to the questions listed below, add all points together, and classify yourself using the norms listed.

During the past 30 days, how often did you feel:

	All of the time (4 pts)	Most of the time (3 pts)	Some of the time (2 pts)	None of the time (0 pts)
so sad that nothing could cheer you up?	☐	☐	☐	☐
nervous?	☐	☐	☐	☐
hopeless?	☐	☐	☐	☐
that everything was an effort?	☐	☐	☐	☐
worthless?	☐	☐	☐	☐

Scoring/Classification

To score the K6, the points are added together, yielding a possible total of 0 to 24 points. A threshold of 13 or more is used to define serious mental illness.

For more information, see Kessler RC, Barker PR, Colpe LJ, Epstein JF, Gfoerer JC, Hiripi E, Howes MJ, Normand S-LT, Manderscheid RW, Walters EE, Zaslavasky AM. Screening for serious mental illness in the general population. *Arch Gen Psychiatry* 60:184–189, 2003.

PHYSICAL FITNESS ACTIVITY 14.8

Do You Have Problems with Sleep?

Insomnia may be keeping you from getting a good night's sleep and affecting the quality of your life. Complete the following self-assessment to determine if you might be at risk for insomnia. Then, learn more about insomnia and talk to your doctor about your sleep.

1. **Are you:**
   - ○ Female
   - ○ Male

It is estimated that approximately one third of Americans experience symptoms of insomnia at some time during their lifetime. Insomnia has been found to be more frequent among women, shift workers, and older adults. Women often have difficulty sleeping during periods of biological change when hormone levels rise and fall, such as menstruation, pregnancy, and menopause.

2. **Are you:**
   - ○ Less than 20 years of age
   - ○ 20–35 years of age
   - ○ 35–55 years of age
   - ○ 55–65 years of age
   - ○ Over 65 years of age

For older people who may have medical conditions, disruptions to their sleep may be caused by discomfort or pain. They may also be more sensitive to noise, light, or temperature and other physical changes that make it difficult to sleep soundly. Establishing a regular bed and wake time and sleeping in a room that is dark, quiet, and comfortable, preferably cool, helps to promote sleep.

3. **How often do you have difficulty falling asleep, frequent awakenings during the night, wake too early and are unable to get back to sleep, or wake feeling unrefreshed?**
   - ○ Every night or almost every night
   - ○ A few nights a week
   - ○ A few nights a month
   - ○ Rarely
   - ○ Never

Insomnia is generally described as an inability to get sufficient sleep or having poor sleep with disturbances for a few nights a week or more. Difficulty falling asleep, especially if it takes 30 minutes or longer, can be due to stress or anxiety caused by a current problem or situation such as a loss (job, loved one), important event coming up, or worry. Establishing a regular, non-alerting bedtime routine can help, but after at least 20 minutes in bed, get out of bed and go to another room. Then, do something relaxing until you feel sleepy enough that you are likely to fall asleep when you return to bed. This routine can be followed if you have frequent awakenings, another sign of insomnia. When waking during the night, if too many thoughts are in your head, try writing them down. Some people also wake too early and find it difficult to get back to sleep. Many older people experience this as well as those who are depressed. In general, it is best to not stay in bed and toss and turn. This can become a habit and you want to associate your bed with sleep and sex only. Another sign of insomnia is to wake feeling groggy or unrefreshed, as if your sleep did not help restore you and help you to become alert when you woke up.

4. **What is your employment status:**

- ❍ Work regular work hours
- ❍ Shift worker
- ❍ Work part-time
- ❍ Unemployed

Shift workers, who work at irregular hours, are unable to get in sync with the body's regular sleep-wake cycle. Getting enough quality sleep at off hours and when it is light is a challenge.

5. **If you answered that you have any of the symptoms listed above for a few nights a week or more, how long have you had these symptoms:**

- ❍ 1–2 weeks
- ❍ 3–4 weeks
- ❍ 1–3 months
- ❍ 3–6 months
- ❍ 6 months or more
- ❍ N/A

Insomnia that is acute or short-term usually lasts 1–2 weeks. However, if it occurs for a few nights a week and continues for a month or longer, it can become chronic or long-term. It is helpful to keep a sleep diary and is important to talk to your doctor, particularly if insomnia becomes long-term. Chronic insomnia may be due to another medical or health problem so you may be asked if you have other symptoms as well. This may also include any mood swings or depression, or questions regarding your health and sleep habits and conditions. Another type of insomnia is called primary and it may occur without any other medical or health problems. It also lasts a long time and is sometimes associated with people who find it difficult to relax or become easily excited. They are often in a hyper state and may find it difficult to sleep well.

6. **Do you use any of the following within 3 hours of bedtime:**

- ❍ Caffeine
- ❍ Alcohol
- ❍ Nicotine
- ❍ None of the above

Make sure you are following NSF's sleep tips that include a relaxing bedtime routine and avoiding alcohol, nicotine, caffeine, and exercise too close to bedtime, and also consider what is keeping you from falling asleep. Use of alcohol or tobacco can also lead to sleep disruptions later in the night.

7. **Do you do any of the following right before bedtime:**

- ❍ Work
- ❍ Watch a dramatic TV program
- ❍ Go to bed hungry or too full
- ❍ None of the above

Having a light nutritious snack before bed is fine as long as you are not too hungry or too full when you go to sleep. It is best to not engage in something that is physically or mentally difficult. If you are thinking about something or are emotionally aroused when trying to fall asleep, follow the tips above. If you are having a physical problem and it takes you a long time to fall asleep or fall back to sleep, talk to your doctor.

8. **If you have difficulty falling asleep, how long does it typically take to get to sleep?**
   - ○ 0–15 minutes
   - ○ 15–20 minutes
   - ○ 20–30 minutes
   - ○ 30 or more minutes

The time it takes to fall asleep is variable. Ten to 20 minutes is common. Falling asleep very quickly can be a sign of insufficient sleep or a sleep disorder. If it takes longer than 30 minutes, you may be experiencing a symptom of insomnia.

9. **How many hours of sleep do you typically get on a weeknight?**
   - ○ Less than 6 hours
   - ○ 6–6.9 hours
   - ○ 7–7.9 hours
   - ○ 8–8.9 hours
   - ○ More than 9 hours

Not getting enough sleep or sleep deprivation is not insomnia. However, when you have difficulty sleeping and have symptoms of insomnia, you are more likely to get less sleep than you need to feel and do your best during wake time. In NSF's *2002 Sleep in America* poll, it was found that adults with insomnia get on average 6.7 hours of sleep per weeknight compared to 7.2 hours of sleep for those who rarely or never experience insomnia.

10. **How would you describe the quality of your sleep?**
    - ○ Excellent
    - ○ Very good
    - ○ Good
    - ○ Fair
    - ○ Poor

Because people with insomnia find it difficult to get continuous sleep without disruptions, the quality of their sleep suffers. They may not be spending enough time in bed actually sleeping. Rather, they are trying to sleep, are uncomfortable, get frequently aroused and wake up, and are tossing and turning in bed. As a result, their sleep may also be lighter because it takes time to go into deeper, restorative sleep and to get enough of it so that the person feels great the next day. In NSF's 2002 poll, those experiencing insomnia symptoms described the quality of their sleep as fair to poor and were not likely to rate it as excellent or very good.

11. **On how many days during a typical week does sleepiness interfere with and make it more difficult to do your daily activities:**
    - ○ Every day or almost every day
    - ○ A few days a week
    - ○ A few days a month
    - ○ Rarely/Never

Because the sleep of people with insomnia is often interrupted, they may not get enough deep sleep and they may not get enough hours of sleep. This leads to sleepiness during wake hours. According to NSF's 2002 poll, 75% of those with insomnia symptoms experience daytime sleepiness so severe it interferes with daily activities. Sleepiness makes it difficult to perform and function at your best. As a result, many people find it hard to concentrate, pay attention, solve problems, listen well, and get along with others, and their productivity suffers. In this same poll, those with symptoms of insomnia were less likely to be full of energy, optimistic, happy, relaxed, satisfied with life, or to feel peaceful. Being sleepy during the day also makes you more prone to accidents, drowsy driving crashes, injury, and illness.

12. How often do you take a nap:

- ❍ Less than 1 a week
- ❍ 1–2 naps a week
- ❍ More than 2 naps a week
- ❍ Every day or almost every day

In general, naps are not a substitute for a good night's sleep and should not become a habit. In NSF's 2005 *Sleep in America* poll, those who napped two or more times a week were more likely to be experiencing symptoms of insomnia. Naps are sometimes taken following a poor night of sleep, but they reduce your need for sleep the next night. If you need to take a nap, it should occur earlier in the day and be limited to 20–30 minutes.

13. Have you been diagnosed by your doctor with any of the following conditions:

- ❍ Cardiovascular disease (e.g. hypertension, heart disease, stroke)
- ❍ Depression
- ❍ Heartburn, GERD, or gastrointestinal problems
- ❍ Arthritis, back pain, or other muscular disorder
- ❍ Anxiety or psychiatric disorder
- ❍ Sleep disorder such as sleep apnea or restless legs syndrome
- ❍ None of the above

Many medical conditions as well as medications can be an underlying cause or contribute to insomnia. A side effect of many medications is sleep disturbance. This more frequently applies to older persons who may be taking medications that lead to poor sleep.

A major psychiatric condition, depression in particular, puts a person at risk for insomnia and vice versa since having symptoms of insomnia can also result in impaired moods and mental problems. For example, 50–70% of those with anxiety disorders also complain of insomnia. There is a similar occurrence of insomnia for those with stress (posttraumatic) and panic disorders. Other symptoms, such as heartburn, breathing disorders, increased heart rate, and general discomfort all contribute to the challenge of getting a good night's sleep without sleep disturbances.

Many studies also show a strong association between insomnia and cardiovascular problems, lung disease, arthritis, heartburn and other sleep disorders such as sleep apnea and restless legs syndrome. In these cases, those with insomnia have been shown to have more medical conditions, and lack of quality sleep can worsen the symptoms and pain of these disorders.

If you have any of these conditions or take any of these medications, talk to your doctor about their effect on your sleep because a good night's sleep can contribute to your overall health.

14. Do you take any of the following medications:

- ❍ Antidepressants
- ❍ Beta blockers
- ❍ Decongestants
- ❍ None of the above

Many medical conditions as well as medications can be an underlying cause or contribute to insomnia. A side effect of many medications is sleep disturbance. This more frequently applies to older persons who may be taking medications that lead to poor sleep.

Medications used for psychiatric problems (including some antidepressants) can contribute to sleep difficulties; some may make you sleepy, but then cause difficulty falling asleep. Beta blockers used for heart problems can also lead to insomnia, as can nasal decongestants.

If you have any of these conditions or take any of these medications, talk to your doctor about their effect on your sleep because a good night's sleep can contribute to your overall health.

From the National Sleep Foundation. www.sleepfoundation.org.

chapter 15

Aging, Osteoporosis, and Arthritis

All parts of the body which have a function, if used in moderation and exercised in labors in which each is accustomed, become thereby healthy, well-developed and age more slowly, but if unused and left idle they become liable to disease, defective in growth, and age quickly.

—Hippocrates

Age is a question of mind over matter. If you don't mind, it doesn't matter.

—Satchel Paige

How old would you be if you didn't know how old you were?

—Satchel Paige

The United States has long thought of itself as a nation of youth, and at least in the mind of Ponce deLeon, the "fountain of youth." Americans idolize youth, yearn for it, and spare no expense to regain it (or at least look the part). Yet scientists now regard this nation as an "aging society." In colonial times, for instance, the average age of the population was 16 years. Today it is 33 years, and it will be 42 years in 2030.[1–6]

The fastest-growing minority in the United States is the *elderly*—those who reach or pass the age of 65[2] (see Figure 15.1). Figure 15.2 shows that there are now nearly 36 million elderly people in the United States, a figure that will climb to 75 million, or 22% of the population, by the year 2040. The 65-and-over group is growing twice as fast as the rest of the population. Most of this growth is due to the fact that the baby-boom generation (people born between 1945

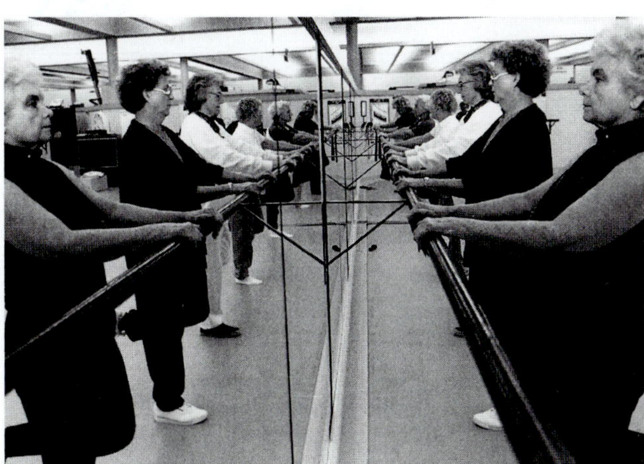

Figure 15.1 The ranks of the elderly are multiplying faster than any other segment of our society.

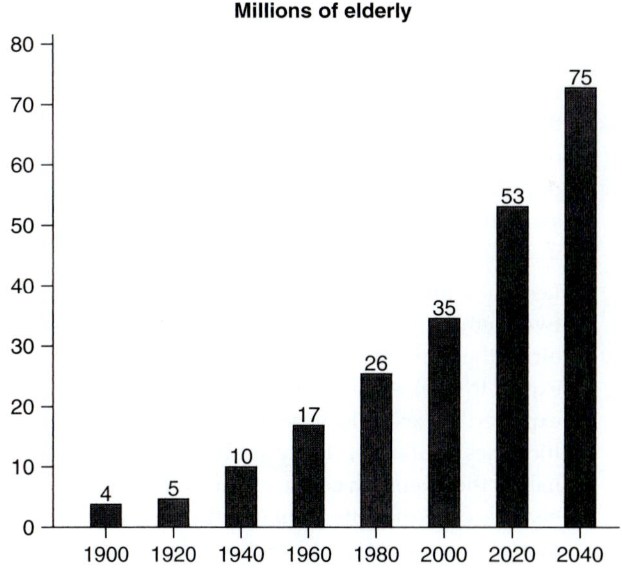

Figure 15.2 The U.S. population of adults aged ≥ 65 years will double during 1995–2030 (33.5 to 69.4 million). Source: Centers for Disease Control and Prevention. Surveillance for selected public health indicators affecting older adults—United States. *MMWR* 48(SS-8), 1999.

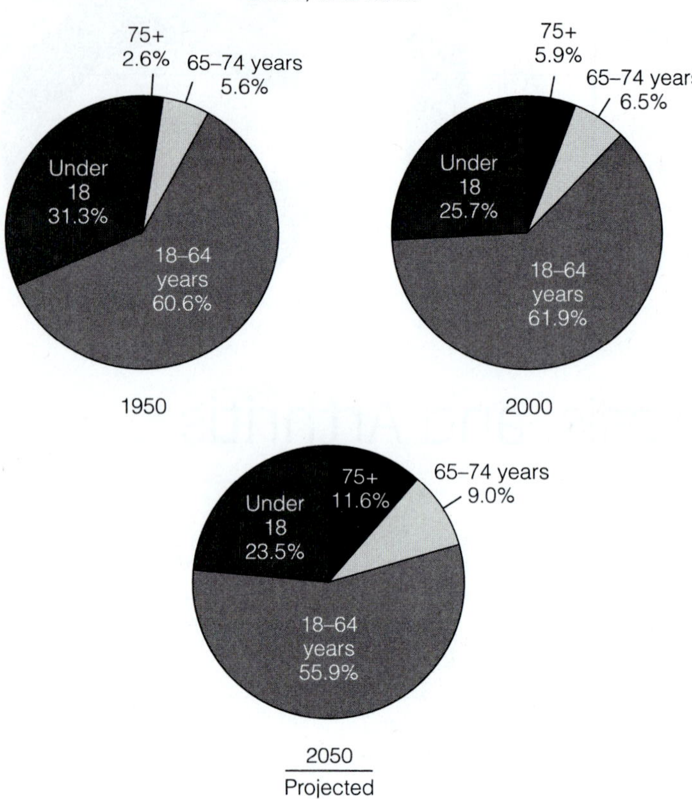

Figure 15.3 In 1950, the elderly comprised 8.2% of the population, a proportion that will climb to 20.6% in 2050. Sources: U.S. Census Bureau, 1950 and 2000 decennial censuses and 2050 interim population projections.

and 1965), which constitutes one third of the U.S. population, is advancing inevitably toward old age (See Figure 15.3.).[2]

Consider these statistics:[1–6]

- It is difficult to comprehend that in 1900, only 40% of American individuals lived beyond age 65, while today approximately 80% survive to age 65, and 50% live to be age 80 (see Figure 15.4). Since the mid-1980s, intense interest has been focused on the 85-and-older population (termed the "very old"). This is projected to be the fastest-growing population segment over the next several decades, swelling from 3.6 million in 1995 to 8.5 million in 2030.
- Length of life has increased remarkably during the twentieth century (see Figure 15.5). *Life expectancy* at birth (the number of years a newborn baby can expect to live) is now 77 years on average and is expected to exceed 82 years by the year 2050. Increases in life expectancy at birth during the first half of the twentieth century occurred mainly because of reductions in infant and childhood mortality and control of infectious disease due to improved sanitation, increased use of preventive health services, and better medical care.[4] These reductions meant that more Americans survived to middle age. By contrast, increases in longevity in recent years have largely resulted from decreasing mortality from chronic diseases (primarily heart disease and stroke) among the middle-aged (45–64) and elderly (65–84) populations. Despite these impressive gains in U.S. life expactancy, we still rank far behind many other nations.

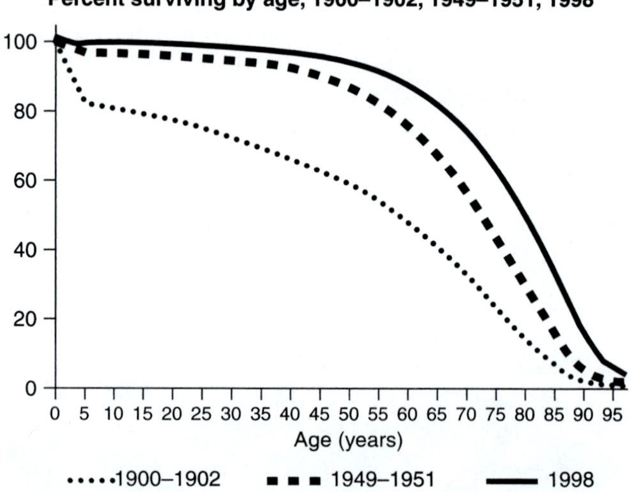

Figure 15.4 Survival curves, 1900–1902, 1949–1951, 1998. A larger proportion of Americans now survive to age 65 years (80%) compared to 1900–1902 (40%). Source: Anderson RN. United States Life Tables, 1998. *National Vital Statistics Reports* 48(18). Hyattsville, MD: National Center for Health Statistics, 2001.

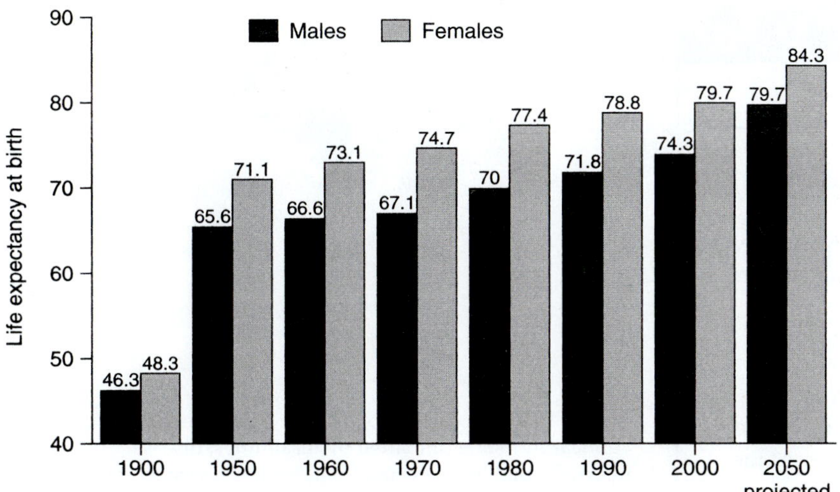

Figure 15.5 Life expectancy has risen since 1900 for both males and females to 77 years. By 2050, life expectancy will rise to about 82 years, on average. Source: National Center for Health Statistics. *Health, United States, 2004.* Hyattsville, MD: 2004.

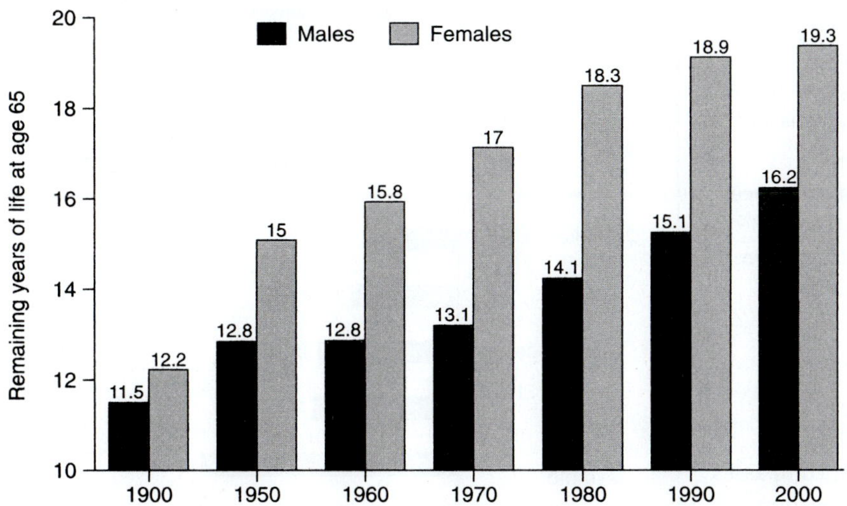

Figure 15.6 Life expectancy at age 65 averages just under 18 years, a gain of 6 years since 1900. Source: National Center for Health Statistics. *Health, United States, 2004.* Hyattsville, MD: 2004.

- Life expectancy at age 65 has increased dramatically since mid-century. From 1900 to 1960, life expectancy at age 65 improved only 2.4 years, as compared with 3.4 years from 1960 to 2000. People who are 65 years of age can now expect to live an extra 18 years (see Figure 15.6).

Although these trends are generally welcome, public health officials have expressed concern about several issues.[1–10]

- The central issue raised by increasing longevity is that of net gain in active functional years versus total years of disability and dysfunction.[1] As reviewed in Box 15.1, one of the major *Healthy People 2010* goals is to increase the quality and years of healthy life. As depicted in Figure 15.7, the National Center for Health Statistics estimates that 17% of the average American's life is spent in an "unhealthy" state (impaired by disabilities, injuries, and/or disease).[1,5] Among the elderly, 5 of their remaining 18 years, on average, will be unhealthy ones. As summarized in Figure 15.8, the prevalence of risk factors and disease is high among the elderly.[1–10] Nearly 9 in 10 elderly individuals have one or more chronic health conditions.[7,8] The average 75-year-old has three chronic conditions and uses five different prescription drugs.[4]
- Cardiovascular diseases (diseases of the heart and stroke combined) and cancers account for about two thirds of all deaths among the elderly.[2] While the good news is that death rates for heart disease and stroke are declining among the elderly, those for cancer are rising, mainly because of lung cancer.[2,6]
- Osteoporosis, defined as a decrease in bone density, is widespread among the elderly. One third of women over age 65 develop fractures of their spinal

Box 15.1

Healthy People 2010

Goal 1: Increase Quality and Years of Healthy Life

The first goal of *Healthy People 2010* is to help individuals of all ages increase life expectancy and improve their quality of life.

Life Expectancy

- Life expectancy is the average number of years people born in a given year are expected to live based on a set of age-specific death rates. At the beginning of the twentieth century, life expectancy at birth was 47.3 years; today, the average life expectancy at birth is 77 years.
- Life expectancy for persons at every age group has also increased during the past century. Individuals aged 65 years can be expected to live an average of 18 more years (total of 83 years).
- Differences in life expectancy between populations, however, suggest a substantial need and opportunity for improvement. At least 18 countries with populations of 1 million or more have life expectancies greater than the United States for both men and women.

Quality of Life

- Quality of life reflects a general sense of happiness and satisfaction with our lives and environment. General quality of life encompasses all aspects of life, including health, recreation, culture, rights, values, beliefs, aspirations, and the conditions that support a life containing these elements.
- Health-related quality of life reflects a personal sense of physical and mental health and the ability to react to factors in the physical and social environments.
- Years of healthy life is a combined measure developed for the *Healthy People 2010* initiative. The difference between life expectancy and years of healthy life reflects the average amount of time spent in less than optimal health because of chronic or acute limitations. After decreasing in the early 1990s, years of healthy life increased to a level in 1996 that was only slightly above that at the beginning of the decade (64.0 years in 1990 to 64.2 years in 1996). During the same period, life expectancy increased a full year.

Source: U.S. Department of Health and Human Services. *Healthy People 2010.* Washington DC: January 2000. www.health.gov/healthypeople.

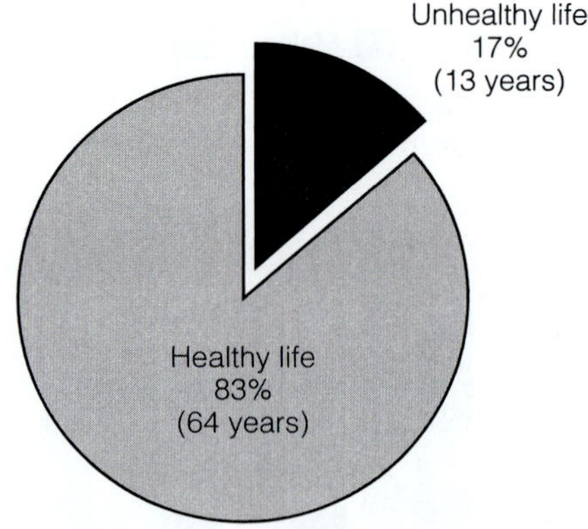

Figure 15.7 Proportion of life that is spent in an "unhealthy" state (impaired by disabilities, disease, injuries), total life expectancy—77 years. Seventeen percent of life is spent in an "unhealthy" state, a proportion that health officials have targeted as a priority issue for the year 2010. Source: Department of Health and Human Services. *Healthy People 2010.* Washington DC: January 2000. www.health.gov/healthypeople.

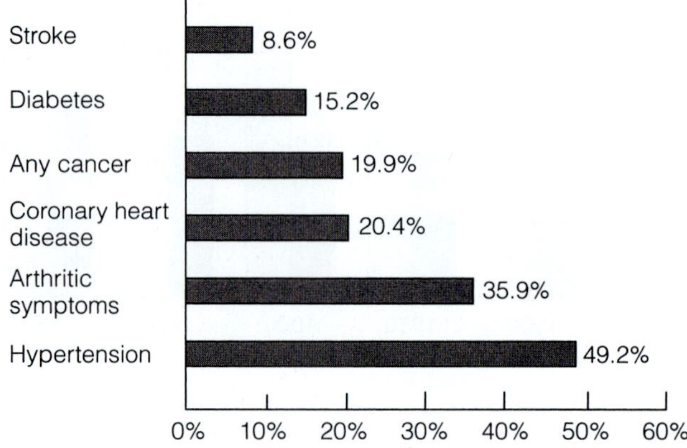

Figure 15.8
Hypertension and arthritic symptoms are the two most common chronic conditions among the elderly. Source: CDC, National Center for Health Statistics, *National Health Interview Survey,* 2000–2001. www.cdc.gov.

bones, and by extreme old age, one of every three women and one of every six men will have had a hip fracture. (This is discussed in more detail later in this chapter.)

- There are several types of senile dementia, the most common form being Alzheimer's disease.[10] Memory loss, especially for recent events, is usually the first sign, followed by more profound and debilitating mental, behavioral, and bodily control impairments. Alzheimer's disease strikes about 10% of people over age 65 and nearly half of those age 85 and older. About 4.5 million Americans have Alzheimer's, a prevalence which is expected to quadruple in the next 50 years. The cost of care for these patients is now $100 billion per year.[10]

- The elderly account for 13% of the population but over one third of health-care spending and prescription drug use and half of physician's visits and half of all hospital stays.[2,4,10,11] The forecasted increase in people 85 years of age and older may lead to a large increase in the use of nursing homes in the future. Financing the health care of the elderly in the future is a serious concern.[2]

THE AGING PROCESS

Aging refers to the normal yet irreversible biological changes that occur throughout a person's lifetime.[12–14] It is a very complex phenomenon and is influenced by genetic, environmental, and lifestyle factors. The aging process takes place at all ages, but for those over 65, it often becomes more manifest, with significant changes in quality of life. There are two major kinds of theories of aging: damage theories and program theories.[12]

Damage theories speculate that with advancing age, we become less able to repair damage caused by internal malfunctions or external assault from oxygen-free radicals to the body. Various biochemical and hormonal changes with aging may finally lead to death. The immune system is less effective in the elderly, and free radicals are less effectively mopped up by scavengers. The body may be less able to combat infection or destroy abnormal body cells.

Program theories of aging suggest that an internal clock starts ticking at conception and is programmed to run just so long. Some researchers feel that human cells can only divide a certain number of times and then stop, leading to death. DNA transcription occurs at lower rates and in significantly altered patterns as cells age.

As a person ages, many changes take place in the body:[7–19]

- *Loss of taste and smell.* The elderly often complain of a decreased ability to taste and enjoy food. Taste buds decrease in number and size, affecting sweet and salty tastes in particular. About 40% of people 80 years or older appear to have difficulty identifying common substances by smell.
- *Periodontal (bone area around the teeth) bone loss.* The majority of the elderly suffer bone loss and disease in the tissues around the teeth as they grow older. As a result, one third of the population over 65 have lost all of their teeth, and about 65% have lost teeth in at least one arch. The end result of this is obvious: Older people tend to choose foods that are easy to chew, leading to a reduced consumption of fresh fruit and vegetables high in dietary fiber.
- *Decrease in gastrointestinal function.* With an increase in age, the stomach cells are less able to secrete digestive juices, interfering with the digestion of protein and vitamin B_{12}. The small intestine becomes less capable of absorbing some nutrients, and there may also be a reduced ability of the intestine to move its contents through the digestive tract, resulting in constipation. Constipation is further exacerbated by lack of dietary fiber.
- *Loss in visual and auditory function.* Visual function starts to decline around age 45 and worsens gradually thereafter. After age 80, less than 15% of the population has 20/20 vision. Gradual hearing loss generally begins at about age 20 and has been estimated to affect as many as 66% of people reaching age 80.
- *Decrease in lean body weight.* The prevalence of obesity is highest in the 55–64 age group, but then falls thereafter. As a person ages, body fat increases, while muscle and bone (or lean body weight) decreases. This leads to a decrease in energy expended during rest, partially explaining why the elderly consume fewer Calories than younger people. The resting metabolic rate decreases by 1–2% per decade starting at about age 20.
- *Loss of bone mineral mass.* As discussed previously, loss of bone (osteoporosis) is an almost universal phenomenon with increasing age. The resulting fractures often mend with difficulty, resulting in long periods of decreased physical activity and social interaction.
- *Mental impairment.* Senility, also called senile dementia or organic brain syndrome, affects about 60% of the elderly. Some of the problems associated with senile dementia include impairment of memory, judgment, feelings, personality, and ability to speak. Senile dementia of the Alzheimer's type accounts for at least half of all dementia in old age.
- *Decreased ability to metabolize drugs.* The elderly account for about one third of all prescription drug consumption, yet they have a decreased ability to absorb, distribute, metabolize, and excrete both prescription and nonprescription drugs. The majority of the elderly are on more than one prescription drug, and these can interact with each other, affecting nutritional status.
- *High prevalence of chronic disease.* As discussed earlier, up to 88% of the elderly suffer from at least one chronic disease. A variety of diseases are more

common among the elderly, including diabetes, cancer, heart disease, high blood pressure, stroke, and arthritis.

- *Neuromuscular changes.* Reaction time, ability to balance, and strength of muscles, tendons, and ligaments decrease with aging, limiting normal activity for many. Accidents increase, and the ability to shop for and prepare food may be hampered.
- *Urinary incontinence.* Up to 20% of the elderly living at home and 75% of those in long-term-care facilities cannot control the muscle that controls urination. This can lead to social isolation, embarrassment, and the decision to live in a nursing home environment.
- *Decrease in liver and kidney function.* The size and function of the liver and kidneys decrease steadily with age, making the removal of metabolic waste products more difficult.
- *Decrease in heart and lung fitness.* With aging, there is a decrease on the order of 8–10% per decade in the ability of the heart and lungs to supply oxygen to the muscles. Most of this is due to the decreasing physical activity of the elderly.

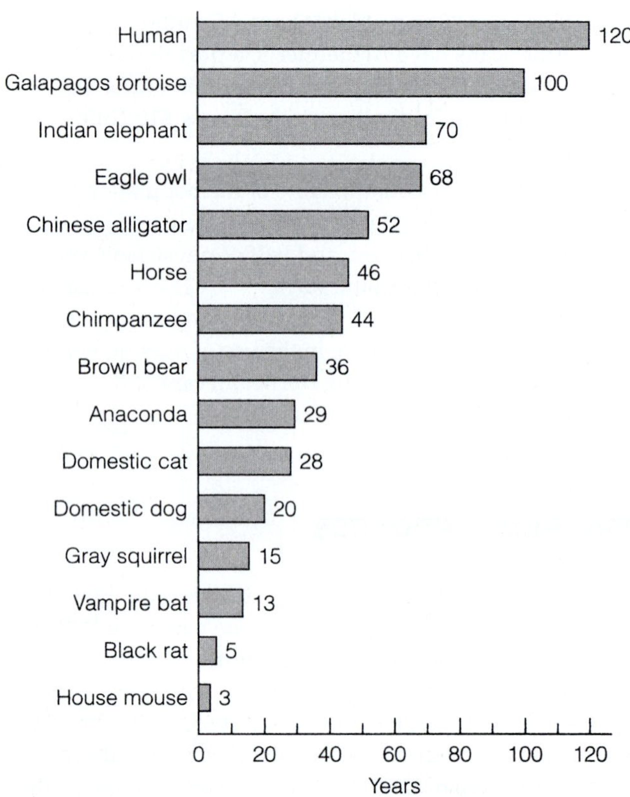

Figure 15.9 Maximum recorded life spans for selected species. The maximum life span varies widely among species. Source: Kirkwood TBL. Comparative life spans of species: Why do species have the life spans they do? *Am J Clin Nutr* 55:1191S–1195S, 1992.

HEALTH HABITS AND AGING

While *life expectancy* is defined as the average number of years of life expected for a population of a given age, *life span* refers to the maximum age obtainable by a particular species. Figure 15.9 shows that the maximum life span varies widely among species and is thought to be 120 for humans (about 43 years higher than the current average American life expectancy).[14] Several humans have lived to 120 years or more. Arthur Reed of Oakland, California, lived to be 124 years of age. Born the year Lincoln was elected president (1860), he rode his bike on his 100th birthday and held a job until age 116. Shigechigo Isumi of Japan died in 1986 and was reported to be 121 years old. Mary Thompson of Orlando, Florida, died in 1996 at the age of 120. In 1997, Jeanne Calment of France died at age 122.[12]

Currently cancer, heart disease, and injuries are the leading causes of "years of potential life" lost before age 75 years[6] (see Figure 11.5). To move life expectancy toward the maximum life span of the human species, these will have to be largely eliminated as major causes of early death. This will require a strong commitment to improved health habits and lifestyles on the part of Americans.

There is much current interest in life-extension strategies including energy restriction (which has been shown to lengthen the life of rodents), hormone supplements, various drugs, antioxidants, and gene manipulation. Much more research is needed to assess effectiveness, safety, and socioeconomic impact.[16,20,21] Health habits are clearly identified as having a major influence on life expectancy and quality of life during old age[22–28] (see Physical Fitness Activities 15.1 and 15.3). Lester Breslow of UCLA, for example, in his study of more than 6,000 people in the San Francisco Bay Area, showed a dramatic difference in death rate between those who followed seven simple health habits (never smoked, moderate alcohol consumption, daily breakfast, no snacking, 7–8 hours of sleep per night, regular exercise, ideal weight) and those who did not.[25–28] Those following all seven health habits were estimated to live 9 years longer than those who did not practice any of them. In addition, the healthful lifestyle followers were only half as likely to have suffered disabilities that kept them from work or limited their day-to-day activities.[25] In other words, habitual healthful living appears not only to promote longevity but also to increase the chance of having the physical ability to enjoy life to its fullest in later years.[22]

Data from large, population-based, prospective studies indicate that keeping major risk factors under control (serum cholesterol, blood pressure, and smoking), and avoiding diabetes, leads to low mortality rates and increased life expectancy.[24,27,28] As summarized in Figure 15.10, young and middle-aged adults that fit this profile experience an increase in life expectancy of 10 and 6 years, respectively.[27] In Japan, more than 8,000 men were followed for 28 years, and the most consistent predictors of healthy aging (low illness and impairment) were low blood pressure, low serum glucose, not smoking cigarettes, and not being obese.[24] Another study of 1,741 university alumni followed for 24 years showed that the onset of disability was postponed by more than 5 years in the low- compared to high-risk group based on avoidance of smoking and obesity and maintaining a regular exercise program.[28] In general, these studies indicate that beyond the biological effects of aging, much of the illness and disability among the elderly is related to risk factors and lifestyle habits present during adulthood.

According to the CDC, three behaviors—smoking, poor diet, and physical inactivity—are the actual causes of almost 35% of U.S. deaths, and underlie the development of four of the five leading causes of death in the elderly: heart disease, cancer, stroke, and diabetes.[4] Adopting healthier behaviors and getting regular screenings (mammograms and colonoscopies, for example) can dramatically reduce an elderly individual's risk for most chronic diseases and improve quality of life. Table 15.1 summarizes 15 indicators related to older adult health status, behaviors, preventive care and screening, and injuries.[4] These indicators were chosen by the CDC because they are each modifiable and present a comprehensive picture of older adult health. Notice that of the nine *Healthy People 2010* targets, four have been met and five still need substantial progress.

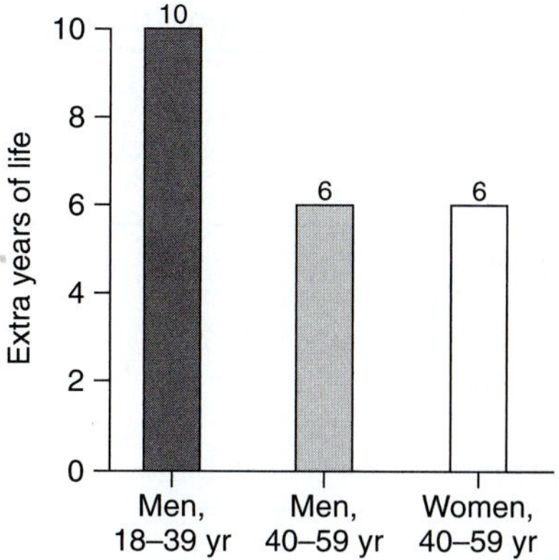

Figure 15.10 Keeping major risk factors under control and avoiding diabetes can lead to lower mortality rates and increased life expectancy.

Figure 15.14 summarizes the physiological changes that take place in the human body with aging. Interestingly, many of the changes that accompany aging are the same types of changes that can be expected with inactivity and weightlessness.[34–37] The identifying characteristics of both aging and the "disuse syndrome" are a decrease in cardiorespiratory function, obesity, musculoskeletal fragility, and premature aging. However, as is emphasized in this section, older individuals adapt to both resistive and endurance exercise training in a fashion similar to young people.[30] In other words, it makes sense that a significant proportion of the deterioration attributed to aging can be explained by the tendency of people to exercise less as they age.

EXERCISE AND AGING

A key ingredient to healthy aging is regular physical activity.[17] Of all age groups, the elderly have the most to gain by being active, including the potential for decreased risk of cardiovascular disease, cancer, high blood pressure, depression, osteoporosis, bone fractures, and diabetes, with improved body composition, fitness, longevity, ability to perform personal-care activities, and management of arthritis or other conditions leading to activity limitations[29–33] (see Figure 15.11). Yet national surveys indicate that among the elderly, 49% of males and 56% of females are physically inactive, more than other age groups[4,31] (see Chapter 1 and Figure 15.12). With increase in age, a vicious cycle can set in—lower physical activity can lead to increased frailty and activity limitations and a further decrease in physical activity[2,6] (see Figure 15.13 and Box 15.2).

$\dot{V}O_{2max}$ and the Aging Process

Researchers who have evaluated the effects of aging on the cardiorespiratory system have focused on work capacity, or $\dot{V}O_{2max}$. The ability of the body to take in oxygen, transport it, and use it for oxidation of fuel is viewed as the single best variable to define the overall functional changes that occur with aging.[30]

$\dot{V}O_{2max}$ normally declines 8–10% per decade for both males and females after 25 years of age[38–43] (see Figure 15.15). From cross-sectional data, the rate of decline in $\dot{V}O_{2max}$ for men and women is about 0.35–0.50 $ml \cdot kg^{-1} \cdot min^{-1}$ per year, starting at age 25 years.

Why does $\dot{V}O_{2max}$ tend to be low among the elderly? Declining physical activity appears to be a major factor, along with the loss in fat-free mass and an increase in fat mass.[44] Two studies of 1,499 men and 409 women have determined that nearly half of the age-related decline in aerobic power is due to changes in body composition and exercise habits.[41,42] Notice in Figure 15.15 that athletic

TABLE 15.1 The National Report Card on Healthy Aging: How Healthy Are America's Seniors?

Indicator	Data for Persons Age 65 or Older* (Data Year)	*Healthy People 2000* Target	Grade (pass/fail)†	*Healthy People 2010* Target
Health Status				
1. Physically unhealthy days (mean number of days in past month)	5.5 (2001)	‡	‡	‡
2. Frequent mental distress (%)[ç]	6.3 (2000-2001)	‡	‡	‡
3. Oral health: Complete tooth loss (%)	22.4 (2002)	20	Fail	20
4. Disability (%)[ƒ]	30.8 (2001)	‡	‡	‡
Health Behaviors				
5. No leisure time physical activity in past month (%)	32.9 (2002)	22	Fail	20
6. Eating 5+ fruits and vegetables daily (%)	32.4 (2002)	50	Fail	N/A[¶]
7. Obesity (%)[#]	19.5 (2002)	‡	‡	15
8. Current smoking (%)	10.1 (2002)	15	Pass	12
Preventive Care & Screening				
9. Flu vaccine in past year (%)	63.0 (2002)	60	Pass	90
10. Ever had pneumonia vaccine (%)	63.0 (2002)	60	Pass	90
11. Mammogram within past 2 years (%)	77.2 (2002)	60	Pass	70
12. Ever had sigmoidoscopy or colonoscopy (%)	58.3 (2002)	40	Pass	50
13. Up to date on select preventive services (%)**				
Men	34.4 (2002)	‡	‡	‡
Women	33.4 (2002)	‡	‡	‡
14. Cholesterol checked within past 5 years (%)	85.4 (2001)	75	Pass	80
Injuries				
15. Hip fracture hospitalizations (per 100,000 persons)	525 (men) 1127 (women) 877 (total) (2002)	607 (total)	Fail	474 (men) 416 (women) N/A (total)††

*Data for Indicators 1–14 were collected by CDC's Behavioral Risk Factor Surveillance System (BRFSS). Data for Indicator 15, hip fracture, hospitalizations, come from CDC's National Center for Health Statistics, National Hospital Discharge Survey.

†Grade is based on the attainment of *Healthy People 2000* targets.

‡Indicators 1, 2, 4, and 13 are more recently developed measures and, as such, do not have *Healthy People 2000* targets. Data related to Indicator 7, obesity, were combined with the overweight category in *Healthy People 2000* and, therefore, obesity has no individual *Healthy People 2000* target.

çFrequent mental distress is defined as having had 14 or more mentally unhealthy days in the previous month. Data from the 2000 and 2001 BRFSS are combined here to get a sufficient sample size.

ƒDisability was defined on the basis of an affirmative response to either of the following two questions on the 2001 BRFSS: "Are you limited in any way in any activities because of physical, mental or emotional problems?" or "Do you have any health problem that requires you to use special equipment, such as a cane, wheelchair, a special bed, or a special telephone?"

¶*Healthy People 2010* segments the nutrition target into multiple categories of fruits and vegetables. See Appendix for a full description of this change.

#*Healthy People 2000* defined a target for overweight, but not obesity. Because current standards separate these two conditions, obesity data are included in this report. The *Healthy People 2010* definition of obesity is a body mass index (BMI) of > 30 kg/m2.

**For men, three services are included: flu vaccine in past year, ever had a pneumonia vaccine, and ever had sigmoidoscopy or colonoscopy. For women, these same three services plus a mammogram within past two years are included.

††*Healthy People 2010* has separate hip fracture hospitalization targets for men and women, and no target for the total number.

Source: CDC. *The State of Aging and Health in America, 2004.* www.cdc.gov/aging.

males who are 65–75 years of age have the $\dot{V}O_{2max}$ of young adult sedentary males. Figure 15.16 shows the results of one study that compared highly conditioned and sedentary septuagenarian women.[45] The highly conditioned elderly women (who competed in state and national senior games endurance competitions and had been training intensively for an average of 11 years) were much leaner and had a $\dot{V}O_{2max}$ 67% higher than their sedentary counterparts and similar to that of sedentary women 35 years of age (Figure 15.17).

Many other studies have shown that elderly people who are vigorous in their exercise possess high aerobic power (similar to that of sedentary young adults) and are capable of performing at levels once thought unattainable.[33,40,45–50] For example, in 1991, 70-year-old Warren Utes of Illinois set an age-group world record of 38:24 for the 10-kilometer race. Sixty-year-old Luciano Acquarone of Italy ran a 2:38 marathon, a pace of 6 minutes a mile, while Derek Turnbull of New Zealand ran 5 kilometers in 16:39 at age 65. At age 49, Evy Palm ran a half-marathon in 1:12:36 in Holland, a time regarded as one of the top-rated, age-graded performances of all time. In 2003, Ed Whitlock of Canada became the first person 70 or older to break 3 hours in a marathon. (See the Sports Medicine Insight at the end of the chapter for a discussion of Mavis Lindgren, who has performed well in extreme old age.)

However, even among athletes who exercise vigorously throughout their lifetimes, $\dot{V}O_{2max}$ still declines at a similar rate to that of sedentary individuals (albeit at a much higher absolute level). Some studies have demonstrated that the rate of decline may be reduced for several years during which vigorous exercise is engaged in (with no decrease in exercise frequency, intensity, or duration), but ultimately, $\dot{V}O_{2max}$ will start falling at normal or accelerated rates

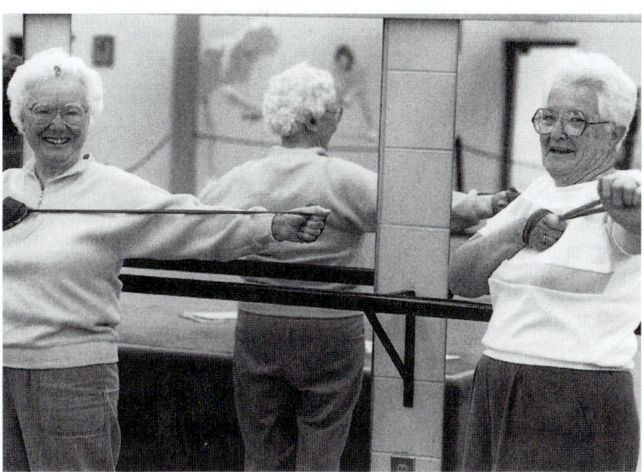

Figure 15.11 Of all age groups, the elderly have the most to gain by being active.

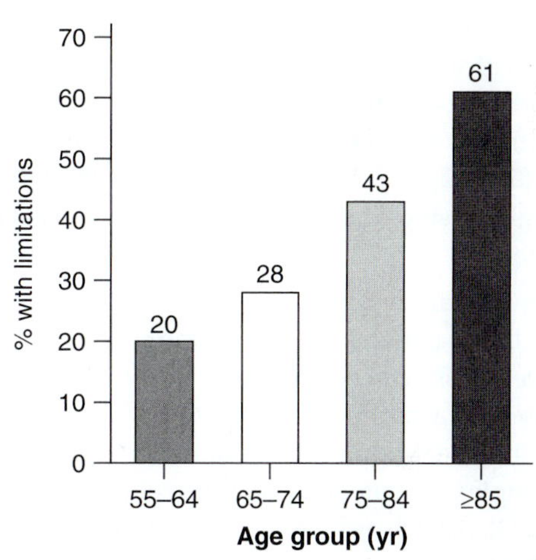

Figure 15.13 Limitations in basic functional skills increase with advancing age. Source: Centers for Disease Control and Prevention. Surveillance for selected public health indicators affecting older adults—United States. *CDC Surveillance Summaries,* December 17, 1999. *MMWR* 48(SS-8), 1999.

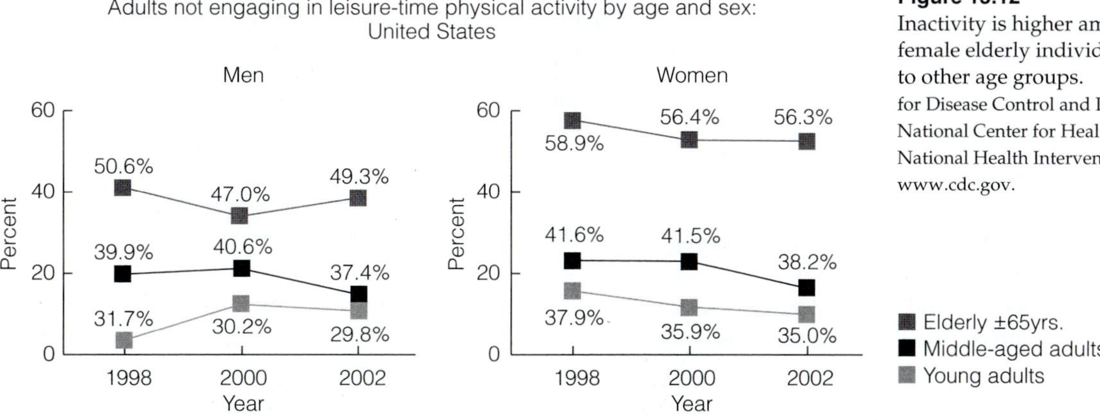

Figure 15.12 Inactivity is higher among male and female elderly individuals compared to other age groups. Source: Centers for Disease Control and Prevention, National Center for Health Statistics, National Health Intervention Survey. www.cdc.gov.

Box 15.2

Health and Aging: Physical Functioning and Disability

- Quality of life in later years may be diminished if illness, chronic conditions, or injuries limit the ability to care for oneself without assistance. Older persons maintain their independence and eliminate costly caregiving services by, among other things, shopping on their own, cooking their meals, bathing and dressing themselves, and walking and climbing stairs without assistance.
- Among noninstitutionalized persons 70 years of age and over, about one third have difficulty performing at least one of nine basic physical activities (see Figure 15.13). Activity limitations increase with age, and women are more likely than men to have a physical limitation. About 18% of women and 12% of men 70 years of age and over are unable to walk a quarter of a mile without assistance. About 11% of women 70 years of age and over are unable to climb a flight of steps, and 15% cannot stoop, crouch, or kneel.
- An indication of functional well-being is the ability to perform certain tasks of daily living. These tasks can be grouped into two categories: essential activities of daily living (ADLs) such as bathing, eating, and dressing; and the more complex instrumental activities of daily living (IADLs), such as making meals, shopping, or cleaning. Among noninstitutionalized people 70 years of age and over, 20% have difficulty performing at least one ADL, and 10% have difficulty performing at least one IADL.
- Recent trends indicate that the proportion of older men and women with functional and ADL limitations is declining.

Source: National Center for Health Statistics. *Health, United States, 1999, and Health and Aging Chartbook.* Hyattsville, MD: 1999.

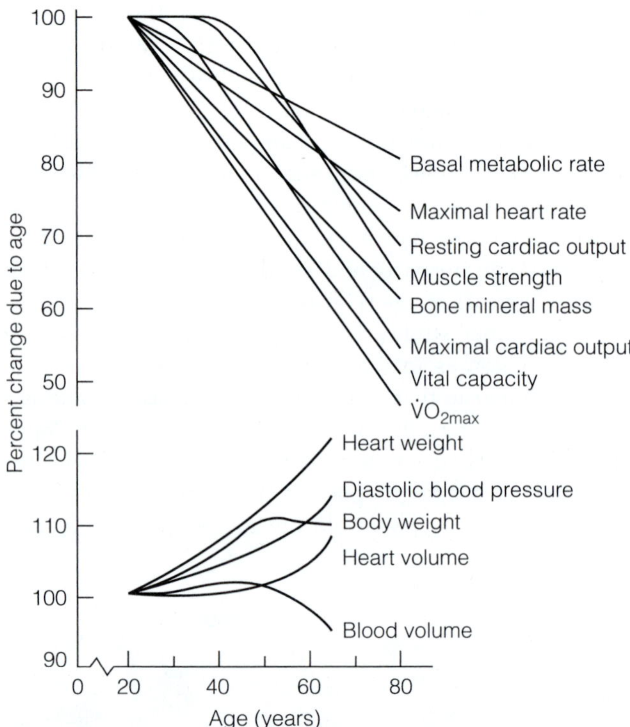

Figure 15.14 Physiological changes with increase in age. Aging is accompanied by a decrease in cardiorespiratory and musculoskeletal functions. Many of these changes also occur during the transition from a trained to an untrained state.

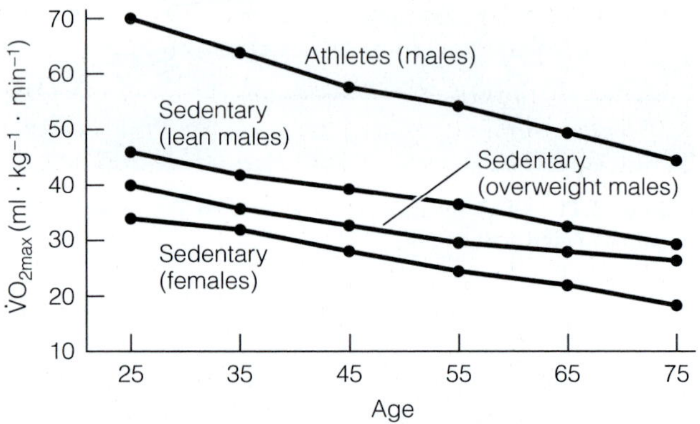

Figure 15.15 Decline in $\dot{V}O_{2max}$ with age in different groups of males and females. $\dot{V}O_{2max}$ decreases by about 8–10% per decade for both males and females, athletes and nonathletes. Sources: Heath GW, Hagberg JM, Ehsani AA, Holloszy JO. A physiological comparison of young and older endurance athletes. *J Appl Physiol* 51:634–640, 1981; Nieman DC, Pover NK, Segebartt KS, Arabatzis K, Johnson M, Dietrich SJ. Hematological, anthropometric, and metabolic comparisons between active and inactive healthy old old to very old women. *Ann Sports Med* 5:2–8, 1990.

later.[45–53] Most scientists now believe that endurance exercise may be effective in reducing the rate for a certain time period, but that the age-related decrease in aerobic power and cardiovascular function cannot be prevented.[30,47–57] A lower stroke volume, heart rate, and arteriovenous oxygen difference all appear to contribute to the age-related decline in $\dot{V}O_{2max}$, even when the individual tries to keep physically active.[55–57]

The bottom line is that at any given age, athletes who exercise vigorously can be fitter than their sedentary counterparts, but because of the aging process, less fit than younger athletes. Studies have confirmed that men achieve peak performance in their 20s for all running and swimming events (e.g., 23 years for sprinting and 28 for marathon running).[58]

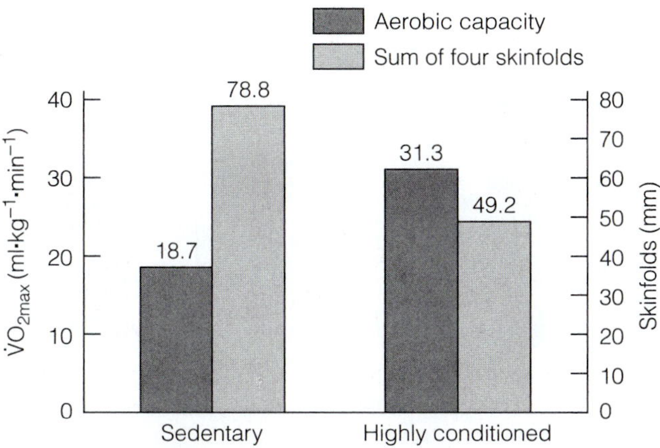

Figure 15.16 Fitness and leanness in highly active elderly women. Septuagenarian women (mean age 73 years) who were highly active, competing in state and national senior games endurance competitions were much leaner and fitter ($\dot{V}O_{2max}$ 67% higher) than their sedentary counterparts.
Source: Warren BJ, Nieman DC, Dobson RG, Adkins CH, O'Donnell KA, Haddock BL, Butterworth DE. Cardiorespiratory responses to exercise training in septuagenarian women. *Int J Sports Med* 14:60–65, 1993.

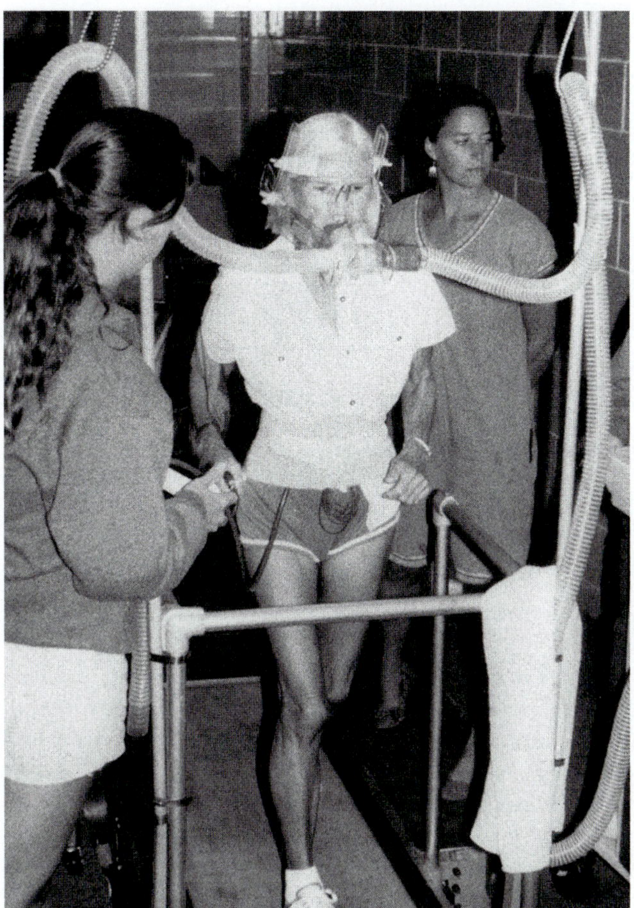

Figure 15.17 This highly conditioned elderly woman (age 67) has a $\dot{V}O_{2max}$ of 35 ml · kg^{-1}· min^{-1}, equal to that of a woman 40 years younger than herself (a subject in study from Figure 15.15).

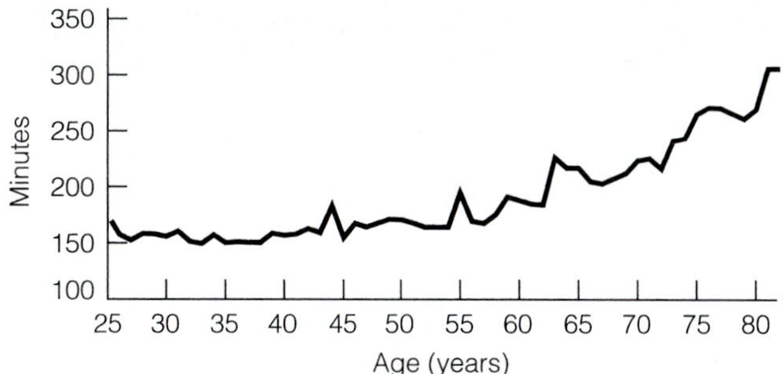

Figure 15.18 John Kelley's Boston marathon times, ages 25–82 years. John Kelley raced the Boston marathon every year between the ages of 25 and 82. Despite intensive training, his race time was about twice as slow in old age, compared to when he was a young adult.

A case in point is the 57-year history of John Kelley, the famous runner who competed in the Boston marathon every year between the ages of 25 and 82. As shown in Figure 15.18, despite intensive training and unusual motivation and tenacity, his race time at age 82 was about twice as slow as it was during his 20s and 30s. Running the marathon at age 82 was a tremendous feat in and of itself (something the vast majority of people worldwide cannot do at any age), but the aging process was strong enough to slow him down considerably.

Physical Training by the Elderly

The studies from the previous section were primarily cross-sectional in nature, with researchers comparing older and younger athletes and nonathletes. A more difficult research design is to randomly divide sedentary subjects into exercise and nonexercise groups and then to compare them before and after several months of training. The question of interest has been whether elderly individuals are capable of improving cardiorespiratory and musculoskeletal fitness, and body composition in a fashion similar to that of younger adults. The answer is "yes," but the absolute level attained after training is lower than can be attained when younger.[30] See Box 15.3 for a summary of the ACSM position stand on exercise training for older adults.[30]

Cardiorespiratory Training

Although earlier studies suggested that older individuals are not as responsive to aerobic training as their younger counterparts, there is now a growing consensus that the relative increase in $\dot{V}O_{2max}$ over an 8–26 week period is similar between young and old adults.[30,45,59–65]

Figure 15.19 shows the result of a randomized controlled study involving women in their 70s.[45] Twelve weeks of brisk walking led to a 12.6% improvement in $\dot{V}O_{2max}$, an increase similar to that reported for younger adults. Notice, however, that $\dot{V}O_{2max}$ was still far below that of younger females or a

Box 15.3

Exercise and Physical Activity for Older Adults—American College of Sports Medicine (ACSM) Position Stand

In 1998, the ACSM published a position statement on exercise training for older adults. Key statements from this publication include the following:

- Participation in a regular exercise program is an effective intervention to reduce and prevent a number of functional declines associated with aging.
- Older individuals (including octo- and nonagenarians) adapt and respond to both endurance and strength training. Endurance training by older individuals elicits the same 10–30% increase in $\dot{V}O_{2max}$ and reduction in body fat as measured in younger adults.
- Endurance training by older individuals maintains and improves cardiovascular function, improves disease risk factors (e.g., hypertension, dyslipidemia, insulin sensitivity), and contributes to an increase in life expectancy.
- Strength training helps offset the loss in muscle mass and strength typically associated with normal aging and increases levels of spontaneous physical activity.
- Regular exercise training also improves bone health, reducing the risk for osteoporosis.
- Postural stability is improved with regular exercise, reducing the risk for falls and related injuries and fractures. Exercise also increases flexibility and joint range of motion in older individuals.
- Some evidence suggests that exercise training provides psychological benefits, including preserved cognitive function, alleviation of depression, and improved self-efficacy.
- In general, regular physical activity contributes to a healthy, independent lifestyle and improves functional capacity and quality of life in older individuals.

Source: Mazzeo RS, Cavanagh P, Evans WJ, Fiatarone M, Hagberg J, McAuley E, Startzell J. Position Stand from the American College of Sports Medicine. Exercise and physical activity for older adults. *Med Sci Sports Exerc* 30:992–1008, 1998.

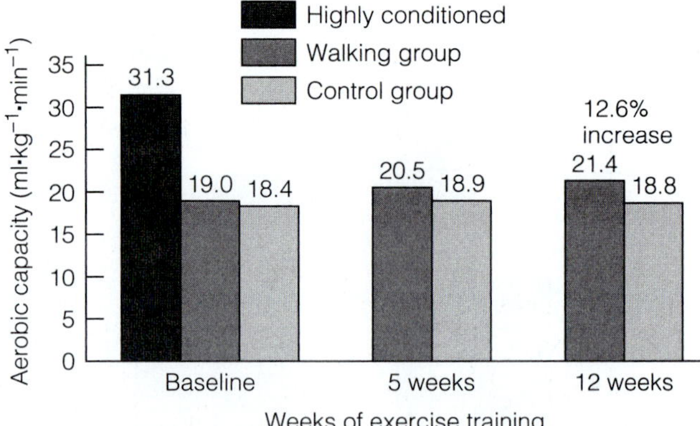

Figure 15.19 Exercise and aerobic capacity in elderly women; highly conditioned subjects had exercised vigorously for an average of 11 years; 12-week training program = 5 days/week, brisk walking, 37 minutes/session at 60% aerobic capacity. Twelve weeks of brisk walking by elderly women led to a 12.6% improvement in $\dot{V}O_{2max}$. The dark bar shows the $\dot{V}O_{2max}$ of a highly conditioned group of elderly women who had been training vigorously for 11 years, competing in state and national senior games competitions. Source: Warren BJ, Nieman DC, Dotson RG, Adkins CH, O'Donnell KA, Haddock BL, Butterworth DE. Cardiorespiratory responses to exercise training in septuagenarian women. *Int J Sports Med* 14:60–65, 1993.

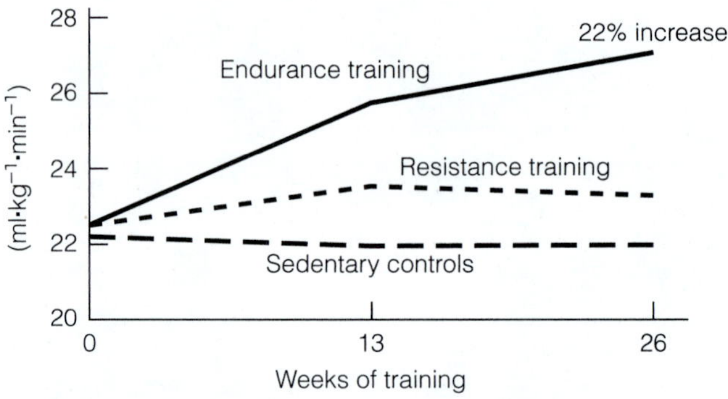

Figure 15.20 Exercise training in 70- to 79-year-olds, endurance training = 3 days/week, 40 minutes/session, 50% increasing to 75–85% $\dot{V}O_{2max}$. After 26 weeks of vigorous endurance training, $\dot{V}O_{2max}$ improved 22% in elderly men and women. Source: Hagberg JM, Graves JE, Limacher M, et al. Cardiovascular responses of 70- to 79-year-old men and women to exercise training. *J Appl Physiol* 66:2589–2594, 1989.

group of elderly female athletes who had been training intensely for an average of 11 years (Figures 15.16 and 15.19).

In another study of septuagenarian subjects, 26 weeks of high-intensity exercise led to even greater gains (22% increase overall) in aerobic power (see Figure 15.20).[62] Men and women between the ages of 70 and 79 were randomly assigned to endurance training, resistance training, or a control group. Subjects in the endurance group trained on treadmills, gradually increasing the intensity of exercise from 50% (walking) to 75–85% (walking/jogging) of $\dot{V}O_{2max}$ for 40 minutes per session, 3 days a week. The researchers concluded that "healthy men and women in their 70s increased their $\dot{V}O_{2max}$ to the same relative degree as would be expected in younger individuals in response to a prolonged and vigorous program of endurance exercise training" and that people in their eighth decade of life "have not lost the ability to adapt to endurance exercise training."[62]

There is some concern about exercise-induced injury rates among the elderly. While walking has been associated

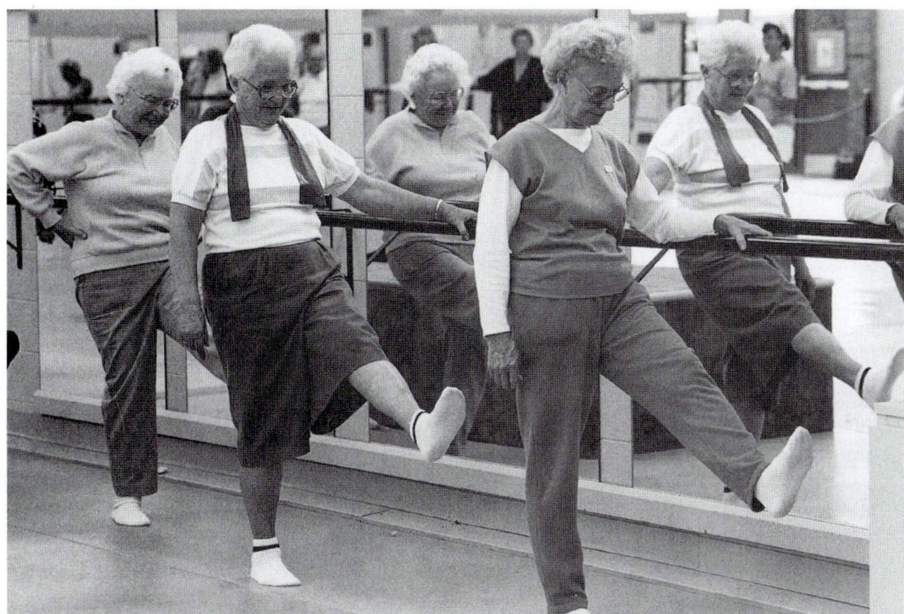

Figure 15.21 The elderly are more fragile and susceptible to musculoskeletal injury during high-impact aerobic activities. Low-impact aerobic dance or other activities such as walking or swimming are preferable to high-impact aerobic dance or jogging.

with low injury rates among the elderly, jogging may induce an unusually high injury rate.[66] Some researchers feel that the elderly, as compared to younger adults, are more fragile and susceptible to musculoskeletal injury during high-impact aerobic activities (such as jogging or aerobic dance) and that such activities as walking, low-impact aerobic dance, or swimming may be preferable (see Figure 15.21).

In general, the same basic exercise prescription principles used for young adults can be applied to the elderly, but with an emphasis on greater caution and slower progression.[30,59] The elderly are frequently divided into three approximate groupings: the young old, 65–73 years of age; the old old, 74–84 years of age; and the very old, greater than 84 years of age.[67] The question of whether regular cardiorespiratory exercise can improve aerobic power in very old individuals has received little attention, and more research is needed to determine their trainability. At this extreme age, the aging process may dominate so powerfully that little improvement in cardiorespiratory fitness may be experienced.[51] In addition, for many people over age 75, health problems and a lack of motivation may prevent them from being able to engage in appropriate amounts of exercise.

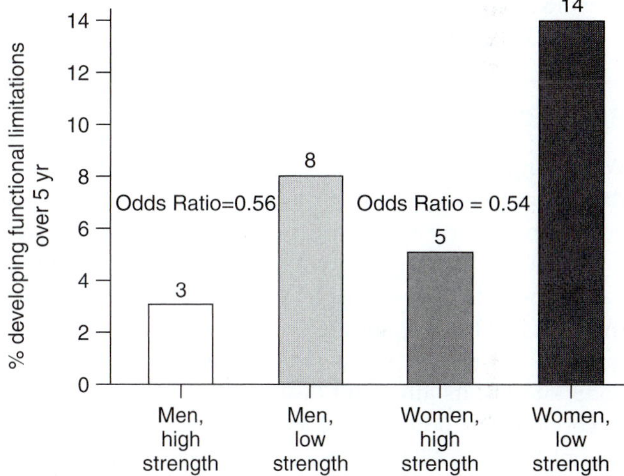

Figure 15.22 Men and women with high compared to low strength developed fewer functional limitations in this 5-year study of 3,069 men and 589 women. Source: Brill PA, Macera CA, Davis DR, Blair SN, Gordon N. Muscular strength and physical function. *Med Sci Sports Exerc* 32:412–416, 2000.

Muscular Strength and Resistance Training

Muscle strength in most individuals is well preserved to about 45 years of age but then deteriorates by about 5–10% per decade thereafter (see Chapter 6).[30,35,68] The average individual will lose about 30% of muscle strength and 40% of muscle size between the second and seventh decades of life.[30,35] The loss in muscle mass appears to be the major reason strength is decreased among the elderly, with the aging process leading to only minor changes in the muscle's ability to generate tension.[69] Muscle atrophy appears to be the result of loss of both the size and number of muscle fibers.[68] The term "sarcopenia" is used to represent the loss of muscle mass and strength that occurs with normal aging.[68]

In older individuals, muscle weakness may compromise common activities of daily living, leading to dependency on others. Also, reduced leg strength may increase the risk of injury through falling. In fact, the capacity of the elderly to remain functionally independent appears to depend less on cardiorespiratory fitness than on muscular fitness. The maintenance of strength throughout the life span has been linked to a reduced likelihood of developing functional limitations. For example, in a 5-year study conducted at the Cooper Institute for Aerobics Research, men and women with high compared to low strength had a lower prevalence of functional limitations as depicted in Figure 15.22.[70] These results support current ACSM guidelines that encourage all adults to improve both aerobic and muscular fitness.[30]

At issue has been whether the elderly can improve muscular strength by engaging in regular resistance training. Many studies have now shown that the elderly respond to progressive resistance training with relative (but not absolute) improvements in muscular strength and size that compare favorably to responses seen in younger adults.[30,35,68–78]

In general, resistance training studies with older individuals support the following findings.[30,68–78] Benefits of resistance training are that it

- Counters sarcopenia because resistance training produces substantial increases in the strength, mass, and power of old skeletal muscle.
- Improves neural activation in trained muscles.
- Helps reduce some disease risk factors, in particular, high blood pressure and insulin resistance.
- Builds fat-free mass and thereby increases resting metabolic rate slightly.
- Reduces risk factors for falls.
- Helps reduce both total and intra-abdominal fat.

Body Composition Changes

With aging, there is an accumulation of fat and a substantial loss of muscle mass.[79] Comparisons between average young and elderly adults suggest a decrease in the fat-free mass of 15–30% by age 80, with the rate and degree of loss varying widely depending on both genetic and lifestyle influences.[35,79] During middle age, there is typically a gain in body fat, and in some individuals, centralization of body fat with its attendant health risks may also occur.[79] In very old age, both fat-free and fat mass are lost as body weight declines. All the various components of the fat-free mass—muscle and bone mineral mass, and total body water—are decreased in older men and women, relative to young adults. The decline in resting metabolic rate with advancing age is primarily due to this decline in fat-free mass.[69,79]

As reviewed in the previous section, resistance exercise can increase muscle mass and strength in the elderly.[35,79] Elderly individuals can also demonstrate a level of body fat somewhat similar to that of younger persons if they have a consistent physical activity history and control their food intake throughout life.[45] (See Figure 15.16.) Although short-term reductions in body fat and gains in muscle mass have been reported in studies with the elderly, the usual age-related changes in body composition may not be completely countered unless aerobic and resistance training are combined. In a study of master athletes, for example, fat weight increased about 2.5 pounds during a 10-year period, while fat-free weight dropped 3–6 pounds, despite heavy endurance training (about 30 miles per week of running).[80]

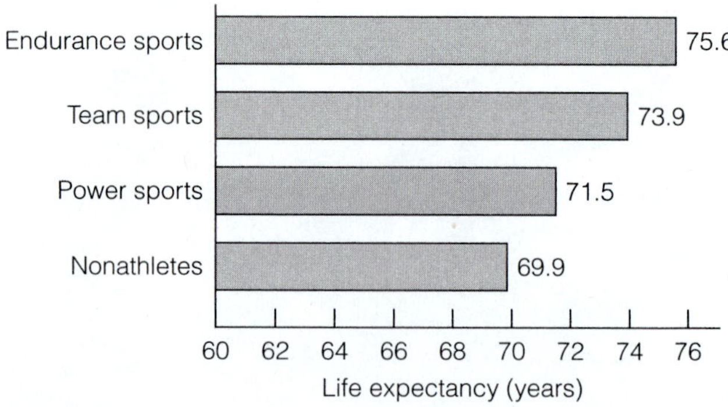

Figure 15.23 Mean life expectancy among athletes versus nonathletes. These cross-sectional data of Finnish male world-class athletes and nonathletes suggest that endurance-sport athletes have a greater life expectancy than athletes from other sports or nonathletes. Source: Sarna S, Sahi T, Koskenvuo M, Kaprio J. Increased life expectancy of world class male athletes. *Med Sci Sports Exerc* 25:237–244, 1993.

Physical Activity and Life Expectancy

With an increasingly aged population, there is an urgent need for health practices that can prolong adult vigor and delay the onset and progression of chronic diseases. In other words, prolonging active life expectancy, not just disabled existence, is an important goal. "Medicated survival" by the elderly is a state to be avoided, and exercise is one factor, along with other lifestyle habits, that can improve the quality of life of the elderly.

Can regular exercise lengthen life expectancy? Do active people live longer? This has been an active area of research, and in general, most studies using both cross-sectional and longitudinal research designs suggest the answer is "yes," for both men and women.[81–89] In general, the combined studies indicate that the most active or fit individuals experience death rates that are 20–50% lower than the rates among those least active or fit.[83,85] This relationship holds true even after genetic and other lifestyle factors are taken into account.[86]

Figure 15.23 shows the results of one interesting cross-sectional study of 2,613 Finnish male world-class athletes who competed during 1920–1965, and 1,712 nonathletes.[81] Using death certificates and other medical records dating up to 1989, the life expectancy of endurance sport athletes (long-distance running and cross-country skiing) was shown to be nearly 6 years greater than that of the nonathletes and 4 years greater than that of power-sport athletes (boxing, wrestling, weight lifting, and throwers in field athletics), with team-sport athletes in an intermediate position (soccer, ice hockey, basketball, jumpers, and sprinters). Many of the athletes (especially the runners and skiers) continued their regular exercise programs throughout life, and both this and genetic selection may have explained their increased life expectancy.

Ralph Paffenbarger of Stanford University showed that Harvard alumni whose weekly energy output in

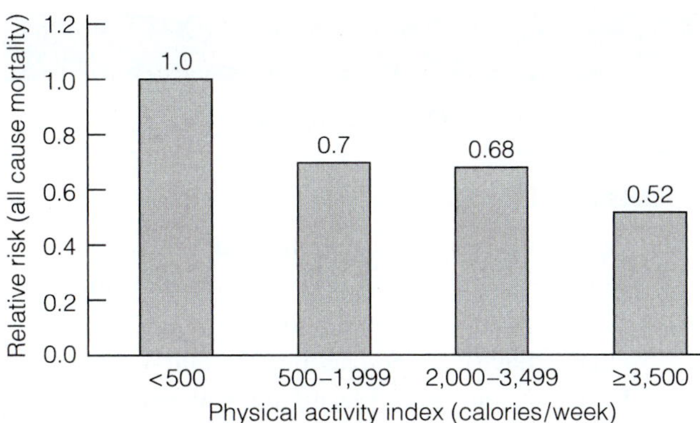

Figure 15.24 Relative risk of death from all causes, among 10,269 Harvard alumni, according to patterns of physical activity. In the Harvard alumni study, the risk of death from all causes was reduced among the physically active. For those exercising at least 2,000 Calories a week, life expectancy was estimated to be about 2 years greater than for the sedentary. Source: Paffenbarger PS, Hyde RT, Wing AL, et al. Physical activity, all-cause mortality, and longevity of college alumni. *N Engl J Med* 314:605–613, 1986.

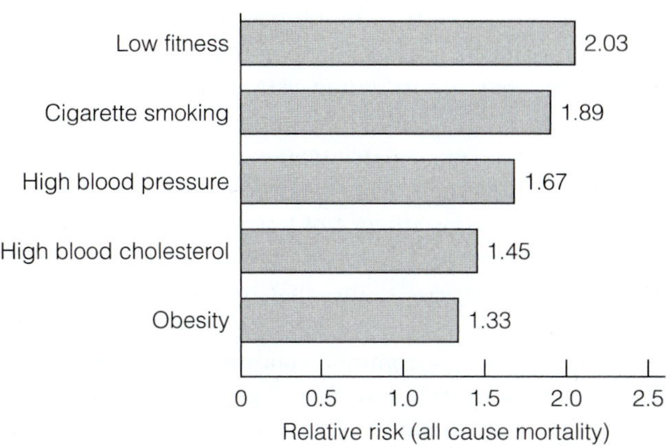

Figure 15.25 Relative risk of death from all causes among 25,341 men, Cooper Institute for Aerobics Research. Low fitness ranks highest as a predictor of early mortality among men. Source: Blair SN, Kampert JB, Kohl HW, et al. Influences of cardiorespiratory fitness and other precursors on cardiovascular disease and all-cause mortality in men and women. *JAMA* 276:205–210, 1996.

walking, stair climbing, and playing sports totaled 2,000 to 3,500 Calories a week experienced a 32% reduction in all-cause death rates[87,88] (see Figure 15.24). For subjects exercising at least 3,500 Calories a week, death rates were about half those of sedentary alumni. In general, life expectancy was found to be about 2 years greater in those exercising at least 2,000 Calories a week. Although this may not seem like much, this is the same impact in epidemiological terms of completely removing cancer from the United States. In practical terms, this improvement in life expectancy can be gained by walking or jogging 8–10 miles a week. A more recent analysis from this same cohort indicates that vigorous activities (≥ 6 METs) are associated with the lowest mortality rates in comparison to light or moderate activities.[84]

Data from the Cooper Institute for Aerobics Research have shown that the least fit of men and women are about twice as likely to die as their fit counterparts.[82] As shown in Figure 15.25, low fitness is one of the strongest risk factors for death from all causes in males and is at least as risky as cigarette smoking.

OSTEOPOROSIS

Osteoporosis is a skeletal disorder characterized by compromised bone strength predisposing to an increased risk of fracture[90–96] (see Figure 15.26). There is no accurate measure of overall bone strength. Bone mineral density is used as a proxy measure and accounts for about 70% of bone strength. The World Health Organization defines osteoporosis as bone density 2.5 standard deviations below the mean for young adult white women.[91,97] *Primary*

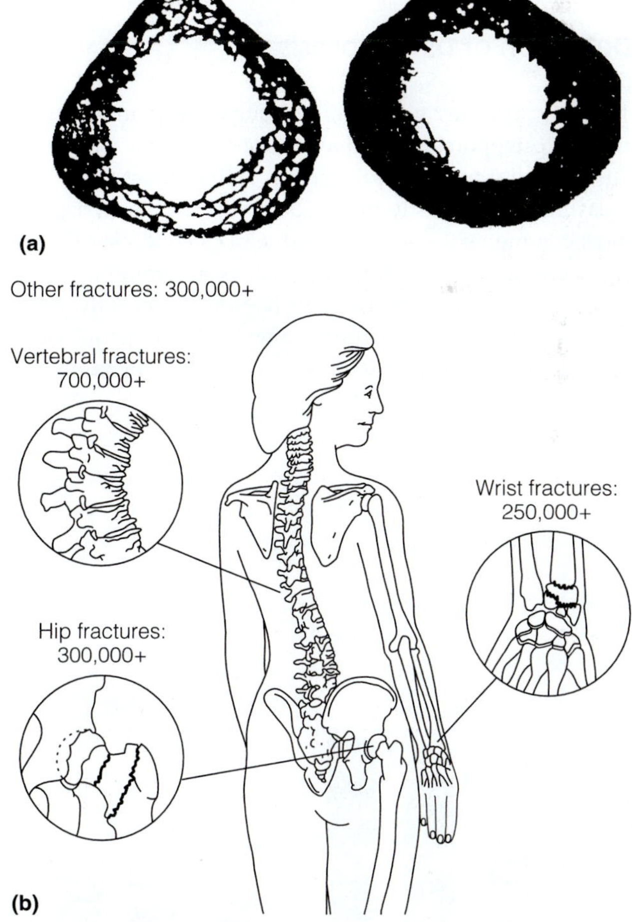

Figure 15.26 Osteoporosis is characterized by a decrease in the amount of bone, often so severe that it leads to fractures after even minimal trauma. (a) Cross-sections of normal and osteoporotic bone; (b) the three most common sites of osteoporosis.

osteoporosis may occur in two types: Type I osteoporosis (postmenopausal), which is the accelerated decrease in bone mass that occurs when estrogen levels fall after menopause; and Type II osteoporosis (age related), which is the inevitable loss of bone mass with age and occurs in both men and women. *Secondary osteoporosis* may develop at any age as a consequence of hormonal, digestive, and metabolic disorders, as well as prolonged bed rest and weightlessness (space flight) that result in loss of bone mineral mass.

Osteoporosis is a common condition afflicting 10 million Americans (8 million women, 2 million men) and causing each year an estimated 1.5 million fractures of the spinal bones, hips, forearms, and other bones in those 45 years of age and older. Loss of bone mineral density (BMD) is an almost universal phenomenon with increasing age among white men and women in the United States (see Box 15.4). Osteoporosis is an important public health problem, exacting an enormous economic and medical burden worldwide. The problem will increase as the number of elderly people grows. See Figure 15.27.

Detection of Osteoporosis

The only sure way to determine bone density and fracture risk for osteoporosis is to have a bone mass measurement (also called bone mineral density or BMD test). The test measures bone density in the spine, hip, and/or wrist, the most common sites of fractures due to osteoporosis. DEXA (dual-energy x-ray absorptiometry) is a commonly used method to measure BMD (see Chapter 5). Recently, bone density tests have been approved by the FDA that measure bone density in the middle finger and the heel or shinbone.

Box 15.4

Osteoporosis

Facts and Figures

- Osteoporosis is a major public health threat for 44 million Americans, 68% of whom are women.
- In the United States today, 10 million individuals already have osteoporosis and 34 million more have low bone mass, placing them at increased risk for this disease.
- One out of every two women and one in four men over 50 will have an osteoporosis-related fracture in their lifetime.
- More than 2 million American men suffer from osteoporosis, and millions more are at risk. Each year, 80,000 men suffer a hip fracture and one third of these men die within a year.
- Osteoporosis can strike at any age.
- Osteoporosis is responsible for more than 1.5 million fractures annually, including 300,000 hip fractures, approximately 700,000 vertebral fractures, 250,000 wrist fractures, and more than 300,000 fractures at other sites.
- Estimated national direct expenditures (hospitals and nursing homes) for osteoporosis and related fractures are $18 billion each year.

Source: National Institutes of Health, Osteoporosis and Related Bone Diseases National Resource Center. www.osteo.org.

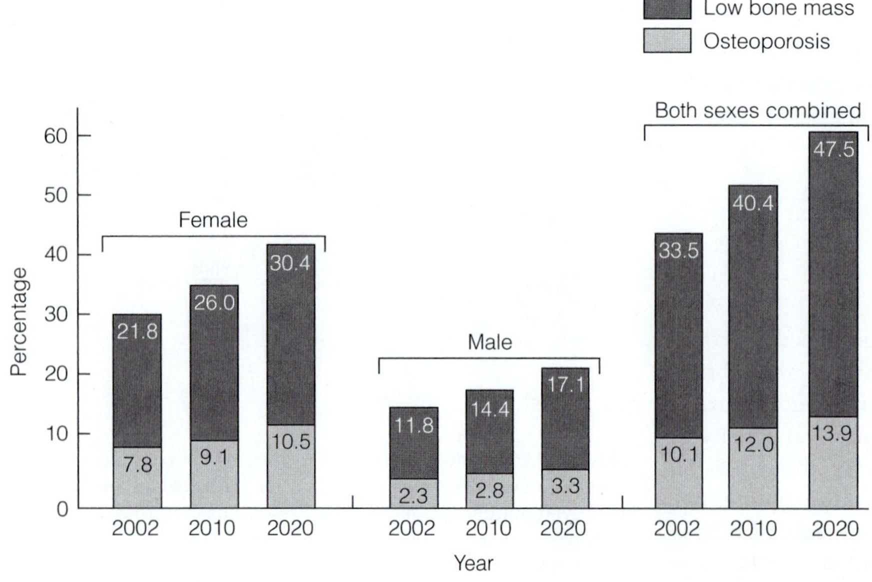

Figure 15.27 Projected prevalence of osteoporosis and/or low bone mass of the hip in women, men, and both sexes, 50 years of age or older. Source: U.S. Department of Health and Human Services. *Bone Health and Osteoporosis: A Report of the Surgeon General.* Rockville, MD: U.S. Department of Health and Human Services, Office of the Surgeon General, 2004.

The National Osteoporosis Foundation (www.nof.org) recommends that BMD testing should be performed on:

- All women aged 65 and older regardless of risk factors.
- Younger postmenopausal women with one or more risk factors (other than being white, postmenopausal, and female).
- Postmenopausal women who have experienced a bone fracture (to confirm the diagnosis and determine disease severity).

Medicare covers BMD testing for individuals aged 65 and older, estrogen-deficient women at clinical risk for osteoporosis, those with vertebral abnormalities, individuals receiving or planning to receive long-term glucocorticoid (steroid) therapy, those with primary hyperparathyroidism, and individuals being monitored to assess the response or efficacy of an approved osteoporosis drug therapy. Medicare permits individuals to repeat BMD testing every 2 years.

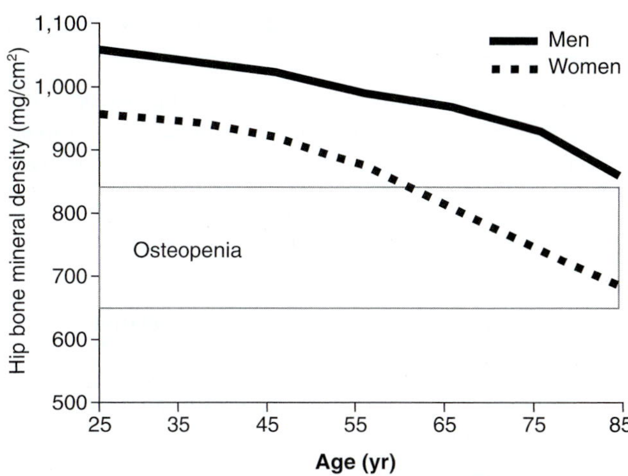

Figure 15.28 Loss of hip bone mineral density with age in U.S. men and women. Osteopenia is defined as a bone mineral density of 648 to 833 mg/cm^2 (1 to 2.5 standard deviations below mean values for young adult white women). Source: Looker AC. Updated data on proximal femur bone mineral levels of US adults. *Osteoporos Int* 8:468–489, 1998.

Risk Factors

Bone is a spongy protein matrix in which crystals of calcium and phosphorus salts are embedded.[95,96] In many bones, there are two distinct regions: an outer, dense shell of compact bone (cortical) and an inner, open, spongelike region of cancellous bone (trabecular). Once produced, bone does not remain as a fixed structure. From birth until death, bone tissue is continually being formed, broken down, and reformed in a process called *remodeling*. The cells that break down bone are called *osteoclasts*, and those that build bone are called *osteoblasts*.

During puberty, rapid increases in bone growth and density occur, with peak bone density achieved between the ages of 20 and 30.[90,95,96] About 98% of the adult bone mineral content is deposited by age 20, and this process is affected by both genetic and lifestyle factors.[90,95,96] The period between ages 9 and 20 is critical in building up an optimal bone density as a safeguard against losses later in life. Osteoporosis is now viewed as a pediatric health problem.[91] Bone mass is approximately 30% higher in men than in women and about 10% higher in blacks than in whites. Once peak bone mass is reached, osteoclast and osteoblast activity remain in balance until about age 45–50, when osteoclast activity becomes greater than that of the osteoblasts, and adults begin to slowly lose bone mass. At menopause, women normally have an accelerated loss of bone mineral mass (2.5–5% per year) for several years[90,98] (see Figure 15.28). During the course of their lifetimes, women lose about 50% of their trabecular bone and 30% of their cortical bone, while men lose about 30% and 20%, respectively.[90–98] Although peak bone mass is an important factor explaining why some individuals develop osteoporosis and bone fractures and others do not, differences in bone architecture and structure also appear to be important.[90,91]

The best strategies for preventing osteoporosis are to build strong bones early in life, and then reduce bone loss in later years (see Physical Fitness Activity 15.2). Several risk factors predict those who should be most concerned about prevention of osteoporosis (see Box 15.5).[91–113] This includes risk factors that cannot be changed—gender, age, body size, ethnicity, family history—and these that can be changed—sex hormones, anorexia, a lifetime diet low in calcium and vitamin D, use of certain medications, an inactive lifestyle, cigarette smoking, and excessive use of alcohol.[91,96]

Medications for Treatment

There is no cure for osteoporosis, but the National Osteoporosis Foundation (www.nof.org) recommends several steps for slowing its progress:

Step 1: A balanced diet rich in calcium and vitamin D

Step 2: Weight-bearing exercise

Step 3: A healthy lifestyle with no smoking or excessive alcohol intake

Step 4: Talking to a health-care professional about bone health

Step 5: Bone density testing and medication when appropriate (see Box 15.6)

As summarized in Box 15.6, alendronate, raloxifene, and risedronate are approved by the U.S. Food and Drug Administration (FDA) for the prevention and treatment

Box 15.5

Risk Factors for Osteoporosis and Prevention Steps

Certain people are more likely to develop osteoporosis than others. Factors that increase the likelihood of developing osteoporosis are called "risk factors." These risk factors include:

- Personal history of fracture after age 45
- Current low bone mass
- History of fracture in a first-degree relative
- Being female
- Being thin and/or having a small frame (weight less than 127 pounds)
- Advanced age
- A family history of osteoporosis
- Estrogen deficiency as a result of early menopause (< age 45) or surgically induced
- Abnormal absence of menstrual periods (amenorrhea)
- Anorexia nervosa
- Low lifetime calcium intake
- Vitamin D deficiency
- Use of certain medications:

  Oral glucocorticoids, excess thyroxine replacement, antiepileptic medications, gonadal hormone suppression, immunosuppressive agents
- Presence of certain chronic medical conditions:

  Hyperthyroidism, chronic lung disease, endometriosis, cancer, chronic liver/kidney disease, hyperparathyroidism, vitamin D deficiency, Cushingís disease, multiple sclerosis, sarcoidosis, hemachromotosis
- Low testosterone levels in men
- An inactive lifestyle and minimal weight-bearing exercise
- Current cigarette smoking
- Excessive use of alcohol
- Being Caucasian or Asian

Prevention

By about age 20, the average woman has acquired 98% of her skeletal mass. Building strong bones during childhood and adolescence can be the best defense against developing osteoporosis later. There are five steps that together can optimize bone health and help prevent osteoporosis. They are:

Step 1: A balanced diet rich in calcium and vitamin D

Step 2: Weight-bearing exercise

Step 3: A healthy lifestyle with no smoking or excessive alcohol intake

Step 4: Talking to a health-care professional about bone health

Step 5: Bone density testing and medication when appropriate.

Sources: National Osteoporosis Foundation, www.nof.org; U.S. Department of Health and Human Services. *Bone Health and Osteoporosis: A Report of the Surgeon General.* Rockville, MD: U.S. Department of Health and Human Services, Office of the Surgeon General, 2004.

Box 15.6

Therapeutic Medications for Osteoporosis Prevention and Treatment

Currently, alendronate, raloxifene, and risedronate are approved by the U.S. Food and Drug Administration (FDA) for the prevention and treatment of postmenopausal osteoporosis. Teriparatide is approved for the treatment of the disease in postmenopausal women and men who are at high risk for fracture. Estrogen/hormone therapy (ET/HT) is approved for the prevention of postmenopausal osteoporosis, and calcitonin is approved for treatment. In addition, alendronate is approved for the treatment of osteoporosis in men, and both alendronate and risedronate are approved for use by men and women with glucocorticoid-induced osteoporosis.

Alendronate. Alendronate (brand name Fosamax®) is a medication from the class of drugs called *bisphosphonates.* Like estrogen and raloxifene, alendronate is approved for both the prevention and treatment of osteoporosis. Alendronate is also used to treat the bone loss from glucocorticoid medications such as prednisone or cortisone and is approved for the treatment of osteoporosis in men. In postmenopausal women with osteoporosis, the bisphosphonate alendronate reduces bone loss, increases bone density in both the spine and hip, and reduces the risk of both spine fractures and hip fractures. Side effects from alendronate are uncommon, but may include abdominal or musculoskeletal pain, nausea, heartburn, or

(continued)

Box 15.6

Therapeutic Medications for Osteoporosis Prevention and Treatment *(continued)*

irritation of the esophagus. The medication should be taken on an empty stomach and with a full glass of water first thing in the morning. After taking alendronate, it is important to wait in an upright position for at least one-half hour, or preferably one hour, before the first food, beverage, or medication of the day.

Risedronate. Risedronate sodium (brand name Actonel®) is approved for the prevention and treatment of osteoporosis in postmenopausal women and for the prevention and treatment of glucocorticoid-induced osteoporosis in both men and women. Risedronate, a bisphosphonate, has been shown to slow or stop bone loss, increase bone mineral density, and reduce the risk of spine and non-spine fractures. In clinical trials, side effects of risedronate were minimal to moderate and those that were reported occurred equally among people taking the medication and those taking a placebo. Risedronate should be taken with a glass of water at least 30 minutes before the first food or beverage of the day other than water. After taking risedronate, it is important to remain in an upright position and refrain from eating for at least 30 minutes.

Raloxifene. Raloxifene (brand name Evista®) is a drug that is approved for the prevention and treatment of postmenopausal osteoporosis. It is from a new class of drugs called Selective Estrogen Receptor Modulators (SERMs) that appear to prevent bone loss at the spine, hip, and total body. Raloxifene has been shown to have beneficial effects on bone mass and bone turnover and can reduce the incidence of vertebral fractures. Though side effects are not common with raloxifene, those reported include hot flashes and deep vein thrombosis, the latter of which is also associated with estrogen therapy. Additional research studies on raloxifene will be ongoing for several more years.

Calcitonin. Calcitonin is a naturally occurring non-sex hormone involved in calcium regulation and bone metabolism. In women who are at least 5 years beyond menopause, calcitonin slows bone loss, increases spinal bone density, and according to anecdotal reports, relieves the pain associated with bone fractures. Calcitonin reduces the risk of spinal fractures and may reduce hip fracture risk as well. Studies on fracture reduction are ongoing. Calcitonin is currently available as an injection or nasal spray. Though it does not affect other organs or systems in the body, injectable calcitonin may cause an allergic reaction and unpleasant side effects including flushing of the face and hands, urinary frequency, nausea, and skin rash. The only side effect reported with nasal calcitonin is a runny nose.

Teriparatide. Teriparatide (brand name Forteo®) is an injectable form of human parathyroid hormone that is approved for postmenopausal women and men with osteoporosis who are at high risk for having a fracture. Teriparatide stimulates new bone formation in both the spine and hip and reduces the risk of vertebral and nonvertebral fractures in postmenopausal women. In men, teriparatide reduces the risk of vertebral fractures but the study was not large enough to examine the effect on nonvertebral fractures. Side effects include nausea, dizziness, and leg cramps. Teriparatide is approved for use for up to 24 months.

Estrogen/Hormone Therapy. Estrogen/hormone therapy (ET/HT) has been shown to reduce bone loss, increase bone density in both the spine and hip, and reduce the risk of hip and spine fractures in postmenopausal women. ET/HT is approved for the prevention of postmenopausal osteoporosis and is most commonly administered in the form of a pill or skin patch. When estrogen (estrogen therapy or ET) is taken alone, it can increase a woman's risk of developing cancer of the uterine lining (endometrial cancer). To eliminate this risk, physicians prescribe the hormone progestin in combination with estrogen (hormone therapy/HT) for those women who have not had a hysterectomy. Side effects of ET/HT include vaginal bleeding, breast tenderness, mood disturbances, venous blood clots, and gallbladder disease. The Women's Health Initiative (WHI), a large government-funded research study, recently demonstrated that HT (Prempro®) is associated with a modest increase in the risk of breast cancer, stroke, and heart attack. The WHI also demonstrated that ET is associated with an increase in the risk of stroke. Another large study from the National Cancer Institute (NCI) indicated that long-term use of ET may be associated with an increase in the risk of ovarian cancer. It is not yet clear whether HT carries a similar risk. Any estrogen therapy should be prescribed for the shortest period of time possible. When used solely for the prevention of postmenopausal osteoporosis, any ET/HT regimen should only be considered for women at significant risk of osteoporosis and nonestrogen medications should be carefully considered.

Source: National Institutes of Health, Osteoporosis and Related Bone Diseases National Resource Center. www.osteo.org.

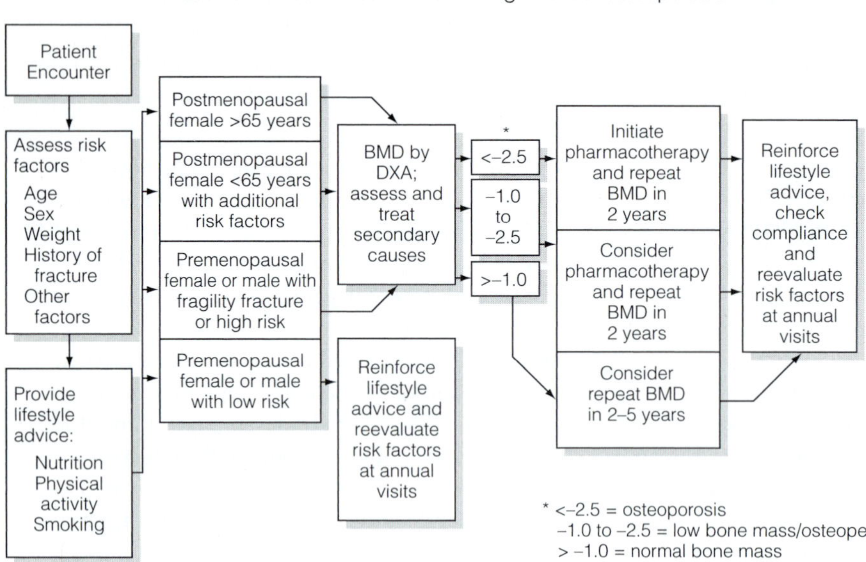

Figure 15.29 This flow chart outlines a broad approach to assessing bone health and preventing bone disease, determining who should have bone density measurements, and deciding on pharmacologic treatment for osteoporosis. Source: U.S. Department of Health and Human Services. *Bone Health and Osteoporosis: A Report of the Surgeon General.* Rockville, MD: U.S. Department of Health and Human Services, Office of the Surgeon General, 2004.

of postmenopausal osteoporosis.[96] Teriparatide is approved for the treatment of the disease in postmenopausal women and men who are at high risk for fracture. Estrogen/hormone therapy (ET/HT) is approved for the prevention of postmenopausal osteoporosis, and calcitonin is approved for treatment. In addition, alendronate is approved for the treatment of osteoporosis in men, and both alendronate and risedronate are approved for use by men and women with glucocorticoid-induced osteoporosis.

Pharmacologic therapy should be considered in older adults who have osteoporosis or who have low bone mass with multiple risk factors, as outlined in Figure 15.29.[96] Selection of therapeutic drugs can be tailored by the health-care professional to meet the severity of the patient's bone loss and other medical conditions. Combinations of medications are more effective than single agents. Medications are not recommended for young and middle-aged adults. Therapy in this age group should focus on maximizing nutrition and lifestyle modifications and addressing any underlying medical conditions.[96]

Nutrition

The recommended diet for optimal bone health is consistent with diets recommended for the prevention of other diseases.[91,96] Since many nutrients are important for bone health, it is important to eat a well-balanced diet containing a variety of foods, including grains, fruits and vegetables, nonfat or low-fat dairy products or other calcium-rich foods, and meat or beans each day.

The most important nutrient for bone health is calcium. Most Americans do not consume recommended levels of calcium, but reaching these levels is a feasible goal.[91,96] (See Figure 15.30.) Calcium intake should be 1,000–1,200 mg per day for adults (see Table 15.2). Significant food sources of calcium include dairy products, calcium-set tofu, canned fishes with bones, and other calcium-fortified foods (see also Physical Fitness Activity 15.4). Approximately three 8-ounce glasses of low-fat milk each day, combined with the calcium from the rest of a normal diet, is enough to meet the recommended daily requirements for most individuals. Foods fortified with calcium and calcium supplements can assist those who do not consume an adequate amount of calcium-rich foods.

Vitamin D is important for bone health. For many, especially elderly individuals, getting enough vitamin D from sunshine is not practical. These individuals should look to boost their vitamin D levels through diet.[91,96] Young adults need 200 IU/day vitamin D, middle-aged adults 400 IU/day, and the elderly 600 IU/day (Figure 15.30). Primary food sources of vitamin D are limited to fortified milk (100 IU per cup), egg yolk (25 IU per yolk), fortified cereals, and fish oils. Vitamin D is also available in supplements for those unable to get enough through sunshine and diet.

The Role of Physical Activity

Can exercise maximize peak bone mass and minimize age-related losses? The use of exercise in the prevention and treatment of osteoporosis has been an active area of research, and although it is now well accepted that physical activity is essential for the maintenance of bone health, further research is needed to understand the role exercise can play in preventing osteoporosis.[96,114–119]

It is well known that humans lose bone mass rapidly when gravitational or muscle forces on the legs are de-

	Calcium (mg/day)	Vitamin D (IU/day)	Physical Activity	Bone Density Testing	Patients at Increased Risk
Infants					Frequent fractures, anorexia, amenorrhea, chronic hepatic, renal, gastrointestinal, autoimmune disease. Medications
0–6 Months	210	200	Interactive play	As clinically indicated in high-risk patients.	
6–12 Months	270				
Children and Adolescents					
1–3 years	500	200	Moderate to vigorous activity at least 60 minutes per day. Emphasize weight-bearing activity.	As clinically indicated in high-risk patients.	
4–8 years	800				
9–18 years	1300				
Adults					
18–50 years	1000	200	Moderate activity at least 30 minutes per day, on most, preferably all, days of the week. Emphasize weight-bearing activity. For prevention programs, modified for the frail elderly and spine fracture patients.	As clinically indicated in high-risk patients.	
51–70 years	1200	400		Bone density testing by DXA in all women over age 65; consider in women under age 65 with risk factors. No consensus on men.	Individuals with risk factors.
>70 years	1200	600			

Figure 15.30 Nutrition, physical activity, and bone testing recommendations for good bone health. Source: U.S. Department of Health and Human Services. *Bone Health and Osteoporosis: A Report of the Surgeon General.* Rockville, MD: U.S. Department of Health and Human Services, Office of the Surgeon General, 2004.

creased or become absent, as in weightlessness, bed rest, or spinal cord injury.[120,121] Healthy individuals who undergo complete bed rest for 4–36 weeks can lose an average of 1% bone mineral content per week, while astronauts in a gravity-free environment can lose bone mass at a monthly rate as high as 4% for trabecular bone and 1% for cortical bone.[122] The bone adapts to imposed stress or lack of stress by forming or losing mass.[119] The bone becomes bigger and denser when stress is applied in excess of normal levels because of stimulation or remodeling. The bone will continue to grow and adapt until it is restructured to handle the new imposed stress. This is one reason why total body weight has been found to be directly related to bone mineral density, with the heaviest people having the greatest bone density.[123]

There are also substantial data showing that athletes have a greater bone density than sedentary controls.[124–130] Weight-bearing activities such as walking, running, and racket sports are more effective in maintaining density of the leg and spinal bones than non-weight-bearing activities such as bicycling and swimming (see Figure 15.31). The athletes with the greatest bone mineral masses are weight lifters, followed by athletes throwing the shotput and discus, then runners, soccer players, and finally swimmers.

A significant relationship exists between lifetime physical activity, bone mineral mass, and lowered risk of hip fracture in men and postmenopausal women.[124,127,131–133] Children who engage in sports that produce significant impact loading on their skeletons (e.g., running, gymnastics, and dance) have greater femoral neck bone density than children in sports producing low-impact loads to the bones (e.g., swimming).[126,128,134] This is considered important because a higher peak bone mass may be experienced in these individuals if exercise is maintained, decreasing the risk of osteoporosis later in life.

These differences between athletes and nonathletes may be due to factors of heredity and self-selection. In other words, people who do well in sports competition tend to have strong, dense bones to begin with. Although this may be true to a certain extent, studies comparing the active and inactive arms of tennis players, for example,

TABLE 15.2 Calcium-Containing Foods by Calcium Content per Serving with 100 mg

Food	Serving Size	Calcium, mg
> 400 mg		
Tofu, regular with calcium sulfate	½ cup	434
Tofu, firm, with calcium sulfate	½ cup	860
Fortified cereal	¾ cup	varies by brand
300–400 mg		
Whole milk	1 cup	291
Milkshake	8 oz.	300
Lowfat yogurt	8 oz.	300
Fortified soy milk	1 cup	300
Fortified rice milk	1 cup	300
Skim, 1%, or 2% milk	1 cup	321
Fortified cereal	¾ cup	varies by brand
Fortified oatmeal	1 pkt	350
200–300 mg		
Cheddar, monterey or provolone cheese	1 oz.	206
Soybeans, roasted	1 cup	237
Spinach (cooked)	1 cup	245
Mixed cheese dish	1 cup	250
Fortified energy bar	1	250
Soybeans (cooked)	1 cup	261
Swiss cheese	1 oz.	272
Plain yogurt	8 oz	274
100–200 mg		
Pizza	1 slice	100
Fortified waffles	2	100
Fortified butter or margarine	1 Tbsp.	100
Sherbet	1 cup	103
Mustard greens (cooked), Bok Choy	1 cup	104
Spaghetti, lasagna	1 cup	125
Cottage cheese	1 cup	138
Baked beans	1 cup	142
Dandelion greens or turnip greens (cooked)	1 cup	147
Ice cream	1 cup	151
Frozen yogurt or pudding	½ cup	152
America, Feta, or Mozzarella cheese	1 oz.	174
Soybeans, boiled	1 cup	175

Source: U.S. Department of Health and Human Services. *Bone Health and Osteoporosis: A Report of the Surgeon General.* Rockville, MD: U.S. Department of Health and Human Services, Office of the Surgeon General, 2004.

show differences in bone density.[135] This suggests that bones adapt to the exercise stresses imposed directly on them.

Among female athletes (especially runners and other endurance athletes) who lose their menstrual periods, bone mineral density typically decreases.[114,115] The loss in bone density occurs even though they engage in vigorous endurance exercise.[136] However, research with amenorrheic female gymnasts has shown that the extremely high stress on their skeletons from tumbling and dismount landings can actually override the negative effects of low reproductive hormones.[137] Thus it appears that in some cases, if the exercise stress is high enough, the bone will strengthen, regardless of the poor hormonal environment. Nonetheless, female endurance athletes who are amenorrheic should attempt to regain their menstrual period or use estrogen therapy to avoid early osteoporosis.[114,115] Running is an insufficient stimulus to counteract the loss of estrogen that occurs with amenorrhea, and few women are willing to undergo the intense gymnastic-like exercise that is necessary to protect bone mass under these conditions.

As emphasized earlier in this section, the foundation for bone health begins early in life. Thus, physical activity that places a load on the bones is essential throughout childhood and the adolescent years.[134] Adolescents who have stronger muscles through regular exercise also have denser bones, which should translate to a reduced risk of osteoporosis later in life.[115,138]

Among older individuals, a history of lifelong physical activity relates to a greater bone mineral mass and, very importantly, a lowered risk of hip fracture.[131,132] Typically, as people age, both bone density and muscular strength decrease, as shown in Figure 15.32.[117,139] Thus, muscular strength has an important influence on bone mineral density at all sites among women. In other words, if women maintain good muscle strength through intensive exercise, bone density should be better preserved even into old age.[139]

Boxes 15.7 and 15.8 summarize physical activity recommendations from the Office of the Surgeon General and ACSM.[96,115] Box 15.9 provides a specific program of exercise to prevent osteoporosis.

Several studies have shown the value of intensive resistance and weight-bearing training in protecting the skeletons of postmenopausal women.[140–149] In a 1-year study of 39 postmenopausal women, subjects engaged in intensive weight training for 45 minutes, two times a week. The weight trainers improved their strength and muscle mass, and also their bone mineral density when compared to the control subjects[141] (see Figure 15.33). In another 1-year study of postmenopausal women (32 women, 60–72 years of age), subjects walked and jogged and climbed stairs vigorously for 50 minutes a session, three to four times a week.

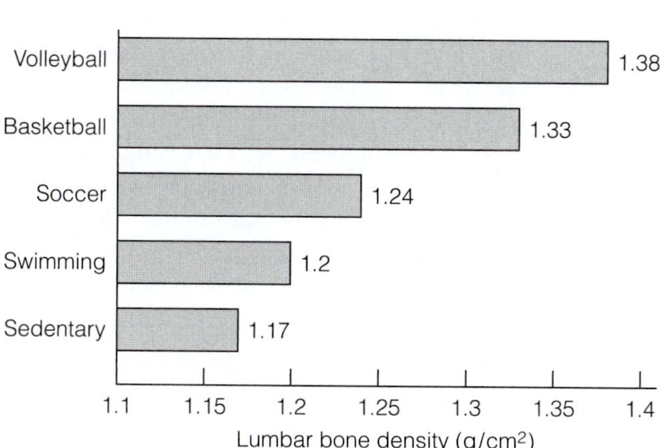

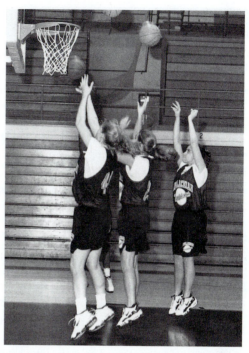

Figure 15.31 Lumbar bone mineral density in female athletes. Sports that require jumping and short bursts of powerful leg movements are associated with the highest bone density in female athletes. Source: Lee EJ, Long KA, Risser WL, Poindexter HBW, Gibbons WE, Goldzieher J. Variations in bone status of contralateral and regional sites in young athletic women. *Med Sci Sports Exerc* 27:1354–1361, 1995.

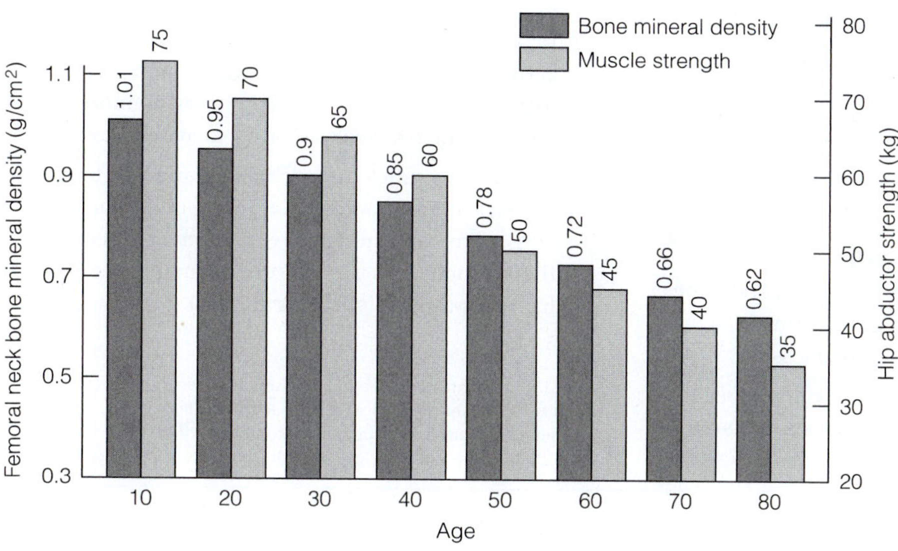

Figure 15.32 Age and bone mineral density and strength in the hip. Typically, as people age, bone density and muscular strength decrease in parallel. Source: Snow CM. Exercise and bone mass in young and premenopausal women. *Bone* 18(suppl):51S–55S, 1996.

Exercise and estrogen therapy together had the greatest effect on lumbar bone density, with about one third of the improvement due to exercise[140] (see Figure 15.34). These results suggest that the efficacy of estrogen therapy is enhanced by combining it with weight-bearing exercise. Other research has indicated that the regimen of intensive exercise must continue indefinitely because just as quickly as the bone mineral density is gained it can be lost through detraining.[149]

A potential benefit of regular exercise by the elderly is a decrease in the risk of falling. Falls and the resulting injuries are among the most serious and common medical

Box 15.7

Physical Activity and Osteoporosis Recommendations from the Office of the Surgeon General

- In addition to meeting recommended guidelines for physical activity (at least 30 minutes a day for adults and 60 minutes for children), specific strength- and weight-bearing activities are critical to building and maintaining bone mass throughout life.
- Because continued physical activity provides a positive stimulus for bone, muscle, and other aspects of health, a lifelong commitment to physical activity and exercise is critical.
- Ending a physical activity regimen will result in bone mass returning to the level that existed before the activity began. Because repetitive programs of physical activity may be discontinued due to lack of motivation or interest, variety and creativity are important if physical activity is to be continued over the long term.
- Physical activity will only affect bone at the skeletal sites that are stressed (or loaded) by the activity. In other words, physical activity programs do not necessarily benefit the whole skeleton, although any type of activity provides more benefit to bone than does no activity at all.
- For bone gain to occur, the stimulus must be greater than that which the bone usually experiences. Static loads applied continuously (such as standing) do not promote increased bone mass.
- Complete lack of activity, such as periods of immobility, causes bone loss. When it is not possible to avoid immobility (e.g., bed rest during sickness), even brief daily weight-bearing movements can help to reduce bone loss.
- General physical activity every day and some weight-bearing, strength-building, and balance-enhancing activities two or more times a week is generally effective for promoting bone health for most persons.
- Any activity that imparts impact (such as jumping or skipping) may increase bone mass more than will low- and moderate-intensity, endurance-type activities, such as brisk walking. However, endurance activities may still play an important role in skeletal health by increasing muscle mass and strength, balance, and coordination, and they may also help prevent falls in the elderly. Endurance activity is also very important for other aspects of health, such as helping to prevent obesity, diabetes, and cardiovascular disease.
- Load-bearing physical activities such as jumping need not be engaged in for long periods of time to provide benefits to skeletal health. In fact, 5–10 minutes daily may suffice. Most adults should begin with weight-bearing exercise and gradually add some skipping and jumping activity. Longer periods (30–45 minutes) may be needed for weight training or walking/jogging. Those who have been inactive should work up to this amount of time gradually using a progressive program; for example, start with shorter times and easier activities (light weights or walking) and then increase time or intensity slowly (by no more than 10 percent each week) in order to avoid injury.
- Physical activities that include a variety of loading patterns (such as strength training or aerobic classes) may promote increased bone mass more than do activities that involve normal or regular loading patterns (such as running).

Source: U.S. Department of Health and Human Services. *Bone Health and Osteoporosis: A Report of the Surgeon General.* Rockville, MD: U.S. Department of Health and Human Services, Office of the Surgeon General, 2004.

problems suffered by the elderly. Each year, about 3 in 10 elderly individuals sustain a fall, with somewhat less than 5% of falls resulting in bone fractures.

Although more research is needed, some studies suggest that exercise directed towards balance and lower extremity strength training may reduce the risk of falling.[150] There is good evidence that physical activity is linked to a 20–40% reduced risk of hip fracture.[150] In other words, regular weight-bearing and resistance exercise has a twofold benefit for the elderly—an improvement in bone mineral density and a reduced likelihood of falling leading to fractures.

Box 15.8

ACSM Guidelines on Physical Activity and Bone Health

- Physical activity appears to play an important role in maximizing bone mass during childhood and the early adult years, maintaining bone mass through the fifth decade, attenuating bone loss with aging, and reducing falls and fractures in the elderly.
- Physical activities that generate relatively high-intensity loading forces, such as plyometrics (e.g., explosive jumping on and off a step), gymnastics, intensive resistance training, and running and jumping sports such as soccer and basketball augment bone accrual in children and adolescents. Children and adolescents should engage in these activities at least 3 days per week for 10 to 20 minutes a session (and two times per day or more may be more effective).
- During adulthood, the primary goal of physical activity should be to maintain bone mass through activities such as weight-bearing endurance activities (e.g., tennis, stair climbing, jogging, sports such as volleyball and basketball that involve jumping, and resistance training). The intensity should be moderate to high (in terms of bone-loading forces). Weight-bearing activities should be engaged in three to five times per week, and resistance exercise two to three times per week. Duration should be 30–60 minutes of a combination of weight-bearing endurance activities, activities that involve jumping, and resistance exercise that targets all major muscle groups.
- The general recommendation that adults maintain a relatively high level of weight-bearing physical activity for bone health does not have an upper age limit, but as age increases, so too does the need for ensuring that physical activities can be performed safely. Exercise programs for elderly women and men should include not only weight-bearing endurance and resistance activities aimed at preserving bone mass, but also activities designed to improve balance and prevent falls.

Source: American College of Sports Medicine. ACSM position stand on physical activity and bone health. *Med Sci Sports Exerc* 36:1985–1996, 2004.

Box 15.9

Exercise Prescription for Prevention of Osteoporosis

A community-based program for postmenopausal women has been developed to improve bone health and prevent osteoporosis by researchers in the Bone, Estrogen, Strength Training (BEST) Study. The BEST exercise program consists of three 60 to 75-minute supervised sessions each week and has the following six components.

1. *Warmup (5–10 minutes).* Walk for 5–10 minutes before beginning other components.
2. *Progressive weight bearing (25 minutes).* This involves several types of activities:
   - Walking while wearing a weighted vest, beginning with 10 pounds and building up to 25 pounds, at a heart rate ranging between 50–80% maximal heart rate.
   - Completing a circuit that includes skipping, jogging, hopping, and jumping at a heart rate ranging between 50–80% maximal heart rate.
   - Stepping or stair climbing, with a weighted vest (10–25 pounds), beginning with 4 sets of 30 steps at a pace of 2 seconds per step (8-inch step height) and progressing to 10 sets of 30 steps.
3. *Resistance exercises with large-muscle groups (20 minutes).* Perform eight resistance exercises using machines and free weights, emphasizing the large-muscle groups of the arms, legs, upper and lower trunk; build to two sets of 6–8 repetitions maximum with 45–60 seconds rest between sets.
4. *Resistance exercises with small-muscle groups (10 minutes).* Perform exercises using a physiotherapy ball, elastic bands, and free weights (1- to 3-pound dumbbells).
5. *Abdominal strengthening (5 minutes).* Train the abdominal muscles with a variety of lower extremity movements with the spine stabilized. Use ankle weights to increase resistance.
6. *Stretching and balance (5 minutes).* Perform a variety of stretching and balance exercises.

Source: Metcalfe L, Lohman T, Going S, Houtkooper L, Ferriera D, Flint-Wagner H, Guido T, Martin J, Wright J, Cussler E. Postmenopausal women and exercise for prevention of osteoporosis. The Bone, Estrogen, Strength Training (BEST) Study. *ACSM's Health & Fitness Journal* 5(3):6–14, 2001.

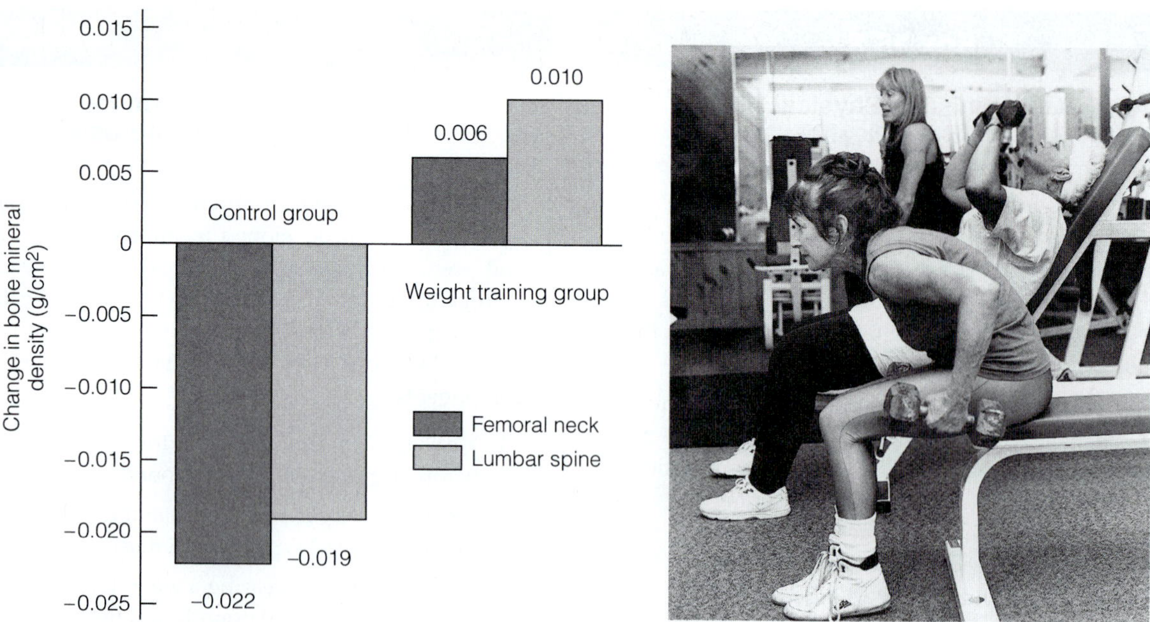

Figure 15.33 Changes in bone mineral density with intensive strength training, 1-year study: two weight training sessions/week, 45 minutes, high intensity. High-intensity weight training improved bone density in postmenopausal women. Source: Nelson ME, Fiatarone MA, Morganti CM, Trice I, Greenberg RA, Evans WJ. Effects of high-intensity strength training on multiple risk factors for osteoporotic fractures: A randomized controlled trial. *JAMA* 272:1909–1914, 1994.

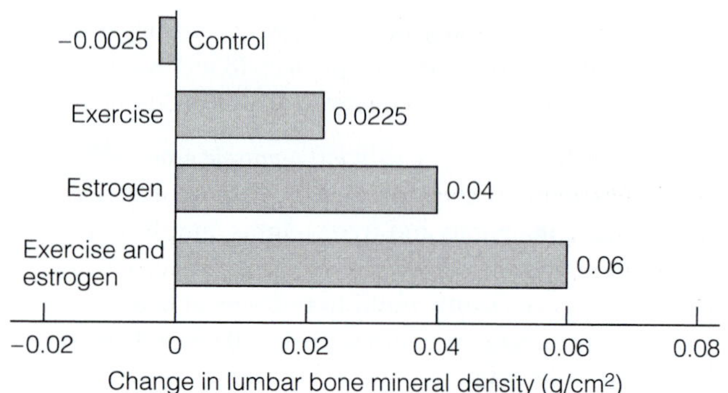

Figure 15.34 Changes in bone with weight-bearing exercise and estrogen, 1-year study: three to four walk/jog/stair-climb sessions/week, 50 minutes/session, high intensity; 32 women, 60–72 years of age. Weight-bearing exercise with estrogen can build lumbar bone density in postmenopausal women. Source: Kohrt WM, Snead DB, Slatopolsky E, Birge SJ. Additive effects of weight-bearing exercise and estrogen on bone mineral density in older women. *J Bone Min Res* 10:1303–1311, 1995.

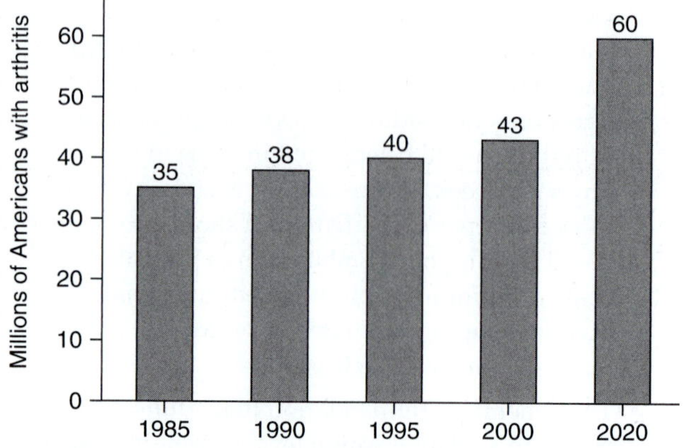

Figure 15.35 The number of Americans with arthritis will increase strongly during the next 2 decades. Source: Lawrence RC, Helmick CG, Arnett FC, et al. Estimates of the prevalence of arthritis and selected musculoskeletal disorders in the United States. *Arthritis and Rheumatism* 41:778–799, 1998.

ARTHRITIS

Arthritis and other rheumatic conditions are among the most prevalent chronic conditions in the United States, affecting an estimated 43 million persons in 2002 (one in five) and a projected 60 million by 2020, according to the Centers for Disease Control and Prevention[151–153] (see Figure 15.35). Another 23 million adults (11%) had possible arthritis but had not been diagnosed by a doctor. Women are affected by arthritis more than men—about 60% of people with arthritis are women and one-half of the elderly have been diagnosed with arthritis (see Figure 15.36). Arthritis is the number one cause of disability in America, and it limits everyday activities such as dressing, climbing stairs, getting in and out of bed, or walking, for about 8 million Americans.

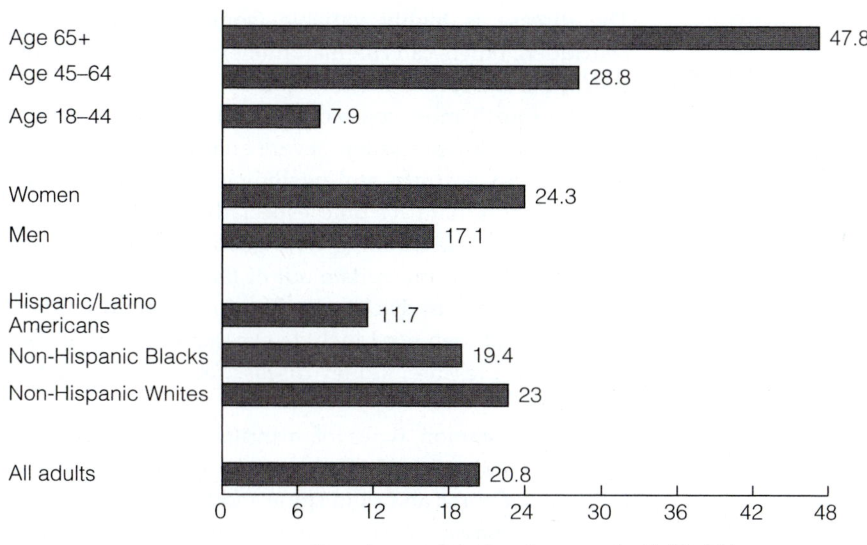

Figure 15.36 Arthritis is highly prevalent among the elderly, females, and whites. Source: CDC. Racial/ethnic differences in the prevalence and impact of doctor-diagnosed arthritis—United States, 2002. *MMWR* 54:119–123, 2005.

Common Types of Arthritis

Arthritis means joint inflammation, a general term that includes over 100 kinds of rheumatic diseases.[152,154,155] Rheumatic diseases are those affecting joints, muscles, and connective tissue, which make up or support various structures of the body. Arthritis is usually chronic and lasts a lifetime. The early warning signs of arthritis include pain, swelling, and limited movement that lasts for more than 2 weeks.

The most common type of arthritis is *osteoarthritis,* affecting about 21 million Americans[151–155] (see Figure 15.37). Although this degenerative joint disease is common among the elderly, it may appear decades earlier. Osteoarthritis begins when joint cartilage breaks down, sometimes eroding entirely to leave a bone-on-bone joint. The joint then loses shape, bone ends thicken, and spurs (bony growths) develop. Any joint can be affected, but the feet, knees, hips, and fingers are most common (see Figure 15.38). Osteoarthritis is not fatal, but it is incurable, with few effective treatments. Symptoms of pain and stiffness can persist for long periods of time, leading to difficulty in walking, stair climbing, rising from a chair, transferring in and out of a car, and lifting and carrying.

The second most common type of arthritis is *Fibromyalgia syndrome,* a condition with generalized muscular pain, fatigue, and poor sleep. It affects about 3.7 million Americans (see Figure 15.37). "Fibromyalgia" means pain in the muscles, ligaments, and tendons. Although it may feel like a joint disease, it is not a true form of arthritis and does not cause deformities of the joints.[154] Instead, fibromyalgia is a form of soft-tissue or muscular rheumatism.

The third most common form of arthritis is *rheumatoid arthritis,* an autoimmune disease that affects 2.1 million Americans, three times more women than men.[151–154,156] It can strike at any age, but usually appears between ages 20 and 50. Rheumatoid arthritis starts slowly over several weeks to months. The small joints of the hands and the knee joint are most commonly affected, but it can affect most joints of the body. Rheumatoid arthritis is frequently related to severe complications and decline in ability to function, with most patients dying 5–15 years earlier than those who are nonafflicted.

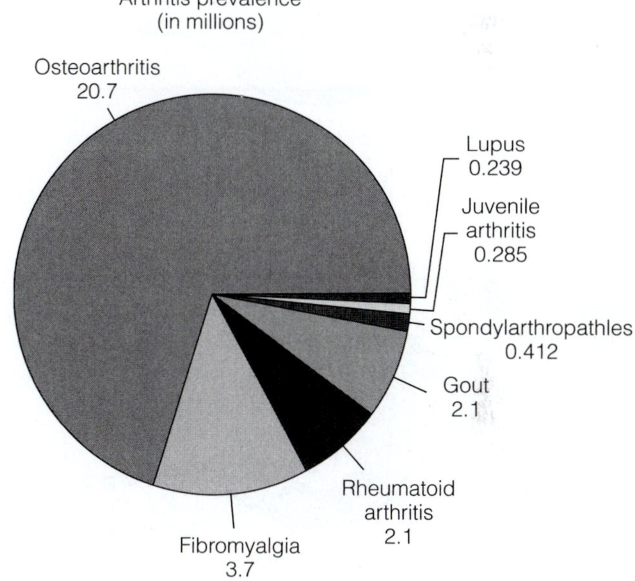

Figure 15.37 Osteoarthritis is the most common type of arthritis. Source: Arthritis Foundation. www.arthritis.org.

Many joints of the body have a tough capsule lined with a synovial membrane that seals the joint and provides a lubricating fluid. In rheumatoid arthritis, inflammation begins in the synovial lining of the joint and can spread to the entire joint. The inflamed joint lining leads to damage of the bone and cartilage. The space between joints diminishes, and the joint loses shape and alignment (see Figure 15.38).

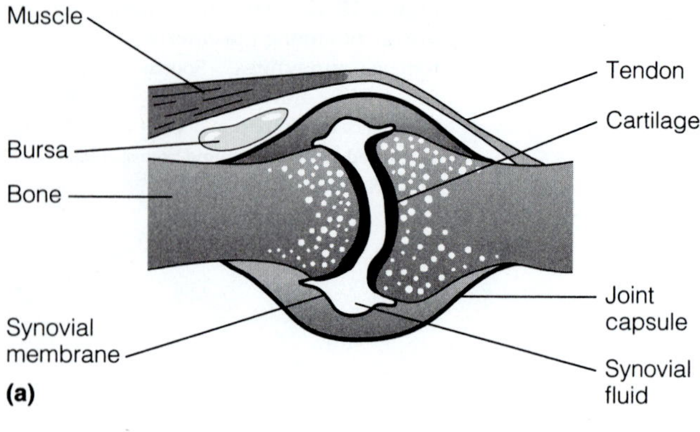

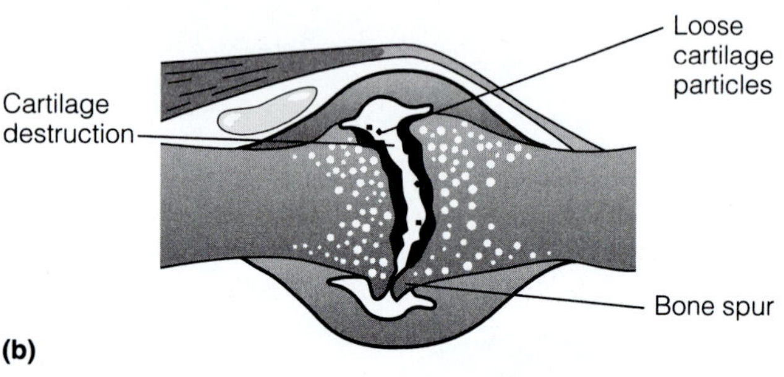

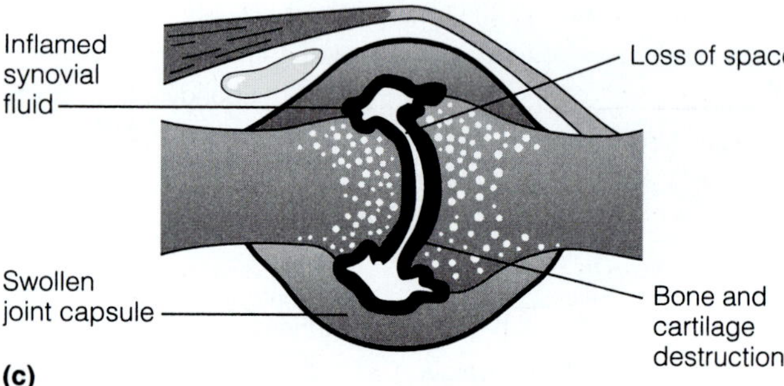

Figure 15.38 A comparison between a normal joint and joints with arthritis. (a) *Normal joint.* In a normal joint (where two bones come together), the muscle, bursa, and tendon support the bone and aid movement. The synovial membrane (an inner lining) releases a slippery fluid into the joint space. Cartilage covers the bone ends, absorbing shocks and keeping the bones from rubbing together when the joint moves. (b) *Osteoarthritis.* In osteoarthritis, cartilage breaks down and the bones rub together. The joint then loses shape and alignment. Bone ends thicken, forming spurs (bony growths). Bits of cartilage or bone float in the joint space. (c) *Rheumatoid arthritis.* In rheumatoid arthritis, inflammation accompanies thickening of the synovial membrane or joint lining, causing the whole joint to look swollen due to swelling in the joint capsule. The inflamed joint lining enters and damages bone and cartilage, and inflammatory cells release an enzyme that gradually digests bone and cartilage. Space between bones diminishes, and the joint loses shape and alignment. Source: Strange CJ. Coping with arthritis in its many forms. *FDA Consumer*, March 1996, 17–21.

The disease is highly variable (some patients become bedridden, others can run marathons) and difficult to control, and it can severely deform joints.

The fourth most common type of arthritis is gout, a disease that causes sudden, severe attacks of pain, tenderness, redness, warmth, and swelling in some joints. It usually affects one joint at a time, especially the joint of the big toe. The pain and swelling with gout are caused by uric acid crystals that precipitate out of the blood and are deposited in the joint. Factors leading to increased levels of uric acid and then gout include excessive alcohol intake, high blood pressure, kidney disease, obesity, and certain drugs.[152,154]

Other common types of arthritis include *ankylosing spondylitis* (inflammatory disease of the spine that can result in fused vertebrae and rigid spine and is a type of spondylarthropy), *juvenile arthritis* (involving 300,000 American children), *psoriatic arthritis* (affects about 5% of people with psoriasis, a chronic skin disease), and *systemic lupus erythematosous* (an autoimmune disorder that can involve skin, kidneys, blood vessels, joints, the nervous system, heart, and other internal organs).[152,154]

Risk Factors for Arthritis

According to the Centers for Disease Control (www.cdc.gov/arthritis), certain factors increase the risk of arthritis. Some of these risk factors are modifiable; others are not.

Nonmodifiable Risk Factors

- **Age:** The risk of developing most types of arthritis increases with age.
- **Gender:** Most types of arthritis are more common in women, accounting for 60% of all cases. Gout is more common in men.
- **Genetic:** Genes have been identified that are associated with a higher risk of certain types of arthritis, such as rheumatoid arthritis and systemic lupus erythematosous.

Modifiable Risk Factors

- **Overweight and Obesity:** Excess weight can contribute to both the onset and progression of knee osteoarthritis.
- **Joint Injuries:** Damage to a joint can contribute to the development of osteoarthritis of that joint.
- **Infection:** Many microbial agents can infect joints and potentially cause the development of various forms of arthritis.
- **Occupation:** Certain occupations involving repetitive knee bending are associated with osteoarthritis of the knee.

No cure for arthritis exists, so growing emphasis is being placed on prevention of arthritis. Obesity is the main preventable risk factor.[157] Obesity produces changes in chondrocytes (cartilage cells) that alter the synthesis and degradation of the hyaline cartilage, and increases levels of inflammatory cytokines that promote osteoarthritis. The National Arthritis Action Plan: A Public Health Strategy organized by the Arthritis Foundation and the Centers for Disease Control has identified weight management as a key strategy for the primary prevention of knee osteoarthritis in the general population (www.cdc.gov).

The link between diet and arthritis is still being investigated. Some studies suggest that higher intakes of red meat and total protein as well as lower intakes of fruit, vegetables, and vitamin C are associated with an increased risk of arthritis, and that the Mediterranean-type diet may have protective effects, but much more research is needed before a consensus can be established.[158]

As will be emphasized later in this chapter, keeping the muscles strong through regular exercise while avoiding traumatic joint injury is also an important preventive strategy. There is growing evidence that individuals who stay lean and fit as they grow older are at a much lower risk for the development of osteoarthritis compared to their obese and unfit counterparts. Thigh muscle weakness has emerged as a predictor of future knee osteoarthritis. As summarized in Figure 15.39, data from the Aerobics Center Longitudinal Study indicate that regular physical activity reduces the risk of hip and knee osteoarthritis, especially among women, after adjustment for age, body mass index, and history of hip and knee joint injury.[159]

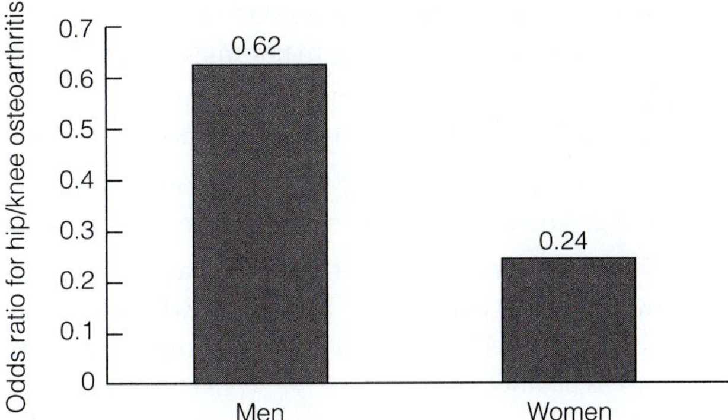

Figure 15.39 Odds ratio for hip/knee osteoarthritis was 38% lower in men and 76% lower in women who experienced moderate to high joint stress from physical activity compared to sedentary controls. Data are from the Aerobics Center Longitudinal Study. Source: Rogers LQ, Macera CA, Hootman JM, Ainsworth BE, Blair SN. The association between joint stress from physical activity and self-reported osteoarthritis: An analysis of the Cooper Clinic data. *Osteoarthritis Cartilage* 10:617–62, 2002.

Treatment

The key to treatment of arthritis is early diagnosis and a plan individualized to the needs of each patient.[152,154–156] Therapeutic treatment of arthritis has four major goals: easing of pain, decrease of painful inflammation, improvement in function, and lessening of joint damage. Most treatment programs include a combination of patient education, medication, exercise, rest, use of heat and cold, joint protection techniques, and sometimes surgery (for example, total hip replacement surgery). Total hip arthroplasty (THA) is commonly used to treat severe osteoarthritis of the hip.[160]

The Arthritis Foundation advises the following treatment options for arthritis (in addition to surgery, when indicated):[154]

- *Lifestyle changes.* Exercise to strengthen muscles, improve joint range of motion, and cardiorespiratory endurance; rest as needed to recover from exercise or during flares; a balanced diet; weight loss to reduce stress on joints.
- *Joint protection.* Learning ways to limit the pressure on involved joints so as not to add to the damage the joints may have already sustained because of disease.
- *Medications.* Many effective drugs are used to treat arthritis (see discussion later in chapter).
- *Physical and occupational therapy.* Therapists work to help people with arthritis make their lives easier (using exercises, applications of heat or cold, and instruction in self-help devices and other ways to make everyday activities easier and reduce joint strain).
- *Patient education.* Inform patients about the disease, provide them with tools to help overcome their pain, and help them adjust to their situation.

Arthritis symptoms come and go, with a worsening or reappearance of the disease called a *flare.* This can be followed by a remission period that brings welcome relief. The normal up-and-down nature of this painful, incurable disease has led to widespread fraud and quackery.[154] People with arthritis spend nearly 2 billion dollars a year on unproven remedies, largely diets and supplements. Arthritis patients have been lured by an astounding array of quack devices, including copper or magnetic bracelets, "electronic" mechanisms, vibrating chairs, pressurized enema devices, snake venom, and countless nutritional supplements, including cod liver oil, alfalfa, pokeberries, vinegar, iodine, and kelp. While some of these remedies seem harmless, they can become hurtful if they cause people to abandon conventional therapy.

Regarding diet, the FDA and American College of Rheumatology advise that until more data are available, patients should continue to follow balanced and healthy diets, be skeptical of "miraculous" claims, and avoid elimination diets and fad nutritional practices.[152] Gout is the only rheumatic disease known to be helped by avoiding certain foods, especially those high in purines such as wine, anchovies, and liver. Diets high in certain types of unsaturated fatty acids (omega-3 fatty acids, found in salmon, cod, halibut, and tuna) tend to lessen inflammation in some people with arthritis.[158] Two controversial nutritional supplements, glucosamine and chondroitin sulfate, are not approved by the FDA but are taken by millions of Americans because of claims that they rebuild joint tissues damaged by osteoarthritis.[152] Both glucosamine and chondroitin sulfate occur in the body naturally and are vital to normal cartilage formation, but there is no consistent evidence that, when ingested, these supplements are absorbed and deposited into the joints.[152,154]

Overweight persons are at high risk of osteoarthritis in the knees, hips, and hands.[157] For example, the heaviest Americans (those in the upper 20% of body weight) have 4–10 times greater risk of developing osteoarthritis of the knee than those of normal weight. Among U.S. adults, the prevalence of arthritis is 43.5% among the obese compared to 25.9% among those that are normal weight.[157] (See Figure 15.40.) Weight control is an important concern for people with arthritis to help decrease the pressure on the knees and hips.

There are many different kinds of drugs used to treat arthritis.[152,154,157] Anti-inflammatory agents generally work by slowing the body's production of prostaglandins, substances that play a role in inflammation. The most familiar anti-inflammatory agent is aspirin, often a good arthritis treatment. Acetaminophen is recommended as a first-line therapy, at doses up to 4,000 mg/day. More than a dozen nonsteroidal anti-inflammatory drugs (NSAIDS) are available, most by prescription only, which fight pain and inflammation. The FDA has approved three NSAIDS for over-the-counter marketing: ibuprofen (marketed as Advil, Nuprin, Motrin, and others), naproxen sodium (sold as Aleve), and ketoprofen (marketed as Actron and Orudis). See Box 15.10 for a review of medications used for arthritis, including an update on COX-2 inhibitors.[152]

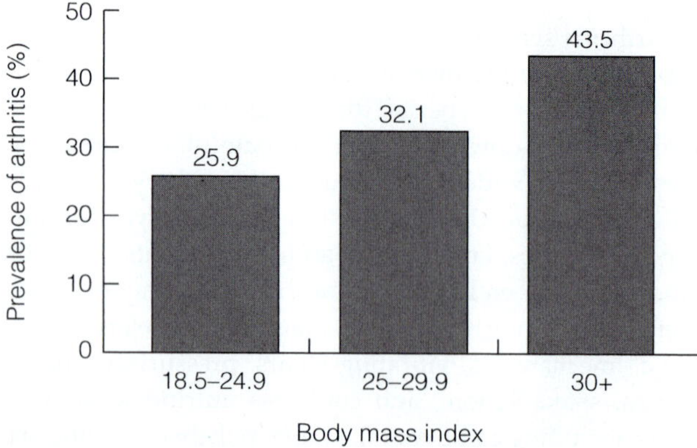

Figure 15.40 The prevalence of arthritis was significantly lower in normal-weight individuals compared to obese individuals. Data are from the Behavioral Risk Factor Surveillance System, with arthritis based on self-report of doctor diagnosis or chronic joint symptoms. Source: Mehrotra C, Naimi TS, Serdula M, Bolen J, Pearson K. Arthritis, body mass index, and professional advice to lose weight: Implications for clinical medicine and public health. *Am J Prev Med* 27:16–21, 2004.

The Role of Exercise

In the past, doctors often advised arthritis patients to rest and avoid exercise.[161–163] Rest remains important, especially during flares, but inactivity can lead to weak muscles, stiff joints, reduced joint range of motion, and decreased energy and vitality. Rheumatologists today routinely advise a balance of physical activity and rest, individualized to meet special patient needs.

Studies have consistently shown that people with arthritis are more physically inactive, have weaker muscles, less joint flexibility and range of motion, and lower aerobic capacity, compared to those without arthritis.[161] In addition, individuals with arthritis have been found to be at higher risk for several other chronic diseases, including coronary heart disease, diabetes mellitus, and osteoporosis. Thus, it makes sense that a well-rounded physical fitness program may be of benefit to those suffering from arthritis. Prior to initiating an exercise program, however, each patient should have an extensive evaluation to assess the severity and extent of joint involvement, presence of systemic involvement, overall functional capacity, and presence of other medical conditions that may interfere with exercise.[161]

The American College of Sports Medicine recommends the following exercise testing program for patients with arthritis:[161]

- *Muscular strength and endurance.* Use isokinetic machines at 90–120° per second to measure the strength and endurance of major muscle groups.
- *Aerobic endurance.* Various walking tests including the 6-minute walk or the 1-mile walk test.
- *Joint flexibility and range of motion.* Use a goniometer to measure joint range of motion. Assess asymmetry.
- *Neuromuscular fitness.* Gait analysis may be necessary for people who have severe disease, altered biomechanics, and a need for orthotics. Also assess balance.
- *Functional capacity.* Assess capacity to accomplish daily activities of living by observing ability to walk with balance and symmetry, ability to sit and then stand up several times, and ability to stand in one place without difficulty.

Individuals with arthritis will often respond to their pain by limiting their physical activity.[164] Over time, this leads to loss of muscle strength and endurance, which further weakens the joints and sets up a vicious cycle that

Box 15.10

U.S. Food and Drug Administration (FDA) Update on Medications for Arthritis

Most arthritis medications fall into three categories: those that relieve pain; those that reduce inflammation or the body process that causes swelling, warmth, and redness; and those that slow the disease process and limit further damage to the joints—so-called disease-modifying agents.[152]

COX-2 Inhibitors: The unsettling news in late 2004 that the popular anti-inflammatory arthritis drugs Vioxx (rofecoxib), Celebrex (celecoxib), and Bextra (valdecoxib) could cause a heart attack or stroke or aggravate high blood pressure has left some patients wondering whether they should keep taking them. Data from clinical trials showed that cyclooxygenase-2 selective agents, better known as COX-2 inhibitors, may be associated with an increased risk of serious cardiovascular problems, especially when used in high doses or for long periods in patients with existing cardiovascular disease, or in very high-risk situations, such as immediately after heart surgery. COX-2 inhibitors are the newest subset of nonsteroidal anti-inflammatory drugs (NSAIDs). COX-2 inhibitors were developed specifically to decrease the well-recognized gastric side effects and intolerance associated with the use of some NSAIDs. The agency has recommended, among other things, that physicians limit the use of COX-2 inhibitors until further review.

Other NSAIDs: Traditional NSAIDs, such as aspirin or ibuprofen, act by blocking the production of a family of chemicals known as prostaglandins, which are not only important in the development of inflammation, but also play an important role in maintaining the integrity of the stomach lining. At least two enzymes are involved in this inflammation, namely cyclooxygenase-1 (COX-1) and cyclooxygenase-2 (COX-2). Traditional NSAIDs inhibit both COX-1 and COX-2. Unfortunately, this nonselective inhibition of both COX enzymes also inhibits those prostaglandins involved in some of the important "housekeeping" functions of the body, such as helping blood to clot and protecting the stomach from ulceration. There is also growing concern that ibuprofen may increase risk of cardiovascular disease, similar to COX-2 inhibitors.

Pain Relivers: Pain relievers such as Tylenol (acetaminophen) and NSAIDs such as Motrin (ibuprofen) are used to reduce the pain caused by many rheumatic conditions. NSAIDs have the added benefit of decreasing the inflammation associated with arthritis.

DMARDs: Depending on the type of arthritis, a person may use a disease-modifying anti-rheumatic drug (DMARD). This category includes several unrelated medications that are intended to slow or stop disease progress and prevent disability and discomfort. DMARDs include Rheumatrex (methotrexate), Azulfidine (sulfasalazine), and Arava (leflunomide). Someone diagnosed with rheumatoid arthritis today is likely to be prescribed a DMARD fairly early in the course of the disease, as doctors have found that starting these drugs early can help prevent irreparable joint damage that might otherwise occur.

Corticosteroids: Corticosteroids, such as prednisone, cortisone, methylprednisolone, and hydrocortisone, are used to treat many rheumatic conditions because they decrease inflammation and suppress the immune system. The dosage of these medications will vary depending on the diagnosis and the patient. Corticosteroids can be given by mouth or by direct injection into a joint or tendon sheath.

Biologic Treatments: Biological products are a relatively new class of drugs used for the treatment of rheumatoid arthritis. Biologics differ from conventional drugs in that they are derived from living sources, such as cell culture systems. Conventional drugs are chemically synthesized. Of the four currently licensed biologics, three help reduce inflammation and structural damage of the joints by blocking a substance called tumor necrosis factor (TNF), a protein involved in immune system responses. Elevated levels of TNF are found in the synovial fluid of rheumatoid and some other arthritis patients. The first biologic to receive FDA approval for patients with moderate-to-severe RA was Enbrel (etanercept). Initially, it was taken twice weekly by injection, but a once-weekly preparation is now available. Enbrel has been shown to decrease pain and morning stiffness and improve joint swelling and tenderness. The two other TNF-blocking products approved to treat rheumatoid arthritis are Remicade (infliximab) and Humira (adalimumab). All three TNF blockers have been demonstrated to improve physical function in studies of at least 2 years in duration.

Source: Rados C. Helpful treatments keep people with arthritis moving. *FDA Consumer Magazine,* March–April, 2005.

accelerates arthritis. There are three objectives of exercise for patients with arthritis:[161–163]

- Preserve or restore range of motion and flexibility around each affected joint
- Increase muscle strength and endurance to enhance joint stability
- Increase aerobic conditioning to improve psychological mood state and decrease risk of disease.

As depicted in Figure 15.41, the exercise program should be organized according to the "exercise pyramid," with exercises to develop joint range of motion and flexibility providing the foundation.

- *Range-of-motion and stretching exercises.* Maintaining joint mobility is very important for all patients with arthritis. Loss of joint range of motion results in a tightening of surrounding tendons, muscles, and other tissues. Acutely inflamed joints should be put through gentle range-of-motion exercises several times per day, with the assistance of a therapist or trained family member. Overzealous stretching or improper technique can have harmful effects on a joint, especially if it is inflamed or is unstable. Utilizing a trained therapist to initially monitor and teach the patient proper technique is recommended. Once the joints become less inflamed, the patient can gradually build up to several sets of 10 repetitions daily of stretching and range-of-motion exercises.
- *Muscle strengthening.* Both isometric and isotonic strengthening exercises are recommended. Isometric exercises can build muscle strength without adverse effects on an acutely inflamed joint. Isotonic exercises (e.g., weight lifting, calisthenics) allow the joints to move through a limited or full range of motion while the muscles are contracting. This type of exercise is recommended when pain and joint inflammation have been controlled and sufficient strength has been achieved through isometric exercise.
- *Aerobic exercise.* In the past, the treatment of arthritis has often excluded aerobic exercise, for fear of increasing joint inflammation and accelerating the disease process. Aerobic exercise, however, has been demonstrated to be a safe and effective treatment for patients who are not in acute flares. Low-impact activities such as swimming, water aerobics, walking, bicycling, low-impact dance aerobics, and rowing can improve aerobic fitness without negatively affecting arthritis. Patients should start with 10–15 minutes of aerobic activity every other day, gradually progressing toward near-daily activity of 30–45 minutes duration at a moderate-to-somewhat-hard intensity. Each aerobic session should begin and end with range-of-motion exercises.
- *Recreational exercise.* Patients with arthritis commonly find golfing, gardening, hiking on gentle terrain, and other hobbies requiring physical activity enjoyable. Many organizations, including the Arthritis Foundation, offer aquatic exercise classes or other group activities. Patients may experience improvements in both fitness and psychological mood state as they engage in group recreational activities.

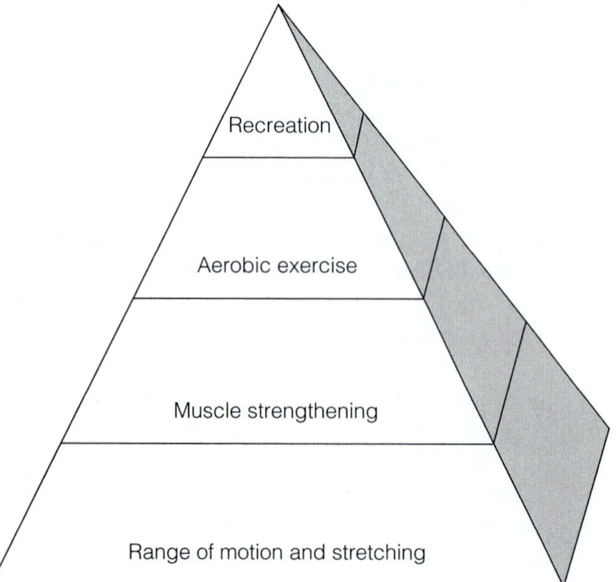

Figure 15.41 Exercise pyramid for patients with arthritis. Exercise treatment for patients with arthritis should be based on the exercise pyramid. Source: Hoffman DF. Arthritis and exercise. *Primary Care* 20:895–910, 1993.

Exercise Benefits

There are many potential benefits of exercise for the individual with arthritis:[161–163]

- Improvement in joint function and range of motion
- Increase in muscular strength and aerobic fitness to enhance activities of daily living
- Elevation of psychological mood state
- Decrease in loss of bone mass
- Decrease in risk of heart disease, diabetes, hypertension, and other chronic diseases

Can regular exercise improve, retard the progression of, or even cure arthritis? While exercise for people with arthritis is important for all the aforementioned reasons, investigators have typically found that exercise training does not improve arthritis, but neither does it worsen the disease process. In other words, exercise does not affect the underlying disease state in people with arthritis one way or the other, but it does improve many other areas of importance to life quality.[165–175]

In one study, researchers randomly divided 102 patients with osteoarthritis of the knee into walking and control groups.[169] Those in the walking group walked up to 30 minutes, three times a week, for 8 weeks. As shown in Figure 15.42, the walkers experienced a strong increase in their performance during a 6-minute walking test, an effect that was achieved without exacerbating pain or triggering flares. In other words, those with osteoarthritis became fitter with the exercise program, but their disease was neither reversed nor progressed.

In the 18-month FAST (Fitness Arthritis and Seniors Trial) study, 439 adults age 60 years or older, with osteoarthritis, were randomly divided into one of three groups: (1) health education (no exercise), (2) aerobic exercise (three 40-minute sessions per week), or (3) resistance exercise (three 40-minute sessions per week, with two sets of 12 repetitions of nine exercises).[167] As shown in Figure 15.43, the mean score on the physical disability questionnaire was significantly improved for both exercise groups. Other tests revealed lower pain scores and improved measures of performance with exercise. The researchers concluded that older disabled persons with osteoarthritis of the knee can experience modest improvements in measures of disability, physical performance, and pain as a result of participating in a regular exercise program.

Other researchers have come to the same conclusion: Patients with arthritis are trainable (i.e., they can get stronger and more aerobically fit), and the exercise can be done safely without detrimental effects on the joints and in most patients with osteoarthritis, symptoms diminish.[165–175] The combination of weight loss and exercise improves function and decreases joint pain better than either intervention alone.[165] However, the results show no effect of training on the disease activity or on the progression of the disease.

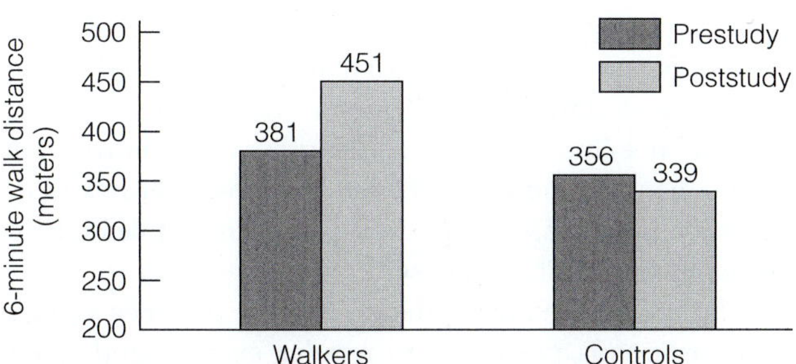

Figure 15.42 Supervised fitness walking in patients with osteoarthritis of the knee, 47 walkers compared to 45 controls after 8 weeks of training (three sessions/week, 90 minutes/session). Exercise training improves walking performance in patients with knee osteoarthritis. Source: Kovar PA, Allegrante JP, MacKenzie R, Peterson MGE, Gutin B, Charlson ME. Supervised fitness walking in patients with osteoarthritis of the knee. *Ann Intern Med* 116:529–534, 1992.

Potential Exercise Training Complications

There are several potential complications of exercise training for patients with arthritis:[161]

- Pain, stiffness, biomechanical inefficiency, and gait abnormalities can increase the metabolic cost of physical activity by as much as 50%. Patients with arthritis tend to be less physically fit than others, and as a result, gradual progression in exercise training is recommended.
- Joint range of motion may be restricted by stiffness, swelling, pain, bony changes, fibrosis, and ankylosis. The exercise program should be adapted to ensure joint protection and safety. The site and severity of joint involvement determines the activity mode for both exercise testing and prescription. Deconditioned and poorly supported joints are at high risk for injury from high-impact or poorly controlled movements.
- Many patients with arthritis are unable to perform rapid, repetitive movements. Exercise modes should be adapted to the individual patient to protect the involved joints.
- Depending on the type of arthritis, consideration should be given to the following complications:

  Osteoarthritis. Spinal stenosis (narrowing) and spondylosis (stiffening or fixation of the spinal bones, causes localized back pain and radiating pain)

  Rheumatoid arthritis. Cervical spine subluxation (cervical instability, spinal cord decompression, numbness, tingling, weakness), foot disease (foot pain and instability), wrist and hand disease (pain, instability, loss of grip strength)

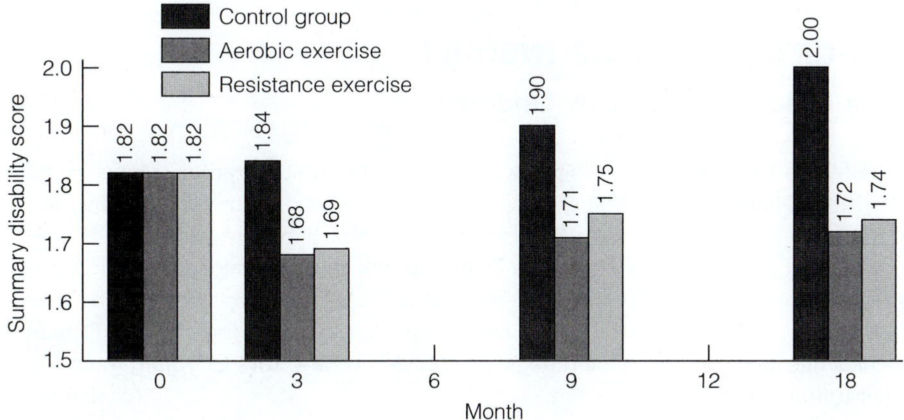

Figure 15.43 Influence of aerobic exercise and resistance exercise on physical disability, 18-month study of 365 older adults with knee osteoarthritis. Physical disability symptoms are reduced in adults with knee osteoporosis who exercise regularly. Source: Ettinger WH, Burns R, Messier SP, et al. A randomized trial comparing aerobic exercise and resistance exercise with a health education program in older adults with knee osteoarthritis: The fitness arthritis and seniors trial (FAST). *JAMA* 277:25–31, 1997.

Lupus. Necrosis (tissue death) of femoral head (hip pain, often associated with long-term corticosteroid use)

Osteoarthritis and Wear and Tear

Some clinicians have defined osteoarthritis as a "wear-and-tear" disease, and fear that high amounts of weight-bearing exercise may increase the risk for osteoarthritis.[163]

Early studies suggested that repetitive trauma to joints during work may lead to arthritis. For example, some studies reported increased osteoarthritis in the elbows and knees of miners, the shoulders and elbows of pneumatic drill operators, the hands of cotton workers and diamond cutters, and the spines of dock workers. However, not all of these studies were carried out to contemporary standards, nor have they been confirmed through replication.[163]

Many athletic endeavors place tremendous stress on joints. Baseball, football, basketball, gymnastics, soccer, wrestling, and ballet dancing have each been studied for their effect on osteoarthritis.[176–179] There are many anecdotal reports of famous athletes developing arthritis. Los Angeles Dodger Sandy Koufax, for example, was forced to retire from pitching in 1966 because of an arthritic elbow. However, most experts now feel that participation in vigorous exercise and sports does not increase the risk of osteoarthritis unless the involved joint has some sort of abnormality or previous major injury.[179] Normal joints are well designed to withstand the repetitive stress that comes with physical activity. Nonetheless, an injury to the joint alters its ability to handle exercise stress. Several studies of athletes with major knee injuries, for example, have shown that they are at increased risk of premature osteoarthritis.[179]

Long-distance runners have been studied more than any other type of athlete because of the long-term and repetitive stress they experience to joints of their legs. During running, two and one-half to three times the body weight is transmitted to the lower limbs at heel strike. The stresses that the feet and ankles do not absorb are shifted to the knees, hips, and spine. Despite the repetitive stress to their feet and legs, long-distance runners who train for many years do not appear to be at increased risk of osteoarthritis unless they have abnormal biomechanical problems or prior injuries in the hips, knees, or ankles.[177,178]

The injury rate among participants in many sports is quite high. Fortunately, most injuries appear to be limited, with no long-term consequences. If the injury leads to long-term joint instability, however, the risk for osteoarthritis climbs sharply.[179]

Knee pain is a common musculoskeletal symptom among adults, with a prevalence of 10 to 60% depending on age and the definition of knee pain.[180] Knee pain often occurs without osteoarthritis, and in one study, only 15% of individuals with knee pain had radiographic evidence of osteoarthritis.[181] Knee pain can be caused by conditions other than osteoarthritis including bursitis, tendinitis, meniscal lesions, and chondromalacia. A study of ~2,500 employees of a large Finnish forestry company showed that significant predictors of knee pain in adults included previous knee injuries (strongest predictor), a body mass index (BMI) of 26 and higher (indicating obesity), smoking, and job dissatisfaction.[180] In this study, neither the amount of general physical exercise nor the practicing of different types of sports was related to knee pain.

In a large prospective study of over 5,000 subjects, participation in physical activity as an adult did not increase the risk of hip or knee osteoarthritis, and among walkers and runners there was no association between the frequency, pace, or weekly training mileage.[182] In that study, older age, previous joint injury and surgery, and higher body mass index were confirmed as independent risk factors for knee/hip osteoarthritis. Another case-control study of 800 men and women in Finland showed that risk of osteoarthritis decreased with increasing cumulative hours of recreational physical exercise.[183]

For most individuals, the cartilage in the knee and hip joints responds positively to regular exercise and grows thicker. A study showed that in the absence of knee pain and injury, vigorous physical activity promotes the growth of articular cartilage.[184]

In summary, normal knee and hip joints (i.e., those without underlying biomechanical problems or prior traumatic injury) respond well to regular physical activity and do not "wear out."

SPORTS MEDICINE INSIGHT

A Case Study of Mavis Lindgren

The author has been gathering data on Mavis Lindgren, an elderly marathon runner, since 1985. Mavis was sedentary most of her life until age 63, when she began walking for her health. After a few months of slow progression, she started jogging 25–30 miles a week, a routine she faithfully kept for 7 years.

At the age of 70, in response to a challenge laid down by her physician son, she increased her training to 40–50 miles per week and ran her first marathon. Mavis found that she enjoyed the challenge of marathon running and the attention it brought her. Between the ages of 70 and 90, she ran 76 marathons and maintained a training distance of 40–50 miles a week. During this time, she became the oldest woman ever to race to the top of Pike's Peak in Colorado and to finish the New York City marathon.

(continued)

SPORTS MEDICINE INSIGHT *(continued)*

A Case Study of Mavis Lindgren

Figure 15.44 plots the race times for these marathons, as well as the results of 11 treadmill $\dot{V}O_{2max}$ tests that were conducted on Mavis between the ages of 77 and 90. There are several interesting points to be made, especially considering the information in this chapter.

- Between the ages of 80 and 83, Mavis's $\dot{V}O_{2max}$ fell rapidly and then plateaued, despite maintaining a training schedule of 40–50 miles a week. $\dot{V}O_{2max}$ decreased 44% between the ages of 77 and 90, which occurred during a period when her marathon race times increased by about 80%. There are probably several reasons explaining this loss of aerobic fitness and racing ability, including effects due to the aging process itself and a decline in ability to sustain a high training intensity despite unusually high motivation.
- Between the ages of 77 and 80, her $\dot{V}O_{2max}$ averaged about 38 ml · kg^{-1} · min^{-1}, an aerobic fitness level equal to that of untrained women in their 20s. Despite significant decreases in her aerobic power since age 77, Mavis still has the $\dot{V}O_{2max}$ of a woman about 25 years of age.

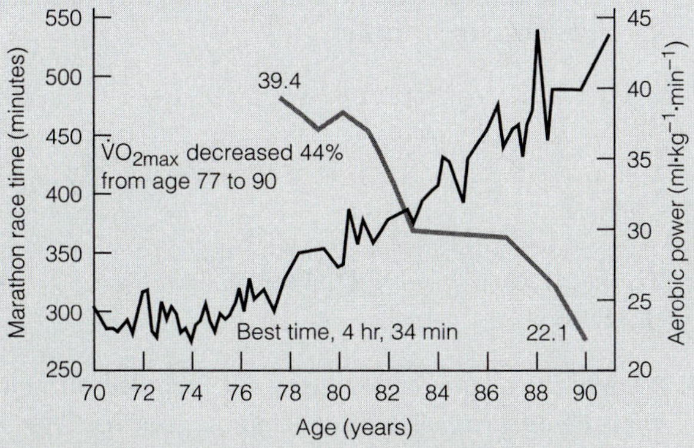

Figure 15.44 Mavis Lindgren's marathon times and aerobic power, 76 marathons from age 70–90; first treadmill test age 77, trained 40–50 miles/week each year since age 70. Mavis Lindgren ran 76 marathons between the ages of 70 and 90. Her race times slowed about 80% during a period in which her measured aerobic power fell 44%.

Mavis has demonstrated that it is never too late to start exercising, and that an unusually high $\dot{V}O_{2max}$ is possible even in old age when there is a motivation to engage in large amounts of exercise.

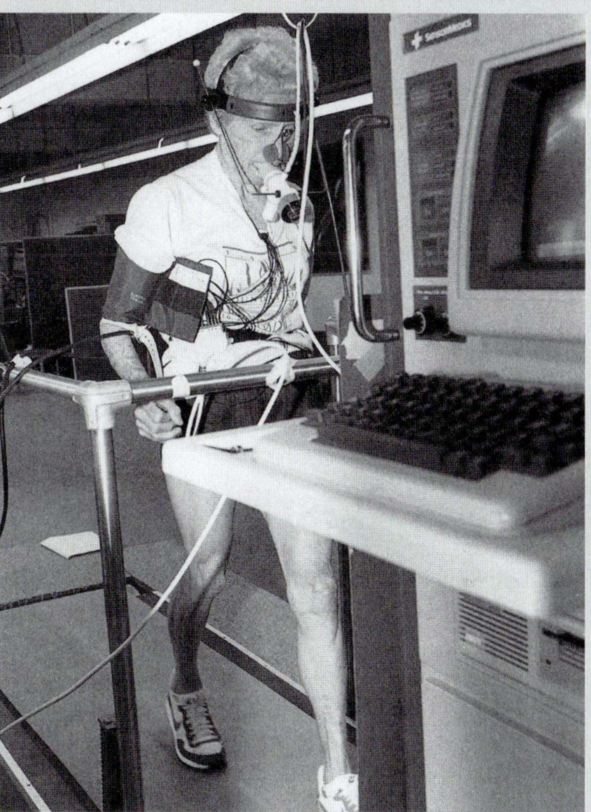

At the age of 80, Mavis Lindgren had the $\dot{V}O_{2max}$ capacity of a women nearly 60 years younger than herself.

SUMMARY

1. The ranks of the aged are increasing rapidly, as heart disease and stroke continue to decrease. The fastest-growing minority in the United States today is the elderly.
2. The average baby born today can expect to live to 77 years of age. Increases in life expectancy at birth during the first half of the twentieth century occurred mainly because of reductions in infant mortality, and recently because of decreasing mortality from chronic diseases.
3. Prominent aging-related concerns include the quality of life in old age, the high prevalence of chronic diseases, osteoporosis, and senile dementia among the elderly, and the financial impact of those problems.
4. Aging refers to the normal yet irreversible biological changes that occur during the total years that a person lives. The maximum life span of the human species is thought to be about 120 years. There are several theories of aging, including the damage and the program

theories. As a person ages, many changes take place in the body (summarized in the text). Health habits have a major influence on life expectancy.

5. There is great similarity between the physiological changes that accompany aging and those that accompany inactivity. The identifying characteristics of both aging and the disuse syndrome are a decrease in cardiorespiratory function, obesity, musculoskeletal fragility, and (among the inactive) premature aging.
6. Most researchers who have evaluated the effects of aging on the cardiorespiratory system have focused on work capacity, or $\dot{V}O_{2max}$. $\dot{V}O_{2max}$ normally declines 8–10% per decade for both males and females after 25 years of age.
7. Declining physical activity and changes in body composition are responsible in part for the low $\dot{V}O_{2max}$ in old age.
8. The elderly can recapture decades worth of $\dot{V}O_{2max}$ with appropriate (gradual) training.
9. The data suggest that the overall rate of loss of cardiorespiratory function is similar for active and inactive people, but that at any given age, the active conserve more function.
10. Several studies suggest that the elderly can respond to physical training over an 8- to 26-week period in a manner expected of younger people.
11. In general, the same basic exercise prescription principles used for younger adults can be applied for the elderly, but with greater caution and slower progression.
12. Regular physical activity can have a beneficial impact on life expectancy by reducing the life-shortening effects of the various chronic diseases.
13. Osteoporosis is characterized by decreased bone mass and increased susceptibility to fractures. The mainstays of treatment include estrogen replacement, adequate lifelong calcium intake, and appropriate exercise.
14. Weightlessness and bed rest can cause a dramatic loss in bone mass. Cross-sectional studies show that athletes have denser bones than sedentary people. Some studies show that postmenopausal women can retard bone mineral mass loss, or even increase bone density, with appropriate exercise, especially resistance training.
15. Arthritis (joint inflammation) includes over 100 kinds of rheumatic diseases. Two common types of arthritis are osteoarthritis and rheumatoid arthritis.
16. Based on existing research, professionals recommend a comprehensive physical fitness program designed to improve joint range of motion and flexibility, muscular strength and endurance, and aerobic endurance, all of which are individualized to the patient's special needs and goals. This program is safe and effective and improves quality of life but does not cure arthritis.

Review Questions

1. *The central issue raised by increasing longevity is that of*

   A. Financing the health care of the elderly
   B. Quality of life
   C. Cardiovascular disease
   D. Cancer

2. *What percent of the average American's life is spent in an unhealthy state (impaired by disabilities, injuries, or disease)?*

   A. 15 B. 5 C. 35 D. 50 E. 25

3. *Which of the following statements regarding $\dot{V}O_{2max}$ is true?*

   A. Decreases with increase in age at approximately similar rates in both sedentary and athletic groups
   B. Can be increased in young but not elderly adults
   C. Can be maintained throughout life
   D. Decreases 1% per decade of life

4. *Muscular strength peaks in the ____ decade of life.*

   A. First B. Second
   C. Third D. Fourth
   E. Fifth

5. *Which one of the following is* **not** *included in the top three leading causes of "years of potential life" lost before age 75 years?*

   A. Cancer B. Heart disease
   C. Injuries D. HIV

6. ____ *osteoporosis may develop at any age as a consequence of hormonal, digestive, and metabolic disorders.*

   A. Primary B. Secondary

7. *Peak bone mass is achieved between the ages of ____.*

   A. 15–20 B. 20–30
   C. 35–40 D. 40–50
   E. 50–60

8. *Osteoporosis afflicts ____ million Americans.*

   A. 2 B. 4
   C. 6 D. 10
   E. 20

9. *Which one of the following is* **not** *considered to be a risk factor that is associated with increased risk of osteoporosis?*

   A. Age **B.** Bed rest
   C. Obesity **D.** Excessive use of alcohol
   E. Removal of ovaries

10. *Which athlete listed is most likely to have the lowest bone density?*

    A. Swimmer **B.** Runner
    C. Weight lifter **D.** Soccer player

11. *Even after menopause when loss of bone mass is greatest, women ____ retard bone mineral mass loss with appropriate levels of vigorous, weight-bearing exercise.*

    A. Cannot **B.** Can

12. *The loss of muscle strength and size that usually accompanies increase in age ____ be reduced or even reversed with appropriate weight training programs.*

    A. Can **B.** Cannot

13. *Which type of person listed would be* **least** *likely to develop osteoporosis?*

    A. Thin, inactive, Caucasian elderly woman who smokes
    B. Obese African American man who exercises and avoids alcohol and tobacco
    C. Obese Caucasian woman
    D. Thin African American woman who exercises

14. *Which type of person listed below would be* **most** *likely to develop osteoporosis?*

    A. Thin, inactive, Caucasian elderly woman who smokes
    B. Obese African American man who exercises and avoids alcohol and tobacco
    C. Obese Caucasian woman
    D. Thin African American woman who exercises

15. *The term ____ is used to represent the loss of muscle mass and strength that occurs with normal aging.*

    A. Osteopenia **B.** Progressive resistance
    C. Sarcopenia **D.** Hypertrophy

16. *Life expectancy at birth is now about ____ years for the average American.*

    A. 57 **B.** 65 **C.** 85 **D.** 91 **E.** 77

17. *Which one of the following is* **not** *true regarding changes in the body with aging?*

    A. Increase in lean body weight
    B. Loss of bone mineral mass
    C. Decrease in gastrointestinal function
    D. Loss of taste and smell
    E. Decrease in heart and lung fitness

18. *$\dot{V}O_{2max}$ normally declines ____% per decade for both males and females.*

    A. 1–2 **B.** 4–6
    C. 8–10 **D.** 15–20
    E. 20–25

19. *Resistance training studies with older individuals support which one of the following findings?*

    A. Counters sarcopenia
    B. Decreases neural activation of trained muscles
    C. Decreases metabolic resting rate
    D. Builds intra-abdominal fat
    E. Increases fall risk

20. *There are several physiological changes that occur with aging. Which one of the following normally increases with age (in contrast to others which decrease)?*

    A. Basal metabolic rate
    B. Taste, smell, hearing, and vision
    C. Muscle strength
    D. Bone mineral mass
    E. Blood pressure

21. *The World Health Organization defines osteoporosis as bone density ____ standard deviations below the mean for young adult Caucasian women.*

    A. 2.5 **B.** 1 **C.** 4 **D.** 2 **E.** 0.5

22. *When a female athlete loses her menstrual period, and then experiences a loss in bone mass, this is classified as ____ osteoporosis.*

    A. Primary, type 1 **B.** Secondary
    C. Primary, type 2 **D.** Tertiary

23. *____ is a type of arthritis with generalized muscular pain, fatigue, and poor sleep, and affects about 3.7 million Americans.*

    A. Osteoarthritis
    B. Fibromyalgia syndrome
    C. Rheumatoid arthritis
    D. Gout
    E. Psoriatic arthritis

24. *Which one of the following is* **not** *a good source of calcium?*

    A. Low-fat dairy products
    B. Red meat
    C. Dark-green vegetables
    D. Nuts and seeds
    E. Legumes

25. *Half of the age-related decline in the aerobic power with age is due to changes in body composition and*

A. Exercise habits B. Gastrointestinal function
C. Sensory loss D. Cognitive decline
E. Depression

26. *The RMR decreases ____% per decade starting at about age 20.*

A. 1–2 B. 5–10 C. 10–15 D. 15–20

27. *About ____% of the elderly suffer from at least one chronic disease.*

A. 25 B. 45 C. 55 D. 75 E. 88

28. *In the Breslow study of 6,000 people in the San Francisco Bay area, those who followed all seven of the health habits had lower death rates and were estimated to live ____ years longer on average than those not following any of them.*

A. 3 B. 9 C. 12 D. 18 E. 25

29. *National surveys indicate that ____% of elderly men are inactive, more than any other age group.*

A. 10 B. 15 C. 49 D. 60 E. 75

30. *____ is the only rheumatic disease known to be helped by avoiding certain foods, especially those high in purines.*

A. Osteoarthritis
B. Fibromyalgia syndrome
C. Rheumatoid arthritis
D. Gout
E. Psoriatic arthritis

31. *Muscle strength in most individuals is well preserved until about ____ years of age, but then deteriorates by about 5–10% per decade thereafter.*

A. 25 B. 35 C. 45 D. 65 E. 80

32. *The loss in ____ appears to be the major reason why strength is decreased among the elderly.*

A. Muscle cell size B. Muscle cell number
C. Neither A or B D. Both A and B

33. *The acceleration of bone loss that occurs when estrogen levels fall after menopause is called ____ osteoporosis.*

A. Secondary B. Primary, type I
C. Primary, type II

34. *Cells that break down bone are called ____.*

A. Osteoclasts B. Osteoblasts

35. *Bone mass is approximately 30% higher in ____ compared to the opposite gender.*

A. Women B. Men

36. *Once peak bone mass is reached, osteoclast and osteoblast activity remain in balance until about age ____.*

A. 30–35 B. 35–45
C. 45–50 D. 50–60
E. 60–70

37. *Which of the following has the greatest effect on bone mass in postmenopausal women?*

A. Calcium supplements
B. Exercise
C. Estrogen replacement therapy

38. *In general, all the studies together indicate that the most active or fit individuals experience death rates that are ____% lower than the rates among those least active or fit.*

A. 20–50 B. 100–200
C. 10–15 D. 75–90
E. 50–75

39. *About ____% of the adult bone mineral content is deposited by the end of adolescence.*

A. 10 B. 25
C. 50 D. 75
E. 98

40. *Children and youth between the ages of 9 and 18 are recommended to take in ____ mg of calcium per day.*

A. 500 B. 1,000
C. 1,300 D. 2,000
E. 2,500

41. *Arthritis is more prevalent among*

A. Men B. Women

42. *The most common type of arthritis is*

A. Rheumatoid arthritis
B. Osteoarthritis
C. Gout
D. Lupus
E. Psoriatic arthritis

43. *Arthritis and other rheumatic conditions are among the most prevalent chronic conditions in the United States, affecting an estimated one in*

A. 7 **B.** 2
C. 10 **D.** 15
E. 20

44. *Any joint can be affected in arthritis, but the feet, knees, ____, and fingers are most commonly affected.*

A. Neck **B.** Hips
C. Toes **D.** Ankles
E. Spine

45. *Which type of arthritis is defined as a metabolic disorder leading to high uric acid and crystal formation in joints?*

A. Ankylosing spondylitis
B. Juvenile arthritis
C. Psoriatic arthritis
D. Gout
E. Systemic lupus erythematosous

46. *Low-fat, high-fiber diets have proven to be very useful in the treatment of all forms of arthritis.*

A. True **B.** False

47. *Overweight persons are at high risk of osteoarthritis in the knee, hips, and hands.*

A. True **B.** False

48. *Studies have consistently shown that people with arthritis have weaker muscles, less joint flexibility and range of motion, and lower aerobic capacity compared to those without arthritis.*

A. True **B.** False

49. *Which one of the following is* **not** *included in the arthritis exercise pyramid?*

A. Competitive sports
B. Range of motion and stretching exercises
C. Muscle strengthening
D. Aerobic exercise
E. Recreational exercise

50. *There are many potential benefits of exercise for the individual with arthritis. Which one of the following is not included?*

A. Improvement in joint function and range of motion
B. Increase in muscular strength and aerobic fitness to enhance activities of daily living
C. Elevation of psychological mood state
D. Cure of autoimmune basis for arthritis
E. Decrease in risk of heart disease, diabetes, hypertension, and other chronic diseases

Answers

1. B	**26.** A
2. A	**27.** E
3. A	**28.** B
4. C	**29.** C
5. D	**30.** D
6. B	**31.** C
7. B	**32.** D
8. D	**33.** B
9. C	**34.** A
10. A	**35.** B
11. B	**36.** C
12. A	**37.** C
13. B	**38.** A
14. A	**39.** E
15. C	**40.** C
16. E	**41.** B
17. A	**42.** B
18. C	**43.** A
19. A	**44.** B
20. E	**45.** D
21. A	**46.** B
22. A	**47.** A
23. B	**48.** A
24. B	**49.** A
25. A	**50.** D

REFERENCES

1. U.S. Department of Health and Human Services. *Healthy People 2010.* Washington DC: January, 2000. http:/www.health.gov/healthypeople/.
2. Centers for Disease Control and Prevention. Surveillance for selected public health indicators affecting older adults—United States. *CDC Surveillance Summaries,* December 17, 1999, *MMWR* 48(No. SS-8), 1999; Public health and aging: Trends in aging—United States and Worldwide. *MMWR* 52(06):101–106, 2003.
3. Arias E. United States life tables, 2002. *National Vital Statistics Reports* 53(6). Hyattsville, MD: National Center for Health Statistics, 2004.
4. CDC and the Merck Institute of Aging and Health. *The State of Aging and Health in America, 2004.* www.cdc.gov/aging; www.miahonline.org. See also: American Association for World Health. *Healthy Aging, Healthy Living—Start Now!* Washington, DC: Author, 1999.
5. Wagener DK, Molla MT, Crimmins EM, Pamuk E, Madans JH. Summary measures of population health: Addressing the first goal of healthy people 2010, improving health expectancy. *Statistical Notes,* no. 22. Hyattsville, MD: National Center for Health Statistics, September, 2001.

6. National Center for Health Statistics. *Health, United States, 1999,* and *Health and Aging Chartbook.* Hyattsville, MD: 1999; *Health United States, 2004.* Hyattsville, MD: 2004.
7. Hoffman C, Rice D, Sung HY. Persons with chronic conditions. Their prevalence and costs. *JAMA* 276:1473–1479, 1996.
8. Liao Y, McGee DL, Cao G, Cooper RS. Quality of the last year of life of older adults: 1986 vs 1993. *JAMA* 283:512–518, 2000.
9. Lubitz J, Beebe J, Baker C. Longevity and medicare expenditures. *N Engl J Med* 332:999–1003, 1995.
10. Hoyert DL, Rosenberg HM. Mortality from Alzheimer's disease: An update. *National Vital Statistics Reports* 47(20). Hyattsville, MD: National Center for Health Statistics, 1999.
11. Willcox SM, Himmelstein DU, Woolhandler S. Inappropriate drug prescribing for the community-dwelling elderly. *JAMA* 272:292–296, 1994.
12. Banks DA, Fossel M. Telomeres, cancer, and aging. Altering the human life span. *JAMA* 278:1345–1348, 1997.
13. Weinert BT, Timiras PS. Invited review: Theories of aging. *J Appl Physiol* 95:1706–1716, 2003.
14. Kirkwood TBL. Comparative life spans of species: Why do species have the life spans they do? *Am J Clin Nutr* 55:1191S-1195S, 1992.
15. Schiffman SS. Taste and smell losses in normal aging and disease. *JAMA* 278:1357–1362, 1997.
16. Wilson MM, Morley JE. Invited review: Aging and energy balance. *J Appl Physiol* 95:1728–1736, 2003.
17. Shiraki K, Sagawa S, Yousef MK. *Physical Fitness and Health Promotion in Active Aging.* Leiden, The Netherlands: Backhuys Publishers, 2001.
18. Russell RM. Changes in gastrointestinal function attributed to aging. *Am J Clin Nutr* 55:1203S–1207S, 1992.
19. Doherty TJ. Invited review: Aging and sarcopenia. *J Appl Physiol* 95:1717–1727, 2003.
20. Bernarducci MP, Owens NJ. Is there a fountain of youth? A review of current life extension strategies. *Pharmacotherapy* 16:183–200, 1996.
21. Heilbronn LK, Ravussin E. Calorie restriction and aging: Review of the literature and implications for studies in humans. *Am J Clin Nutr* 78:361–369, 2003.
22. LaCroix AZ, Guralnik JM, Berkman LF, Wallace RB, Satterfield S. Maintaining mobility in late life. II. Smoking, alcohol consumption, physical activity, and body mass index. *Am J Epidemiol* 137:858–869, 1993.
23. Campbell AJ, Busby WJ, Robertson MC. Over 80 years and no evidence of coronary heart disease: Characteristics of a survivor group. *J Am Geriatr Soc* 41:1333–1338, 1993.
24. Reed DM, Foley DJ, White LR, Heimovitz H, Burchfiel CM, Masaki K. Predictors of healthy aging in men with high life expectancies. *Am J Public Health* 88:1463–1468, 1998.
25. Breslow L, Breslow N. Health practices and disability: Some evidence from Alameda County. *Prev Med* 22:86–95, 1993.
26. Enstrom JE, Kanim LE, Breslow L. The relationship between vitamin C intake, general health practices, and mortality in Alameda County, California. *Am J Public Health* 76:1124–1130, 1986.
27. Stamler J, Stamler R, Neaton JD, Wentworth D, Daviglus ML, Garside D, Dyer AR, Liu K, Greenland P. Low risk-factor profile and long-term cardiovascular and noncardiovascular mortality and life expectancy. Findings for 5 large cohorts of young adult and middle-aged men and women. *JAMA* 282:2012–2018, 1999.
28. Vita AJ, Terry RB, Hubert HB, Fries JF. Aging, health risks, and cumulative disability. *N Engl J Med* 338:1035–1041, 1998.
29. Paffenbarger RS, Lee IM. Physical activity and fitness for health and longevity. *Res Quart Exerc Sport* 67(suppl):11–28, 1996.
30. Mazzeo RS, Cavanagh P, Evans WJ, Fiatarone M, Hagberg J, McAuley E, Startzell J. Position Stand from the American College of Sports Medicine. Exercise and physical activity for older adults. *Med Sci Sports Exerc* 30:992–1008, 1998.
31. Yusuf HR, Croft JB, Giles WH, Anda RF, Casper ML, Caspersen CJ, Jones DA. Leisure-time physical activity among older adults. United States, 1990. *Arch Intern Med* 156:1321–1326, 1996.
32. DiPetro L. The epidemiology of physical activity and physical function in older people. *Med Sci Sports Exerc* 28:596–600, 1996.
33. Shephard RJ, Kavanagh T, Mertens DJ, Qureshi S, Clark M. Personal health benefits of masters athletics competition. *Br J Sport Med* 29:35–40, 1995.
34. Convertino VA, Bloomfield SA, Greenleaf JE. An overview of the issues: Physiological effects of bed rest and restricted physical activity. *Med Sci Sports Exerc* 29:187–190, 1997.
35. Nair KS. Aging muscle. *Am J Clin Nutr* 81:953–963, 2005.
36. Westerterp KR. Daily physical activity and aging. *Curr Opin Clin Nutr Metab Care* 3:485–488, 2000.
37. Elia M, Ritz P, Stubbs RJ. Total energy expenditure in the elderly. *Eur J Clin Nutr* 54(suppl 3):S92–S103, 2000.
38. Heath GW, Hagberg JM, Ehsani AA, Holloszy JO. A physiological comparison of young and older endurance athletes. *J Appl Physiol* 51:634–640, 1981.
39. Nieman DC, Pover NK, Segebartt KS, Arabatzis K, Johnson M, Dietrich SJ. Hematological, anthropometric, and metabolic comparisons between active and inactive healthy old old to very old women. *Ann Sports Med* 5:2–8, 1990.
40. Wilson TM, Tanaka H. Meta-analysis of the age-associated decline in maximal aerobic capacity in men: Relation to training status. *Am J Physiol Heart Circ Physiol* 278:H829–H834, 2000.
41. Jackson AS, Beard EF, Wier LT, Ross RM, Stuteville JE, Blair SN. Changes in aerobic power of men, ages 25–70 yr. *Med Sci Sports Exerc* 27:113–120, 1995.
42. Jackson AS, Wier LT, Ayers GW, Beard EF, Stuteville JE, Blair SN. Changes in aerobic power of women, ages 20–64 yr. *Med Sci Sports Exerc* 28:884–891, 1996.
43. Fitzgerald MD, Tanaka H, Tran ZV, Seals DR. Age-related declines in maximal aerobic capacity in regularly exercising vs. sedentary women: A meta-analysis. *J Appl Physiol* 83:160–165, 1997.
44. Joth MJ, Gardner AW, Ades PA, Poehlman ET. Contribution of body composition and physical activity to age related decline in peak $\dot{V}O_{2max}$ in men and women. *J Appl Physiol* 77:647–652, 1994.
45. Warren BJ, Nieman DC, Dotson RG, Adkins CH, O'Donnell KA, Haddock BL, Butterworth DE. Cardiorespiratory responses to exercise training in septuagenarian women. *Int J Sports Med* 14:60–65, 1993.
46. Paterson DH, Cunningham DA, Koval JJ, St. Croix CM. Aerobic fitness in a population of independently living men and women aged 55–86 years. *Med Sci Sports Exerc* 31:1813–1820, 1999.
47. Lemura LM, Von Duvillard SP, Mookerjee S. The effects of physical training on functional capacity in adults. Ages 46 to 90: A meta-analysis. *J Sports Med Phys Fitness* 40:1–10, 2000.

48. Trappe SW, Costill DL, Vukovich MD, Jones J, Melham T. Aging among elite distance runners: A 22–yr longitudinal study. *J Appl Physiol* 80:285–290, 1996.
49. Pollock ML, Mengelkoch LJ, Graves JE, Lowenthal DT, Limacher MC, Foster C, Wilmore JH. Twenty-year follow-up of aerobic power and body composition of older track athletes. *J Appl Physiol* 82:1508–1516, 1997.
50. Hagerman FC, Fielding RA, Fiatarone MA, Gault JA, Kirkendall DT, Ragg KE, Evans WJ. A 20–yr longitudinal study of olympic oarsmen. *Med Sci Sports Exerc* 28:1150–1156, 1996.
51. Stevenson ET, Davy KP, Seals DR. Maximal aerobic capacity and total blood volume in highly trained middle-aged and older female endurance athletes. *J Appl Physiol* 77:1691–1696, 1994.
52. Tanaka H, Seals DR. Age and gender interactions in physiological functional capacity: Insight from swimming performance. *J Appl Physiol* 82:846–851, 1997.
53. Green JS, Crouse SF. The effects of endurance training on functional capacity in the elderly: A meta-analysis. *Med Sci Sports Exerc* 27:920–926, 1995.
54. Jubrias SA, Esselman PC, Price LB, Cress ME, Conley KE. Large energetic adaptations of elderly muscle to resistance and endurance training. *J Appl Physiol* 90:1663–1670, 2001.
55. Wiebe CG, Gledhill N, Jamnik VK, Ferguson S. Exercise cardiac function in young through elderly endurance trained women. *Med Sci Sports Exerc* 31:684–691, 1999.
56. Hawkins SA, Marcell TJ, Jaque SV, Wiswell RA. A longitudinal assessment of change in $\dot{V}O_{2max}$ and maximal heart rate in master athletes. *Med Sci Sports Exerc* 33:1744–1750, 2001.
57. Tanaka H, Seals DR. Invited review: Dynamic exercise performance in Masters athletes: Insight into the effects of primary human aging on physiological functional capacity. *J Appl Physiol* 95:2152–2162, 2003.
58. Schultz R, Curnow C. Peak performance and age among superathletes: Track and field, swimming, baseball, tennis, and golf. *J Gerontol* 43:P113–120, 1988.
59. deJong AA, Franklin BA. Prescribing exercise for the elderly: Current research and recommendations. *Curr Sports Med Rep* 3:337–343, 2004. See also: Mazzeo RS, Tanaka H. Exercise prescription for the elderly: Current recommendations. *Sports Med* 31:809–818, 2001.
60. Gass G, Gass E, Wicks J, Browning J, Bennett G, Morris N. Rate and amplitude of adaptation to two intensities of exercise in men aged 65–75 yr. *Med Sci Sports Exerc* 36:1811–1818, 2004.
61. MaKrides L, Heigenhauser GJF, Jones NL. High-intensity endurance training in 20- to 30- and 60- to 70-yr-old healthy men. *J Appl Physiol* 69:1792–1798, 1990.
62. Hagberg JM, Graves JE, Limacher M, et al. Cardiovascular responses of 70- to 79-yr-old men and women to exercise training. *J Appl Physiol* 66:2589–2594, 1989.
63. Kohrt WM, Malley MT, Coggan AR, et al. Effects of gender, age, and fitness level on response of $\dot{V}O_{2max}$ to training in 60–71 yr olds. *J Appl Physiol* 71:2004–2011, 1991.
64. Coudert J, Van Praagh E. Endurance exercise training in the elderly: Effects on cardiovascular function. *Curr Opin Clin Nutr Metab Care* 3:479–483, 2000.
65. Spina RJ, Ogawa T, Kohrt WM, Martin WH, Holloszy JO, Ehsani AA. Differences in cardiovascular adaptations to endurance exercise training between older men and women. *J Appl Physiol* 75:849–855, 1993.
66. Pollock ML, Carroll JF, Graves JE, et al. Injuries and adherence to walk/jog and resistance training programs in the elderly. *Med Sci Sports Exerc* 23:1194–1200, 1991.
67. Zauber N, Zauber A. Hematologic data of healthy very old people. *JAMA* 257:2181–2184, 1987.
68. Vandervoot AA, Symons TB. Functional and metabolic consequences of sarcopenia. *Can J Appl Physiol* 26:90–101, 2001.
69. Going S, Williams D, Lohman T. Aging and body composition: Biological changes and methodological issues. *Exerc Sport Sci Rev* 23:411–455, 1995.
70. Brill PA, Macera CA, Davis DR, Blair SN, Gordon N. Muscular strength and physical function. *Med Sci Sports Exerc* 32:412–416, 2000.
71. Hurley BF, Roth SM. Strength training in the elderly. Effects on risk factors for age-related diseases. *Sports Med* 30:249–268, 2000.
72. Seynnes O, Fiatarone Singh MA, Hue O, Pras P, Legros P, Bernard PL. Physiological and functional responses to low-moderate versus high-intensity progressive resistance training in frail elders. *J Gerontol A Biol Sci Med Sci* 59:503–509, 2004.
73. Meuleman JR, Brechue WF, Kulilis PS, Lowenthal DT. Exercise training in the debilitated aged: Strength and functional outcomes. *Arch Phys Med Rehabil* 81:312–318, 2000.
74. Hunter GR, Wetzstein CJ, Fields DA, Brown A, Bamman MM. Resistance training increases total energy expenditure and free-living physical activity in older adults. *J Appl Physiol* 89:977–984, 2000.
75. Henwood TR, Taaffe DR. Improved physical performance in older adults undertaking a short-term programme of high-velocity resistance training. *Gerontology* 51:108–115, 2005.
76. Fiatarone MA, Marks EC, Ryan ND, Meredith CN, Lipsitz LA, Evans WJ. High-intensity strength training in nonagenarians. *JAMA* 263:3029–3034, 1990.
77. Hagerman FC, Walsh SJ, Staron RS, Hikida RS, Gilders RM, Murray TF, Toma K, Ragg KE. Effects of high-intensity resistance training on untrained older men. I. Strength , cardiovascular, and metabolic responses. *J Gerontol A Biol Sci Med* 55:B336–B346, 2000.
78. Trappe S, Williamson D, Godard M, Porter D, Rowden G, Costill D. Effect of resistance training on single muscle fiber contractile function in older men. *J Appl Physiol* 89:143–152, 2000.
79. Going SB, Williams DP, Lohman TG, Hewitt MJ. Aging, body composition, and physical activity: A review. *J Aging Phys Act* 2:38–66, 1994.
80. Pollock ML, Foster C, Knapp D, Rod JL, Schmidt DH. Effect of age and training on aerobic capacity and body composition of master athletes. *J Appl Physiol* 62:725–731, 1987.
81. Sarna S, Sahi T, Koskenvuo M, Kaprio J. Increased life expectancy of world class male athletes. *Med Sci Sports Exerc* 25:237–244, 1993.
82. Blair SN, Kampert JB, Kohl HW, et al. Influences of cardiorespiratory fitness and other precursors on cardiovascular disease and all-cause mortality in men and women. *JAMA* 276:205–210, 1996.
83. Lee IM, Skerrett PJ. Physical activity and all-cause mortality: What is the dose-response relation? *Med Sci Sports Exerc* 33(suppl):S459–S471, 2001.
84. Lee IM, Paffenbarger RS. Associations of light, moderate, and vigorous intensity physical activity with longevity. The Harvard Alumni Health Study. *Am J Epidemiol* 151:293–299, 2000.
85. Lee IM, Paffenbarger RS. Do physical activity and physical fitness avert premature mortality? *Exerc Sports Sci Rev* 24:135–169, 1996.
86. Kujala UM, Kaprio J, Sarna S, Koskenvuo M. Relationship of leisure-time physical activity and mortality. The Finnish Twin Cohort. *JAMA* 279:440–444, 1998.

87. Paffenbarger PS, Hyde RT, Wing AL, et al. Physical activity, all-cause mortality, and longevity of college alumni. *N Engl J Med* 314:605–613, 1986.
88. Paffenbarger RS, Hyde RT, Wing AL, Lee I-M, Jung DL, Kampert JB. The association of changes in physical-activity level and other lifestyle characteristics with mortality among men. *N Engl J Med* 328:538–545, 1993.
89. Gregg EW, Cauley JA, Stone K, Thompson TJ, Bauer DC, Cummings SR, Ensrud KE. Relationship of changes in physical activity and mortality among older women. *JAMA* 289:2379–2386, 2003.
90. Kenny AM, Prestwood KM. Osteoporosis. Pathogenesis, diagnosis, and treatment in older adults. *Rheum Dis Clin North Am* 26:569–591, 2000.
91. National Institutes of Health Consensus Development Panel on Osteoporosis Prevention, Diagnosis, and Therapy. Osteoporosis prevention, diagnosis, and therapy. *JAMA* 285:785–795, 2001.
92. South-Paul JE. Osteoporosis: Part I. Evaluation and assessment. *Am Fam Physician* 63:897–904, 2001. Osteoporosis: Part II. Nonpharmacologic and pharmacologic treatment. *Am Fam Physician* 63:1121–1128, 2001.
93. McClung MR. Prevention and management of osteoporosis. *Best Pract Res Clin Endocrinol Metab* 17:53–71, 2003.
94. Van der Voort DJ, Geusens PP, Dinant GJ. Risk factors for osteoporosis related to their outcomes: Fractures. *Osteoporos Int* 12:630–638, 2001.
95. Parsons LC. Osteoporosis: Incidence, prevention, and treatment of the silent killer. *Nurs Clin North Am* 40:119–133, 2005.
96. U.S. Department of Health and Human Services. *Bone Health and Osteoporosis: A Report of the Surgeon General.* Rockville, MD: U.S. Department of Health and Human Services, Office of the Surgeon General, 2004.
97. Kanis JA, and the WHO Study Group. Assessment of fracture risk and its application to screening for postmenopausal osteoporosis: Synopsis of a WHO report. *Osteoporosis Int* 4:268–381, 1994.
98. Looker AC. Updated data on proximal femur bone mineral levels of US adults. *Osteoporos Int* 8:468–489, 1998.
99. Cauley JA, Lucas LL, Kuller LH, Vogt MT, Browner WS, Cummings SR. Bone mineral density and risk of breast cancer in older women: The study of osteoporotic fractures. *JAMA* 276:1404–1408, 1996.
100. Schneider DL, Barrett-Connor EL, Morton DJ. Timing of postmenopausal estrogen for optimal bone mineral density. The Rancho Bernardo study. *JAMA* 277:543–547, 1997.
101. Villareal DT, Binder EF, Williams DB, Schechtman KB, Yarasheski KE, Kohrt WM. Bone mineral density response to estrogen replacement in frail elderly women. A randomized controlled trial. *JAMA* 286:815–820, 2001.
102. Cummings SR, Nevitt MC, Browner WS, et al. Risk factors for hip fracture in white women. *N Engl J Med* 332:767–773, 1995.
103. Ensrud KE, Cauley J, Lipschutz R, Cummings SR. Weight change and fractures in older women. *Arch Intern Med* 157:857–863, 1997.
104. LeBoff MS, Kohlmeier L, Hurwitz S, Franklin J, Wright J, Glowacki J. Occult vitamin D deficiency in postmenopausal US women with acute hip fracture. *JAMA* 281:1505–1511, 1999.
105. Col NF, Eckman MH, Karas RH, et al. Patient-specific decisions about hormone replacement therapy in postmenopausal women. *JAMA* 277:1140–1147, 1997.
106. Hollenbach KA, Barrett-Connor E, Edelstein SL, Holbrook T. Cigarette smoking and bone mineral density in older men and women. *Am J Public Health* 83:1265–1270, 1993.
107. Hernandez-Avila M, Colditz GA, Stampfer MJ, et al. Caffeine, moderate alcohol intake, and risk of fractures of the hip and forearm in middle-aged women. *Am J Clin Nutr* 54:157–163, 1991.
108. Lin JD, Chen JF, Chang HY, Ho C. Evaluation of bone mineral density by quantitative ultrasound of bone in 16,862 subjects during routine health examination. *Br J Radiol* 74:602–606, 2001.
109. Reid IR, Ames RW, Evans MC, Gamble GD, Sharpe SJ. Effect of calcium supplementation on bone loss in postmenopausal women. *N Engl J Med* 328:460–464, 1993.
110. Chapuy MC, Arlot ME, Duboeuf F, et al. Vitamin D_3 and calcium to prevent hip fractures in elderly women. *N Engl J Med* 327:1637–1642, 1992.
111. Dawson-Hughes B, Harris SS, Krall EA, Dallal GE. Effect of calcium and vitamin D supplementation on bone density in men and women 65 years of age and older. *N Engl J Med* 337:670–676, 1997.
112. Stevenson M, Lloyd Jones M, De Nigris E, Brewer N, Davis S, Oakley J. A systematic review and economic evaluation of alendronate, etidronate, risedronate, raloxifene and teriparatide for the prevention and treatment of postmenopausal osteoporosis. *Health Technol Assess* 9:1–160, 2005.
113. Gallagher JC. Role of estrogens in the management of postmenopausal bone loss. *Rheum Dis Clin North* 27:143–162, 2001.
114. Drinkwater BL. Physical fitness, activity and osteoporosis. In Bouchard C, Shephard RJ (eds.). *Exercise, Fitness, and Health: A Consensus of Current Knowledge.* Champaign, IL: Human Kinetics, 1994.
115. American College of Sports Medicine. ACSM position stand on physical activity and bone health. *Med Sci Sports Exerc* 36:1985–1996, 2004.
116. Beck BR, Snow CM. Bone health across the lifespan—exercising our options. *Exerc Sport Sci Rev* 31:117–122, 2003.
117. Marcus R. Role of exercise in preventing and treating osteoporosis. *Rheum Dis Clin North Am* 27:131–141, 2001.
118. Cullen DM, Smith RT, Akhter MP. Time course for bone formation with long-term external mechanical loading. *J Appl Physiol* 88:1943–1948, 2000.
119. Clarke MS. The effects of exercise on skeletal muscle in the aged. *J Musculoskelet Neuronal Interact* 4:175–178, 2004.
120. Zernicke RF, Vailas AC, Salem GJ. Biomechanical response of bone to weightlessness. *Exerc Sports Sci Rev* 18:167–192, 1990.
121. Bloomfield SA. Changes in musculoskeletal structure and function with prolonged bed rest. *Med Sci Sports Exerc* 29:197–206, 1997.
122. Bailey DA, McCulloch RG. Bone tissue and physical activity. *Can J Sport Sci* 15:229–239, 1990.
123. Edelstein SL, Barrett-Connor E. Relation between body size and bone mineral density in elderly men and women. *Am J Epidemiol* 138:160–169, 1993.
124. Dook JE, James C, Henderson NK, Price RI. Exercise and bone mineral density in mature female athletes. *Med Sci Sports Exerc* 29:291–296, 1997.
125. Lee EJ, Long KA, Risser WL, Poindexter HBW, Gibbons WE, Goldzieher J. Variations in bone status of contralateral and regional sites in young athletic women. *Med Sci Sports Exerc* 27:1354–1361, 1995.
126. Dyson K, Blimkie CJR, Davison KS, Webber CE, Adachi JD. Gymnastic training and bone density in pre-adolescent females. *Med Sci Sports Exerc* 29:443–450, 1997.
127. Creighton DL, Morgan AL, Boardley D, Brolinson PG. Weight-bearing exercise and markers of bone turnover in female athletes. *J Appl Physiol* 90:565–570, 2001.

128. Nichols DL, Sanborn CF, Bonnick SL, Ben-Ezra V, Gench B, DiMarco NM. The effects of gymnastics training on bone mineral density. *Med Sci Sports Exerc* 26:1220–1226, 1994.

129. Suominen H. Bone mineral density and long term exercise: An overview of cross-sectional athlete studies. *Sports Med* 16:316–330, 1993.

130. Andreoli A, Monteleone M, Van Loan M, Promenzio L, Tarantion U, De Lorenzo A. Effects of different sports on bone density and muscle mass in highly trained athletes. *Med Sci Sports Exerc* 33:507–511, 2001.

131. Devine DA, Dhaliwal SS, Dick IM, Bollerslev J, Prince RL. Physical activity and calcium consumption are important determinants of lower limb bone mass in older women. *J Bone Miner Res* 19:1634–1639, 2004.

132. Kujala UM, Kaprio J, Kannus P, Sarna S, Koskenvuo M. Physical activity and osteoporotic hip fracture risk in men. *Arch Intern Med* 160:705–708, 2000.

133. Lloyd T, Petit MA, Lin HM, Beck TJ. Lifestyle factors and the development of bone mass and bone strength in young women. *J Pediatr* 144:776–782, 2004.

134. Vicente-Rodriguez G, Ara I, Perez-Gomez J, Serrano-Sanchez JA, Dorado C, Calbet JAL. High femoral bone mineral density accretion in prepubertal soccer players. *Med Sci Sports Exerc* 36:1789–1795, 2004.

135. Kontulainen S, Kannus P, Haapasalo H, Sievanen H, Pasanen M, Heinonen A, Oja P, Vuori I. Good maintenance of exercise-induced bone gain with decreased training of female tennis and squash players: A prospective 5-year follow-up study of young and old starters and controls. *J Bone Miner Res* 16:195–201, 2001.

136. Micklesfield LK, Lambert EV, Fataar AB, Noakes TD, Myburgh KH. Bone mineral density in mature, premenopausal ultramarathon runners. *Med Sci Sports Exerc* 27:688–696, 1995.

137. Keay N, Fogelman I, Blake G. Bone mineral density in professional female dancers. *Br J Sports Med* 31:143–147, 1997.

138. Fuchs RK, Bauer JJ, Snow CM. Jumping improves hip and lumbar spine bone mass in prepubescent children: A randomized controlled trial. *J Bone Miner Res* 16:148–156, 2001.

139. Witzke KA, Snow CM. Lean body mass and leg power best predict bone mineral density in adolescent girls. *Med Sci Sports Exerc* 31:1558–1563, 1999.

140. Kohrt WM, Snead DB, Slatopolsky E, Birge SJ. Additive effects of weight-bearing exercise and estrogen on bone mineral density in older women. *J Bone Min Res* 10:1303–1311, 1995.

141. Nelson ME, Fiatarone MA, Morganti CM, Trice I, Greenberg RA, Evans WJ. Effects of high-intensity strength training on multiple risk factors for osteoporotic fractures: A randomized controlled trial. *JAMA* 272:1909–1914, 1994.

142. Rhodes EC, Martin AD, Taunton JE, Donnelly M, Warren J, Elliot J. Effects of one year of resistance training on the relation between muscular strength and bone density in elderly women. *Br J Sports Med* 34:18–22, 2000.

143. Layne JE, Nelson ME. The effects of progressive resistance training on bone density: A review. *Med Sci Sports Exerc* 31:25–30, 1999.

144. Vincent KR, Braith RW. Resistance exercise and bone turnover in elderly men and women. *Med Sci Sports Exerc* 34:17–27, 2002.

145. Nichols DL, Sanborn CF, Love AM. Resistance training and bone mineral density in adolescent females *J Pediatr* 139: 494–500, 2001.

146. Kerr D, Ackland T, Maslen B, Morton A, Prince R. Resistance training over 2 years increases bone mass in calcium-replete postmenopausal women. *J Bone Miner Res* 16:175–181, 2001.

147. Villareal DT, Binder EF, Yarasheski KE, Williams DB, Brown M, Sinacore DR, Kohrt WM. Effects of exercise training added to ongoing hormone replacement therapy on bone mineral density in frail elderly women. *J Am Geriatr Soc* 51:985–990, 2003.

148. Kelley GA, Kelley KS, Tran ZV. Resistance training and bone mineral density in women: A meta-analysis of controlled trials. *Am J Phys Med Rehabil* 80:65–77, 2001.

149. Winters KM, Snow CM. Detraining reverses positive effects of exercise on the musculoskeletal system in premenopausal women. *J Bone Miner Res* 15:2495–2503, 2000.

150. Gregg EW, Pereira MA, Caspersen CJ. Physical activity, falls, and fractures among older adults: A review of the epidemiologic evidence. *J Am Geriatr Soc* 48:883–893, 2000.

151. Lawrence RC, Helmick CG, Arnett FC, et al. Estimates of the prevalence of arthritis and selected musculoskeletal disorders in the United States. *Arthritis & Rheumatism* 41:778–799, 1998.

152. Rados C. Helpful treatments keep people with arthritis moving. *FDA Consumer Magazine,* March–April, 2005. See also: Lewis C. Arthritis. Timely treatments for an ageless disease. *FDA Consumer Magazine,* May–June, 2000.

153. CDC. Racial/ethnic differences in the prevalence and impact of doctor-diagnosed arthritis—United States, 2002. *MMWR* 54:119–123, 2005. See also: CDC. Prevalence of arthritis—United States, 1997. *MMWR* 50:334–336, 2001; CDC. Prevalence of self-reported arthritis or chronic joint symptoms among adults—United States, 2001. *MMWR* 51:948–950, 2002; CDC. Prevalence of disabilities and associated health conditions among adults—United States, 1999. *MMWR* 50:120–125, 2001.

154. Arthritis Foundation. Arthritis fact sheet. Author: http:/www.arthritis.org, 2005.

155. Manek NJ. Medical management of osteoarthritis. *Mayo Clin Proc* 76:533–539, 2001.

156. Bykerk VP, Keystone EC. What are the goals and principles of management in the early treatment of rheumatoid arthritis? *Best Pract Res Clin Rheumatol* 19:147–161, 2005.

157. Mehrotra C, Naimi TS, Serdula M, Bolen J, Pearson K. Arthritis, body mass index, and professional advice to lose weight: Implications for clinical medicine and public health. *Am J Prev Med* 27:16–21, 2004.

158. Choi HK. Dietary risk factors for rheumatic diseases. *Curr Opin Rheumatol* 17:141–146, 2005.

159. Rogers LQ, Macera CA, Hootman JM, Ainsworth BE, Blair SN. The association between joint stress from physical activity and self-reported osteoarthritis: An analysis of the Cooper Clinic data. *Osteoarthritis Cartilage* 10:617–622, 2002.

160. Altman RD, Abadie E, Avouac B, Bouvenot G, Branco J, Bruyere O, Calvo G, Devogelaer JP, Dreiser RL, Herrero-Beaumont G, Kahan A, Kreutz G, Laslop A, Lemmel EM, Menkes CJ, Pavelka K, Van De Putte L, Vanhaelst L, Reginster JY; Group for Respect of Excellence and Ethics in Science (GREES). Total joint replacement of hip or knee as an outcome measure for structure modifying trials in osteoarthritis. *Osteoarthritis Cartilage* 13:13–19, 2005.

161. American College of Sports Medicine. *ACSM's Exercise Management for Persons with Chronic Diseases and Disabilities.* Champaign, IL: Human Kinetics, 1997.

162. Brandt KD. The importance of nonpharmacologic approaches in management of osteoarthritis. *Am J Med* 105(1B):39S–44S, 1998.

163. Panush RS. Physical activity, fitness, and osteoarthritis. In Bouchard C, Shephard RJ, Stephens T (eds.). *Physical Activity, Fitness, and Health: International Proceedings and Consensus Statement.* Champaign, IL: Human Kinetics, 1994, pp. 712–722.

164. Fontaine KR, Heo M, Bathon J. Are US adults with arthritis meeting public health recommendations for physical activity?

Arthritis Rheum 50:624–628, 2004. See also: CDC. Prevalence of leisure-time physical activity among persons with arthritis and other rheumatic conditions—United States, 1990–1991. *MMWR* 46:389–393, 1997.

165. Messier SP, Loeser RF, Miller GD, Morgan TM, Rejeski WJ, Sevick MA, Ettinger WH, Pahor M, Williamson JD. Exercise and dietary weight loss in overweight and obese older adults with knee osteoarthritis: The Arthritis, Diet, and Activity Promotion Trial. *Arthritis Rheum* 50:1501–1510, 2004.
166. Ettinger WH, Afable RF. Physical disability from knee osteoarthritis: The role of exercise as an intervention. *Med Sci Sports Exerc* 26:1435–1440, 1994.
167. Ettinger WH, Burns R, Messier SP, et al. A randomized trial comparing aerobic exercise and resistance exercise with a health education program in older adults with knee osteoarthritis. The Fitness Arthritis and Seniors Trial (FAST). *JAMA* 277:25–31, 1997.
168. Van den Ende CH, Vliet Vlieland TP, Munneke M, Hazes JM. Dynamic exercise therapy in rheumatoid arthritis: A systematic review. *Br J Rheumatol* 37:677–687, 1998.
169. Kovar PA, Allegrante JP, MacKenzie R, Peterson MGE, Gutin B, Charlson ME. Supervised fitness walking in patients with osteoarthritis of the knee. *Ann Intern Med* 116:529–534, 1992.
170. OíGrady M, Fletcher J, Ortez S. Therapeutic and physical fitness exercise prescription for older adults with joint disease: An evidence-based approach. *Rheum Dis Clin North Am* 26:617–646, 2000.
171. American Geriatrics Society Panel on Exercise and Osteoarthritis. Exercise prescription for older adults with osteoarthritis pain: Consensus practice recommendations. A supplement to the ACS Clinical Practice Guidelines on the management of chronic pain in older adults. *J Am Geriatr Soc* 49:808–823, 2001.
172. Vuori IM. Dose-response of physical activity and low back pain, osteoarthritis, and osteoporosis. *Med Sci Sports Exerc* 33(suppl):S551–S586, 2001.
173. Deyle GD, Henderson NE, Matekel RL, Ryder MG, Garber MB, Allison SC. Effectiveness of manual physical therapy and exercise in osteoarthritis of the knee. *Ann Intern Med* 132:173–181, 2000.
174. Van Gool CH, Penninx BW, Kempen GI, Rejeski WJ, Miller GD, Van Eijk JT, Pahor M, Messier SP. Effects of exercise adherence on physical function among overweight older adults with knee osteoarthritis. *Arthritis Rheum* 53:24–32, 2005.
175. Roddy E, Zhang W, Doherty M. Aerobic walking or strengthening exercise for osteoarthritis of the knee? A systematic review. *Ann Rheum Dis* 64:544–548, 2005.
176. Buckwalter JA. Sports, joint injury, and posttraumatic osteoarthritis. *J Orthop Sports Phys Ther* 33:578–588, 2003. See also: Saxon L, Finch C, Bass S. Sports participation, sports injuries and osteoarthritis: Implications for prevention. *Sports Med* 28:123–135, 1999.
177. Lane NE, Michel B, Bjorkengren A, Oehlert J, Shi H, Bloch DA, Fries JF. The risk of osteoarthritis with running and aging: A 5-year longitudinal study. *J Rheumatol* 20:461–468, 1993.
178. Lane NE, Buckwalter JA. Exercise: A cause of osteoarthritis? *Rheumatic Dis Clin N Am* 19:617–633, 1993.
179. Rangger C, Kathrein A, Klestil T, Glotzer W. Partial meniscectomy and osteoarthritis. Implications for treatment of athletes. *Sports Med* 23:61–68, 1997.
180. Miranda H, Viikari-Juntura E, Martikainen R, Riihimaki H. A prospective study on knee pain and its risk factors. *Osteoarthritis Cartilage* 10:623–630, 2002.
181. Hannan MT, Felson DT, Pincus T. Analysis of the discordance between radiographic changes and knee pain in osteoarthritis of the knee. *J Rheumatol* 27:1513–1517, 2000.
182. Hootman JM, Macera CA, Helmick CG, Blair SN. Influence of physical activity-related joint stress on the risk of self-reported hip/knee osteoarthritis: A new method to quantify physical activity. *Prev Med* 36:636–644, 2003.
183. Manninen P, Riihimaki H, Heliovaara M, Suomalainen O. Physical exercise and risk of severe knee osteoarthritis requiring arthroplasty. *Rheumatology* (Oxford) 40:432–437, 2001.
184. Jones G, Ding C, Glisson M, Hynes K, Ma D, Cicuttini F. Knee articular cartilage development in children: A longitudinal study of the effect of sex, growth, body composition, and physical activity. *Pediatr Res* 54:230–236, 2003.

PHYSICAL FITNESS ACTIVITY 15.1

Health Check

As reviewed in this chapter, health habits have a significant impact on life expectancy. In this activity, you can conduct a comprehensive review of your health habits to determine your overall risk for mortality. Note the points given by each of your answers, total them, and then apply them to the norms listed at the end of this activity.

Name: ______________________________ Today's Date: ______________

Your age? _______ years Sex: ❑ Male ❑ Female How tall are you (without shoes)? _______ feet _______ inches

If male ≥50 yr or female ≥55 yr = 4 points; all others, 0

How much do you weigh (minimal clothing and without shoes)? _______ pounds

Calculate BMI (kg/m²):

Points		
2	**<18.5**	**Too lean**
0	**18.5–24.9**	**Desirable**
2	**25–29.9**	**Overweight** (may be due to extra muscle mass)
3	**30–40**	**Mild to Moderate obesity**
4	**>40**	**Severe obesity**

What is the most you have ever weighed? _______ pounds

If ± 20% or more from present weight = 2 points; if within ± 20% = 0 points.

Please check the appropriate box for each question.

Yes No

4 0 Points

❑ ❑ 1. Has your father or brother had a heart attack or died suddenly of heart disease before age 55 years; has your mother or sister experienced these heart problems before age 65 years?

4 0

❑ ❑ 2. Has a doctor told you that you have high blood pressure (more than 140/90 mm Hg), or are you on medication to control your blood pressure?

OR 2a. If you know your blood pressure, please check the appropriate category:

0 ❑ Less than 120/80 mm Hg	**3** ❑ 140/90 to 159/99	**0** ❑ Do not know
1 ❑ 120/80 to 129/84	**4** ❑ 160/100 to 180/110	
2 ❑ 130/85 to 139/89	**5** ❑ More than 180/110	

Yes No

4 0

❑ ❑ 3. Is your total blood cholesterol greater than 240 mg/dl, or has a doctor told you that your cholesterol is at a high risk level?

OR 3a. If you know your blood cholesterol, please check the appropriate category:

0 ❑ Less than 160 mg/dl	**2** ❑ 200–219	**5** ❑ More than 260
0 ❑ 160–179	**3** ❑ 200–239	**0** ❑ Do not know
1 ❑ 180–199	**4** ❑ 240–260	

4 0

❑ ❑ 4. Do you have diabetes?

3 0

❑ ❑ 5. During the past year, would you say that you experienced enough stress, strain, and pressure to have a significant effect on your health?

4 0

❑ ❑ 6. Do you eat foods nearly every day that are high in fat and cholesterol such as fatty meats, cheese, fried foods, butter, whole milk, ice cream, or eggs?

7. In general, compared to other persons your age, rate how healthy you are:

1❑	2❑	3❑	3❑	4❑	5❑	6❑	7❑	8❑	9❑	10❑
Not at all healthy					Somewhat healthy					Extremely healthy

1,2 = 3 points; 3,4 = 2 points; 5,6,7 = 1 point; 8,9,10 = 0 points

8. Outside of your normal work or daily responsibilities, how often do you engage in exercise that at least moderately increases your breathing and heart rate, and makes you sweat, for at least 20 minutes (such as brisk walking, cycling, swimming, jogging, aerobic dance, stair climbing, rowing, basketball, racquetball, vigorous yard work, etc.)?

   0 ❑ 5 or more times per week **1** ❑ 3 to 4 times per week **2** ❑ 1 to 2 times per week

   3 ❑ Less than 1 time per week **4** ❑ Seldom or never

9. On average, how many servings of fruit and vegetables do you eat per day? (one serving = 1 medium fruit, ½ cup of chopped, cooked, or canned fruit or vegetable, ¾ cup of fruit or vegetable juice).

   4 ❑ none **3** ❑ 1–2 **2** ❑ 3–4 **1** ❑ 5–6 **0** ❑ 7–8 **0** ❑ 9 or more

10. On average, how many servings of bread, cereal, rice, or pasta do you eat per day? (one serving = 1 slice of bread, 1 ounce of ready-to-eat cereal, ½ cup of cooked cereal, rice, or pasta).

    3 ❑ None **3** ❑ 1–2 **2** ❑ 3–5 **1** ❑ 6–8 **0** ❑ 9–11 **0** ❑ 12 or more

11. How have you been feeling in general during the past month?

    0 ❑ In excellent spirits **1** ❑ In good spirits mostly **2** ❑ In low spirits mostly

    0 ❑In very good spirits **1** ❑ I've been up and down in spirits a lot **3** ❑ In very low spirits

12. On average, how many hours of sleep do you get in a 24-hour period?

    2 ❑ Less than 5 **1** ❑ 5 to 6.9 **0** ❑ 7 to 9 **0** ❑ More than 9

13. How would you describe your cigarette smoking habits?

    0 ❑ Never smoked

    0 ❑ Used to smoke

    How many years has it been since you smoked? (Check appropriate box.)

    3 ❑ Less than 1 year **1** ❑ 6–15

    2 ❑ 1–5 **0** ❑ More than 15

    ❑ Still smoke

    How many cigarettes a day do you smoke on average?

    3 ❑ 1–10 **4** ❑ 21–30 **5** ❑ More than 40

    3 ❑ 11–20 **4** ❑ 31–40

14. How many alcoholic drinks do you consume? (A "drink" is a glass of wine, a wine cooler, a bottle or can of beer, a shot glass of liquor, or a mixed drink.)

    0 ❑ Never use alcohol **0** ❑ Less than 1 per week **0** ❑ 1 to 6 per week

    0 ❑ 1 per day **3** ❑ 2 to 3 per day **4** ❑ More than 3 per day

15. When driving or riding in a car, do you wear a seat belt:

    0 ❑ All or most of the time **1** ❑ Some of the time **2** ❑ Once in awhile **3** ❑ Rarely or never

---

Norms

Total Points	Classification
0–7	Excellent health habits may increase life expectancy 6 to 12 years
8–15	Good, but some improvement needed
16–24	Fair, improvement needed
25 or more	Poor, at high risk for disease

PHYSICAL FITNESS ACTIVITY 15.2

Osteoporosis—Are You at Risk for Weak Bones?

Learn more about this bone-thinning disease that causes debilitating fractures of the hip, spine, and wrist. Complete the following questionnaire to determine your risk for developing osteoporosis.

Check any of these that apply to you.

- ❑ I'm older than 65.
- ❑ I've broken a bone after age 50.
- ❑ My close relative has osteoporosis or has broken a bone.
- ❑ My health is "fair" or "poor."
- ❑ I smoke.
- ❑ I am underweight for my height.
- ❑ I started menopause before age 45.
- ❑ I've never gotten enough calcium.
- ❑ I have more than two drinks of alcohol several times a week.
- ❑ I have poor vision, even with glasses.
- ❑ I sometimes fall.
- ❑ I'm not active.
- ❑ I have one of these medical conditions:
  - Hyperthyroidism
  - Chronic lung disese
  - Cancer
  - Inflammatory bowel disease
  - Chronic hepatic or renal disease
  - Hyperparathyroidism
  - Vitamin D deficiency
  - Cushing's disease
  - Multiple sclerosis
  - Rheumatoid arthritis
- ❑ I take one of these medicines:
  - Oral glucocorticoids (steroids)
  - Cancer treatments (radiation, chemotherapy)
  - Thyroid medicine
  - Antiepileptic medications
  - Gonadal hormone suppression
  - Immunosuppressive agents

If you have any of these "red flags," you could be at high risk for weak bones. Talk to your doctor, nurse, pharmacist, or other health-care professional.

Source: U.S. Department of Health and Human Services. *Bone Health and Osteoporosis: A Report of the Surgeon General.* Rockville, MD: U.S. Department of Health and Human Services, Office of the Surgeon General, 2004.

PHYSICAL FITNESS ACTIVITY 15.3

Health Risk Appraisal on the Internet

As emphasized in this chapter, successful aging is tightly linked to personal lifestyle habits. Health risk appraisal is the process of tabulating your health habits, producing a total score with recommendations for improvement, and estimating how many years of life are subtracted or added. Choose one of the three Internet sites listed below, print out your report, and turn it in to your instructor.

Here are three Internet sites that provide comprehensive health risk appraisals:

1. Wellmed *(www.wellmed.com)*

   Go to the site, click on New Member, fill in the information requested, and then click on Checkup HQ. The program will ask a series of questions concerning your health habits, estimate a "health quotient," and compare your score to that of others your age. Information is also provided on 13 risk factors and diseases.

2. YouFirst *(www.youfirst.com)*

   Go to the site, click on Free Personal Health Assessment, and then answer questions to determine your health age and receive a report.

3. RealAge *(www.realage.com)*

   Go to the site, click on The Real Age Test, register, and fill in answers to a long list of questions, and then print out your "age reduction planner."

PHYSICAL FITNESS ACTIVITY 15.4

Calculating Your Calcium Intake

Directions: Think about your average daily food intake. Use the list below to add up your calcium points based on your average day.

Calcium Calculator

Help your bones. Choose foods that are high in calcium. Here are some examples.

Food	Calcium (mg)	Points
Fortified oatmeal, 1 packet	350	3
Sardines, canned in oil, with edible bones, 3 oz.	324	3
Cheddar cheese, 1½ oz. shredded	306	3
Milk, nonfat, 1 cup	302	3
Milkshake, 1 cup	300	3
Yogurt, plain, low-fat, 1 cup	300	3
Soybeans, cooked, 1 cup	261	3
Tofu, firm, with calcium, ½ cup	204	2
Orange juice, fortified with calcium, 6 oz.	200–260 (varies)	2–3
Salmon, canned, with edible bones, 3 oz.	181	2
Pudding, instant, (chocolate, banana, etc.) made with 2% milk, ½ cup	153	2
Baked beans, 1 cup	142	1
Cottage cheese, 1% milk fat, 1 cup	138	1
Spaghetti, lasagna, 1 cup	125	1
Frozen yogurt, vanilla, soft-serve, ½ cup	103	1
Ready-to-eat cereal, fortified with calcium, 1 cup	100–1000 (varies)	1–10
Cheese pizza, 1 slice	100	1
Fortified waffles, 2	100	1
Turnip greens, boiled, ½ cup	99	1
Broccoli, raw, 1 cup	90	1
Ice cream, vanilla, ½ cup	85	1
Soy or rice milk, fortified with calcium, 1 cup	80–500 (varies)	1–5

Points Needed:
babies/toddlers (ages 0–3) need 2–5
children (ages 4–8) need 8
teens need 23
adults under 50 need....................................10
adults over 50 need 12

How do you rate: Total calcium points ______

Source: U.S. Department of Health and Human Services. *Bone Health and Osteoporosis: A Report of the Surgeon General.* Rockville, MD: U.S. Department of Health and Human Services, Office of the Surgeon General, 2004.

chapter 16

Exercise Risks

The athlete's habit of body neither produces a good condition for the general purposes of civic life, nor does it encourage ordinary health and the procreation of children. Some amount of exertion is essential for the best habit, but it must be neither violent nor specialized, as is the case with the athlete. It should rather be a general exertion, directed to all the activities of a free man.

—Aristotle

The modern-day fitness movement is not yet 40 years old. It was given its first great impetus in 1968, when Kenneth Cooper, a physician for the Air Force, published his book *Aerobics* (see Chapter 1). In this book, Cooper challenged Americans to take personal charge of their lifestyles and counter the "epidemics" of heart disease, obesity, and rising health-care costs. Millions took up the "aerobic challenge" and began jogging, cycling, walking, and swimming their way to better health—thus starting the new fitness revolution.

Americans are now exercising more than at any other time in our modern era. Exercise is suddenly prestigious. With the prestige, however, have come some real problems.

One product of the added prestige is "overzealousness." Excessive exercise appears to be America's newest elixir in that endless search for the "fountain of youth." Some people, allured by the media reports, and perhaps overreacting to health problems, job dissatisfaction, boredom, marital difficulties, and a fear of growing old, have seized on exercise as a panacea. As many recent articles in the medical literature have shown, excessive training has brought a host of problems.[1] This chapter reviews the major risks of carrying exercise too far.

MUSCULOSKELETAL INJURIES

This section places emphasis on running, aerobic dance, bicycling, and swimming, fitness activities that are popular among Americans, yet have been associated with significant risk for injury when certain conditions are exceeded. Figure 16.1 summarizes the number of emergency room visits for a variety of sports (this information on sport injury will not be emphasized in this chapter). Walking and gardening are the two most prevalent forms of physical activity (see Chapter 1), and one study showed that injury rates are extremely low for these two activity modes.[2]

Running Injuries

The muscles, joints, and supporting ligaments and tendons of the legs and feet respond poorly to excessive exercise, especially activities that require running and jumping.

Many studies have explored the relationship between running and musculoskeletal injuries, and several excellent literature reviews are available. More injury information has been gathered on runners than on any other mode of exercise, due in large part to the rate of injury.[3–16]

The Extent of the Problem

Depending on the study, the 1-year injury incidence rate for runners in the general population varies from 2% to 77% or 2.5–12 injuries per 1,000 hours of running.[3,4] One of the earliest studies conducted by the Centers for Disease Control and Prevention evaluated the injury rates for 2,500 male and female runners for 1 year.[6–9] Thirty-seven percent developed orthopedic injuries serious enough to reduce weekly running mileage. Of these, 38% sought medical consultation for their injuries. The risk of injury increased with weekly running mileage, with 53% injured when running

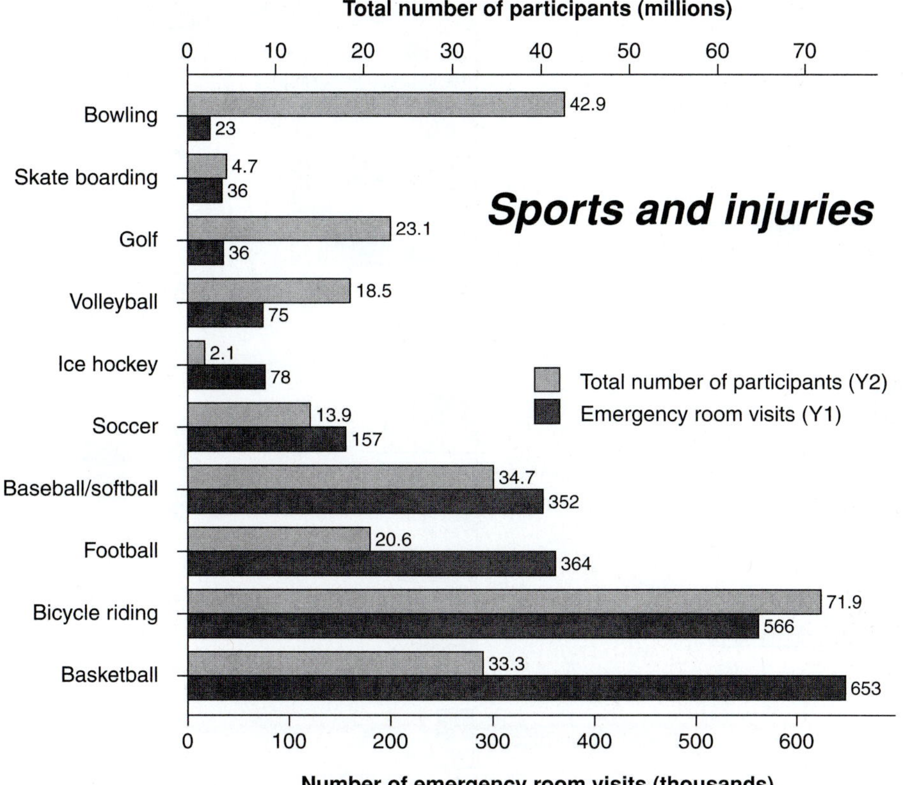

Figure 16.1 This chart compares number of emergency room visits and prevalence of participants. Source: National Safety Council.

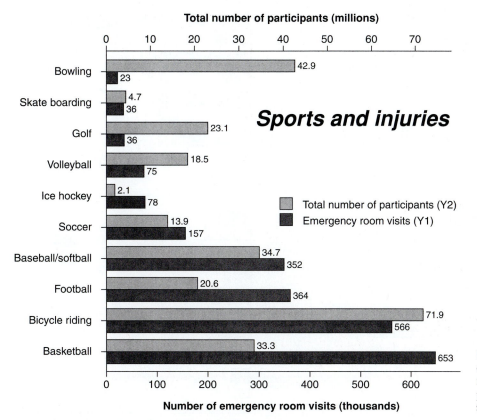

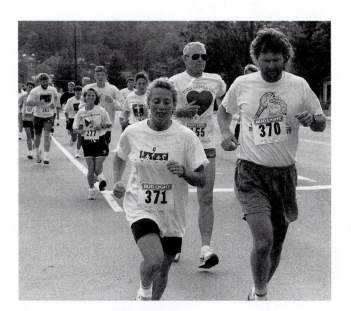

Figure 16.2 According to the Centers for Disease Control and Prevention, the average recreational runner has a one-in-three chance of being injured within any given year.

30–39 miles per week, and 65% injured when running more than 50 miles per week.

Sixty percent of the injuries involved the knee and foot areas. The researchers concluded that the average runner has a one-in-three chance of being injured within any given year, and a one-in-ten likelihood of incurring an injury that will require medical attention (see Figure 16.2). A person running 15 miles a week can count on one injury every 2 years. In a 10-year follow-up study of this cohort of runners, the CDC reported that 53% had at least one injury.[9] As shown in Figures 16.3 and 16.4, injury rates increased with running distance (except for the ≥50 mile/week category), with the knee and foot identified as the most common sites. Almost half of the cohort of runners had quit running, with injury cited as a common cause.[9]

In one of the largest studies ever conducted on running injuries, a study of 4,358 male and 428 female joggers in Switzerland, researchers reported that 45.8% and 40%, respectively, had sustained a jogging injury during the preceding year.[10,11] Because of injuries, 1 in 7 male joggers sought medical treatment, and 1 out of 40 missed work. One in five male runners was forced to fully interrupt his exercise routine. Frequency of jogging injuries increased with increase in weekly distance jogged (see Figure 16.5).

Factors Associated with Injuries

Many potential factors have been suggested as influencing risk of injury for runners. These are usually divided into two general categories: personal characteristics of the runner (gender, age, running experience, previous injury, body composition, and psychological factors) and training habits (weekly mileage, frequency, speed, racing activity, warm-up, time of run, stretching, and running surface).[3,15] Of these, the most consistent predictors are excessive weekly running

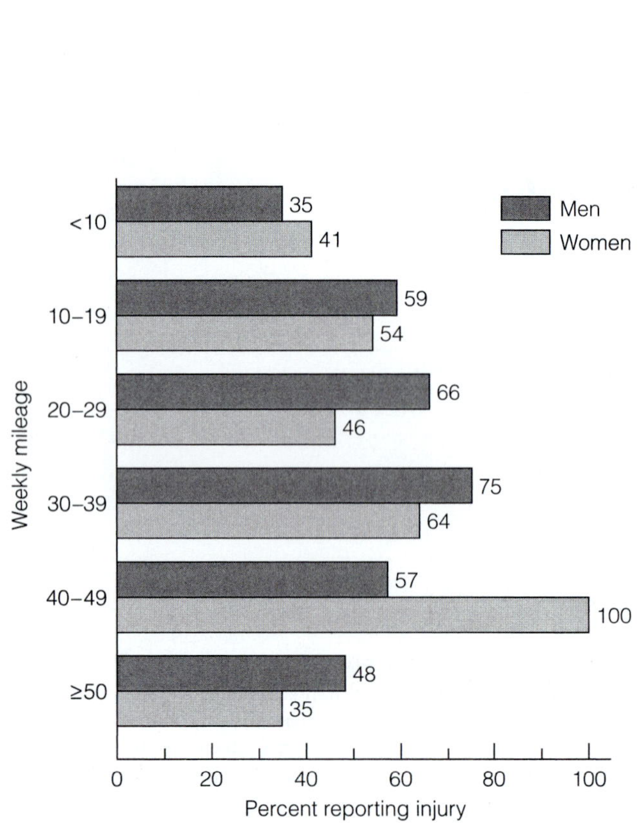

Figure 16.3 Percentage of runners injured by running distance among 326 men and 209 women during 10 years. Except for the highest-mileage runners, injury rates tend to rise with increases in weekly running mileage. Source: Koplan JP, Rothenberg RB, Jones EL. The natural history of exercise: A 10-yr follow-up of a cohort of runners. *Med Sci Sports Exerc* 27: 1180–1184, 1995.

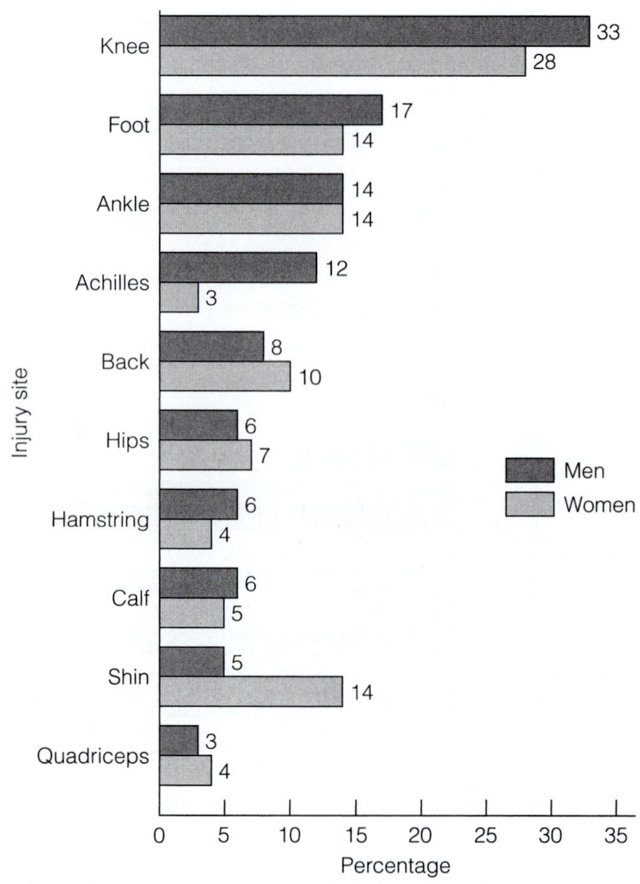

Figure 16.4 Injury sites in runners over a 10-year period among 326 men and 209 women. The knee is the most common site of injury in runners. Source: Koplan JP, Rothenberg RB, Jones EL. The natural history of exercise: A 10-yr follow-up of a cohort of runners. *Med Sci Sports Exerc* 27:1180–1184, 1995.

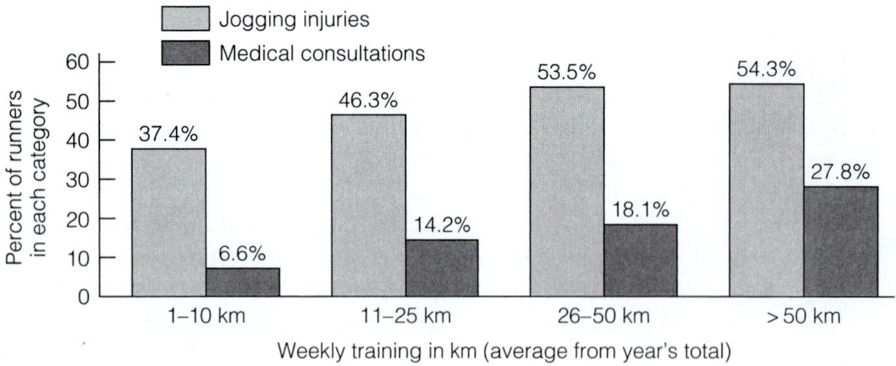

Figure 16.5 Percentage of Swiss male runners injured during previous 12 months. Frequency of jogging injuries and medical consultations as a result of jogging injuries increased according to weekly training distance of Swiss male runners. Source: Marti B, Vader JP, Minder CE, Abelin T. On the epidemiology of running injuries. *Am J Sports Med* 16:285–294, 1998.

distance, previous injury, lack of running experience, and running to compete[3,4,5,15] (see Figure 16.6). Factors not apparently associated with running injuries are age, gender, stretching routines, type of running surface, type of terrain, and speed of training. Although some exercise physiologists have theorized that muscle tightness (lack of flexibility) may be related to injuries, support for this theory is lacking.[17]

Running is a traumatic form of exercise for the musculoskeletal system of the human body. Studies of triathletes have found that relatively few of their injuries involve their bicycling and swimming—most are from running. In one study, 72% of the injuries sustained by 58 triathletes occurred during running.[18]

The sudden impact of the foot with the running surface causes a force equal to 1.5 to 5 times one's body weight.[15] The human body appears to be able to handle moderate amounts of running, but when running is excessive or when distances are suddenly increased, injuries become common.

The injuries most frequently associated with running are those classified as *overuse syndromes,* especially common among runners who run excessive distances in their training.[19]

Overtraining creates an imbalance between training and recovery.[1,19] It can cause staleness as the physical and emotional stress of the exercise program exceeds the individual's coping capacity (ability to respond to stress) (see Figure 16.7 and Box 16.1 for an overview of the terms and the signs and symptoms associated with overtraining).[1] One of the most effective ways of avoiding overtraining is to follow a well-balanced, progressive training schedule.

The running style (biomechanical factors) and anatomical structure of runners have been associated with running injuries, but the data are far from conclusive.[16,20–23] In one study, 48 trained runners with runner's knee were examined, treated, and followed for 8 months to identify the causes and response to treatment.[22] Most were found to have anatomic malalignment of the lower limb. Sixty-nine percent were also predisposed to runner's knee because of suddenly increased running distance, hill running, interval training, or racing too often. Other researchers have found that the "Q angle" (the angle at which the femur comes down to the knee) is important in predicting who gets knee pain from running.[20] Other researchers, however, have been unable to establish that lower-extremity alignment is a risk factor for running injuries.[16] One review concluded that runners who have developed stride patterns that incorporate relatively low levels of impact forces and a moderately rapid rate of pronation are at a reduced risk of incurring overuse running injuries.[5]

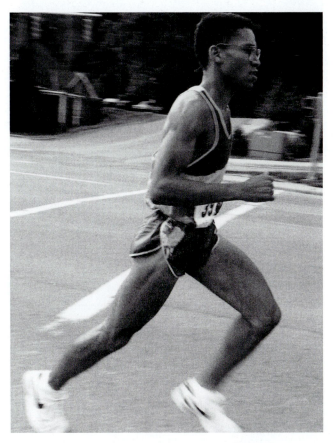

Figure 16.6 The most consistent predictors of running injuries are excessive weekly running distance, previous injury, lack of running experience, and running to compete.

Aerobic-Dance Injuries

Aerobic dance is among the most popular organized fitness activity for women in the United States (see Figure 16.8 and Chapter 1). Aerobic dance traces its origins to Jacki Sorenson, the wife of a naval pilot, who began conducting exercise classes at a U.S. Navy base in Puerto Rico in 1969.[24] The growth of aerobic dance has been enhanced by the availability of dance exercise programs on video and DVD.

The original aerobic-dance programs consisted of an eclectic combination of various dance forms, including ballet, modern jazz, disco, and folk, as well as calisthenic-type exercises. More recent innovations include water aerobics in a swimming pool, nonimpact or low-impact aerobics (one foot on the ground at all times), specific dance aerobics, step aerobics, and "assisted" aerobics with weights worn on the wrists and/or ankles.

Exercise physiologists were concerned initially that the early aerobic-dance programs were conceived by people with little or no background in medicine, kinesiology, or exercise physiology. In addition, some of the activities and positions utilized in the aerobic-dance programs were potentially injurious. Today, most of the popular videotapes with entertainment stars are designed using professional

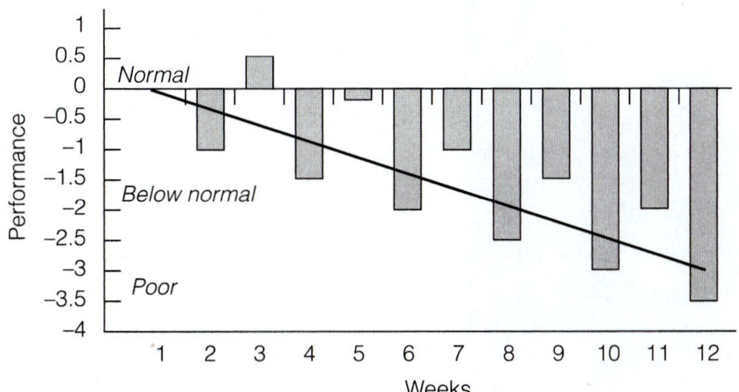

Figure 16.7 Overtraining syndrome. Schematic of training overload resulting in decreased performance. Source: Data from Kreider RB, Fry AC, O'Toole ML. *Overtraining in Sport.* Champaign, IL: Human Kinetics, 1998.

Box 16.1

Overreaching and Overtraining

Overreaching

Overreaching involves an accumulation of training or nontraining stress, resulting in a *short-term* decrement in performance capacity, with or without related physiological and psychological signs and symptoms of overtraining, in which restoration of performance capacity may take from several days to several weeks.

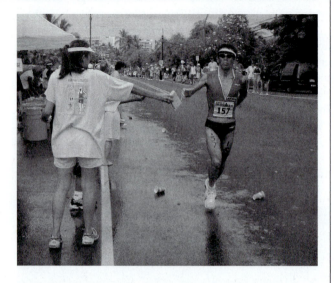

Overtraining

Overtraining involves an accumulation of training or nontraining stress, resulting in a *long-term* decrement in performance capacity, with or without related physiological and psychological signs and symptoms of overtraining, in which restoration of performance capacity may take several weeks or months.

Signs and Symptoms of Overtraining

Psychosocial

- Apathy
- Lethargy
- Sleep disturbance
- Lowered self-esteem
- Mood changes
- Feelings of depression
- Difficulty in concentrating
- Fear of competition

Performance

- Decreased performance
- Lack of desire to train
- Inability to meet previously attained performance
- Chronic fatigue
- Increased heart rate and RPE at set workload
- Decreased muscular strength
- Reduced toleration of pain during training
- Prolonged recovery following training

Physiological

- Immune suppression, with increased rates of infection
- Depressed muscle glycogen concentration
- Decreased body iron stores
- Elevated cortisol levels
- Decreased testosterone levels
- Loss of appetite and decreased body weight
- Amenorrhea or oligomenorrhea
- Gastrointestinal disturbances

Source: Kreider RB, Fry AC, O'Toole ML. *Overtraining in Sport.* Champaign, IL: Human Kinetics, 1998.

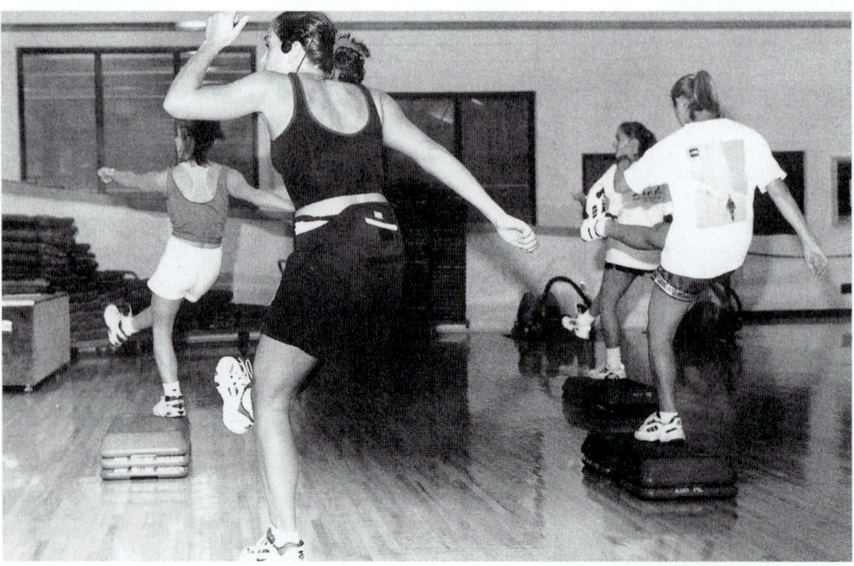

Figure 16.8 Aerobic dance is a popular activity, especially for millions of females.

consultants who try to keep the various movements safe and within the range of most people.

The early major studies examining the injury potential of aerobic dance found that about 45% of students and 75% of instructors reported injuries.[24–28] Rates of injury for students were about 1 per 100 hours of dancing, and for instructors, about 1 per 400 hours. Most of these injuries, however, were mild, causing some pain and some disruption in participation, but generally not leading participants to stop dancing or to seek professional medical assistance. The lower extremities accounted for about 80% of all injuries.

What factors were associated with increased risk of aerobic-dance injuries? In one study of 1,123 female and 164 male aerobics students, those who exercised more than three times per week, wore improper shoes, and exercised on nonresilient surfaces suffered the most injuries.[28] The lower-leg injuries were the result of excessive physical trauma.

Since these studies were published during the mid-1980s, much has been done to reduce the injury risk of aerobic dancing. In particular, low-impact aerobic routines have been substituted for the high-impact (jumping and dancing on the balls of the feet) variety. In low-impact dance aerobics, the common denominator is that at least one foot is touching the floor throughout the aerobic portion of the workout. Movements are not ballistic, but focus on large-muscle upper-body and arm movements, combined with leg kicks, high-powered steps, side-to-side movements, and lunges, often with steps or small weights.

Although no large-scale studies have yet been published on the injury risk of low-impact aerobics, there is every reason to believe that it is much lower than during the early history of the aerobic-dance movement.

Bicycling Injuries

Bicyclers also suffer their share of injuries, but they are usually caused by accidents. Actual rates of injuries due to the cycling exercise itself appear to be quite low, although pain in the hands, seat, neck, and back are commonly reported.[29] Among cyclists in the United States, there are about 1,000 deaths and 600,000 emergency room visits each year.[30,31] Head injuries account for approximately two thirds of bicycling deaths and bicycle-related hospital admissions. The large increase in off-road or mountain bicycling has increased the need for safety, with injuries reported by 50–90% of participants each year.[32]

Bicycle helmets have been shown to provide substantial protection against head injuries for cyclists of all ages involved in crashes[33] (see Figure 16.9). The Injury Prevention Program of the World Health Organization has been coordinating a worldwide initiative to increase the use of bicycle helmets, and in the United States, there is a push for legislation to mandate their use.[34,35] Also, because helmets are costly ($25 to $65), the requirement of a helmet with new bicycle purchases may prove helpful, especially when combined with legislation and education.

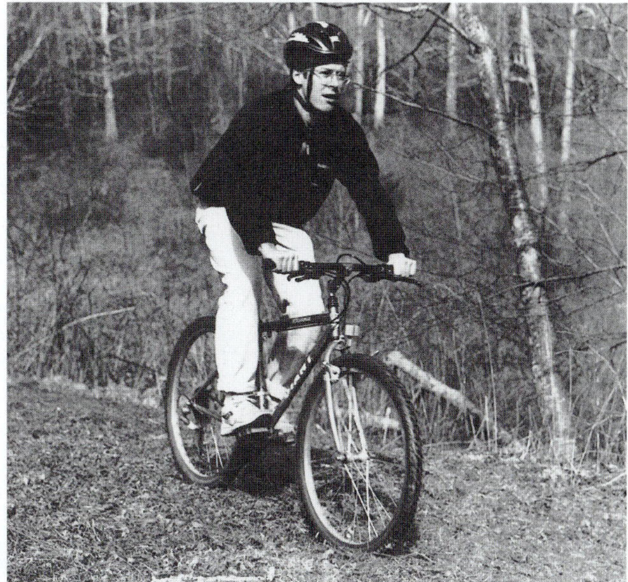

Figure 16.9 Bicycle helmets provide substantial protection against head injuries for cyclists of all ages.

Swimming Injuries

Competitive swimmers may swim 8,000–20,000 yards per day, 5–7 days each week. Shoulder pain is the most common musculoskeletal complaint, usually resulting from supraspinatus or biceps tendonitis and impingement of subacromial tissues.[36,37] Symptoms include point tenderness on the anterior part of the tip of the shoulder. (It is painful to raise the bent arm overhead.) In severe cases, total rest may be necessary to alleviate the pain. Physical therapy may be helpful.

Knee pain can occur among breaststroke swimmers (involving pain and tenderness in the medial aspect of the knee joint, apparently related to the breaststroke "whip kick").[38] Leg strengthening and flexibility exercises may be helpful, and coaching on proper technique should be emphasized.

However, among competitive swimmers, about three in four breaststroke specialists report a history of "breaststroker's knee," indicating that regardless of technique, the breaststroke kick itself may be too stressful for the average human knee.[38]

Management of Overuse Injuries

Figure 16.10 and Box 16.2 summarize the various steps that can be used in the diagnosis and management of overuse injuries by a multidisciplinary, sports-medicine team.[39] The pyramid plan provides a functional approach to injuries and pain that offers patients the best chance for recovering from injury. Treatment of musculoskeletal pain and injury during the first 72 hours centers around rest, ice, compression, and elevation (RICE).[39–42] Additional therapy includes the use of ultrasound and orally administered analgesics and anti-inflammatory agents such as ibuprofen

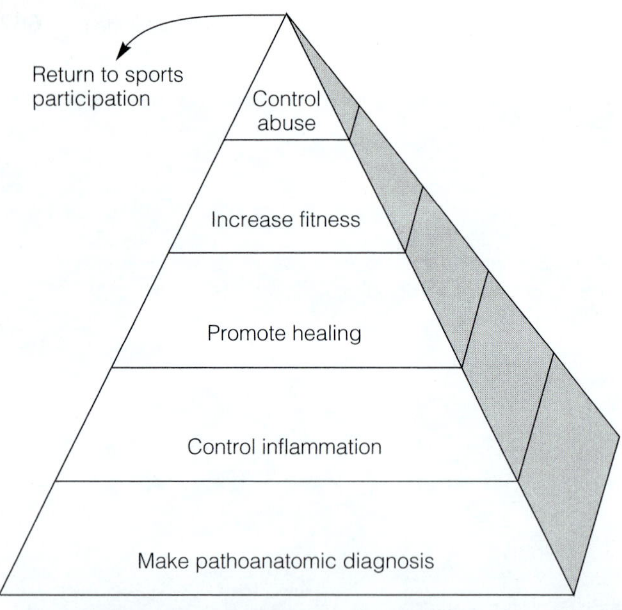

Figure 16.10 Management pyramid for overuse injuries. Management of overuse injuries is organized into five separate phases. Source: O'Connor FG, Howard TM, Fieseler CM, Nirschl RP. Managing overuse injuries: A systematic approach. *Physician Sportsmed* 25(5):88–113, 1997.

Box 16.2

Management of Overuse Injuries

The diagnosis and management of overuse injuries require a multidisciplinary approach involving the sports-medicine physician, physical therapists, orthotists, athletic trainers, and coaches. Follow the five-step approach shown in the management pyramid (see Figure 16.10). Diagnosis should focus on the quality of the athlete's pain, based on a complete physical examination.

Nirschl Pain Phase Scale of Athletic Overuse Injuries

Phase 1. Stiffness or mild soreness after activity. Pain is usually gone within 24 hours.

Phase 2. Stiffness or mild soreness before activity that is relieved by warm-up. Symptoms are not present during activity but return afterward, lasting up to 48 hours.

Phase 3. Stiffness or mild soreness before specific sport or occupational activity. Pain is partially relieved by warm-up. It is minimally present during activity but does not cause the athlete to alter activity.

Phase 4. Similar to phase 3 pain but more intense, causing the athlete to alter performance of the activity. Mild pain occurs with activities of daily living but does not cause a major change in them.

Phase 5. Significant (moderate or greater) pain before, during, and after activity, causing alteration of activity. Pain occurs with activities of daily living but does not cause a major change in them.

Phase 6. Phase 5 pain that persists even with complete rest. Pain disrupts simple activities of daily living and prohibits doing household chores.

Phase 7. Phase 6 pain that also disrupts sleep consistently. Pain is aching in nature and intensifies with activity.

Recommendations Based on Pain Phase

Phases 1, 2, and 3. Avoid intensive exercise that could make the injury worse. Moderate exercise with appropriate warm-up and cool-down is recommended.

Phases 3 and 4. Mild-to-moderate exercise only, with duration and frequency cut in half to allow appropriate rest for healing. Control inflammation with RICE (rest, ice, compression, and elevation) and medications. Consider duplicating land workouts in a swimming pool.

Phases 5, 6, and 7. Control inflammation with RICE and medications. Promote healing with site-specific rehabilitation exercise under the care of a physical therapist or certified athletic trainer (early exercise enhances tissue oxygenation and nutrition, minimizes unnecessary atrophy, and aligns collagen fibers to meet eventual sports-induced stresses). Also incorporate exercises for general body conditioning. During the healing process, control force loads to the rehabilitated tissue area by bracing or taping the injured part, controlling the intensity and duration of the activity, appropriately modifying equipment, and improving the athlete's sports technique.

Source: Data from O'Connor FG, Howard TM, Fieseler CM, Nirschl RP. Managing overuse injuries: A systematic approach. *Phys Sportsmed* 25(5):88–113, 1997.

(Advil, Motrin IB, Nuprin) and aspirin (Bayer, Empirin, Norwich).[41] (Acetaminophen, e.g., Tylenol, does not reduce inflammation.) Controlling the *edema* (accumulation of fluid) and swelling that accompany the injury is of the utmost importance. Control of edema brings about more rapid and complete healing, allowing more normal joint function and reducing pain and necrotic tissue buildup.

Compression of the area appears to be the most effective deterrent to swelling. Applying external compression inhibits the seepage of fluid into underlying tissue spaces and disperses excess fluid.

Initial rest for the injured area is also important. Movement that causes severe pain should be avoided (athletes who want to continue exercising should engage in some form of substitute activity that does not cause pain).

POTENTIAL PROBLEMS OF EXCESS EXERCISE FOR WOMEN

While exercise is widely viewed as beneficial for women of all ages, for some the pressure to succeed in competitive sports leads them to train excessively and restrict eating in order to achieve unrealistically low body weights.[43–45] Certain susceptible women may develop *amenorrhea* (absence of menstruation for 3 to 6 consecutive cycles), leading to osteoporosis. This syndrome of disordered eating (and excessive exercising), amenorrhea, and osteoporosis is called the "female athlete triad" (see Figure 16.11).[45]

The Female Athlete Triad

Large volumes of exercise have been associated with increased rates of *oligomenorrhea* (scanty or infrequent menstrual flow) and amenorrhea. Whereas only 2–5% of the sedentary population has this problem, approximately 5–20% of women who exercise regularly and vigorously and up to 50% of competitive athletes in sports that emphasize leanness may develop it.[43–47] Another common problem among highly active young females in endurance or "appearance" sports (gymnastics, for example) is delayed menarche (>16 years).[48]

The rates vary widely, depending on the type of athlete and the amount of training. Runners and ballet dancers, for example, have much higher rates than swimmers and cyclists. Nearly half of female runners who train 80 or more miles per week are amenorrheic, compared to only about 5–10% of runners who run more moderate distances. Moderate amounts of exercise have little effect on menstrual function[49,50] (see Figure 16.12).

Although all physically active girls and women could be at risk for developing one or more components of the female athlete triad (see Box 16.3), participation in the following sports is a major risk factor:[43]

- Sports in which performance is subjectively scored (dance, figure skating, diving, gymnastics, aerobics)
- Endurance sports emphasizing a low body weight (distance running, cycling, cross-country skiing)
- Sports requiring body-contour-revealing clothing for competition (volleyball, swimming, diving, cross-country running, cross-country skiing, track, cheerleading)
- Sports using weight categories for participation (horse racing, some martial arts, wrestling, rowing)
- Sports emphasizing a prepubertal body habitus for performance success (figure skating, gymnastics, diving)

The female athlete triad syndrome is associated with increased risk of musculoskeletal problems and decreased bone mass. Researchers have reported that spinal bone mass is 20–30% lower for women with amenorrhea, with a high prevalence of stress fractures and musculoskeletal injuries[51–55] (see Figure 16.13).

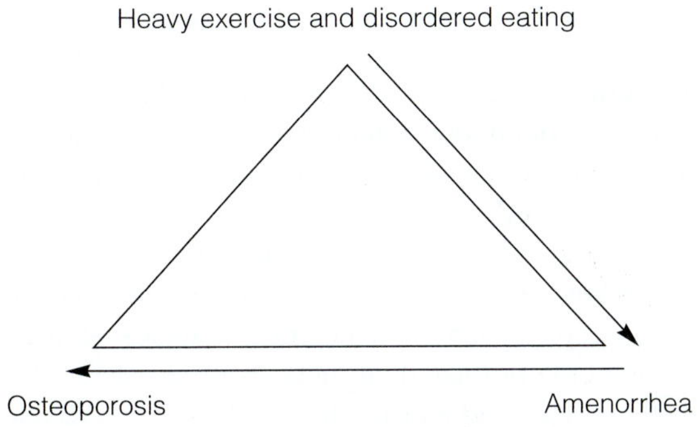

Heavy exercise and disordered eating

Osteoporosis

Amenorrhea

Figure 16.11 The female athlete triad. Female athletes with disordered eating habits and heavy exercise habits may be susceptible to amenorrhea, potentially leading to osteoporosis. Source: Yeager KK, Agostini R, Nattiv A, Drinkwater B. The female athlete triad: Disordered eating, amenorrhea, osteoporosis. *Med Sci Sports Exerc* 25:775–777, 1993.

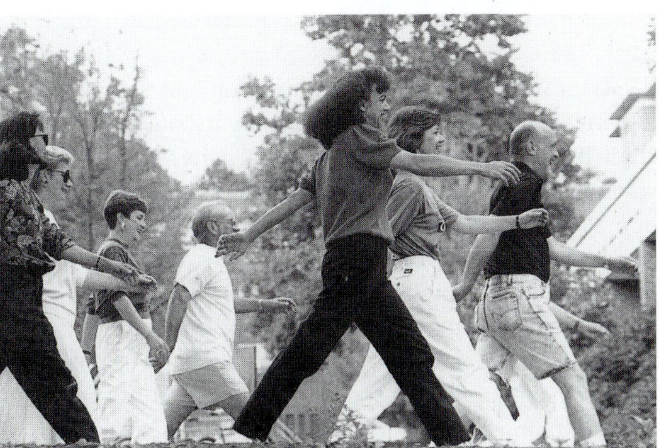

Figure 16.12 Moderate amounts and intensity of exercise, such as with brisk walking, have not been found to impair normal menstrual cycle function.

Box 16.3

The Female Athlete Triad: ACSM Position Stand

Based on a comprehensive literature survey, research studies, case reports, and the consensus of experts, it is the position of the American College of Sports Medicine that:

1. The female athlete triad is a serious syndrome consisting of disordered eating, amenorrhea, and osteoporosis. The components of the Triad are interrelated in etiology, pathogenesis, and consequences. Because of the recent definition of the triad, prevalence studies have not yet been completed. However, it occurs not only in elite athletes but also in physically active girls and women participating in a wide range of physical activities. The triad can result in declining physical performance, as well as medical and psychological morbidity and mortality.
2. Internal and external pressures placed on girls and women to achieve or maintain unrealistically low body weight underlies the development of these disorders.
3. The triad is often denied, not recognized, and underreported. Sports-medicine professionals need to be aware of the interrelated pathogenesis and the varied presentation of components of the triad. They should be able to recognize, diagnose, and treat or refer women with any one component of the triad.
4. Women with one component of the triad should be screened for the other components. Screening for the triad can be done at the time of the preparticipation examination and during clinical evaluation of the following: menstrual change, disordered eating patterns, weight change, cardiac arrhythmias including bradycardia, depression, or stress fracture.
5. All sports-medicine professionals, including coaches and trainers, should learn about preventing and recognizing the symptoms and risks of the triad. All individuals working with active girls and women should participate in athletic training that is medically and psychologically sound. They should avoid pressuring girls and women about losing weight. They should know basic nutrition information and have referral sources for nutritional counseling and medical and mental health evaluation.
6. Parents should avoid pressuring their daughters to diet and lose weight. Parents should be educated about the warning signs of the triad and initiate medical care for their daughters if signs are present.
7. Sports-medicine professionals, athletic administrators, and officials of sport governing bodies share a responsibility to prevent, recognize, and treat the triad. The sport governing bodies should work toward offering opportunities for educational programs for coaches to educate them and to lead them toward professional certification. They should work toward developing programs to monitor coaches and others to ensure safe training practices.
8. Physically active girls and women should be educated about proper nutrition, safe training practices, and the warning signs and risks of the triad. They should be referred for medical evaluation at the first sign of any of the components of the triad.
9. Further research is needed into the prevalence, causes, prevention, treatment, and sequelae of the triad.

Source: Adapted from ACSM Position Stand on the Female Athlete Triad. *Med Sci Sports Exerc* 29:i–ix, 1997.

The causes of menstrual dysfunction and the associated loss in bone mineral mass are still hotly debated but may include the direct effect of exercise itself on the sex hormones or some indirect effect of exercise, such as psychological stress, or malnutrition.[43–47,55–62] The most widely accepted hypothesis is that heavily exercising female athletes do not eat enough to match caloric expenditure (called "energy drain").[46] This causes the hypothalamus to release less gonadotropin-releasing hormone. There are many parallels between the amenorrhea induced by anorexia nervosa and by strenuous athletic training, with both causing an increased secretion of antireproductive hormones, which inhibit the normal pulsatile secretion pattern of gonadotropins.[47,60]

Although the percentage of athletic women with disordered eating habits is not known for certain, estimates range from 30% to 65%.[45,61,62] Whatever the percentages, the net result of athletic amenorrhea is that estrogen levels drop to postmenopausal levels, leading to a rapid loss of bone in the spine.[43,45]

All women who stop menstruating or menstruate irregularly because of their exercise program should be examined by a physician. Amenorrheic athletes should be encouraged to optimize their diets, increase calcium intake to 1,500 mg/day, and modify their exercise to avoid energy drain.[43,45] Amenorrhea appears to be rapidly reversible upon increase in eating and moderation of hard training.[63–66] Even the loss of bone mineral mass has been found to be reversible (though not always completely so) when runners reduce their running distances, gain weight, and resume regular menses.[63–65]

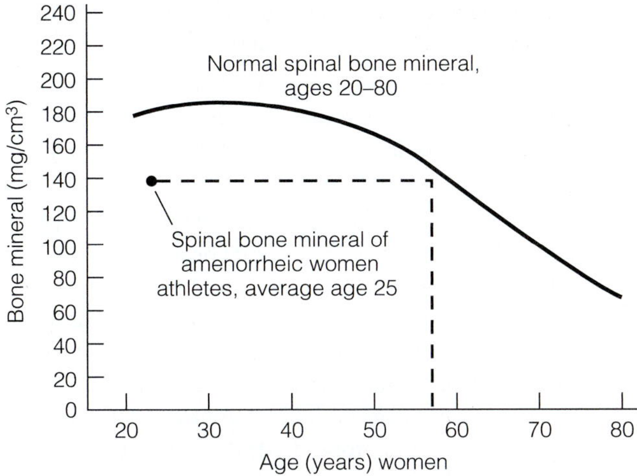

Figure 16.13 Several researchers have found that the spinal bone mineral mass of amenorrheic women athletes at age 25 is equal to that of women twice their age. Source: Drinkwater BL, Nilson K, Chestnut CH, et al. Bone mineral content of amenorrheic and eumenorrheic athletes. *N Engl J Med* 311:277–281, 1984.

Exercise and Pregnancy

During much of the 1900s, pregnant women were urged to reduce physical activity and stop working, especially during the later stages of pregnancy.[67] Exercise was thought to increase the risk of early labor by stimulating uterine activity. Today, concerns have been raised regarding female athletes who continue intensive training throughout their pregnancies. Ingride Kristiansen, the famous runner from Norway, for example, ran to the day of labor and delivered a healthy baby boy. Five months later, she ran a 2:27 marathon, and then a few months later, a 2:24, and within 2 years held the world records for the 5K, 10K, and marathon. *Runner's World* magazine reported the story of a woman who ran up to 40 miles a week throughout her pregnancy. Nine days before giving birth, she completed a marathon race. The day before giving birth to a healthy baby boy, she competed in a 24-hour race, running 62.5 miles.

Many athletes have the attitude expressed by Joan Ullyot, a physician and marathon runner who has observed, "Gazelles run when they're pregnant. Why should it be any different for women?" These types of stories have concerned many experts and doctors who provide health care for women.[67–71]

Pregnancy stresses the body more than any other physiological event in a healthy woman's life.[67] A variety of cardiovascular, metabolic, hormonal, respiratory, and musculoskeletal adaptations take place during the 9 months of pregnancy. Can regular, moderate physical activity provide benefits to the mother and fetus? On the other hand, could high volumes of intensive exercise pose potential risks for pregnancy outcome?

Moderate amounts of exercise during pregnancy are recommended for the health and fitness of the mother and baby.[67–74] One large-scale study of some 2,000 women in Missouri showed that those who largely avoided exercise during pregnancy were more likely to give birth to very low birth weight infants (who are more prone to sickness and death).[73] In another study of some 400 pregnant women, aerobic exercise throughout pregnancy led to fewer discomforts later on.[74] A few studies even suggest that fit mothers gain less unnecessary body fat during pregnancy, experience shorter labor, and have fewer cesarean births.[67,70–72] There is limited evidence that moderate exercise during pregnancy may be a useful treatment for gestational diabetes.[75] In general, 30–45 minutes of moderate aerobic activity on a near-daily basis does not appear to expose the mother to serious metabolic consequences that might adversely affect her or the fetus.

Debate still centers on whether intense and prolonged exercise by the pregnant mother can cause harm to the growing fetus.[67,69,76,77] Concern has been expressed that during heavy exertion, body temperature may rise to high levels, while blood flow, glucose supply, and oxygen delivery to the fetus may be decreased, affecting normal development. In other words, the dual stresses of pregnancy and intense exercise may create conflicting physiological demands that could adversely affect pregnancy outcome.[67]

In 1985, the American College of Obstetricians and Gynecologists (ACOG) released guidelines for exercise during pregnancy.[78] The ACOG took a cautious approach, urging that pregnant women exercise moderately for only 15 minutes at a time, keeping the heart rate below 140 beats per minute. These guidelines caused an outcry among some experts, who claimed they were too conservative. In one review of the medical literature, researchers concluded that exercise performed for up to 40–45 minutes, three times a week at a heart rate of up to 140–145 beats per minute did not appear to adversely affect the mother or the fetus.[71]

In 1994, the ACOG released new guidelines, which removed the heart rate guideline.[79] According to the ACOG, "There are no data in humans to indicate that pregnant women should limit exercise intensity and lower target heart rates because of potential adverse effects." However, the ACOG did urge that regular, moderate exercise is sufficient to derive health benefits, and that pregnant women should listen to their bodies, stop exercising when fatigued, and not exercise to exhaustion.

In 2002, the ACOG reiterated that "recreational and competitive athletes with uncomplicated pregnancies can stay active during pregnancy while modifying their usual exercise routines as medically indicated. Because information on strenuous exercise in pregnancy is scarce, women who participate in such activities should be closely medically supervised. . . . In the absence of either medical or obstetric complications, 30 minutes or more of moderate exercise a day on most, if not all, days of the week is recommended for pregnant women."[68]

Here is a summary of current guidelines for exercise during pregnancy that is consistent with ACOG recommendations:[67,68]

- All women with uncomplicated pregnancies should participate in aerobic and strength-conditioning exercises as part of a healthy lifestyle. Exercising at least 30 minutes on most, if not all, days of the week has multiple health and fitness benefits for the pregnant woman, including improvement in energy and mood state, promotion of muscle and aerobic fitness, and prevention of gestational diabetes. Despite the fact that pregnancy is associated with profound anatomical and physiological changes, there are few instances that should preclude otherwise healthy pregnant women from following the same physical activity recommendations provided for the general adult population.

- Reasonable goals of aerobic conditioning in pregnancy should be to maintain a good fitness level throughout pregnancy without trying to reach peak fitness or train for an athletic competition.
- Recommended physical activities during pregnancy include brisk walking, stationary cycling, cross-country skiing, swimming, and water aerobics. If one is accustomed to running, this routine can be continued during pregnancy, but the exercise intensity should be at a moderate to "somewhat hard" level. Avoid activities such as scuba diving, horseback riding, downhill skiing, and gymnastics that may put the fetus at risk of harm due to loss of balance and accidents, and risk of abdominal trauma.
- Despite a lack of clear evidence that musculoskeletal injuries are increased during pregnancy, this possibility should be considered when prescribing exercise in pregnancy, with special attention given to the increased weight in pregnancy and increase in ligamentous laxity.
- Supine positions should be avoided as much as possible during rest and exercise.
- Warning signs to terminate exercise while pregnant include vaginal bleeding, difficulty in breathing before exercise, dizziness, headache, chest pain, muscle weakness, calf pain or swelling, preterm labor, decreased fetal movement, and amniotic fluid leakage.
- Women with abnormal pregnancies should seek qualified medical advice before making a decision to exercise. Relative contraindications to aerobic exercise during pregnancy include severe anemia, chronic bronchitis, poorly controlled type 1 diabetes, extreme morbid obesity, extreme underweight, history of extremely sedentary lifestyle, poorly controlled hypertension/preeclampsia, orthopaedic limitations, heavy smoker, and poorly controlled thyroid disease and seizure disorder. Absolute contraindications should be determined by a medical doctor, and may include heart and lung disease, persistent second or third trimester bleeding, premature labor, ruptured membranes, and pregnancy-induced hypertension.
- Pregnant women who have been sedentary before pregnancy should follow a gradual progression of up to 30 minutes a day. Pregnancy is not a time for greatly improving physical fitness.
- Women who attained a high level of fitness before pregnancy should exercise caution in engaging in higher levels of fitness activities during pregnancy. Further, they should expect overall activity and fitness levels to decline somewhat as pregnancy progresses.
- Given the variability in maternal heart rate responses to exercise, target heart rates cannot be used to monitor exercise intensity in pregnancy. Ratings of perceived exertion are recommended, with a target of 12–14 (somewhat hard). Exercise should be performed in a thermoneutral environment, with attention given to proper hydration and appropriate energy intake (300 extra Calories per day after the 13th week of pregnancy, and additional caloric intake as needed to compensate for extra physical activity).
- Nonstrenuous exercise during the postpartum period has been shown to reduce postpartum depression, and does not interfere with milk supply through breastfeeding. A gradual return to former activities is advised.

HEAT INJURIES

Heat-related illnesses cause about 240 deaths per year in the United States. Almost all of these deaths occur in persons over 50 years of age and are not related to exertional activities. The actual incidence of heat illness in sports is unknown but is thought to number in the thousands each year.

The American College of Sports Medicine has advised athletes that heat exhaustion and heat strokes are their number one enemies.[80] Risk factors for heat illness are listed in Box 16.4.[80–86] The four major forms of heat illness—heat cramps, heat exhaustion, heat stroke, and exertional rhabdomyolysis—are reviewed in this section (see Chapter 9 for a review of exercise in the heat). Box 16.5 summarizes ACSM guidelines for conducting race events.[80]

Heat Cramps

Heat cramps involve muscular pains and spasms and are associated with weakness, fatigue, nausea, vomiting, and a high heart rate. First aid includes moving the victim to a cool place, having the person lie down, and administering one or two glasses of liquid with ¼ teaspoon of salt added to each glass. The cause is most likely a salt deficit from heavy sweating during prolonged strenuous exercise.[82]

Heat Exhaustion

Heat exhaustion, primarily body fluid depletion due to lack of salt or water deprivation, is characterized by fatigue, weakness, and collapse. Heat exhaustion is the most common form

Box 16.4

Risk Factors and Symptoms for Heat Illness

Because of the potentially grave consequences of heat illness, all athletes and fitness professionals should be alert to these risk factors and symptoms.

Risk Factors

1. Obesity (or high body mass index)
2. Low degree of physical fitness
3. Dehydration
4. Lack of heat acclimatization
5. Previous history of heat stroke
6. Sleep deprivation
7. Certain medications, including diuretics and antidepressants
8. Sweat-gland dysfunction or sunburn
9. Sickness with fever, respiratory tract infection, diarrhea

Symptoms

1. Clumsiness
2. Stumbling
3. Headache
4. Nausea
5. Dizziness
6. Apathy
7. Confusion
8. Impairment of consciousness

Source: Adapted from American College of Sports Medicine. Position stand on heat and cold illnesses during distance running. *Med Sci Sports Exerc* 27:i–x, 1996.

of heat injury among athletes and soldiers.[82] There is profuse sweating, and the skin is often pale and clammy, while body temperature is usually close to normal. First aid includes moving the victim to the coolest possible place, removing clothing, and cooling (with cold water applications, fans to create a draft, or ice packs). Care should be taken to avoid chilling the victim. Oral electrolyte solutions will suffice for most cases, but some athletes may need 3–4 liters after prolonged exercise. Intravenous solutions most commonly used are 5% dextrose in 0.45% NaCl.[84] Salt tablets are not recommended.

Box 16.5

ACSM Recommendations for Race Managers and Medical Directors of Community Race Events

The American College of Sports Medicine advises that the following recommendations be employed by race managers and medical directors of community events that involve prolonged or intense exercise in mild and stressful environments.

1. *Race organization.* Distance races should be scheduled to avoid extremely hot and humid and very cold months. Summer events should be scheduled in the early morning or the evening. The heat stress index should be measured at the race site, using the wet bulb globe temperature (WBGT). If the WBGT is above 82°F, consideration should be given to canceling or postponing the race. An adequate supply of fluid must be available before the start of the race, along the race course, and at the end of the event. Encourage athletes to drink 150–300 ml every 15 minutes. Cool or cold (ice) water immersion is the most effective means of cooling a collapsed hyperthermic athlete. Race officials should be aware of the warning signs of heat illness and should warn athletes to slow down or stop if they appear to be in difficulty. Radio communication or cellular phones should be available throughout the race course for emergency responses.
2. *Medical director.* A sports-medicine physician should work closely with the race director to enhance overall safety and provide adequate medical care for all participants.
3. *Medical support.* The medical director should alert local hospitals and ambulance services. Medical support staff and facilities must be available at the race site.
4. *Competitor education.* Race organizers should conduct clinics and publish articles in the local media to educate runners about heat illness and measures to take to reduce risk. Signs at the race event should caution athletes about the environmental heat stress.

Source: Adapted from American College of Sports Medicine. Position stand on heat and cold illnesses during distance running. *Med Sci Sports Exerc* 27:i–x, 1996.

Heat Stroke

Heat stroke is distinguished by extremely high body temperature (≥ 104°F) and disturbance of the sweating mechanism. The skin is hot, red, and dry (although sweating may persist), the pulse is rapid and strong, and the victim may be unconscious (or disoriented). First aid includes moving the victim to a cool place, removing clothing, and cooling as fast as possible with all available means, including cold water, ice, fans, or rubbing alcohol (ice water baths are best).[85] Speed is of the essence. Heat stroke is a life-threatening situation and is linked to a mortality of 10–80%.

Exertional Rhabdomyolysis

Exertional rhabdomyolysis is the degeneration of skeletal muscle caused by excessive unaccustomed exercise on hot days. Symptoms include muscle pain, weakness, and swelling; dark urine (from a muscle pigment called myoglobin); and increased levels of muscle enzymes and chemicals in the blood. In rare cases, the myoglobin can precipitate in the kidneys, causing renal failure and death. Severe incidents of rhabdomyolysis tend to occur at the start of a training program when exercise is excessive and accompanied by heat stress and dehydration.

Measuring Temperature for Exercise Risk

The "apparent temperature" table from the National Weather Service is derived from measurements of the relative humidity and air temperature and can be adjusted for shaded and light wind conditions (see Figure 16.14). The simplest measurement of environmental heat stress is the *wet bulb temperature* (WBT). It is obtained by putting a wick around the bulb of a thermometer, wetting it, and then blowing air by it with a fan, to determine the effects of evaporation on the temperature reading. Because evaporation is affected by humidity, the WBT will help provide a guide to the degree of environmental stress. A WBT of 78°F or higher requires that exercise be postponed.

The *wet bulb globe temperature* (WBGT) consists of a dry bulb temperature reading, a wet bulb temperature reading, and a black globe temperature reading. The black globe, which is simply a thermometer placed with its bulb inside a copper toilet float painted black, measures the effect of radiant heat from the sun. All readings are taken in the open, allowing 30 minutes of exposure before readings are taken. To compute WBGT, use the following formula:

$$\text{WBGT (°F)} = (0.7 \times \text{wb}) + (0.2 \times \text{g}) + (0.1 \times \text{db})$$

where wb = wet bulb temperature; g = globe temperature; and db = dry bulb temperature (°F).

The following standards have been developed primarily for mass-participation runs:[80]

<65 WBGT	Low risk
65–73 WBGT	Moderate risk (warn the runners that conditions may worsen)
73–82 WBGT	High risk (warn runners; those at high risk should not run)
>82 WBGT	Very high risk (postpone race)

ENVIRONMENTAL POLLUTION

Air pollution has long been suspected of causing ill health and increased risk of lung cancer and other pulmonary diseases.[87–90] In 1952, 4,000 excess deaths occurred in London due to a thick accumulation of air pollutants emitted from burning fossil fuels and blocked by a severe temperature inversion layer.[87] Similar episodes have occurred in Belgium and Pennsylvania. In a 15-year study of more than 8,000 adults in six U.S. cities, Harvard researchers showed that death from lung cancer and cardiopulmonary disease was 26% higher in those living in the most polluted areas.[88] Mortality was most strongly associated with fine particulates including soot, acid condensates, and sulfate and nitrate particles that can be breathed deep into the lungs, posing a risk to health. According to the Centers for Disease Control (CDC) and Prevention,

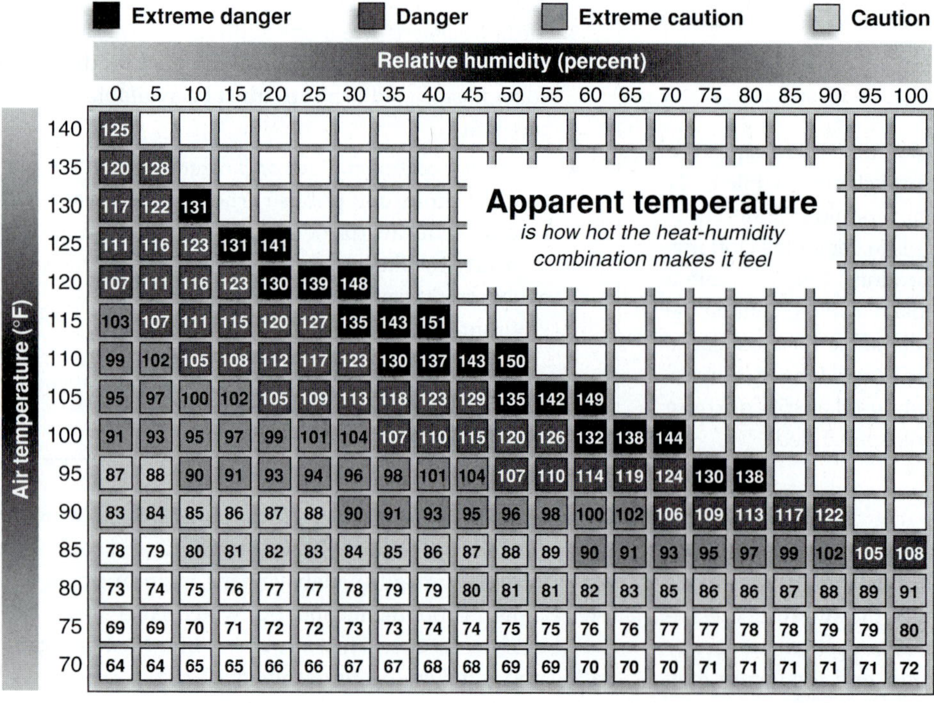

Air temperature (°F)	0	5	10	15	20	25	30	35	40	45	50	55	60	65	70	75	80	85	90	95	100
140	125																				
135	120	128																			
130	117	122	131																		
125	111	116	123	131	141																
120	107	111	116	123	130	139	148														
115	103	107	111	115	120	127	135	143	151												
110	99	102	105	108	112	117	123	130	137	143	150										
105	95	97	100	102	105	109	113	118	123	129	135	142	149								
100	91	93	95	97	99	101	104	107	110	115	120	126	132	138	144						
95	87	88	90	91	93	94	96	98	101	104	107	110	114	119	124	130	138				
90	83	84	85	86	87	88	90	91	93	95	96	98	100	102	106	109	113	117	122		
85	78	79	80	81	82	83	84	85	86	87	88	89	90	91	93	95	97	99	102	105	108
80	73	74	75	76	77	77	78	79	79	80	81	81	82	83	85	86	86	87	88	89	91
75	69	69	70	71	72	72	73	73	74	74	75	75	76	76	77	77	78	78	79	79	80
70	64	64	65	65	66	66	67	67	68	68	69	69	70	70	70	71	71	71	71	71	72

Figure 16.14 Apparent temperature is based on both air temperature and relative humidity. The "caution" and "danger" zones are recommendations given for all people engaged in daily activities (not intense exercise). Source: National Oceanic and Atmospheric Administration.

Box 16.6

Air Quality Index

Air Quality	Weather Conditions	Health Advisory
Good (0.00–0.064 parts per million [ppm] ozone)	Cool summer temperatures Windy and/or cloudy Recent rain or cool front	None
Moderate (0.065–0.084 ppm ozone)	Mild summer temperatures Light/moderate winds High-pressure system, or partly cloudy skies	Extremely sensitive individuals, usually with respiratory disease, should limit prolonged exertion outdoors
Unhealthy for Sensitive Groups (0.085–0.104 ppm ozone)	Temperature upper 80s or above Light winds Sunny skies	People with respiratory disease and other sensitive individuals should limit prolonged exertion outdoors
Unhealthy (0.105–0.124 ppm ozone)	Hazy, hot, and humid	People with respiratory disease and other sensitive individuals should avoid exertion outdoors. Others should limit prolonged or vigorous outdoor exercise
Very unhealthy to hazardous (0.125–0.374 ppm ozone)	Continuing hot, stagnant weather	People with respiratory disease and other sensitive individuals should avoid outdoor activity. Others should limit or avoid exertion outdoors

You may have seen air quality reports in the newspaper or heard them on the radio. The air quality index is a measure of ozone, the main component of smog. Ozone forms when sunlight reacts with hydrocarbons emitted by cars and various commercial and industrial sources.

A beneficial layer of ozone exists naturally in the upper levels of the atmosphere and protects us from the harmful rays of the sun. But the ozone in smog can irritate our lungs, causing shortness of breath, wheezing, and coughing. The first people to feel the effects of high ozone, the so-called sensitive groups, include children, the elderly, people with breathing problems such as asthma, and adults who work or exercise outdoors.

The U.S. Environmental Protection Agency recently revised the air quality index to include precautionary measures for these sensitive groups.

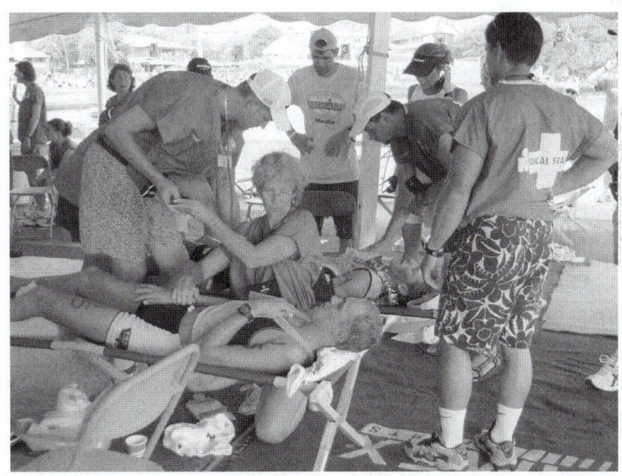

Source: U.S. Environmental Protection Agency.

66% of the U.S. population is at risk for excessive exposure to "inhalable particles" from air pollution.[89]

The CDC has listed exercisers as "an important group at risk" for the effects of ozone and other air pollutants.[89] The long-term effect of exercising in air with fine particulates is unknown, but common sense would urge caution, especially on days with high levels.

During rest, the average human ventilates only 6 liters of air per minute. During heavy exercise, women can ventilate 60–90 liters of air per minute, and males 100–130 liters of air per minute. Obviously, the dosage of air pollutants entering the body is increased, and exercise can exaggerate the normal pulmonary effects of air pollution.[91]

There are two kinds of air pollutants: primary and secondary. *Primary air pollutants* include carbon monoxide (CO), carbon dioxide (CO_2), sulfur dioxide (SO_2), nitrogen oxide (NO), and particulate material such as lead, graphite carbon, and fly ash. *Secondary air pollutants* are formed by the chemical action of the primary pollutants and the natural chemicals in the atmosphere. Examples include ozone (O_3), sulfuric acid (H_2SO_4), nitric acid (HNO_3), peroxyacetyl nitrate, and a host of other inorganic and organic compounds.

Ozone is produced by the photochemical reaction of sunlight and hydrocarbons and nitrogen dioxide from car exhaust. Box 16.6 summarizes new air quality index values and health advisories set by the U.S. Environmental

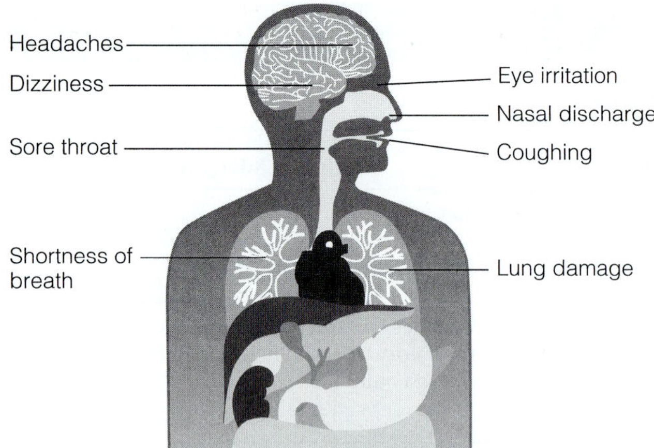

Figure 16.15 Ozone symptoms. Ozone reacts rapidly, causing multiple symptoms. *Ground-level ozone* is the main ingredient in urban smog. Naturally occurring ozone in the upper atmosphere protects life by filtering the ultraviolet radiation from the sun. Ground-level ozone is produced by vehicle or industrial emissions combining with sunlight and heat during times of little or no wind. *Health hazard:* High concentrations of ozone can cause inflammation and irritation of the respiratory tract. Ozone can increase asthma and allergy problems and susceptibility to lung infections. Ozone damage to lungs can continue days after exposure has ended. *Most vulnerable people:* Those most likely to suffer ozone pollution effects include people with lung diseases, the elderly, children and healthy adults who exercise outdoors. Children are especially vulnerable because they often play outside and, in muggy heat, breathe more rapidly and inhale more air pollution.

Protection Agency. In the Los Angeles area, ozone levels reach 0.2 ppm levels for 1 hour or more on about 180 days per year.[91]

Ozone's toxicity is due to its action as an oxidant.[91–96] It is extremely reactive, affecting the pulmonary membranes. Ozone has been shown to cause tissue injury and lung inflammation and reacts rapidly.[94] Symptoms include chest tightness, coughing, headache, dyspnea, nausea, throat irritation, and burning of the eyes (see Figure 16.15).

Heavy exercise in air polluted with ozone impairs the ability to exercise and reduces lung function, at least temporarily.[91–97] Statistically significant impairment of exercise performance can occur at 0.2 ppm. Individuals vary widely, however, in their response to ozone. Reported subjective symptoms have included shortness of breath, coughing, excess sputum, raspy throat, and wheezing.

Interestingly, sensitivity to ozone has been found to diminish with repeated exposure.[95] Results show that by the end of 4-day periods of repeated exercise in polluted air, significant improvements are experienced in $\dot{V}O_{2max}$ and performance time, with decreased subjective symptoms. Although habituation may benefit competitive performance, the long-term consequences of repeated exposures may be undesirable. There are data suggesting that high exposure to ozone over 10–20 years does impair pulmonary function.[97]

SUDDEN DEATH FROM HEART ATTACK

Of all the potential problem areas associated with exercise, the one that has caused the most controversy is the effect on the heart.

The Saga of Jim Fixx

In northern Vermont, late on the afternoon of Friday, July 20, 1984, a passing motorcyclist discovered a man lying dead beside the road. He was clad only in shorts and Nike running shoes. The man was Jim Fixx, author of *The Complete Book of Running*. This amazingly successful book had stayed on the best-seller list for nearly 2 years, helping to accelerate the running boom of the late 1970s. Jim Fixx had become one of the leading spokespersons on the health benefits of running. Now he lay dead—with his running shoes on—and this is why so many Americans were disturbed. Jim Fixx died of cardiac arrest pounding the pavement to gain the fitness and health he advocated for all.[98]

On autopsy, it was discovered that all of Jim Fixx's blood vessels were partially or nearly completely blocked from atherosclerotic plaque buildup. The left circumflex coronary artery was 99% occluded, and scar tissue indicated that three other heart attacks had occurred within 2 months of his death. How could a man in seemingly peak condition, having run 60–70 miles per week for more than 12 years, be stricken by a disease most strongly associated with a sedentary life?

Jim Fixx, despite his running, was at extremely high risk for heart disease—yet he chose to ignore the warning signals. Jim's father had died of a heart attack at age 43. (Family history of heart disease, especially before age 55 for men, is an extremely potent risk factor; see Chapter 10.)

Up to his mid-30s, Jim Fixx was smoking two packs of cigarettes per day, was a "steak-and-potatoes" man, weighed 220 pounds, and had a high-stress, executive job. At age 35, he suddenly tried to turn his life around by running a lot of miles. He lost weight and soon began racing marathons. He decided there was no need to see a doctor, however, even when experiencing heart disease warning signals such as throat and chest tightness. (Six months before Fixx's death, Ken Cooper had invited Fixx to undergo a stress test, but he declined.) In addition, Fixx was not handling well the strain, stress, and pressure of notoriety.

Seventeen years later, at age 52, Jim Fixx lay dead by the side of that Vermont back road, dead of a heart attack. Running may have lengthened his life a bit, but it probably ended up killing him as well.

Exercise and Heart Attack: A Double-Edged Sword

There's probably not a single fitness enthusiast in America who has not read the reports of famous athletes dying on basketball courts, runners found dead with their running shoes

Normal heart

Aorta
Left atrium
Right atrium
Left ventricle
Right ventricle

Heart with hypertrophic cardiomyopathy

- Often affects the left ventricle, which pumps blood to the aorta. The blood then goes through the aorta to the rest of the body.
- Often is hereditary.
- Condition usually develops before age 20.
- Considered cause of death in 36% of all cases of sudden deaths in athletes.

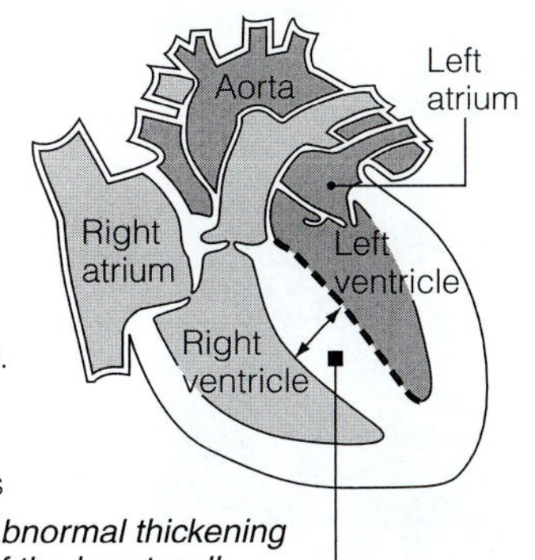

Abnormal thickening of the heart wall

Figure 16.16 Hypertrophic cardiomyopathy is an abnormal thickening of the left ventricle muscle wall that typically goes undetected during routine physical exams and can cause sudden death in young athletes. Medical experts consider hypertrophic cardiomyopathy the most common fatal heart defect among young athletes. An athlete with this condition can compete for years without showing any symptoms and suddenly suffer a heart attack.

on, executives discovered slumped over their treadmills, or middle-aged fathers unearthed alongside their snow shovels. Examples besides Jim Fixx include basketball stars Reggie Lewis, "Pistol Pete" Maravich, and Hank Gathers, and MCI chair Bill McGowan. During the "blizzard of the century" in 1993, scores of people along the eastern seaboard died of sudden heart attack while shoveling their driveways.

Yet, as reviewed in Chapter 10, people who exercise regularly are less likely to die of heart disease than those who refrain (relative risk for inactivity is about 1.9). According to the Centers for Disease Control and Prevention, when all the evidence is considered, lack of exercise is just as responsible for the epidemic of heart disease in America as is high blood pressure, high blood cholesterol, and smoking.[99]

Whether exercise is beneficial or hazardous to the heart appears to depend on who the person is. In one study of 158 athletes who died young (average age 17) and in their prime, 134 of them had heart or blood vessel defects that were present at birth.[100] Most common was hypertrophic cardiomyopathy, a thickening of the heart's main pumping muscle (see Figure 16.16). In other words, when a young athlete dies during or shortly after exercise, it is most often due to a birth defect of the cardiovascular system. There are renewed calls by many experts that despite the relative rarity of these types of deaths and the cost of testing, young athletes should be examined prior to sport participation[101,102] (see Chapter 3).

For most individuals over age 30, however, who die during or shortly after exercise, the cause is entirely different—a narrowing of the coronary blood vessels of the heart because of cholesterol and fat deposits called *atherosclerosis* (as in Jim Fixx).[102–105] Between 4% and 15% of heart attacks occur during or soon after vigorous exertion, making exertion one of the most common triggers of accute heart attack.[105] It appears that when people with these narrowed coronary blood vessels exert themselves heavily during exercise, the increase in heart rate and blood pressure may disrupt the deposits, setting in motion a chain of events that cause a complete blockage and heart attack.[102–105] In other words, middle-aged and older adults who die during exercise tend to be people who already have heart disease. They are at high risk to begin with, and then the vigorous exercise triggers a heart attack.

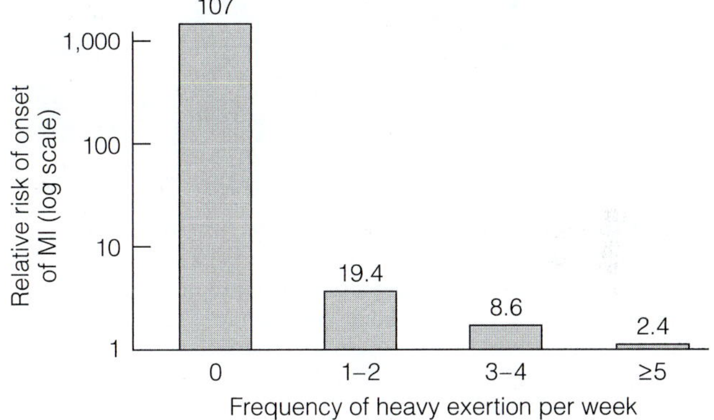

Figure 16.17 Risk of myocardial infarction after heavy exertion. During the hour after heavy exertion, the relative risk of myocardial infarction is much higher for sedentary people than for those who exercise frequently. Source: Data from Kreider RB, Fry AC, O'Tolle ML. Overtraining in Sport. Champagin, IL: *Human Kinetics*, 1998.

Researchers from Harvard University studied the heart attack episodes of 1,228 men and women and found that the risk was 5.9 times higher after heavy versus lighter or no exertion.[103] As shown in Figure 16.17, heavy physical exertion was especially risky for people who were habitually inactive. In other words, people who usually exercised very little, and then went out and exercised vigorously (e.g., shoveling snow), were much more likely to suffer a heart attack than those who were accustomed to exercise (see Figure 16.18). These researchers concluded that every year in the United States, 75,000 Americans suffer a heart attack after vigorous exercise and that these victims tend to be sedentary and at high risk for heart attack to begin with. Another study, from Germany, has also concluded that "a period of strenuous physical activity is associated with a temporary increase in the risk of having a myocardial infarction, particularly among patients who exercise infrequently."[104] A study of 640 patients with acute heart attack showed that exertion-related heart attacks occur in habitually inactive people with multiple heart disease risk

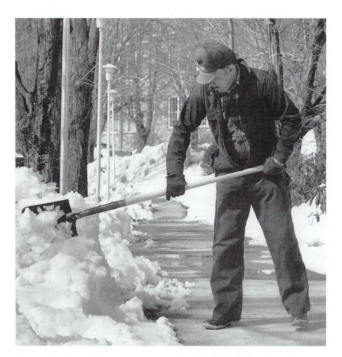

Figure 16.18 People who usually exercise very little and are at high risk for heart disease are much more likely to suffer a heart attack during exercise than are low-risk individuals accustomed to regular exercise.

RPE	Description	Category
6		**Light exercise** Some health benefits, but minimal fitness improvement
7	Very, very light	
8		
9	Very light	
10		
11	Fairly light	
12		**Moderate exercise** Both health and fitness benefits with minimal risk
13	Somewhat hard	
14		
15	Hard	**Intense exercise** For those who desire high fitness. Can precipitate heart attack in high-risk individuals.
16		
17	Very hard	
18		
19	Very, very hard	
20	Maximal	

Figure 16.19 Exercise risk versus benefit using the rating of perceived exertion. The rating of perceived exertion scale can be used to guide exercisers according to their personal goals and fitness levels. Risk for heart attack is greatest when the perceived exertion is "hard" to "maximal."

factors.[105] These patients may benefit from moderate exercise training and aggressive risk-factor modification before they perform vigorous physical activity.

In one study of 36 marathon runners who had died suddenly or suffered a heart attack, researchers found that in most of the cases, a strong family history of heart disease, high blood cholesterol, or early warning symptoms (e.g., chest pain) were present.[106] Most of the runners had symptoms of heart disease but denied they had them and continued training and racing until they finally had a heart attack or died, as did Jim Fixx.[107]

It is important to understand that the risk of a heart attack during exercise is a rare event despite the media reports. Most researchers have found that in a given year, fewer than 10 out of 100,000 men will have a heart attack during exercise.[102,107–109] These victims tend to be men who were sedentary, already had heart disease or were at high risk for it, and then exercised too hard for their fitness level. If an individual is at low risk for heart disease, has not experienced any symptoms, and exercises moderately, risk is extremely low, and overall, risk for heart disease should be lowered because of the regular exercise program.

People at high risk for heart disease should avoid heavy exertion until being cleared by their physicians after taking a maximal treadmill ECG test (see Chapter 3). Even after clearance, they should avoid intense exercise until fitness has been gradually improved and heart disease risk factors have been brought under control. Figure 16.19 outlines recommendations for intensity of exercise using the rating of perceived exertion scale.

RISK FOR UPPER RESPIRATORY TRACT INFECTION

People who exercise report fewer colds than their sedentary peers.[110,111] For example, a 1989 *Runner's World* survey revealed that 61% of 700 recreational runners reported fewer colds since beginning to run, while only 4% felt they had experienced more. In another survey of 170 runners who had been training for 12 years, 90% reported that they definitely or mostly agreed with the statement that they "rarely get sick." A survey of 750 master athletes (ranging in age from 40 to 81 years) showed that 76% perceived themselves as less vulnerable to viral illnesses than their sedentary peers.

Very few studies have been carried out in the area of moderate exercise and colds, and more research is certainly needed to investigate this interesting question. A few randomized, controlled studies with young adult and elderly women have been conducted.[112,113] In these studies, women in the exercise groups walked briskly 35–45 minutes, 5 days a week, for 12–15 weeks during the winter/spring or fall, while the control groups remained physically inactive. The results were in the same direction reported by fitness enthusiasts—walkers experienced about half the days with cold symptoms as the sedentary controls did.

Other research has shown that during moderate exercise, several positive changes occur in the immune system.[111,114,115] Stress hormones, which can suppress immunity, are not elevated during moderate exercise. Although the immune system returns to pre-exercise levels very quickly after the exercise session is over, each session represents a boost that appears to reduce the risk of infection over the long term. Although public health recommendations must be considered tentative, the data on the relationship between moderate exercise and lowered risk of sickness are

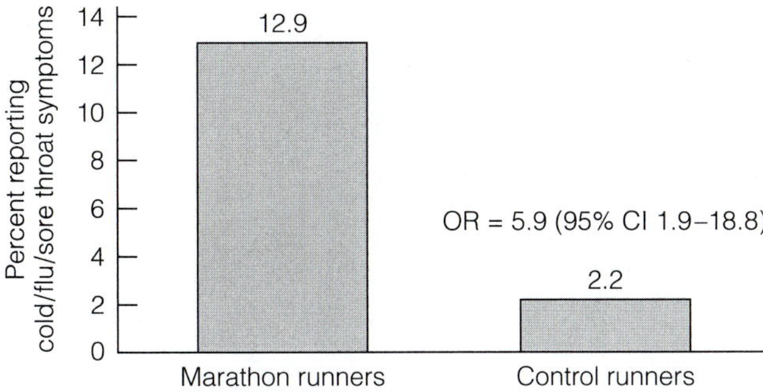

Figure 16.20 Risk of upper respiratory tract infection increases during the week after a marathon race. During the week after the Los Angeles marathon (March 1987), the odds for reporting an upper respiratory tract infection among runners who ran the race were 5.9 times greater than for those who applied but did not run. Source: Nieman DC, Johansen LM, Lee JW, Cermak J, Arabatzis K. Infectious episodes in runners before and after the Los Angeles marathon. *J Sports Med Phys Fit* 30:316–328, 1990.

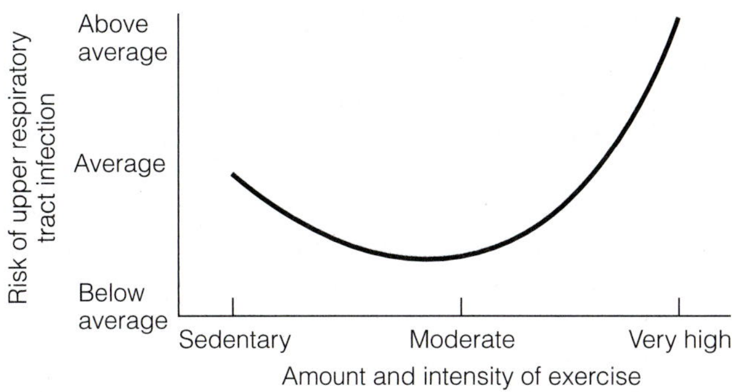

Figure 16.21 Whereas moderate physical activity may decrease the risk for upper respiratory tract infection, heavy exertion may increase this risk. Source: Nieman DC. Exercise, upper respiratory tract infection, and the immune system. *Med Sci Sports Exerc* 26:128–139, 1994.

consistent with guidelines urging the general public to engage in near-daily brisk walking.[111]

In contrast, among elite athletes and their coaches, a common perception is that heavy exertion lowers resistance to colds.[111,116] For example, Liz McColgan, one of the best female runners in Scotland, blamed overtraining "which led to a cold and two subsequent illnesses" as the major reason for her poor performance in the 1992 World Cross Country Championships. Uta Pippig, winner of the 1994 Boston Marathon, caught a cold the week before the race, after training 140 miles a week for 10 weeks at high altitude. Claimed Pippig, "when you are on such a high level you can so quickly fall off." Alberto Salazar, once one of the best marathon runners in the world, reported that while training for the 1984 Olympic marathon, he caught 12 colds in 12 months. "My immune system was totally shot," he recalls. "I caught everything. I felt like I should have been living in a bubble." During the winter and summer Olympic Games, it has been regularly reported by clinicians that "upper respiratory infections abound" and that "the most irksome troubles with the athletes were infections."[111]

To determine whether these anecdotal reports were true, researchers studied a group of 2,311 marathon runners who ran the 1987 Los Angeles marathon.[117] During the week following the race, one out of seven runners came down sick, which was nearly six times the rate of runners who trained for but did not run the marathon (see Figure 16.20). During the 2-month period before the race, runners training more than 60 miles a week doubled their odds for sickness, compared to those training less than 20 miles a week. Researchers in South Africa have also confirmed that after marathon-type exertion, runners are at high risk for sickness.[118,119]

The immune systems of marathon runners have been studied under laboratory conditions before and after running 2–3 hours.[116,120] A steep drop in immune function occurs, which lasts a half day or more depending on the immune measure. Much of this immune suppression appears to be related to the elevation of stress hormones, which are secreted in high quantity during and following heavy exertion. Several exercise immunologists believe this allows viruses to spread and gain a foothold.[111,114,116]

Together, these studies on the relationship between exercise and infection have potential implications for public health, and for the athlete, they may mean the difference between being able to compete or performing at a subpar level or missing the event altogether because of illness. The relationship between exercise and infection may be modeled in the form of a "J" curve.[111] This model suggests that although the risk of infection may decrease below that of a sedentary individual when one engages in moderate exercise training, risk may rise above average during periods of excessive amounts of high-intensity exercise (see Figure 16.21).

Athletes must train hard to prepare for competition. Although this increases the risk for infection if the training becomes too intensive, there are several practical recommendations the athlete can follow to minimize the impact of other stressors on the immune system:[111]

- Keep other life stresses to a minimum. Mental stress in and of itself has been linked to an increased risk of upper respiratory tract infection.
- Eat a well-balanced diet to keep vitamin and mineral pools in the body at optimal levels.
- Avoid overtraining and chronic fatigue.
- Obtain adequate sleep on a regular schedule. Sleep disruption has been linked to suppressed immunity.
- Avoid rapid weight loss (which has also been linked to negative immune changes).
- Avoid putting hands to the eyes and nose (primary routes of introducing viruses into the body). Before important race events, avoid sick people and large crowds when possible.
- For athletes competing during the winter months, flu shots are recommended.
- Use carbohydrate beverages before, during, and after marathon-type race events or unusually heavy training bouts. This may lower the impact of stress hormones on the immune system.

Athletes and fitness enthusiasts are often uncertain of whether they should exercise or rest during sickness. Human studies are lacking to provide definitive answers.[111] Animal studies, however, generally support the finding that one or two periods of exhaustive exercise following injection of the animal with certain types of viruses or bacteria lead to more frequent appearance of infection and more severe symptoms.

With athletes, it is well established that the ability to compete is reduced during sickness. Also, several case histories have shown that sudden and unexplained downturns in athletic performance can sometimes be traced to a recent bout of sickness.[111] In some athletes, exercising when sick can lead to a severely debilitating state known as "post-viral fatigue syndrome." The symptoms can persist for several months and include weakness, inability to train hard, easy fatigability, frequent infections, and depression.

Concerning exercising when sick, most clinical authorities in the area of exercise immunology recommend[111,114,116]

- If one has common cold symptoms (e.g., runny nose and sore throat without fever or general body aches and pains), intensive exercise training may be safely resumed a few days after the resolution of symptoms.
- Mild-to-moderate exercise (e.g., walking) when sick with the common cold does not appear to be harmful. In two studies using nasal sprays of a rhinovirus leading to common cold symptoms, subjects were able to engage in exercise during the course of the illness without any negative effects on severity of symptoms or performance capability.
- With symptoms of fever, extreme tiredness, muscle aches, and swollen lymph glands, 2–4 weeks should probably be allowed before resumption of intensive training.

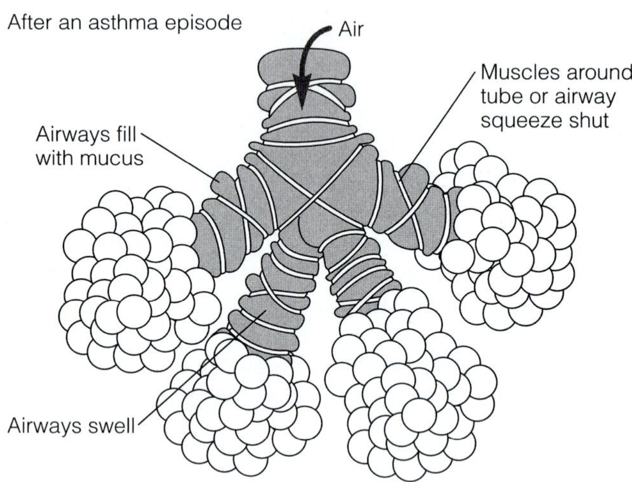

Figure 16.22 During an asthma episode, the muscles around the airways tighten, and the lining swells and produces mucus. Source: Flieger K. Controlling asthma. *FDA Consumer,* November 1996, 19–23.

EXERCISE-INDUCED ASTHMA

Of the various triggers for asthma, physical activity is one of the most common.[121–128] More than 80% of children and 60% of adult asthmatics get exercise-induced asthma (EIA) during or after exercise. In the 1972 Olympic Games, EIA gained considerable attention when an American swimmer lost a gold medal due to the use of a banned drug to treat asthma.[121] Recognition that EIA could be controlled with proper medication and education grew, following reports of the success of U.S. Olympians. Of 597 U.S. athletes in the 1984 Olympic summer games in Los Angeles, 11% reported a history of EIA. These athletes still won 41 medals. In the 1988 Olympic Games in Seoul, about 8% of U.S. athletes were confirmed asthmatics and won, proportionately, as many medals as did athletes without asthma. At the 1998 Olympic Winter Games in Nagano, Japan, 22% of U.S. athletes had asthma, but rates varied widely among the sports.[126]

Prevalence of Asthma

Asthma (Greek, "to pant") is an inflammation of the lungs that causes airways to narrow, making it difficult to breathe. Inflammation makes the airways sensitive to allergens, chemical irritants, tobacco smoke, cold air, or exercise.[129–135] When exposed to these stimuli, an asthma attack can occur, causing the muscles around the windpipes to tighten, making the opening smaller. The lining of the windpipe swells (becomes inflamed) and produces mucus. This leads to coughing, wheezing, chest tightness, and difficulty in breathing, particularly at night or in the early morning (see Figure 16.22). Asthma symptoms come and go; they can last for a few moments or for days. Asthma attacks can be mild or severe and sometimes fatal.

Each year in America, close to 5,000 people die from asthma, with rates twice as high among blacks compared

Box 16.7

Asthma Facts

Prevalence

- More Americans than ever before say they are suffering from asthma. This chronic lung disease is characterized by inflammation of the air passages, which results in the temporary narrowing of the airways that transport air from the nose and mouth to the lungs. It is this country's most common and costly illness.
- The prevalence of asthma has been increasing since the early 1980s across all age, sex, and racial groups. However, the prevalence of asthma is higher among children than adults, and higher among blacks than whites.
- An estimated 20 million Americans suffer from asthma; nearly 5 million are under age 18. It is the most common chronic childhood disease, affecting more than 1 child in 20.

Deaths

- Asthma is the only chronic disease, besides AIDS and tuberculosis, with an increasing death rate. Each day 14 Americans die from asthma.
- From 1980, asthma death rates increased 50% overall. The death rate for children 19 years and younger increased by 80% since 1980.
- More females die of asthma than males and more blacks die of asthma than whites.
- Certain factors indicate that many asthma-related deaths and hospitalizations are preventable when asthma is properly managed. For instance, people with asthma need to avoid environmental factors that make asthma worse, recognize early warning signs of worsening asthma, recognize the severity of an asthma episode, take appropriate medications as prescribed, and seek prompt medical help when problems occur.

The Costs

- The cost of asthma in 2005 was estimated to be $18 billion. Direct costs accounted for $10 billion, and indirect costs were $5 billion. Hospitalizations accounted for the single largest portion of the cost.
- Among children ages 5–17, asthma is the leading cause of school absences from a chronic illness. It accounts for an annual loss of more than 14 million school days per year and more hospitalizations than any other childhood disease.
- For adults, asthma is the fourth leading cause of work loss, resulting in 15 million lost workdays each year.
- Asthma also accounts for about 2 million emergency room visits and 10 million doctor office visits each year.
- Asthma results in about a half million hospitalizations each year. More women are hospitalized for asthma than men, and blacks are hospitalized from asthma three times more than whites.

Ethnic Differences

- Asthma tends to affect the lives of more blacks and Hispanics. Blacks are three times as likely as whites to be hospitalized from asthma and three times as likely to die from the disease.
  - The racial differences in asthma prevalence, morbidity, and mortality are highly correlated with poverty, urban air quality, indoor allergens, and lack of patient education and inadequate medical care.

Source: Asthma and Allergy Foundation of America (AAFA). 1233 20th Street, NW, Suite 402, Washington, DC, 20036. www.aafa.org.

to whites.[134] See Box 16.7 for a summary of facts and figures on asthma. Asthma is a major public health problem, affecting more than 100 million people worldwide and 7% of Americans (about 20 million).[129,130,134] In the United States, about 1 child in every 20 has asthma. Since 1980 for unknown reasons, asthma rates rose 50%, a problem also recognized in many other nations. According to experts of the Global Initiative for Asthma, "this may be linked to factors including housing with reduced ventilation, exposure to indoor allergens (such as domestic dust mites in bedding, carpets, and stuffed furnishings, and animals with fur, especially cats), tobacco smoke, viral infections, air pollution, and chemical irritants."[133]

Prevention Guidelines

Asthma episodes can be prevented, but more studies are needed to determine whether development of the underlying inflammatory disease can be averted.[133,134] Controlling exposure to environmental allergens, irritants, and pollution may help prevent asthma. Asthma is no longer considered a condition with isolated and periodic attacks. Rather, asthma is now understood to be a chronic inflammatory affliction of the airways.[132–135] Inflammation makes the airways hypersensitive to a wide variety of irritants. Causes of the initial tendency toward inflammation in the airways are not yet known for certain, but one of the strongest risk factors is an inherited tendency to have allergic reactions.

Common allergens that are risk factors for developing asthma include dust mites, animals with fur, cockroaches, pollens, and molds.[133] Exposure to tobacco smoke, especially in infants, is a strong risk factor. Chemicals or air pollutants in the workplace can also lead to the development of asthma. Viral respiratory infections, small size at birth, and diet (e.g., certain foods such as shellfish, peanuts, eggs, and chocolate) may also contribute.

Many of these risk factors for developing asthma also aggravate it and are known as triggers because they provoke asthma attacks. Other triggers include wood smoke from open fires or stoves, physical activity, extreme emotional expressions (e.g., laughing or crying hard), cold air or weather changes, certain food additives (e.g., metabisulphite, monosodium glutamate), and aspirin. By avoiding triggers, a person with asthma lowers the risk of irritating the sensitive airways. The risk can be further reduced by taking medications that decrease airway inflammation.[133,134]

Although asthma cannot be cured, it can be controlled by establishing a lifelong management plan with a physician.[133,134] Patients can be educated to avoid triggers and to use appropriate medications. Various quick-relief and long-term preventive medications should be considered. The quick-relief medications include short-acting bronchodilators (e.g., inhaled beta$_2$-agonists) that act quickly to relieve airway tightness and acute symptoms such as coughing, chest tightness, and wheezing. Long-term preventive medications (e.g., inhaled corticosteroids) help control the inflammation that causes attacks. Many asthma medications are delivered by metered dose inhalers, which are highly effective.

The best way to stop asthma attacks is prevention. Identifying and controlling triggers is essential for successful control of asthma. The common triggers include[131,133,134]

- *Dust mites.* These are often a major component of house dust and feed on human skin sheddings. They are found in mattresses, blankets, rugs, soft toys, and stuffed furniture. Exposure to mite allergens in early childhood contributes strongly to the development of asthma. Hot laundering, airtight covers, removal of carpets, and avoiding fabric-covered furniture are recommended.
- *Allergens from animals with fur.* These furry animals include small rodents, cats, and dogs and can trigger asthma. Animals should be removed from the home.
- *Tobacco smoke.* This is a trigger whether the patient smokes or breathes in the smoke from others.
- *Cockroach allergen.* A common trigger in some locations. Infested homes should be cleaned thoroughly and regularly.
- *Mold and other fungal spores and pollens.* These are particles from plants. Windows and doors should be closed, and those with asthma are advised to stay indoors when pollen and mold counts are highest. Air conditioning can be helpful.
- *Smoke from wood-burning stoves and other indoor air pollutants.* These produce irritating particles. Vent all furnaces and stoves to the outdoors, and keep rooms well ventilated.
- *Colds or viral respiratory infections.* These can trigger asthma, especially in children. Give an influenza vaccination every year to patients with moderate-to-severe asthma. At the first sign of a cold, use asthma medications to control symptoms.
- *Physical activity.* Intense activity is a common trigger for most people with asthma.

Exercise-Induced Asthma Symptoms and Phases

Although not entirely understood, most clinicians feel that EIA is triggered as the lining cells of the airway are cooled and dried during exercise.[134] As air is taken into the lungs, it is warmed and humidified, resulting in a cooling and drying of the airway lining. Certain chemicals are then released by the lining cells, causing the airways to tighten. This cooling and drying are worsened by several factors, including exercising in cool and dry air, a switch from nasal to mouth breathing, and fast and deep breathing from intense exercise. If pollutants and pollen are in the air, the risk of EIA is increased.[121–128]

EIA symptoms do not generally occur during the exercise bout itself or the first few minutes after exercise (see Figure 16.23). Following exercise, EIA goes through at least three phases:[121,124,125]

- *Early phase response.* Within several minutes after stopping exercise, the airways begin to tighten, leading to difficulty in breathing, wheezing, coughing, and chest tightness. The symptoms are most severe within 5–10 minutes after exercise. The EIA attack generally lasts 5–15 minutes.

  In the laboratory, clinicians diagnose EIA if the ability to exhale a certain amount of air from the

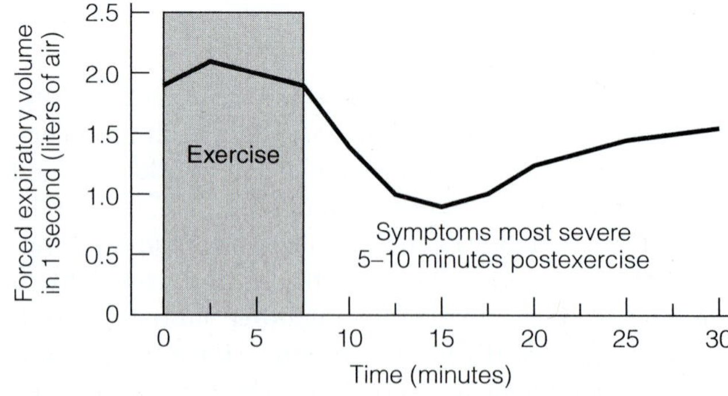

Figure 16.23 Pattern of exercise-induced asthma. EIA is diagnosed if FEV$_1$ falls by 15% or more following 6–8 minutes of high-intensity exercise. Source: Hendrickson CD, Lynch JM, Gleeson K. Exercise induced asthma: A clinical perspective. *Lung* 172:1–14, 1993.

lungs quickly (within 1 second) falls by 15% or more following 6–8 minutes of high-intensity exercise (90% of the maximal heart rate)[134] (see Box 16.8). Many asthmatics now use peak-flow meters, which are small devices that measure how well air moves out of the airways. Asthmatics should avoid exercising vigorously until the peak-flow reading returns to or exceeds 80% of the personal-best peak-flow reading.

- *Spontaneous recovery.* EIA symptoms gradually diminish, usually within 45–60 minutes.
- *Refractory period.* If the individual exercises again within 30–90 minutes of the first bout, the airway tightening is markedly less, and fewer EIA symptoms are experienced.

Some individuals with EIA appear to experience a late asthmatic attack about 3–6 hours after the first one. This late response is still debated, and many factors other than exercise may be responsible.[133,134]

Despite the fact that exercise may trigger asthma, the benefits that come from regular physical training are so important that most asthma experts urge that it be included as an important part of the management strategy of the asthmatic.[134] Regular exercise improves the overall physical fitness level of the individual with asthma, improves psychological mood state, decreases the risk for other chronic diseases, and improves heart and lung function. Also, several researchers have shown that as the individual with asthma becomes physically fit, EIA attacks are less frequent.

Box 16.8

National Institutes of Health Guidelines for Exercise-Induced Asthma

Exercise-induced asthma, which untreated can limit and disrupt otherwise normal lives, should be anticipated in all asthma patients. EIA is a bronchospastic event that is caused by a loss of heat, water, or both from the lungs during exercise because of hyperventilation of air that is cooler and dryer than that of the respiratory tree. EIA usually occurs during or minutes after vigorous activity, reaches its peak 5–10 minutes after stopping the activity, and usually resolves in another 20–30 minutes.

Exercise may be the only precipitant of asthma symptoms for some patients. These patients should be monitored regularly to ensure that they have no symptoms of asthma or reductions in peak expiratory flow (PEF) in the absence of exercise because EIA is often a marker of inadequate asthma management and responds well to regular anti-inflammatory therapy.

Diagnosis

A history of cough, shortness of breath, chest pain or tightness, wheezing, or endurance problems during exercise suggests EIA. An exercise challenge can be used to establish the diagnosis. This can be performed in a formal laboratory setting or as a free-run challenge sufficiently strenuous to increase the baseline heart rate to 80% of maximum for 4–6 minutes. Alternatively, the patient may simply undertake the task that previously caused the symptoms. A 15% decrease in PEF or FEV_1 (forced expiratory volume in 1 second) (measurements taken before and after exercise at 5-minute intervals for 20–30 minutes) is compatible with EIA.

Management Strategies

One goal of management is to enable patients to participate in any activity they choose without experiencing asthma symptoms. EIA should not limit either participation or success in vigorous activities. Recommended treatments include the following:

Beta$_2$-agonists will prevent EIA in more than 80% of patients.

- Short-acting inhaled beta$_2$-agonists used shortly before exercise (or as close to exercise as possible) may be helpful for 2–3 hours.
- Salmeterol has been shown to prevent EIA for 10–12 hours.

Cromolyn and nedocromil, taken shortly before exercise, are also acceptable for preventing EIA.

A lengthy warm-up period before exercise may benefit patients who can tolerate continuous exercise with minimal symptoms. The warm-up may preclude a need for repeated medications.

Long-term-control therapy, if appropriate, may affect EIA. There is evidence that appropriate long-term control of asthma with anti-inflammatory medication will reduce airway responsiveness, and this is associated with a reduction in the frequency and severity of EIA.

Teachers and coaches need to be notified that a child has EIA, should be able to participate in activities, and may need inhaled medication before activity. Individuals involved in competitive athletics need to be aware that their medication use should be disclosed and should adhere to standards set by the U.S. Olympic Committee. The U.S. Olympic Committee's Drug Control Hotline is 800-233-0393.

Source: U.S. Department of Health and Human Services, PHS, NIH, NHLBI. *Guidelines for the Diagnosis and Management of Asthma,* NIH Publication No. 97-4051. Bethesda, MD: National Heart, Lung, and Blood Institute, 1997.

Many famous athletes have coped with asthma, including Jackie Joyner-Kersee, Bill Koch, Greg Louganis, Dominique Wilkins, Jim Ryun, Tom Dolan, and Nancy Hogshead.[127] Each learned how to follow her or his own personal asthma management plan, which included a mix of proper medications and control of asthma triggers. Individuals who follow their asthma management plans and keep their asthma under control can usually participate vigorously in the full range of sports and physical activities. Proper management of EIA includes[133,134] (see Box 16.8):

- Monitoring airflow with a peak-flow meter
- Avoiding allergic triggers
- Using medication before exercise
- Modifying exercise habits and practices

Asthma symptoms can change a lot. They are often worse at night than during the day. They may be more intense in the winter or during "allergy seasons" when pollen counts are high. To help monitor airflow, the new National Heart, Lung, and Blood Institute guidelines recommend that people with moderate-to-severe asthma use a peak-flow meter twice a day.[134] Often, decreases in airflow can provide an early warning of an asthma attack.

Drugs that relax the muscle spasm in the wall of the airways and help to open them (e.g., bronchodilators) are often the first line of treatment in preventing EIA.[134] Doctors recommend using the medication (typically $beta_2$-agonist) from 5 minutes to 1 hour before exercise. $Beta_2$-agonist medications will control EIA in more than 80% of asthmatics and are helpful for several hours. However, because effectiveness does decrease with time, it is preferable to take the medication just before exercise. If breathing problems develop during exercise, a second dose may be needed.

Cromolyn sodium is often prescribed to treat athletes who have EIA.[132–134] This drug, which is also an inhalant, prevents the lining of the airways from swelling in response to cold air or allergic triggers. Cromolyn sodium can be used up to 15 minutes before engaging in physical activity. Corticosteroids should be used as preventive medicine, usually on an ongoing basis, to help control the underlying inflammation.[132–135]

In addition to proper medications, control of triggers, and use of peak-flow meters, several modifications to the exercise program have proven valuable:[121–128]

- *Adequate warm-up and cool-down periods.* These help prevent or lessen episodes of EIA. The warm-up helps asthmatics take advantage of the refractory period when episodes of EIA are reduced.
- *Type of exercise.* This plays a critical role in determining the degree of EIA. Outdoor running is regarded as most conducive to EIA, followed by treadmill running, cycling, walking, and swimming. Swimming rarely leads to EIA because warm and humid air near the surface of the water prevents cooling and drying of the airways.
- *Length of exercise.* Long, intense, continuous exercise (e.g., running and cycling) causes more EIA than repeated short bursts of exercise (generally less than 5 minutes each). Stop-and-go sports such as tennis, volleyball, or football may lead to less EIA for some asthmatics.
- *Intensity of exercise.* High-intensity exercise (above 80–90% of the maximal heart rate) causes more EIA than does exercise at more moderate levels (e.g., walking).
- *Nasal breathing.* Breathe slowly through the nose whenever possible. Nasal breathing warms and humidifies the air better than breathing through the mouth. Interestingly, research has shown that while breathing through the nose only, most people can reach an exercise intensity great enough to improve aerobic fitness.
- *Wear a mask or scarf in cold weather.* This can increase the temperature and humidity of the inhaled air, reducing cooling and drying of the airway lining.
- *Monitor the environment for potential allergens and irritants.* Examples include a recently mowed field, refinished gym floor, smoke in the air, or high pollen counts during a spring morning. If an allergen or irritant is present, a temporary change in time of day or location should be considered because the presence of irritants can trigger more severe EIA attacks.

SPORTS MEDICINE INSIGHT

Risks versus Benefits—A Summary

Broad claims have been made regarding the health benefits of physical activity—but claiming too much can ruin the message.[136–140] Many of the benefit claims are not supported by all researchers. In addition, benefits must be balanced against the risks, which rise exponentially with excessive exercise.

Table 16.1 is a summary of the major benefits of exercise described in Chapters 10–15, balanced against the potential risks outlined in this chapter. The summary represents the author's evaluation of present evidence and published data. The "surety rating" is an estimate of the strength of the data.

(continued)

SPORTS MEDICINE INSIGHT *(continued)*

Risks versus Benefits—A Summary

Notice from Table 16.1 that the highest "surety ratings" indicate that regular physical activity improves health in the following ways:

- Reduces the risk of dying prematurely (i.e., improves life expectancy)
- Reduces the risk of dying from coronary heart disease
- Reduces the risk of developing type 2 diabetes
- Helps prevent and treat high blood pressure
- Reduces the risk of developing colon cancer
- Reduces feelings of depression and anxiety, while improving mood state and self-esteem
- Helps control body weight
- Helps build and maintain healthy bones and muscles, and improves heart and lung fitness
- Improves the life quality of older adults, patients with disease, and people of all ages

Also notice that in some health and disease areas, very little evidence exists to support a prevention or treatment role for regular physical activity. As summarized in Table 16.1, there are few or no physical activity research data supporting the treatment or prevention of type 1 diabetes, arthritis, asthma, and most types of cancer. Regular exercise has also not been shown to slow the progression of HIV infection to AIDS. When change in dietary habits and weight loss is controlled, physical exercise has not been consistently linked to a decrease in LDL cholesterol. Also, more research is needed to confirm whether physical activity can promote regression of atherosclerosis, prevent stroke or hormone-dependent cancers such as breast and prostate cancer, treat osteoporosis, prevent and treat low-back pain, improve diet quality, enhance success in quitting cigarette smoking, improve immunity, and protect against the common cold.

Figure 16.24 depicts the relationship between exercise and risks versus benefits. The greatest gain in the risk–benefit relationship occurs at the lower end of the activity spectrum. In other words, the greatest benefits of exercise are gained by previously sedentary people just beginning moderate exercise programs. Risks are low at the lower levels of activity, but become increasingly frequent and severe at higher levels. Thus, such activities as brisk walking are highly recommended, producing many benefits with few risks.

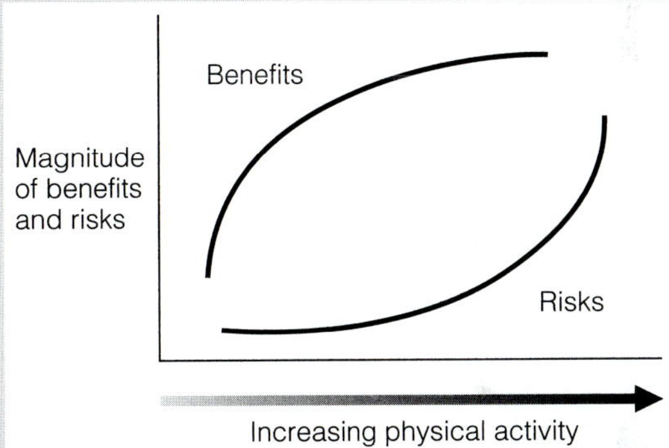

Figure 16.24 The increase in benefits from regular exercise are greatest at low levels and diminish with increasing activity. Risks, on the other hand, are low at lower levels and become increasingly frequent and severe at higher levels.

TABLE 16.1 The Health Benefits and Risks of Regular Physical Activity[a]

Physical Activity Benefit/Risk	Surety Rating
Fitness of body	
Improved heart and lung fitness	****
Improved muscular strength/size	****
Risk: Musculoskeletal injury	****
Risk: Heat injury	****
Cardiovascular disease	
Coronary heart disease prevention	****
Regression of atherosclerosis	**
Treatment of heart disease	***
Prevention of stroke	**
Risk: Heart attack for those at high risk	****
Arthritis	
Prevention of arthritis	*
Treatment/cure of arthritis	*
Improvement of life quality/fitness	****
High blood pressure	
Prevention of high blood pressure	****
Treatment of high blood pressure	****
Asthma	
Prevention/treatment of asthma	*
Improvement in asthmatic's life quality	***
Risk: Exercise-induced asthma	****

(continued)

TABLE 16.1 *(continued)*

Physical Activity Benefit/Risk	Surety Rating
Cancer	
Prevention of colon cancer	****
Prevention of breast cancer	***
Prevention of uterine cancer	**
Prevention of prostate cancer	**
Prevention of other cancers	*
Treatment of cancer	*
Improvement in life quality of cancer patients	***
Osteoporosis	
Helps build up bone density	****
Prevention of osteoporosis	***
Treatment of osteoporosis	**
Blood cholesterol/lipoproteins	
Lowers total blood cholesterol	*
Lowers LDL cholesterol	*
Lowers triglycerides	***
Raises HDL cholesterol	***
Low-back pain	
Prevention of low-back pain	**
Treatment of low-back pain	**
Nutrition and diet quality	
Improvement in diet quality	**
Increase in total energy intake	***
Risk: Iron deficiency	***
Cigarette smoking	
Improves success in quitting	**
Diabetes	
Prevention of type 2	****
Treatment of type 2	***
Treatment of type 1	*
Improvement of diabetic life quality	****
Risk: Hypoglycemia, type 1	****
Infection and Immunity	
Prevention of the common cold	**
Improve overall immunity	**
Slow progression of HIV to AIDS	*
Improve life quality of HIV-infected	***
Risk: Immune suppression, infection	***
Sleep	
Improvement in sleep quality	***
Risk: Sleep disturbance from overtraining, overexertion	***
Weight management	
Prevention of weight gain	****
Treatment of obesity	**
Helps maintain weight loss	****
Risk: Musculoskeletal injury	****
Children and youths	
Prevention of obesity	***
Control of disease risk factors	***
Reduction of unhealthy habits	**
Improves odds of adult activity	**
Elderly and the aging process	
Improvement in physical fitness	****
Counter loss in heart/lung fitness	**
Counter loss of muscle	***
Counter gain in fat	***
Improvement in life expectancy	****
Improvement in life quality	****
Psychological well-being	
Elevation in mood	****
Buffers effects of mental stress	***
Alleviate/prevent depression	****
Anxiety reduction	****
Improvement in self-esteem	****
Risk: Exercise addiction	***
Risk: Mood disturbance, overtraining	***
Special issues for women	
Improves total body fitness	****
Improves fitness while pregnant	****
Improves birthing experience	**
Improves health of fetus	**
Risk: Female athlete triad	****
Risk: Harm to fetus	**

[a]Table is based on a total physical fitness program that includes physical activity designed to improve both aerobic and musculoskeletal fitness.

[****]Strong consensus, with little or no conflicting data

[***]Most data are supportive, but more research is needed for clarification

[**]Some data are supportive, but much more research is needed

[*]Little or no data support

SUMMARY

1. This chapter surveyed some of the risks involved with exercise, especially when performed excessively. These include musculoskeletal injuries, disruption of normal reproductive function of women, possible problems for women who are pregnant, heat injury, effects of air pollution on performance, sudden death from heart attack, increased risk of infectious episodes and exercise-induced asthma.
2. The potential for musculoskeletal injury was reviewed for running, aerobic dance, bicycling, and swimming. Most of the injuries are related to overtraining and accidents. The muscles, joints, and supporting ligaments and tendons of the legs and feet respond very poorly to excessive exercise, especially activities that require running and jumping.
3. Running is associated with a high rate of musculoskeletal injuries, with 24–77% of runners reporting injuries within a given year. Although most of the runners usually do not seek medical help, the pain is frequently serious enough to disrupt the running routine.
4. Researchers have tried to measure the factors responsible for the high prevalence of injuries among runners and have looked at both personal factors and training habits. Overtraining is a common cause of injury.
5. The major studies examining the injury potential of aerobic dance have found that about 45% of students and 75% of instructors report injuries. Most of these injuries, however, are mild, causing some pain and some disruption in participation, but generally falling short of leading participants to cease aerobic-dance activities or to seek professional medical assistance.
6. Studies have shown that exercise increases the rates of oligomenorrhea and amenorrhea; they vary widely, however, depending on the type of athlete and the amount of training. The causes are still hotly debated. Loss of bone mineral mass is a problem for oligomenorrheic athletes. The female athlete triad is the syndrome of disordered eating habits and heavy exercise leading to amenorrhea and osteoporosis.
7. Moderate exercise during pregnancy serves to maintain the fitness of the mother and has been associated with several favorable pregnancy outcomes.
8. The American College of Sports Medicine has advised athletes that the risk of heat exhaustion and heat stroke during high temperature and humidity is greatly increased. Heat injury is a major cause of death among exercising athletes, and appropriate measures should be taken, including postponing the exercise.
9. The air pollutant regarded as the most detrimental to athletic performance is ozone. Heavy exercise in air polluted with ozone has been shown to impair the ability to exercise and decrease lung function at least temporarily.
10. The principal cause of death among adults over 30 years of age during exercise is coronary heart attack. It happens rarely, however, and more often to those with underlying heart disease and those unaccustomed to exercise. Congenital forms of cardiovascular disease are the leading cause of athletic death in younger athletes.
11. Excessive exercise has been associated with increased risk of infectious health problems. Moderate exercise may be protective, but little research has been conducted so far to verify this.
12. During and following strenuous exercise, the majority of asthmatics experience exercise-induced asthma (EIA). EIA can be controlled with appropriate medications and exercise techniques.
13. The risks of exercise must be balanced with all of its documented benefits. The greatest gain in the risk–benefit relationship occurs at the lower end of the activity spectrum.

Review Questions

1. *____ injuries account for the vast majority of bicycling deaths.*

   A. Head **B.** Chest
   C. Abdominal **D.** Liver

2. *Exercise should be postponed when the wet bulb temperature rises above a threshold of ____ °F.*

   A. 45 **B.** 78 **C.** 90 **D.** 100

3. *When a young adult dies suddenly during exercise, this is usually related to*

   A. Coronary heart disease
   B. Congenital defects of the heart or its vessels
   C. Heat stroke

4. *The most common cause of injury in runners is*

   A. Biomechanical imbalances
   B. Overuse syndrome
   C. Poor shoes
   D. Running style
   E. Stretching before running

5. *Three body sites are most often injured in runners. Which one of the following is* **not** *included?*

   A. Foot
   B. Leg
   C. Knee
   D. Lower back

6. *Which of the following statements regarding oligomenorrhea and amenorrhea in women is true?*

   A. Prevalence rates tend to decrease with increasing amounts of intense running.
   B. Bone densities in these women are greater compared to those in women with normal menstrual cycles.
   C. Oligomenorrhea and amenorrhea are usually reversible upon cessation of hard training and resumption of normal energy intake.
   D. Oligomenorrhea and amenorrhea occur in the majority of recreational runners.

7. *Which of the following is* **not** *included in the 2002 ACOG exercise guidelines for pregnant women?*

   A. Avoid exercise in the supine position after the first trimester.
   B. Do not exercise to the point of exhaustion.
   C. Augment heat dissipation by ensuring adequate hydration, appropriate clothing, and optimal environmental surroundings during exercise.
   D. Avoid any type of exercise involving the potential for even mild abdominal trauma to the abdomen.
   E. Weight-bearing exercise is recommended to decrease risk of injury and facilitate continuation of exercise during pregnancy.

8. *When an older adult dies suddenly during exercise, this is usually related to*

   A. Coronary heart disease
   B. Congenital defects of the heart or its vessels
   C. Heat stroke

9. *Which one of the following is a sign of overtraining?*

   A. Decreased exercise heart rate at a certain workload
   B. Lack of desire to train
   C. Increased appetite
   D. Weight gain
   E. Elevated testosterone levels

10. *Absence of menstrual flow is called*

    A. Amenorrhea **B.** Oligomenorrhea

11. *Moderate exercise during pregnancy ____ pose harm to the growing fetus.*

    A. Does not **B.** Does

12. *When the skin is hot, red, and dry, with the pulse strong and rapid, the victim has ____.*

    A. Heat exhaustion **B.** Heat stroke

13. *The greatest health benefits of exercise are gained by*

    A. Athletes who step up their training for competition
    B. Sedentary people who initiate a regular physical activity program
    C. Walkers who initiate a running program
    D. Cyclers who switch to a swimming program

14. *There is good evidence that muscle tightness and lack of flexibility ____ the risk for injury with exercise training.*

    A. Increase **B.** Decrease
    C. Are not related to

15. *Which one of the following is* **not** *included in the RICE treatment for pain and injury?*

    A. Rest **B.** Intense stretching
    C. Compression **D.** Exercise

16. *The female athlete triad does* **not** *include*

    A. Disordered eating **B.** Osteoporosis
    C. Depression

17. *The loss of bone mass has been found to be reversible (although not always completely) when runners reduce their running distances, gain weight, and resume regular menses.*

    A. True **B.** False

18. *An estimated ____ million Americans suffer from asthma.*

    A. 5 **B.** 8 **C.** 10 **D.** 13 **E.** 20

19. *____ are three times as likely as whites to be hospitalized from asthma and three times as likely to die from the disease.*

    A. Hispanics **B.** Asians
    C. Blacks **D.** Native Americans

20. *____ is the degeneration of skeletal muscle caused by excessive unaccustomed exercise on hot days.*

    A. Exertional rhabdomyolysis
    B. Heat exhaustion
    C. Heat stroke
    D. Sarcopenia
    E. Osteopenia

21. *Which one of the following is* **not** *a secondary air pollutant?*

    A. Carbon monoxide **B.** Ozone
    C. Sulfuric acid **D.** Nitric acid
    E. Peroxyacetyl nitrate

22. *Heavy exercise in air polluted with ozone ____ been found to impair the ability to exercise.*

    A. Has **B.** Has not

23. *Heavy physical exertion can cause sudden death in some people, especially*

    A. Those who are habitually inactive
    B. Older athletes

C. Obese teenagers
D. Middle-aged women

24. *Marathon runners have been found to be immune from heart attacks.*

A. True B. False

25. *Athletes engaging in marathon-type events are at ____ risk of upper respiratory tract infection.*

A. Increased B. Decreased

26. *Immune function is ____ during recovery from heavy exertion.*

A. Stimulated B. Suppressed

27. *EIA is often induced by exercising at ____% $\dot{V}O_{2max}$ for 5–8 minutes.*

A. 50 B. 65 C. 75 D. 85

28. *EIA can be controlled by following several guidelines. Which one of the following is* **not** *included?*

A. Exercise in a cold, dry environment
B. Exercise in repeated spurts of less than 5 minutes each
C. Exercise at intensities below 85%
D. Use appropriate medications
E. Warm-up before training or competing

29. *Which one of the following benefits of regular exercise has the strongest and most consistent research support?*

A. Improved quality of dietary habits
B. Prevention of colon cancer
C. Prevention of type 2 diabetes
D. Treatment of osteoporosis among the elderly
E. Prevention of heart disease

30. *Which one of the following risks of excessive or inappropriate exercise has the strongest and most consistent research support?*

A. Iron deficiency
B. Musculoskeletal injury
C. Risk to fetus of pregnant woman
D. Suppression of immune function
E. Vitamin and mineral deficiencies

31. *Which benefit of regular aerobic exercise listed has the weakest research support?*

A. Lengthens life span
B. Improves cardiorespiratory fitness
C. Improves glycemic control of type 2 diabetics
D. Prevention of obesity
E. Control of hypertension in hypertensives

32. *When ozone is at 0.105–0.124 ppm, the air quality index is*

A. Good
B. Moderate
C. Unhealthy for sensitive groups
D. Unhealthy
E. Very unhealthy to hazardous

33. *Which one of the following is* **not** *a risk factor for heat illness?*

A. Obesity
B. High degree of physical fitness
C. Sleep deprivation
D. Use of diuretic medication
E. Respiratory tract infection

34. *Which one of the following is* **not** *a trigger for asthma attacks?*

A. Dust mites
B. Tobacco smoke
C. Cockroach allergen
D. Smoke from wood-burning stoves
E. Physical inactivity

35. *In the laboratory, EIA is diagnosed if the FEV_1 (forced expiratory volume in 1 second) falls by at least ____% following 6–8 minutes of high-intensity exercise.*

A. 5 B. 10 C. 15 D. 25 E. 50

36. *EIA symptoms gradually diminish after intensive exercise, usually within ____ minutes.*

A. 5–10 B. 15–30
C. 60–90 D. 120–150
E. 45–60

37. *Several modifications to the exercise program have proven valuable for controlling EIA. Which one of the following is* **not** *included?*

A. Avoid use of a mask or scarf in cold weather.
B. Lower intensity of exercise to moderate level.
C. Have adequate warm-up and cool-down.
D. Breathe through nose whenever possible.
E. When possible, swim instead of run.

Answers

1. A	**12.** B	**23.** A	**34.** E
2. B	**13.** B	**24.** B	**35.** C
3. B	**14.** C	**25.** A	**36.** E
4. B	**15.** B	**26.** B	**37.** A
5. D	**16.** C	**27.** D	
6. C	**17.** A	**28.** A	
7. E	**18.** E	**29.** E	
8. A	**19.** C	**30.** B	
9. B	**20.** A	**31.** A	
10. A	**21.** A	**32.** D	
11. A	**22.** A	**33.** B	

REFERENCES

1. Kreider RB, Fry AC, O'Toole ML. *Overtraining in Sport.* Champaign, IL: Human Kinetics, 1998.
2. Powell KE, Heath GW, Kresnow MJ, Sacks JJ, Branche CM. Injury rates from walking, gardening, weightlifting, outdoor bicycling, and aerobics. *Med Sci Sports Exerc* 30:1246–1249, 1998.
3. Pate RR, Macera CA. Risk of exercising: Musculoskeletal injuries. In Bouchard C, Shephard RJ (eds.). *Exercise, Fitness, and Health: A Consensus of Current Knowledge.* Champaign, IL: Human Kinetics Books, 1994.
4. Van Mechelen W. Running injuries: A review of the epidemiological literature. *Sports Med* 14:320–335, 1992.
5. Hreljac A. Impact and overuse injuries in runners. *Med Sci Sports Exerc* 36:845–849, 2004.
6. Koplan JP, Powell KE, Sikes RK, Shirley RW, Campbell GC. An epidemiologic study of the benefits and risks of running. *JAMA* 248:3118–3121, 1982.
7. Koplan JP, Siscovick DS, Goldbaum GM. The risks of exercise: A public health view of injuries and hazards. *Pub Health Rep* 100:189–195, 1985.
8. Powell KE, Kohl HW, Caspersen CJ, Blair SN. An epidemiological perspective on the causes of running injuries. *Physician Sportsmed* 14(6):100–114, 1986.
9. Koplan JP, Rothenberg RB, Jones EL. The natural history of exercise: A 10-yr follow-up of a cohort of runners. *Med Sci Sports Exerc* 27:1180–1184, 1995.
10. Marti B, Vader JP, Minder CE, Abelin T. On the epidemiology of running injuries. *Am J Sports Med* 16:285–294, 1988.
11. Marti B. Benefits and risks of running among women: An epidemiologic study. *Int J Sports Med* 9:92–98, 1988.
12. Kennedy JG, Knowles B, Dolan M, Bohne W. Foot and ankle injuries in the adolescent runner. *Curr Opin Pediatr* 17:34–42, 2005.
13. Macera CA, Pate RR, Power KE, et al. Predicting lower-extremity injuries among habitual runners. *Arch Intern Med* 149:2565–2568, 1989.
14. Walter SD, Hart LE, McIntosh JM, Sutton JR. The Ontario cohort study of running-related injuries. *Arch Intern Med* 149:2561–2564, 1989.
15. Van Mechelen W. Can running injuries be effectively prevented? *Sports Med* 19:161–165, 1995.
16. Wen DY, Puffer JC, Schmalzried TP. Lower extremity alignment and risk of overuse injuries in runners. *Med Sci Sports Exerc* 29:1291–1298, 1997.
17. Jones BH, Knapik JJ. Physical training and exercise-related injuries. Surveillance, research and injury prevention in military populations. *Sports Med* 27:111–125, 1999.
18. Clements K, Yates B, Curran M. The prevalence of chronic knee injury in triathletes. *Br J Sports Med* 33:214–216, 1999.
19. Halson SL, Jeukendrup AE. Does overtraining exist? An analysis of overreaching and overtraining research. *Sports Med* 34:967–981, 2004.
20. Messier SP, Davis SE, Curl WW, Lowery RB, Pack RJ. Etiologic factors associated with patellofemoral pain in runners. *Med Sci Sports Exerc* 23:1008–1015, 1991.
21. Duffey MJ, Martin DF, Cannon DW, Craven T, Messier SP. Etiologic factors associated with anterior knee pain in distance runners. *Med Sci Sports Exerc* 32:1825–1832, 2000.
22. Pretorius DM, Noakes TD, Irving G, Allerton K. Runner's knee: What is it and how effective is conservative management? *Phys Sportsmed* 14(12):71–81, 1986.
23. Hreljac A, Marshall MN, Hume PA. Evaluation of lower extremity overuse injury potential in runners. *Med Sci Sports Exerc* 32:1635–1641, 2000.
24. Garrick JG, Requa RK. Aerobic dance: A review. *Sports Med* 6:169–179, 1988.
25. Garrick JG, Gillien DM, Whiteside P. The epidemic of aerobic dance injuries. *Am J Sports Med* 14:67–72, 1986.
26. Rothenberger LA, Chang JI, Cable TA. Prevalence and types of injuries in aerobic dancers. *Am J Sports Med* 16:403–407, 1988.
27. Mutoh Y, Sawai S, Takanashi Y, Skurko L. Aerobic dance injuries among instructors and students. *Physician Sportsmed* 16:81–88, 1988.
28. Richie DH, Kelso SF, Bellucci PA. Aerobic dance injuries: A retrospective study of instructors and participants. *Physician Sportsmed* 13:130–140, 1985.
29. Puder DR, Visintainer P, Spitzer D, Casal D. A comparison of the effect of different bicycle helmet laws in 3 New York City suburbs. *Am J Public Health* 89:1736–1738, 1999.
30. Sacks JJ, Holmgreen P, Smith SM, Sosin DM. Bicycle-associated head injuries and deaths in the United States from 1984 through 1988. How many are preventable? *JAMA* 266:3016–3018, 1991.
31. Thompson DC, Patterson MQ. Cycle helmets and the prevention of injuries. Recommendations for competitive sport. *Sports Med* 25:213–219, 1998.
32. Kronisch RL, Pfeiffer RP, Chow TK. Acute injuries in cross-country and downhill off-road bicycle racing. *Med Sci Sports Exerc* 28:1351–1355, 1996.
33. Thompson DC, Rivara FP, Thompson RS. Effectiveness of bicycle safety helmets in preventing head injuries. *JAMA* 276:1968–1973, 1996.
34. Dannenberg AL, Vernick JS. A proposal for the mandatory inclusion of helmets with new children's bicycles. *Am J Public Health* 83:644–646, 1993.
35. Royal S, Kendrick D, Coleman T. Non-legislative interventions for the promotion of cycle helmet wearing by children. *Cochrane Database Syst Rev* 18(2):CD003985, 2005.
36. Johnson JE, Sim FH, Scott SG. Musculoskeletal injuries in competitive swimmers. *Mayo Clin Proc* 62:289–304, 1987.
37. Koehler SM, Thorson DC. Swimmer's shoulder. *Physician Sportsmed* 24(11):39–50, 1996.
38. Vizsolyi P, Taunton J, Robertson G, et al. Breaststroker's knee: An analysis of epidemiological and biochemical factors. *Am J Sports Med* 15:63–71, 1987.
39. O'Connor FG, Howard TM, Fieseler CM, Nirschl RP. Managing overuse injuries. A systematic approach. *Physician Sportsmed* 25(5):88–113, 1997.
40. Rizzo TD. Using RICE for injury relief. *Physician Sportsmed* 24(10):33–34, 1996.
41. Hasson SM, Daniels JC, Divine JG, et al. Effect of ibuprofen use on muscle soreness, damage, and performance: A preliminary investigation. *Med Sci Sports Exerc* 25:9–17, 1993.
42. Meeusen R, Van der Veen P, Harley S. Cold and compression in the treatment of athletic injuries. *Am J Med Sports* 3:166–170, 2001.
43. ACSM position stand on the female athlete triad. *Med Sci Sports Exerc* 29:i–ix, 1997.
44. Adams Hillard PJ, Deitch HR. Menstrual disorders in the college-age female. *Pediatr Clin North Am* 52(1):179–197, 2005.

45. Birch K. Female athlete triad. *BMJ* 330(7485):244–246, 2005.
46. Loucks AB. Energy availability, not body fatness, regulates reproductive function in women. *Exerc Sport Sci Rev* 31:144–148, 2003. See also: Loucks AB, Verdun M, Heath EM. Low energy availability, not stress of exercise, alters LH pulsatility in exercising women. *J Appl Physiol* 84:37–46, 1998.
47. Harber VJ. Menstrual dysfunction in athletes: An energetic challenge. *Exerc Sport Sci Rev* 28:19–23, 2000.
48. Merzenich H, Boeing H, Wahrendorf J. Dietary fat and sports activity as determinants for age at menarche. *Am J Epidemiol* 138:217–224, 1993.
49. Bonen A. Recreational exercise does not impair menstrual cycles: A prospective study. *Int J Sports Med* 13:110–120, 1992.
50. Rogol AD, Weltman A, Weltman JY, et al. Durability of the reproductive axis in eumenorrheic women during 1 yr of endurance training. *J Appl Physiol* 74:1571–1580, 1992.
51. Rencken ML, Chesnut CH, Drinkwater BL. Bone density at multiple skeletal sites in amenorrheic athletes. *JAMA* 276:238–240, 1996.
52. Lloyd T, Triantafyllou SJ, Baker ER, et al. Women athletes with menstrual irregularity have increased musculoskeletal injuries. *Med Sci Sports Exerc* 18:374–379, 1986.
53. Barrow GW, Saha S. Menstrual irregularity and stress fractures in collegiate female distance runners. *Am J Sports Med* 16:209–216, 1988.
54. Drinkwater BL, Nilson K, Chesnut CH, et al. Bone mineral content of amenorrheic and eumenorrheic athletes. *N Eng J Med* 311:277–281, 1984.
55. Cobb KL, Bachrach LK, Greendale G, et al. Disordered eating, menstrual irregularity, and bone mineral density in female runners. *Med Sci Sports Exerc* 35:711–719, 2003.
56. Torstveit MK, Sundgot-Borgen J. The female athlete triad: Are elite athletes at increased risk? *Med Sci Sports Exerc* 37:184–193, 2005.
57. De Souza MJ. Menstrual disturbances in athletes: A focus on luteal phase defects. *Med Sci Sports Exerc* 35:1553–1563, 2003.
58. Williams NI, Young JC, McArthur JW, Bullen B, Skrinar GS, Turnbull B. Strenuous exercise with caloric restriction: Effect on luteinizing hormone secretion. *Med Sci Sports Exerc* 27:1390–1398, 1995.
59. Dueck CA, Manore MM, Matt KS. Role of energy balance in athletic menstrual dysfunction. *Int J Sport Nutr* 6:165–190, 1996.
60. Keizer HA, Rogol AD. Physical exercise and menstrual cycle alterations: What are the mechanisms? *Sports Med* 10:218–235, 1990.
61. Williams NI, Bullen BA, McArthur JW, Skrinar GS, Turnbull BA. Effects of short-term strenuous endurance exercise upon corpus luteum function. *Med Sci Sports Exerc* 31:949–958, 1999.
62. Zanker CL, Swaine IL. Relation between bone turnover, oestradiol, and energy balance in women distance runners. *Br J Sports Med* 32:167–171, 1998.
63. Lindberg JS, Powell MR, Hunt MM, et al. Increased vertebral bone mineral in response to reduced exercise in amenorrheic runners. *West J Med* 146:39–42, 1987.
64. Drinkwater BL, Nilson K, Ott S, Chesnut CH. Bone mineral density after resumption of menses in amenorrheic athletes. *JAMA* 256:380–382, 1986.
65. Dueck CA, Matt KS, Manore MM, Skinner JS. Treatment of athletic amenorrhea with a diet and training intervention program. *Int J Sport Nutr* 6:24–40, 1996.
66. Cumming DC. Exercise-associated amenorrhea, low bone density, and estrogen replacement therapy. *Arch Intern Med* 156:2193–2195, 1996.
67. Artal R, O'Toole M. Guidelines of the American College of Obstetricians and Gynecologists for exercise during pregnancy and the postpartum period. *Br J Sports Med* 37:6–12, 2003.
68. ACOG Committee opinion. Number 267, January 2002: Exercise during pregnancy and the postpartum period. ACOG Committee Obstetric Practice. *Obstet Gynecol* 99:171–173, 2002.
69. Paisley TS, Joy EA, Price RJ. Exercise during pregnancy: A practical approach. *Curr Sports Med Rep* 2:325–330, 2003.
70. Bloom SL, McIntire DD, Kelly MA, Beimer HL, Burpo RH, Garcia MA, Leveno KJ. Lack of effect of walking on labor and delivery. *N Engl J Med* 339:76–79, 1998.
71. Lokey EA, Tran ZT, Wells CL, Myers BC, Tran AC. Effects of physical exercise on pregnancy outcomes: A meta-analytic review. *Med Sci Sports Exerc* 23:1234–1239, 1991.
72. Clapp JF, Little KD. Effect of recreational exercise on pregnancy weight gain and subcutaneous fat deposition. *Med Sci Sports Exerc* 27:170–177, 1995.
73. Schramm WF, Stockbauer JW, Hoffman HJ. Exercise, employment, other daily activities, and adverse pregnancy outcomes. *Am J Epidemiol* 143:211–218, 1996.
74. Sternfeld B, Quesenberry CP, Eskenazi B, Newman LA. Exercise during pregnancy and pregnancy outcome. *Med Sci Sports Exerc* 27:634–640, 1995.
75. Artal R. Exercise: An alternative therapy for gestational diabetes. *Physician Sportsmed* 24(3):54–66, 1996.
76. Wolfe LA, Ohtake PJ, Mottola MF, McGrath MJ. Physiological interactions between pregnancy and aerobic exercise. *Exerc Sport Sci Rev* 17:295–351, 1989.
77. Clapp JF, Dickstein S. Endurance exercise and pregnancy outcome. *Med Sci Sports Exerc* 16:556–562, 1984.
78. American College of Obstetricians and Gynecologists. *Exercise during Pregnancy and the Postnatal Period (ACOG Home Exercise Programs).* Washington, DC: ACOG, 1985.
79. American College of Obstetricians and Gynecologists. *Exercise during Pregnancy and the Postpartum Period.* Technical Bulletin No. 189. Washington, DC: Author, 1994.
80. American College of Sports Medicine. Position stand on heat and cold illnesses during distance running. *Med Sci Sports Exerc* 27:i–x, 1996.
81. CDC. Heat-related deaths—United States, 1993. *MMWR* 42:558–560, 1993.
82. Coris EE, Ramirez AM, Van Durme DJ. Heat illness in athletes. The dangerous combination of heat, humidity, and exercise. *Sports Med* 34:9–16, 2004.
83. Watts SA. Prevention and treatment of dehydration in athletes. *Am J Med Sports* 3:286–293, 2001.
84. Galloway SDR, Maughan RJ. Effects of ambient temperature on the capacity to perform prolonged cycle exercise in man. *Med Sci Sports Exerc* 29:1240–1249, 1997.
85. Dallam GM, Jonas S, Miller TK. Medical considerations in triathlon competition: Recommendations for triathlon organizers, competitors, and coaches. *Sports Med* 35:143–161, 2005.
86. Wallace RF, Kriebel D, Punnett L, Wegman DH, Wenger CB, Gardner JW, Gonzalez RR. The effects of continuous hot weather training on risk of exertional heat illness. *Med Sci Sports Exerc* 37:84–90, 2005.

87. Bernstein JA, Alexis N, Barnes C, Bernstein IL, Bernstein JA, Nel A, Peden D, Diaz-Sanchez D, Tarlo SM, Williams PB. Health effects of air pollution. *J Allergy Clin Immunol* 114:1116–1123, 2004.

88. Dockery DW, Pope A, Xu X, et al. An association between air pollution and mortality in six U.S. cities. *N Engl J Med* 329:1753–1759, 1993.

89. CDC. Populations at risk from air pollution—United States, 1991. *MMWR* 42:301–304, 1993.

90. Borja-Aburto VH, Loomis DP, Bangdiwala SI, Shy CM, Rascon-Pacheco RA. Ozone, suspended particulates, and daily mortality in Mexico City. *Am J Epidemiol* 145:258–268, 1997.

91. Adams WC. Effects of ozone exposure at ambient air pollution episode levels on exercise performance. *Sports Med* 4:395–424, 1987.

92. Hazucha MJ, Bates DV, Dromberg PA. Mechanisms of action of ozone on the human lung. *J Appl Physiol* 67:1535–1541, 1989.

93. Carlisle AJ, Sharp NC. Exercise and outdoor ambient air pollution. *Br J Sports Med* 35:214–222, 2001.

94. Frank R, Liu MC, Spannhake EW, Mlynarek S, Macri K, Weinmann GG. Repetitive ozone exposure of young adults. Evidence of persistent small airway dysfunction. *Am J Respir Crit Care Med* 164:1253–1260, 2001.

95. Foxcroft WJ, Adams WC. Effects of ozone exposure on four consecutive days on work performance and $\dot{V}O_{2\ max}$. *J Appl Physiol* 61:960–966, 1986.

96. Korrick SA, Neas LM, Dockery DW, Gold DR, Allen GA, Hill LB, Kimball KD, Rosner BA, Speizer FE. Effects of ozone and other pollutants on the pulmonary function of adult hikers. *Environ Health Perspect* 106:93–99, 1998.

97. Kunzli N, Lurmann F, Segal M, Ngo L, Balmes J, Tager IB. Association between lifetime ambient ozone exposure and pulmonary function in college freshmen—results of a pilot study. *Environ Res* 72:8–23, 1997.

98. Cooper KH. *Running without Fear.* New York: Bantam Books, 1985.

99. Powell KE, Thompson PD, Caspersen CJ, Kendrick JS. Physical activity and the incidence of coronary heart disease. *Ann Rev Public Health* 8:253–287, 1987.

100. Maron BJ, Chaitman BR, Ackerman MJ, Bayes de Luna A, Corrado D, Crosson JE, Deal BJ, Driscoll DJ, Estes NA, Araujo CG, Liang DH, Mitten MJ, Myerburg RJ, Pelliccia A, Thompson PD, Towbin JA, Van Camp SP; Working Groups of the American Heart Association Committee on Exercise, Cardiac Rehabilitation, and Prevention; Councils on Clinical Cardiology and Cardiovascular Disease in the Young. Recommendations for physical activity and recreational sports participation for young patients with genetic cardiovascular diseases. *Circulation* 109:2807–2816, 2004.

101. Wingfield K, Matheson GO, Meeuwisse WH. Preparticipation evaluation: An evidence-based review. *Clin J Sport Med* 14:109–122, 2004.

102. Futterman LG, Myerburg R. Sudden death in athletes. An update. *Sports Med* 26:335–350, 1998.

103. Mittleman MA, Maclure M, Tofler GH, Sherwood JB, Goldberg RJ, Muller JE. Triggering of acute myocardial infarction by heavy physical exertion: Protection against triggering by regular exertion. *N Engl J Med* 329:1677–1683, 1993.

104. Willich SN, Lewis M, Löwel H, Arntz H-R, Schubert F, Schröder R. Physical exertion as a trigger of acute myocardial infarction. *N Engl J Med* 329:1684–1690, 1993.

105. Giri S, Thompson PD, Kiernan FJ, Clive J, Fram DB, Mitchel JF, Hirst JA, McKay RG, Waters DD. Clinical and angiographic characteristics of exertion-related acute myocardial infarction. *JAMA* 282:1731–1736, 1999.

106. Noakes TD. Heart disease in marathon runners: A review. *Med Sci Sports Exerc* 19:187–194, 1987.

107. Maron BJ, Poliac LC, Roberts WO. Risk for sudden cardiac death associated with marathon running. *J Am Coll Cardiol* 28:428–431, 1996.

108. Albert CM, Mittleman MA, Chae CU, Lee IM, Hennekens CH, Manson JE. Triggering of sudden death from cardiac causes by vigorous exertion. *N Engl J Med* 343:1355–1361, 2000.

109. Maron BJ, Araujo CGS, Thompson PD, et al. Recommendations for preparticipation screening and the assessment of cardiovascular disease in masters athletes. *Circulation* 103:327–334, 2001.

110. Nieman DC. Does exercise alter immune function and respiratory infections? *President's Council on Physical Fitness and Sports, Research Digest,* Series 3, No. 13, June, 2001.

111. Nieman DC. Is infection risk linked to exercise workload? *Med Sci Sports Exerc* 32 (suppl 7):S406–S411, 2000.

112. Nieman DC, Nehlsen-Cannarella SL, Henson DA, Koch AJ, Butterworth DE, Fagoaga OR, Utter A. Immune response to exercise training and/or energy restriction in obese females. *Med Sci Sports Exerc* 30:679–686, 1998.

113. Nieman DC, Henson DA, Gusewitch G, Warren BJ, Dotson RC, Butterworth DE, Nehlsen-Cannarella SL. Physical activity and immune function in elderly women. *Med Sci Sports Exerc* 25:823–831, 1993.

114. Nieman DC, Henson DA, Austin MD, Brown VA. The immune response to a 30-minute walk. *Med Sci Sports Exerc* 37:57–62, 2005.

115. Nieman DC. Current perspective on exercise immunology. *Curr Sports Med Rep* 2:239–242, 2003.

116. Nieman DC, Dumke CL, Henson DA, McAnulty SR, McAnulty LS, Lind RH, Morrow JD. Immune and oxidative changes during and following the Western States Endurance Run. *Int J Sports Med* 24:541–547, 2003.

117. Nieman DC, Johansen LM, Lee JW, Cermak J, Arabatzis K. Infectious episodes in runners before and after the Los Angeles Marathon. *J Sports Med Phys Fit* 30:316–328, 1990.

118. Peters EM, Bateman ED. Respiratory tract infections: An epidemiological survey. *S Afr Med J* 64:582–584, 1983.

119. Peters EM, Goetzsche JM, Grobbelaar B, et al. Vitamin C supplementation reduces the incidence of postrace symptoms of upper-respiratory-tract infection in ultramarathon runners. *Am J Clin Nutr* 57:170–174, 1993.

120. Nieman DC, Henson DA, McAnulty SR, McAnulty LS, Morrow JD, Ahmed A, Heward CB. Vitamin E and immunity after the Kona Triathlon World Championship. *Med Sci Sports Exerc* 36:1328–1335, 2004.

121. Storms WW. Review of exercise-induced asthma. *Med Sci Sports Exerc* 35:1464–1470, 2003; See also: Mahler DA. Exercise-induced asthma. *Med Sci Sports Exerc* 25:554–561, 1993.

122. Cerny FJ, Maxwell PJ. Control of exercise-induced asthma. Triggers, medications, warm-ups. *ACSM's Health & Fitness Journal* 4(1):17–24, 2000.

123. Randolph C. Exercise-induced asthma: Pathophysiology, diagnosis, and management for the primary care provider. *Am J Med Sports* 2:383–394, 2000.

124. Giesbrecht GG, Younes M. Exercise- and cold-induced asthma. *Can J Appl Physiol* 20:300–314, 1995.

125. Anderson SD, Kippelen P. Exercise-induced bronchoconstriction: Pathogenesis. *Curr Allergy Asthma Rep* 5:116–122, 2005.

126. Weiler JM, Ryan EJ. Asthma in United States Olympic athletes who participated in the 1998 Olympic Winter Games. *J Allergy Clin Immunol* 106:267–271, 2000.

127. Meadows M. Breathing better. *FDA Consumer,* March–April, 2003; See also: Papazian R. Being a sport with exercise-induced asthma. *FDA Consumer,* January–February, pp. 30–33, 1994.

128. Tan RA, Spector SL. Exercise-induced asthma. *Sports Med* 25:1–6, 1998.

129. CDC. Self-reported asthma prevalence and control among adults—United States, 2001. *MMWR* 52:382–384, 2003; See also: CDC. Surveillance for asthma—United States, 1960–1995. *MMWR* 47(No.SS-1), 1998.

130. Weiss KB, Wagener DK. Changing patterns of asthma mortality: Identifying target populations at high risk. *JAMA* 264:1683–1687, 1990.

131. CDC. Asthma prevalence and control characteristics by race/ethnicity—United States, 2002. *MMWR* 53:145–148, 2004; See also: CDC. Self-reported asthma prevalence among adults—United States, 2000. *MMWR* 50(32):682–686, 2001.

132. U.S. Department of Health and Human Services, PHS, NIH, NHLBI. *Asthma and Physical Activity in the School.* NIH Publication No. 95-3651. Bethesda, MD: National Heart, Lung, and Blood Institute Information Center, 1995.

133. U.S. Department of Health and Human Services, PHS, NIH, NHLBI. *Asthma Management and Prevention, Global Initiative for Asthma: A Practical Guide for Public Health Officials and Health Care Professionals.* NIH Publication No. 96-3659A. Bethesda, MD: National Heart, Lung, and Blood Institute, 1995. See also: CDC. Key clinical activities for quality asthma care. Recommendations of the National Asthma Education and Prevention Program. *MMWR* 52(RR-6):1–8, 2003.

134. NHLBI, National Asthma Education and Prevention Program. *Quick Reference for the NAEPP Expert Panel Report: Guidelines for the Diagnosis and Management of Asthma—Update on Selected Topics 2002.* Publication No. 02-5075. Bethesda, MD: US Department of Health and Human Services, National Institutes of Health, 2002. See also: NHLBI, National Asthma Education and Prevention Program. *Guidelines for the Diagnosis and Management of Asthma.* NIH Publication No. 97-4051. Bethesda, MD: National Heart, Lung, and Blood Institute, 1997.

135. Kemp JP, Kemp JA. Management of asthma in children. *Am Fam Physician* 63:1341–1348, 1353–1354, 2001.

136. Powell KE, Paffenbarger RS. Workshop on epidemiologic and public health aspects of physical activity: A summary. *Public Health Rep* 100:118–126, 1985.

137. U.S. Department of Health and Human Services. *Physical Activity and Health: A Report of the Surgeon General.* Atlanta, GA: U.S. Department of Health and Human Services, Centers for Disease Control and Prevention, National Center for Chronic Disease Prevention and Health Promotion, 1996.

138. Elrick H. Exercise is medicine. *Physician Sportsmed* 24(2):72–78, 1996.

139. Roberts CK, Barnard RJ. Effects of exercise and diet on chronic disease. *J Appl Physiol* 98:3–30, 2005.

140. Nieman DC. *The Exercise–Health Connection.* Champaign, IL: Human Kinetics, 1998.

PHYSICAL FITNESS ACTIVITY 16.1

Benefits versus Risks of Exercise

As noted at the end of this chapter, though heavy amounts of exercise are associated with various risks, moderate exercise can bring many health benefits. Not exercising at all is worse than too much exercise, and moderate exercise is a virtue. The well-documented benefits of moderate exercise are too valuable to be ignored.

Major benefits of regular, moderate exercise include the following:

1. Improved heart and lung fitness
2. Lower resting heart rate
3. Firmer, toned muscles
4. Reduced body fat (especially when dietary fat is low)
5. Reduced risk of high blood pressure
6. Increased high-density lipoprotein cholesterol, reduced triglycerides
7. Reduced risk of cancer
8. Reduced risk of heart disease
9. Reduced risk of diabetes
10. Elevation of psychological mood state, and reduced anxiety and depression
11. Increased self-esteem
12. Increased density of bones, and lowered risk of osteoporosis
13. Improved quality of life even into old age
14. Increased life expectancy
15. Less fatigue, increased energy for work, leisure, and emergencies

Review this list carefully, and then, drawing on your own experience, list five benefits that *you* personally feel are most valuable to you. List the benefit, and then explain why you chose it. List the benefits in order of importance, beginning with the most important.

1. ____

____

2. ____

____

3. ____

____

4. ____

____

5. ____

____

Review the chapter again carefully. List three risks that *you* personally feel have been most bothersome for you. In other words, drawing on your own experience, what risks have caused you the most pain and grief? List the risk, and then explain why you chose it. Again, list in order of importance.

1. ____

____

2. ____

____

3. ____

____

 **PHYSICAL FITNESS ACTIVITY 16.2**

Rate Your Foot and Ankle Health

How healthy are your feet and ankles? Take this self-assessment quiz from the Foot Health Foundation of America. See below for scoring.

1. How much time do you spend on your feet each day?
   - **a.** Less than 2 hours. 0
   - **b.** 2–4 hours 1
   - **c.** 5–7 hours 2
   - **d.** 8 hours or more 3
2. How old are you?
   - **a.** Under 40 0
   - **b.** 40–59 1
   - **c.** 60 or older. 2
3. How would you describe your weight?
   - **a.** Ideal to 20 pounds over 0
   - **b.** 20–39 pounds over 2
   - **c.** 40 or more pounds over 3
4. Have foot or ankle problems stopped you from leisure or sports activities?
   - **a.** Yes 2
   - **b.** No 0

   Work?
   - **a.** Yes 3
   - **b.** No 0
5. Have you received medical treatment for feet or ankles?
   - **a.** Yes 3
   - **b.** No 0
6. Do you regularly wear heels 2 or more inches high?
   - **a.** Yes 2
   - **b.** No 0
7. What types of exercise do you do or plan soon? Check all that apply.
   - **a.** Walking. 1
   - **b.** Field sports—softball, golf. 2
   - **c.** Winter sports like skiing 2
   - **d.** Court sports like tennis 3
   - **e.** Aerobics 3
   - **f.** Running 3
   - **g.** None

   (If you answer g, skip to number 12)
8. Do you have the right shoes for your sport?
   - **a.** Yes 0
   - **b.** No 3
9. Do you have foot or ankle pain walking or exercising?
   - **a.** Rarely 1
   - **b.** Sometimes 2

c. Often 3
d. Never. 0

10. Do you exercise in shoes more than 1 year old or that are hand-me-downs?
a. Yes 3
b. No 0

11. Do you stretch properly after exercising?
a. Yes 0
b. No 3

12. Do you have diabetes?
a. Yes 3
b. No 0

13. Do you have a family history of diabetes?
a. Yes 2
b. No 0

14. Do you have numbness or burning in your feet?
a. Yes 3
b. No 0

15. Do you sprain your ankles often, or are they weak?
a. Yes 2
b. No 0

16. Do you have flat feet or very high arches?
a. Yes 2
b. No 0

17. Do you have Achilles' tendon pain, heel pain, or shinsplints?
a. Yes 2
b. No 0

18. Do you have corns, calluses, bunions, or hammertoes?
a. Yes 3
b. No 0

19. Do you have arthritis or joint pain in your feet?
a. Yes 3
b. No 0

20. Do you have poor circulation or leg cramps?
a. Yes 3
b. No 0

Classification

Total the numbers at the right of each answer:

0 to 20 Congratulations. Your feet and ankles are very healthy.

21 to 40 Pay attention. You are in the moderate risk category. Consider professional help.

41 or higher. Caution. You are at high risk for long-term problems. Get help.

APPENDIX **A**

Physical Fitness Test Norms

Section 1. Physical Fitness Test Norms for Children, Adolescents, and College Students

NATIONAL CHILDREN AND YOUTH FITNESS STUDY I (NCYFS I)

In 1984, the Public Health Service (Office of Disease Prevention and Health Promotion, U.S. Department of Health and Human Services), in response to the landmark government report *Promoting Health/Preventing Disease: Objectives for the Nation,* launched the National Children and Youth Fitness Study to determine how fit and how active first- through twelfth-grade students actually are. Data on 10- to 18-year-olds were collected from a random sample of 10,275 students from 140 public and private schools in 19 states between February and May 1984. The NCYFS I was the first nationwide assessment of the physical fitness of American young people in nearly a decade and the most rigorous study of fitness among our youths ever conducted in the United States.

Test items of the NCYFS I include*

- Triceps and subscapular skinfolds for body composition
- Walk/run (1 mile) for cardiorespiratory endurance
- Sit-and-reach test for lower back–hamstring flexibility
- Pull-up for upper-body muscular strength and endurance
- Bent-knee sit-ups (1 minute) for abdominal strength/endurance

Interpretations of norms: <25% = unacceptable or poor; 25–50% = minimal or fair; 50–75% = acceptable or good; >75% = optimal or excellent.

**Note:* See description of methods in Chapters 4–6.

Source: Public Health Service. Summary of findings from National Children and Youth Fitness Study. *JOPHER*/January 1985, 44–90.

TABLE 1 Sum of Triceps and Subscapular Skinfolds—Boys (total mm)

Age	10	11	12	13	14	15	16	17	18
99%	9	9	9	9	9	10	10	10	11
90	12	12	12	11	12	12	12	13	13
80	13	13	13	13	13	13	13	14	14
75	14	14	14	13	13	14	14	14	15
70	15	15	15	14	14	14	14	15	15
60	16	16	16	15	15	15	15	16	17
50	17	18	17	17	17	17	17	17	18
40	20	20	20	19	18	18	18	19	19
30	22	23	22	21	21	20	20	21	22
25	24	25	24	23	22	22	22	22	24
20	25	26	28	25	25	24	23	24	25
10	35	36	38	34	33	32	30	30	30

TABLE 2 Sum of Triceps and Subscapular Skinfolds—Girls (total mm)

Age	10	11	12	13	14	15	16	17	18
99%	10	11	11	12	12	13	13	16	14
90	13	14	15	15	17	19	19	20	19
80	15	16	17	18	19	21	21	22	21
75	16	17	18	19	20	23	22	23	22
70	17	18	18	20	21	24	23	24	23
60	18	19	21	22	24	26	24	26	25
50	20	21	22	24	26	28	26	28	27
40	22	24	24	26	28	30	28	31	28
30	25	28	27	29	31	33	32	34	32
25	27	30	29	31	33	34	33	36	34
20	29	33	31	34	35	37	35	37	36
10	36	40	40	43	40	43	12	42	42

TABLE 3 Chin-Ups—Boys (hands in underhand position, palms toward subject)

Age	10	11	12	13	14	15	16	17	18
99%	13	12	13	17	18	18	20	20	21
90	8	8	8	10	12	14	14	15	16
80	5	5	6	8	9	11	12	13	14
75	4	5	5	7	8	10	12	12	13
70	4	4	5	7	8	10	11	12	12
60	2	3	4	5	6	8	10	10	11
50	1	2	3	4	5	7	9	9	0
40	1	1	2	3	4	6	8	8	9
30	0	0	1	1	3	5	6	6	7
25	0	0	0	1	2	4	6	5	6
20	0	0	0	0	1	3	5	4	5
10	0	0	0	0	0	1	2	2	3

TABLE 4 Chin-Ups—Girls (hands in underhand position, palms toward subject)

Age	10	11	12	13	14	15	16	17	18
99%	8	8	8	5	8	6	8	7	6
90	3	3	2	2	2	2	2	2	2
80	2	1	1	1	1	1	1	1	1
75	1	1	1	1	1	1	1	1	1
70	1	1	1	0	1	1	1	1	1
60	0	0	0	0	0	0	0	0	0
50	0	0	0	0	0	0	0	0	0
40	0	0	0	0	0	0	0	0	0
30	0	0	0	0	0	0	0	0	0
20	0	0	0	0	0	0	0	0	0
10	0	0	0	0	0	0	0	0	0

TABLE 5 Bent-Knee Sit-Ups—Boys (number in 1 minute; arms crossed on chest)

Age	10	11	12	13	14	15	16	17	18
99%	60	60	61	62	64	65	65	68	67
90	47	48	50	52	52	53	55	56	54
80	43	43	46	48	49	50	51	51	50
75	40	41	44	46	47	48	49	50	50
70	38	40	43	45	45	46	48	49	48
60	36	38	40	41	43	44	45	46	44
50	34	36	38	40	41	42	43	43	43
40	32	34	35	37	39	40	41	41	40
30	30	31	33	34	37	37	39	39	38
25	28	30	32	32	35	36	38	37	36
20	26	28	30	31	34	35	36	35	35
10	22	22	25	28	30	31	32	31	31

TABLE 6 Bent-Knee Sit-Ups—Girls (number in 1 minute; arms crossed on chest)

Age	10	11	12	13	14	15	16	17	18
99%	50	53	66	58	57	56	59	60	65
90	43	42	46	46	47	45	49	47	47
80	39	39	41	41	42	42	42	41	42
75	37	37	40	40	41	40	40	40	40
70	36	36	39	39	40	39	39	39	40
60	33	34	36	35	37	36	37	37	38
50	31	32	33	33	35	35	35	36	35
40	30	30	31	31	32	32	33	33	33
30	27	28	30	28	30	30	30	31	30
25	25	26	28	27	29	30	30	30	30
20	24	24	27	25	27	28	28	29	28
10	20	20	21	21	23	24	23	24	24

TABLE 7 Sit-and-Reach, Flexibility Test—Boys (footline set at 0; measurement in inches, plus or minus)

Age	10	11	12	13	14	15	16	17	18
99%	6	6.5	6.5	7.5	8	9.5	10	9.5	10
90	4	4.5	4	4.5	5.5	6	7	7.5	7.5
80	3	3.5	3	3	4	5	6	6	6
75	2.5	3	3	3	3.5	4.5	5	5.5	5.5
70	2.5	2.5	2.5	2.5	3	4	5	5	5
60	2	2	1.5	1.5	2	3	4	4	4
50	1.5	1	1	1	1.5	2	3	3.5	3
40	0.5	1.5	0	0.5	1	1.5	2	2.5	2.5
30	0	0	−0.5	0	0	0.5	1.5	1.5	1.5
25	−0.5	−0.5	−1	−1	−1	0	1	1	1
20	−1	−1	−1.5	−1.5	−1	−0.5	0	−0.5	−0.5
10	−2	−2.5	−3.5	−3	−3	−2.5	−2	−1.5	−2

TABLE 8 Sit-and-Reach, Flexibility Test—Girls (footline set at 0; measurement in inches, plus or minus)

Age	10	11	12	13	14	15	16	17	18
99%	8.5	8.5	9	10	10	11	11	11	10.5
90	5.5	6	7	8	7.5	8	8.5	8.5	8.5
80	4.5	5	6	7	7	7	7.5	7.5	7.5
75	4.5	4.5	5	6	6.5	7	7	7	7
70	4	4.5	5	5.5	6	6.5	7	7	6.5
60	3	3.5	4	5	5.5	6	6	6	6
50	2.5	3	3.5	4	5	5	5.5	6	5.5
40	2	2	3	3.5	4	5	5	5	5
30	1	1.5	2.5	2.5	3	4	4.5	4	4
25	1	1	2	2	3	3.5	4	3.5	3.5
20	0	1	1.5	1.5	2	3	3.5	3	3
10	−1.5	−0.5	0	0	0.5	1.5	2	1.5	1

TABLE 9 1-Mile Run—Boys (min:sec)

Age	10	11	12	13	14	15	16	17	18
99%	6:55	6:21	6:21	5:59	5:43	5:40	5:31	5:14	5:33
90	8:13	7:25	7:13	6:48	6:27	6:23	6:13	6:08	6:10
80	8:35	7:52	7:41	7:07	6:58	6:43	6:31	6:31	6:33
75	8:48	8:02	7:53	7:14	7:08	6:52	6:39	6:40	6:42
70	9:02	8:12	8:03	7:24	7:18	7:00	6:50	6:46	6:57
60	9:26	8:38	8:23	6:46	7:34	7:13	7:07	7:10	7:15
50	9:52	9:03	8:48	8:04	7:51	7:30	7:27	7:31	7:35
40	10:15	9:25	9:17	8:26	8:14	7:50	7:48	7:59	7:53
30	10:44	10:17	9:57	8:54	8:46	8:18	8:04	8:24	8:12
20	11:25	10:55	10:38	9:20	9:28	8:50	8:34	8:55	9:10
10	12:27	12:07	11:48	10:38	10:34	10:13	9:36	10:43	10:50

TABLE 10 1-Mile Run—Girls (min:sec)

Age	10	11	12	13	14	15	16	17	18
99%	7:55	7:14	7:20	7:08	7:01	6:59	7:03	6:52	6:58
90	9:09	8:45	8:34	8:27	8:11	8:23	8:28	8:20	8:22
80	9:56	9:52	9:30	9:13	8:49	9:04	9:06	9:10	9:27
75	10:09	9:56	9:52	9:30	9:16	9:28	9:25	9:26	9:31
70	10:27	10:10	10:05	9:48	9:31	9:49	9:41	9:41	9:36
60	10:51	10:35	10:32	10:22	10:04	10:20	10:15	10:16	10:08
50	11:14	11:15	10:58	10:52	10:32	10:46	10:34	10:34	10:51
40	11:54	11:46	11:26	11:22	10:58	11:20	11:08	10:59	11:27
30	12:27	12:33	12:03	11:55	11:35	11:53	11:49	11:43	11:58
25	12:52	12:54	12:33	12:17	11:49	12:18	12:10	12:03	12:14
20	13:12	13:17	12:53	12:43	12:10	12:48	12:32	12:30	12:37
10	14:20	14:35	14:07	13:45	13:13	14:07	13:42	13:46	15:18

NATIONAL CHILDREN AND YOUTH FITNESS STUDY II (NCYFS II)

As described in Chapter 1, the second National Children and Youth Fitness Study (NCYFS II) was launched to study the physical fitness and physical activity habits of 4,678 children ages 6–9. The study was the first to assess the fitness and activity patterns of 6- to 9-year-olds.

Test items of the NCYFS II include*

- Triceps, subscapular, and medial calf skinfolds for body composition
- Walk/run for cardiorespiratory endurance (1 mile, age 8 or 9; or 1/2 mile, age 6 or 7)
- Sit-and-reach test for lower back–hamstring flexibility
- Modified pull-up for upper-body muscular strength and endurance
- Bent-knee sit-ups (1 minute) for abdominal strength/endurance

Interpretations of norms: <25% = unacceptable or poor; 25–50% = minimal or fair; 50–75% = acceptable or good; >75% = optimal or excellent.

**Note:* See description of methods in Chapters 4–6.

Source: Ross JG, Pate RR, Delpy LA, Gold RS, Svilar M. New health-related fitness norms. *JOPERD*, November/December 1987, 66–70.

TABLE 11 Triceps Skinfold (mm)

	Age							
	Boys				Girls			
Percentile	6	7	8	9	6	7	8	9
99	5	5	5	5	5	6	6	6
95	6	5	6	6	7	7	7	7
90	6	6	6	6	8	7	8	8
85	7	7	7	7	8	8	8	9
80	7	7	7	7	9	8	9	10
75	7	7	7	8	9	9	9	10
70	7	7	8	8	9	9	10	11
65	8	8	8	9	10	10	10	11
60	8	8	8	10	10	10	11	12
55	8	8	9	10	11	11	12	12
50	8	9	9	10	11	11	12	13
45	9	9	10	11	12	12	13	14
40	9	10	10	12	12	12	14	14
35	10	10	11	13	13	13	15	15
30	10	11	12	14	13	13	16	16
25	10	11	13	15	14	14	17	18
20	11	12	14	16	14	15	18	19
15	12	14	15	18	15	17	19	21
10	13	16	19	21	17	19	21	22
5	16	20	23	23	20	22	25	25

TABLE 12 Subscapular Skinfold (mm)

	Age							
	Boys				Girls			
Percentile	6	7	8	9	6	7	8	9
99	4	4	4	4	4	4	4	4
95	4	4	4	4	4	4	5	5
90	4	4	4	5	5	5	5	5
85	4	5	5	5	5	5	5	5
80	5	5	5	5	5	5	5	6
75	5	5	5	5	5	5	6	6
70	5	5	5	5	5	5	6	6
65	5	5	5	6	6	6	6	6
60	5	5	5	6	6	6	6	7
55	5	5	6	6	6	6	7	7
50	5	5	6	6	6	6	7	8
45	5	6	6	7	6	7	7	8
40	6	6	6	7	7	7	8	9
35	6	6	6	7	7	7	8	9
30	6	6	7	8	7	8	9	10
25	6	7	7	9	8	9	10	12
20	7	7	8	10	8	10	12	15
15	7	8	10	12	10	11	15	17
10	8	10	14	15	12	13	17	21
5	12	16	19	20	16	19	21	25

TABLE 13 Sum of Triceps and Medial Calf Skinfolds (mm)

	Age							
	Boys				Girls			
Percentile	6	7	8	9	6	7	8	9
99	9	9	9	9	11	11	11	12
95	11	11	11	11	13	13	14	14
90	12	12	12	12	15	15	15	16
85	12	13	13	13	16	16	16	18
80	13	13	13	14	17	17	18	19
75	14	14	14	15	18	18	19	20
70	14	14	15	16	18	18	20	21
65	15	16	17	18	20	20	22	23
60	15	16	17	18	20	20	22	23
55	16	16	17	19	21	21	23	25
50	16	17	18	21	21	22	24	26
45	17	18	19	22	22	23	26	27
40	17	19	20	23	23	24	27	29
35	18	20	21	25	24	25	29	30
30	20	21	23	27	25	26	31	32
25	20	22	24	29	27	28	33	35
20	22	24	27	31	28	31	35	37
15	23	27	31	35	30	33	38	41
10	27	32	37	40	33	37	43	45
5	33	39	44	47	38	43	49	52

TABLE 14 Modified Pull-Ups (number completed)

	Age							
	Boys				Girls			
Percentile	6	7	8	9	6	7	8	9
99	25	27	38	35	24	27	25	30
95	18	20	21	25	17	20	20	20
90	15	19	20	20	13	16	17	17
85	12	15	17	20	11	14	14	15
80	11	13	15	17	10	12	12	13
75	10	13	14	15	9	11	11	12
70	9	12	13	14	9	10	11	11
65	8	11	12	13	7	9	10	10
60	7	10	11	12	7	8	9	10
55	7	9	10	11	6	8	9	9
50	6	8	10	10	6	7	8	9
45	6	8	9	10	5	7	7	8
40	5	7	8	9	5	6	6	7
35	5	6	8	7	4	4	5	5
30	4	5	7	7	4	4	5	5
25	3	4	6	6	3	4	4	4
20	3	4	5	5	2	3	4	4
15	2	3	4	4	1	2	3	2
10	1	1	3	3	0	1	1	1
5	0	0	1	2	0	0	0	0

The child is positioned on his or her back with the shoulders directly below a bar that is set at a height 1 or 2 inches beyond the child's reach. An elastic band is suspended across the uprights parallel to and about 7–8 inches below the bar. In the start position, the child's buttocks are off the floor, the arms and legs are straight, and only the heels are in contact with the floor. An overhand grip (palm away from the body) is used, and the thumbs are placed around the bar. A pull-up is completed when the chin is hooked over the elastic band. The movement should be accomplished using only the arms, and the body must be kept rigid and straight (see Chapter 6).

TABLE 15 Timed Bent-Knee Sit-Ups (number in 1 minute)

	Age							
	Boys				Girls			
Percentile	6	7	8	9	6	7	8	9
99	36	42	43	48	36	40	44	43
95	31	35	38	42	31	35	37	39
90	28	32	35	39	28	33	34	36
85	26	30	33	36	26	30	32	34
80	25	29	32	35	24	28	30	32
75	24	28	30	33	23	27	29	31
70	22	27	29	32	22	26	28	30
65	21	26	28	31	21	24	27	29
60	20	25	27	30	20	23	26	28
55	19	24	26	29	19	22	25	26
50	19	23	26	28	18	21	25	26
45	17	21	24	26	17	20	23	24
40	17	21	24	26	17	20	23	24
35	16	20	23	24	15	17	20	22
30	15	19	21	24	15	17	20	22
25	14	18	20	23	14	16	19	21
20	12	16	19	22	12	15	17	19
15	11	14	17	19	10	13	16	17
10	9	12	15	16	6	11	13	15
5	4	7	11	13	1	7	9	10

Note: See Chapter 6 for details on methods.

TABLE 16 Sit-and-Reach, Flexibility Test (in inches; footline set at zero)

	Age							
	Boys				Girls			
Percentile	6	7	8	9	6	7	8	9
99	5.5	6.0	6.0	5.5	6.5	6.0	7.0	7.0
95	4.5	4.5	4.5	4.0	5.5	5.5	5.5	6.0
90	4.0	4.0	4.0	3.5	4.5	5.0	5.0	5.0
85	3.5	4.0	3.5	3.0	4.0	4.5	4.5	4.5
80	3.0	3.5	3.0	2.5	4.0	4.0	4.0	4.0
75	3.0	3.0	2.5	2.5	3.5	4.0	4.0	4.0
70	2.5	2.5	2.5	2.0	3.0	3.0	3.0	3.0
65	2.0	2.0	2.0	2.0	3.0	3.0	3.0	3.0
60	2.0	2.0	2.0	1.5	3.0	3.0	3.0	3.0
55	1.5	1.5	1.5	1.0	2.5	3.0	2.5	2.5
50	1.5	1.5	1.5	1.0	2.0	2.5	2.0	2.0
45	1.0	1.0	1.0	0.5	2.0	2.5	2.0	2.0
40	0.5	0.5	0.5	0.0	2.0	2.0	1.5	2.0
35	0.5	0.5	0.5	0.0	1.5	2.0	1.5	1.5
30	0.0	0.0	0.0	−0.5	1.0	1.5	1.0	1.0
25	0.0	−0.5	−0.5	−1.0	0.5	1.0	0.5	0.5
20	−0.5	−0.5	−1.0	−1.5	0.0	0.5	0.0	0.0
15	−1.0	−1.0	−1.5	−2.0	0.0	0.0	−0.5	−0.5
10	−1.5	−2.0	−2.5	−2.5	−0.5	−0.5	−1.0	−1.0
5	−2.0	−3.0	−3.5	−4.0	−1.5	−1.5	−2.0	−3.0

TABLE 17 Distance Walk/Run (1 mile for children age 8 or 9; ½ mile for children age 6 or 7; min:sec)

	Age							
	Boys				Girls			
	Half Mile		Mile		Half Mile		Mile	
Percentile	6	7	8	9	6	7	8	9
99	3:53	3:34	7:42	7:31	4:05	4:03	8:18	8:06
95	4:15	3:56	8:18	7:54	4:29	4:18	9:14	8:41
90	4:27	4:11	8:46	8:10	4:46	4:32	9:39	9:08
85	4:35	4:22	9:02	8:33	4:57	4:38	9:55	9:26
80	4:45	4:28	9:19	8:48	5:07	4:46	10:08	9:40
75	4:52	4:33	9:29	9:00	5:13	4:54	10:23	9:50
70	4:59	4:40	9:40	9:13	5:20	5:00	10:35	10:15
65	5:04	4:46	9:52	9:29	5:25	5:06	10:46	10:31
60	5:10	4:50	10:04	9:44	5:31	5:11	10:59	10:41
55	5:17	4:54	10:16	9:58	5:39	5:18	11:14	10:56
50	5:23	5:00	10:39	10:10	5:44	5:25	11:32	11:13
45	5:28	5:05	11:00	10:27	5:49	5:32	11:46	11:30
40	5:33	5:11	11:14	10:41	5:55	5:39	12:03	11:46
35	5:41	5:17	11:30	10:59	6:00	5:46	12:14	12:09
30	5:50	5:28	11:51	11:16	6:07	5:55	12:37	12:26
25	5:58	5:35	12:14	11:44	6:14	6:01	12:59	12:45
20	6:09	5:46	12:39	12:02	6:27	6:10	13:26	13:13
15	6:21	6:06	13:16	12:46	6:39	6:20	14:18	13:44
10	6:40	6:20	14:05	13:37	6:51	6:38	14:48	14:31
5	7:15	6:50	15:24	15:15	7:16	7:09	16:35	15:40

THE 1985 SCHOOL POPULATION FITNESS SURVEY, PRESIDENT'S COUNCIL ON PHYSICAL FITNESS AND SPORTS*

As described in Chapter 1, the President's Council on Physical Fitness and Sports School Population Fitness Survey was conducted in 1985. Data were collected to assess the physical fitness status of American public school children ages 6–17. A four-stage probability sample was designed to select approximately 19,200 boys and girls from 57 school districts and 187 schools.

The test was not designed to measure all of the health-related fitness components (body composition was not assessed). In addition, several skill-related tests were included. Nine test items were selected for both boys and girls. Norms are given for boys and girls ages 6–17.

- Pull-ups
- Flexed-arm hang
- Curl-ups
- 1-mile run/walk
- V-sit reach
- Shuttle run
- 2-mile walk
- 50-yard dash
- Standing long jump

**Source:* Youth Physical Fitness in 1985. *The President's Council on Physical Fitness and Sports School Population Fitness Survey.* President's Council on Physical Fitness and Sports. 450 Fifth St., NW, Suite 7103, Washington, DC 20001.

Suggested Interpretation of Norms

90–100% Excellent

75–85% Very good

60–70% Good

45–55% Average

30–40% Fair

15–25% Poor

0–10% Very poor

The results from this survey form the basis for the norms used in the "President's Challenge" (see norms next page and discussion in Chapters 3 and 4). Those youngsters reaching the 85th percentile or above on all five items of the test become eligible to receive the Presidential Physical Fitness Award. The National Physical Fitness Award was added in 1987 and recognizes those who score at or above the 50th percentile for all five test items. The Participant Award, introduced in 1991, recognizes those who attempt all test items but whose scores fall below the 50th percentile on one or more of them. The award standards were validated by means of comparison with a nationwide sample in 1994.

Source: President's Council on Physical Fitness and Sports. *Get Fit: A Handbook for Youth Ages 6–17.* Washington, DC: Author, 1998-1999.

TABLE 18 The Presidential Physical Fitness Awards

The Presidential Physical Fitness Award

Age	Curl-Ups (# in 1 min)	OR Partial* Curl-Ups (#)	Shuttle Run (sec)	V-Sit Reach (in)	OR Sit and Reach (cm)	One-Mile Run (min:sec)	OR Distance Option† (min:sec) 1/4 mile	Distance Option† (min:sec) 1/2 mile	Pull-Ups (#)	OR RT. Angle* Push-Ups (#)
Boys										
6	33	22	12.1	+3.5	31	10:15	1:55		2	9
7	36	24	11.5	+3.5	30	9:22	1:48		4	14
8	40	30	11.1	+3.0	31	8:48		3:30	5	17
9	41	37	10.9	+3.0	31	8:31		3:30	5	18
10	45	35	10.3	+4.0	30	7:57			6	22
11	47	43	10.0	+4.0	31	7:32			6	27
12	50	64	9.8	+4.0	31	7:11			7	31
13	53	59	9.5	+3.5	33	6:50			7	39
14	56	62	9.1	+4.5	36	6:26			10	40
15	57	75	9.0	+5.0	37	6:20			11	42
16	56	73	8.7	+6.0	38	6:08			11	44
17	55	66	8.7	+7.0	41	6:06			13	53
Girls										
6	32	22	12.4	+5.5	32	11:20	2:00		2	9
7	34	24	12.1	+5.0	32	10:36	1:55		2	14
8	38	30	11.8	+4.5	33	10:02		3:58	2	17
9	39	37	11.1	+5.5	33	9:30		3:53	2	18
10	40	33	10.8	+6.0	33	9:19			3	20
11	42	43	10.5	+6.5	34	9:02			3	19
12	45	50	10.4	+7.0	36	8:23			2	20
13	46	59	10.2	+7.0	38	8:13			2	21
14	47	48	10.1	+8.0	40	7:59			2	20
15	48	38	10.0	+8.0	43	8:08			2	20
16	45	49	10.1	+9.0	42	8:23			1	24
17	44	58	10.0	+8.0	42	8:15			1	25

(continued)

TABLE 18 *(continued)*

The National Physical Fitness Award

Age	Curl-Ups (# in 1 min)	OR	Partial* Curl-Ups (#)	Shuttle Run (sec)	V-Sit Reach (in)	OR	Sit and Reach (cm)	One-Mile Run (min:sec)	OR	Distance Option† (min:sec) 1/4 mile	Distance Option† (min:sec) 1/2 mile	Pull-Ups (#)	OR	RT. Angle* Push-Ups (#)	OR	Flexed-Arm Hang (sec)
Boys																
6	22		10	13.3	+1.0		26	12:36		2:21		1		7		6
7	28		13	12.8	+1.0		25	11:40		2:10		1		8		8
8	31		17	12.2	+0.5		25	11:05			4:22	1		9		10
9	32		20	11.9	+1.0		25	10:30			4:14	2		12		10
10	35		24	11.5	+1.0		25	9:48				2		14		12
11	37		26	11.1	+1.0		25	9:20				2		15		11
12	40		32	10.6	+1.0		26	8:40				2		18		12
13	42		39	10.2	+0.5		26	8:06				3		24		14
14	45		40	9.9	+1.0		28	7:44				5		24		20
15	45		45	9.7	+2.0		30	7:30				6		30		30
16	45		37	9.4	+3.0		30	7:10				7		30		28
17	44		42	9.4	+3.0		34	7:04				8		37		30
Girls																
6	23		10	13.8	+2.5		27	13:12		2:26		1		6		5
7	25		13	13.2	+2.0		27	12:56		2:21		1		8		6
8	29		17	12.9	+2.0		28	12:30			4.56	1		9		8
9	30		20	12.5	+2.0		28	11:52			4:50	1		12		8
10	30		24	12.1	+3.0		28	11:22				1		13		8
11	32		27	11.5	+3.0		29	11:17				1		11		7
12	35		30	11.3	+3.5		30	11:05				1		10		7
13	37		40	11.1	+3.5		31	10:23				1		11		8
14	37		30	11.2	+4.5		33	10:06				1		10		9
15	36		26	11.0	+5.0		36	9:58				1		15		7
16	35		26	10.9	+5.5		34	10:31				1		12		7
17	34		40	11.0	+4.5		35	10:22				1		16		7

The Participant Physical Fitness Award

Boys and girls who attempt all five test items but whose scores fall below the 50th percentile on one or more of them are eligible to receive the Participant Award.

*Norms from Canada Fitness Award Program, Health Canada, Government of Canada, used with permission.

†1/4 and 1/2 mile norms from Amateur Athletic Union Physical Fitness Program, used with permission.

Note: Award standards were most recently validated by means of comparison with a large nationwide sample in 1994.

TABLE 19 The Fitnessgram® Standards for Healthy Fitness Zone (HFZ)*

Boys

Age	$\dot{V}O_{2max}$		One Mile Run		PACER		Walk Test $\dot{V}O_{2max}$		Percent Fat		Body Mass Index	
			min:sec		*# laps*		*ml/kg/min*					
5									10	25	14.7	20
6			*Completion of distance. Time standards not recommended.*		*Participate in run. Lap count standards not recommended.*				10	25	14.7	20
7									10	25	14.9	20
8									10	25	15.1	20
9									7	25	13.7	20
10	42	52	11:30	9:00	23	61			7	25	14.0	21
11	42	52	11:00	8:30	23	72			7	25	14.3	21
12	42	52	10:30	8:00	32	72			7	25	14.6	22
13	42	52	10:00	7:30	41	83	42	52	7	25	15.1	23
14	42	52	9:30	7:00	41	83	42	52	7	25	15.6	24.5
15	42	52	9:00	7:00	51	94	42	52	7	25	16.2	25
16	42	52	8:30	7:00	61	94	42	52	7	25	16.6	26.5
17	42	52	8:30	7:00	61	106	42	52	7	25	17.3	27
17+	42	52	8:30	7:00	72	106	42	52	7	25	17.8	27.8

Age	Curl-Up		Trunk Lift		Push-Up		Modified Pull-Up		Flexed Arm Arm Hang		Back Saver Sit & Reach**	Shoulder Stretch
	# completed		*inches*		*# completed*		*# completed*		*seconds*		*inches*	
5	2	10	6	12	3	8	2	7	2	8	8	Healthy Fitness Zone = Touching fingertips together behind the back on both right and left sides
6	2	10	6	12	3	8	2	7	2	8	8	
7	4	14	6	12	4	10	3	9	3	8	8	
8	6	20	6	12	5	13	4	11	3	10	8	
9	9	24	6	12	6	15	5	11	4	10	8	
10	12	24	9	12	7	20	5	15	4	10	8	
11	15	28	9	12	8	20	6	17	6	13	8	
12	18	36	9	12	10	20	7	20	10	15	8	
13	21	40	9	12	12	25	8	22	12	17	8	
14	24	45	9	12	14	30	9	25	15	20	8	
15	24	47	9	12	16	35	10	27	15	20	8	
16	24	47	9	12	18	35	12	30	15	20	8	
17	24	47	9	12	18	35	14	30	15	20	8	
17+	24	47	9	12	18	35	14	30	15	20	8	

(continued)

TABLE 19 *(continued)*

Girls													
Age	$\dot{V}O_{2max}$		One Mile Run		PACER		Walk Test $\dot{V}O_{2max}$		Percent Fat		Body Mass Index	
5			*min:sec*		*# laps*		*ml/kg/min*		17	32	16.2	21
6			*Completion of distance. Time standards not recommended.*		*Participate in run. Lap count standards not recommended.*				17	32	16.2	21
7									17	32	16.2	22
8									17	32	16.2	22
9									13	32	13.5	23
10	39	47	12:30	9:30	7	41			13	32	13.7	23.5
11	38	46	12:00	9:00	15	41			13	32	14.0	24
12	37	45	12:00	9:00	15	41			13	32	14.5	24.5
13	36	44	11:30	9:00	23	51	36	44	13	32	14.9	24.5
14	35	43	11:00	8:30	23	51	35	43	13	32	15.4	25
15	35	43	10:30	8:00	32	51	35	43	13	32	16.0	25
16	35	43	10:00	8:00	32	61	35	43	13	32	16.4	25
17	35	43	10:00	8:00	41	61	35	43	13	32	16.8	26
17+	35	43	10:00	8:00	41	72	35	43	13	32	17.2	27.3

Age	Curl-Up		Trunk Lift		90° Push-Up		Modified Pull-Up		Flexed Arm Arm Hang		Back Saver Sit & Reach**	Shoulder Stretch
	# completed		*inches*		*# completed*		*# completed*		*seconds*		*inches*	
5	2	10	6	12	3	8	2	7	2	8	9	Healthy Fitness Zone = Touching fingertips together behind the back on both right and left sides
6	2	10	6	12	3	8	2	7	2	8	9	
7	4	14	6	12	4	10	3	9	3	8	9	
8	6	20	6	12	5	13	4	11	3	10	9	
9	9	22	6	12	6	15	4	11	4	10	9	
10	12	26	9	12	7	15	4	13	4	10	9	
11	15	29	9	12	7	15	4	13	6	12	10	
12	18	32	9	12	7	15	4	13	7	12	10	
13	18	32	9	12	7	15	4	13	8	12	10	
14	18	32	9	12	7	15	4	13	8	12	10	
15	18	35	9	12	7	15	4	13	8	12	12	
16	18	35	9	12	7	15	4	13	8	12	12	
17	18	35	9	12	7	15	4	13	8	12	12	
17+	18	35	9	12	7	15	4	13	8	12	12	

*Number on left is lower end of HFZ; number on right is upper end of HFZ.

**Test scored Pass/Fail; must reach this distance to pass.

Source: © 2004, The Cooper Institute, Dallas, Texas.

AAHPERD NORMS FOR COLLEGE STUDENTS

The American Association of Health, Physical Education, Recreation, and Dance (AAHPERD) released the results of it's new testing program for college students in 1985. The study population consisted of 5,158 young adults in colleges from all geographic regions of the United States. The data for the study were collected under the supervision of 24 coinvestigators. The test items, in order, are as follows:

- Two-site skinfold test (triceps and subscapular)
- Mile run or 9-minute run for cardiorespiratory endurance
- Sit-and-reach test for flexibility
- Timed (1 minute) sit-ups for abdominal muscular endurance

AAHPERD allows authors to publish only a limited part of the norms. The reader is urged to purchase the book from AAHPERD, listed in the source note.*

TABLE 20a Health-Related Physical Fitness Test Items—Males

%	Mile Run	Sit-Ups	Sit and Reach	Sum of Skinfold	% Body Fat
99	5:06	68	26	10	2.9
75	6:12	50	16	16	6.6
50	6:49	44	11	21	9.4
25	7:32	38	6	26	13.1
5	9:47	30	−4	40	20.4

TABLE 20b Health-Related Physical Fitness Test Items—Females

%	Mile Run	Sit-Ups	Sit and Reach	Sum of Skinfold	% Body Fat
99	6:04	61	28	11	7.9
75	8:15	42	18	24	19.0
50	9:22	35	14	30	22.8
25	10:41	0	9	37	27.1
5	12:43	21	1	51	33.7

Mile run: Run 1 mile in the fastest possible time.
Sit-ups: As many correctly executed sit-ups as possible in 60 seconds.
Sit and reach: Footline is set at 0 cm. Score is cm beyond feet when legs are straight.
Sum of skinfolds: Triceps plus subscapular skinfolds.
See Chapters 4–6 for details on how to administer tests.

Source (Tables 20a and b): AAHPERD. *Norms for College Students: Health Related Physical Fitness Test.* 1985. Reprinted by permission of the American Alliance for Health, Physical Education, Recreation, and Dance, 1900 Association Dr., Reston, VA 22091.

Section 2. Cardiorespiratory Test Norms for Adults

See Chapter 4 for instructions.

TABLE 21 YMCA Norms for Resting Heart Rate (beats/min)

Age (yr)	18–25		26–35		36–45		46–55		56–65		>65	
Gender	M	F	M	F	M	F	M	F	M	F	M	F
Excellent	40–54	42–57	36–53	39–57	37–55	40–58	35–56	43–58	42–56	42–59	40–55	49–59
Good	57–59	59–63	55–59	60–62	58–60	61–63	58–61	61–64	59–61	61–64	57–61	60–64
Above average	61–65	64–67	61–63	64–66	62–64	65–67	63–65	65–69	63–65	65–68	62–65	66–68
Average	66–69	68–71	65–67	68–70	66–69	69–71	66–70	70–72	68–71	69–72	66–69	70–72
Below average	70–72	72–76	69–71	72–74	70–72	72–75	72–74	73–76	72–75	73–77	70–73	73–76
Poor	74–78	77–81	74–78	77–81	75–80	77–81	77–81	77–82	76–80	79–81	74–79	78–83
Very poor	82–103	84–104	81–102	84–102	83–101	83–102	84–103	85–104	84–103	84–103	83–103	86–97

Source: Reprinted and adapted with permission of the YMCA of the USA, 101 N. Wacker Drive, Chicago, IL 60606.

TABLE 22 YMCA 3-Minute Step Test Postexercise 1-Minute Heart Rate (beats/min)

Age (yr)	18–25		26–35		36–45		46–55		56–65		>65	
Gender	M	F	M	F	M	F	M	F	M	F	M	F
Excellent	50–76	52–81	51–76	58–80	49–76	51–84	56–82	63–91	60–77	60–92	59–81	70–92
Good	79–84	85–93	79–85	85–92	80–88	89–96	87–93	95–101	86–94	97–103	87–92	96–101
Above average	88–93	96–102	88–94	95–101	92–98	100–104	95–101	104–110	97–100	106–111	94–102	104–111
Average	95–100	104–110	96–102	104–110	100–105	107–112	103–111	113–118	103–109	113–118	104–110	116–121
Below average	102–107	113–120	104–110	113–119	108–113	115–120	113–119	120–124	111–117	119–127	114–118	123–126
Poor	111–119	122–131	114–121	122–129	116–124	124–132	121–126	126–132	119–128	129–135	121–126	128–133
Very poor	124–157	135–169	126–161	134–171	130–163	137–169	131–159	137–171	131–154	141–174	130–151	135–155

Note: Pulse is to be counted for 1 full minute following 3 minutes of stepping at 24 steps/minute on a 12-inch bench. See Chapter 4 for further instructions.
Source: Reprinted and adapted with permission of the YMCA of the USA, 101 N. Wacker Drive, Chicago, IL 60606.

TABLE 23a Aerobic Power Tests—Men

	Ages 20–29				Ages 30–39				
%	Balke Treadmill (time)	$\dot{V}O_{2max}$ (ml/kg/min)	12-Minute Run (miles)	1.5-Mile Run (time)	Balke Treadmill (time)	$\dot{V}O_{2max}$ (ml/kg/min)	12-Minute Run (miles)	1.5-Mile Run (time)	
99	30:20	58:79	1.94	7:29	29:00	58.86	1.89	7:11	S
95	27:00	53.97	1.81	8:13	26:00	52.53	1.77	8:44	
90	25:11	51.35	1.74	9:09	24:30	50.36	1.71	9:30	
85	24:00	49.64	1.69	9:45	23:00	48.20	1.65	10:16	
80	23:00	48.20	1.65	10:16	22:00	46.75	1.61	10:47	E
75	22:10	46.99	1.62	10:42	21:00	45.31	1.57	11:18	
70	22:00	46.75	1.61	10:47	20:30	44.59	1.55	11:34	
65	21:00	45.31	1.57	11:18	20:00	43.87	1.53	11:49	
60	20:15	44.23	1.54	11:41	19:00	42.42	1.49	12:20	G
55	20:00	43.87	1.53	11:49	18:25	41.58	1.47	12:38	
50	19:03	42.49	1.50	12:18	18:00	40.98	1.45	12:51	
45	19:00	42.42	1.49	12:20	17:00	39.53	1.41	13:22	
40	18:00	40.98	1.45	12:51	16:32	38.86	1.39	13:36	F
35	17:30	40.26	1.43	13:06	16:00	38.09	1.37	13:53	
30	17:00	39.53	1.41	13:22	15:30	37.37	1.35	14:08	
25	16:00	38.09	1.37	13:53	15:00	36.65	1.33	14:24	
20	15:20	37.13	1.34	14:13	14:06	35.35	1.29	14:52	P
15	15:00	36.65	1.33	14:24	13:10	34.00	1.25	15:20	
10	13:30	34.48	1.27	15:10	12:09	32.53	1.21	15:52	
5	11:30	31.57	1.19	16:12	11:00	30.87	1.17	16:27	VP
1	8:23	27.09	1.06	17:48	8:00	26.54	1.13	18:00	
	n = 1675				*n* = 7094				

(continued)

TABLE 23a ***(continued)***

	Ages 40–49				Ages 50–59				
%	Balke Treadmill (time)	$\dot{V}O_{2max}$ (ml/kg/ min)	12-Minute Run (miles)	1.5-Mile Run (time)	Balke Treadmill (time)	$\dot{V}O_{2max}$ (ml/kg/ min)	12-Minute Run (miles)	1.5-Mile Run (time)	
99	28:00	55.42	1.85	7:42	26:00	52.53	1.77	8:44	S
95	24:30	50.36	1.71	9:30	22:15	47.11	1.62	10:40	
90	23:00	48.20	1.65	10:16	21:00	45.31	1.57	11:18	
85	21:00	45.31	1.57	11:18	19:00	42.42	1.49	12:20	
80	20:10	44.11	1.54	11:44	18:00	40.98	1.45	12:51	E
75	20:00	43.89	1.53	11:49	17:00	39.53	1.41	13:22	
70	18:32	41.75	1.47	12:34	16:15	38.45	1.38	13:45	
65	18:00	40.98	1.45	12:51	15:40	37.61	1.35	14:03	
60	17:15	39.89	1.42	13:14	15:00	36.65	1.33	14:24	G
55	17:00	39.53	1.41	13:22	14:30	36.10	1.31	14:40	
50	16:00	38.09	1.37	13:53	14:00	35.20	1.29	14:55	
45	15:30	37.37	1.35	14:08	13:15	34.12	1.26	15:08	
40	15:00	36.69	1.33	14:29	13:00	33.76	1.25	15:26	F
35	14:15	35.56	1.30	14:47	12:07	32.48	1.22	15:53	
30	13:57	35.13	1.29	14:56	12:00	32.31	1.21	15:57	
25	13:00	33.76	1.25	15:26	11:08	31.06	1.17	16:23	
20	12:30	33.04	1.23	15:41	10:30	30.15	1.15	16:43	P
15	12:00	32.31	1.21	15:57	10:00	29.43	1.13	16:58	
10	10:59	30.85	1.17	16:28	9:00	27.98	1.09	17:29	
5	6:21	28.29	1.10	17:23	7:00	25.09	1.01	18:31	VP
1	6:21	24.15	.98	18:51	4:54	22.06	.92	19:36	

n = 6837 (Ages 40–49); n = 7094 (Ages 50–59)

	Age 60+				
%	Balke Treadmill (time)	$\dot{V}O_{2max}$ (ml/kg/ min)	12-Minute Run (miles)	1.5-Mile Run (time)	
99	24:29	50.39	1.71	9:30	S
95	20:56	45.21	1.57	11:20	
90	19:00	42.46	1.49	12:20	
85	17:00	39.53	1.41	13:22	
80	16:00	38.09	1.37	13:53	E
75	15:00	36.65	1.30	14:24	
70	14:04	35.30	1.29	14:53	
65	13:22	39.29	1.26	15:19	
60	12:53	33.59	1.24	15:29	G
55	12:03	32.39	1.21	15:55	
50	11:40	31.83	1.19	16:07	
45	11:00	30.87	1.17	16:27	
40	10:30	30.15	1.15	16:43	F
35	10:00	29.43	1.13	16:58	
30	9:30	28.70	1.11	17:14	
25	8:54	27.89	1.08	17:32	
20	8:00	26.54	1.05	18:00	P
15	7:00	25.09	1.01	18:31	
10	5:35	23.05	.95	19:15	
5	4:00	20.76	.89	20:04	VP
1	2:17	18.28	.82	20:57	

Note: n = 1005; S-superior; E-excellent; G-good; F-fair; P-poor; VP-very poor.

TABLE 23b Aerobic Power Tests—Women

	Ages 20–29				Ages 30–39				
%	Balke Treadmill (time)	$\dot{V}O_{2max}$ (ml/kg/min)	12-Minute Run (miles)	1.5-Mile Run (time)	Balke Treadmill (time)	$\dot{V}O_{2max}$ (ml/kg/min)	12-Minute Run (miles)	1.5-Mile Run (time)	
99	26:21	53.03	1.78	8:33	23:22	48.73	1.66	10:05	S
95	22:00	46.75	1.61	10:47	20:00	43.87	1.53	11:49	
90	20:12	44.15	1.54	11:43	18:00	40.98	1.45	12:51	
85	19:00	42.42	1.49	12:20	17:30	40.26	1.43	13:06	
80	18:00	40.98	1.45	12:51	16:20	38.57	1.38	13:43	E
75	17:00	39.53	1.41	13:22	15:30	37.37	1.35	14:08	
70	16:00	38.09	1.37	13:53	15:00	36.65	1.33	14:24	
65	15:30	37.37	1.35	14:08	14:10	35.44	1.29	14:50	
60	15:00	36.65	1.33	14:24	13:35	34.60	1.27	15:08	G
55	14:39	36.14	1.31	14:35	13:10	33.85	1.26	15:20	
50	14:00	35.20	1.29	14:55	13:00	33.76	1.25	15:26	
45	13:30	34.48	1.27	15:10	12:10	32.41	1.22	15:47	
40	13:00	33.76	1.25	15:26	12:00	32.31	1.21	15:57	F
35	12:17	32.72	1.22	15:48	11:09	31.09	1.17	16:23	
30	12:00	32.31	1.21	15:57	10:45	30.51	1.16	16:35	
25	11:03	30.94	1.17	16:26	10:00	29.93	1.13	16:58	
20	10:50	30.63	1.16	16:33	9:30	28.70	1.11	17:14	P
15	10:00	29.43	1.13	16:58	9:00	27.98	1.09	17:29	
10	9:17	28.39	1.10	17:21	8:00	26.54	1.05	18:00	
5	7:33	25.89	1.03	18:14	7:00	25.09	1.01	18:31	VP
1	5:15	22.57	.94	19:25	5:12	22.49	.93	19:27	
	n = 764				*n* = 2049				

	Ages 40–49				Ages 50–59				
%	Balke Treadmill (time)	$\dot{V}O_{2max}$ (ml/kg/min)	12-Minute Run (miles)	1.5-Mile Run (time)	Balke Treadmill (time)	$\dot{V}O_{2max}$ (ml/kg/min)	12-Minute Run (miles)	1.5-Mile Run (time)	
99	22:00	46.75	1.61	10:47	18:44	42.04	1.48	12:28	S
95	18:00	40.98	1.45	12:51	15:07	36.81	1.33	14:20	
90	17:00	39.53	1.41	13:22	14:00	35.20	1.29	14:55	
85	15:35	37.49	1.35	14:06	12:53	33.59	1.24	15:29	
80	14:45	36.28	1.32	14:31	12:00	32.31	1.21	15:57	E
75	13:56	35.11	1.29	14:57	11:43	39.90	1.20	16:05	
70	13:00	33.76	1.25	15:16	11:00	30.87	1.17	16:27	
65	12:30	33.04	1.23	15:41	10:14	29.76	1.14	16:51	
60	12:00	32.31	1.21	15:57	10:00	29.43	1.13	16:58	G
55	11:30	31.59	1.19	16:12	9:30	28.70	1.11	17:14	
50	11:00	30.87	1.17	16:27	9:10	28.22	1.10	17:24	
45	10:48	30.58	1.16	16:34	9:00	27.98	1.09	17:29	
40	10:01	29.45	1.13	16:58	8:13	26.85	1.06	17:55	F
35	10:00	29.43	1.12	16:59	7:43	26.13	1.04	18:09	
30	9:11	28.25	1.10	17:24	7:16	25.48	1.02	18:23	
25	9:00	27.98	1.09	17:29	7:00	25.09	1.01	18:31	
20	8:00	26.54	1.05	18:00	6:25	24.25	.98	18:49	P
15	7:20	25.57	1.02	18:21	6:00	23.65	.97	19:02	
10	7:00	25.09	1.01	18:31	5:05	22.33	.93	19:30	
5	5:55	23.53	.96	19:05	4:14	21.10	.90	19:57	VP
1	4:00	20.76	.89	20:04	2:36	18.74	.83	20:47	
	n = 1630				*n* = 7094				

(continued)

TABLE 23b *(continued)*

	Age 60+				
%	Balke Treadmill (time)	$\dot{V}O_{2max}$ (ml/kg/min)	12-Minute Run (miles)	1.5-Mile Run (time)	
99	20:25	44.47	1.55	11:36	S
95	15:34	37.46	1.35	14:06	
90	14:00	35.20	1.29	14:55	
85	12:00	32.31	1.21	15:57	
80	11:15	31.23	1.18	16:20	E
75	11:00	30.87	1.17	16:27	
70	10:00	29.43	1.13	16:58	
65	9:00	27.98	1.09	17:29	
60	8:28	27.21	1.07	17:46	G
55	8:00	26.54	1.05	18:00	
50	7:30	25.82	1.03	18:16	
45	7:00	25.09	1.01	18:31	
40	6:35	24.49	.99	18:44	F
35	6:16	24.03	.98	18:54	
30	6:08	23.80	.97	18:59	
25	6:00	23.65	.97	19:02	
20	5:24	22.78	.94	19:21	P
15	5:00	22.21	.93	19:33	
10	4:00	20.76	.89	20:04	
5	3:15	19.68	.86	20:23	VP
1	2:00	17.87	.81	21:06	

Note: n = 202; S = superior; E = excellent; G = good; F = fair; P = poor; VP = very poor.

Source (Tables 23a and b): Data provided by the Institute for Aerobics Research, Dallas, TX, 2005. Reprinted by permission of the Cooper Institute for Aerobics Research, Dallas, TX.

TABLE 24 $\dot{V}O_{2max}$ Norms

	Low	Fair	Avg	Good	High	Athletic	Olympic
Women							
20–29	<28	29–34	35–43	44–48	49–53	54–59	60+
30–39	<27	28–33	34–41	42–47	48–52	53–58	59+
40–49	<25	26–31	32–40	41–45	46–50	51–56	57+
50–65	<21	22–28	29–36	37–41	42–45	46–49	50+
Men							
20–29	<38	39–43	44–51	52–56	57–62	63–69	70+
30–39	<34	35–39	40–47	48–51	52–57	58–64	65+
40–49	<30	31–35	36–43	44–47	48–53	54–60	61+
50–59	<25	26–31	32–39	40–43	44–48	49–44	56+
60–69	<21	22–26	27–35	36–39	40–44	45–49	50+

Note: $\dot{V}O_{2max}$ is expressed in tables as milliliters of oxygen per kilogram of body weight per minute.

Source: Adapted from Astrand, *ACTA Physiol Scand* 49(suppl):169,1960. Reprinted with permission from Blackwell Scientific Publications LTD.

TABLE 25 $\dot{V}O_{2max}$ Norms

Maximal Oxygen Uptake of Male and Female Athletes					
Athletic Group	**Sex**	**Age (yr)**	**Height (cm)**	**Weight (kg)**	**$\dot{V}O_{2max}$ (ml/kg/min)**
Baseball/softball					
	Male	21	182.7	83.3	52.3
	Male	28	183.6	88.1	52.0
	Female	19–23	—	—	55.3
Basketball					
	Female	19	167.0	63.9	42.3
	Female	19	169.1	62.6	42.9
	Female	19	173.0	68.3	49.6
Centers	Male	28	214.0	109.2	41.9
Forwards	Male	25	200.6	96.9	45.9
Guards	Male	25	188.0	83.6	50.0
Bicycling (competitive)					
	Male	24	182.0	74.5	68.2
	Male	24	180.4	79.2	70.3
	Male	25	180.0	72.8	67.1
	Male	—	180.3	67.1	74.0
	Male	—	—	—	74.0
	Male	—	—	—	69.1
	Female	20	165.0	55.0	50.2
	Female	—	167.7	61.3	57.4
Canoeing/paddling					
	Male	19	173.0	64.0	60.0
	Male	22	190.5	80.7	67.7
	Male	24	182.0	79.6	66.1
	Male	26	181.0	74.0	56.8
	Female	18	166.0	57.3	49.2
Dancing					
Ballet	Male	24	177.5	68.0	48.2
	Female	24	165.6	49.5	43.7
General	Female	21	162.7	51.2	41.5
Football					
	Male	19	186.8	93.1	56.5
	Male	20	184.9	96.4	51.3
Defensive backs	Male	25	182.5	84.8	53.1
Offensive backs	Male	25	183.8	90.7	52.2
Linebackers	Male	24	188.6	102.2	52.1
Offensive linemen	Male	25	193.0	112.6	49.9
Defensive linemen	Male	26	192.4	117.1	44.9
Quarterbacks/kickers	Male	24	185.0	90.1	49.0
Gymnastics					
	Male	20	178.5	69.2	55.5
	Female	15	159.7	48.8	49.8
	Female	19	163.0	57.9	36.3
Ice hockey					
	Male	11	140.5	35.5	56.6
	Male	22	179.0	77.3	61.5
	Male	24	179.3	81.8	54.6
	Male	26	180.1	86.4	53.6

(continued)

TABLE 25 ***(continued)***

Athletic Group	Sex	Age (yr)	Height (cm)	Weight (kg)	$\dot{V}O_{2max}$ (ml/kg/min)
Jockeys					
	Male	31	158.2	50.3	53.8
Orienteering					
	Male	25	179.7	70.3	71.1
	Male	31	—	72.2	61.6
	Male	52	176.0	72.7	50.7
	Female	23	165.8	60.0	60.7
	Female	29	—	58.1	46.1
Pentathlon					
	Female	21	175.4	65.4	45.9
Racquetball/handball					
	Male	24	183.7	81.3	60.0
	Male	25	181.7	80.3	58.3
Rowing					
	Male	—	—	—	65.7
	Male	23	192.7	89.9	62.6
	Male	25	189.9	86.9	66.9
Heavyweight	Male	23	192.0	88.0	68.9
Lightweight	Male	21	186.0	71.0	71.1
	Female	23	173.0	68.0	60.3
Skating					
Speed	Male	20	175.5	73.9	56.1
	Male	21	181.0	76.5	72.9
	Male	25	183.1	82.4	64.6
	Female	20	168.1	65.4	52.0
	Female	21	164.5	60.8	46.1
Figure	Male	21	166.9	59.6	58.5
	Female	17	158.8	48.6	48.9
Skiing					
Alpine	Male	16	173.1	65.5	65.6
	Male	21	176.0	70.1	63.8
	Male	22	177.8	75.5	66.6
	Male	26	176.6	74.8	62.3
	Female	19	165.1	58.8	52.7
Cross-country	Male	21	176.0	66.6	63.9
	Male	25	180.4	73.2	73.9
	Male	26	174.0	69.3	78.3
	Male	23	176.2	73.2	73.0
	Male	—	—	—	72.8
	Female	20	163.4	55.9	61.5
	Female	24	163.0	59.1	68.2
	Female	25	165.7	60.5	56.9
	Female	—	—	—	58.1
Nordic	Male	23	176.0	70.4	72.8
	Male	22	181.7	70.4	67.4
Ski jumping					
	Male	22	174.0	69.9	61.3

(continued)

TABLE 25 ***(continued)***

Athletic Group	Sex	Age (yr)	Height (cm)	Weight (kg)	$\dot{V}O_{2max}$ (ml/kg/min)
Soccer					
	Male	26	176.0	75.5	58.4
Swimming					
	Male	12	150.4	41.2	52.5
	Male	13	164.8	52.1	52.9
	Male	15	169.6	59.8	56.6
	Male	15	166.8	59.1	56.8
	Male	20	181.4	76.7	55.7
	Male	20	181.0	73.0	50.4
	Male	21	182.9	78.9	62.1
	Male	21	181.0	78.3	69.9
	Male	22	182.3	79.1	56.9
	Male	22	182.3	79.7	55.9
	Female	12	154.8	43.3	46.2
	Female	13	160.0	52.1	43.4
	Female	15	164.8	53.7	40.5
Sprint	Male	19	181.1	75.0	58.3
Middle distance	Male	22	178.0	74.6	55.4
Long distance	Male	21	179.0	74.9	65.4
	Female	19	168.0	63.8	37.6
Tennis					
	Male	42	179.6	77.1	50.2
	Female	39	163.3	55.7	44.2
Track and field					
Run	Male	21	180.6	71.6	66.1
	Male	22	177.4	64.5	64.0
	Male	23	177.0	69.5	72.4
Sprint	Male	17–22	—	—	51.0
	Male	46	177.0	74.1	47.2
Middle distance	Male	25	180.1	67.8	70.1
	Male	25	179.0	72.3	69.8
Long distance	Male	10	144.3	31.9	56.6
	Male	17–22	—	—	65.5
	Male	26	176.1	64.5	72.2
	Male	26	178.9	63.9	77.4
	Male	26	177.0	66.2	78.1
	Male	27	178.7	64.9	73.2
	Male	32	177.3	64.3	70.3
	Male	35	174.0	63.1	66.6
	Male	36	177.3	69.6	65.1
	Male	40–49	180.7	71.6	57.5
	Male	55	174.5	63.4	54.4
	Male	50–59	174.7	67.2	54.4
	Male	60–69	175.7	67.1	51.4
	Male	70–75	175.6	66.8	40.0
	Male	—	—	—	72.5
	Female	16	162.6	48.6	63.2
	Female	16	163.3	50.9	50.8
	Female	21	170.2	58.6	57.5
	Female	32	169.4	57.2	59.1
	Female	44	161.5	53.8	43.4
	Female	—	—	—	58.2

(continued)

TABLE 25 (continued)

Athletic Group	Sex	Age (yr)	Height (cm)	Weight (kg)	$\dot{V}O_{2max}$ (ml/kg/min)
Race walking	Male	27	178.7	68.5	62.9
Jumping	Male	17–22	—	—	55.0
Shot/discus	Male	17–22	—	—	49.5
	Male	26	190.8	110.5	42.8
	Male	27	188.2	112.5	42.6
	Male	28	186.1	104.7	47.5
Volleyball					
	Male	25	187.0	84.5	56.4
	Male	26	192.7	85.5	56.1
	Female	19	166.0	59.8	43.5
	Female	20	172.2	64.1	56.0
	Female	22	183.7	73.4	41.7
	Female	22	178.3	70.5	50.6
Weight lifting					
	Male	25	171.0	81.3	40.1
	Male	25	166.4	77.2	42.6
Power	Male	26	176.1	92.0	49.5
Olympic	Male	25	177.1	88.2	50.7
Bodybuilding	Male	27	178.8	88.1	46.3
	Male	29	172.4	83.1	41.5
Wrestling					
	Male	21	174.8	67.3	58.3
	Male	23	—	79.2	50.4
	Male	24	175.6	77.7	60.9
	Male	26	177.0	81.8	64.0
	Male	27	176.0	75.7	54.3

Source: Wilmore JH. Design issues and alternatives in assessing physical fitness among apparently healthy adults in a health examination survey of the general population. In Drury TF (ed.), National Center for Health Statistics. *Assessing Physical Fitness and Physical Activity in Population-Based Surveys.* DHHS Pub. No. (PHS) 89-1253. Public Health Service. Washington, DC: U.S. Government Printing Office, 1989.

Section 3. Body Composition

TABLE 26 Disease Risk Associated with Body Mass Index and Waist Circumference

Classification	Obesity Class	BMI (kg/m^2)	Disease Risk Relative to Normal Weight and Waist Circumference*	
			Men ≤40 in Women ≤35 in	>40 in >35 in
Underweight		<18.5		
Normal		18.5–24.9		
Overweight		25.0–29.9	Increased	High
Obesity	I	30.0–34.9	High	Very high
	II	35.0–39.9	Very high	Very high
Extreme obesity	III	≥40	Extremely high	Extremely high

*Disease risk for type 2 diabetes, hypertension, and cardiovascular disease.

Source: NHLBI Obesity Education Initiative Expert Panel. *Clinical Guidelines on the Identification, Evaluation, and Treatment of Overweight and Obesity in Adults.* National Heart, Lung, and Blood Institute: www.nhlbi.nih.gov/nhlbi/1998.

TABLE 27a Number Examined, Mean, Standard Error of Mean, and Triceps Skinfold Thickness for Males for Selected Percentiles, by Age: United States, 1999–2002

Race or ethnicity and age	Number of examined persons	Mean	Standard error of mean	Percentile 5th	10th	15th	25th	50th	75th	85th	90th	95th
				Millimeters								
Male												
2 months	16	*	*	*	*	*	*	*	*	*	*	*
3–5 months	106	11.2	0.35	*	*	8.2	9.6	11.1	12.3	13.6	*	*
6–8 months	117	11.3	0.28	*	*	8.9	9.7	11.1	12.4	13.5	*	*
9–11 months	121	10.9	0.29	*	*	8.4	9.1	10.5	12.1	13.1	*	*
1 year	287	10.0	0.26	*	7.2	7.7	8.2	9.5	11.2	12.2	13.0	*
2 years	247	9.7	0.28	*	6.9	7.1	7.8	9.1	10.9	12.3	13.8	*
3 years	211	9.4	0.18	*	6.3	6.8	7.5	8.9	10.4	11.9	12.4	*
4 years	173	9.4	0.21	*	6.5	6.8	7.2	9.0	10.8	11.8	12.1	*
5 years	150	9.8	0.54	*	*	6.4	7.0	8.5	10.7	12.7	*	*
6 years	184	9.9	0.21	*	6.0	6.2	7.1	9.0	11.7	13.3	14.4	*
7 years	185	10.3	0.37	*	6.2	6.7	7.4	9.1	11.3	14.4	15.0	*
8 years	211	12.3	0.70	*	5.7	6.3	7.3	10.7	14.3	19.4	22.2	*
9 years	173	13.4	0.74	*	6.9	7.0	7.7	10.5	15.0	21.4	25.8	*
10 years	184	14.0	0.59	*	7.3	8.1	8.7	12.6	16.3	20.4	24.0	*
11 years	182	13.8	0.65	*	7.1	8.0	8.6	11.6	18.2	22.3	24.7	*
12 years	298	14.6	0.74	*	7.0	7.6	8.9	12.1	19.0	22.8	26.1	*
13 years	289	13.4	0.73	*	6.6	7.1	7.8	10.5	17.9	21.6	24.3	*
14 years	264	13.7	0.59	*	6.8	7.1	8.0	11.0	17.9	21.0	24.3	*
15 years	281	12.0	0.50	*	6.1	6.5	7.1	9.3	15.2	18.8	20.8	*
16 years	301	13.5	0.71	*	6.0	6.8	7.8	11.2	17.1	21.9	25.3	*
17 years	304	12.4	0.60	5.0	5.3	5.9	6.9	10.4	15.8	20.1	23.3	27.9
18 years	280	12.5	0.50	*	6.1	7.0	7.8	10.4	15.7	18.8	21.9	*
19 years	263	12.9	0.79	*	6.1	6.6	7.4	10.0	15.4	21.7	24.9	*

(continued)

TABLE 27a ***(continued)***

Race or Ethnicity and Age	Number of Examined Persons	Mean	Standard Error of Mean	Percentile								
				5th	10th	15th	25th	50th	75th	85th	90th	95th
				Millimeters								
All race or ethnicity groups												
20 years and over	4,148	14.3	0.11	5.9	7.0	7.9	9.5	12.9	17.4	21.1	23.6	27.8
20–29 years	683	13.8	0.28	5.1	6.2	7.0	8.1	12.4	17.3	21.7	23.9	28.1
30–39 years	670	13.8	0.28	5.4	6.4	7.2	8.9	12.1	17.3	20.8	24.0	28.5
40–49 years	738	13.9	0.19	6.1	7.1	8.7	9.9	12.6	16.5	20.0	22.4	25.2
50–59 years	569	15.3	0.34	6.7	7.7	8.4	10.1	13.8	18.9	22.3	24.8	30.0
60–69 years	671	15.5	0.33	7.6	8.4	9.2	10.6	13.8	19.2	22.1	24.7	28.9
70–79 years	508	14.2	0.22	6.9	8.3	9.1	10.3	13.1	16.6	20.0	21.4	24.5
80 years and over	309	13.6	0.42	6.7	7.9	8.7	9.4	12.4	16.2	18.1	20.6	24.5
Non-Hispanic white												
20 years and over	2,064	14.6	0.15	6.3	7.3	8.3	9.9	13.2	17.9	21.5	23.9	27.9
20–39 years	574	14.1	0.29	5.4	6.5	7.2	8.6	12.5	17.4	21.8	24.3	28.5
40–59 years	648	14.9	0.22	6.9	8.2	9.0	10.4	13.4	17.9	21.6	23.6	27.1
60 years and over	842	15.0	0.23	7.4	8.5	9.2	10.6	13.5	18.2	21.2	23.1	27.8
Non-Hispanic black												
20 years and over	762	13.3	0.25	4.7	5.5	6.2	7.5	11.6	16.7	20.6	23.4	28.4
20–39 years	252	12.7	0.36	4.6	5.3	6.1	7.4	11.1	15.7	19.3	22.1	27.1
40–59 years	267	13.5	0.40	4.8	5.4	6.0	7.2	11.8	17.1	21.3	24.0	30.3
60 years and over	243	14.5	0.43	5.0	6.5	8.0	9.4	12.6	18.2	21.8	25.5	28.4
Mexican American												
20 years and over	994	13.2	0.31	5.8	6.9	7.8	9.1	11.9	15.7	19.2	21.2	25.1
20–39 years	383	13.3	0.38	5.6	6.7	7.5	9.0	12.0	15.8	20.0	22.0	25.1
40–59 years	294	12.9	0.42	5.8	7.2	8.0	9.4	11.5	15.3	18.0	19.8	24.5
60 years and over	317	13.3	0.33	6.6	7.6	8.3	9.4	12.0	16.0	18.6	20.2	24.3

Source: McDowell MA, Fryar CD, Hirsch R, Ogden CL. Anthropometric reference data for children and adults: U.S. population, 1999–2002. Advance data from vital and health statistics; no. 361. Hyattsville, MD: National Center for Health Statistics, 2005.

TABLE 27b Number Examined, Mean, Standard Error of Mean, and Triceps Skinfold Thickness for Females for Selected Percentiles, by Race or Ethnicity and Age: United States, 1999–2002

Race or Ethnicity and Age	Number of Examined Persons	Mean	Standard Error of Mean	Percentile								
				5th	10th	15th	25th	50th	75th	85th	90th	95th
				Millimeters								
Female												
0–2 months	14	*	*	*	*	*	*	*	*	*	*	*
3–5 months	116	11.4	0.25	*	*	8.5	9.4	10.9	12.9	14.1	*	*
6–8 months	99	11.2	0.30	*	*	*	9.4	10.8	13.0	*	*	*
9–11 months	109	10.5	0.35	*	*	7.6	8.2	9.9	12.0	13.3	*	*
1 year	230	10.1	0.26	*	6.9	7.5	8.1	9.9	11.5	12.5	14.0	*
2 years	236	10.1	0.22	*	7.0	7.4	8.0	9.7	11.5	12.2	13.1	*
3 years	169	10.0	0.18	*	7.4	7.9	8.6	9.8	11.2	11.7	12.4	*
4 years	183	10.3	0.38	*	7.1	7.6	7.9	9.6	11.6	13.0	14.0	*
5 years	185	11.0	0.45	*	6.5	6.9	7.9	10.2	13.0	15.0	15.6	*
6 years	169	11.1	0.58	*	6.6	7.3	8.3	10.1	12.7	13.6	15.2	*

(continued)

TABLE 27b ***(continued)***

Race or Ethnicity and Age	Number of Examined Persons	Mean	Standard Error of Mean	Percentile								
				5th	10th	15th	25th	50th	75th	85th	90th	95th
				Millimeters								
Female *(continued)*												
7 years	195	11.5	0.42	*	7.3	7.5	7.9	10.1	13.3	16.8	18.1	*
8 years	180	14.3	0.72	*	8.1	8.4	9.6	12.1	17.3	22.9	24.8	*
9 years	184	15.4	0.52	*	8.0	9.2	9.7	13.7	19.7	21.7	23.4	*
10 years	163	15.5	0.58	*	8.1	8.7	9.7	12.9	19.4	23.1	25.0	*
11 years	189	16.7	0.70	*	9.3	10.0	11.0	14.1	20.9	24.8	27.9	*
12 years	306	16.7	0.60	7.6	8.9	9.8	11.5	15.3	21.0	24.3	26.6	30.2
13 years	310	18.0	0.65	8.1	8.9	9.2	11.8	17.0	22.5	26.7	30.9	33.4
14 years	314	18.7	0.67	9.0	10.3	10.9	13.6	17.0	23.2	26.2	28.2	31.5
15 years	258	18.3	0.79	*	10.2	11.0	12.7	17.2	22.9	26.1	27.6	*
16 years	264	19.6	0.57	*	11.0	11.6	14.1	18.3	25.2	28.3	29.8	*
17 years	244	18.9	0.57	*	11.0	11.3	13.2	18.2	23.6	25.9	28.0	*
18 years	234	20.3	0.58	*	11.9	12.7	13.7	19.2	24.4	28.4	31.5	*
19 years	214	21.0	0.72	*	10.8	11.9	13.8	20.3	27.3	30.9	32.6	*
All race or ethnicity groups												
20 years and over	3,820	23.6	0.20	11.4	13.7	15.3	18.1	23.4	28.9	31.9	33.8	36.1
20–29 years	596	22.5	0.39	10.5	12.6	14.3	16.7	22.1	27.8	30.4	32.4	35.4
30–39 years	614	23.5	0.39	10.3	12.6	14.7	16.9	23.4	29.6	32.7	34.2	36.5
40–49 years	670	24.3	0.40	12.1	14.1	15.9	18.9	24.5	29.0	32.7	34.4	36.8
50–59 years	515	24.9	0.35	13.0	15.7	17.4	19.8	24.7	30.0	32.7	34.2	36.4
60–69 years	638	25.1	0.35	14.6	16.0	17.5	19.3	25.0	30.1	33.0	35.0	36.8
70–79 years	455	22.3	0.37	11.0	13.2	14.9	17.4	21.9	26.8	29.0	31.2	33.6
80 years and over	332	19.4	0.57	8.7	10.8	12.4	14.4	18.6	23.7	26.9	28.6	31.1
Non-Hispanic white												
20 years and over	1,845	23.3	0.25	11.1	13.3	15.2	17.9	23.1	28.5	31.7	33.7	36.0
20–39 years	510	22.7	0.36	10.1	12.4	14.2	16.7	22.2	28.4	31.7	33.1	35.5
40–59 years	542	24.2	0.40	12.1	14.1	15.9	18.9	24.1	29.1	32.7	34.2	36.7
60 years and over	793	22.8	0.25	11.4	13.7	15.2	17.6	22.5	27.9	30.3	32.9	35.4
Non-Hispanic black												
20 years and over	704	24.8	0.39	10.9	14.2	15.3	18.4	25.6	30.9	33.1	34.6	36.9
20–39 years	241	23.9	0.59	10.4	12.9	14.8	16.3	24.3	30.9	33.0	34.8	36.8
40–59 years	232	26.3	0.50	12.2	15.6	18.3	21.9	26.8	31.5	33.7	35.3	36.6
60 years and over	231	23.9	0.60	9.6	12.9	15.3	18.1	24.4	29.6	31.9	33.2	37.1
Mexican American												
20 years and over	930	23.9	0.38	12.5	14.7	16.1	18.4	24.0	28.8	31.8	33.9	36.2
20–39 years	333	23.2	0.51	12.4	14.0	15.5	17.4	23.4	27.9	30.4	33.3	35.4
40–59 years	294	25.7	0.35	14.3	16.3	17.9	20.2	25.9	30.3	32.8	34.8	37.3
60 years and over	303	22.6	0.52	10.8	13.4	15.6	17.0	22.0	26.9	31.0	32.9	36.0

Note: Pregnant women are excluded.

Source: McDowell MA, Fryar CD, Hirsch R, Ogden CL. Anthropometric reference data for children and adults: U.S. population, 1999–2002. Advance data from vital and health statistics; no. 361. Hyattsville, MD: National Center for Health Statistics, 2005.

TABLE 27c Number Examined, Mean, Standard Error of Mean, and Standing Height for Males Aged 20 Years and Over for Selected Percentiles, by Race or Ethnicity and Age: United States, 1999–2002

Race or Ethnicity and Age	Number of Examined Persons	Mean	Standard Error of Mean	Percentile 5th	10th	15th	25th	50th	75th	85th	90th	95th
				Inches								
All race or ethnicity groups												
20 years and over	4,341	69.3	0.05	64.1	65.4	66.2	67.3	69.3	71.3	72.3	73.1	74.2
20–29 years	724	69.6	0.11	64.1	65.7	66.5	67.5	69.6	71.4	72.6	73.5	74.6
30–39 years	717	69.5	0.10	64.2	65.7	66.3	67.4	69.3	71.6	72.6	73.3	74.4
40–49 years	784	69.7	0.13	65.1	66.1	66.7	67.7	69.6	71.7	72.6	73.2	74.4
50–59 years	601	69.2	0.13	64.0	65.4	66.2	67.2	69.3	71.4	72.3	73.0	73.9
60–69 years	702	68.8	0.13	64.4	65.1	65.8	67.0	68.9	70.7	71.7	72.3	73.1
70–79 years	519	68.0	0.17	63.0	64.3	64.9	65.9	68.1	70.1	71.0	71.5	72.5
80 years and over	294	67.2	0.17	62.8	63.7	64.5	65.4	67.1	69.0	70.0	70.6	71.7
Non-Hispanic white												
20 years and over	2,136	69.8	0.07	65.0	66.2	66.9	67.9	69.7	71.7	72.6	73.3	74.4
20–39 years	604	70.2	0.09	65.6	66.5	67.4	68.4	70.1	71.9	73.0	73.9	74.8
40–59 years	677	70.0	0.13	65.5	66.4	67.2	68.1	70.1	72.0	72.8	73.5	74.4
60 years and over	855	68.6	0.08	64.3	65.0	65.7	66.8	68.7	70.4	71.4	72.1	73.1
Non-Hispanic black												
20 years and over	826	69.6	0.07	65.1	66.2	66.7	67.8	69.5	71.4	72.3	73.3	74.2
20–39 years	278	70.0	0.15	65.8	66.5	67.2	68.1	69.8	71.7	73.1	73.6	74.8
40–59 years	293	69.6	0.15	65.0	66.0	66.8	68.0	69.8	71.5	72.1	72.8	73.7
60 years and over	255	68.6	0.18	63.8	65.0	65.8	66.7	68.5	70.4	71.4	72.1	73.1
Mexican American												
20 years and over	1,039	66.8	0.11	62.0	63.2	63.9	64.9	66.8	68.5	69.6	70.1	71.1
20–39 years	409	66.8	0.16	62.0	62.9	63.7	64.9	66.8	68.6	69.6	70.2	71.7
40–59 years	313	66.9	0.19	62.2	63.6	64.3	65.1	66.9	68.4	69.4	70.1	70.8
60 years and over	317	66.3	0.16	62.1	63.1	63.7	64.6	66.3	68.0	68.9	69.4	69.9

Source: McDowell MA, Fryar CD, Hirsch R, Ogden CL. Anthropometric reference data for children and adults: U.S. population, 1999–2002. Advance data from vital and health statistics: no. 361. Hyattsville, MD: National Center for Health Statistics, 2005.

TABLE 27d Number Examined, Mean, Standard Error of Mean, and Standing Height for Females Aged 20 Years and Over for Selected Percentiles, by Race or Ethnicity and Age: United States, 1999–2002

Race or Ethnicity and Age	Number of Examined Persons	Mean	Standard Error of Mean	Percentile 5th	10th	15th	25th	50th	75th	85th	90th	95th
				Inches								
All race or ethnicity groups												
20 years and over	4,888	63.8	0.06	59.4	60.3	61.0	62.0	63.8	65.6	66.5	67.3	68.2
20–29 years	1,034	64.1	0.12	59.9	60.5	61.4	62.3	64.1	65.8	67.0	67.5	68.4
30–39 years	909	64.2	0.11	59.9	60.8	61.5	62.4	64.2	65.9	66.9	67.5	68.6
40–49 years	799	64.3	0.09	59.9	60.8	61.5	62.5	64.3	66.1	67.0	67.6	68.7
50–59 years	604	63.9	0.14	59.7	60.6	61.3	62.1	63.9	65.5	66.4	67.2	68.1
60–69 years	723	63.2	0.10	59.0	59.9	60.7	61.6	63.2	64.9	65.8	66.5	67.1
70–79 years	482	62.6	0.12	58.4	59.1	59.9	61.0	62.6	64.1	65.3	65.8	66.6
80 years and over	337	61.3	0.13	57.4	58.1	58.9	59.8	61.4	62.8	63.7	64.4	65.6

(continued)

TABLE 27d (continued)

Race or Ethnicity and Age	Number of Examined Persons	Mean	Standard Error of Mean	Percentile 5th	10th	15th	25th	50th	75th	85th	90th	95th
All race or ethnicity groups				Inches								
Non-Hispanic white												
20 years and over	2,325	64.1	0.06	59.9	61.0	61.5	62.4	64.2	65.8	66.8	67.4	68.4
20–39 years	847	64.7	0.10	60.7	61.5	62.1	63.2	64.5	66.2	67.3	67.8	68.6
40–59 years	635	64.6	0.10	60.8	61.5	62.1	63.1	64.6	66.1	67.1	67.8	68.7
60 years and over	843	62.8	0.07	58.5	59.5	60.2	61.2	62.8	64.5	65.4	66.1	66.8
Non-Hispanic black												
20 years and over	941	64.2	0.08	60.2	61.0	61.5	62.4	64.2	65.9	66.8	67.4	68.4
20–39 years	372	64.5	0.13	60.5	61.3	61.7	62.8	64.5	66.1	67.1	67.6	68.5
40–59 years	294	64.3	0.13	60.3	61.3	61.7	62.4	64.1	65.9	66.5	67.4	68.5
60 years and over	275	63.2	0.14	58.6	59.8	60.5	61.4	63.2	65.2	66.0	66.7	67.9
Mexican American												
20 years and over	1,175	62.0	0.12	57.8	58.8	59.4	60.3	61.9	63.6	64.5	65.3	66.2
20–39 years	513	62.2	0.18	58.3	59.1	59.8	60.5	62.1	63.8	64.7	65.3	66.2
40–59 years	338	61.9	0.16	57.7	58.5	59.3	60.2	61.8	63.5	64.6	65.5	66.3
60 years and over	324	60.7	0.13	56.1	57.1	57.9	59.2	60.7	62.2	63.4	64.0	64.5

Source: McDowell MA, Fryar CD, Hirsch R, Ogden CL. Anthropometric reference data for children and adults: U.S. population, 1999–2002. Advance data from vital and health statistics; no. 361. Hyattsville, MD: National Center for Health Statistics, 2005.

TABLE 27e Number Examined, Mean, Standard Error of Mean, and Weight for Males Aged 20 Years and Over for Selected Percentiles, by Race or Ethnicity and Age: United States, 1999–2002

Race or Ethnicity and Age	Number of Examined Persons	Mean	Standard Error of Mean	Percentile 5th	10th	15th	25th	50th	75th	85th	90th	95th
All race or ethnicity groups				Pounds								
20 years and over	4,314	190.4	0.92	133.1	143.4	150.4	162.3	184.0	212.1	230.1	243.0	267.1
20–29 years	712	183.8	1.55	125.2	136.7	142.9	152.3	176.7	205.8	224.4	238.7	268.0
30–39 years	704	189.5	1.99	130.2	142.3	149.1	161.2	183.2	208.8	227.6	242.1	278.2
40–49 years	776	196.4	1.61	140.3	149.1	158.6	168.3	188.9	217.1	237.1	247.9	273.9
50–59 years	598	195.8	2.06	139.1	149.2	156.5	169.4	190.6	219.2	235.8	243.1	264.1
60–69 years	691	194.4	1.61	139.5	147.3	156.7	168.8	190.5	216.2	235.8	247.2	262.2
70–79 years	524	182.4	1.56	132.7	141.6	148.1	160.3	179.1	204.2	214.4	224.4	239.7
80 years and over	309	167.5	1.46	128.2	136.6	141.7	148.9	164.6	181.6	195.3	202.6	221.5
Non-Hispanic white												
20 years and over	2,136	193.8	1.02	138.4	146.5	154.5	165.9	187.3	214.7	231.8	244.0	266.8
20–39 years	598	189.9	1.86	131.7	142.5	149.2	160.3	182.7	210.8	227.8	241.9	275.1
40–59 years	672	199.8	1.54	143.5	153.9	162.7	173.6	191.7	220.6	239.4	247.5	270.3
60 years and over	866	189.2	0.98	139.3	146.1	155.1	164.4	184.4	209.9	226.7	238.2	254.6
Non-Hispanic black												
20 years and over	813	190.0	1.43	127.9	139.3	146.1	157.8	182.6	212.4	235.3	252.5	275.4
20–39 years	273	189.7	2.71	129.7	139.5	147.8	155.8	178.1	212.7	235.8	255.5	275.5
40–59 years	288	191.4	2.62	128.0	139.5	145.4	159.5	187.4	211.9	236.4	251.8	274.5
60 years and over	252	187.3	2.53	124.3	135.4	142.8	158.2	182.0	211.8	227.6	248.5	266.8
Mexican American												
20 years and over	1,027	176.3	1.48	124.5	136.3	142.0	150.7	172.2	195.6	208.3	219.2	241.3
20–39 years	399	172.9	2.16	122.1	131.4	139.7	146.3	167.6	191.3	207.0	216.9	236.7
40–59 years	310	184.0	1.98	128.9	144.8	151.8	159.6	178.7	200.8	215.7	230.4	252.7
60 years and over	318	176.0	2.45	133.5	139.5	143.5	151.4	172.4	193.5	206.0	218.1	239.8

Source: McDowell MA, Fryar CD, Hirsch R, Ogden CL. Anthropometric reference data for children and adults: U.S. population, 1999–2002. Advance data from vital and health statistics; no. 361. Hyattsville, MD: National Center for Health Statistics, 2005.

TABLE 27f Number Examined, Mean, Standard Error of Mean, and Weight for Females Aged 20 Years and Over for Selected Percentiles, by Race or Ethnicity and Age: United States, 1999–2002

Race or Ethnicity and Age	Number of Examined Persons	Mean	Standard Error of Mean	Percentile 5th	10th	15th	25th	50th	75th	85th	90th	95th
				Pounds								
All race or ethnicity groups												
20 years and over	4,299	163.3	1.02	109.8	117.6	123.4	132.5	154.8	184.6	206.1	220.8	243.0
20–29 years	656	156.8	1.98	104.4	112.5	119.6	127.5	149.2	178.9	198.0	212.2	235.0
30–39 years	699	163.4	2.00	110.6	117.6	122.3	131.0	151.7	185.0	209.7	228.8	248.5
40–49 years	787	168.6	2.41	113.2	119.9	124.7	134.0	159.9	192.5	211.8	226.2	258.2
50–69 years	593	169.5	2.53	116.4	123.7	129.0	137.8	161.9	190.4	214.2	228.6	249.4
60–69 years	728	168.1	1.68	114.1	124.4	130.3	139.6	162.0	189.2	208.7	226.8	244.0
70–79 years	486	156.4	1.68	108.6	117.8	123.9	133.3	153.4	176.3	191.8	201.5	213.5
80 years and over	350	140.5	2.90	99.9	103.1	109.2	118.3	137.5	157.2	171.0	175.8	201.2
Non-Hispanic white												
20 years and over	2,052	162.2	1.16	109.8	117.4	123.2	131.9	154.0	183.7	205.3	218.5	239.6
20–39 years	564	158.6	1.97	108.2	115.6	121.6	128.5	149.5	180.3	200.5	214.5	239.2
40–59 years	628	167.9	2.20	113.4	120.2	124.7	134.1	160.0	192.3	212.0	226.0	252.4
60 years and over	860	158.3	1.17	107.2	116.3	123.0	133.6	152.9	176.4	195.8	206.5	228.8
Non-Hispanic black												
20 years and over	861	182.8	1.53	117.2	128.3	134.3	147.6	174.8	208.0	232.5	247.8	278.7
20–39 years	297	179.6	3.00	115.8	123.3	131.0	140.6	167.7	206.9	233.2	250.4	283.2
40–59 years	292	189.3	2.75	124.0	134.2	143.0	152.3	177.4	215.4	233.7	247.9	284.4
60 years and over	272	177.2	3.32	113.2	126.2	133.8	146.1	174.7	201.2	223.1	239.9	253.0
Mexican American												
20 years and over	1,019	157.0	1.62	109.7	115.7	123.0	131.2	150.5	177.1	194.6	203.5	224.9
20–39 years	358	153.2	2.20	107.7	114.7	121.2	129.0	146.6	170.8	188.4	198.9	222.3
40–59 years	332	165.9	2.61	114.9	123.2	128.6	138.4	161.8	184.9	202.0	215.1	232.6
60 years and over	329	151.0	2.65	96.9	109.3	117.3	128.2	148.0	170.2	184.6	196.2	206.9

Note: Pregnant women are excluded.

Source: McDowell MA, Fryar CD, Hirsch R, Ogden CL. Anthropometric reference data for children and adults: U.S. population, 1999–2002. Advance data from vital and health statistics; no. 361. Hyattsville, MD: National Center for Health Statistics, 2005.

TABLE 28 Relative Body Fat in Male and Female Athletes

Athletic Group	Sex	Age (yr)	Height (cm)	Weight (kg)	Relative Fat
Baseball					
	Male	20.8	182.7	83.3	14.2
	Male	—	—	—	11.8
	Male	27.4	183.1	88.0	12.6
Basketball					
	Female	19.1	169.1	62.6	20.8
	Female	19.4	167.0	63.9	26.9
Centers	Male	27.7	214.0	109.2	7.1
Forwards	Male	25.3	200.6	96.9	9.0
Guards	Male	25.2	188.0	83.6	10.6
Canoeing					
	Male	23.7	182.0	79.6	12.4
Football					
	Male	20.3	184.9	96.4	13.8
	Male	—	—	—	13.9
Defensive backs	Male	17–23	178.3	77.3	11.5
	Male	24.5	182.5	84.8	9.6
Offensive backs	Male	17–23	179.7	79.8	12.4
	Male	24.7	183.8	90.7	9.4
Linebackers	Male	17–23	180.1	87.2	13.4
	Male	24.2	188.6	102.2	14.0
Offensive linemen	Male	17–23	186.0	99.2	19.1
	Male	24.7	193.0	112.6	15.6
Defensive linemen	Male	17–23	186.6	97.8	18.5
	Male	25.7	192.4	117.1	18.2
Quarterbacks, kickers	Male	24.1	185.0	90.1	14.4
Gymnastics					
	Male	20.3	178.5	69.2	4.6
	Female	20.0	158.5	51.5	15.5
	Female	14.0	—	—	17.0
	Female	23.0	—	—	11.0
	Female	23.0	—	—	9.6
Ice hockey					
	Male	26.3	180.3	86.7	15.1
	Male	22.5	179.0	77.3	13.0
Jockeys					
	Male	30.9	158.2	50.3	14.1
Orienteering					
	Male	31.2	—	72.2	16.3
	Female	29.0	—	58.1	18.7
Pentathlon					
	Female	21.5	175.4	65.4	11.0
Racquetball					
	Male	25.0	181.7	80.3	8.1
Rowing					
Heavyweight	Male	23.0	192.0	88.0	11.0
Lightweight	Male	21.0	186.0	71.0	8.5
	Female	23.0	173.0	68.0	14.0

(continued)

TABLE 28 ***(continued)***

Athletic Group	Sex	Age (yr)	Height (cm)	Weight (kg)	Relative Fat
Skiing					
Alpine	Male	21.2	176.0	70.1	14.1
	Male	21.8	177.8	75.5	10.2
	Female	19.5	165.1	58.8	20.6
Cross-country	Male	21.2	176.0	66.6	12.5
	Male	25.6	174.0	69.3	10.2
	Male	22.7	176.2	73.2	7.9
	Female	24.3	163.0	59.1	21.8
	Female	20.2	163.4	55.9	15.7
Nordic combination	Male	22.9	176.0	70.4	11.2
	Male	21.7	181.7	70.4	8.9
Ski jumping					
	Male	22.2	174.0	69.9	14.3
Soccer					
	Male	26.0	176.0	75.5	9.6
Speed skating					
	Male	21.0	181.0	76.5	11.4
Swimming					
	Male	21.8	182.3	79.1	8.5
	Male	20.6	182.9	78.9	5.0
	Female	19.4	168.0	63.8	26.3
Sprint	Female	—	165.1	57.1	14.6
Middle distance	Female	—	166.6	66.8	24.1
Long distance	Female	—	166.3	60.9	17.1
Tennis					
	Male	—	—	—	15.2
	Male	42.0	179.6	77.1	16.3
	Female	39.0	163.3	55.7	20.3
Track and field					
	Male	21.3	180.6	71.6	3.7
	Male	—	—	—	8.8
Run	Male	22.5	177.4	64.5	6.3
Long distance	Male	26.1	175.7	64.2	7.5
	Male	26.2	177.0	66.2	8.4
	Male	40–49	180.7	71.6	11.2
	Male	55.3	174.5	63.4	18.0
	Male	50–59	174.7	67.2	10.9
	Male	60–69	175.7	67.1	11.3
	Male	70–75	175.6	66.8	13.6
	Male	47.2	176.5	70.7	13.2
	Female	19.9	161.3	52.9	19.2
	Female	32.4	169.4	57.2	15.2
Middle distance	Male	24.6	179.0	72.3	12.4
Sprint	Female	20.1	164.9	56.7	19.3
	Male	46.5	177.0	74.1	16.5
Discus	Male	28.3	186.1	104.7	16.4
	Male	26.4	190.8	110.5	16.3
	Female	21.1	168.1	71.0	25.0
Jumping and hurdling	Female	20.3	165.9	59.0	20.7

(continued)

TABLE 28 ***(continued)***

Athletic Group	Sex	Age (yr)	Height (cm)	Weight (kg)	Relative Fat
Shot-put	Male	27.0	188.2	112.5	16.5
	Male	22.0	191.6	126.2	19.6
	Female	21.5	167.6	78.1	28.0
Volleyball					
	Female	19.4	166.0	59.8	25.3
	Female	19.9	172.2	64.1	21.3
Weight lifting					
	Male	24.9	166.4	77.2	9.8
Power	Male	26.3	176.1	92.0	15.6
Olympic	Male	25.3	177.1	88.2	12.2
Bodybuilding	Male	29.0	172.4	83.1	8.4
	Male	27.6	178.7	88.1	8.3
Wrestling					
	Male	26.0	177.8	81.8	9.8
	Male	27.0	176.0	75.7	10.7
	Male	22.0	—	—	5.0
	Male	23.0	—	79.3	14.3
	Male	19.6	174.6	74.8	8.8
	Male	15–18	172.3	66.3	6.9
	Male	20.6	174.8	67.3	4.0

Source: Wilmore JH. Design issues and alternatives in assessing physical fitness among apparently healthy adults in a health examination survey of the general population. In Drury TF (ed.), National Center for Health Statistics. *Assessing Physical Fitness and Physical Activity in Population-Based Surveys.* DHHS Pub. No. (PHS) 89-1253. Public Health Service. Washington, DC: U.S. Government Printing Office, 1989.

Section 4. Musculoskeletal Test Norms for Adults

See descriptions given with each test. Also review Chapter 6.

TABLE 29 Push-Up Norms by Age Groups and Gender

Age (yr)	15–19		20–29		30–39		40–49		50–59		60–69	
Gender	M	F	M	F	M	F	M	F	M	F	M	F
Excellent	≥39	≥33	≥36	≥30	≥30	≥27	≥25	≥24	≥21	≥21	≥18	≥17
Very good	29–38	25–32	29–35	21–29	22–29	20–26	17–24	15–23	13–20	11–20	11–17	12–16
Good	23–28	18–24	22–28	15–20	17–21	13–19	13–16	11–14	10–12	7–10	8–10	5–11
Fair	18–22	12–17	17–21	10–14	12–16	8–12	10–12	5–10	7–9	2–6	5–7	1–4
Needs improvement	≤17	≤11	≤16	≤9	≤11	≤7	≤9	≤4	≤6	≤1	≤4	≤1

Procedures: Males—The participant lies on his stomach, legs together. His hands, pointing forward, are positioned under the shoulders. The participant pushes up from the mat by fully straightening the elbows and using the toes as the pivotal point. The upper body must be kept in a straight line. The participant returns to the starting position, chin to the mat. Neither the stomach nor the thighs should touch the mat. *Females*—Same as for males, except the knees are the pivotal point. The lower legs remain in contact with the mat, ankles plantarflexed.

Source: The Canadian Physical Activity, Fitness & Lifestyle Appraisal: CSEP-Health & Fitness Programs Health-Related Appraisal and Counselling Strategy, 3rd Edition. © 2003. Reprinted with permission of the Canadian Society for Exercise Physiology.

TABLE 30 Grip-Strength (kg) Norms by Age Groups and Gender for Combined Right and Left Hand

Age (yr)	15–19		20–29		30–39		40–49		50–59		60–69	
Gender	M	F	M	F	M	F	M	F	M	F	M	F
Excellent	≥108	≥68	≥115	≥70	≥115	≥71	≥108	≥69	≥101	≥61	≥100	≥54
Very Good	98–107	60–67	104–114	63–69	104–114	63–70	97–107	61–68	92–100	54–60	91–99	48–53
Good	90–97	53–59	95–103	58–62	95–103	58–62	88–96	54–60	84–91	49–53	84–90	45–47
Fair	79–89	48–52	84–94	52–57	84–94	51–57	80–87	49–53	76–83	45–48	73–83	41–44
Needs improvement	≥78	≥47	≥83	≥51	≥83	≥50	≥79	≥48	≥75	≥44	≥72	≥40

Procedures: Have the participant grasp the dynamometer in the right hand first. Adjust the grip of the dynamometer so the second joint of the fingers fits snugly under the handle. The participant holds the dynamometer in line with the forearm at the level of the thigh. The dynamometer is then squeezed vigorously so as to exert maximum force. During the test, neither the hand nor the dynamometer should touch the body or any other object. Measure both hands alternately, allowing two trials per hand. Record the scores for each hand to the nearest kilogram. Combine the maximum score for each hand.

Source: The Canadian Physical Activity, Fitness & Lifestyle Appraisal: CSEP-Health & Fitness Programs Health-Related Appraisal and Counselling Strategy, 3rd Edition. © 2003. Reprinted with permission of the Canadian Society for Exercise Physiology.

TABLE 31 Age Group and Gender Classifications for Partial Curl-Ups

Age	Excellent	Very Good	Good	Fair	Needs Improvement
15–19					
Male	25	23–24	21–22	16–20	≤15
Female	25	22–24	17–21	12–16	≤11
20–29					
Male	25	21–24	16–20	11–15	≤10
Female	25	18–24	14–17	5–13	≤4
30–39					
Male	25	18–24	15–17	11–14	≤10
Female	25	19–24	10–18	6–9	≤5
40–49					
Male	25	18–24	13–17	6–12	≤5
Female	25	19–24	11–18	4–10	≤3
50–59					
Male	25	17–24	11–16	8–10	≤7
Female	25	19–24	10–18	6–9	≤5
60–69					
Male	25	16–24	11–15	6–10	≤5
Female	25	17–24	8–16	3–7	≤2

Instructions:

1. Apply masking tape and string across a gym mat in two parallel lines 10 cm apart.
2. The individual to be tested should lie in a supine position with the head resting on the mat, arms straight and fully extended at the sides and parallel to the trunk, palms of the hands in contact with the mat, and the middle fingertip of both hands at the 0 mark line. The knees should be bent at a 90° angle. The heels must stay in contact with the mat, and the test is performed with the shoes on.
3. Set a metronome to a cadence of 50 beats per minute. The subject performs as many consecutive curl-ups as possible, without pausing, at a rate of 25 per minute. The test is terminated after 1 minute. During each curl-up, the upper spine should be curled up so that the middle fingertips of both hands reach the 10 cm mark. During the curl-up the palms and heels must remain in contact with the mat. Anchoring of the feet is not permitted. On the return, the shoulder blades and head must contact the mat, and the fingertips of both hands must touch the 0 mark. The movement is performed in a slow, controlled manner at a rate of 25 per minute.
4. The test is terminated before 1 minute if subjects experience undue discomfort, are unable to maintain the required cadence, or are unable to maintain the proper curl-up technique (e.g., heels come off the floor) over two consecutive repetitions despite cautions by the test supervisor.

Source: The Canadian Physical Activity, Fitness & Lifestyle Appraisal: CSEP-Health & Fitness Programs Health-Related Appraisal and Counselling Strategy, 3rd Edition. © 2003. Reprinted with permission of the Canadian Society for Exercise Physiology.

TABLE 32a Sit-and-Reach Test for Lower Back–Hamstring Flexibility Norms by Age Groups and Gender for Trunk Forward Flexion (cm)

Age (yr)	15–19		20–29		30–39		40–49		50–59		60–69	
Gender	M	F	M	F	M	F	M	F	M	F	M	F
Excellent	≥39	≥43	≥40	≥41	≥38	≥41	≥35	≥38	≥35	≥39	≥33	≥35
Very good	34–38	38–42	34–39	37–40	33–37	36–40	29–34	34–37	28–34	33–38	25–32	31–34
Good	29–33	34–37	30–33	33–36	28–32	32–35	24–28	30–33	24–27	30–32	20–24	27–30
Fair	24–28	29–33	25–29	28–32	23–27	27–31	18–23	25–29	16–23	25–29	15–19	23–26
Needs improvement	≤23	≤28	≤24	≤27	≤22	≤26	≤17	≤24	≤15	≤24	≤14	≤23

Procedures: Have the participant warm up for this test by performing slow aerobic activities and then stretching movements. The participant, barefoot, sits with legs fully extended with the soles of the feet placed flat against the flexibility box (see Chapter 6). Keeping knees fully extended, arms evenly stretched, palms down, the participant bends and reaches forward without jerking, pushing the sliding marker along the scale with the fingertips as far as possible. The position of maximum flexion must be held for approximately 2 seconds. The test is repeated twice. The footline is set at 26 cm.

TABLE 32b

Classification	Sit and Reach (inches; footline at 0)
Excellent	≥ +7
Good	+4–6.75
Average	+0–3.75
Fair	−3–0.25
Poor	< −3

Note: There is some feeling that flexibility should not decrease with age if regular range-of-motion exercise is engaged in. The preceding norms are proposed.

Source (Tables 33a and b): The Canadian Physical Activity, Fitness & Lifestyle Appraisal: CSEP-Health & Fitness Programs Health-Related Appraisal and Counselling Strategy, 3rd Edition. © 2003. Reprinted with permission of the Canadian Society for Exercise Physiology.

TABLE 33a Push-Up Norms—Men

	Age					
%	20–29	30–39	40–49	50–59	60+	
99	100	86	64	51	39	S
95	62	52	40	39	28	
90	57	46	36	30	26	
85	51	41	34	28	24	
80	47	39	30	25	23	E
75	44	36	29	24	22	
70	41	34	26	21	21	
65	39	31	25	20	20	
60	37	30	24	19	18	G
55	35	29	22	17	16	
50	33	27	21	15	15	
45	31	25	19	14	12	
40	29	24	18	13	10	F
35	27	21	16	11	9	
30	26	20	15	10	8	
25	24	19	13	9.5	7	
20	22	17	11	9	6	P
15	19	15	10	7	5	
10	18	13	9	6	4	
5	13	9	5	3	2	VP
n =	1045	790	364	172	26	

Total n = 2397.

TABLE 33b Modified Push-Up Norms—Women

	Age					
%	20–29	30–39	40–49	50–59	60+	
99	70	56	60	31	20	S
95	45	39	33	28	20	
90	42	36	28	25	17	
85	39	33	26	23	15	
80	36	31	24	21	15	E
75	34	29	21	20	15	
70	32	28	20	19	14	
65	31	26	19	18	13	
60	30	24	18	17	12	G
55	29	23	17	15	12	
50	26	21	15	13	8	
45	25	20	14	13	6	
40	23	19	13	12	5	F
35	22	17	11	10	4	
30	20	15	10	9	3	
25	19	14	9	8	2	
20	17	11	6	6	2	P
15	15	9	4	4	1	
10	12	8	2	1	0	
5	9	4	1	0	0	VP
n =	579	411	246	105	12	

Total n = 1353; S = superior; E = excellent; G = good; F = fair; P = poor; VP = very poor.

Push-Up Test Procedures for Measurement of Muscular Endurance:

1. The push-up test is administered with male subjects in the standard "up" position (hands shoulder-width apart, back straight, head up) and female subjects in the modified "knee push-up" position (ankles crossed, knees bent at 90° angle, back straight, hands shoulder-width apart, head up).
2. When testing male subjects, the tester places a fist on the floor beneath the subject's chest, and the subject must lower the body to the floor until the chest touches the tester's fist. The fist method is not used for female subjects, and no criteria are established for determining how much the torso must be lowered to count as a proper push-up.
3. For both men and women, the subject's back must be straight at all times and the subject must push up to a straight-arm position.
4. The maximal number of push-ups performed consecutively without rest is counted as the score.

Source (Tables 34a and b): Data provided by the Institute for Aerobics Research, Dallas, TX, 2005. Reprinted by permission of the Cooper Institute for Aerobics Research, Dallas, TX.

TABLE 34a Muscular Endurance—Men

1-Minute Sit-Up (number)*

%	Age <20	20–29	30–39	40–49	50–59	60+	
99	>62	>55	>51	>47	>43	>39	S
95	62	55	51	47	43	39	
90	55	52	48	43	39	35	
85	53	49	45	40	36	31	
80	51	47	43	39	35	30	E
75	50	46	42	37	33	28	
70	48	45	41	36	31	26	
65	48	44	40	35	30	24	
60	47	42	39	34	28	22	G
55	46	41	37	32	27	21	
50	45	40	36	31	26	20	
45	42	39	36	30	25	19	
40	41	38	35	29	24	19	F
35	39	37	33	28	22	18	
30	38	35	32	27	21	17	
25	37	35	31	26	20	16	
20	36	33	30	24	19	15	P
15	34	32	28	22	17	13	
10	33	30	26	20	15	10	
5	27	27	23	17	12	7	VP
1	<27	<27	<23	<17	<12	<7	
n =	46	312	1431	1558	919	205	

Total *n* = 4471.

*Knees bent, with arms crossed over chest and feet held by a partner; sit up and touch elbows to knees.

TABLE 34b Muscular Endurance—Women

1-Minute Sit-Up (number)*

%	Age <20	20–29	30–39	40–49	50–59	60+	
99	>55	>51	>42	>38	>30	>28	S
95	55	51	42	38	30	28	
90	54	49	40	34	29	26	
85	49	45	38	32	25	20	
80	46	44	35	29	24	17	E
75	40	42	33	28	22	15	
70	38	41	32	27	22	12	
65	37	39	30	25	21	12	
60	36	38	29	24	20	11	G
55	35	37	28	23	19	10	
50	34	35	27	22	17	8	
45	34	34	26	21	16	8	
40	32	32	25	20	14	6	F
35	30	31	24	19	12	5	
30	29	30	22	17	12	4	
25	29	28	21	16	11	4	
20	28	27	20	14	10	3	P
15	27	24	18	13	7	2	
10	25	23	15	10	6	1	
5	25	18	11	7	5	0	VP
1	<25	<18	<11	<7	<5	<0	
n =	15	144	289	249	137	26	

Total *n* = 860; S = superior; E = excellent; G = good; F = fair; P = poor; VP = very poor.

Source (Tables 35a and b): Data provided by the Institute for Aerobics Research, Dallas, TX, 2005. Reprinted by permission of the Cooper Institute for Aerobics Research, Dallas, TX.

TABLE 35a Upper-Body Strength—Men

1-Repetition Maximum Bench Press

$$\text{Bench Press Weight Ratio} = \frac{\text{Weight Pushed}}{\text{Body Weight}}$$

	Age						
%	<20	20–29	30–39	40–49	50–59	60+	
99	>1.76	>1.63	>1.35	>1.20	>1.05	>.94	S
95	1.76	1.63	1.35	1.20	1.05	.94	
90	1.46	1.48	1.24	1.10	.97	.89	
85	1.38	1.37	1.17	1.04	.93	.84	
80	1.34	1.32	1.12	1.00	.90	.82	E
75	1.29	1.26	1.08	.96	.87	.79	
70	1.24	1.22	1.04	.93	.84	.77	
65	1.23	1.18	1.01	.90	.81	.74	
60	1.19	1.14	.98	.88	.79	.72	G
55	1.16	1.10	.96	.86	.77	.70	
50	1.13	1.06	.93	.84	.75	.68	
45	1.10	1.03	.90	.82	.73	.67	
40	1.06	.99	.88	.80	.71	.66	F
35	1.01	.96	.86	.78	.70	.65	
30	.96	.93	.83	.76	.68	.63	
25	.93	.90	.81	.74	.66	.60	
20	.89	.88	.78	.72	.63	.57	P
15	.86	.84	.75	.69	.60	.56	
10	.81	.80	.71	.65	.57	.53	
5	.76	.72	.65	.59	.53	.49	VP
1	<.76	<.72	<.65	<.59	<.53	<.49	
n =	60	425	1909	2090	1279	343	

Total n = 6106.

TABLE 35b Upper-Body Strength—Women

1-Repetition Maximum Bench Press

$$\text{Bench Press Weight Ratio} = \frac{\text{Weight Pushed}}{\text{Body Weight}}$$

	Age						
%	<20	20–29	30–39	40–49	50–59	60+	
99	>.88	>1.01	>.82	>.77	>.68	>.72	S
95	.88	1.01	.82	.77	.68	.72	
90	.83	.90	.76	.71	.61	.64	
85	.81	.83	.72	.66	.57	.59	
80	.77	.80	.70	.62	.55	.54	E
75	.76	.77	.65	.60	.53	.53	
70	.74	.74	.63	.57	.52	.51	
65	.70	.72	.62	.55	.50	.48	
60	.65	.70	.60	.54	.48	.47	G
55	.64	.68	.58	.53	.47	.46	
50	.63	.65	.57	.52	.46	.45	
45	.60	.63	.55	.51	.45	.44	
40	.58	.59	.53	.50	.44	.43	F
35	.57	.58	.52	.48	.43	.41	
30	.56	.56	.51	.47	.42	.40	
25	.55	.53	.49	.45	.41	.39	
20	.53	.51	.47	.43	.39	.38	P
15	.52	.50	.45	.42	.38	.36	
10	.50	.48	.42	.38	.37	.33	
5	.41	.44	.39	.35	.31	.26	VP
1	<.41	<.44	<.39	<.35	<.31	<.26	
n =	20	191	379	333	189	42	

Total n = 1154; S = superior; E = excellent; G = good; F = fair; P = poor; VP = very poor.

Instructions:

1. Have your client warm up by completing 5–10 repetitions of the exercise at 40–60% of the estimated 1-RM.
2. During a 1-minute rest, have the client stretch the muscle group. This is followed by 3–5 repetitions of the exercise at 60–80% of the estimated 1-RM.
3. Then increase the weight conservatively and have the client attempt the 1-RM lift. If the lift is successful, the client should rest 3–5 minutes before attempting the next weight increment. Follow this procedure until the client fails to complete the lift. The 1-RM typically is achieved within three to five trials.
4. Record the 1-RM value as the maximum weight lifted for the last successful trial.

Source (Tables 36a and b): Data provided by the Institute for Aerobics Research, Dallas, TX, 2005. Reprinted with permission from the Cooper Institute for Aerobics Research, Dallas, TX.

TABLE 36a Leg Strength—Men

1-Repetition Maximum Leg Press

$$\text{Leg Press Weight Ratio} = \frac{\text{Weight Pushed}}{\text{Body Weight}}$$

%	Age <20	20–29	30–39	40–49	50–59	60+	
99	>2.82	>2.40	>2.20	>2.02	>1.90	>1.80	S
95	2.82	2.40	2.20	2.02	1.90	1.80	
90	2.53	2.27	2.07	1.92	1.80	1.73	
85	2.40	2.18	1.99	1.86	1.75	1.68	
80	2.28	2.13	1.93	1.82	1.71	1.62	E
75	2.18	2.09	1.89	1.78	1.68	1.58	
70	2.15	2.05	1.85	1.74	1.64	1.56	
65	2.10	2.01	1.81	1.71	1.61	1.52	
60	2.04	1.97	1.77	1.68	1.58	1.49	G
55	2.01	1.94	1.74	1.65	1.55	1.46	
50	1.95	1.91	1.71	1.62	1.52	1.43	
45	1.93	1.87	1.68	1.59	1.50	1.40	
40	1.90	1.83	1.65	1.57	1.46	1.38	F
35	1.89	1.78	1.62	1.54	1.42	1.34	
30	1.82	1.74	1.59	1.51	1.39	1.30	
25	1.80	1.68	1.56	1.48	1.36	1.27	
20	1.70	1.63	1.52	1.44	1.32	1.25	P
15	1.61	1.58	1.48	1.40	1.28	1.21	
10	1.57	1.51	1.43	1.35	1.22	1.16	
5	1.46	1.42	1.34	1.27	1.15	1.08	VP
1	<1.46	<1.42	<1.34	<1.27	<1.15	<1.08	
n =	60	424	1909	2089	1286	347	

Total n = 6115.

TABLE 36b Leg Strength—Women

1-Repetition Maximum Leg Press

$$\text{Leg Press Weight Ratio} = \frac{\text{Weight Pushed}}{\text{Body Weight}}$$

%	Age <20	20–29	30–39	40–49	50–59	60+	
99	>1.88	>1.98	>1.68	>1.57	>1.43	>1.43	S
95	1.88	1.98	1.68	1.57	1.43	1.43	
90	1.85	1.82	1.61	1.48	1.37	1.32	
85	1.81	1.76	1.52	1.40	1.31	1.32	
80	1.71	1.68	1.47	1.37	1.25	1.18	E
75	1.69	1.65	1.42	1.33	1.20	1.16	
70	1.65	1.58	1.39	1.29	1.17	1.13	
65	1.62	1.53	1.36	1.27	1.12	1.08	
60	1.59	1.50	1.33	1.23	1.10	1.04	G
55	1.51	1.47	1.31	1.20	1.08	1.01	
50	1.45	1.44	1.27	1.18	1.05	.99	
45	1.42	1.40	1.24	1.15	1.02	.97	
40	1.38	1.37	1.21	1.13	.99	.93	F
35	1.33	1.32	1.18	1.11	.97	.90	
30	1.29	1.27	1.15	1.08	.95	.88	
25	1.25	1.26	1.12	1.06	.92	.86	
20	1.22	1.22	1.09	1.02	.88	.85	P
15	1.19	1.18	1.05	.97	.84	.80	
10	1.09	1.14	1.00	.94	.78	.72	
5	1.06	.99	.96	.85	.72	.63	VP
1	<1.06	<.99	<.96	<.85	<.72	<.63	
n =	20	192	281	337	192	44	

Total n = 1166; S = superior; E = excellent; G = good; F = fair; P = poor; VP = very poor.

Instructions:

1. Have your client warm up by completing 5–10 repetitions of the exercise at 40–60% of the estimated 1-RM.
2. During a 1-minute rest, have the client stretch the muscle group. This is followed by 3–5 repetitions of the exercise at 60–80% of the estimated 1-RM.
3. Then increase the weight conservatively and have the client attempt the 1-RM lift. If the lift is successful, the client should rest 3–5 minutes before attempting the next weight increment. Follow this procedure until the client fails to complete the lift. The 1-RM typically is achieved within three to five trials.
4. Record the 1-RM value as the maximum weight lifted for the last successful trial.

Source (Tables 37a and b): Data provided by the Institute for Aerobics Research, Dallas, TX, 2005. Reprinted with permission from the Cooper Institute for Aerobics Research, Dallas, TX.

TABLE 37 YMCA Endurance Bench-Press Test—Total Lifts

Age (yr)	18–25		26–35		36–45		46–55		56–65		>65	
Gender	M	F	M	F	M	F	M	F	M	F	M	F
Excellent	44–64	42–66	41–61	40–62	36–55	33–57	28–47	29–50	24–41	24–42	20–36	18–30
Good	34–41	30–38	30–37	29–34	26–32	26–30	21–25	20–24	17–21	17–21	12–16	12–16
Above average	29–33	25–28	26–29	24–28	22–25	21–24	16–20	14–18	12–14	12–14	10	8–10
Average	24–28	20–22	21–24	18–22	18–21	16–20	12–14	10–13	9–11	8–10	7–8	5–7
Below average	20–22	16–18	17–20	14–17	14–17	12–14	9–11	7–9	5–8	5–6	4–6	3–4
Poor	13–17	9–13	12–16	9–13	9–12	6–10	5–8	2–6	2–4	2–4	2–3	0–2
Very poor	0–10	0–6	0–9	0–6	0–6	0–4	0–2	0–1	0–1	0–1	0–1	0

Note: See Chapter 6 for instructions. Women use a 35-pound bar; men, 80 pounds. Maximum repetitions in time to metronome at 30 lifts per minute.

Source: Reprinted from *YMCA Fitness Testing Assessment Manual,* 2000 edtion, with permission of the YMCA of the USA, 101 N. Wacker Drive, Chicago, IL 60606.

TABLE 38 Pull-Ups

Classification	Number of Pull-Ups
Excellent	15+
Good	12–14
Average	8–11
Fair	5–7
Poor	0–4

Note: See Chapter 6 for instructions. Norms are for college men.

Source: Johnson BL, Nelson JK. *Practical Measurement for Evaluation in Physical Education.* Minneapolis: Burgess Publishing Co., 1979. Reprinted with permission of Pearson Custom Publishing.

TABLE 39 Parallel Bar Dips

Classification	Number of Bar Dips
Excellent	25+
Good	18–24
Average	9–17
Fair	4–8
Poor	0–3

Note: See Chapter 6 for instructions.

Source: Adapted from Johnson BL, Nelson JK. *Practical Measurement for Evaluation in Physical Education.* Minneapolis: Burgess Publishing Co., 1979. Reprinted with permission of Pearson Custom Publishing.

TABLE 40 Serum Total Cholesterol of Males 4 Years of Age and Older by Age: Mean and Selected Percentiles, United States, 1988–94

	Number of Examined Persons	Mean	Standard Deviation	Standard Error of the Mean	Selected Percentiles								
					5th	10th	15th	25th	50th	75th	85th	90th	95th
Age in years													
4 years and older, crude	11,200	192	41.9	0.63	131	142	149	162	189	220	237	248	266
4 years and older, age adjusted		191											
4–5 years	846	161	24.3	1.33	123	133	136	144	159	175	185	192	203
6–8 years	695	166	26.4	1.59	127	135	140	147	165	183	191	203	212
9–11 years	757	172	28.4	1.64	135	140	145	153	171	189	196	209	227
12–15 years	703	158	27.5	1.65	117	124	130	140	158	174	184	192	203
16–19 years	668	158	29.7	1.82	117	123	127	138	156	175	190	200	214
20 years and older, crude	7,531	202	41.0	0.75	139	151	160	173	200	228	244	255	273
20 years and older, age adjusted		202											
20–74 years	6,587	202	41.0	0.80	139	151	160	173	200	228	244	255	273
20–74 years, age adjusted		201											
20–29 years	1,551	180	36.2	1.46	127	137	145	155	177	200	216	225	242
30–39 years	1,389	201	39.3	1.68	139	153	162	171	199	228	244	253	267
40–49 years	1,169	211	39.2	1.82	147	164	173	186	209	236	249	261	275
50–59 years	829	216	40.8	2.25	154	166	177	191	214	240	257	270	286
60–69 years	1,137	217	39.2	1.85	152	169	177	190	215	241	256	270	285
70–79 years	812	208	39.2	2.18	148	159	169	180	205	233	248	256	275
80+ years	644	201	41.0	2.56	140	152	158	170	198	226	244	253	270

Source: NHANES III, 1988–94.

TABLE 41 Serum Total Cholesterol of Females 4 Years of Age and Older by Age: Mean and Selected Percentiles, United States, 1988–94

	Number of Examined Persons	Mean	Standard Deviation	Standard Error of the Mean	Selected Percentiles								
					5th	10th	15th	25th	50th	75th	85th	90th	95th
Age in years													
4 years and older, crude	12,361	197	45.1	0.61	135	145	153	165	191	224	244	257	278
4 years and older, age adjusted		195											
4–5 years	861	164	25.9	1.32	126	134	140	146	163	179	190	197	206
6–8 years	672	166	26.5	1.53	127	136	143	150	165	181	190	196	203
9–11 years	731	169	26.7	1.48	131	137	143	149	167	185	196	205	219
12–15 years	799	164	29.8	1.58	123	130	135	143	160	182	192	201	218
16–19 years	767	171	39.8	2.16	118	128	136	145	164	189	203	217	238
20 years and older, crude	8,531	206	44.7	0.73	143	153	161	175	201	233	251	265	284
20 years and older, age adjusted		206											
20–74 years	7,429	204	44.2	0.77	142	152	160	173	199	231	249	262	282
20–74 years, age adjusted		204											
20–29 years	1,760	183	37.2	1.33	131	141	147	157	179	205	217	229	244
30–39 years	1,750	189	34.7	1.24	138	147	153	166	186	209	226	234	250
40–49 years	1,300	204	38.2	1.59	150	158	164	177	201	225	245	254	277
50–59 years	962	228	43.8	2.12	166	177	184	199	224	255	273	284	304
60–69 years	1,109	235	45.5	2.05	170	183	193	205	230	258	278	290	309
70–79 years	934	233	44.8	2.20	164	177	188	200	233	262	277	287	309
80+ years	716	228	43.3	2.43	165	177	183	196	224	254	270	285	305

Source: NHANES III, 1988–94.

TABLE 42 Serum High-Density Lipoprotein (HDL) Cholesterol of Males 4 Years of Age and Older by Age: Mean and Selected Percentiles, United States, 1988–94

			Selected Percentiles										
	n[1]	Mean	SD[2]	SEM[3]	5th	10th	15th	25th	50th	75th	85th	90th	95th
Age in years													
4 years and older, crude	11,123	47	13.4	0.21	28	32	34	38	45	54	60	64	72
4 years and older, age adjusted		47											
4–5 years	845	50	11.9	0.69	31	36	38	42	49	56	63	66	72
6–8 years	692	53	12.3	0.78	33	38	40	44	52	61	65	68	74
9–11 years	752	54	12.7	0.77	37	39	42	44	53	62	67	71	76
12–15 years	697	48	11.3	0.71	33	36	37	40	47	55	60	63	68
16–19 years	664	46	11.1	0.72	30	33	36	38	45	52	57	61	67
20 years and older, crude	7,473	46	13.7	0.26	28	31	34	37	44	53	58	63	72
20 years and older, age adjusted		46											
20–74 years	6,535	46	13.6	0.28	28	30	33	37	44	53	58	62	72
20–74 years, age adjusted		46											
20–29 years	1,541	47	12.5	0.53	29	33	35	39	45	54	60	63	69
30–39 years	1,379	46	13.3	0.60	27	32	34	37	44	52	58	61	70
40–49 years	1,152	45	14.8	0.73	26	30	32	36	43	51	58	64	74
50–59 years	823	44	13.9	0.81	27	30	32	36	42	51	56	61	75
60–69 years	1,130	46	13.7	0.68	28	31	32	36	43	53	58	63	72
70–79 years	808	46	14.9	0.87	28	31	33	36	44	53	59	63	74
80+ years	640	47	14.2	0.94	29	31	34	38	44	55	63	66	74

[1]Number of examined persons.

[2]Standard deviation.

[3]Standard error of the mean.

Source: Nhanes III, 1988–94.

TABLE 43 Serum High-Density Lipoprotein (HDL) Cholesterol of Females 4 Years of Age and Older by Age: Mean and Selected Percentiles, United States, 1988–94

	n[1]	Mean	SD[2]	SEM[3]	Selected Percentiles 5th	10th	15th	25th	50th	75th	85th	90th	95th
Age in years													
4 years and older, crude	12,286	54	14.8	0.20	34	38	40	44	53	63	68	73	80
4 years and older, age adjusted		54											
4–5 years	852	48	11.3	0.58	30	35	37	40	47	55	59	62	68
6–8 years	670	50	11.2	0.65	33	38	40	43	49	58	61	65	70
9–11 years	727	51	11.3	0.63	33	38	40	42	50	58	61	66	70
12–15 years	797	51	11.6	0.61	34	37	40	43	50	59	63	66	70
16–19 years	762	52	12.0	0.66	34	38	40	44	52	60	63	67	73
20 years and older, crude	8,478	55	15.5	0.25	34	38	41	44	54	64	70	75	83
20 years and older, age adjusted		55											
20–74 years	7,382	55	15.4	0.27	34	38	41	45	53	64	70	75	83
20–74 years, age adjusted		55											
20–29 years	1,751	55	14.8	0.53	35	38	41	45	53	64	70	75	84
30–39 years	1,744	54	15.0	0.54	33	37	40	44	53	64	69	74	81
40–49 years	1,282	55	14.0	0.59	36	38	41	45	53	64	68	72	79
50–59 years	955	57	17.2	0.83	34	38	41	45	54	65	73	78	87
60–69 years	1,104	56	17.2	0.78	32	37	40	44	53	65	72	78	87
70–79 years	929	56	16.4	0.81	32	36	40	45	55	64	71	75	84
80+ years	713	56	15.9	0.89	33	37	40	44	54	65	71	76	85

[1]Number of examined persons.

[2]Standard deviation.

[3]Standard error of the mean.

Source: NHANES III, 1988–94.

APPENDIX **B**

Calisthenics for Development of Flexibility and Muscular Strength and Endurance

FLEXIBILITY EXERCISES

The key to developing good flexibility is to hold each of the following positions just short of pain for 15–30 seconds. *Relax* totally, letting your muscles slowly go limp as the tension of the stretched muscle area slowly subsides. After the tension has subsided, it is a good idea to stretch just a bit farther to better develop your flexibility (hold this "developmental stretch" also for 15–30 seconds). Be sure that you do not stretch to the point of pain, for flexibility cannot be developed while the stretched muscle is in pain.

Flexibility exercises should be conducted *following* the aerobic phase. Research has shown that stretching is safer and more effective when done with warm muscles and joints. You can stretch farther without injury more often following stimulating aerobics than before.

Do not be worried if you seem "tighter" than other people in many of the following stretches. Flexibility is an individual matter, and each person should "make the most" of what she or he has, realizing there are genetic differences.

Flexibility 1

Lower Back–Hamstring Rope Stretch

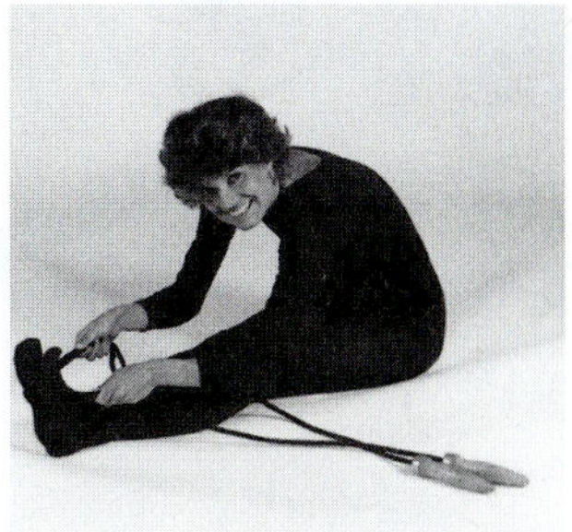

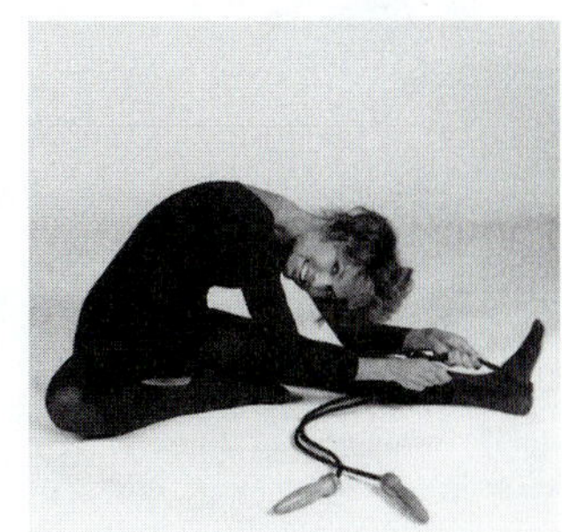

Start by sitting on the floor, one leg straight, the other relaxed off to the side (some people like the other leg bent at a 90° angle, foot against the other leg, some like it straight off to the side a bit, others slightly bent and loose). The rope should be doubled over the heel. (This exercise can also be done with both legs at one time.)

Stretch by reaching down the rope toward your foot with both hands until you feel a good tension in the back of your leg (some feel tension in the lower back also). Relax, breathe easily, letting the tension slowly subside; then reach a bit farther, holding this for 15–30 seconds also. Repeat with the other leg.

Benefits: This is perhaps the best stretch for the lower back and hamstrings (muscles on the back of your thigh). Your goal is to slowly work toward your foot as the weeks pass until you can at least hold on to your foot with one hand.

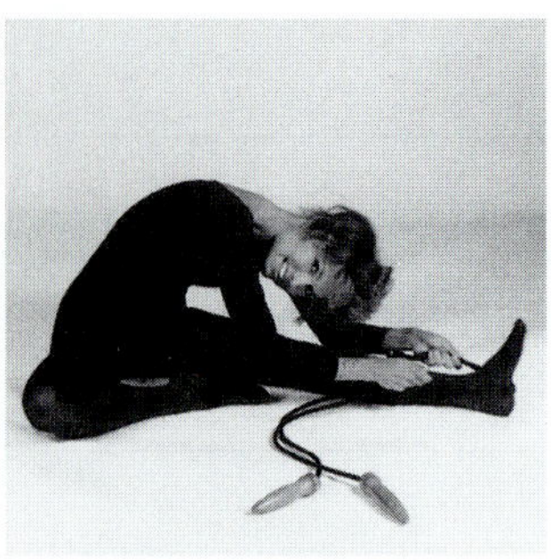

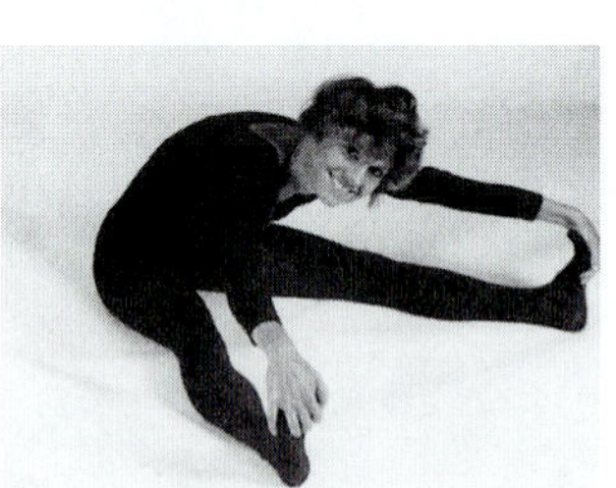

Flexibility 2

Calf Rope Stretch

Start just the same as for the lower back–hamstring rope stretch, but put the rope on the ball of your foot.

Stretch by pulling your upper foot (easy does it) toward your body until you feel a good tension in the top of your calf muscle. Relax and hold this position for 15–30 seconds; then reach a bit farther down the rope for a second 15- to 30-second stretch. Repeat with the other leg.

Benefits: Stretches the calf muscle.

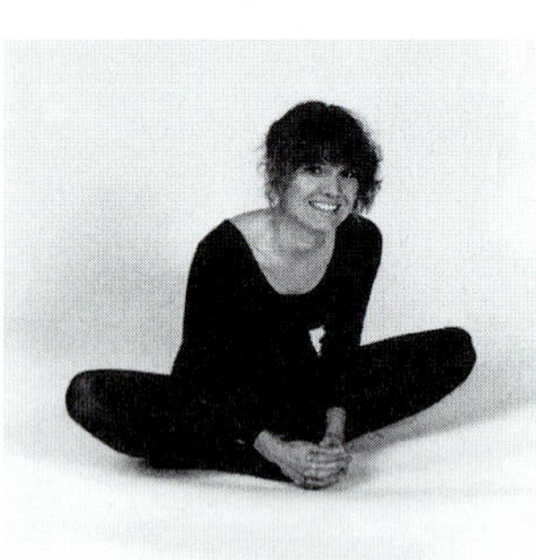

Flexibility 3

Groin Stretch

Start by sitting on the floor with the soles of your feet together, legs bent, knees up and out.

Stretch by pulling your feet with your hands to within a few inches of your crotch. Hold this position as you lean forward from the waist, keeping your chin up, and knees down as far as possible. Feel a good tension in the groin area, and hold. Be careful that you do not overstretch.

Benefits: Stretches the muscles in the groin area.

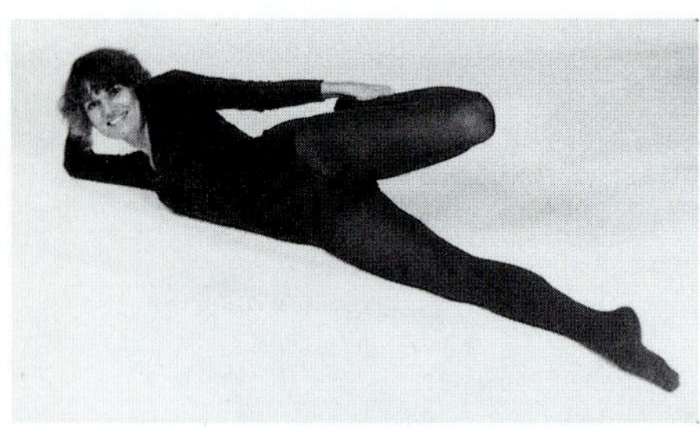

Flexibility 4

Quad Stretch

Start by lying on your right side, right hand supporting your head.

Stretch by bending your left leg, pulling the heel to your seat with the left hand grasping the ankle. Slowly move the entire left leg somewhat behind you until there is a good tension in front of the thigh, and hold. Repeat with the other leg.

Benefits: The muscles of the front of the thigh (quadriceps) are stretched in this exercise.

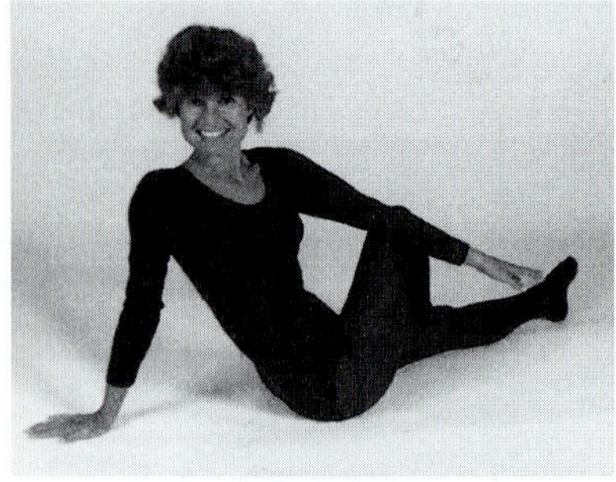

Flexibility 5

Spinal Twist

Start by sitting with your left leg straight out in front of you, your right leg bent, right foot crossed over the left knee.

Stretch by placing your left elbow on the outside of your right knee, pushing the right knee inward. At the same time, place your right hand on the ground behind you, and twist looking over your right shoulder. Keep pushing with your left elbow and twisting with your head over your right shoulder until you feel a good tension along your spine and hip, and hold for 15–30 seconds. Repeat on the other side.

Benefits: Stretches the muscles along the spine and side of the hips. Some people find this a hard stretch to coordinate. You may have to practice carefully with the pictures until you get used to all the important details.

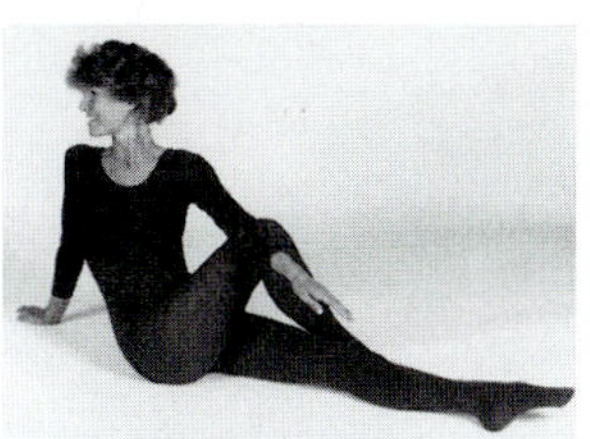

Flexibility 6

Downward Dog

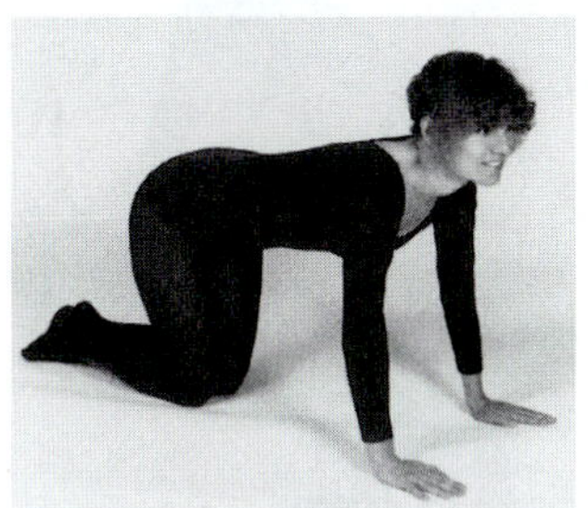

Start by getting on hands and knees.

Stretch by humping your seat straight up, with legs straight. Walk in with your hands toward your feet until your hands and feet are about 3 feet apart. Then try to keep your heels on the ground as you lean somewhat backward, keeping your legs straight, hands on the floor, and head down. You should feel a good tension all along your posterior leg. Hold for 15–30 seconds until the tension slowly subsides. The key is to keep the heels on the ground, but be careful not to hold a painful position, as this could injure your legs.

Benefits: This is an excellent stretch for the hamstrings and calves of your legs, as well as the lower back. Running tends to tighten the posterior leg muscles, and this exercise helps to counter this.

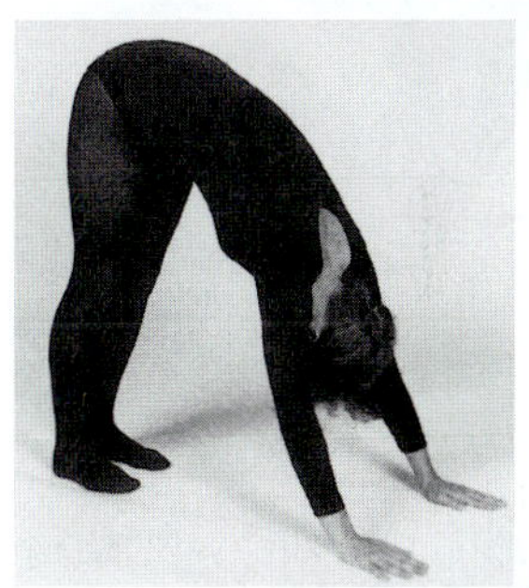

Flexibility 7

Upper-Body Stretch

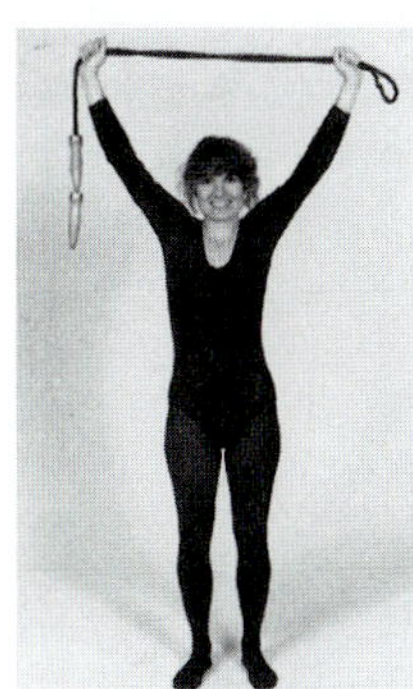

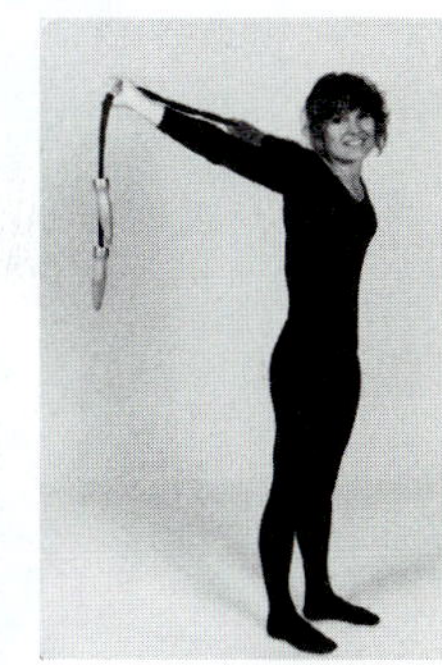

Start by grasping a rope or towel with your hands 2–4 feet apart.

Stretch by keeping your arms perfectly straight and slowly circling them up and behind you. Move slowly, feeling the tension in the front of your chest and shoulders. If you cannot keep your arms straight, or if the pain is too intense, put your hands farther apart. Repeat several times.

Benefits: Running tends to tighten the muscles in the front of the chest. This exercise helps to stretch those muscles, improving your posture.

Flexibility 8

Standing Side Stretch

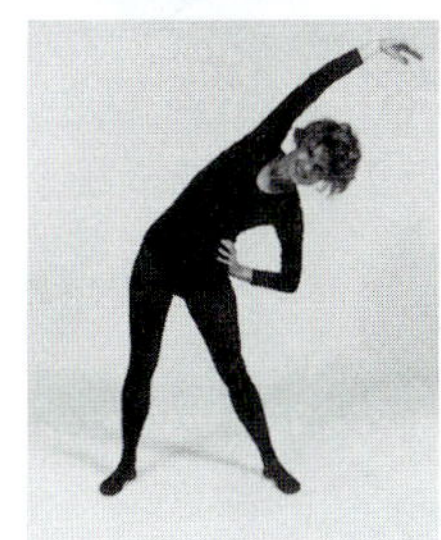

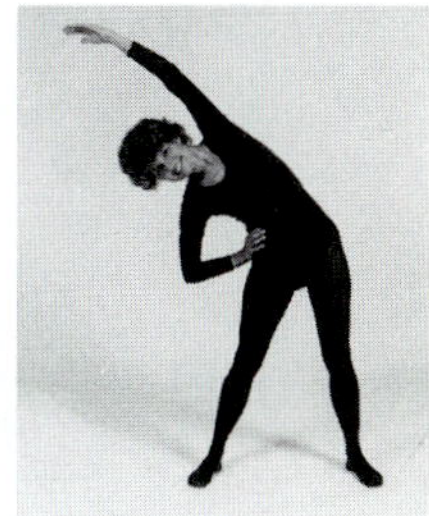

Start by standing with your feet 3 feet apart, hands on your hips.

Stretch by raising your right hand up and over your head as you lean way over to the left side. Keep your legs straight and lean straight to the side. Hold the position, feeling the stretch along your right side and inner left thigh. Repeat with the other side. If you do not feel a stretch in your thighs, put your feet farther apart.

Benefits: This exercise stretches the muscles along both sides and inner thighs.

MUSCLE ENDURANCE AND STRENGTH EXERCISES

The following exercises localize movement to specific muscle groups, developing the strength and muscle endurance in each of these areas. Do 5–15 reps of each (remembering that a rep = one–one, two, three; two–one, two, three; etc.).

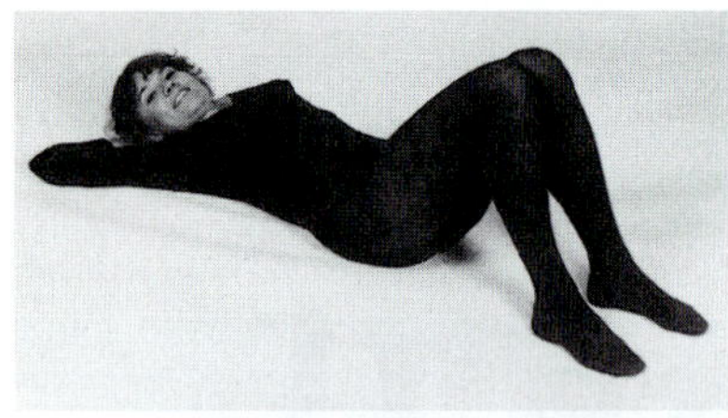

Abdomen 1

Bent-Knee Sit-Ups

Start by lying on the ground, knees bent at a 90° angle. Most people need to tuck their feet under either another person or an object. If you are in good shape, you can put your hands behind your head. If your abdominal muscles are not in good shape, you can put your arms straight out in front of you (and even pull on your knees if you need to).

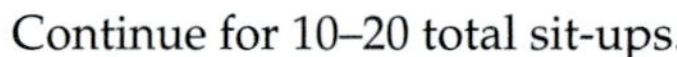

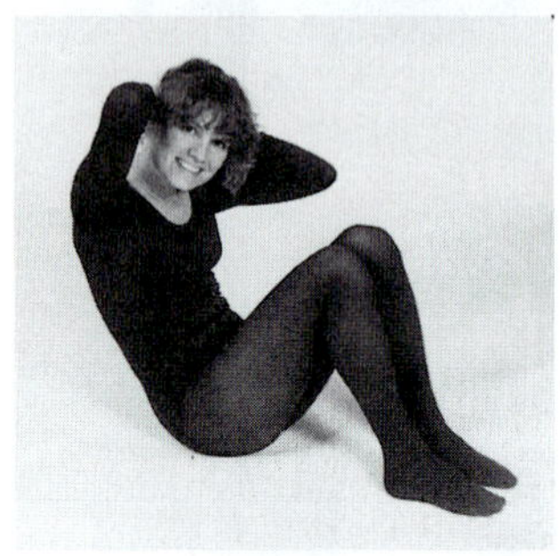

1. Sit up by flexing your abdominal muscles, and touch your elbows to your knees. If you need to, keep your arms out in front of you.
2. Lie back down, keeping your knees bent.

Repeat.

Continue for 10–20 total sit-ups.

Benefits: The bent-knee sit-up is an excellent exercise for toning up the abdominal muscles. The knees are bent so that the strong hip flexors will have minimal action, allowing the abdominal muscles to act.

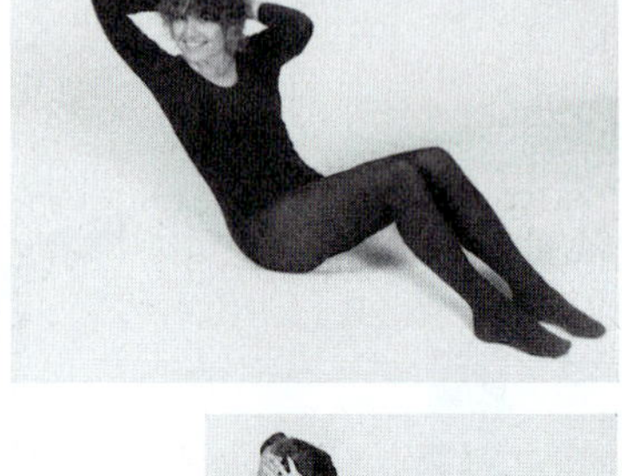

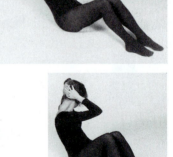

Abdomen 2

Ab-Curl Twisters

Start in the same basic position as the sit-up, except that you should have your torso two thirds the way up toward your knees.

1. Keeping your body in a two-thirds sit-up position, twist to your left.
2. Next twist to your right.

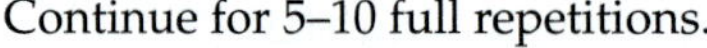

Keep twisting back and forth, right and left, while leaning back, feeling a good tension in your abdominal area. If the movement becomes too hard, move closer to your knees.

Continue for 5–10 full repetitions.

Benefits: The sides of the abdomen are given a great workout, as well as the middle abdominal muscles.

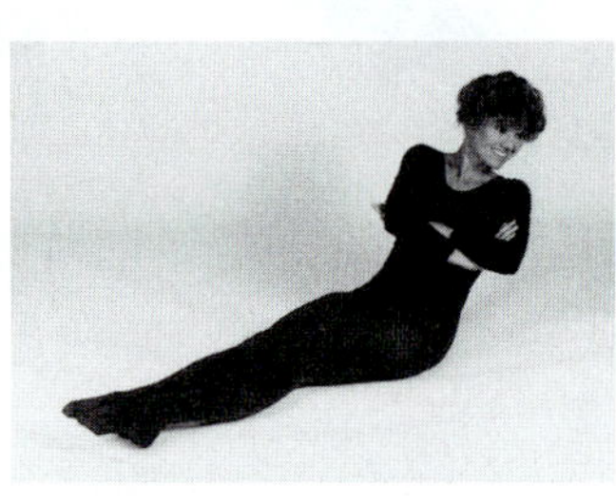

Abdomen 3

Straight-Leg Ab-Twisters

Start by sitting with your legs together, straight out in front of you, arms crossed over your chest.

1. Lean back at least one third of the way to the floor, hold this position throughout, and twist to the left, looking to the ground on the left side.
2. Next do the same to the right side.

Repeat, twisting left and right while leaning back, legs straight.

Continue for 5–10 repetitions.

Benefits: This exercise also gives the sides of the abdomen a good workout while developing the muscle endurance of the middle abdominals as well.

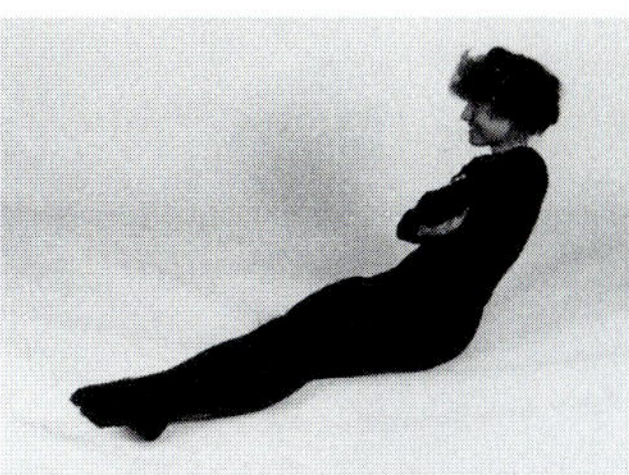

Abdomen 4

Steam Engine

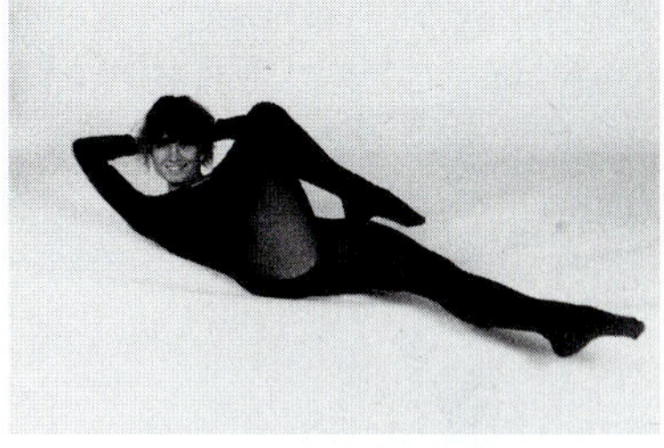

Start by lying on your back, hands behind the head. Then lift the head off the ground and touch your left elbow to your right knee. The right leg is bent, foot off the ground, while the left leg is straight, off the ground as well.

1. While maintaining the basic starting position, twist your torso to the left while bending the left leg and straightening the right leg. Touch in one smooth movement your right elbow to your left knee.
2. Return to the starting position, twisting your torso to the right.

Repeat, twisting right and left, touching the elbow on each side to the knee of the opposite bent leg. The alternating leg should be straight and off the ground.

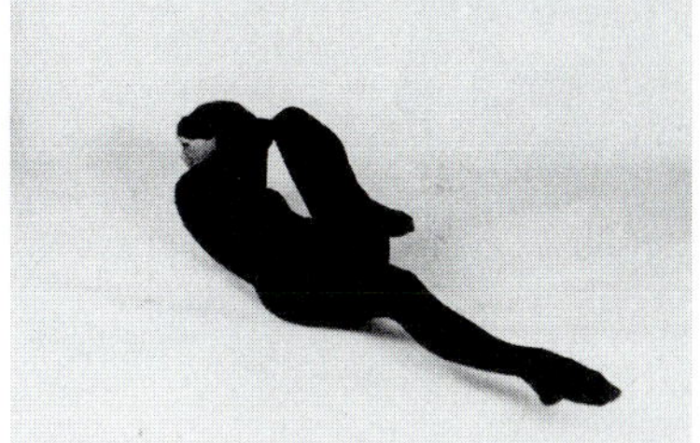

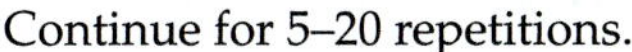

Continue for 5–20 repetitions.

Benefits: This is probably the best abdominal exercise because the entire abdominal area is given a great workout. The abdominal muscles are best developed when the trunk is curled and twisted, as here.

Abdomen 5

Wringer

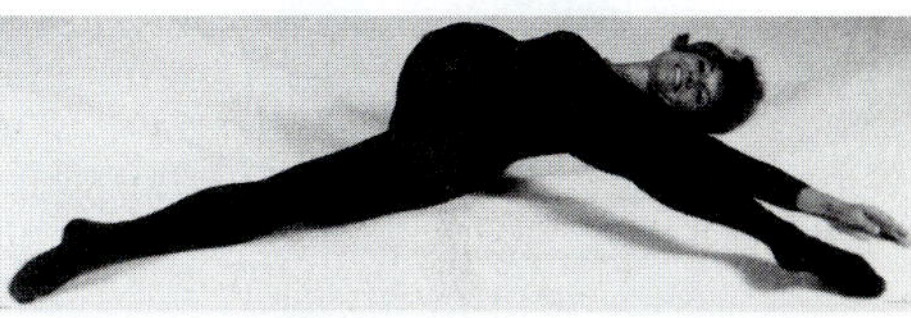

Start by lying on the ground, legs straight and together, but arms straight and out to the sides.

1. Lift your leg up and over to your outstretched right hand. Try to keep your leg straight, plus keep your left shoulder as close to the ground as possible.
2. Return your left leg to the starting position.
3. Repeat with your right leg, once again lifting it up and over to your left hand, which is straight out perpendicular from your body.
4. Return your right leg to the starting position.

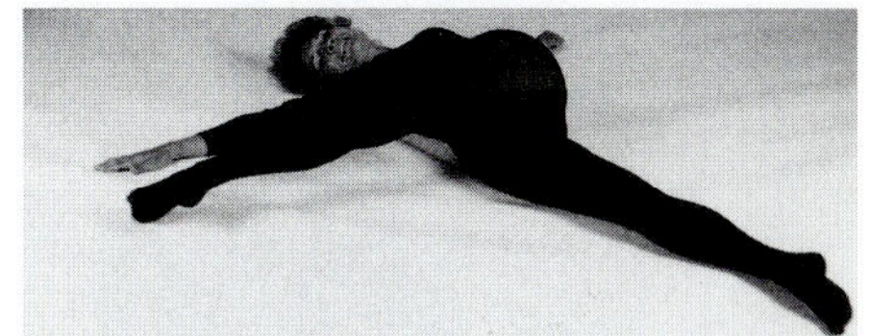

Continue for 10–15 full repetitions.

Benefits: This exercise will not only develop the muscular endurance of the hip flexors and abdominal muscles, but also stretch the muscles along the sides of the body.

Abdomen 6

Gut Tucks

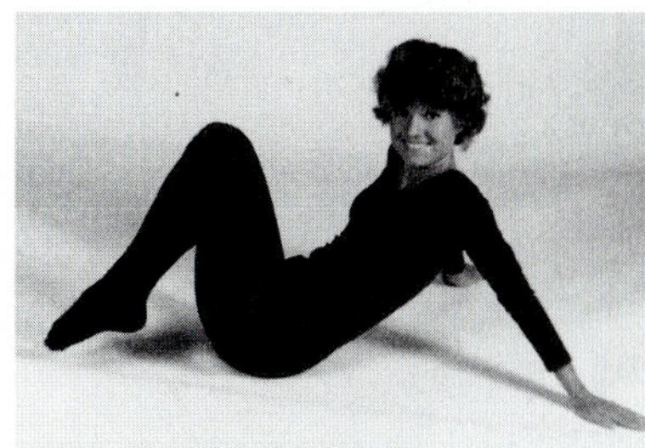

Start by sitting in a tuck position, with your legs drawn up close to your body and hands on the floor slightly behind you for balance and support.

1. Lift your feet several inches off the ground as you straighten your legs halfway. It is important not to straighten the legs all the way because this places too great a strain on the lower back.

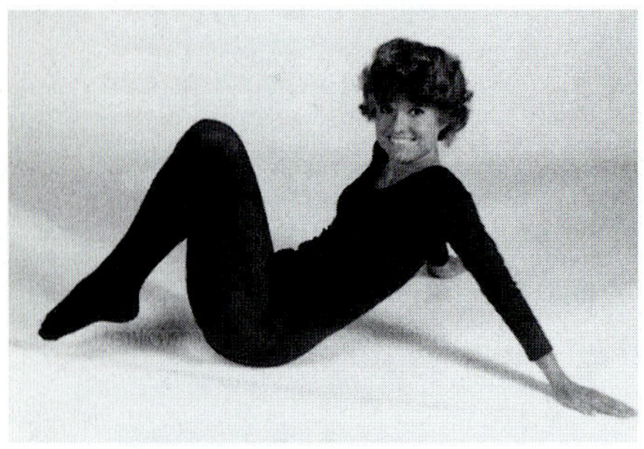

2. Return your legs to the tuck position, with your legs drawn up close to your body, and hands on the floor slightly behind you for balance and support.

Repeat, half straightening your legs and then tucking them back in, keeping the feet off the ground as you support yourself with your hands, leaning back slightly.

Continue for 5–10 repetitions.

Benefits: This is an excellent abdominal exercise, firming up the muscles in the lower abdominal area especially.

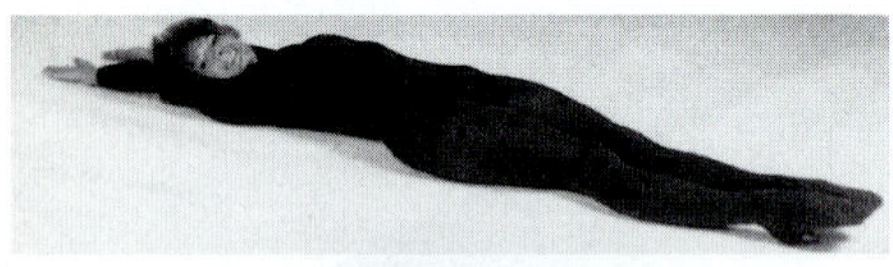

Abdomen 7

Half-Pike Sit-Ups

Start by lying on the ground on your back, body fully stretched out, legs together, and arms together over your head.

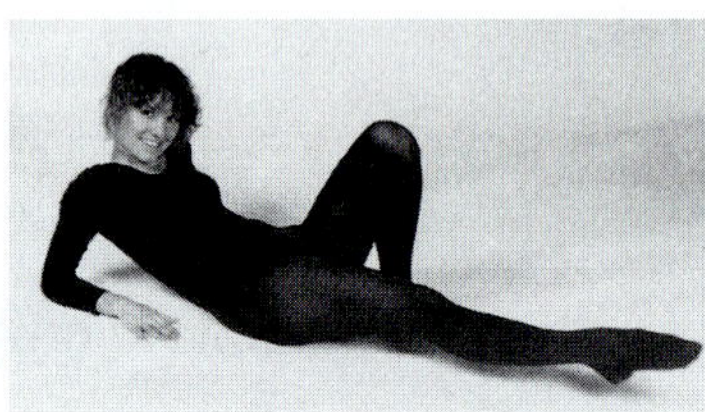

1. Lift your right leg up straight off the floor while lifting your arms, head, and shoulders up until you can touch your hands to your ankle or foot.
2. Return to the starting position.
3. Repeat with your left leg.

Continue for 10 repetitions.

Benefits: The hip flexors are given a good workout, while the abdominals are developed to a lesser extent because there is little abdominal curling going on.

Abdomen 8

Single Leg Lifts

Start by supporting yourself on your elbows and seat, with your left leg bent, right leg straight.

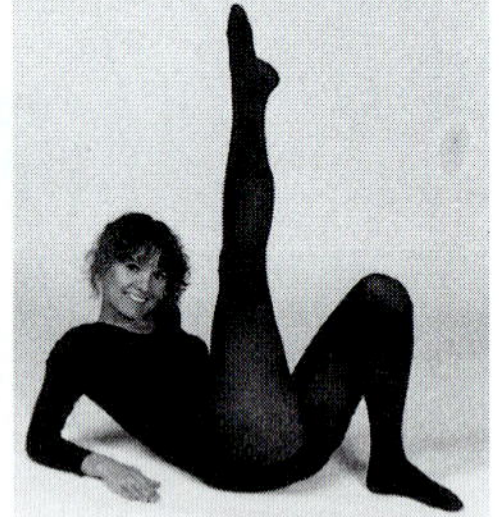

1. Lift your right leg, keeping it straight, up off the ground as high as you can.
2. Return your right leg to the starting position, but keep it several inches off the ground.

Repeat for 5–10 repetitions; then do the same with your left leg.

Continue lifting the straight leg up and down while keeping the other leg bent, supporting yourself with your elbows. It is important to stay in this position to prevent lower-back strain from lifting the straight leg.

Benefits: This exercise is especially good for the hip flexors, and secondarily for lower abdominal muscles.

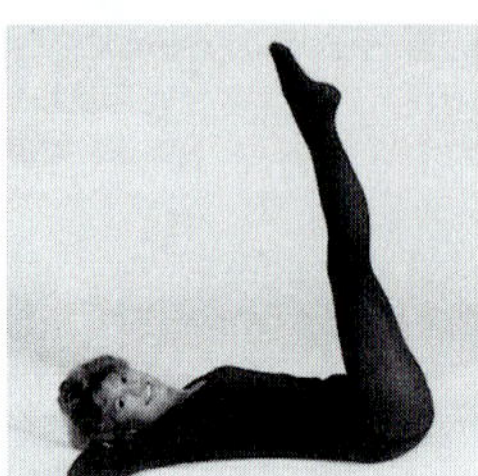

Abdomen 9

Extended Leg Sit-Ups

Start by lying on your back, legs straight up in a "pike" position, with your hands joined together behind your head, elbows out.

1. Lift your head, arms, and shoulders up as high as you can off the ground, making sure to keep the elbows out.
2. Return to the starting position.

Repeat, curling your upper body up and then down while keeping the legs straight up off the ground.

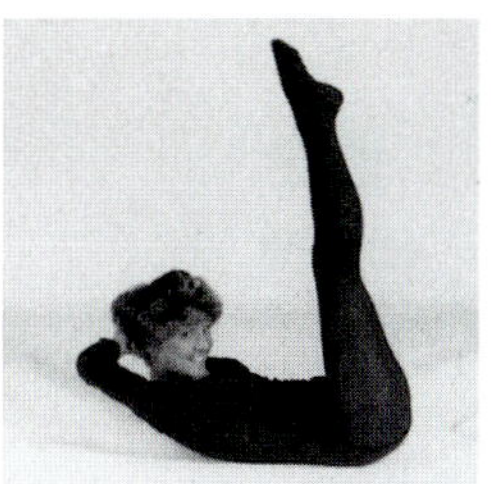

Continue for 5–10 repetitions.

Benefits: This is one of the best abdominal exercises you can do to develop a "flat tummy." The hip flexors are not involved because of the straight-leg-pike position which forces the abdominal muscles to curl your head and shoulders up.

Abdomen 10

Rowing

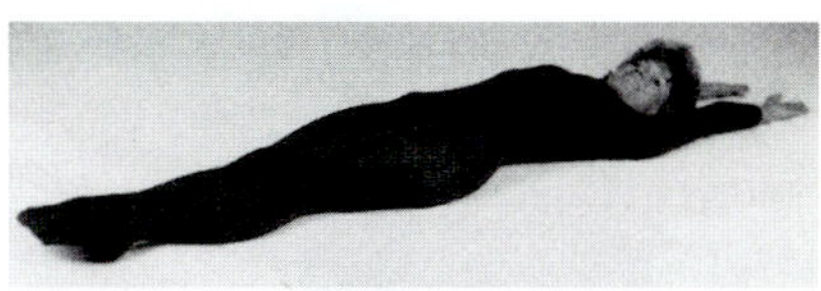

Start by lying on your back, arms and legs fully stretched and together.

1. Draw your legs up to your body in a tuck position as you lift your upper body forward, reaching past your bent knees with your straight arms.
2. Return to the starting position.

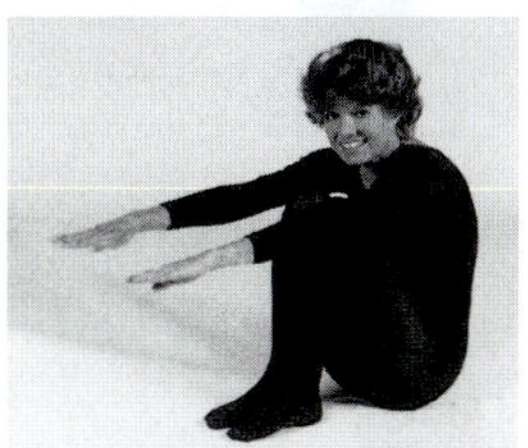

Repeat, tucking your body into a tight ball, then returning to the starting position.

Continue for 5–10 repetitions.

Benefits: This is another excellent exercise for the abdominals and hip flexors. The tighter the ball you draw yourself into, the better.

Arms–Shoulders 1

Push-Ups

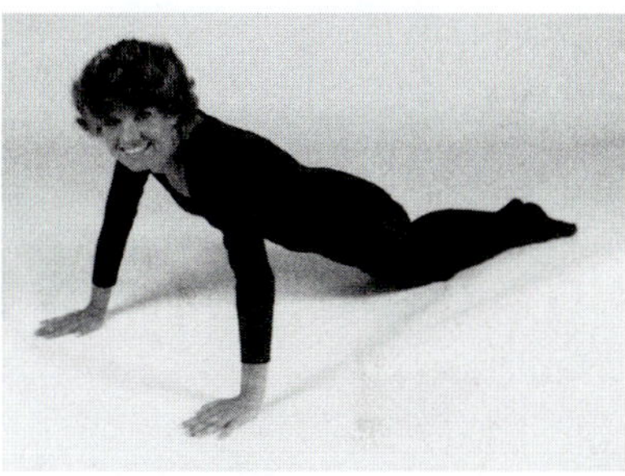

Start by supporting yourself on your knees and hands. It is important that your back be straight, seat not humped up. Your shoulders should be over your hands, arms straight. You should feel that you are supporting a good part of your weight on your hands. *Note:* If you are strong enough, support yourself between your feet and hands, keeping the trunk of your body perfectly straight and rigid. This can strain the lower back, so be certain that you possess sufficient strength.

1. Lower yourself down to within a few inches off the ground, keeping your back rigid and straight, weight equally distributed between knees and hands.
2. Straighten your arms up, once again keeping the back rigid and straight. Avoid sagging or humping.

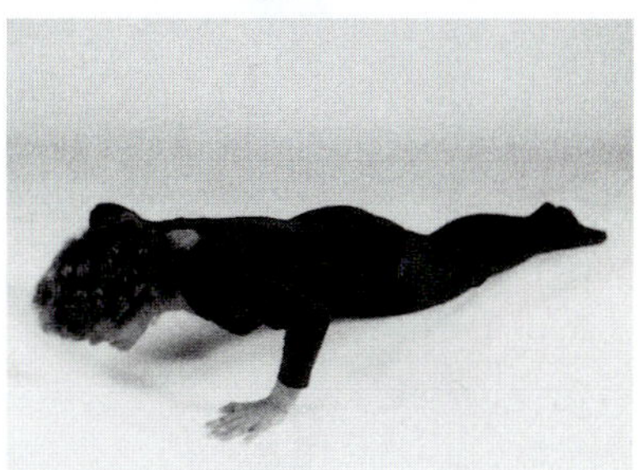

Repeat, lowering your body down and then pushing up, while the trunk is straight, and weight well felt on your arms and hands.

Continue for 5–15 repetitions (10–30 single push-ups).

Benefits: This exercise develops muscular strength and endurance of the muscles of the front of the chest (pectorals) and back of the upper arm (triceps). The muscles of the trunk are also developed as the body is kept in a straight and rigid position throughout the exercise.

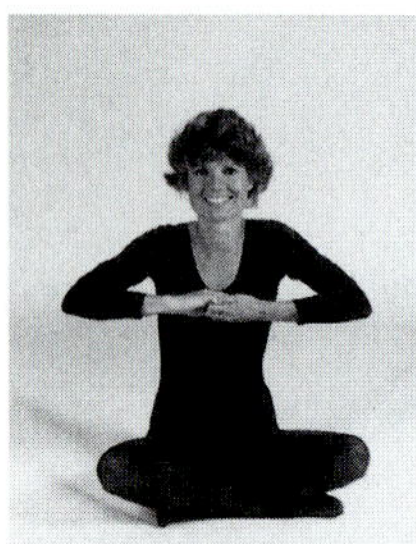

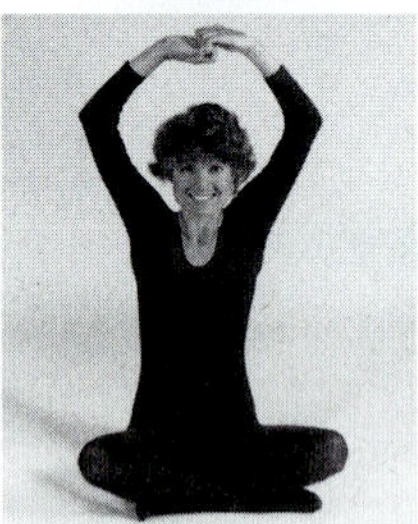

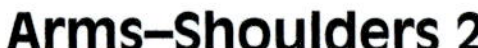

Arms–Shoulders 2

Sitting Hand Pull Raises

Start by sitting with your legs crossed, hands clasped together in the "Indian grip" (fingers hooked, hands opposite). Elbows should be out.

1. Pull hands apart, keeping them together with hooked fingers as you lift your hands and arms above your head. Keep pulling the hands hard the entire time.
2. Return the hands and arms to the starting position, still pulling hard.

Repeat, lifting the hands up and down as you try to pull them apart.

Continue for 5–10 repetitions.

Benefits: This calisthenic especially develops the muscles between the shoulder blades, the rhomboids. The muscles of the upper back and neck, the trapezius in particular, are also developed. The overall benefit is to improve back posture.

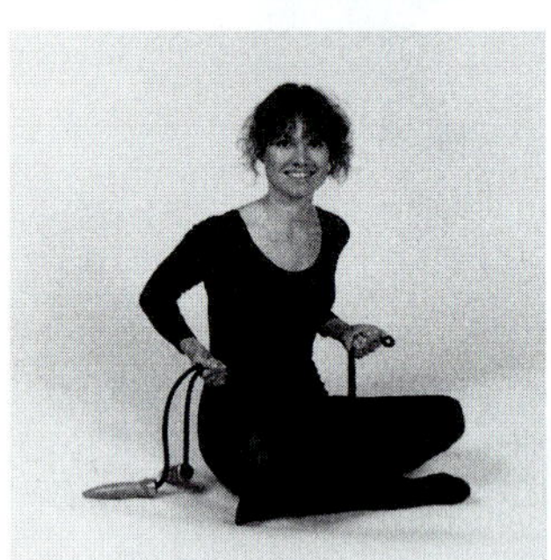

Arms–Shoulders 3

Isometric Rope Curls

Start by sitting with legs crossed. Sit on top of your jumping rope and grasp the rope with both hands, palms up, arms at a 90° angle.

Forcefully lift up, contracting your arm muscles as tightly as possible. Hold for 5 seconds and then relax. *Isometric* means that there is muscle contraction without movement.

Repeat 3–5 times, contracting as forcefully as you can each time.

Benefits: This develops the biceps, the muscles on the front of your upper arms, plus other muscles of the forearm. This simple exercise will increase the strength of your arms.

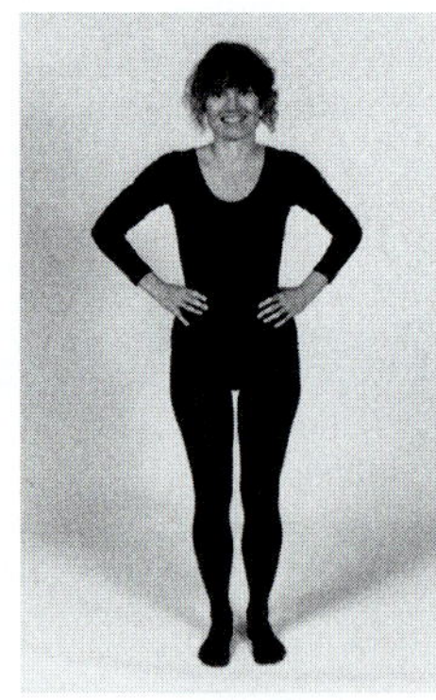

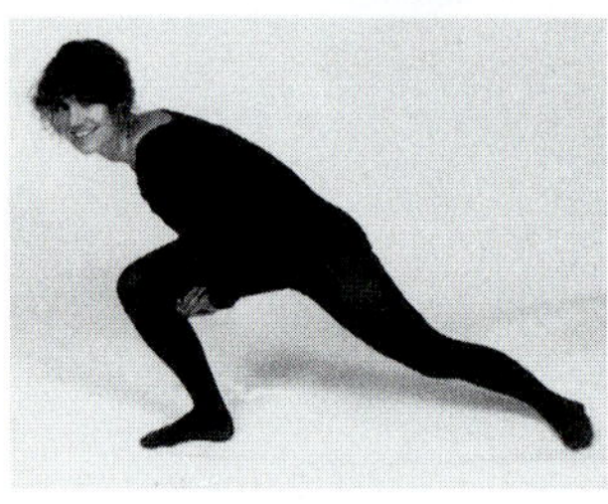

Hips–Thighs–Lower Back 1

Bear Hugs

Start by standing in a normal position, feet together.

1. Keeping your left foot in the same spot, step out straight to your right side, pointing your right foot in that direction. Reach out far enough so that your left leg remains straight, but your right leg is well bent. Wrap your arms around your right thigh as you finish stepping out to the right.
2. Return to the starting position.
3. Repeat with the left side.

Continue stepping out to each side, hugging your thigh, and then returning back to the starting position. Be careful not to overdo the first several times, for this movement can cause quite a bit of soreness.

Continue for 5–10 repetitions.

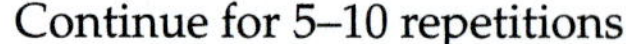

Benefits: The hamstrings and gluteus maximus (back of upper thigh and buttock muscles) are well developed in this exercise. This exercise also develops the quadricep muscles in the front of your thigh.

Hips–Thighs–Lower Back 2

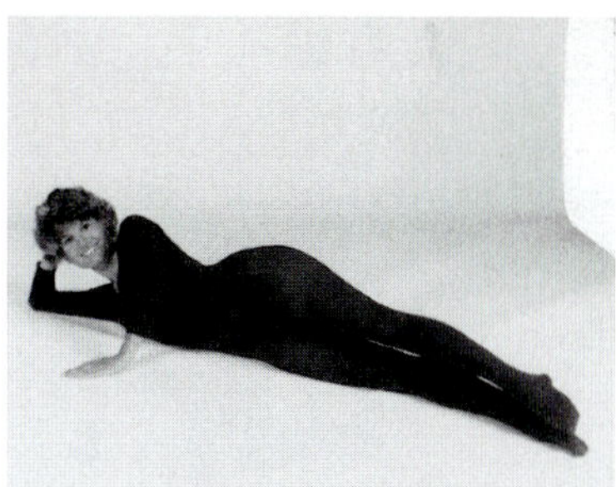

Lateral Leg Raises

Start by lying on your right side, your head held propped up with your right hand, your left leg lying on top of your right leg.

1. Lift your left leg up as high as you can. Keep the leg straight.

2. Return the leg to the down position.

Repeat. Keep lifting the leg up, then down, concentrating on a full range of motion. Repeat with the other leg.

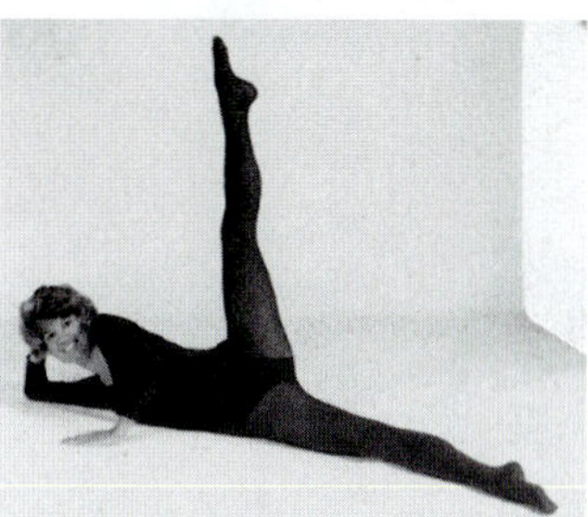

Continue for 5–10 repetitions.

Benefits: Develops the muscles on the side of your hip, the abductors. As the muscles here are developed, you will lose inches from your hip measurement.

Hips–Thighs–Lower Back 3

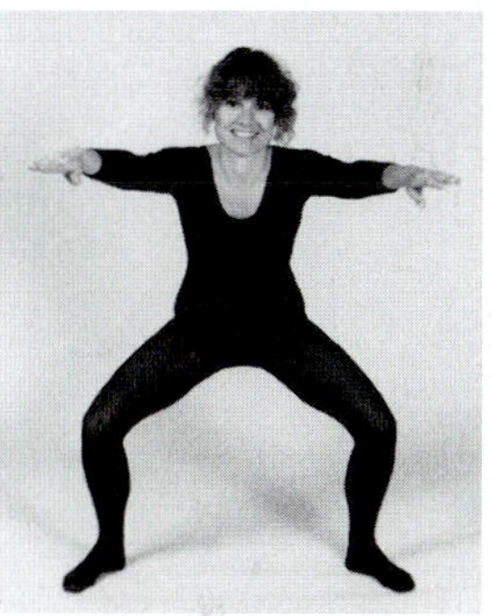

Ballet Squats

Start by standing with your feet 3 feet apart, toes pointing out at a 45° angle. The arms should be straight, parallel to the ground, and out to the sides or angled forward.

1. Squat down until the thighs are parallel to the ground.

2. Straighten your legs only halfway. Do not stand all the way up, but keep the knees well bent.

Repeat, moving up and down between a half-squat and three-quarters squat position. The arms should be straight the entire time. The movement should be quick and almost bouncy.

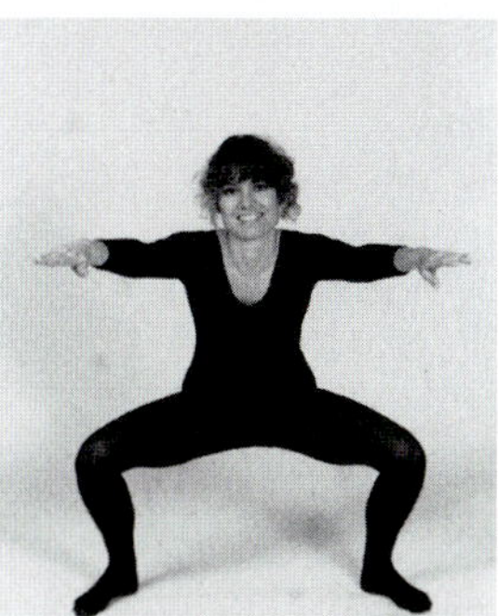

Continue for 5–10 repetitions.

Benefits: The quadriceps, the muscles on the front of the thigh, are highly developed in this exercise. The buttock muscles also get a good workout.

Hips–Thighs–Lower Back 4

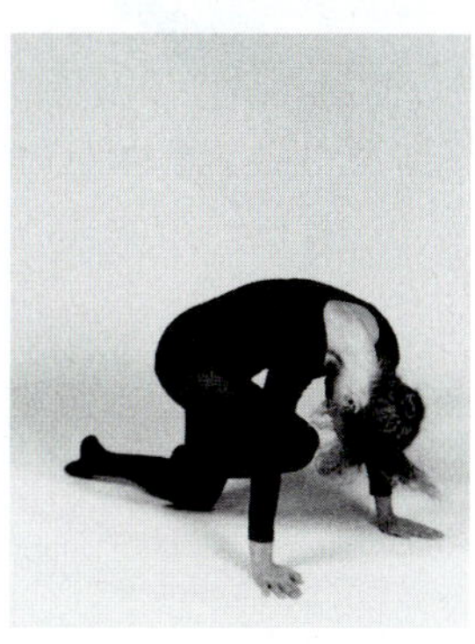

Kneeling Leg Raises

Start by getting on hands and knees.

1. Lift your right leg slightly up and move it forward as you curl your head down, curling up the right side of your body. Your right knee should be close to your head.

2. Next lift your head up high as you also straighten and lift your right leg up high, arching your back.

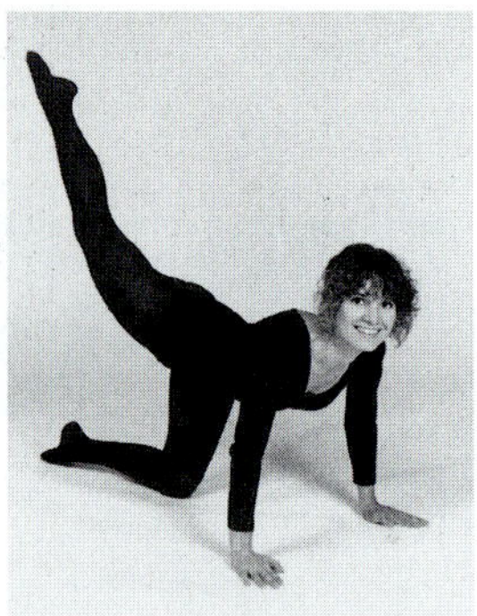

Repeat, alternating curling and arching on one side of your body and then the other. Be careful not to strain your lower back by lifting your leg too high.

Continue for 5–10 repetitions.

Benefits: The major benefit is to the muscles of your back, especially near the neck and hip areas.

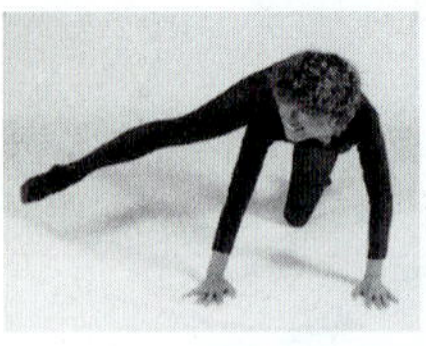

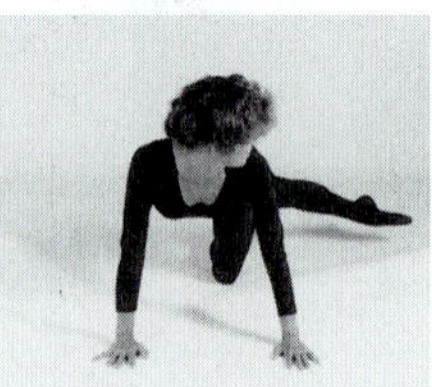

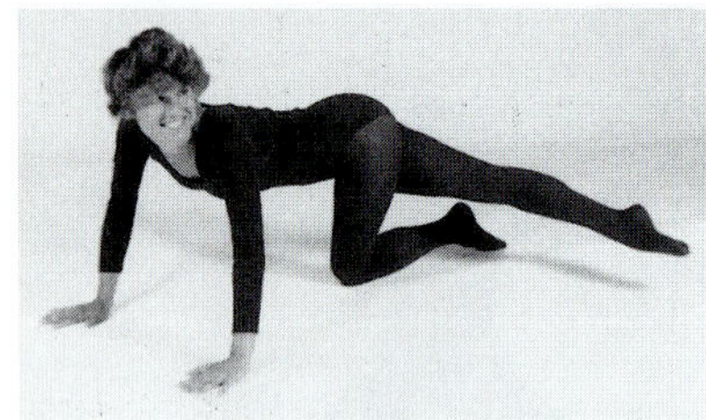

Hips–Thighs–Lower Back 5

Kneeling Leg Swings

Start by getting on hands and knees.

1. Straighten your right leg and swing it out to the side. Keep your leg straight, about 6–12 inches off the ground. Move your head and look right.
2. Next swing your right leg behind you and cross over to the left side as far as you can while looking left. Your leg should still be straight and off the ground 6–12 inches.

Repeat, swinging the leg back and forth, far to the right, and then crossing behind, while moving your head right, then left.

Repeat with the left leg.

Continue for 5–10 repetitions.

Benefits: This is an excellent exercise for developing the muscles along the sides of the abdomen and in the lower back. In addition, the muscles along the sides of the trunk are given a good stretch each time the head and leg curl to the opposite side.

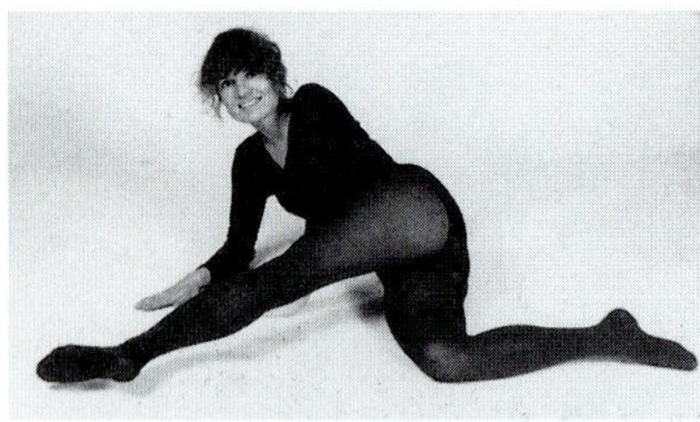

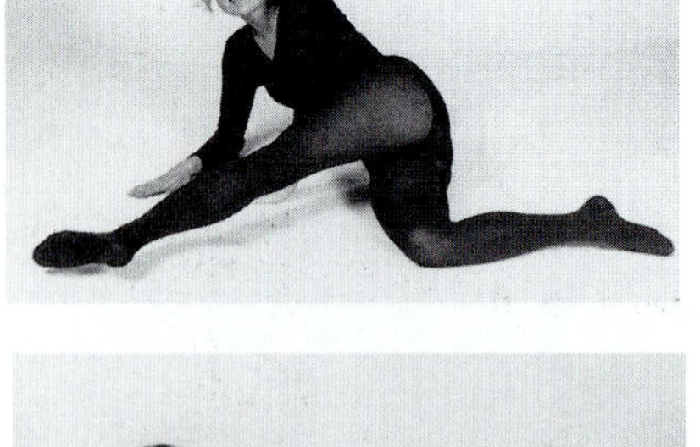

Hips–Thighs–Lower Back 6

Leg Pumps

Start by supporting yourself on your right side: right elbow, right hand, and bent right leg. Also put your left hand on the ground in front of you for support and balance. Your left leg should be straight, on top of the right.

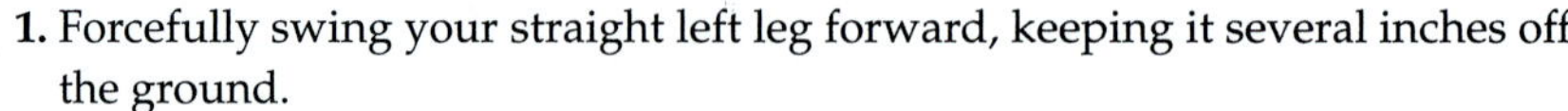

1. Forcefully swing your straight left leg forward, keeping it several inches off the ground.
2. Next swing your leg way back behind you (keep it straight, off the ground several inches).

Repeat, swinging your leg forward and back over your bent right leg. Keep the top leg straight.

Repeat with the other leg.

Continue for 5–10 repetitions.

Benefits: This calisthenic develops the muscles on the side of the hip, the abductors, which will help to reduce the measurement of the hips. The muscles of the abdomen and lower back are also developed.

Hips–Thighs–Lower Back 7

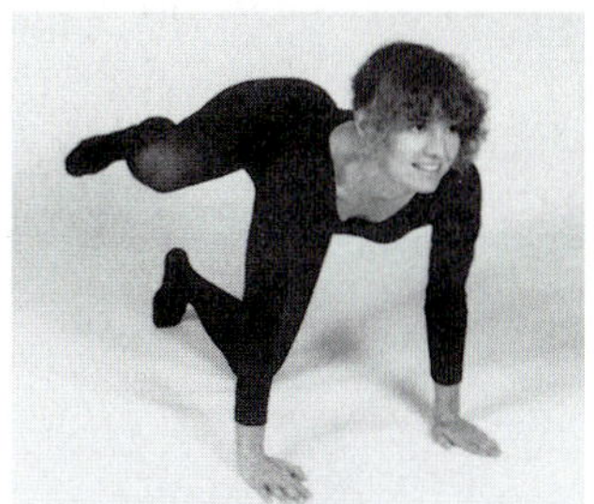

Kneeling Bent-Leg Raises

Start by supporting yourself on your hands and knees.

1. Lift your right leg, keeping it bent at a 90° angle, straight up to your side until it is parallel to the ground. Look at your leg with your head turned to the right side.
2. Return to the starting position.

Repeat, raising the bent leg up while looking right, and then returning to the starting position.

Do the same on the left side.

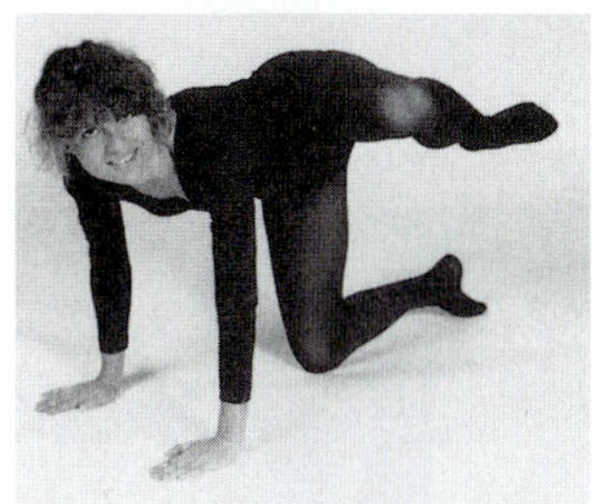

Continue for 5 repetitions on each leg.

Benefits: The muscles on the sides of the hips, the abductors, are developed in this exercise.

Hips–Thighs–Lower Back 8

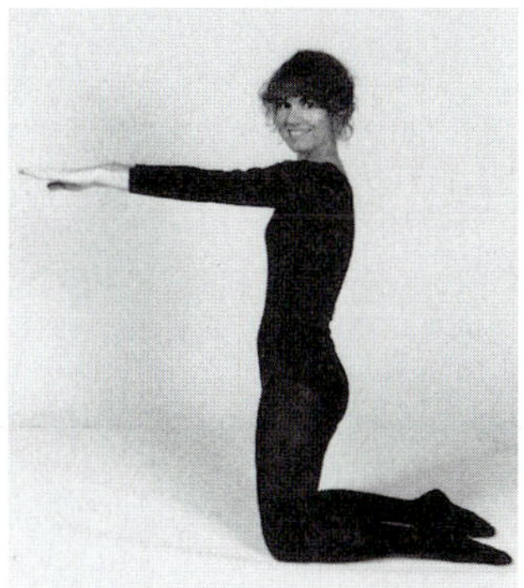

Knee Leans

Start by kneeling, keeping your upper body straight, arms straight and reaching forward.

1. Keeping your body rigid and straight, lean back over your heels.
2. Return to the starting position.

Repeat, leaning back and then going forward, keeping the trunk rigid. To get the full effect, it is important that you do not bend at the waist. Be careful that you do not overdo the first several times, for these muscles can easily get sore with this movement.

Continue for 5–10 repetitions.

Benefits: This is an excellent exercise for developing the *quadricep muscles,* the big muscles on the front of your thighs.

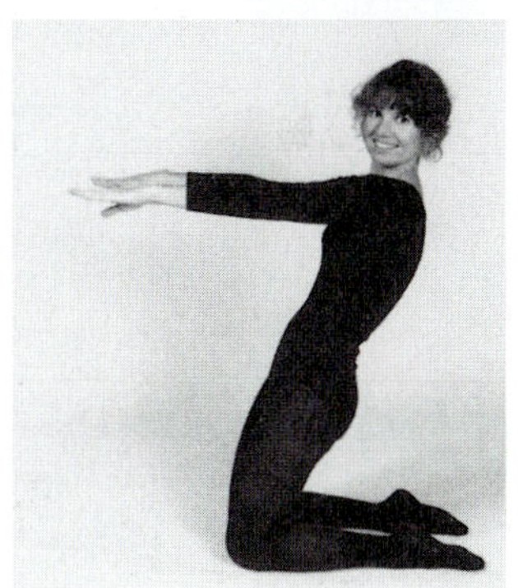

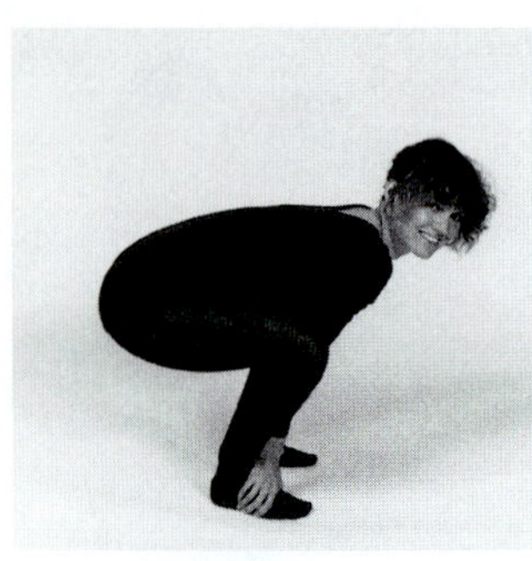

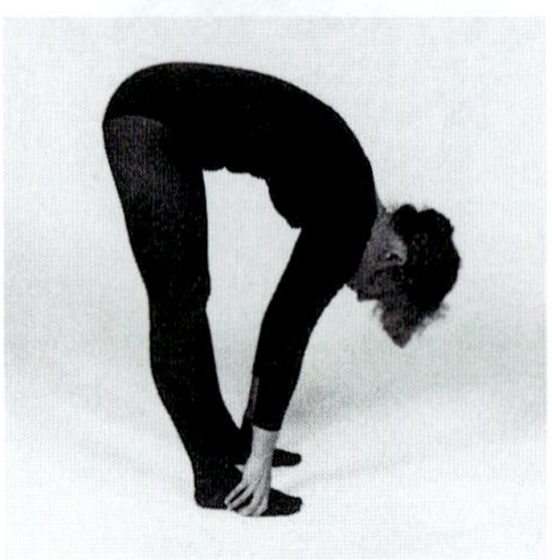

Hips–Thighs–Lower Back 9

Bent-over Squats

Start by squatting down, hands holding your feet (or if you are a stiff person, your ankles).

1. While holding your feet or ankles, straighten your legs so that your seat humps up above you. You should feel a good stretch as you straighten your legs.
2. Return to the starting position.

Repeat, straightening and bending the legs as you keep gripping your feet or ankles. Be careful that you do not overstretch. The movement should be slow and methodical.

Continue for 5–10 repetitions.

Benefits: This exercise does two things well—it develops the muscle endurance and strength of the quadricep muscles (front of the thigh), plus helps to stretch the muscles in the lower back and posterior leg.

APPENDIX **C**

Major Bones, Muscles, and Arteries of the Human Body

MAJOR BONES OF THE SKELETON

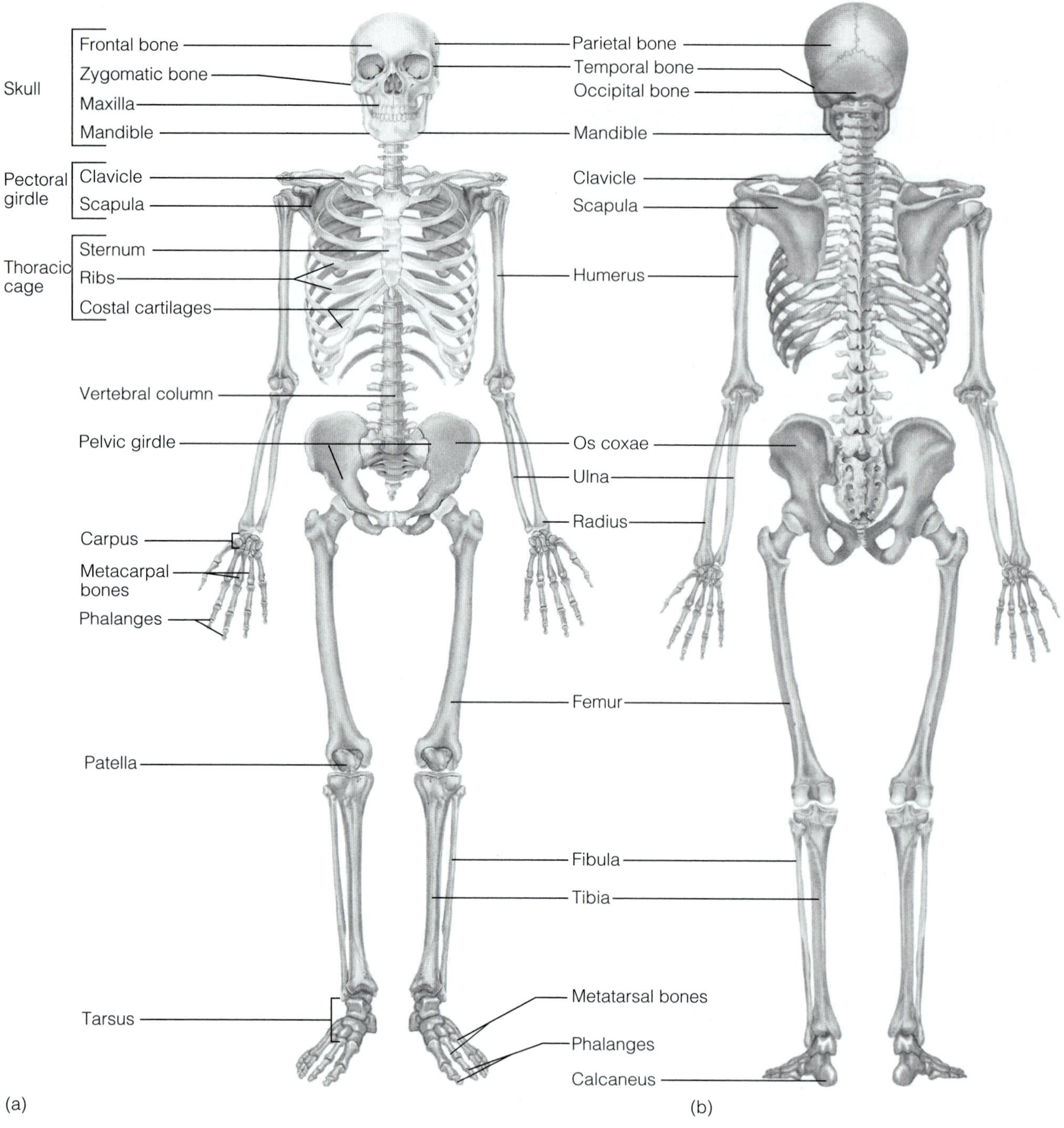
Skull
Frontal bone
Zygomatic bone
Maxilla
Mandible
Pectoral girdle
Clavicle
Scapula
Thoracic cage
Sternum
Ribs
Costal cartilages
Vertebral column
Pelvic girdle
Carpus
Metacarpal bones
Phalanges
Patella
Tarsus
Parietal bone
Temporal bone
Occipital bone
Mandible
Clavicle
Scapula
Humerus
Os coxae
Ulna
Radius
Femur
Fibula
Tibia
Metatarsal bones
Phalanges
Calcaneus
(a)
(b)

MAJOR MUSCLES OF THE BODY

(Anterior)

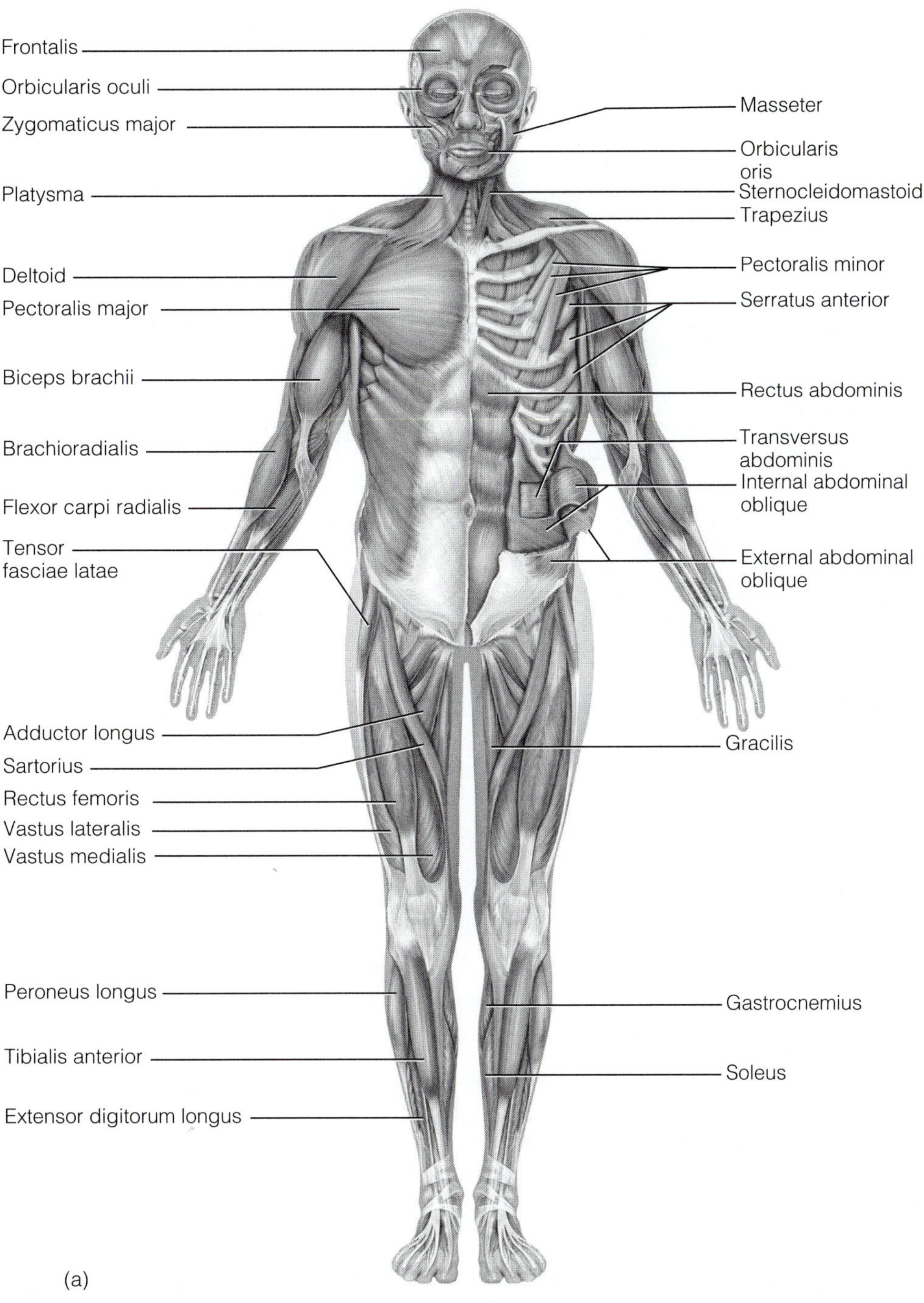
Frontalis
Orbicularis oculi
Zygomaticus major
Platysma
Deltoid
Pectoralis major
Biceps brachii
Brachioradialis
Flexor carpi radialis
Tensor fasciae latae
Adductor longus
Sartorius
Rectus femoris
Vastus lateralis
Vastus medialis
Peroneus longus
Tibialis anterior
Extensor digitorum longus
Masseter
Orbicularis oris
Sternocleidomastoid
Trapezius
Pectoralis minor
Serratus anterior
Rectus abdominis
Transversus abdominis
Internal abdominal oblique
External abdominal oblique
Gracilis
Gastrocnemius
Soleus

(a)

MAJOR MUSCLES OF THE BODY

(Posterior)

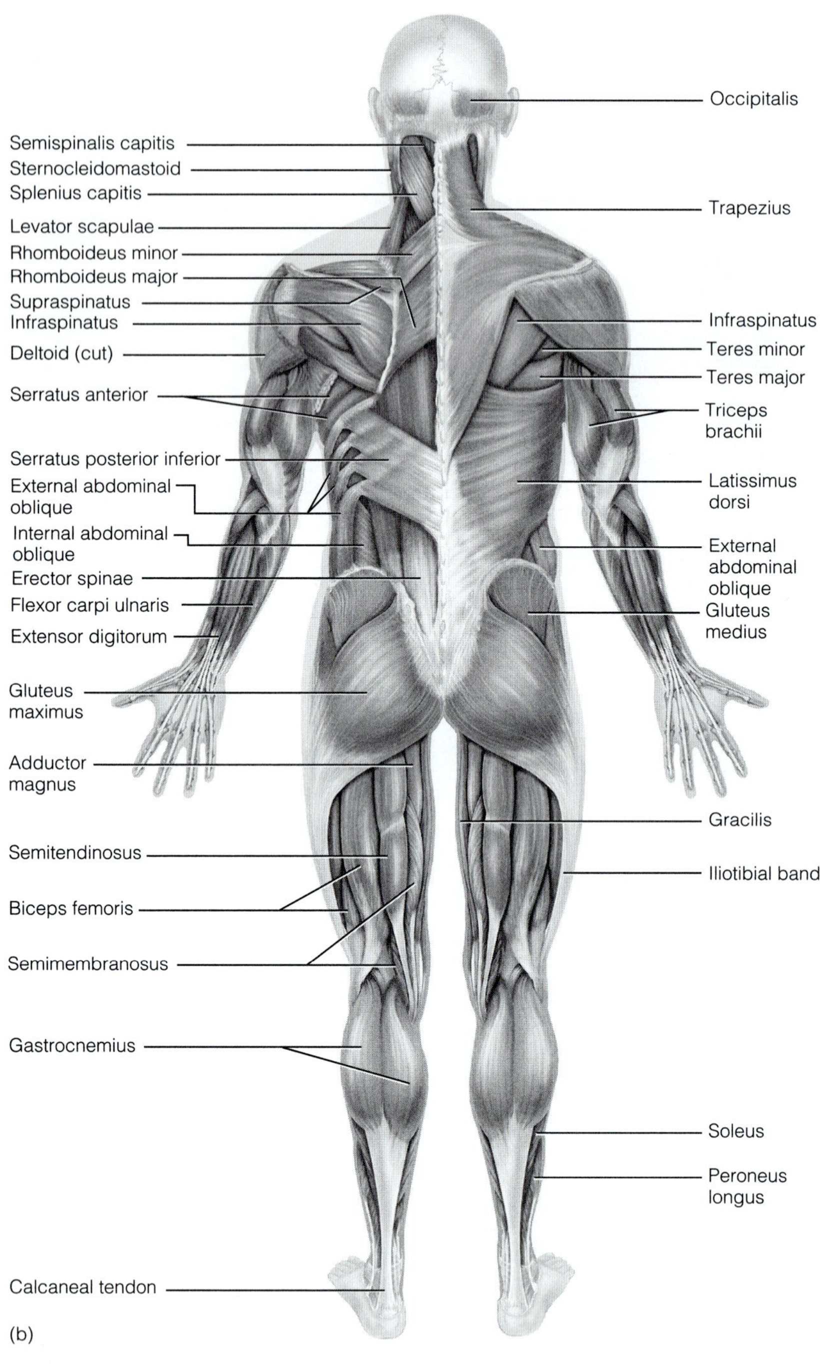
Occipitalis
Semispinalis capitis
Sternocleidomastoid
Splenius capitis
Trapezius
Levator scapulae
Rhomboideus minor
Rhomboideus major
Supraspinatus
Infraspinatus
Infraspinatus
Teres minor
Deltoid (cut)
Teres major
Serratus anterior
Triceps brachii
Serratus posterior inferior
External abdominal oblique
Latissimus dorsi
Internal abdominal oblique
External abdominal oblique
Erector spinae
Flexor carpi ulnaris
Gluteus medius
Extensor digitorum
Gluteus maximus
Adductor magnus
Gracilis
Semitendinosus
Iliotibial band
Biceps femoris
Semimembranosus
Gastrocnemius
Soleus
Peroneus longus
Calcaneal tendon

(b)

MAJOR ARTERIES OF THE CIRCULATORY SYSTEM

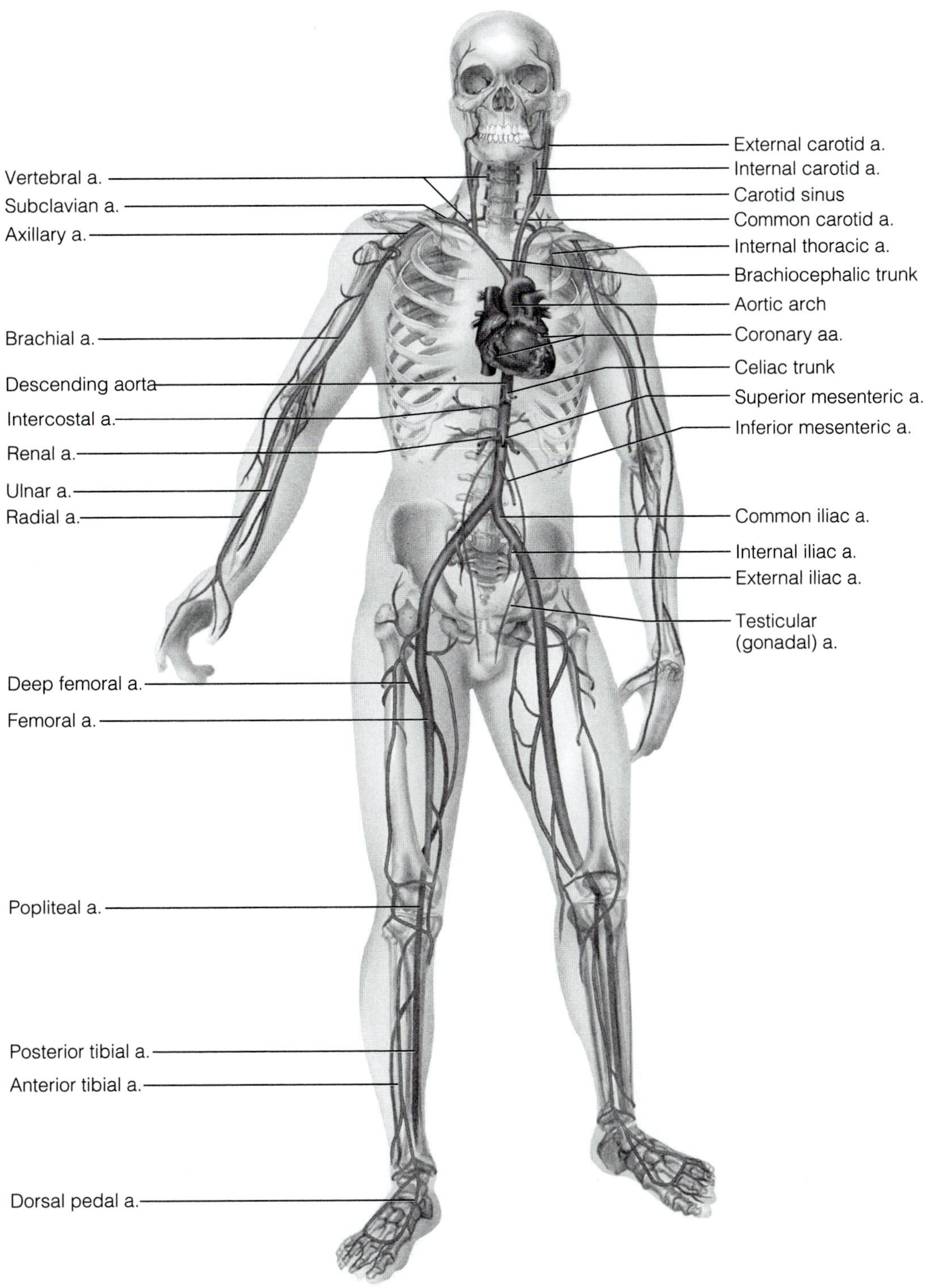
Vertebral a.
Subclavian a.
Axillary a.
Brachial a.
Descending aorta
Intercostal a.
Renal a.
Ulnar a.
Radial a.
Deep femoral a.
Femoral a.
Popliteal a.
Posterior tibial a.
Anterior tibial a.
Dorsal pedal a.
External carotid a.
Internal carotid a.
Carotid sinus
Common carotid a.
Internal thoracic a.
Brachiocephalic trunk
Aortic arch
Coronary aa.
Celiac trunk
Superior mesenteric a.
Inferior mesenteric a.
Common iliac a.
Internal iliac a.
External iliac a.
Testicular
(gonadal) a.

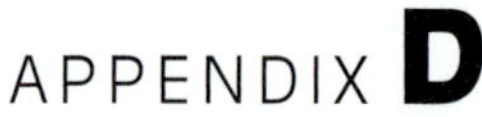

Compendium of Physical Activities

This "compendium of physical activities" was developed to provide researchers and practitioners with a comprehensive coding scheme and energy cost classification for a wide variety of human physical activities. MET values are listed beside the code number for each activity description. To determine energy cost in Calories per hour, multiply the MET value times the kilogram body weight of the individual. For example, bicycling at 14–15.9 mph (activity code #01040) demands 10 METs for a 70-kg individual, 700 Calories per hour.

Section 1. Codes and MET Values of Physical Activities

Code	MET	Specific Activity	Examples
01009	8.5	Bicycling	Bicycling, BMX or mountain
01010	4.0	Bicycling	Bicycling, <10 mph, leisure, to work or for pleasure (Taylor Code 115)
01015	8.0	Bicycling	Bicycling, general
01020	6.0	Bicycling	Bicycling, 10–11.9 mph, leisure, slow, light effort
01030	8.0	Bicycling	Bicycling, 12–13.9 mph, leisure, moderate effort
01040	10.0	Bicycling	Bicycling, 14–15.9 mph, racing or leisure, fast, vigorous effort
01050	12.0	Bicycling	Bicycling, 16–19 mph, racing/not drafting or >19 mph drafting, very fast, racing general
01060	16.0	Bicycling	Bicycling, ≥20 mph, racing, not drafting
01070	5.0	Bicycling	Unicycling
02010	7.0	Conditioning exercise	Bicycling, stationary, general
02011	3.0	Conditioning exercise	Bicycling, stationary, 50 watts, very light effort
02012	5.5	Conditioning exercise	Bicycling, stationary, 100 watts, light effort
02013	7.0	Conditioning exercise	Bicycling, stationary, 150 watts, moderate effort
02014	10.5	Conditioning exercise	Bicycling, stationary, 200 watts, vigorous effort
02015	12.5	Conditioning exercise	Bicycling, stationary, 250 watts, very vigorous effort
02020	8.0	Conditioning exercise	Calisthenics (e.g., push-ups, sit-ups, pull-ups, jumping jacks), heavy, vigorous effort
02030	3.5	Conditioning exercise	Calisthenics, home exercise, light or moderate effort, general (example: back exercises), going up & down from floor (Taylor Code 150)
02040	8.0	Conditioning exercise	Circuit training, including some aerobic movement with minimal rest, general
02050	6.0	Conditioning exercise	Weight lifting (free weight, Nautilus or Universal-type), power lifting or body building, vigorous effort (Taylor Code 210)

Code	MET	Specific Activity	Examples
02060	5.5	Conditioning exercise	Health club exercise, general (Taylor Code 160)
02065	9.0	Conditioning exercise	Stair-treadmill ergometer, general
02070	7.0	Conditioning exercise	Rowing, stationary ergometer, general
02071	3.5	Conditioning exercise	Rowing, stationary, 50 watts, light effort
02072	7.0	Conditioning exercise	Rowing, stationary, 100 watts, moderate effort
02073	8.5	Conditioning exercise	Rowing, stationary, 150 watts, vigorous effort
02074	12.0	Conditioning exercise	Rowing, stationary, 200 watts, very vigorous effort
02080	7.0	Conditioning exercise	Ski machine, general
02090	6.0	Conditioning exercise	Slimnastics, jazzercise
02100	2.5	Conditioning exercise	Stretching, hatha yoga
02101	2.5	Conditioning exercise	Mild stretching
02110	6.0	Conditioning exercise	Teaching aerobic exercise class
02120	4.0	Conditioning exercise	Water aerobics, water calisthenics
02130	3.0	Conditioning exercise	Weight lifting (free, Nautilus, or Universal-type), light or moderate effort, light workout, general
02135	1.0	Conditioning exercise	Whirlpool, sitting
03010	4.8	Dancing	Ballet or modern, twist, jazz, tap, jitterbug
03015	6.5	Dancing	Aerobic, general
03016	8.5	Dancing	Aerobic, step, with 6–8 inch step
03017	10.0	Dancing	Aerobic, step, with 10–12 inch step
03020	5.0	Dancing	Aerobic, low impact
03021	7.0	Dancing	Aerobic, high impact
03025	4.5	Dancing	General, Greek, Middle Eastern, hula, flamenco, belly, swing
03030	5.5	Dancing	Ballroom, fast (Taylor Code 125)
03031	4.5	Dancing	Ballroom, fast (disco, folk, square), line dancing, Irish step dancing, polka, contra, country
03040	3.0	Dancing	Ballroom, slow (e.g., waltz, foxtrot, slow dancing), samba, tango, 19th century, mambo, chacha
03050	5.5	Dancing	Anishinaabe Jingle Dancing or other traditional American Indian dancing
04001	3.0	Fishing and hunting	Fishing, general
04010	4.0	Fishing and hunting	Digging worms, with shovel
04020	4.0	Fishing and hunting	Fishing from river bank and walking
04030	2.5	Fishing and hunting	Fishing from boat, sitting
04040	3.5	Fishing and hunting	Fishing from river bank, standing (Taylor Code 660)
04050	6.0	Fishing and hunting	Fishing in stream, in waders (Taylor Code 670)
04060	2.0	Fishing and hunting	Fishing, ice, sitting
04070	2.5	Fishing and hunting	Hunting, bow and arrow or crossbow
04080	6.0	Fishing and hunting	Hunting, deer, elk, large game (Taylor Code 710)
04090	2.5	Fishing and hunting	Hunting, duck, wading
04100	5.0	Fishing and hunting	Hunting, general
04110	6.0	Fishing and hunting	Hunting, pheasants or grouse (Taylor Code 680)
04120	5.0	Fishing and hunting	Hunting, rabbit, squirrel, prairie chick, raccoon, small game (Taylor Code 690)
04130	2.5	Fishing and hunting	Pistol shooting or trap shooting, standing
05010	3.3	Home activities	Carpet sweeping, sweeping floors
05020	3.0	Home activities	Cleaning, heavy or major (e.g., wash car, wash windows, clean garage), vigorous effort
05021	3.5	Home activities	Mopping
05025	2.5	Home activities	Multiple household tasks all at once, light effort
05026	3.5	Home activities	Multiple household tasks all at once, moderate effort
05027	4.0	Home activities	Multiple household tasks all at once, vigorous effort
05030	3.0	Home activities	Cleaning, house or cabin, general
05040	2.5	Home activities	Cleaning, light (dusting, straightening up, changing linen, carrying out trash)
05041	2.3	Home activities	Wash dishes—standing or in general (not broken into stand/walk components)
05042	2.5	Home activities	Wash dishes; clearing dishes from table—walking
05043	3.5	Home activities	Vacuuming
05045	6.0	Home activities	Butchering animals
05050	2.0	Home activities	Cooking or food preparation—standing or sitting or in general (not broken into stand/walk components), manual appliances

Code	MET	Specific Activity	Examples
05051	2.5	Home activities	Serving food, setting table—implied walking or standing
05052	2.5	Home activities	Cooking or food preparation—walking
05053	2.5	Home activities	Feeding animals
05055	2.5	Home activities	Putting away groceries (e.g., carrying groceries, shopping without a grocery cart), carrying packages
05056	7.5	Home activities	Carrying groceries upstairs
05057	3.0	Home activities	Cooking Indian bread on an outside stove
05060	2.3	Home activities	Food shopping, with or without a grocery cart, standing or walking
05065	2.3	Home activities	Non-food shopping, standing or walking
05070	2.3	Home activities	Ironing
05080	1.5	Home activities	Sitting—knitting, sewing, light wrapping (presents)
05090	2.0	Home activities	Implied standing—laundry, fold or hang clothes, put clothes in washer or dryer, packing suitcase
05095	2.3	Home activities	Implied walking—putting away clothes, gathering clothes to pack, putting away laundry
05100	2.0	Home activities	Making bed
05110	5.0	Home activities	Maple syruping/sugar bushing (including carrying buckets, carrying wood)
05120	6.0	Home activities	Moving furniture, household items, carrying boxes
05130	3.8	Home activities	Scrubbing floors, on hands and knees, scrubbing bathroom, bathtub
05140	4.0	Home activities	Sweeping garage, sidewalk, or outside of house
05146	3.5	Home activities	Standing—packing/unpacking boxes, occasional lifting of household items—light–moderate effort
05147	3.0	Home activities	Implied walking—putting away household items—moderate effort
05148	2.5	Home activities	Watering plants
05149	2.5	Home activities	Building a fire inside
05150	9.0	Home activities	Moving household items upstairs, carrying boxes or furniture
05160	2.0	Home activities	Standing—light (pump gas, change light bulb, etc.)
05165	3.0	Home activities	Walking—light, noncleaning (readying to leave, shut/lock doors, close windows, etc.)
05170	2.5	Home activities	Sitting—playing with child(ren)—light, only active periods
05171	2.8	Home activities	Standing—playing with child(ren)—light, only active periods
05175	4.0	Home activities	Walk/run—playing with child(ren)—moderate, only active periods
05180	5.0	Home activities	Walk/run—playing with child(ren)—vigorous, only active periods
05181	3.0	Home activities	Carrying small children
05185	2.5	Home activities	Child care: sitting/kneeling—dressing, bathing, grooming, feeding, occasional lifting of child—light effort, general
05186	3.0	Home activities	Child care: standing—dressing, bathing, grooming, feeding, occasional lifting of child—light effort
05187	4.0	Home activities	Elder care, disabled adult, only active periods
05188	1.5	Home activities	Reclining with baby
05190	2.5	Home activities	Sit, playing with animals, light, only active periods
05191	2.8	Home activities	Stand, playing with animals, light, only active periods
05192	2.8	Home activities	Walk/run, playing with animals, light, only active periods
05193	4.0	Home activities	Walk/run, playing with animals, moderate, only active periods
05194	5.0	Home activities	Walk/run, playing with animals, vigorous, only active periods
05195	3.5	Home activities	Standing—bathing dog
06010	3.0	Home repair	Airplane repair
06020	4.0	Home repair	Automobile body work
06030	3.0	Home repair	Automobile repair
06040	3.0	Home repair	Carpentry, general, workshop (Taylor Code 620)
06050	6.0	Home repair	Carpentry, outside house, installing rain gutters, building a fence (Taylor Code 640)
06060	4.5	Home repair	Carpentry, finishing or refinishing cabinets or furniture

Code	MET	Specific Activity	Examples
06070	7.5	Home repair	Carpentry, sawing hardwood
06080	5.0	Home repair	Caulking, chinking log cabin
06090	4.5	Home repair	Caulking, except log cabin
06100	5.0	Home repair	Cleaning gutters
06110	5.0	Home repair	Excavating garage
06120	5.0	Home repair	Hanging storm windows
06130	4.5	Home repair	Laying or removing carpet
06140	4.5	Home repair	Laying tile or linoleum, repairing appliances
06150	5.0	Home repair	Painting, outside house (Taylor Code 650)
06160	3.0	Home repair	Painting, papering, plastering, scraping, inside house, hanging Sheetrock, remodeling
06165	4.5	Home repair	Painting (Taylor Code 630)
06170	3.0	Home repair	Put on and removal of tarp—sailboat
06180	6.0	Home repair	Roofing
06190	4.5	Home repair	Sanding floors with a power sander
06200	4.5	Home repair	Scrape and paint sailboat or powerboat
06210	5.0	Home repair	Spreading dirt with a shovel
06220	4.5	Home repair	Washing and waxing hull of sailboat, car, powerboat, airplane
06230	4.5	Home repair	Washing fence, painting fence
06240	3.0	Home repair	Wiring, plumbing
07010	1.0	Inactivity, quiet	Lying quietly and watching television
07011	1.0	Inactivity, quiet	Lying quietly, doing nothing, lying in bed awake, listening to music (not talking or reading)
07020	1.0	Inactivity, quiet	Sitting quietly and watching television
07021	1.0	Inactivity, quiet	Sitting quietly, sitting smoking, listening to music (not talking or reading), watching a movie in a theater
07030	0.9	Inactivity, quiet	Sleeping
07040	1.2	Inactivity, quiet	Standing quietly (standing in a line)
07050	1.0	Inactivity, light	Reclining—writing
07060	1.0	Inactivity, light	Reclining—talking or talking on phone
07070	1.0	Inactivity, light	Reclining—reading
07075	1.0	Inactivity, light	Meditating
08010	5.0	Lawn and garden	Carrying, loading or stacking wood, loading/unloading or carrying lumber
08020	6.0	Lawn and garden	Chopping wood, splitting logs
08030	5.0	Lawn and garden	Clearing land, hauling branches, wheelbarrow chores
08040	5.0	Lawn and garden	Digging sandbox
08050	5.0	Lawn and garden	Digging, spading, filling garden, composting (Taylor Code 590)
08060	6.0	Lawn and garden	Gardening with heavy power tools, tilling a garden, chain saw
08080	5.0	Lawn and garden	Laying crushed rock
08090	5.0	Lawn and garden	Laying sod
08095	5.5	Lawn and garden	Mowing lawn, general
08100	2.5	Lawn and garden	Mowing lawn, riding mower (Taylor Code 550)
08110	6.0	Lawn and garden	Mowing lawn, walk, hand mower (Taylor Code 570)
08120	5.5	Lawn and garden	Mowing lawn, walk, power mower
08125	4.5	Lawn and garden	Mowing lawn, power mower (Taylor Code 590)
08130	4.5	Lawn and garden	Operating snow blower, walking
08140	4.5	Lawn and garden	Planting seedlings, shrubs
08150	4.5	Lawn and garden	Planting trees
08160	4.3	Lawn and garden	Raking lawn
08165	4.0	Lawn and garden	Raking lawn (Taylor Code 600)
08170	4.0	Lawn and garden	Raking roof with snow rake
08180	3.0	Lawn and garden	Riding snow blower
08190	4.0	Lawn and garden	Sacking grass, leaves
08200	6.0	Lawn and garden	Shoveling snow, by hand (Taylor Code 610)
08210	4.5	Lawn and garden	Trimming shrubs or trees, manual cutter
08215	3.5	Lawn and garden	Trimming shrubs or trees, power cutter, using leaf blower, edger
08220	2.5	Lawn and garden	Walking, applying fertilizer or seeding a lawn
08230	1.5	Lawn and garden	Watering lawn or garden, standing or walking
08240	4.5	Lawn and garden	Weeding, cultivating garden (Taylor Code 580)
08245	4.0	Lawn and garden	Gardening, general
08246	3.0	Lawn and garden	Picking fruit off trees, picking fruits/vegetables, moderate effort
08250	3.0	Lawn and garden	Implied walking/standing—picking up yard, light, picking flowers or vegetables
08251	3.0	Lawn and garden	Walking, gathering gardening tools
09010	1.5	Miscellaneous	Sitting—card playing, playing board games
09020	2.3	Miscellaneous	Standing—drawing (writing), casino gambling, duplicating machine

Code	MET	Specific Activity	Examples
09030	1.3	Miscellaneous	Sitting—reading, book, newspaper, etc.
09040	1.8	Miscellaneous	Sitting—writing, desk work, typing
09050	1.8	Miscellaneous	Standing—talking or talking on the phone
09055	1.5	Miscellaneous	Sitting—talking or talking on the phone
09060	1.8	Miscellaneous	Sitting—studying, general, including reading, and/or writing
09065	1.8	Miscellaneous	Sitting—in class, general, including note-taking or class discussion
09070	1.8	Miscellaneous	Standing—reading
09071	2.0	Miscellaneous	Standing—miscellaneous
09075	1.5	Miscellaneous	Sitting—arts and crafts, light effort
09080	2.0	Miscellaneous	Sitting—arts and crafts, moderate effort
09085	1.8	Miscellaneous	Standing—arts and crafts, light effort
09090	3.0	Miscellaneous	Standing—arts and crafts, moderate effort
09095	3.5	Miscellaneous	Standing—arts and crafts, vigorous effort
09100	1.5	Miscellaneous	Retreat/family reunion activities involving sitting, relaxing, talking, eating
09105	2.0	Miscellaneous	Touring/traveling/vacation involving walking and riding
09110	2.5	Miscellaneous	Camping involving standing, walking, sitting, light-to-moderate effort
09115	1.5	Miscellaneous	Sitting at a sporting event, spectator
10010	1.8	Music playing	Accordion
10020	2.0	Music playing	Cello
10030	2.5	Music playing	Conducting
10040	4.0	Music playing	Drums
10050	2.0	Music playing	Flute (sitting)
10060	2.0	Music playing	Horn
10070	2.5	Music playing	Piano or organ
10080	3.5	Music playing	Trombone
10090	2.5	Music playing	Trumpet
10100	2.5	Music playing	Violin
10110	2.0	Music playing	Woodwind
10120	2.0	Music playing	Guitar, classical, folk (sitting)
10125	3.0	Music playing	Guitar, rock and roll band (standing)
10130	4.0	Music playing	Marching band, playing an instrument, baton twirling (walking)
10135	3.5	Music playing	Marching band, drum major (walking)
11010	4.0	Occupation	Bakery, general, moderate effort

Code	MET	Specific Activity	Examples
11015	2.5	Occupation	Bakery, light effort
11020	2.3	Occupation	Bookbinding
11030	6.0	Occupation	Building road (including hauling debris, driving heavy machinery)
11035	2.0	Occupation	Building road, directing traffic (standing)
11040	3.5	Occupation	Carpentry, general
11050	8.0	Occupation	Carrying heavy loads, such as bricks
11060	8.0	Occupation	Carrying moderate loads up stairs, moving boxes (16–40 lb)
11070	2.5	Occupation	Chambermaid, making bed (nursing)
11080	6.5	Occupation	Coal mining, drilling coal, rock
11090	6.5	Occupation	Coal mining, erecting supports
11100	6.0	Occupation	Coal mining, general
11110	7.0	Occupation	Coal mining, shoveling coal
11120	5.5	Occupation	Construction, outside, remodeling
11121	3.0	Occupation	Custodial work—buffing the floor with electric buffer
11122	2.5	Occupation	Custodial work—cleaning sink and toilet, light effort
11123	2.5	Occupation	Custodial work—dusting, light effort
11124	4.0	Occupation	Custodial work—feathering arena floor, moderate effort
11125	3.5	Occupation	Custodial work—general cleaning, moderate effort
11126	3.5	Occupation	Custodial work—mopping, moderate effort
11127	3.0	Occupation	Custodial work—take out trash, moderate effort
11128	2.5	Occupation	Custodial work—vacuuming, light effort
11129	3.0	Occupation	Custodial work—vacuuming, moderate effort
11130	3.5	Occupation	Electrical work, plumbing
11140	8.0	Occupation	Farming, baling hay, cleaning barn, poultry work, vigorous effort
11150	3.5	Occupation	Farming, chasing cattle, nonstrenuous (walking), moderate effort
11151	4.0	Occupation	Farming, chasing cattle or other livestock on horseback, moderate effort
11152	2.0	Occupation	Farming, chasing cattle or other livestock, driving, light effort
11160	2.5	Occupation	Farming, driving harvester, cutting hay, irrigation work

Code	MET	Specific Activity	Examples
11170	2.5	Occupation	Farming, driving tractor
11180	4.0	Occupation	Farming, feeding small animals
11190	4.5	Occupation	Farming, feeding cattle, horses
11191	4.5	Occupation	Farming, hauling water for animals, general hauling water
11192	6.0	Occupation	Farming, taking care of animals (grooming, brushing, shearing sheep, assisting with birthing, medical care, branding)
11200	8.0	Occupation	Farming, forking straw bales, cleaning corral or barn, vigorous effort
11210	3.0	Occupation	Farming, milking by hand, moderate effort
11220	1.5	Occupation	Farming, milking by machine, light effort
11230	5.5	Occupation	Farming, shoveling grain, moderate effort
11240	12.0	Occupation	Fire fighter, general
11245	11.0	Occupation	Fire fighter, climbing ladder with full gear
11246	8.0	Occupation	Fire fighter, hauling hoses on ground
11250	17.0	Occupation	Forestry, ax chopping, fast
11260	5.0	Occupation	Forestry, ax chopping, slow
11270	7.0	Occupation	Forestry, barking trees
11280	11.0	Occupation	Forestry, carrying logs
11290	8.0	Occupation	Forestry, felling trees
11300	8.0	Occupation	Forestry, general
11310	5.0	Occupation	Forestry, hoeing
11320	6.0	Occupation	Forestry, planting by hand
11330	7.0	Occupation	Forestry, sawing by hand
11340	4.5	Occupation	Forestry, sawing, power
11350	9.0	Occupation	Forestry, trimming trees
11360	4.0	Occupation	Forestry, weeding
11370	4.5	Occupation	Furriery
11380	6.0	Occupation	Horse grooming
11390	8.0	Occupation	Horse racing, galloping
11400	6.5	Occupation	Horse racing, trotting
11410	2.6	Occupation	Horse racing, walking
11420	3.5	Occupation	Locksmith
11430	2.5	Occupation	Machine tooling, machining, working sheet metal
11440	3.0	Occupation	Machine tooling, operating lathe
11450	5.0	Occupation	Machine tooling, operating punch press
11460	4.0	Occupation	Machine tooling, tapping and drilling
11470	3.0	Occupation	Machine tooling, welding
11480	7.0	Occupation	Masonry, concrete
11485	4.0	Occupation	Masseur, masseuse (standing)
11490	7.5	Occupation	Moving, pushing heavy objects, 75 lb or more (desks, moving van work)
11495	12.0	Occupation	Skindiving or SCUBA diving as a frogman (Navy Seal)
11500	2.5	Occupation	Operating heavy duty equipment/automated, not driving
11510	4.5	Occupation	Orange grove work
11520	2.3	Occupation	Printing (standing)
11525	2.5	Occupation	Police, directing traffic (standing)
11526	2.0	Occupation	Police, driving a squad car (sitting)
11527	1.3	Occupation	Police, riding in a squad car (sitting)
11528	4.0	Occupation	Police, making an arrest (standing)
11530	2.5	Occupation	Shoe repair, general
11540	8.5	Occupation	Shoveling, digging ditches
11550	9.0	Occupation	Shoveling, heavy (more than 16 lb/min)
11560	6.0	Occupation	Shoveling, light (less than 10 lb/min)
11570	7.0	Occupation	Shoveling, moderate (10–15 lb/min)
11580	1.5	Occupation	Sitting—light office work, general (chemistry lab work, light use of hand tools, watch repair or microassembly, light assembly/repair), sitting, reading, driving at work
11585	1.5	Occupation	Sitting—meetings, general, and/or with talking involved, eating at a business meeting
11590	2.5	Occupation	Sitting; moderate (heavy levers, riding mower/forklift, crane operation), teaching stretching or yoga
11600	2.3	Occupation	Standing; light (bartending, store clerk, assembling, filing, duplicating, putting up Christmas tree), standing and talking at work, changing clothes when teaching physical education
11610	3.0	Occupation	Standing; light/moderate (assemble/repair heavy parts, welding, stocking, auto repair, pack boxes for moving, etc.), patient care (as in nursing)
11615	4.0	Occupation	Lifting items continuously, 10–20 lb, with limited walking or resting

Code	MET	Specific Activity	Examples
11620	3.5	Occupation	Standing; moderate (assembling at fast rate, intermittent, lifting 50 lb, hitch/twisting ropes)
11630	4.0	Occupation	Standing; moderate/heavy (lifting more than 50 lb, masonry, painting, paper hanging)
11640	5.0	Occupation	Steel mill, fettling
11650	5.5	Occupation	Steel mill, forging
11660	8.0	Occupation	Steel mill, hand rolling
11670	8.0	Occupation	Steel mill, merchant mill rolling
11680	11.0	Occupation	Steel mill, removing slag
11690	7.5	Occupation	Steel mill, tending furnace
11700	5.5	Occupation	Steel mill, tipping molds
11710	8.0	Occupation	Steel mill, working in general
11720	2.5	Occupation	Tailoring, cutting
11730	2.5	Occupation	Tailoring, general
11740	2.0	Occupation	Tailoring, hand sewing
11750	2.5	Occupation	Tailoring, machine sewing
11760	4.0	Occupation	Tailoring, pressing
11765	3.5	Occupation	Tailoring, weaving
11766	6.5	Occupation	Truck driving, loading and unloading truck (standing)
11770	1.5	Occupation	Typing, electric, manual or computer
11780	6.0	Occupation	Using heavy power tools such as pneumatic tools (jackhammers, drills, etc.)
11790	8.0	Occupation	Using heavy tools (not power) such as shovel, pick, tunnel bar, spade
11791	2.0	Occupation	Walking on job, less than 2.0 mph (in office or lab area), very slow
11792	3.3	Occupation	Walking on job, 3.0 mph, in office, moderate speed, not carrying anything
11793	3.8	Occupation	Walking on job, 3.5 mph, in office, brisk speed, not carrying anything
11795	3.0	Occupation	Walking, 2.5 mph, slowly and carrying light objects less than 25 lb
11796	3.0	Occupation	Walking, gathering things at work, ready to leave
11800	4.0	Occupation	Walking, 3.0 mph, moderately and carrying light objects less than 25 lb
11805	4.0	Occupation	Walking, pushing a wheelchair
11810	4.5	Occupation	Walking, 3.5 mph, briskly and carrying objects less than 25 lb
11820	5.0	Occupation	Walking or walk downstairs or standing, carrying objects about 25–49 lb
11830	6.5	Occupation	Walking or walk downstairs or standing, carrying objects about 50–74 lb
11840	7.5	Occupation	Walking or walk downstairs or standing, carrying objects about 75–99 lb
11850	8.5	Occupation	Walking or walk downstairs or standing, carrying objects about 100 lb or over
11870	3.0	Occupation	Working in scene shop, theater actor, backstage, employee
11875	4.0	Occupation	Teach physical education, exercise, sports classes (nonsport play)
11876	6.5	Occupation	Teach physical education, exercise, sports classes (participate in the class)
12010	6.0	Running	Jog/walk combination (jogging component of less than 10 minutes) (Taylor Code 180)
12020	7.0	Running	Jogging, general
12025	8.0	Running	Jogging, in place
12027	4.5	Running	Jogging on a mini-tramp
12030	8.0	Running	Running, 5 mph (12 min/mile)
12040	9.0	Running	Running, 5.2 mph (11.5 min/mile)
12050	10.0	Running	Running, 6 mph (10 min/mile)
12060	11.0	Running	Running, 6.7 mph (9 min/mile)
12070	11.5	Running	Running, 7 mph (8.5 min/mile)
12080	12.5	Running	Running, 7.5 mph (8 min/mile)
12090	13.5	Running	Running, 8 mph (7.5 min/mile)
12100	14.0	Running	Running, 8.6 mph (7 min/mile)
12110	15.0	Running	Running, 9 mph (6.5 min/mile)
12120	16.0	Running	Running, 10 mph (6 min/mile)
12130	18.0	Running	Running, 10.9 mph (5.5 min/mile)
12140	9.0	Running	Running, cross-country
12150	8.0	Running	Running (Taylor Code 200)
12170	15.0	Running	Running, stairs, up
12180	10.0	Running	Running, on a track, team practice
12190	8.0	Running	Running, training, pushing a wheelchair
13000	2.0	Self care	Standing—getting ready for bed, in general
13009	1.0	Self care	Sitting on toilet

Code	MET	Specific Activity	Examples
13010	1.5	Self care	Bathing (sitting)
13020	2.0	Self care	Dressing, undressing (standing or sitting)
13030	1.5	Self care	Eating (sitting)
13035	2.0	Self care	Talking and eating or eating only (standing)
13036	1.0	Self care	Taking medication, sitting or standing
13040	2.0	Self care	Grooming (washing, shaving, brushing teeth, urinating, washing hands, putting on make-up), sitting or standing
13045	2.5	Self care	Hairstyling
13046	1.0	Self care	Having hair or nails done by someone else, sitting
13050	2.0	Self care	Showering, toweling off (standing)
14010	1.5	Sexual activity	Active, vigorous effort
14020	1.3	Sexual activity	General, moderate effort
14030	1.0	Sexual activity	Passive, light effort, kissing, hugging
15010	3.5	Sports	Archery (nonhunting)
15020	7.0	Sports	Badminton, competitive (Taylor Code 450)
15030	4.5	Sports	Badminton, social singles and doubles, general
15040	8.0	Sports	Basketball, game (Taylor Code 490)
15050	6.0	Sports	Basketball, nongame, general (Taylor Code 480)
15060	7.0	Sports	Basketball, officiating (Taylor Code 500)
15070	4.5	Sports	Basketball, shooting baskets
15075	6.5	Sports	Basketball, wheelchair
15080	2.5	Sports	Billiards
15090	3.0	Sports	Bowling (Taylor Code 390)
15100	12.0	Sports	Boxing, in ring, general
15110	6.0	Sports	Boxing, punching bag
15120	9.0	Sports	Boxing, sparring
15130	7.0	Sports	Broomball
15135	5.0	Sports	Children's games (hopscotch, 4-square, dodge ball, playground apparatus, t-ball, tetherball, marbles, jacks, arcade games)
15140	4.0	Sports	Coaching: football, soccer, basketball, baseball, swimming, etc.
15150	5.0	Sports	Cricket (batting, bowling)
15160	2.5	Sports	Croquet
15170	4.0	Sports	Curling
15180	2.5	Sports	Darts, wall or lawn
15190	6.0	Sports	Drag racing, pushing or driving a car
15200	6.0	Sports	Fencing
15210	9.0	Sports	Football, competitive
15230	8.0	Sports	Football, touch, flag, general (Taylor Code 510)
15235	2.5	Sports	Football or baseball, playing catch
15240	3.0	Sports	Frisbee playing, general
15250	8.0	Sports	Frisbee, ultimate
15255	4.5	Sports	Golf, general
15265	4.5	Sports	Golf, walking and carrying clubs
15270	3.0	Sports	Golf, miniature, driving range
15285	4.3	Sports	Golf, walking and pulling clubs
15290	3.5	Sports	Golf, using power cart (Taylor Code 070)
15300	4.0	Sports	Gymnastics, general
15310	4.0	Sports	Hacky sack
15320	12.0	Sports	Handball, general (Taylor Code 520)
15330	8.0	Sports	Handball, team
15340	3.5	Sports	Hang gliding
15350	8.0	Sports	Hockey, field
15360	8.0	Sports	Hockey, ice
15370	4.0	Sports	Horseback riding, general
15380	3.5	Sports	Horseback riding, saddling horse, grooming horse
15390	6.5	Sports	Horseback riding, trotting
15400	2.5	Sports	Horseback riding, walking
15410	3.0	Sports	Horseshoe pitching, quoits
15420	12.0	Sports	Jai alai
15430	10.0	Sports	Judo, jujitsu, karate, kick boxing, tae kwan do
15440	4.0	Sports	Juggling
15450	7.0	Sports	Kickball
15460	8.0	Sports	Lacrosse
15470	4.0	Sports	Motor-cross
15480	9.0	Sports	Orienteering
15490	10.0	Sports	Paddleball, competitive
15500	6.0	Sports	Paddleball, casual, general (Taylor Code 460)
15510	8.0	Sports	Polo
15520	10.0	Sports	Racketball, competitive
15530	7.0	Sports	Racketball, casual, general (Taylor Code 470)
15535	11.0	Sports	Rock climbing, ascending rock
15540	8.0	Sports	Rock climbing, rapelling
15550	12.0	Sports	Rope jumping, fast
15551	10.0	Sports	Rope jumping, moderate, general
15552	8.0	Sports	Rope jumping, slow
15560	10.0	Sports	Rugby
15570	3.0	Sports	Shuffleboard, lawn bowling
15580	5.0	Sports	Skateboarding
15590	7.0	Sports	Skating, roller (Taylor Code 360)
15591	12.5	Sports	Roller blading (in-line skating)

Code	MET	Specific Activity	Examples
15600	3.5	Sports	Sky diving
15605	10.0	Sports	Soccer, competitive
15610	7.0	Sports	Soccer, casual, general (Taylor Code 540)
15620	5.0	Sports	Softball or baseball, fast or slow pitch, general (Taylor Code 440)
15630	4.0	Sports	Softball, officiating
15640	6.0	Sports	Softball, pitching
15650	12.0	Sports	Squash (Taylor Code 530)
15660	4.0	Sports	Table tennis, ping pong (Taylor Code 410)
15670	4.0	Sports	Tai chi
15675	7.0	Sports	Tennis, general
15680	6.0	Sports	Tennis, doubles (Taylor Code 430)
15685	5.0	Sports	Tennis, doubles
15690	8.0	Sports	Tennis, singles (Taylor Code 420)
15700	3.5	Sports	Trampoline
15710	4.0	Sports	Volleyball (Taylor Code 400)
15711	8.0	Sports	Volleyball, competitive, in gymnasium
15720	3.0	Sports	Volleyball, noncompetitive, 6–9 member team, general
15725	8.0	Sports	Volleyball, beach
15730	6.0	Sports	Wrestling (one match = 5 min)
15731	7.0	Sports	Wallyball, general
15732	4.0	Sports	Track and field (shot, discus, hammer throw)
15733	6.0	Sports	Track and field (high jump, long jump, triple jump, javelin, pole vault)
15734	10.0	Sports	Track and field (steeplechase, hurdles)
16010	2.0	Transportation	Automobile or light truck (not a semi) driving
16015	1.0	Transportation	Riding in a car or truck
16016	1.0	Transportation	Riding in a bus
16020	2.0	Transportation	Flying airplane
16030	2.5	Transportation	Motor scooter, motorcycle
16040	6.0	Transportation	Pushing plane in and out of hangar
16050	3.0	Transportation	Driving heavy truck, tractor, bus
17010	7.0	Walking	Backpacking (Taylor Code 050)
17020	3.5	Walking	Carrying infant or 15-lb load (e.g., suitcase), level ground or downstairs
17025	9.0	Walking	Carrying load upstairs, general
17026	5.0	Walking	Carrying 1–15 lb load, upstairs
17027	6.0	Walking	Carrying 16–24 lb load, upstairs
17028	8.0	Walking	Carrying 25–49 lb load, upstairs
17029	10.0	Walking	Carrying 50–74 lb load, upstairs
17030	12.0	Walking	Carrying 74+ lb load, upstairs
17031	3.0	Walking	Loading/unloading a car
17035	7.0	Walking	Climbing hills with 0–9 lb load
17040	7.5	Walking	Climbing hills with 10–20 lb load
17050	8.0	Walking	Climbing hills with 21–42 lb load
17060	9.0	Walking	Climbing hills with 42+ lb load
17070	3.0	Walking	Downstairs
17080	6.0	Walking	Hiking, cross country (Taylor Code 040)
17085	2.5	Walking	Bird watching
17090	6.5	Walking	Marching, rapidly, military
17100	2.5	Walking	Pushing or pulling stroller with child or walking with children
17105	4.0	Walking	Pushing a wheelchair, nonoccupational setting
17110	6.5	Walking	Race walking
17120	8.0	Walking	Rock or mountain climbing (Taylor Code 060)
17130	8.0	Walking	Up stairs, using or climbing up ladder (Taylor Code 030)
17140	5.0	Walking	Using crutches
17150	2.0	Walking	Walking, household
17151	2.0	Walking	Walking, less than 2.0 mph, level ground, strolling, very slow
17152	2.5	Walking	Walking, 2.0 mph, level, slow pace, firm surface
17160	3.5	Walking	Walking for pleasure (Taylor Code 010)
17161	2.5	Walking	Walking from house to car or bus, from car or bus to go places, from car or bus to and from the worksite
17162	2.5	Walking	Walking to neighbor's house or family's house for social reasons
17165	3.0	Walking	Walking the dog
17170	3.0	Walking	Walking, 2.5 mph, firm surface
17180	2.8	Walking	Walking, 2.5 mph, downhill
17190	3.3	Walking	Walking, 3.0 mph, level, moderate pace, firm surface
17200	3.8	Walking	Walking, 3.5 mph, level, brisk, firm surface, walking for exercise

Code	MET	Specific Activity	Examples
17210	6.0	Walking	Walking, 3.5 mph, uphill
17220	5.0	Walking	Walking, 4.0 mph, level, firm surface, very brisk pace
17230	6.3	Walking	Walking, 4.5 mph, level, firm surface, very, very brisk
17231	8.0	Walking	Walking, 5.0 mph
17250	3.5	Walking	Walking, for pleasure, work break
17260	5.0	Walking	Walking, grass track
17270	4.0	Walking	Walking, to work or class (Taylor Code 015)
17280	2.5	Walking	Walking to and from an outhouse
18010	2.5	Water activities	Boating, power
18020	4.0	Water activities	Canoeing, on camping trip (Taylor Code 270)
18025	3.3	Water activities	Canoeing, harvesting wild rice, knocking rice off the stalks
18030	7.0	Water activities	Canoeing, portaging
18040	3.0	Water activities	Canoeing, rowing, 2.0–3.9 mph, light effort
18050	7.0	Water activities	Canoeing, rowing, 4.0–5.9 mph, moderate effort
18060	12.0	Water activities	Canoeing, rowing, >6 mph, vigorous effort
18070	3.5	Water activities	Canoeing, rowing, for pleasure, general (Taylor Code 250)
18080	12.0	Water activities	Canoeing, rowing, in competition, or crew or sculling (Taylor Code 260)
18090	3.0	Water activities	Diving, springboard or platform
18100	5.0	Water activities	Kayaking
18110	4.0	Water activities	Paddle boat
18120	3.0	Water activities	Sailing, boat and board sailing, windsurfing, ice sailing, general (Taylor Code 235)
18130	5.0	Water activities	Sailing, in competition
18140	3.0	Water activities	Sailing, Sunfish/Laser/Hoby Cat, Keel boats, ocean sailing, yachting
18150	6.0	Water activities	Skiing, water (Taylor Code 220)
18160	7.0	Water activities	Skimobiling
18180	16.0	Water activities	Skindiving, fast
18190	12.5	Water activities	Skindiving, moderate
18200	7.0	Water activities	Skindiving, SCUBA diving, general (Taylor Code 310)
18210	5.0	Water activities	Snorkeling (Taylor Code 320)
18220	3.0	Water activities	Surfing, body or board
18230	10.0	Water activities	Swimming laps, freestyle, fast, vigorous effort
18240	7.0	Water activities	Swimming laps, freestyle, slow, moderate or light effort
18250	7.0	Water activities	Swimming, backstroke, general
18260	10.0	Water activities	Swimming, breaststroke, general
18270	11.0	Water activities	Swimming, butterfly, general
18280	11.0	Water activities	Swimming, crawl, fast (75 yards/min), vigorous effort
18290	8.0	Water activities	Swimming, crawl, slow (50 yards/min), moderate or light effort
18300	6.0	Water activities	Swimming, lake, ocean, river (Taylor Code 280, 295)
18310	6.0	Water activities	Swimming, leisurely, not lap swimming, general
18320	8.0	Water activities	Swimming, sidestroke, general
18330	8.0	Water activities	Swimming, synchronized
18340	10.0	Water activities	Swimming, treading water, fast vigorous effort
18350	4.0	Water activities	Swimming, treading water, moderate effort, general
18355	4.0	Water activities	Water aerobics, water calisthenics
18360	10.0	Water activities	Water polo
18365	3.0	Water activities	Water volleyball
18366	8.0	Water activities	Water jogging
18370	5.0	Water activities	Whitewater rafting, kayaking, or canoeing
19010	6.0	Winter activities	Moving ice house (set up/drill holes, etc.)
19020	5.5	Winter activities	Skating, ice, 9 mph or less
19030	7.0	Winter activities	Skating, ice, general (Taylor Code 360)
19040	9.0	Winter activities	Skating, ice, rapidly, more than 9 mph
19050	15.0	Winter activities	Skating, speed, competitive
19060	7.0	Winter activities	Ski jumping (climb up carrying skis)
19075	7.0	Winter activities	Skiing, general
19080	7.0	Winter activities	Skiing, cross country, 2.5 mph, slow or light effort, ski walking
19090	8.0	Winter activities	Skiing, cross country, 4.0–4.9 mph, moderate speed and effort, general
19100	9.0	Winter activities	Skiing, cross country, 5.0–7.0 mph, brisk speed, vigorous effort
19110	14.0	Winter activities	Skiing, cross country, >8.0 mph, racing
19130	16.5	Winter activities	Skiing, cross country, hard snow, uphill, maximum, snow mountaineering

Code	MET	Specific Activity	Examples
19150	5.0	Winter activities	Skiing, downhill, light effort
19160	6.0	Winter activities	Skiing, downhill, moderate effort, general
19170	8.0	Winter activities	Skiing, downhill, vigorous effort, racing
19180	7.0	Winter activities	Sledding, tobogganing, bobsledding, luge (Taylor Code 370)
19190	8.0	Winter activities	Snow shoeing
19200	3.5	Winter activities	Snowmobiling
20000	1.0	Religious activities	Sitting in church, in service, attending a ceremony, sitting quietly
20001	2.5	Religious activities	Sitting, playing an instrument at church
20005	1.5	Religious activities	Sitting in church, talking or singing, attending a ceremony, sitting, active participation
20010	1.3	Religious activities	Sitting, reading religious materials at home
20015	1.2	Religious activities	Standing in church (quietly), attending a ceremony, standing quietly
20020	2.0	Religious activities	Standing, singing in church, attending a ceremony, standing, active participation
20025	1.0	Religious activities	Kneeling in church/at home (praying)
20030	1.8	Religious activities	Standing, talking in church
20035	2.0	Religious activities	Walking in church
20036	2.0	Religious activities	Walking less than 2.0 mph, very slow
20037	3.3	Religious activities	Walking, 3.0 mph, moderate speed, not carrying anything
20038	3.8	Religious activities	Walking, 3.5 mph, brisk speed, not carrying anything
20039	2.0	Religious activities	Walk/stand combination for religious purposes, usher
20040	5.0	Religious activities	Praise with dance or run, spiritual dancing in church
20045	2.5	Religious activities	Serving food at church
20046	2.0	Religious activities	Preparing food at church
20047	2.3	Religious activities	Washing dishes/cleaning kitchen at church
20050	1.5	Religious activities	Eating at church
20055	2.0	Religious activities	Eating/talking at church or standing eating, American Indian Feast days
20060	3.0	Religious activities	Cleaning church
20061	5.0	Religious activities	General yard work at church
20065	2.5	Religious activities	Standing—moderate (lifting 50 lb, assembling at fast rate)
20095	4.0	Religious activities	Standing—moderate/heavy work
20100	1.5	Religious activities	Typing, electric, manual, or computer
21000	1.5	Volunteer activities	Sitting—meeting, general, and/or with talking involved
21005	1.5	Volunteer activities	Sitting—light office work, in general
21010	2.5	Volunteer activities	Sitting—moderate work
21015	2.3	Volunteer activities	Standing—light work (filing, talking, assembling)
21016	2.5	Volunteer activities	Sitting, child care, only active periods
21017	3.0	Volunteer activities	Standing, child care, only active periods
21018	4.0	Volunteer activities	Walk/run play with children, moderate, only active periods
21019	5.0	Volunteer activities	Walk/run play with children, vigorous, only active periods
21020	3.0	Volunteer activities	Standing—light/moderate work (pack boxes, assemble/repair, set up chairs/furniture)
21025	3.5	Volunteer activities	Standing—moderate (lifting 50 lb, assembling at fast rate)
21030	4.0	Volunteer activities	Standing—moderate/heavy work
21035	1.5	Volunteer activities	Typing, electric, manual, or computer
21040	2.0	Volunteer activities	Walking, less than 2.0 mph, very slow
21045	3.3	Volunteer activities	Walking, 3.0 mph, moderate speed, not carrying anything
21050	3.8	Volunteer activities	Walking, 3.5 mph, brisk speed, not carrying anything
21055	3.0	Volunteer activities	Walking, 2.5 mph slowly and carrying objects less than 25 lb
21060	4.0	Volunteer activities	Walking, 3.0 mph moderately and carrying objects less than 25 lb, pushing something
21065	4.5	Volunteer activities	Walking, 3.5 mph, briskly and carrying objects less than 25 lb
21070	3.0	Volunteer activities	Walk/stand combination, for volunteer purposes

Section 2. Guidelines for Assigning Activities by Major Purpose or Intent

1. *Conditioning exercises* include activities with the intent of improving physical condition. This includes stationary ergometers (bicycling, rowing machines, treadmills, etc.), health-club exercise, calisthenics, and aerobics.
2. *Home repair* includes all activity associated with the repair of a house and does not include housework. This is not an occupational task.
3. Sleeping, lying, sitting, and standing are classified as *inactivity*.
4. *Home activities* include all activities associated with maintaining the inside of a house and include house cleaning, laundry, grocery shopping, and cooking.
5. *Lawn and garden* includes all activity associated with maintaining the yard and includes yardwork, gardening, and snow removal.
6. *Occupation* includes all job-related physical activity where one is paid (gainful employment). Specific activities may be cross-referenced in other categories (such as reading, writing, driving a car, walking) and should be coded in this major heading if related to employment. Housework is occupational only if the person is earning money for the task.
7. *Self-care* includes all activity related to grooming, eating, bathing, etc.
8. *Transportation* includes energy expended for the primary purpose of going somewhere in a motorized vehicle.

Section 3. Guidelines for Coding Specific Activities

A. General guidelines: All activities should be coded as "general" if no other information about the activity is given. This applies primarily to intensity ratings. If any additional information is given, activities should be coded accordingly.

B. Specific guidelines

1. Bicycling
   - **a.** Stationary cycling using cycle ergometers (all types), wind trainers, or other conditioning devices should be classified under the major heading of Conditioning Exercise, stationary cycling specific activities (codes 02010 to 02015).
   - **b.** The list does not account for differences in wind conditions.
   - **c.** If bicycling is performed in a race, classify it as general racing if no descriptions are given about drafting (code 01050). If information is given about the speed or drafting, code as 01050 (bicycling, 16–19 mph, racing/not drafting or >19 mph drafting, very fast) or 01060 (bicycling, ≥ 20 mph, racing, not drafting).
   - **d.** Using a mountain bike in the city should be classified as bicycling, general (code 01010). Cycling on mountain trails or on a BMX course is coded 01009.
2. Conditioning Exercises
   - **a.** If a calisthenics program is described as a light or moderate type of activity (e.g., performing back exercises) but indicates a vigorous effort on the part of the participant, code the activity as calisthenics, general (code 02030).
   - **b.** Exercise performed at a health club that is not described should be classified as health club, general (code 02060). Other activities performed at a health club (e.g., weight lifting, aerobic dance, circuit training, treadmill running, etc.) should be classified under separate major headings.
   - **c.** Regardless of whether aerobic dance, conditioning, circuit training, or water calisthenics programs are described by their component parts (i.e., 10 min jogging in place, 10 min sit-ups, 10 min stretching, etc.), code the activity as one activity (e.g., water aerobics, code 02120).
   - **d.** Effort, speed, or intensity breakdowns for the specific activities of stair–treadmill ergometer (code 02065), ski machine (code 02080), water aerobics or water calisthenics (code 02120), circuit training (code 02040), and slimnastics (code 02090) are not given. Code these as general, even though effort or intensities may vary in the descriptions of the activity.

3. Dancing
   a. If the type of dancing performed is not described, code it as dancing, general (code 03025).
4. Home Activities
   a. House cleaning should be coded as light (code 05040) or heavy (code 05020). Examples for each are given in the description of the specific activities.
   b. Making the bed on a daily basis is coded 05100. Changing the bed sheets is coded as cleaning, light (code 05040).
5. Home Repair
   a. Any painting outside of the house (i.e., fence, the house, barn) is coded, painting, outside house (code 60150).
6. Inactivity
   a. Sitting and reading a book or newspaper is listed under the major heading of Miscellaneous, reading, book, newspaper, etc. (code 09030).
   b. Sitting and writing is listed under the major heading of Miscellaneous, writing (code 09040).
7. Lawn and Garden
   a. Working in the garden with a specific type of tool (e.g., hoe, spade) is coded as digging, spading, filling garden (code 08050).
   b. Removing snow may be done by one of three methods: shoveling snow by hand (code 08200), walking and operating a snow blower (code 08130), or riding a snow blower (code 08180).
8. Music Playing
   a. Most variation in music playing will be according to the setting (i.e., rock and roll band, orchestra, marching band, concert band, standing on the stage, performance, practice, in a church, etc.). The compendium does not consider differences in the setting (except for marching band and guitar playing).
9. Occupation
   a. Types of occupational activities not listed separately under specific activities (e.g., chemistry laboratory experiments) should be placed into the types of energy expenditure classifications best describing the activity. See sitting: light (code 11580), sitting: moderate (code 11590), standing: light (code 11600), standing: light to moderate (code 11610), standing: moderate (code 11620), standing: moderate to heavy (code 11630).
   b. Driving an automobile or a light truck for employment (taxi cab, salesperson, contractor, ambulance driver, bus driver) should be listed under the major heading of Transportation, automobile or light truck (not a semi) driving (code 06010).
   c. Performing skin or SCUBA diving as an occupation is listed under the major heading of Water Activities, and the specific activity of skindiving or SCUBA diving as a frogman (code 18170).
10. Running
    a. Running is not classified as treadmill or outdoor running. Running on a treadmill or outdoors should be coded by the speed of the run (codes 12030 to 12130). If speed is not given, code it as running, general (code 12150).
11. Self-care
    a. The compendium does not account for effort ratings. All items are considered to be general.
12. Transportation
    a. Being a passenger in an automobile is coded under the major heading of Inactivity, sitting quietly (code 07020).
13. Walking
    a. Household walking is coded 17150, regardless of whether the subject identified a walking speed.
    b. If the walking speed is unidentified, use 3.0 mph, level, moderate, firm surface as the standard speed (code 17190). This should not be used for household walking.
    c. Walking during a household move, shopping, or for household work is coded under the major heading of Home Activities. Walking for job-related activities is coded under Occupational Activities.
    d. If a subject is backpacking, regardless of descriptors attached, the code is backpacking, general (code 17010).
    e. The compendium does not account for variations in speed or effort while carrying luggage or a child.
    f. Mountain climbing should be classified as general (rock or mountain climbing, code 17120) if no descriptors are given. If the weight of the load is described, code the activity as climbing hills with the appropriate load (codes 17030 to 17060).
    g. Walking on a grassy area (golf course, in a park, etc.) should be coded as walking, grass track (code 17260). The compendium does not

account for variations in walking speed on a grassy area, so ignore recordings of walking speed or effort. If the walking is not on a grassy area, code the activity according to the walking speed (codes 17150 to 17230).

h. Walking to work or to class should be coded as 17270. The compendium does not account for walking speed or effort in this activity. Even though a speed or effort is given for the walking, do not code walking to work or to class in any other walking category.

i. Hiking and cross-country walking (code 17080) should be used only if the walking activity lasted 3 hours or more. Do not use this category for backpacking, but for day hikes.

14. Water Activities

a. Swimming should be coded as leisurely, not lap swimming, general (code 18310) if descriptors about stroke, speed, or swimming location are not given.

b. Lap swimming should be coded as swimming laps, freestyle, slow (code 18240) if the activity is described as lap swimming, light or moderate effort, but stroke or speed are not indicated. Swimming laps should be coded as swimming, laps, freestyle, fast (code 18230) if the activity is described as lap swimming, vigorous effort, but stroke or speed are not indicated.

c. Swimming crawl should be coded as swimming, crawl, slow (50 yards $\cdot$ min^{-1}) if speed is not given and the effort is rated light or moderate (code 18290). Swimming crawl should be coded as swimming, crawl, fast (75 yards $\cdot$ min^{-1}) if speed is not given, but the effort is rated as vigorous (code 18280).

d. The swimming strokes of backstroke (code 18250), breaststroke (code 18260), butterfly (code 18270), and sidestroke (code 18230) are coded as general for speed and intensity.

e. If a swimming activity is not identified as lake, ocean, or river swimming (code 18300), assume that the swimming was performed in a swimming pool.

f. If canoeing is related to a canoe trip, code as canoeing, on a camping trip (code 18020). Otherwise, code it according to the speed and effort listed.

Source: Ainsworth BE, Haskell WL, Whitt MC, Irwin ML, Swartz AM, Strath SJ, O'Brien WL, Bassett DR, Schmitz KH, Emplaincourt PO, Jacobs DR, Leon AS. Compendium of physical activities: An update of activity codes and MET intensities. *Med Sci Sports Exerc* 32(9 suppl):S498–S516, 2000. Used with permission, Lippincott Williams & Wilkens.

Glossary

acclimatization The body's gradual adaptation to a changed environment, such as higher temperatures.

acromegaly A chronic disease caused by excess production of growth hormone, leading to elongation and enlargement of bones of the extremities and certain head bones.

acute Sudden, short-term.

acute muscle soreness Occurs during and immediately following exercise; the muscular tension developed during exercise, which reduces blood flow to the active muscles, causing lactic acid and potassium to build up, stimulating pain receptors.

adenosine triphosphate (ATP) Energy released from the separation of high-energy phosphate bonds; the immediate energy source for muscular contraction.

adherence Sticking to something; used to describe a person's continuation in an exercise program.

adipose tissue Fat tissue.

aerobic Using oxygen.

aerobic activities Activities using large-muscle groups at moderate intensities, which permit the body to use oxygen to supply energy and to maintain a steady state for more than a few minutes.

aerobic dance The original aerobic-dance programs consisted of an eclectic combination of various dance forms, including ballet, modern jazz, disco, and folk, as well as calisthenic-type exercises; more recent innovations include water aerobics (done in a swimming pool), nonimpact or low-impact aerobics (one foot on the ground at all times), specific dance aerobics, and "assisted" aerobics, whereby weights are worn on the wrists and/or ankles.

aerobic power See *maximal oxygen uptake.*

agility Relates to the ability to rapidly change the position of the entire body in space, with speed and accuracy.

aging Refers to the normal yet irreversible biological changes that occur during the total years that a person lives.

alcohol dependent Dependency on alcohol, which leads to negative consequences such as arrest, accident, or impairment of health or job performance.

alcoholism A chronic, progressive, and potentially fatal disease characterized by *tolerance* (brain adaptation to the presence of alcohol) and *physical dependency* (withdrawal symptoms occur when consumption of alcohol is decreased); alcohol-related problems may include symptoms of alcohol dependence such as memory loss, inability to stop drinking until intoxicated, inability to cut down on drinking, binge drinking, and withdrawal symptoms.

alveoli Air sacs of the lung.

Alzheimer's disease Disease that progresses from short-term memory loss to a final stage requiring total care; a form of senile dementia, associated with atrophy of parts of the brain.

amenorrhea Absence of menstruation.

amino acid An organic compound that makes up protein; 20 amino acids are necessary for metabolism and growth, but only 11 are "essential" in that they must be provided from the food eaten.

anabolic The building up of a body substance.

anabolic steroids A group of synthetic, testosterone-like hormones that promote anabolism, including muscle hypertrophy; their use in athletics is considered unethical and carries numerous serious health risks.

anaerobic Not using oxygen.

anaerobic activities Activities using muscle groups at high intensities that exceed the body's capacity to use oxygen to supply energy, thereby creating an oxygen debt by using energy produced without oxygen; see *oxygen debt.*

anaerobic threshold The point at which blood lactate concentrations start to rise above resting values; can be expressed as a percent of $\dot{V}O_{2max}$.

androgenic Causing masculinization.

android A type of obesity characterized by the predominance of body fat in the upper half of the body.

anemia Low hemoglobin concentration in the blood.

aneurysm Localized abnormal dilatation of a blood vessel due to weakness of the wall.

angina A gripping, choking, or suffocating pain in the chest (angina pectoris) caused most often by insufficient flow of oxygen to the heart muscle during exercise or excitement.

anorexia (anorexia nervosa) Lack of appetite; a psychological and physiological condition characterized by inability or refusal to eat, leading to severe weight loss, malnutrition, hormone imbalances, and other potentially life-threatening biological changes.

anthropometry The science dealing with the measurement (size, weight, proportions) of the human body.

anticipatory response Prior to exercise, heart rates can rise due to anticipation of the exercise bout.

apoprotein The protein part of the lipoprotein; important in activating or inhibiting certain enzymes involved in the metabolism of fats.

aquacise Aerobic dance in the water.

arrhythmia Any abnormal rate or rhythm of the heart beat.

arteriosclerosis Commonly called hardening of the arteries; includes a variety of conditions that cause the artery walls to thicken and lose elasticity.

arteriovenous oxygen difference ($\bar{a}-\bar{v}O_2$ difference) The difference between the oxygen content of arterial blood and that of venous blood.

artery Vessel that carries blood away from the heart to the tissues of the body.

asthma A disease characterized by wheezing caused by a spasm of the bronchial tubes or by swelling of their mucous membranes.

atherosclerosis A very common form of arteriosclerosis in which the arteries are narrowed by deposits of cholesterol and other material in the inner walls of the artery.

atrioventricular (AV) node A small mass of specialized conducting tissue at the bottom of the right atrium, through which the electrical impulse stimulating the heart to contract must pass to reach the ventricles.

auscultation Process of listening for sounds within the body using a stethoscope.

balance Relates to the maintenance of equilibrium while stationary or moving.

ballistic movement A flexibility exercise movement in which a part of the body is sharply moved against the resistance of antagonist muscles or against the limits of a joint.

basal metabolic rate The minimum energy required to maintain the body's life functions at rest; usually expressed in Calories per day.

bee pollen A substance gleaned from honey, which is claimed by some to have unusual nutritional qualities enhancing performance; double-blind placebo studies do not support this claim.

behavior modification Considers in great detail the eating behavior to be changed, events that trigger the eating, and the behavior's consequences.

binge eating The consumption of large quantities of rich foods within short periods of time.

blood doping An ergogenic procedure wherein an athlete's own blood is infused, or type-matched donor blood is transfused, to enhance endurance performance.

blood pressure The pressure exerted by the blood on the wall of the arteries; measures are in millimeters of mercury (such as 120/80 mm Hg).

bodybuilding An activity in which competitors work to develop the mass, definition, and symmetry of their muscles, rather than the strength, skill, or endurance required for more common athletic events.

body composition The proportions of fat, muscle, and bone making up the body; usually expressed as percent of body fat and percent of lean body mass.

body density The specific gravity of the body, which can be tested by underwater weighing; compares the weight of the body to the weight of the same volume of water; result can be used to estimate the percentage of body fat.

body mass index (BMI) Calculation of body weight and height indices for determining degree of obesity.

bradycardia Slow heartbeat of less than 60 beats per minute at rest.

branched-chain amino acids Valine, isoleucine, leucine.

BTPS The volume of air at the temperature and pressure of the body, and 100% saturated with water vapor.

bundle of His A bundle of fibers of the impulse-conducting system of the heart; from its origin in the AV node, enters the interventricular septum, where it divides into two branches (bundle branches), the fibers of which pass to the right and left ventricles, becoming continuous with the Purkinje fibers of the ventricles.

caffeine A methylxanthine found in many plants; has unpredictable effects on endurance performance, but may increase muscle utilization of free fatty acids, sparing muscle glycogen stores.

calisthenics A system of exercise movements, without equipment, for the building of muscular strength and endurance, and flexibility; the Greeks formed the word from *kalos* (beautiful) and *sthenos* (strength).

caloric cost The number of Calories burned to produce the energy for a task; usually measured in Calories (kilocalories) per minute.

calorie The energy required to raise the temperature of 1 kilogram of water 1° Celsius; used as a unit of metabolism (as in diet and energy expenditure); 1 Calorie equals 1,000 calories (spelled with a capital C to make that distinction); also called a kilocalorie (kcal).

cancer A large group of diseases characterized by uncontrolled growth and spread of abnormal cells.

carbohydrate Chemical compound of carbon, oxygen, and hydrogen, usually with the hydrogen and oxygen in the right proportions to form water; common forms are starches, sugars, and dietary fibers.

carbohydrate loading A dietary scheme emphasizing high amounts of carbohydrate to increase muscle glycogen stores before long-endurance events.

carbon dioxide A colorless, odorless gas formed in the tissues by the oxidation of carbon and eliminated by the lungs.

carbon monoxide Produced mainly during combustion of fossil fuels such as coal and gasoline; a tasteless, odorless, colorless gas.

cardiac output The volume of blood pumped out by the heart in a given unit of time; equals the stroke volume times the heart rate.

cardiac rehabilitation A program to prepare cardiac patients to return to productive lives with a reduced risk of recurring health problems.

cardiopulmonary resuscitation (CPR) A first-aid method to restore breathing and heart action through mouth-to-mouth breathing and rhythmic chest compressions; CPR instruction is offered by local American Heart Association and American Red Cross units and is a minimum requirement for most fitness-instruction certifications.

cardiorespiratory endurance The same as aerobic endurance; can be defined as the ability to continue or persist in strenuous tasks involving large-muscle groups for extended periods of time; the ability of the circulatory and respiratory systems to adjust to and recover from the effects of whole-body exercise or work.

cardiovascular Pertaining to the heart and blood vessels.

carotid artery The principal artery in both sides of the neck. A convenient place to detect a pulse.

catecholamine Epinephrine and norepinephrine hormones.

cellulite A commercially created name for lumpy fat deposits; actually behaves no differently from other fat; distinguished by straining against irregular bands of connective tissue.

cerebral thrombosis Clot that forms inside the cerebral artery.

cholesterol An alcohol steroid found in animal fats; a pearly, fat-like substance implicated in the narrowing of the arteries in atherosclerosis; all Americans are being urged to decrease their serum cholesterol levels to less than 200 mg/dl.

chronic Continuing over time.

chronic diseases Lifestyle-related diseases, such as heart disease, cancer, and stroke, and also accidents, which together account for 75% of all deaths in America.

circuit training A series of exercises, performed one after the other, with little rest between.

circuit weight training programs Involve 8–12 repetitions with various weight machines at 7–14 stations, moving quickly from one station to the next.

citric acid cycle See *Krebs cycle.*

collateral circulation Blood circulation through small side branches that can supplement (or substitute for) the main vessel's delivery of blood to certain tissues.

compliance Staying with a prescribed exercise program.

concentric action Muscle action in which the muscle is shortening under its own power; commonly called "positive" work or, redundantly, "concentric contraction."

continuous passive motion (CPM) Motorized machines that continuously move isolated muscle groups through their range of motion without requiring any effort by the user.

contraindication Any condition indicating that a particular course of action (or exercise) would be inadvisable.

cool-down A gradual reduction of the intensity of exercise to allow physiological processes to return to normal; also called warm-down.

coordination Relates to the ability to use the senses, such as sight and hearing, together with body parts in performing motor tasks smoothly and accurately.

coronary arteries The arteries circling the heart like a crown, which supply blood to the heart muscle; three major branches.

coronary heart disease (CHD) Atherosclerosis of the coronary arteries.

cortical bone Compact outer shaft bone.

creatine phosphokinase (CPK) A muscle enzyme that can rise dramatically in the blood after unaccustomed exercise, indicating considerable muscle cell damage.

cross-sectional study A study made at one point in time (cf. *longitudinal study*).

cryokinetics A treatment that alternates cold and exercise for rehabilitation of traumatic musculoskeletal injuries in athletes.

dehydration Condition resulting from the excessive loss of body water.

delayed-onset muscle soreness (DOMS) Occurs from 1 to 5 days following unaccustomed or severe exercise, involving actual damage to the muscle cells.

detraining The process of losing the benefits of training by returning to a sedentary life.

DHEA An unapproved drug (dehydroepiandrosterone or dehydroandrosterone) derived from human urine and other sources; manufacturers tout DHEA as a "natural" weight-loss product, but this claim has not been substantiated.

diabetes mellitus A group of disorders that share glucose intolerance (high serum levels of glucose) in common; there are two common types: type 1 and type 2. Type 1 can occur at any age, but especially in the young, and is characterized by an abrupt onset of symptoms and a need for insulin to sustain life; type 2 is most common, usually occurring in people who are obese and over age 40.

diastolic blood pressure The blood pressure when the heart is resting between beats.

dietary fiber Complex plant cell-wall materials that cannot be digested by the enzymes in the human small intestine; examples include cellulose, hemicellulose, pectin, mucilages, and lignin.

diuretic Any agent that increases the flow of urine, ridding the body of water.

drug dependence Criteria are highly controlled or compulsive use, psychoactive effects, and drug-reinforced behavior.

dry bulb thermometer An ordinary instrument for indicating temperature. Does not take into account humidity and other factors that combine to determine the heat stress experienced by the body.

duration The time spent in a single exercise session; frequency, intensity, and duration (time) are the F.I.T. factors, which affect improvement of cardiorespiratory endurance.

dynamometer A device for measuring force; common dynamometers include devices to test hand, leg, and back strength.

dyspnea Difficult or labored breathing.

eccentric action Muscle action in which the muscle resists while it is forced to lengthen; commonly called "negative" work, or "eccentric contraction," but because the muscle is lengthening, the word "contraction" is misapplied.

ECG lead A pair of electrodes placed on the body and connected to an electrocardiograph (ECG recorder).

economy Refers to ease of administration, the use of inexpensive equipment, the need for little time, and the simplicity of the test so that the person taking it can easily understand the purpose and results.

ectomorphic A lean, thin, and linear body type.

efficiency The ratio of energy consumed to the work accomplished.

elderly Individuals who reach or pass the age of 65; this group now represents the fastest-growing minority in the United States.

electrical muscle stimulators (EMS) EMS devices give a painless electrical stimulation to the muscle; manufacturers claim that muscles are toned without exercise; other claimed benefits include face lifts without surgery, slimming and trimming, weight loss, bust development, spot reducing, and removal of cellulite; the Food and Drug Administration considers claims for EMS devices promoted for such purposes to be misbranded and fraudulent.

electrocardiogram (ECG, EKG) A graph of the electrical activity caused by the stimulation of the heart muscle; the millivolts of electricity are detected by electrodes on the body surface and recorded by an electrocardiograph.

electrolyte Scientists call minerals like sodium, chloride, and potassium "electrolytes" because, in water, they can conduct electrical currents; sodium and potassium ions carry positive charges, while chloride ions are negatively charged.

electron transport system An additional metabolic pathway from which the products of the Krebs cycle enter and yield ATP; this cycle requires oxygen.

embolus A blood clot that breaks loose and travels to smaller arterial vessels, where it may lodge and block the blood flow.

endurance The capacity to continue a physical performance over a period of time.

enzyme Complex proteins that induce and accelerate the speed of chemical reactions without being changed themselves; present in digestive juices, enzymes act on food substances, breaking them down into simpler molecules.

epidemiological studies Statistical study of the relationships among various factors that determine the frequency and distribution of disease in human populations.

epinephrine A hormone primarily excreted from the adrenal medulla; also called a catecholamine; involved in many important body functions, including the elevation of blood glucose levels during exercise or stress.

ergogenic aids A physical, mechanical, nutritional, psychological, or pharmacological substance or treatment that either directly improves physiological variables associated with exercise performance or removes subjective restraints that may limit physiological capacity.

ergometer A device that can measure work consistently and reliably; stationary exercise cycles were the first widely available devices equipped with ergometers.

estrogen replacement One of the mainstays of prevention and management of osteoporosis, especially for women who are postmenopausal; also effective in preventing cardiovascular disease.

ethyl alcohol (ethanol) Grain alcohol; a social drug that is called a "sedative–hypnotic" because of its dramatic effects on the brain; ethanol (CH_3CH_2OH) is a small water-soluble molecule that is absorbed rapidly and completely from the stomach and small intestine.

exercise Physical exertion of sufficient intensity, duration, and frequency to achieve or maintain fitness or other health or athletic objectives.

exercise-induced bronchospasm (EIB) Defined as a diffuse bronchospastic response in both large and small airways following heavy exercise; postexercise symptoms include difficulty in breathing, coughing, shortness of breath, and wheezing.

exercise oxygen economy The oxygen cost of exercise, usually expressed as $\dot{V}O_2$ at a certain running or exercise pace.

exercise prescription A recommendation for a course of exercise to meet desirable individual objectives for fitness;

includes activity types, as well as duration, intensity, and frequency of exercise.

exercise program director Certification by the American College of Sports Medicine indicates the competency to design, implement, and administer preventive and rehabilitative exercise programs, to educate staff in conducting tests and leading physical activity, and to educate the community about such programs; must have all the competencies of fitness instructor, exercise technologist, and exercise specialist.

exercise specialist Certified by the American College of Sports Medicine as having the competency and skill to supervise preventive and rehabilitative exercise programs and prescribe activities for patients; must also pass the ACSM standards for exercise technologist.

exercise technologist Certified by the American College of Sports Medicine as competent to administer graded exercise tests, calculate the data, and implement any needed emergency procedures; must have current CPR certification.

expiratory reserve volume (ERV) The amount of air that can be pushed out of the lung following an expired resting tidal volume.

extension Moving the two ends of a jointed body part away from each other, as in straightening the arm.

extensor A muscle that extends a jointed body part.

extracellular Outside of the body cell.

Fartlek training Similar to interval training; a free form of training done on trails or roads.

fast-twitch fibers Muscle fiber type that contracts quickly and is used most in intensive, short-duration exercises, such as weight lifting or sprints; also called Type II fibers.

fat cell theory A theory that may explain obesity; fat cell number can increase two to three times normal if an individual ingests excessive Calories; once formed, the extra fat cells cannot be removed by the body; this can happen any time during the life span of an individual but appears to be particularly important during infancy when fat cells are still dividing.

fat-free weight Lean body mass or bone, muscle, and water.

fatigue A loss of power to continue a given level of physical performance.

fats Serve as a source of energy; in food, the fat molecule is formed from one molecule of glycerol and is combined with three of fatty acids; a high caloric value, yielding about 9 Calories per gram, as compared with 4 Calories for carbohydrates and proteins; *saturated fats* have no double bonds, are generally hard at room temperature, and have been associated with increased risk of heart disease; *monounsaturated fats* and *polyunsaturated fats* have one and two double bonds, respectively, are generally liquid at room temperature, and have been associated with decreased risk of heart disease.

fitness See *physical fitness.*

fitness instructor Directs classes or individuals in the performance of exercise; certification by the American College of Sports Medicine indicates the competency to identify risk factors, conduct submaximal exercise tests, recommend exercise programs, lead classes, counsel exercisers, and work with persons without known disease; CPR certification is required.

flexibility The range of motion around a joint.

flexion Moving the two ends of a jointed body part closer to each other, as in bending the arm.

food supplements Substances or pills that are added to the diet; most reputable nutritionists state that vitamin or mineral supplementation is unwarranted for people eating a balanced diet.

forced vital capacity (FVC) The total amount of air that can be breathed into the lung on top of the residual volume.

frame size Elbow breadth measurement for determination of small, medium, or large skeletal mass.

frequency How often a person repeats a complete exercise session (e.g., three times per week); frequency, along with duration and intensity, affects the cardiorespiratory response to exercise.

functional capacity See *maximal oxygen uptake.*

functional residual capacity (FRC) The combined expiratory reserve volume and residual volume.

gastric stapling Surgery to radically reduce the volume of the stomach to less than 50 ml.

genetic factors One theory advanced to explain the high prevalence of obesity in western countries; some studies have demonstrated that certain people are more prone to obesity than others due to genetic factors; such people have to be unusually careful in their dietary and exercise habits to counteract these inherited tendencies.

glucagon A hormone that is secreted by the pancreas; helps to raise blood glucose levels by stimulating the breakdown of liver glycogen.

gluconeogenesis The formation of glucose and glycogen from noncarbohydrate sources such as amino acids, glycerol, and lactate.

glucose Blood sugar; the transportable form of carbohydrate, which reaches the cells.

glucose polymers Four to six glucose units produced by partial breakdown of corn starch.

glycogen The storage form of carbohydrate; used in the muscles for the production of energy.

glycolysis A metabolic pathway that converts glucose to lactic acid to produce energy in the form of ATP.

glycosuria Glucose in the urine.

Golgi tendon organ Organs at the junction of muscle and tendon which send inhibitory impulses to the muscle when the muscle's contraction reaches certain levels; the purpose may be to protect against separating the tendon from bone when a contraction is too great.

graded exercise test (GXT) A treadmill or cycle-ergometer test with the workload gradually increased until exhaustion or a predetermined endpoint.

grapefruit pills For several decades, grapefruit has been promoted as having special fat-burning properties; this myth has spread far and wide; grapefruit pills contain grapefruit extract, diuretics, and bulk-forming agents, and some contain phenylpropanolamine (PPA), along with herbs or other ingredients.

growth hormone A hormone released from the pituitary, which elevates blood glucose; as its name indicates, this hormone helps regulate growth.

growth hormone releasers Various products sold with the claim that if they are taken before retiring, weight loss will occur overnight due to the increased release of growth hormone from the amino acids arginine and ornithine contained in the products—an erroneous concept.

gynoid A form of obesity characterized by excess body fat in the lower half of the body, especially the hips, buttocks, and thighs.

haptoglobin A mucoprotein to which hemoglobin released into plasma is bound; increased in certain inflammatory conditions, and decreased during hemolysis.

HDL-C:TC The ratio of HDL-C to total cholesterol, which has been found to be highly predictive of heart disease.

health The World Health Organization has defined *health* as a state of complete physical, mental, and social well-being, and not merely the absence of disease.

health fraud Defined as the promotion, for financial gain, of fraudulent or unproven devices, treatments, services, plans, or products (including, but not limited to, diets and nutritional supplements) that alter or claim to alter the human condition.

health promotion The science and art of helping people change their lifestyle to move toward optimal health.

health-related fitness Elements of fitness such as cardiorespiratory fitness, muscular strength and endurance, flexibility, and body composition that are related to improvement of health.

heart attack Also called myocardial infarction; often occurs when a clot blocks an atherosclerotic coronary blood vessel.

heart rate Number of heart beats per minute.

heart rate reserve The difference between the resting heart rate and the maximal heart rate.

heat cramps Muscle twitching or painful cramping, usually following heavy exercise with profuse sweating; the legs, arms, and abdominal muscles are the most often affected.

heat exhaustion Caused by dehydration; symptoms include a dry mouth, excessive thirst, loss of coordination, dizziness, headaches, paleness, shakiness, and cool and clammy skin.

heat stroke A life-threatening illness when the body's temperature-regulating mechanisms fail; body temperature may rise to over 104°F, skin appears red, dry, and warm to the touch; the victim has chills, sometimes nausea and dizziness, and may be confused or irrational; seizures and coma may follow unless temperature is brought down to 102° within an hour.

Hegsted formula Used to predict change in serum cholesterol from saturated fats (S) and polyunsaturated fats (P) and cholesterol in the diet: change in serum cholesterol = $(2.16 \times \text{change in S}) - (1.65 \times \text{change in P}) + (0.097 \times \text{change in dietary cholesterol})$.

hematocrit Expressed as the percentage of total blood volume, consisting of red blood cells and other solids.

heme iron Forty percent of the iron in animal products is called heme iron; the remaining 60% of the iron in animal products and all the iron in vegetable products are called nonheme iron; heme iron is more easily absorbed by the body.

hemoconcentration Increase in the thickness of blood due to loss of plasma volume.

hemoglobin The iron-containing pigment of the red blood cells; its function is to carry oxygen from the lungs to the tissues. Low levels of hemoglobin is called anemia.

hemolysis Breakdown of red blood cells, with liberation of hemoglobin, and loss through the kidneys.

hemorrhage Abnormal internal or external discharge of blood.

hepatic lipase (HL) An enzyme of the liver that removes HDL from circulation.

high blood pressure See *hypertension.*

high-density lipoprotein cholesterol (HDL-C) Cholesterol is carried by the high-density lipoprotein to the liver; the liver then uses the cholesterol to form bile acids, which are finally excreted in the stool; thus, high levels of HDL-C have been associated with low cardiovascular disease risk.

homeostasis State of equilibrium of the internal environment of the body.

hormone A substance secreted from an organ or gland, which is transported by the blood to another part of the body.

human growth hormone Hormone that is liberated by the anterior pituitary and is important for regulating growth.

hypercholesterolemia High blood cholesterol levels.

hyperglycemia Excessive levels of glucose in the blood.

hyperplastic obesity A high number of fat cells, two to three times normal.

hypertension A condition in which the blood pressure is chronically elevated above optimal levels; diagnosis in adults is confirmed when the average of two or more diastolic measurements on at least two separate visits is 90 mm Hg or higher; if the diastolic blood pressure is below 90 mm Hg, systolic hypertension is diagnosed when the average of multiple systolic blood pressure measurements on two or more separate visits is consistently greater than 140 mm Hg.

hyperthermia Body temperatures exceeding normal.

hypertonic Describes a solution concentrated enough to draw water out of body cells.

hypertriglyceridemia High blood triglyceride levels.

hypertrophy An enlargement of a muscle by the increase in size of the cells.

hypochromic Condition of the red blood cells in which they have a reduced hemoglobin content.

hypoglycemia Blood sugar levels below 50 mg/dl, accompanied by symptoms of dizziness, nausea, trembling, irritation, and so on.

hyponatremia Low sodium levels in the bloodstream, which can be caused by excessive sweating and inadequate electrolyte replacement during ultramarathons.

hypothalamus A portion of the brain lying below the thalamus; secretions from the hypothalamus are important in the control of important body functions, including the regulation of water balance, appetite, and body temperature.

hypothermia Body temperature below normal; usually due to exposure to cold temperatures, especially after exhausting ready energy supplies.

hypotonic Describes a solution dilute enough to allow its water to be absorbed by body cells.

hypoxia Insufficient oxygen flow to the tissues.

iliac crest The upper, wide portion of the hip bone.

impaired glucose tolerance Borderline hyperglycemia (between 115 and 140 mg/dl).

indirect calorimetry Measurement of energy expenditure by analysis of expired air.

infarction Death of a section of tissue due to the obstruction of blood flow (ischemia) to the area.

informed consent A procedure for obtaining a client's signed consent to a fitness center's testing and exercise program; includes a description of the objectives and procedures, with associated benefits and risks, stated in plain language, with a consent statement and signature line in a single document.

inspiration Breathing air into the lungs.

inspiratory reserve volume (IRV) The amount of air that can be breathed into the lung on top of a resting inspired tidal volume.

insulin A hormone secreted by special cells (beta cells) in the pancreas; essential for the maintenance of blood glucose levels.

intensity The level of exertion during exercise; intensity, duration, and frequency are important for improving cardiorespiratory endurance.

interval training An exercise session in which the intensity and duration of exercise are consciously alternated between harder and easier work; often used to improve aerobic capacity and/or anaerobic endurance in exercisers who already have a base of endurance in training.

intima The inner layer of arteries.

intracellular Inside the cell.

iron deficiency The most common single nutritional deficiency in the world today; characterized by low iron stores in the body; severe iron deficiency or anemia is characterized by low blood hemoglobin.

iron-deficient erythropoiesis Stage 2 of iron deficiency, following the exhaustion of bone marrow iron stores, and characterized by a diminishing iron supply to developing red blood cells; iron-deficient erythropoiesis (formation of red blood cells) occurs and is measured by increased total iron-binding capacity and reduced serum iron and percent saturation (<16% is abnormal).

ischemia Inadequate blood flow to a body part, caused by constriction or obstruction of a blood vessel, leading to insufficient oxygen supply.

isokinetic contraction A muscle contraction against a resistance that moves at a constant velocity, so that the maximum force of which the muscle is capable throughout the range of motion may be applied.

isometric action Muscle action in which the muscle attempts to contract against an immovable object; sometimes called "isometric contraction," although there is not appreciable shortening of the muscle.

isotonic contraction A muscle contraction against a constant resistance, as in lifting a weight.

Karvonen formula A method to calculate the training heart rate using a percentage of the heart rate reserve, which is the difference between the maximal and resting heart rates.

ketosis An elevated level of ketone bodies in the tissues; seen in sufferers of starvation or diabetes, and a symptom brought about in dieters on very-low-carbohydrate diets.

kilocalorie (kcal) A measure of the heat required to raise the temperature of 1 kilogram of water 1° Celsius; a Calorie, used in diet and metabolism measures, equals 1 kilocalorie or 1,000 calories.

kilogram (kg) A unit of weight equal to 1,000 grams; (2.204623 pounds).

kilogram-meters (kgm) The amount of work required to lift 1 kilogram 1 meter.

kilopond-meters (kpm) Equivalent to kilogram-meters, in normal gravity.

Korotkoff sounds Blood pressure sounds.

Krebs cycle Final common metabolic pathway for fats, proteins, and carbohydrates, which yields additional ATP; carbon dioxide and water are produced.

lactate Lactic acid.

lactate dehydrogenase (LDH) A muscle enzyme that can leak out of ruptured muscle cells into the blood.

lactate system Exercise of 1–3 minutes duration; depends on the lactate system or anaerobic glycolysis for ATP.

lactic acid The end product of the metabolism of glucose (glycolysis) for the anaerobic production of energy.

late-onset (PEL) hypoglycemia Typically, PEL hypoglycemia happens during the night and occurs 6–15 hours after the completion of unusually strenuous exercise or play in diabetics.

law of diminishing returns Appears to be a certain amount of training that most humans will respond quickly and fruitfully to, but every step beyond that level brings less return for the time and effort invested.

L-carnitine An amine responsible for transporting fatty acids into the mitochondria for oxidation; L-carnitine supplements have been claimed to increase the amount of fatty acid oxidation during exercise, sparing the glycogen; however, L-carnitine supplements have never been shown in reputable, double-blind, controlled studies to improve the athletic performance of a healthy individual.

lean body weight The weight of the body, less the weight of its fat.

lecithin:cholesterol acyltransferase (LCAT) An enzyme from the liver that "matures" incomplete HDL by connecting fatty acids to the free cholesterol in the HDL particle. The incomplete HDL (HDL_3) swells into a mature sphere (HDL_3); the LCAT enzyme then grabs more cholesterol from the tissues and other circulating lipoproteins to form even bigger HDL particles (HDL_2).

life expectancy The average number of years of life expected in a population at a specific age, usually at birth.

life span The maximal obtainable age by a particular member of the species, which is primarily related to one's genetic makeup.

lipid A general term used for several different compounds, which include both solid fats and liquid oils; the three major classes of lipids are triglycerides, phospholipids, and sterols.

lipoprotein A soluble aggregate of cholesterol, phospholipids, triglycerides, and protein; this package allows for easy transport through the blood; the four types of lipoproteins are chylomicrons, low-density lipoprotein (LDL), very-low-density lipoprotein (VLDL), and high-density lipoprotein (HDL).

lipoprotein lipase (LPL) An enzyme that breaks down VLDL, providing fatty acids for the muscle or adipose tissue.

longitudinal study A study that observes the same subjects over a period of time (cf. *cross-sectional study*).

lordosis Forward pelvis tilt, often caused from weak abdominals and inflexible posterior thigh muscles, allowing the pelvis to tilt forward, causing curvature in the lower back.

low-back pain (LBP) Pain in the lower back, often caused from weak abdominal muscles and tight lower back and hamstring muscles.

low-density lipoprotein (LDL) Transports cholesterol from the liver to other body cells; often referred to as "bad" cholesterol because it may be taken up by muscle cells in arteries and has been implicated in the development of atherosclerosis.

low-impact aerobics At least one foot is touching the floor throughout exercising.

lumen Inside opening of an artery.

lung diffusion The rate at which gases diffuse from the lung air sacs to the blood in the pulmonary capillaries.

Mason-Likar The 12-lead exercise ECG system.

maximal anaerobic power The ability to exercise for a short time period at high power levels; important for various sports where sprinting and power movements are common.

maximal heart rate The highest heart rate of which an individual is capable; a broad rule of thumb for estimating maximal heart rate is 220 (beats per minute) minus the person's age (in years).

maximal oxygen uptake The highest rate of oxygen consumption of which a person is capable; usually expressed in milliliters of oxygen per kilogram of body weight per minute; also called maximal aerobic power, maximal oxygen consumption, maximal oxygen intake.

mean arterial pressure Equals ⅓ (systolic blood pressure − diastolic blood pressure) + diastolic blood pressure.

mean corpuscular volume Stage 3 iron-deficient anemia, characterized by a drop in hemoglobin; the bone marrow produces an increasing number of smaller and less brightly colored red blood cells; measured when the mean corpuscular volume (MCV) falls below 80 fl.

media Middle layer of muscle in artery wall.

medical history A list of a person's previous illnesses, present conditions, symptoms, medications, and health risk factors; used to help classify an individual as apparently healthy, at risk for disease, or with known disease.

mesomorphic An athletic, muscular body type.

MET A measure of energy output equal to the basal metabolic rate of a resting subject; assumed to be equal to an oxygen uptake of 3.5 milliliters per kilogram of body weight per minute, or approximately 1 kilocalorie per kilogram of body weight per hour.

microcyte A small red blood cell.

mild obesity Defined as being 20–40% overweight.

mineral Of the nearly 45 dietary nutrients known to be necessary for human life, 17 are minerals; although mineral elements represent only a small fraction of human body weight, they play important roles throughout the body; they help form hard tissues such as bones and teeth, aid in normal muscle and nerve activity, act as catalysts in many enzyme systems, help control body water levels, and are integral parts of organic compounds such as hemoglobin and the hormone thyroxine; evidence is growing that certain minerals are related to prevention of disease and proper immune system function.

minute ventilation The volume of air that is breathed into the body each minute.

mitochondria The slender filaments or rods inside of cells, containing enzymes important to producing energy from fat and carbohydrates.

mode Type of exercise.

moderate obesity Defined as being 40–100% overweight.

monosaccharides The simplest carbohydrate, containing only one molecule of sugar; glucose, fructose, and galactose are the primary monosaccharides.

monounsaturated fatty acids See *fats.*

motor neuron A nerve cell that conducts impulses from the central nervous system to a group of muscle fibers, producing movement.

motor unit A motor neuron and the muscle fibers activated by it.

muscle glycogen supercompensation The practice of exercise tapering, combined with a high-carbohydrate diet, that stores very high levels of glycogen in the muscles before long endurance events.

muscle spindle Organ in a muscle that senses changes in the muscle's length, especially stretches; rapid stretching of a muscle results in messages being sent to the nervous system to contract the muscle, thereby limiting the stretch.

muscular endurance Defined as the ability of the muscles to apply a submaximal force repeatedly or to sustain a muscular contraction for a certain period of time.

musculoskeletal fitness Comprises three components: flexibility, muscular strength, and muscular endurance.

myocardial infarction A common form of heart attack in which the blockage of a coronary artery causes the death of a part of the heart muscle.

myofilaments Within the muscle cell; actin and myosin protein fibers are myofilaments.

myoglobin A muscle protein molecule that contains iron; carries oxygen from the blood to the muscle cell.

net energy expenditure Equals the Calories expended during the exercise session minus the Calories expended for the resting metabolic rate and other activities that would have occupied the individual had the person not been formally exercising.

nonpharmacological approaches Use of nondrug methods to treat hypertension, hypercholesterolemia, or other health problems.

non-weight-bearing activities Activities such as bicycling, swimming, and brisk walking, which do not overstress the musculoskeletal system.

norms Represent the average achievement level of a particular group to which the measured scores can be compared.

nutritional assessment Involves the use of a wide variety of clinical and biochemical methods to assess the state of health as characterized by body composition, tissue function, and metabolic activity.

obesity Excessive accumulation of body fat.

oligomenorrhea Scanty or infrequent menstrual flow.

omega-3 fatty acids A type of fat found in fish oils and associated with lower blood cholesterol levels, lower blood pressure, and reduced blood clotting.

one-repetition maximum (1-RM) The maximum resistance with which a person can execute one repetition of an exercise movement.

oral glucose tolerance test (OGTT) The OGTT is a 75-gram glucose solution given after an overnight fast of 10–16 hours.

osmolarity The concentration of a solution participating in osmosis.

osteoarthritis A noninflammatory joint disease of older persons; cartilage in the joint wears down, and bone grows at the edges of the joints; results in pain and stiffness, especially after prolonged exercise.

osteoblasts Bone cells that build bone.

osteoclasts Bone cells that break down bone.

osteoporosis Defined as an age-related disorder characterized by decreased bone mineral content and increased risk of fractures.

overload Subjecting a part of the body to efforts greater than it is accustomed to, in order to elicit a training response; increases may be in intensity or duration.

overuse Excessive repeated exertion or shock, which results in injuries such as stress fractures of bones or inflammation of muscles and tendons.

oxygen debt The oxygen required to restore the capacity for anaerobic work after an effort has used those reserves; measured by the extra oxygen that is consumed during the recovery from the work.

oxygen deficit The energy supplied anaerobically while oxygen uptake has not yet reached the steady state that matches energy output; becomes oxygen debt at end of exercise.

oxygen uptake The amount of oxygen used up at the cellular level during exercise; can be measured by determining the amount of oxygen exhaled (in carbon dioxide), as compared to the amount inhaled, or estimated by indirect means.

ozone In the lower atmosphere, produced by the photochemical reaction of sunlight on hydrocarbons and nitrogen dioxide from car and industrial exhaust.

pangamic acid So-called vitamin B_{15}, which is claimed to enhance performance; reputable nutritionists do not support this claim or even the fact that a vitamin B_{15} exists.

parasympathetic The craniosacral division of the autonomic nervous system.

parcourse An outdoor circuit system that combines calisthenics with running.

passive smoking Breathing of air that has cigarette smoke in it.

pellagra A disease of niacin deficiency.

percentage of total Calories Concept used by nutritionists to represent the percentage of protein, carbohydrate, and fat Calories present in the diet; calculated from the fact that 1 gram of carbohydrate, protein, and fat equals 4 Calories, 4 Calories, and 9 Calories, respectively.

percent saturation During iron-deficient erythropoiesis (stage 2 iron deficiency), percent saturation falls (<16 percent is abnormal).

phenylpropanolamine (PPA) The active ingredient in most nonprescription weight-control products; related to amphetamines and has similar side effects, such as nervousness, insomnia, headaches, nausea, tinnitus (ringing in the ears), and elevated blood pressure.

phospholipids Substances found in all body cells; similar to lipids, but containing only two fatty acids and one phosphorus-containing substance.

physical activity Any form of muscular movement.

physical fitness A dynamic state of energy and vitality that enables one to carry out daily tasks, to engage in active leisure-time pursuits, and to meet unforeseen emergencies without undue fatigue; in addition, physically fit individuals have a decreased risk of hypokinetic diseases and are more able to function at the peak of intellectual capacity while experiencing joie de vivre.

physical work capacity (PWC) An exercise test that measures the amount of work done at a given, submaximal heart rate; work is measured in oxygen uptake, kilogrammeters per minute, or other units, and can be used to estimate maximal heart rate and oxygen uptake.

placebo An inactive substance given to satisfy a patient's demand for medicine.

platelets The clotting material in the blood.

polarized Charged heart cells in the resting state (negative ions inside the cell, positive outside); when electrically stimulated, they depolarize (positive ions inside the heart cell, negative ions outside) and contract.

polydipsia Excessive thirst.

polyphagia Unsatisfied hunger.

polyunsaturated fat Dietary fat comprising molecules that have more than one double bond open to receive more hydrogen; found in safflower oil, corn oil, soybeans, sesame seeds, sunflower seeds.

polyuria Excessive urination.

power Work performed per unit of time; measured by the formula: work equals force times distance divided by time; a combination of strength and speed.

pre-event meal A meal eaten 3–5 hours before an exercise event, emphasizing low-fiber, high-carbohydrate foods.

premature ventricular contraction (PVC) One of the most common ECG abnormalities during the exercise test, where a spot on the ventricle becomes the pacemaker, superseding the SA node.

primary air pollutants Include carbon monoxide (CO), carbon dioxide (CO_2), sulfur dioxide (SO_2), nitrogen oxide (NO), and particulate material such as lead, graphite carbon, and fly ash.

primary osteoporosis May occur in two types: Type I osteoporosis (postmenopausal), which is the accelerated decrease in bone mass that occurs when estrogen levels fall after menopause; and Type II osteoporosis (age-related), which is the inevitable loss of bone mass with age in both men and women.

progressive resistance exercise Exercise in which the amount of resistance is increased to further stress the muscle after it has become accustomed to handling a lesser resistance.

pronation Of the body, assuming a face-down position; of the hand, turning the palm backward or downward; of the foot, lowering the inner (medial) side of the foot so as to flatten the arch; the opposite of supination.

proprioceptive neuromuscular facilitation (PNF) stretch Muscle stretches that use the proprioceptors (muscle spindles) to send inhibiting (relaxing) messages to the muscle that is to be stretched; for example, the contraction of an agonist muscle sends inhibiting signals that relax the antagonist muscle, allowing it to stretch.

protein A complex nitrogen-carrying compound that occurs naturally in plants and animals and yields amino acids when broken down; the component amino acids are essential for the growth and repair of living tissue; also a source of heat and energy for the body.

protoporphyrin A derivative of hemoglobin; formed from heme by deletion of an atom of iron.

prudent diet Defined in this book as the diet adhering to the 1988 *Surgeon General's Report on Nutrition and Health.*

puberty The period in life when one becomes functionally capable of reproduction.

P wave Transmission of electrical impulse through the atria.

QRS complex Impulse through the ventricles.

Quetelet index Body weight in kilograms, divided by height in meters, squared; the most widely accepted body mass index.

radial pulse The pulse at the wrist.

rating of perceived exertion (RPE) A means to quantify the subjective feeling of the intensity of an exercise; Borg scales, charts that describe a range of intensity from resting to maximal energy outputs, are used as a visual aid to exercisers in keeping their efforts in the effective training zone.

reaction time Relates to the time elapsed between stimulation and the beginning of the reaction to it.

recommended dietary allowance (RDA) Established by the National Research Council of the National Academy of Sciences; the premier nutrient standard worldwide; used for nutrition policies and decision making; also used for purposes ranging from development of new food products to setting standards for federal nutrition assistance programs.

relative risk An expression of disease risk that usually compares death rates from groups varying in a certain health-related practice.

relative weight The body weight divided by the midpoint value of the weight range.

relaxation therapy A treatment that involves teaching a patient to accomplish a state of both muscular and mental deactivation by the systematic use of relaxation or meditation exercises to reduce high blood pressure.

reliability Deals with how consistently a certain element is measured by the particular test.

residual volume The volume of air remaining in the lungs after a maximum expiration; must be calculated in the formula for determining body composition through underwater weighing.

respiratory exchange ratio (R) The ratio between the amount of carbon dioxide produced and the amount of oxygen consumed by the body during exercise.

resting metabolic rate (RMR) Represents the energy expended by the body to maintain life and normal body functions, such as respiration and circulation.

R.I.C.E. Recommended treatment of musculoskeletal pain and injury during the first 48–72 hours; stands for rest, ice, compression, and elevation.

risk factors Characteristics associated with higher risk of developing a specific health problem.

sarcolemma The membrane of the muscle cell.

sarcomere The smallest functional skeletal muscle subunit capable of contraction.

satiety The feeling of fullness and satisfaction.

saturated fat Dietary fat comprising molecules saturated with hydrogen; usually hard at room temperature and readily converted into cholesterol in the body; sources include animal products as well as hydrogenated vegetable oils.

scurvy A disease of vitamin C deficiency.

secondary air pollutants Formed by chemical action of the primary pollutants and the natural chemicals in the atmosphere; examples include ozone (O_3), sulfuric acid (H_2SO_4), nitric acid (HNO_3), peroxyacetyl nitrate, and a host of other inorganic and organic compounds.

secondary osteoporosis A loss of bone mineral mass that may develop at any age, as a consequence of hormonal, digestive, and metabolic disorders, as well as prolonged bed rest and weightlessness (space flight).

senile dementia A form of organic brain syndrome, a mental disorder associated with impaired brain function in the elderly.

serum erythropoietin A hormone that regulates red blood cell production.

serum iron During iron-deficient erythropoiesis (stage 2 iron deficiency) serum iron levels fall.

set A group of repetitions of an exercise movement done consecutively, without rest, until a given number, or momentary exhaustion, is reached.

severe obesity Defined as more than 100% overweight.

skeletal muscle Muscle connected to a bone.

skill-related fitness Elements of fitness such as agility, balance, speed, and coordination; important for participation in various dual and team sports but has little significance for the day-to-day tasks of Americans or their general health.

skinfold measurements The most widely used method for determining obesity: calipers are used to measure the thickness of a double fold of skin at various sites.

slow-twitch fibers Muscle fiber type that contracts slowly and is used most in moderate-intensity, endurance exercises, such as distance running; also called Type I fibers.

smokeless tobacco Use of smokeless tobacco takes two forms: (1) dipping—placing a pinch of moist or dry powdered tobacco (snuff) between the cheek or lip and the lower gum; (2) chewing—placing a golfball-size amount of looseleaf tobacco between the cheek and lower gum, where it is sucked and chewed.

sodium An electrolyte that is the major cation (positive ion) of fluids outside the body cells; sodium and chloride ions tend to concentrate outside of body cell walls (extracellular), while potassium tends to concentrate inside of body cell walls (intracellular); this arrangement is essential in maintaining the balance of tissue fluids inside and outside of cells; sodium, potassium, and chloride work with bicarbonate in regulating the acid–base balance of the body; has an important role in regulating normal muscle tone; the Food and Nutrition Board has established safe and adequate daily dietary intakes for sodium of 1,100–3,300 mg.

sodium bicarbonate A substance used by some athletes to enhance performance in events lasting 1–3 minutes; sodium bicarbonate ingestion increases the pH of the body, allowing greater lactic acid to be produced and buffered.

sodium-to-potassium ratio (Na:K) A ratio of the dietary sodium-to-potassium intake, which may be important as an indicator of hypertension risk.

specificity The principle that the body adapts very specifically to the training stimuli it is required to deal with; the body will perform best at the specific speed, type of contraction, using the muscle group and energy source it has been accustomed to in training.

speed Relates to the ability to perform a movement within a short period of time.

sphygmomanometer Blood pressure measurement device; consists of an inflatable compression bag enclosed in an unyielding covering called the cuff, plus an inflating bulb, a manometer from which the pressure is read, and a controlled exhaust to deflate the system during measurement of blood pressure.

spirulina A dark green powder or pill derived from marine algae; has been promoted as a weight-loss product.

spot reducing An effort to reduce fat at one location on the body by concentrating exercise, manipulation, wraps, and so forth on that location; research indicates that any fat loss is generalized over the body, however.

stadiometer A vertical ruler with a horizontal headboard that can be brought into contact with the most superior (highest) point on the head.

starch A polysaccharide made up of glucose monosaccharides.

starch blockers An enzyme inhibitor claimed to block the digestion and absorption of ingested carbohydrate; several studies have shown these not only to be ineffective, but also a possible risk to health.

step-care therapy An approach with lifestyle techniques and various drugs to treat hypertension.

sterols A type of lipid such as cholesterol, estrogen, testosterone, and vitamin D.

stethoscope Device for amplifying physiological sounds (e.g., heart and lungs); made up of rubber tubing attached to a device that amplifies sounds, such as blood passing through the blood vessels during measurement of blood pressure. (See *auscultation.*)

strength The amount of muscular force that can be exerted.

stress The general physical and psychological response of an individual to any real or perceived adverse stimulus, internal or external, that tends to disturb the individual's homeostasis.

stretching Lengthening a muscle to its maximum extension; moving a joint to the limits of its extension.

stroke A form of cardiovascular disease that affects the blood vessels supplying oxygen and nutrients to the brain.

stroke volume The volume of blood pumped out of the heart (by the ventricles) in one contraction.

ST segment depression An indication of atherosclerotic blockage in the coronary arteries.

submaximal Less than maximum; submaximal exercise requires less than one's maximum oxygen uptake, heart rate, or anaerobic power; usually refers to intensity of the exercise, but may be used to refer to duration.

sugars Categorized as *monosaccharides* (glucose, fructose, galactose) and *disaccharides* (lactose, mannose, sucrose).

supination Assuming a horizontal position facing upward; in the case of the hand, it also means turning the palm forward; the opposite of pronation.

supplementation Use of vitamin or mineral pills to supplement the regular diet.

systolic blood pressure The pressure of the blood upon the walls of the blood vessels when the heart is contracting; a normal systolic blood pressure ranges between 90 and 139 mm Hg; when the systolic blood pressure is measured on more than one occasion to be more than 140 mm Hg, high blood pressure is diagnosed.

tachycardia Excessively rapid heart rate. Usually describes a pulse of more than 100 beats per minute at rest.

target heart rate (THR) The heart rate at which one aims to exercise. For example, the American College of Sports Medicine recommends that healthy adults exercise at a THR of 60–90% of maximum heart rate reserve; also called training heart rate.

testosterone An androgen hormone produced by the testicles and adrenal cortex; accelerates growth in tissues.

thermic effect of food (TEF) The increase in energy expenditure above the resting metabolic rate that can be measured for several hours after a meal.

thrombosis Formation or existence of a blood clot within the blood vessel system.

tidal volume The amount of air per breath.

total iron-binding capacity (TIBC) During iron-deficient erythropoiesis (inadequate formation of red blood cells), total iron-binding capacity is increased.

total lung capacity (TLC) Represents the total amount of air in the lung.

total peripheral resistance The sum of all the forces that oppose blood flow in the body's blood vessel system. During exercise, total peripheral resistance decreases because the blood vessels in the active muscles increase in size.

trabecular bone Spongy, internal end bone.

triglyceride A type of fat made of glycerol with three fatty acids; most animal and vegetable fats are triglycerides.

T wave Electrical recovery or repolarization of the ventricles.

type 1 diabetes mellitus The form of diabetes mellitus in which the pancreas does not make or secrete insulin; the patient must use an external source of insulin to sustain life; also called insulin-dependent diabetes mellitus (IDDM) or juvenile-onset diabetes.

type 2 diabetes mellitus See *diabetes mellitus.*

underwater weighing The most widely used laboratory procedure for measuring body density; in this procedure, whole-body density is calculated from body volume according to Archimedes' principle of displacement, which states that an object submerged in water is buoyed up by the weight of the water displaced.

US-RDA A set of standards developed by the Food and Drug Administration (FDA) for use in regulating nutrition labeling; although these standards were taken from the RDA, they are based on very few categories, and only 19 vitamins and minerals were chosen.

validity Refers to the degree to which a test measures what it was designed to measure.

Valsalva maneuver A strong exhaling effort against a closed glottis, which builds pressure in the chest cavity, interfering with the return of blood to the heart; may deprive the brain of blood and cause fainting.

vasoconstriction The narrowing of a blood vessel to decrease blood flow to a body part.

vasodilation The enlarging of a blood vessel to increase blood flow to a body part.

very-low-calorie diet (VLCD) Also called the protein-sparing modified fast; provides 400–700 Calories per day for weight loss; protein is emphasized to help avoid loss of muscle tissue; patients can use either special formula beverages or natural foods such as fish, fowl, or lean meat (along with mineral and vitamin supplements).

very-low-density lipoproteins (VLDL) Transport triglycerides to body tissues.

vital capacity The amount of air that can be expired after a maximum inspiration; the maximum total volume of the lungs, less the residual volume.

vitamin Nutrients essential for life itself; the body uses these organic substances to accomplish much of its work; do not supply energy but do help release energy from carbohydrates, fats, and proteins; play a vital role in chemical reactions throughout the body; there are two types of vitamins—fat-soluble (A,D,E,K) and water-soluble (eight B vitamins and vitamin C); 13 vitamins have been discovered, the most recent in 1948.

$\dot{V}O_{2max}$ Maximum volume of oxygen consumed per unit of time. In scientific notation, a dot appears over the V to indicate "per unit of time."

waist-to-hip circumference ratio (WHR) Ratio of waist and hip circumferences. A relatively high WHR predicts increased complications from obesity.

warm-up A gradual increase in the intensity of exercise to allow physiological processes to prepare for greater energy outputs; changes include rise in body temperature, cardiorespiratory changes, increase in muscle elasticity and contractility, and so on.

watt A measure of power equal to 6.12 kilogram-meters per minute.

weight-reducing clothing Special weight-reducing clothing, including heated belts, rubberized suits, and oilskins, rely chiefly on dehydration and localized pressure.

wet bulb thermometer A thermometer, the bulb of which is enclosed in a wet wick, so that evaporation from the wick will lower the temperature reading more in dry air than in humid air; the comparison of wet and dry bulb readings can be used to calculate relative humidity.

wet globe temperature A temperature reading that approximates the heat stress that the environment will impose on the human body; takes into account not only temperature and humidity, but also radiant heat from the sun and cooling breezes that would speed evaporation and convection of heat away from the body; reading is provided by an instrument that encloses a thermometer in a wetted, black copper sphere (cf. *dry-bulb thermometer, wet-bulb thermometer*).

white blood cells Immune system cells that circulate in the blood, including monocytes, neutrophils, basophils, eosinophils, and lymphocytes.

Index

Note: Italicized page numbers indicate illustrations.